FOURTH EDITION

Breastfeeding Management *for the* Clinician

Using the Evidence

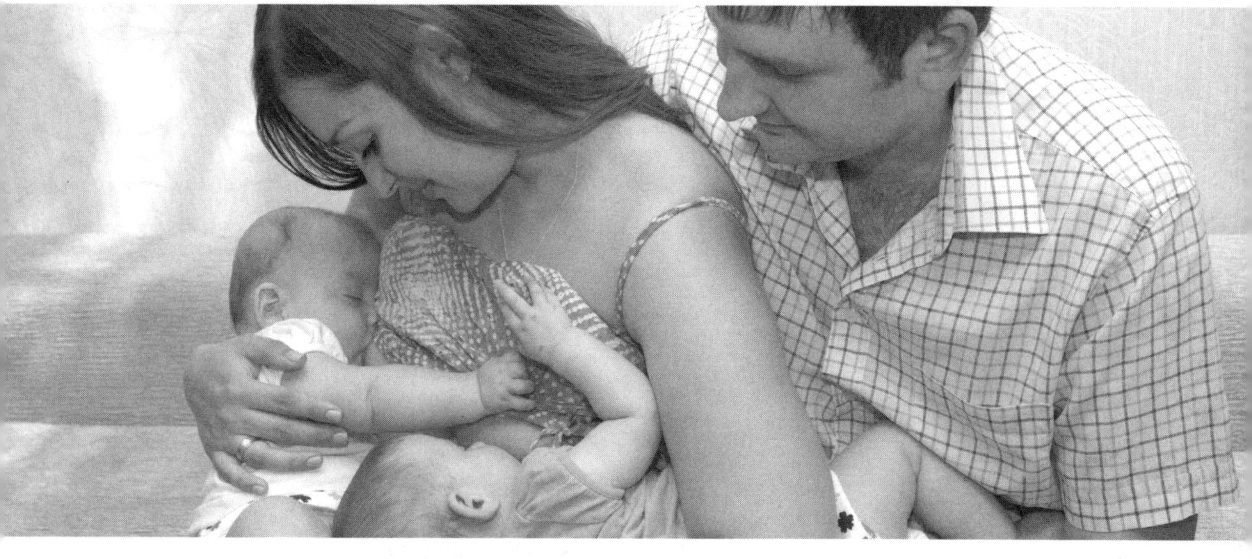

Marsha Walker, RN, IBCLC
Independent Lactation Consultant
Weston, Massachusetts

JONES & BARTLETT
LEARNING

World Headquarters
Jones & Bartlett Learning
5 Wall Street
Burlington, MA 01803
978-443-5000
info@jblearning.com
www.jblearning.com

Jones & Bartlett Learning books and products are available through most bookstores and online booksellers. To contact Jones & Bartlett Learning directly, call 800-832-0034, fax 978-443-8000, or visit our website, www.jblearning.com.

Substantial discounts on bulk quantities of Jones & Bartlett Learning publications are available to corporations, professional associations, and other qualified organizations. For details and specific discount information, contact the special sales department at Jones & Bartlett Learning via the above contact information or send an email to specialsales@jblearning.com.

Production Credits
VP, Executive Publisher: David D. Cella
Executive Editor: Amanda Martin
Acquisitions Editor: Teresa Reilly
Associate Editor: Danielle Bessette
Associate Production Editor: Juna Abrams
Marketing Communications Manager: Katie Hennessy
Product Fulfillment Manager: Wendy Kilborn
Composition: S4Carlisle Publishing Services
Cover Design: Kristin E. Parker
Rights & Media Specialist: Merideth Tumasz
Media Development Editor: Troy Liston
Cover Image: © Vitalinka/Shutterstock
Printing and Binding: Edwards Brothers Malloy
Cover Printing: Edwards Brothers Malloy

Library of Congress Cataloging-in-Publication Data
Names: Walker, Marsha, author.
Title: Breastfeeding management for the clinician : using the evidence / Marsha Walker.
Description: Fourth edition. | Burlington, Massachusetts : Jones & Bartlett Learning, [2017] | Includes bibliographical references and index.
Identifiers: LCCN 2016000926 | ISBN 9781284091045 (alk. paper)
Subjects: | MESH: Breast Feeding | Lactation--physiology | Evidence-Based Medicine
Classification: LCC RJ216 | NLM WS 125 | DDC 649/.33—dc23
LC record available at https://lccn.loc.gov/2016000926

6048

Printed in the United States of America
20 19 18 17 16   10 9 8 7 6 5 4 3 2

As always, my work is dedicated to my growing family: Hap, my husband, for his unlimited patience and support (especially with IT); Shannon, my daughter, wife to Tom, and mother of breastfed Haley, Sophie, and Isabelle; Justin, my son, husband to Sarina and father of Ella and Andrew. I can't ask for more than this.

Contents

Preface

It is the goal of the fourth edition of *Breastfeeding Management for the Clinician* to provide current and relevant information on breastfeeding and lactation, blended with clinical suggestions for best outcomes in the mothers and infants entrusted to our care. Although lactation is a robust process, predating placental gestation, it has become fraught with barriers: Human lactation is only occasionally taught in nursing and medical schools, leaving a gap in healthcare providers' ability to provide appropriate lactation care and services.

With minimal staffing on maternity units, short hospital stays, delays in community follow-up, and the resulting time crunches, breastfeeding often falls through the cracks. Absent or inappropriate care results in reduced initiation, duration, and exclusivity of breastfeeding. This text is intended to provide busy clinicians with options for clinical interventions and the rationale behind them.

Designed as a practical reference rather than a thick textbook, it is hoped that this approach provides quick access to—and help with—the more common as well as some less frequently seen conditions that clinicians are called upon to address. It is my sincere desire that the use of this book as a clinical tool results in the best outcomes for all breastfeeding mothers and infants the reader encounters.

I

The Context of Lactation and Breastfeeding

PRELUDE: INFLUENCE OF THE POLITICAL AND SOCIAL LANDSCAPE ON BREASTFEEDING

Breastfeeding and the provision of human milk define a relatively short window of opportunity to provide the foundation for a person's lifelong health. Increasing the rate of breastfeeding in the United States has been a public health priority for more than a century. For three decades, the U.S. Department of Health and Human Services (HHS) has promulgated breastfeeding goals for the nation through the Healthy People initiative, which provides science-based, 10-year national objectives for improving the health of all Americans. The breastfeeding objectives for 2020 include improving the breastfeeding initiation and duration rates, raising the exclusive breastfeeding rates, increasing the number of employers who have worksite lactation support programs, reducing the proportion of newborns who receive formula supplementation in the hospital, and increasing the number of infants born in hospitals that provide optimal lactation care (HHS, 2010).

Currently, 79.2% of mothers in the United States initiate breastfeeding, with 40.7% exclusively breastfeeding at 3 months (Centers for Disease Control and Prevention [CDC], 2014). A great deal of progress has been made in the political and social environment surrounding breastfeeding (**Box I-1**). Contributing to the progress seen in breastfeeding support over the last 25 years has been the increase in

Box I-1 Timeline of Breastfeeding Progress, 1996–2015

1996	The Loving Support campaign from Food and Nutrition Service is formed to increase the number of breastfeeding mothers in the WIC program.
1997	The American Academy of Pediatrics releases its first policy statement on breastfeeding.
1998	The U.S. Breastfeeding Committee is formed.
1999	The Right to Breastfeed Act (H.R. 1848) by Representative Carolyn Maloney (D-NY) is passed, ensuring a woman's right to breastfeed on all federal property.
2000	The *Healthy People 2010* guidelines for the nation are released with breastfeeding objectives.
2003	The National Breastfeeding Awareness Campaign is conducted, aimed at increasing breastfeeding among first-time parents. Of note, it used a risk-based format and was significantly watered down by interference from the infant formula industry.
2005	• The *Healthy People 2010* mid-course review adds exclusive breastfeeding targets. • HHS issues *Blueprint for Action on Breastfeeding*, which positions breastfeeding as a public health issue, not just an individual choice.
2007	The CDC conducts the first Maternity Practices in Infant Nutrition and Care (mPINC) survey, which highlights hospital practices related to breastfeeding. The results demonstrated how poorly many hospitals were supporting breastfeeding and has led many hospitals to improve their practices.
2008	With the creation of the Business Case for Breastfeeding program, the Maternal and Child Health Bureau and Health Resources and Services Administration involve employers in supporting breastfeeding mothers by providing a package of information on how best to provide lactation accommodations in the worksite.
2009	WIC food packages are revised to better promote breastfeeding.
2010	• The Joint Commission establishes the Perinatal Core Measure Set, which measures, among other things, the number of infants exclusively fed breastmilk upon discharge from the hospital. • The Patient Protection and Affordable Care Act of 2010 (P.L.111-148, Sec. 4207 [2010]) introduces specific worksite protections for breastfeeding employees on a national level. • A presidential memorandum orders the creation of appropriate workplace accommodations for nursing mothers who are federal civilian employees. • The *Healthy People 2020* goals add three more breastfeeding objectives, (1) increase the proportion of employers that have worksite lactation support programs, (2) reduce the proportion of breastfed newborns who receive formula supplementation within the first 2 days of life, and (3) increase the proportion of births that occur in facilities that provide recommended care for lactating mothers and their babies.
2011	• The Surgeon General issues *The Call to Action to Support Breastfeeding.* • The Internal Revenue Service allows breastfeeding equipment to be reimbursed from flexible health spending accounts.

- The Patient Protection and Affordable Care Act states that health insurers will be required to pay for a range of preventive care services specifically aimed at women, including "comprehensive lactation support and counseling, by a trained provider during pregnancy and/or in the postpartum period, and costs for renting breastfeeding equipment."

2012
- The Joint Commission mandates that all birthing hospitals with more than 1,100 deliveries per year must participate in its Perinatal Care Core Measure Set to remain accredited.
- Rhode Island and Massachusetts are the first and second states to achieve the elimination of formula discharge bag distribution in all of their birthing hospitals.
- A CDC grant to the National Institute for Children's Healthcare Quality is made to facilitate 90 hospitals achieving the Baby-Friendly designation.

2014 The TRICARE Moms Improvement Act is signed into law. The law makes breastfeeding supplies, services, and counseling available to military family members covered under the federal Tricare health insurance program.

2015
- Births in Baby-Friendly designated facilities exceed the *Healthy People 2020* goal. More than 17% of births occur in Baby-Friendly designated facilities; the *Healthy People 2020* goal is 8.1%.
- A revised meal pattern is proposed related to the Healthy, Hunger-Free Kids Act of 2010. As an incentive for encouraging breastfeeding and to better align program rules, this proposed rule would allow reimbursement for meals served to infants younger than 6 months of age when the mother directly breastfeeds her child at the childcare facility. Meals containing breastmilk or iron-fortified infant formula supplied by the parent or the facility are already eligible for CACFP reimbursement.

---

employers who provide time and space to express milk at work, the increase in state legislation mandating worksite support for breastfeeding employees and laws protecting the right to breastfeed in public, the expansion in breastfeeding education and training opportunities for healthcare providers, the increase in the interest and number of hospitals obtaining the Baby-Friendly designation, the availability of advanced lactation support and services from international board certified lactation consultants (IBCLCs), and increased research on breastfeeding and human lactation.

While steady progress has been made, there remain many challenges and gaps in care that prevent mothers from meeting their breastfeeding goals. The prevalence of breastfeeding among African American mothers is consistently lower than that among mothers of other races and ethnicities (CDC, 2013). This persistent gap in breastfeeding rates between black women and women of other races and ethnicities might indicate that black women are more likely to encounter unsupportive cultural norms, perceptions that breastfeeding is inferior to formula feeding, lack of partner support, lack of self-efficacy, inadequate care from healthcare providers, social media influence, and an unsupportive work environment (Johnson, Kirk, Rosenblum, & Muzik, 2015).

The Surgeon General's Call to Action to Support Breastfeeding outlines 20 steps that can be taken to remove some of the obstacles faced by women who wish to breastfeed their infants (HHS, 2011) (**Box I-2**).

BOX I-2 Action Items from *The Surgeon General's Call to Action to Support Breastfeeding*

Actions for Mothers and Their Families

1. Give mothers the support they need to breastfeed their babies.
2. Develop programs to educate fathers and grandmothers about breastfeeding.

Actions for Communities

3. Strengthen programs that provide mother-to-mother support and peer counseling.
4. Use community-based organizations to promote and support breastfeeding.
5. Create a national campaign to promote breastfeeding.
6. Ensure that the marketing of infant formula is conducted in a way that minimizes its negative impacts on exclusive breastfeeding.

Actions for Health Care

7. Ensure that maternity care practices around the United States are fully supportive of breastfeeding.
8. Develop systems to guarantee continuity of skilled support for lactation between hospitals and healthcare settings in the community.
9. Provide education and training in breastfeeding for all health professionals who care for women and children.
10. Include basic support for breastfeeding as a standard of care for midwives, obstetricians, family physicians, nurse practitioners, and pediatricians.
11. Ensure access to services provided by IBCLCs.
12. Identify and address obstacles to greater availability of safe banked donor milk for fragile infants.

Actions for Employment

13. Work toward establishing paid maternity leave for all employed mothers.
14. Ensure that employers establish and maintain comprehensive, high-quality lactation support programs for their employees.
15. Expand the use of programs in the workplace that allow lactating mothers to have direct access to their babies.
16. Ensure that all child care providers accommodate the needs of breastfeeding mothers and infants.

Actions for Research and Surveillance

17. Increase funding of high-quality research on breastfeeding.
18. Strengthen existing capacity and develop future capacity for conducting research on breastfeeding.
19. Develop a national monitoring system to improve the tracking of breastfeeding rates as well as the policies and environmental factors that affect breastfeeding.

Action for Public Health Infrastructure

20. Improve national leadership on the promotion and support of breastfeeding.

Each step includes implementation strategies and places responsibility for breastfeeding improvement on all stakeholders.

Social attitudes toward breastfeeding contribute to shaping and influencing a mother's view on breastfeeding. The HealthStyles survey has been conducted since 1995, asking adults 18 years and older questions about their health orientations and practices (CDC, 2010). Progress has not been made in some areas; for example, in the 2010 survey, 32% believed that it is embarrassing to breastfeed in front of others compared with 29% in the 2000 survey. However, progress can be seen in other areas; for example, 59% in 2010 believed that women should have the right to breastfeed in public places compared with 43% who agreed with this statement in 2001. It is disappointing to see that certain misperceptions have become more prevalent; for example, in 2000, 44% thought that mothers had to give up too many lifestyle habits like favorite foods, cigarette smoking, and drinking alcohol, and in 2010, over 48% still thought that mothers had to give up personal preferences or change their lives in order to breastfeed. This attitude, plus other societal constraints such as lack of paid maternity leave, uncooperative employers, being asked to leave public places while breastfeeding, and a lack of understanding regarding the outcomes of not breastfeeding, place barriers in front of mothers that clinicians must address if a mother is to meet her breastfeeding goals.

Some of these barriers are being addressed through state and federal legislation. All states in the United States have at least one breastfeeding law on the books. The National Conference of State Legislatures (2015) catalogs and summarizes all of the state breastfeeding laws. The first state breastfeeding law was passed in New York in 1984, exempting breastfeeding from public indecency offenses. Laws vary from state to state, with some laws encouraging or requiring employer accommodations for breastfeeding mothers, permitting mothers to breastfeed in public, exempting breastfeeding from public indecency laws, allowing breastfeeding mothers to postpone or be excused from jury duty, or outlining some other special or unique requirements. One study showed that the most robust laws associated with increased infant breastfeeding at 6 months were an enforcement provision for workplace pumping laws (odds ratio [OR], 2.0; 95% confidence interval [CI], 1.6–2.6) and a jury duty exemption for breastfeeding mothers (OR, 1.7; 95% CI, 1.3–2.1). Having a private area in the workplace to express breastmilk (OR, 1.3; 95% CI, 1.1–1.7) and having break time to breastfeed or pump (OR, 1.2; 95% CI, 1.0–1.5) were also important for infant breastfeeding at 6 months (Smith-Gagen, Hollen, Tashiro, Cook, & Yang, 2014). When scrutinizing these laws relative to African American mothers, however, it appears that the laws were significantly less helpful to African American mothers compared with Hispanic and white mothers (Smith-Gagen, Hollen, Walker, Cook, & Yang, 2014). For example, most laws that mandate break-time provisions for expressing breastmilk require that it be unpaid break time. Many African American mothers may not be able to afford the income lost during unpaid breaks.

While these laws protect breastfeeding mothers to varying degrees, most lack any penalties for their violation, and large numbers of mothers are not protected by comprehensive laws. Laws that protect all breastfeeding mothers are extremely variable in their coverage and are made less effective by lack of knowledge of their existence and the absence of penalties (Nguyen & Hawkins, 2012). Informing mothers of their breastfeeding rights within their state may help them address various public challenges they encounter. For example, the Massachusetts Breastfeeding Coalition has a "license to breastfeed," which is a two-sided card that states the law regarding breastfeeding in public and where to file a grievance if a mother is harassed for breastfeeding in public (**Figure I-1**). Mothers carry these cards with them and

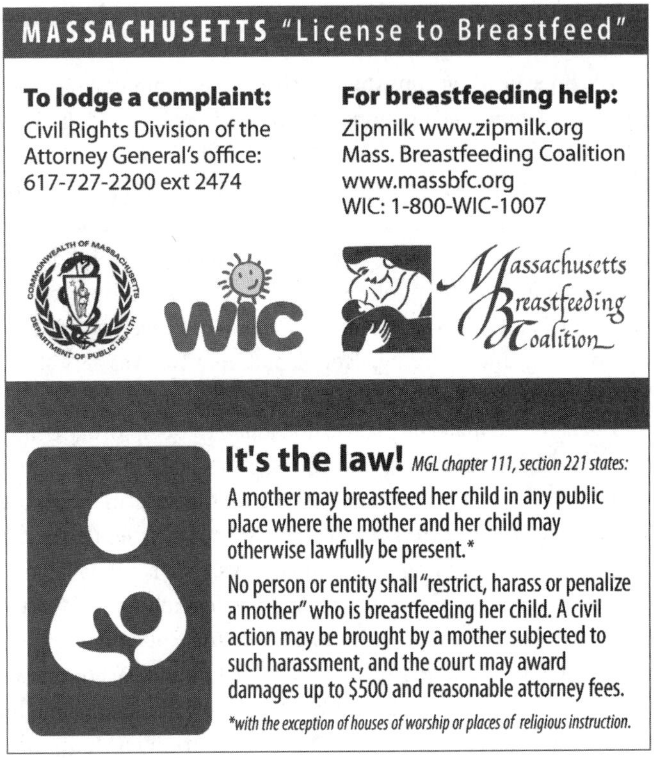
MASSACHUSETTS "License to Breastfeed"
To lodge a complaint:
Civil Rights Division of the Attorney General's office: 617-727-2200 ext 2474
For breastfeeding help:
Zipmilk www.zipmilk.org
Mass. Breastfeeding Coalition www.massbfc.org
WIC: 1-800-WIC-1007
WIC
Massachusetts Breastfeeding Coalition
It's the law! MGL chapter 111, section 221 states:
A mother may breastfeed her child in any public place where the mother and her child may otherwise lawfully be present.*
No person or entity shall "restrict, harass or penalize a mother" who is breastfeeding her child. A civil action may be brought by a mother subjected to such harassment, and the court may award damages up to $500 and reasonable attorney fees.
*with the exception of houses of worship or places of religious instruction.

Figure I-1 "License to breastfeed" to help mothers know their rights.

Courtesy of the Massachusetts Breastfeeding Coalition, http://massbreastfeeding.org. Retrieved from http://massbreastfeeding.org/2011/06/21/get-your-license-to-breastfeed-2/

present the card to anyone who harasses them for breastfeeding in public. These cards can be distributed to breastfeeding mothers by healthcare providers or downloaded from the coalition's website. Laws cannot protect mothers if mothers are unaware of their rights.

Set against the landscape of variable legal protections for breastfeeding mothers came section 4207 of the Patient Protection and Affordable Care Act of 2010 (PL 111-148). This act was the second piece of federal (not state) legislation that offered legal protection for an aspect of breastfeeding (Murtagh & Moulton, 2011). The first piece of federal legislation was section 647 of the Treasury and General Government Appropriations Act (1999), which affirmed that a woman may breastfeed her child at any federal building or federal location where she is authorized to be (Public Law no. 106-058). The Affordable Care Act requires all employers to provide reasonable break time to express milk for a child up to 1 year of age in a private location other than a bathroom. Employers of less than 50 employees who can demonstrate hardship may be exempted from the law. This law applies only to employees who work for hourly wages and does not apply to salaried workers and certain other classes of employees such as administrative employees, school teachers, and many agricultural workers. If a state has a stronger worksite protection law, it takes precedence over the federal law. While this law covers only a portion of employed breastfeeding mothers, it has proven to be a start toward eliminating or reducing employment-related barriers to breastfeeding.

Also under the Affordable Care Act, health insurers will be required to pay for a range of preventive care services specifically aimed at women. These services include "comprehensive lactation support and counseling, by a trained provider during pregnancy and/or in the postpartum period, and costs for renting breastfeeding equipment." While this provision is well intended, the HHS did not provide implementation guidelines for insurers, leaving them to determine for themselves how to interpret the law. This has resulted in some mothers being provided with inappropriate breast pumps and inadequate lactation care and services. See the Resources section for samples of best practices for insurers regarding the Affordable Care Act's breastfeeding provisions. Clinicians are of great importance as a source for informing mothers and employers of the laws and providing help in securing the services to which mothers are entitled.

REFERENCES

Centers for Disease Control and Prevention (CDC). (2010). HealthStyles survey—Breastfeeding practices: 2010. Retrieved from http://www.cdc.gov/breastfeeding/data/healthstyles_survey/survey_2010.htm

Centers for Disease Control and Prevention (CDC). (2013). Progress in increasing breastfeeding and reducing racial/ethnic differences—United States, 2000–2008 births. *Morbidity and Mortality Weekly, 62,* 77–80. Retrieved from http://www.cdc.gov/mmwr/preview/mmwrhtml/mm6205a1.htm?s_cid=mm6205a1_w

Centers for Disease Control and Prevention (CDC). (2014). Breastfeeding report card—United States, 2014. Retrieved from http://www.cdc.gov/breastfeeding/pdf/2014breastfeedingreportcard.pdf

Johnson, A., Kirk, R., Rosenblum, K. L., & Muzik, M. (2015). Enhancing breastfeeding rates among African American women: A systematic review of current psychosocial interventions. *Breastfeeding Medicine, 10,* 45–62.

Murtagh, L., & Moulton, A. D. (2011). Working mothers, breastfeeding, and the law. *American Journal of Public Health, 101,* 217–223.

National Conference of State Legislatures. (2015). Breastfeeding laws, updated May 2015. Retrieved from http://www.ncsl.org/research/health/breastfeeding-state-laws.aspx

Nguyen, T. T., & Hawkins, S. S. (2012). Current state of US breastfeeding laws. *Maternal and Child Nutrition, 9,* 350–358.

Smith-Gagen, J., Hollen, R., Tashiro, S., Cook, D. M., & Yang, W. (2014). The association of state law to breastfeeding practices in the US. *Maternal Child Health Journal, 18,* 2034–2043.

Smith-Gagen, J., Hollen, R., Walker, M., Cook, D. M., & Yang, W. (2014). Breastfeeding laws and breastfeeding practices by race and ethnicity. *Women's Health Issues, 24-1,* e11–e19.

U.S. Department of Health and Human Services. (2010). *Healthy People 2020: Topics and objectives.* Washington, DC: Author. Retrieved from http://healthypeople.gov/2020/topicsobjectives2020/objectiveslist.aspx?topicId=26

U.S. Department of Health and Human Services. (2011). *The Surgeon General's call to action to support breastfeeding.* Washington, DC: Office of the Surgeon General. Retrieved from http://www.surgeongeneral.gov/library/calls/breastfeeding/index.html

RESOURCES

Sample best practices for insurers

Government of the District of Columbia, Department of Health Care Finance. (2014). Policy regarding Medicaid coverage to promote breastfeeding. Retrieved from http://osse.dc.gov/sites/default/files/dc/sites/dhcf/publication/attachments/Transmittal%2014-21.pdf

U.S. Breastfeeding Committee, National Breastfeeding Center. (2014). *Model policy: Payer coverage of breastfeeding support and counseling services, pumps and supplies.* (2nd ed.). Washington, DC: Author. Retrieved from http://nebula.wsimg.com/a8f135dc425654414662d18cc110b5d1?AccessKeyId=824D247BD163CE1574F8&disposition=0&alloworigin=1

Differentiation of providers of lactation care and services

Massachusetts Breastfeeding Coalition. The landscape of breastfeeding support. (2014). Retrieved from http://massbreastfeeding.org/wp-content/uploads/2013/06/Landscape-of-Breastfeeding-Support-03-31-14.pdf

National WIC Association. (2016). Enhancing breastfeeding support in WIC: The case for increasing the number of International Board Certified Lactation Consultants. Retrieved from https://s3.amazonaws.com/aws.upl/nwica.org/ibclc-cc.pdf

U.S. Lactation Consultant Association. (2015). Who's who in lactation? Retrieved from http://uslca.org/wp-content/uploads/2015/12/Whos-Who-Watermark.pdf

Chapter 1

Influence of the Biospecificity of Human Milk

INTRODUCTION

Effective breastfeeding management requires a general understanding of the structure and function of human milk itself. Many of the recommendations for successful breastfeeding and optimal infant health outcomes are based on using what the clinician knows about the components of human milk, what they do, and how they work. This chapter and Appendix 1-1 provide an overview of the components of breastmilk and of breastfeeding management based on milk function and composition.

Human milk is a highly complex and unique fluid that is strikingly different from the milks of other species, including the cow. Aggressive marketing of infant formula has blurred the public's perception of the differences between human milk and infant formula. Data from the HealthStyles survey, an annual national mail survey to U.S. adults, were examined to understand changes in public attitudes toward breastfeeding. The 1999 and 2003 HealthStyles surveys (Li, Rock, & Grummer-Strawn, 2007) included four breastfeeding items related to public attitudes toward breastfeeding in public and toward differences between infant formula and breastmilk. The percentage of respondents in agreement with the statement, "Infant formula is as good as breastmilk," increased significantly, from 14.3% in 1999 to 25.7% in 2003 (Li et al., 2007). In 2010, 20% of respondents still agreed that infant formula is as good as breastmilk, and over 30% neither agreed nor disagreed (Centers for Disease Control and Prevention, 2010). This figure has improved over time, with 15.52% currently agreeing that infant formula is as good as breastmilk and 26.28% neither agreeing nor disagreeing (Centers for Disease Control and Prevention, 2014a). This finding probably suggests that many people may still be sufficiently confused regarding the similarity or difference between infant formula and breastmilk that they cannot form an opinion. Lack of clarity regarding the difference between formula and breastmilk can be caused by clever marketing of infant formula, by contradictory Internet resources, and by social media postings that leave mothers vulnerable to marketing claims and peer opinions. Many of these interwoven resources are typically not evidence based and prey on vulnerabilities of new mothers, resulting in mothers who may be less likely to initiate or sustain breastfeeding. Hundreds of human milk components interact synergistically to fulfill the dual function of breastmilk, nourishing and protecting infants and young children who are breastfed or who receive human milk. The addition of ingredients into infant formula derived from nonhuman sources and pre- and probiotics cannot duplicate the health, cognitive, and developmental outcomes seen in infants fed human milk, no matter what formula advertising might claim.

Lactation is an ancient process that is thought to predate placental gestation and mammals themselves. It appears to have evolved in incremental steps as part of the innate immune system and over time acquired its nutritional function. The mammary gland is thought to have first developed as a mucous skin gland that secreted antimicrobial substances to protect the surface of the egg and skin of the newborn (**Figure 1-1**). Oftedal (2002) suggests that these glands evolved from the role of providing primarily moisture and antimicrobials to parchment-shelled eggs to the role of supplying nutrients for offspring. Fossil evidence indicates that some of the therapsids (mammal-like reptiles) and the mammaliaformes ("mammal-shaped," a branch of life that contains the mammals and their closest extinct relatives), which were present during the Triassic period more than 200 million years ago, produced a nutrient-rich milk-like secretion. Much later, due to gene sharing and gene duplication events, two antimicrobial enzymes (lysozyme and xanthine oxidoreductase) evolved new functions within the mammary epithelium, which allowed the secretion of fat, whey protein, sugar, and water, resulting in the unique and complex fluid we call milk (Vorbach, Capecchi, & Penninger, 2006).

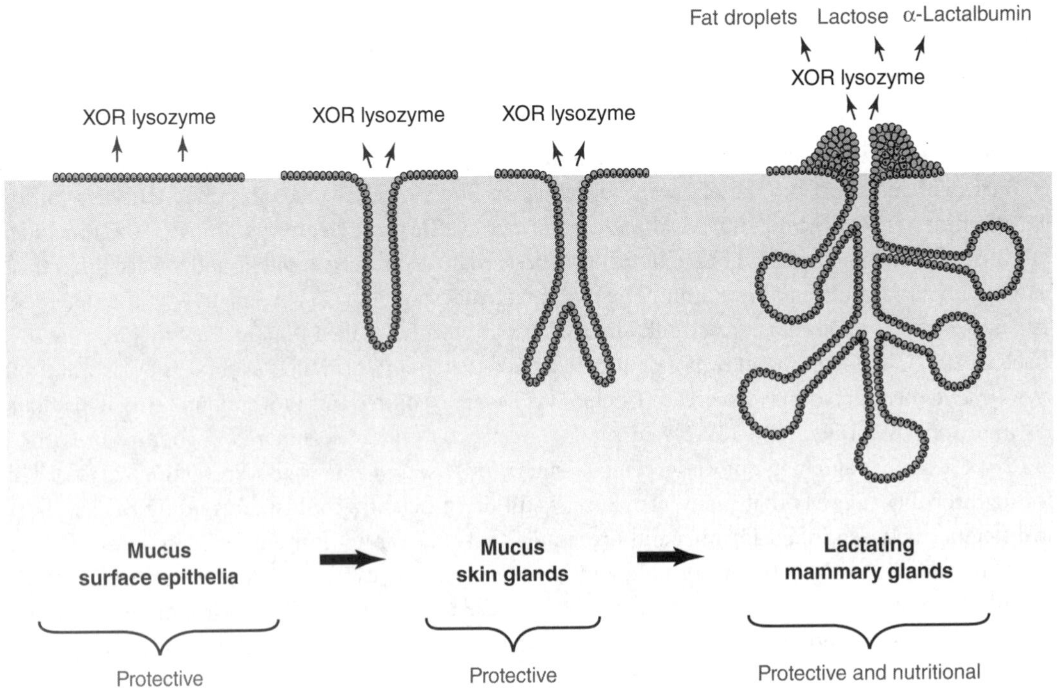

Figure 1-1 Proposed evolution of the mammary gland from a mucus-secreting epithelial gland.

Vorbach, C., Capecchi, M. R., & Penninger, J. M. (2006). Evolution of the mammary gland from the innate immune system? *BioEssays, 28*, 606–616. BioEssays by International Council of Scientific Unions; Company of Biologists. Reproduced with permission of John Wiley & Sons Ltd.

Milk composition and the length of lactation have been modified and adapted to meet the needs of each particular species. Generally, the protein content of milk varies with the rate of growth of the offspring. In many species, including humans, low-solute milk with relatively low concentrations of protein is related to a pattern of frequent feedings. Researchers often refer to species that manifest or practice this concept as "continuous contact" species. Calorie-dense milk with a high fat concentration can be associated with both the size of the species and low environmental temperatures. For example, marine mammals have fat concentrations of 50% or more in their milk to enable their young to lay down a thick insulating layer of fat. Each species has features (e.g., an organ, a behavior, a body system) that serve as major focal points for determining the type, variety, and interactions of the milk components fed to the young. In humans, these focal points include the brain, the immune system, and the acquisition of affiliative behavior.

Human milk composition is not static or uniform like infant formula. Breastmilk is a living dynamic fluid that represents an elegant interplay between the needs and vulnerabilities of the infant and the rapid adaptability of the mother's body to provide milk components to meet those needs and support those vulnerabilities:

- Colostrum (1–5 days) evolves through transitional milk (6–13 days) to mature milk (14 days and beyond).
- During early lactation, a few hours can show a significant change in milk composition. Lactoferrin, for example, decreases significantly over the first 3 days of lactation.
- Milk composition changes during each feeding as the breast drains and the fat content rises.
- Milk composition changes during each day and over the course of the entire lactation.
- Milk of preterm mothers differs from that of mothers delivering at term.
- More than 200 components have been identified in human milk, with some having still unknown roles.
- Hundreds of thousands of immune cells in breastmilk are ingested by the breastfed infant every day.
- Human milk contains stem cells that are involved in the regulation of mammary gland development and tumorigenesis (Thomas, Zeps, Cregan, Hartmann, & Martin, 2011). These stem cells can migrate to different organs to provide active immunity and boost infant development in early life (Hassiotou & Hartmann, 2014).
- Infant formula is an inert nutritional medium with no growth factors, hormones, or live cells like those found in breastmilk.
- Human milk is a biological mediator, carrying a rich variety of bioactive substances intended to grow a brain, construct an immune system, and facilitate affiliative behavior.

COLOSTRUM

Colostrum, the first milk, is present in the breasts from about 12–16 weeks into the pregnancy onward. This thick fluid's yellowish color comes from beta-carotene. It differs from mature milk both in the nature of its components and in their relative proportions. Colostrum has a mean energy value of 67 kcal/dL (18.76 kcal/oz), compared with mature milk's mean energy value of 75 kcal/dL (21 kcal/oz). The volume of colostrum per feeding during the first 3 days ranges from 2 to 20 mL and sometimes more. Colostrum is higher in protein, sodium, chloride, potassium, and fat-soluble vitamins such as vitamin A (3 times higher on day 3 than in mature milk), vitamin E (3 times higher than in mature milk), and carotenoids (10 times higher than in mature milk). It is lower in carbohydrates, lipids (2%), potassium, and lactose.

During the early days following delivery, the tight junctions between the mammary epithelial cells are relatively open and allow the transport of many bioactive immune substances from the mother's circulation into her colostrum (Kelleher & Lonnerdal, 2001). This enrichment of the early milk helps compensate for the relatively naïve neonatal immune system. Colostrum is rich in antioxidants, antibodies, and immunoglobulins, especially secretory immunoglobulin A (sIgA). Colostrum contains a high concentration of sIgA, approximately 10 g/L compared with approximately 1 g/L in mature milk. It contains interferon, which has strong antiviral activity, and fibronectin, which makes certain phagocytes more aggressive so that they ingest microbes even when not tagged by an antibody. Colostrum contains pancreatic secretory trypsin inhibitor (PSTI), a peptide found in the pancreas that protects it from damage by the digestive enzymes that it produces. PSTI is also found in mature breastmilk, but it is seven times more concentrated in colostrum. Marchbank, Weaver, Nilsen-Hamilton, and Playford (2009) found that PSTI stimulated cell migration and proliferation by threefold and reduced apoptosis (cell death) in damaged intestinal cells by 70–80%. PSTI both protects and repairs the delicate intestines of the newborn, readying the organ for processing future foods. Feeding infants colostrum establishes and maintains gut integrity, an important advantage over infant formula, because PSTI is not found in artificial milks. The newborn infant is deficient in CD14, part of a complex that can activate the innate immune system and that is important for protection against pathogen invasion. CD14 is present in human milk, with the highest concentration being present in colostrum. Colostrum's potent cocktail of components also includes specific oligosaccharides that change in concentration over the first 3 days to meet the physiological demands of the infant (Asakuma et al., 2007). They serve as a decoy to inhibit the attachment of pathogenic microorganisms, helping to protect newborns during an especially vulnerable time. Not only is colostrum replete with anti-infective properties, but the colostrum of mothers delivering preterm is more highly enriched with potent disease protectors than the colostrum of mothers delivering at term.

Preterm infants consuming their own mother's colostrum can benefit from ingestion of up to twice as many macrophages, lymphocytes, and total cells compared with those which are present in term colostrum (Mathur, Dwarkadas, Sharma, Saha, & Jain, 1990). They also receive more IgA, lysozymes, lactoferrin, and neutrophils than if they were receiving term colostrum. However, the colostrum of mothers delivering very preterm infants has lower concentrations of secretory IgA and several cytokines than the colostrum of mothers delivering after 30 weeks of gestation (Castellote et al., 2011). The degree of prematurity may affect the immunological composition of breastmilk, with earlier colostrum and milk showing reduced concentrations of some anti-infective factors. Infant formula, however, contains none of these formidable fighters of infection, leaving infants who are not fed colostrum or human milk much more vulnerable to infections and diseases prevented or reduced by breastfeeding or the provision of expressed colostrum and milk.

Colostrum of diabetic mothers is subject to biochemical and immunological alterations that affect the levels of some of its components. The protein expression involved in immunity and nutrition differs between the colostrum of mothers with gestational diabetes and that of mothers without gestational diabetes (Grapov et al., 2015). The colostrum of diabetic mothers is higher in glucose, lower in secretory IgA and secretory IgG, lower in C3 protein, lower in amylase, and higher in lipase (Morceli et al., 2011).

Colostrum of mothers who smoke has a significantly lower antioxidant capacity than the colostrum of mothers who do not smoke (Zagierski et al., 2011). This impairs the colostrum's ability to protect the infant from free radicals that contribute to conditions related to oxidative stress to which preterm infants are so vulnerable, such as necrotizing enterocolitis (NEC) and retinopathy of prematurity.

Maternal smoking alters the colostrum levels of a number of cytokines, which in turn increases the susceptibility of the newborn to infections (Piskin, Karavar, Arasli, & Ermis, 2012). In addition, the mode of delivery affects the antioxidant capacity of colostrum. The colostrum of mothers who deliver by cesarean section is lower in its antioxidative status than the colostrum of mothers who deliver vaginally (Simsek, Karabiyik, Polat, Duran, & Polat, 2014), potentially impeding the ability of colostrum to protect the infant from cellular damage caused by oxidative stress. Cesarean delivery can reduce the volume and prolactin concentration of colostrum as well as decrease the fatty acid levels.

Colostrum contributes to the establishment of bifidus flora in the digestive tract. The composition and volume of colostrum are in keeping with the needs and stores of a newborn human baby. Its primary function is anti-infective, but its biochemical composition has a laxative effect on meconium. It also provides a concentrated dose of certain nutrients such as zinc.

Genetic and environmental features may contribute to the compositional diversity seen in the colostrum of mothers worldwide. Musumeci and Musumeci (2013) reported the compositional differences between the colostrum of mothers living in Sicily and those living in Burkina Faso, one of the poorest countries of the African sub-Saharan area. The colostrum of the African mothers was richer in growth factors (IGF-I) that favor intestinal maturation; endorphins and S100B, which protect the brain from the consequences of asphyxia under difficult childbirth conditions; and chitotriosidase (an enzyme produced by activated macrophages), which is protective against gut pathogens, *Candida albicans*, and nematodes. It is thought that these components are present in higher quantities in African mothers' colostrum due to the precarious conditions of living in Africa, which exert a selective pressure to preserve the newborn.

Given the potential stressors on the composition of colostrum, it would seem prudent to assure maximum intake of colostrum for infants who are born by cesarean section, who experienced a difficult or precarious delivery, whose mothers smoke or have been exposed to secondhand smoke, whose mothers are diabetic, or who are born preterm.

CLINICAL IMPLICATIONS: ALLERGY AND DISEASE

It has long been thought that the gut (gastrointestinal [GI] tract) of a term fetus is sterile and that the bacterial colonization of the newborn gut occurs only following transit through the birth canal, where maternal vaginal and fecal bacteria become the first residents of the neonate's gut. More recent research, however, has shown that infants could develop their original gut microbiome well before birth. Researchers have reported that the meconium of term infants is not sterile, revealing that gut colonization actually starts prior to delivery (Jimenez et al., 2008). Bacteria have been isolated from amniotic fluid without any clinical or histological evidence of infection or inflammation in either the mother or the infant. Given that the fetus continuously swallows amniotic fluid in utero, bacteria present in that amniotic fluid from the maternal digestive tract may be the origin of the first infant gut colonizers. This suggests that the bacterial composition of the maternal gut could affect the bacterial content seen in infant meconium and serve as the pioneer bacteria colonizing the fetal gut.

Further influences and additions to the infant's gut microbiome occur during and after delivery through several mechanisms and routes:

- Method of delivery: During a vaginal delivery, bacteria from the maternal vaginal and intestinal microbiota colonize the infant gut. In a cesarean delivery, infants avoid contact with the maternal vaginal microbiota, leading to a deficiency of strict anaerobes such as *E. coli*, *Bacteroides*, and *Bifidobacterium* and a higher presence of facultative anaerobes such as *Clostridium* species, compared with vaginally born infants (Adlerberth & Wold, 2009). The cesarean-born infant's initial bacterial exposure is more likely to be from environmental microbes in the air, other infants, and the nursing staff, all of which serve as vectors for transfer. Infants born by cesarean section prior to the rupture of the amnion membrane are not exposed to the maternal flora in the birth canal. These infants are also subject to longer separations from their mother, longer hospital stays, and a shorter duration of breastfeeding—all of which increase the likelihood of significant alterations in the colonization of the infant's intestine.
- Gestational age: The pattern of gut colonization in preterm infants differs from that in healthy term infants. The aberration in colonization is due to a number of factors, including the use of sterile infant formula and the common administration of antibiotics, which could also contribute to feeding intolerance and the development of NEC (Neu & Walker, 2011). Preterm infants are also often born by cesarean section, are colonized with fewer bacteria, are separated from their mother, and are exposed to pathogenic institutional organisms.
- Feeding modality: Newborns receive gut-colonizing bacteria from their mother's milk. Breastmilk is thought to be one of the most important postpartum elements modulating the metabolic and immunological programming of a child's health (Aaltonen et al., 2011). Breastmilk is not sterile, nor is it meant to be. In fact, researchers have identified more than 700 bacterial species in human milk that vary from mother to mother depending on the mode of delivery and the obesity status of the mother. Colostrum has an even higher diversity of bacterial species than does transitional or mature milk (Cabrera-Rubio et al., 2012). The conditions of maternal overweight and obesity have been associated with an inflammation-prone aberrant gut microbiota that can be transferred to the infant, provoking unfavorable metabolic development in the baby (Collado, Isolauri, Laitinen, & Salminen, 2010). Divergence or deviation from breastmilk-directed microbial colonization during the early weeks and months of life interferes with many functions in the gut. This departure from the norm provokes a slower postnatal maturation of epithelial cell barrier functions, which alters the permeability of the gut and facilitates invasion of pathogens and foreign or harmful antigens (Perrier & Corthesy, 2011). The perinatal period, therefore, is a critical window of time where "set points" are imprinted in the neonatal gut. The nature of the microbiota acquired during the perinatal period is crucial in determining the intestinal immune response and tolerance. Alterations of the gut environment are directly responsible for mucosal inflammation and disease, autoimmunity conditions, and allergic disorders in childhood and adulthood (Gronlund, Arvilommi, Kero, Lehtonen, & Isolauri, 2000). The lower the percentage of breastmilk intake (less than 88%), the greater the risk of gut inflammation (Moodley-Govender, Mulol, Stauber, Manary, & Coutsoudis, 2015).

The bacterial composition of breastmilk also exerts an influence on the health of the maternal breast itself. The composition of the bacterial communities in the breastmilk are unique to each mother and could influence whether a woman develops mastitis or recurrent mastitis, or never develops mastitis at all (Hunt et al., 2011). It is thought that bacterial competition for nutrients or production of bacteriocins (toxins produced by bacteria that inhibit the growth of similar or closely related bacterial strains) might reduce or eliminate potential pathogens and prevent or remove subsequent signs and symptoms of mastitis (Heikella & Saris, 2003).

The effects of the composition of the first bacterial colonizers of the newborn gut are not confined to the newborn period, but rather endure well into adulthood. If intestinal flora develop on an alternate trajectory as caused by a cesarean delivery and/or feeding with infant formula, the development of the immune system might also be different, leaving it vulnerable to a number of diseases and conditions, including autoimmune disorders. For example, atopic diseases appear more often in infants who have experienced a cesarean delivery compared with those delivered vaginally. One meta-analysis found a 20% increase in the subsequent risk of asthma in children who had been delivered by cesarean section (Thavagnanam, Fleming, Bromley, Shields, & Cardwell, 2008). Cardwell et al. (2008) showed a 20% increase in the risk of childhood type 1 diabetes after cesarean delivery. There is also an increased risk for children born by cesarean delivery to acquire celiac disease (Decker et al., 2010). Cesarean delivery may cause a shift in the gut to a more inflammation-prone environment and an increase in intestinal permeability leading to a higher risk for diseases and conditions caused by inflammatory conditions and pathogenic microorganisms (Decker, Hornef, & Stockinger, 2011). Chronic immune disorders such as asthma, systemic connective tissue disorders, juvenile arthritis, inflammatory bowel diseases, immune deficiencies, and leukemia have all been found to be significantly increased in children delivered by cesarean section (Sevelsted, Stokholm, Bennelykke, & Bisgaard, 2015). The primary gut flora in cesarean-born infants may be disturbed for as long as 6 months after birth (Gronlund, Lehtonen, Eerola, & Kero, 1999). Coinciding with cesarean deliveries is the delayed onset of lactogenesis II (Dewey, 2003; Evans, Evans, Royal, Esterman, & James, 2003; Scott, Binns, & Oddy, 2007), leaving these infants without the early support of breastmilk for the colonization and physiological development of their intestinal flora. Infants at highest risk of colonization by undesirable microbes, or when transfer from maternal sources cannot occur, are cesarean-delivered babies, preterm infants, full-term infants requiring intensive care, or infants separated from their mothers. Infants requiring intensive care acquire intestinal organisms slowly and the establishment of bifidobacterial flora is retarded. Such a delayed bacterial colonization of the gut with a limited number of bacterial species tends to be virulent.

Control and manipulation of the neonatal gut with human milk can be used as a strategy to prevent and treat intestinal diseases (Dai & Walker, 1999). Major ecological disturbances are observed in newborn infants treated with antimicrobial agents. If several infants in a hospital nursery are treated with antibiotics, the intestinal colonization pattern of other infants in the same nursery may be disturbed, with the intestinal microflora returning to normal after several weeks (Tullus & Burman, 1989). One way of minimizing ecological disturbances in the neonatal intensive care unit (NICU) is to provide these infants with fresh breastmilk (Zetterstrom, Bennet, & Nord, 1994). Infants treated with a broad-spectrum antibiotic during the first 4 days of life show reduced colonization of the gut with *Bifidobacterium* and unusual colonization of *Enterococcus* in the first week compared with infants who have not been treated with antibiotics. Overgrowth of enterococci and arrested growth of *Bifidobacterium* occurred in antibiotic-treated infants (Tanaka, Kobayashi, et al., 2009). At 1 month of age, infants treated with antibiotics had a higher intestinal population of Enterobacteriaceae than untreated infants. Infants of mothers who had received a broad-spectrum antibiotic prior to cesarean delivery showed weaker but similar gut alterations.

Breastfed and formula-fed infants have different gut flora (Mountzouris, McCartney, & Gibson, 2002). Breastfed infants have a lower gut pH (acidic environment) of approximately 5.1–5.4 throughout the first 6 weeks, which is dominated by *Bifidobacterium* with reduced pathogenic (disease-causing) microbes such as *Escherichia coli*, *Bacteroides*, *Clostridia*, and streptococci. Flora with a diet-dependent pattern are present from the 4th day of life, with breastmilk-fed guts showing a 47% *Bifidobacterium* level and formula-fed guts showing a 15% level. In comparison, enterococci prevail in formula-fed infants (Rubaltelli, Biadaioli, Pecile, & Nicoletti, 1998). Infants fed formula have a high gut pH of approximately 5.9–7.3 characterized by a variety of putrefactive bacterial species. In infants fed breastmilk and formula supplements, the mean pH is approximately 5.7–6.0 during the first 4 weeks after birth, falling to 5.45 by the 6th week. Supplementation with formula induces a rapid shift in the bacterial pattern of a breastfed infant. The dominance of bifidobacteria during exclusive breastfeeding decreases when infant formula is added to the diet (Favier, Vaughan, De Vos, & Akkermans, 2002). When formula supplements are given to breastfed infants during the first 7 days of life, the production of a strongly acidic environment is delayed and its full potential may never be reached. Breastfed infants who receive formula supplements develop gut flora and behavior like those of formula-fed infants. This effect can be seen well beyond the early days. The infant intestinal microbiome at 6 weeks of age is significantly associated with both delivery mode and feeding method. The supplementation of breastfed infants with infant formula is associated with a gut microbiome composition at 6 weeks, which resembles that of infants who are exclusively formula-fed (Madan et al., 2016). This immediately increases the risk of gut inflammation and disease during a very vulnerable period of time. Another bacterial group found in breastfed infants that is almost as widespread as bifidobacteria is the genus *Ruminococcus* (Morelli, 2008). *Ruminococcus* has a protective function because it produces ruminococcin, which inhibits the development of many of the pathological species of *Clostridium* (Dabard et al., 2001). One notable difference between the microflora of breastfed and formula-fed infants is the low presence of clostridia in breastfed infants as compared with formula-fed infants. New molecular biology techniques have detected the presence of the genus *Desulfovibrio* mainly in formula-fed infants (Hopkins, Macfarlane, Furrie, Fite, & Macfarlane, 2005; Stewart, Chadwick, & Murray, 2006). These organisms have been linked with the development of inflammatory bowel disease.

Free fatty acids created during the digestion of infant formula (but not breastmilk) have been shown to cause cellular death that may contribute to NEC in preterm infants. NEC is much more likely to develop in preterm infants who are fed formula. Penn et al. (2012) "digested" infant formulas and breastmilk in vitro and tested for free fatty acids and whether these fatty acids killed off three types of cells involved in NEC: epithelial cells that line the intestine, endothelial cells that line blood vessels, and neutrophils that respond to inflammation. The digestion of formula lead to cell death in less than 5 minutes in some cases, while breastmilk did not. Digestion of infant formula caused death in 47% to 99% of neutrophils while only 6% of them died as a result of breastmilk digestion. This overwhelming cytotoxicity of infant formula should signal clinicians that every effort should be made for breastmilk to be fed to all infants, but especially preterm infants.

Breastmilk can contain up to 10^9 microbes/L in healthy mothers (West, Hewitt, & Murphy, 1979). Breastmilk from overweight mothers or those who put on more weight than recommended during pregnancy has been found to contain fewer species of bacteria, and mothers who had a planned cesarean delivery have been noted to have fewer species of bacteria in their breastmilk than those who had a vaginal birth (Cabrera-Rubio et al., 2012). The diversity of bacteria in a mother's milk can thus be affected by a number of factors that influence the initial colonization of the infant's gut. *Weisella*, *Leuconostoc*, *Staphylococcus*, *Streptococcus*, and *Lactococcus* were predominant in colostrum samples in the Cabrera-Rubio study, whereas in 1- and 6-month milk samples, the typical inhabitants of the oral cavity (e.g., *Veillonella*, *Leptotrichia*, and *Prevotella*) increased significantly. Frequently encountered bacterial groups in human milk also include staphylococci, streptococci, corynebacteria, lactobacilli, micrococci, propionibacteria, and bifidobacteria. These bacteria can originate from the maternal nipple and areola, the surrounding skin, as well as perhaps the milk ducts within the breast. The mother's nipple, areola, and surrounding skin and the infant's oral cavity represent their own ecological niche, with breastmilk being a relevant source of lactobacilli for the newborn. Allergic mothers have significantly lower amounts of bifidobacteria in their breastmilk compared with nonallergic mothers, which can alter the infant's intestinal microbiota in an infant already at a higher risk for the development of allergies (Gronlund et al., 2007).

Differences in intestinal microbiota may precede the development of overweight and obesity, as data are accumulating that implicate systemic low-grade inflammation and local gut microbiota as contributing factors to overnutrition (Backhed et al., 2004; Fantuzzi, 2005). High levels of *Bacteroides* in the gut microbiota in animal models were shown to predispose toward increased energy storage and obesity (Backhed et al., 2004; Ley et al., 2005). Alteration of gut microbiota in infants during a critical developmental window has been linked to a number of inflammatory conditions (Kalliomaki et al., 2001), creating an environment ripe with the potential for the acquisition of health challenges that have inflammatory origins. Kalliomaki, Collado, Salminen, and Isolauri (2008) demonstrated that bifidobacterial numbers were higher in infancy and *Staphylococcus* aureus was lower in infancy for children remaining at normal weight at 7 years than in children developing overweight. This finding implies that high numbers of bifidobacteria and low numbers of *S. aureus* during infancy as seen in breastfed infants may confer a degree of protection against overweight and obesity. Because adiposity is characterized by low-grade inflammation, the provision of breastmilk with its control of inflammatory pathways contributes to the protection of infants from the development of overweight and obesity. Infant formula has a different effect on the architecture, hydrolysis, and absorption functions in the intestine compared with breastmilk. Infant formula has a trophic or accelerated growth effect on the intestine with gut hypertrophy and acceleration of hydrolytic capacities. This may happen as a result of an adaptive reaction of the intestine to match the nutrient composition of formulas with their high protein content. The result appears as a higher absorption rate of nutrients in formula-fed infants compared to those fed breastmilk for the same food intake (Le Huerou-Luron, Blat, & Boudry, 2010). It could be speculated that this effect also could prime the body for overweight or obesity.

Food intolerances during infancy are common and thought to be related to the failure of adequately developed tolerance to antigens (Field, 2005). The incidence of cow's milk allergy in early childhood is approximately 2–3% in developed countries. Clinical reactions to cow's milk protein in breastmilk have been reported in 0.5% of breastfed infants. Tolerance contributes to reduced incidences of food-related allergies in breastfed infants (van Odijk et al., 2003) as a result of an active process whereby dietary antigens present in breastmilk combine with immunosuppressive cytokines to induce tolerance to dietary and microflora antigens (Brandtzaeg, 2003). Breastmilk contains components that significantly affect the efficiency of the induction of immune tolerance. For example, transforming growth factor beta (TGF-β) is a growth factor that helps inhibit inflammation and promotes T-cell tolerance. Neonates have low levels of TGF-β in the intestine; the high amounts of this factor in breastmilk compensate for this temporary deficiency. The amount of TGF-β in breastmilk is inversely correlated with the risk of allergy development in breastfed children. Specific deviations of the gut flora such as atypical composition and decreased numbers of bifidobacteria (Kalliomaki et al., 2001) can predispose infants to allergic disease (Salminen, Gueimonde, & Isolauri, 2005), inflammatory gut disease, and rotavirus diarrhea (Lee & Puong, 2002).

Immune physiology has been shown to differ between breastfed and formula-fed infants. In a study looking at key cytokines (cell messengers and regulators of inflammatory responses) and antibody-secreting cells in breastfed and formula-fed infants, Kainonen, Rautava, & Isolauri (2013) found that anti-inflammatory cytokine levels were significantly higher in breastfed infants compared to formula-fed babies. Pro-inflammatory cytokines (TNF-alpha and IL-2) were significantly higher in formula-fed infants, with elevated concentrations of these seen throughout the first year of life. TNF-alpha has the ability to disrupt mucosal barrier function. In breastfed infants, the anti-inflammatory TGF-beta2 was significantly higher, which modulates immune response and enhances mucosal barrier function by inducing IgA production. This type of immune physiology in the breastfed infants contributes to the reduced risk of atopic disease and healthy immune function.

Infants have a functionally immature and immunonaïve gut at birth. The tight junctions of the GI mucosa take many weeks to mature and close the gut to whole proteins and pathogens. Intestinal permeability decreases faster in breastfed infants than in formula-fed infants (Catassi, Bonucci, Coppa, Carlucci, & Giorgi, 1995), with human milk accelerating the maturation of the gut barrier function while formula does not (Newburg & Walker, 2007). The open junctions and immaturity of the GI tract's mucosal barrier play a role in the acquisition of NEC, diarrheal disease, and allergy. Preterm infants experience a high risk for acquiring NEC due to their lower gastric acid production, reduced ability to break down toxins, and low levels of sIgA, which increases bacterial adherence to the intestinal mucosa. Preterm infants cannot fully digest carbohydrates and proteins. Undigested casein, the protein in infant formula, can function as a chemoattractant for neutrophils, exacerbating the inflammatory response and opening the tight junctions between intestinal epithelial cells, disrupting the integrity of the epithelium barrier, and allowing the delivery of whole bacteria, endotoxin, and viruses directly into the bloodstream (Claud & Walker, 2001). Feeding preterm infants with infant formula may produce colonization of the intestine with pathogenic bacteria, resulting in an exaggerated inflammatory response. The sIgA from colostrum, transitional milk, and mature milk coats the gut, preventing attachment and invasion of pathogens by competitively binding and neutralizing bacterial antigens. This passively provides immunity during a time of reduced neonatal gut immune function. Mothers' milk sIgA is antigen specific; that is, the antibodies are targeted against pathogens in the infant's immediate surroundings. The mother synthesizes antibodies when she ingests, inhales, or otherwise comes in contact with disease-causing microbes. When the mother is exposed to a pathogen, M cells of the Peyer's patch in her gut-associated lymphoid tissue or tracheobronchial tree mucosa acquire the pathogen, after which the M cell presents its antigen to the B cell. The B cell migrates to the mammary epithelial cell, which secretes IgA with the antibody to the particular pathogen. The IgA enters the breastmilk and is consumed by the infant. The sIgA binds the pathogen in the infant's intestine, inhibiting its ability to infect the infant. These antibodies ignore useful bacteria normally found in the gut and ward off disease without causing inflammation.

It is important to keep the mother and her newborn baby together during their hospital stay. This practice allows the mother to enrich her milk with antibodies against bacteria and viruses to which both she and her baby are exposed. Separating mother and baby interferes with this disease defense mechanism. Feeding artificial baby milk to a newborn infant removes this protection.

The prudent clinician can avoid giving a baby infant formula in the hospital or before gut closure occurs. Once dietary supplementation begins, the bacterial profile of breastfed infants resembles that of formula-fed infants; namely, bifidobacteria are no longer dominant and obligate anaerobic bacterial populations develop (Mackie, Sghir, & Gaskins, 1999). Breastmilk ingestion creates and maintains a low intestinal pH and a microflora in which bifidobacteria are predominant and Gram-negative enteric organisms are almost completely absent. Relatively small amounts of formula supplementation of breastfed infants (1 supplement per 24 hours) result in shifts from a breastfed to a formula-fed gut flora pattern (Bullen, Tearle, & Stewart, 1977). With the introduction of supplementary formula, the flora becomes almost indistinguishable from normal adult flora within 24 hours (Gerstley, Howell, & Nagel, 1932). If breastmilk were again given exclusively, it would take 2–4 weeks for the intestinal environment to return to a state favoring the Gram-positive flora (Brown & Bosworth, 1922; Gerstley et al., 1932). Interestingly, optimal microflora in the infant might have long-term benefits if the flora of the adult is determined by events occurring in the critical period of gut colonization (Edwards & Parrett, 2002).

Other events and exposures that occur during the critical window of immune system development may combine to increase the risk and incidence of allergic disease later in life, such as cesarean delivery, prolonged labor, and infant multivitamin supplementation (Milner & Gergen, 2005). A higher incidence of atopy and allergic rhinitis was observed in adults who had received vitamin D supplementation during their first year of life (Hypponen et al., 2004). These data provide additional support for the importance of exclusive breastfeeding (Host & Halken, 2005) during the first half year of life and the avoidance of adding solid foods, infant formula, additives, supplements, or beverages to an infant's diet before maturation of the gut.

There is a strong relationship between allergic diseases and genetic and environmental factors. Differences in immune function are evident at birth, leading to the concept that prenatal factors such as maternal microbial exposure, diet, and pollutants such as cigarette smoke can modify early immune gene expression through heritable changes in genetic makeup. Certain maternal exposures may disrupt normal gene activation or silencing patterns required for normal newborn immune responses (Prescott & Nowak-Wegrzyn, 2011). The first month of life is a period of rapid maturation of the neonatal immune system and offers a window of opportunity for interventions aimed at prevention of allergy. Innate immune responses are markedly different between neonates who are exclusively breastfed during the first month of life and those who are not. Breastmilk-mediated modulation of the developing innate immune system programs for protection from subsequent disease, asthma, and atopy (Belderbos et al., 2012).

It is thought that initial sensitization to food allergens in the exclusively breastfed infant may occur from external sources such as a single feeding of infant formula. In susceptible families, breastfed infants can be sensitized to cow's milk protein by the giving of "just one bottle" (inadvertent supplementation, unnecessary supplementation, or planned supplementation) in the newborn nursery during the first 3 days of life (Cantani & Micera, 2005; Host, 1991; Host, Husby, & Osterballe, 1988). As early as 1935, Ratner recommended that isolated exposure to cow's milk be avoided in infants fed breastmilk (Ratner, 1935). Small doses of allergens can serve to sensitize an infant to subsequent challenges compared with large doses, which induce tolerance. Infants' risk of developing atopic disease has been calculated as 37% if one parent has atopic disease and as 62–85% if both parents are affected, dependent on whether the parents have similar or dissimilar clinical disease. Those infants showing elevated levels of IgE in cord blood irrespective of family history are also considered to be at high risk (Chandra, 2000). The incidence of cow's milk protein allergy is lower in exclusively breastfed infants compared with formula-fed or mixed-fed infants, with about 0.5% of exclusively breastfed infants showing reproducible clinical reactions to cow's milk protein (Vandenplas et al., 2007). In breastfed infants at risk, exclusive breastfeeding for at least 4 months or breastfeeding with hypoallergenic formulas if medically needed to supplement breastfeeding decreases the risk of atopic dermatitis (Greer, Sicherer, & Burks, 2008).

If atopic disease associated with cow's milk allergy occurs, partially hydrolyzed formula is not recommended because it contains potentially allergenic cow's milk peptides. Different hydrolysates have differing effects on atopic disease. Extensively hydrolyzed casein-based formula may be more advantageous if needed as a supplement for infants at risk for allergy development (von Berg et al., 2003). Miniello et al. (2008) recommend that if supplemental formula feeding is needed, infants from atopic families should be supplemented with a hydrolyzed infant formula for the first 6 months of life. High-risk infants without a history of eczema in a primary relative may receive a protective effect from less expensive partially hydrolyzed formula. Those infants who have first-degree relatives with eczema should receive an extensively hydrolyzed formula. Soy formula is not recommended for the prevention of atopy in infants at high risk of developing allergy (Osborn & Sinn, 2006). Rozenfeld, Docena, Añón, and Fossati (2002) demonstrated that a monoclonal antibody specific to casein (a bovine milk protein) displayed affinity to a component of glycinin, an ingredient in soy-based formulas.

Cross-sensitization between protein sources is well established. Among infants with cow's milk protein allergy, 13–20% have allergies to beef (Martelli, De Chiara, Corvo, Restani, & Fiocchi, 2002). Solid foods should not be introduced until 6 months of age; the introduction of dairy products should be delayed until 1 year of age; and the mother should consider eliminating peanuts, tree nuts, cow's milk, eggs, and fish from her diet (American Academy of Pediatrics [AAP], Committee on Nutrition, 2000; Zeiger, 1999). A 7-day washout of milk proteins is required when instituting a restricted diet, delaying the expected clinical response by the infant (Brill, 2008). A maternal elimination diet may also need to include the elimination of beef and may need to be continued for at least 2 weeks, and up to 4 weeks in cases of atopic dermatitis or allergic colitis. If symptoms improve or disappear during the elimination diet, one food per week can be reintroduced to the mother's diet. If symptoms do not reappear upon reintroduction of a particular food, the mother should begin consuming it again. If symptoms reappear, it should continue to be eliminated from her diet during the course of breastfeeding.

In susceptible families, early exposure to cow's milk proteins or the absence of breastfeeding can increase the risk of the infant or child developing insulin-dependent diabetes mellitus (type 1, or IDDM) (Karjalainen et al., 1992; Mayer et al., 1988) and type 2 diabetes mellitus (Young et al., 2002). Type 1 diabetes is one of the most common chronic diseases in childhood. It results from the autoimmune destruction of the insulin-producing beta cells in the pancreas following a variable subclinical length of time where autoantibodies against the beta cells antigens are present. Breastfeeding for 12 months or longer predicts a lower risk of type 1 diabetes as well as a lower risk of progression from islet autoimmunity to type 1 diabetes in susceptible infants (Lund-Blix et al., 2015).

The human insulin content in breastmilk is significantly higher than the content of bovine insulin in cow's milk. Insulin content in infant formulas is extremely low to absent. Insulin supports gut maturation. In animal models, oral administration of human insulin stimulates the intestinal immune system, thereby generating active cellular mechanisms that suppress the development of autoimmune diabetes. The lack of human insulin in infant formulas may break the tolerance to insulin and lead to the development of type 1 diabetes (Vaarala, Paronen, Otokoski, & Akerblom, 1998). The avoidance of cow's milk protein during the first several months of life may reduce the later development of IDDM or delay its onset in susceptible individuals (AAP, Work Group on Cow's Milk Protein and Diabetes Mellitus, 1994). Infants who are exclusively breastfed for at least 4 months have a lower risk of seroconversion leading to beta-cell autoimmunity. Short-term breastfeeding (less than 2–3 months) and the early introduction of cow's milk-based infant formula may predispose young children who are genetically susceptible to type 1 diabetes to progressive signs of beta-cell autoimmunity (Kimpimaki et al., 2001). Holmberg and coworkers (2007) concluded that positivity for beta-cell autoantibodies in children from the general population was associated with a short duration of both total and exclusive breastfeeding as well as an early introduction of formula. Sensitization and development of immune memory to cow's milk protein is the initial step in the etiology of IDDM (Kostraba et al., 1993). Sensitization can occur with very early exposure to cow's milk before gut cellular tight junction closure takes place. It can also occur with exposure to cow's milk during an infection-caused GI alteration when the mucosal barrier becomes compromised, allowing antigens to cross and initiate immune reactions. Sensitization can take place if the presence of cow's milk protein in the gut damages the mucosal barrier, inflames the gut, or destroys binding components of cellular junctions or if another early insult with cow's milk protein leads to sensitization (Savilahti, Tuomilehto, Saukkonen, Virtala, & Akerblom, 1993). Of further importance is the fact that exposure to infant cereal during the first 3 months of life in genetically predisposed infants significantly increases the risk of developing diabetes (Norris et al., 2003; Ziegler, Schmid, Huber, Hummel, & Bonifacio, 2003).

The IgG immune complexes found in breastmilk function as potent inducers of tolerance to airborne aerosolized antigens to which the mother has been sensitized, providing antigen-specific protection from asthma in the infant (Mosconi et al., 2010). Silvers and colleagues (2012) analyzed 1,105 infants over 6 years focusing on breastfeeding, wheezing, and asthma. Each month of exclusive breastfeeding was associated with significant reductions in current asthma from 2 to 6 years, as was any amount of breastfeeding. The protective effect of breastfeeding against asthma was of even more importance in atopic children, in whom exclusive breastfeeding for 3 or more months reduced asthma at ages 4, 5, and 6 years by 62%, 55%, and 59%, respectively. Dogaru and colleagues (2012) found that breastfeeding had a positive

Table 1-1 Correlation of Number of Feedings in First 24 Hours and Bilirubin Levels

Number of Feedings	Bilirubin Levels at 6 Days of Age
4 times in first 24 h	26% with elevated bilirubin levels on day 6 (12–14 mg/dL)
7–8 times in first 24 h	12% with elevated bilirubin levels on day 6
> 9 times in first 24 h	None with elevated bilirubin levels on day 6

Data from Yamauchi, Y., & Yamanouchi, H. (1990). Breastfeeding frequency during the first 24 hours after birth in fullterm neonates. *Pediatrics*, 86, 171–175.

effect on lung function in school-aged children. There was no detrimental effect of breastfeeding on children whose mothers had asthma. In fact, children of asthmatic mothers had better lung function if they had been breastfed, with a dose–response relationship with the duration of breastfeeding. Breastfeeding may have a direct positive effect on lung growth.

Avoid giving the infant extra formula, water, or sugar water in an attempt to influence bilirubin levels. In the hospital it is important to ensure 8–12 feedings each 24 hours. Bilirubin levels correlate inversely with the number of feedings during the first 24 hours (**Table 1-1**) (Yamauchi & Yamanouchi, 1990). Bilirubin levels also correlate inversely with the number of feedings over the first 3 days of life (DeCarvalho, Klaus, & Merkatz, 1982), as in the following examples:

- If the average number of feedings per day is 6, day 3 bilirubin levels would be at 11 mg/dL.
- If the average number of feedings per day is 6.8, day 3 bilirubin levels would be at 9.3 ± 3.5 mg/dL.
- If the average number of feedings per day is 10.1, day 3 bilirubin levels would be at 6.5 ± 4.0 mg/dL.
- If the average number of feedings per day is 11, day 3 bilirubin levels would be at 5 mg/dL.

Further, bilirubin levels correlate inversely with the amount of water or glucose water given to breastfed newborns (Nicoll, Ginsburg, & Tripp, 1982). The more water or sugar water given to breastfed infants, the higher the bilirubin levels on day 3. Bilirubin functions as an antioxidant to protect cell membranes. Breastfed infants have higher levels of bilirubin than formula-fed infants because they are supposed to. Artificially lowering normally elevated bilirubin levels when feeding babies infant formula has not been shown to be beneficial.

NUTRITIONAL COMPONENTS

Water

Water makes up the majority (87.5%) of human milk. All other components are dissolved, dispersed, or suspended in water. An infant receiving adequate amounts of breastmilk will automatically consume his or her entire water requirement. Even in hot arid or humid climates, human milk provides 100% of water needs (Ashraf, Jalil, Aperia, & Lindblad, 1993).

Clinical Implications

Because human milk with its low solute load provides all the water an infant needs, breastfed infants do not require additional water. Consuming more water than needed can suppress the infant's appetite (especially if the water contains dextrose) and reduce the number of calories the infant receives, placing him or her at risk for hyperbilirubinemia and early weight loss. Sterile water has no calories; 5% dextrose water has 5 calories per ounce, whereas colostrum has 18 calories per ounce. An infant receiving an ounce of sugar water in place of an ounce of colostrum will experience a two-thirds deficit in calories.

Large amounts of low-solute water given to an infant over a short period of time can contribute to oral water intoxication, swelling of the brain, and seizures (Keating, Shears, & Dodge, 1991). Infants under one month of age have a lower glomerular filtration rate and cannot excrete a water load rapidly, making them more susceptible to oral water intoxication when given large water supplements. Oral water intoxication is more commonly seen in formula-fed infants whose caregivers use water bottles to extend the time between feedings or dilute formula supplies to make them last longer. This condition, however, can also occur in breastfed infants. A combination of factors can place the infant at risk for water intoxication, such as administration of large amounts of hypotonic intravenous (IV) solutions to laboring mothers (Tarnow-Mordi, Shaw, Liu, Gardner, & Flynn, 1981), addition of oxytocin by IV (Singhi, Chookang, Hall, & Kalghangi, 1985), and a large oral intake of fluid during labor (Johansson, Lindow, Kapadia, & Norman, 2002). A fluid shift to the fetus plus the birth-related surge in circulating vasopressin (the antidiuretic hormone) in the infant (Leung et al., 1980) can contribute to a water-sparing reaction or water retention in the infant. Excessive water in the infant can artificially inflate the birth weight, causing undue concern about large weight losses as the infant experiences diuresis or eliminates this excess water.

The mistaken belief that breastfed infants need supplemental water to prevent dehydration, hyperbilirubinemia, hypoglycemia, and weight loss disrupts breastfeeding, and the water is often offered simply for convenience (Williams, 2006). Glover and Sandilands (1990) reported that infants who received glucose water supplementation in the hospital lost more weight and stayed in hospital longer than infants who did not receive supplementation. Ruth-Sanchez and Greene (1997) described a 3-day-old breastfed infant who was given 675 mL (22.8 oz) of dextrose water by nurses and the mother in the 24 hours before NICU admission for resulting seizure activity. Infants who are breastfeeding adequately should not be offered additional water no matter what the climate (Almroth & Bidinger, 1990; Cohen, Brown, Rivera, & Dewey, 2000; Sachdev, Krishna, Puri, Satyanarayana, & Kumar, 1991).

Despite data discouraging the practice, giving water or sugar water to breastfed infants persists. In 2007, to characterize maternity practices related to breastfeeding, the CDC (2007) conducted the first national Maternity Practices in Infant Nutrition and Care (mPINC) survey. Survey responses were received from 2,687 hospitals and birthing facilities. When asked whether healthy, full-term, breastfed infants who receive supplements are given glucose water or water, 30% of facilities reported giving feedings of glucose water and 15% reported giving water, practices that are not supportive of breastfeeding. This practice is still prevalent in hospitals, with results from the 2009 mPINC survey showing that 25% of hospitals persist in engaging in the non-evidence-based practice of giving sterile water or glucose water to newborn breastfed infants. The 2013 mPINC survey, however, showed that this practice is now decreasing: An average of 12% of the surveyed hospitals reported giving healthy breastfed infants water or glucose water. Nevertheless, this rate was much higher—more than 20%—in the West North Central and East South Central regions of the United States (Centers for Disease Control and Prevention, 2014b). Data from the Infant Feeding Practices Study II (a survey of mother-reported infant feeding patterns) revealed that 13% of infants received sugar water while in the hospital and 10% of the infants were receiving plain water at the age of 1 month (Grummer-Strawn, Scanlon, & Fein, 2008), even when findings show that infants who do not consume solid foods have no need of solute-free water (Scariati, Grummer-Strawn, & Fein, 1997).

Mothers with low confidence levels with regard to their ability to breastfeed are vulnerable to the plethora of advice offered to them, even if the advice is misguided or incorrect, such as suggestions to offer supplementary or complementary water feedings (Blyth et al., 2002). If they perceive this advice as an indication of insufficient milk, they are significantly more likely to wean. Early water supplementation is associated with the increased likelihood that water-supplemented infants will receive infant formula during the first month of life. Mixed feedings often herald early weaning from the breast and reduce the disease-protective abilities found with exclusive breastfeeding. Giugliani, Santo, de Oliveira, and Aerts (2008) found that infants who received water or herbal teas in the first 7 days of life were more likely to have infant formula introduced during the first month. Wojcicki and colleagues (2011) reported similar outcomes. Infants who received water or teas in the first 7 days of life were 3 times more likely than other infants to receive non-breastmilk fluids by 4 weeks of age.

Mulder and Gardner (2015) proposed a newborn hydration model for understanding newborn hydration immediately following birth (**Figure 1-2**). It has been common practice to supplement a breastfed infant when newborn weight loss reaches more than 7% of birth weight because that has been the threshold used as an indicator of a water deficit or dehydration. Using only this indicator during the first 24–60 hours following birth does not take into account the normal process of newborn diuresis, especially if the mother has received large amounts of IV fluids during labor. During pregnancy, the mother may retain as much as 6 to 8 liters of water, causing the fetus to be "over-hydrated" because the fetus remains in fluid and electrolyte balance with the mother. Following birth, the infant's high levels of arginine vasopressin (which increases water retention) abruptly decrease, heralding the start of physiological diuresis. This point may be clinically apparent in infants with more than a 7% weight loss when they demonstrate significantly more voids than newborns with smaller losses. Researchers have shown that infants with higher weight losses produced more voids during the early hours and days following birth (Chantry, Nommsen-Rivers, Peerson, Cohen, & Dewey, 2011; Mulder, Johnson, & Baker, 2010). Newborns with

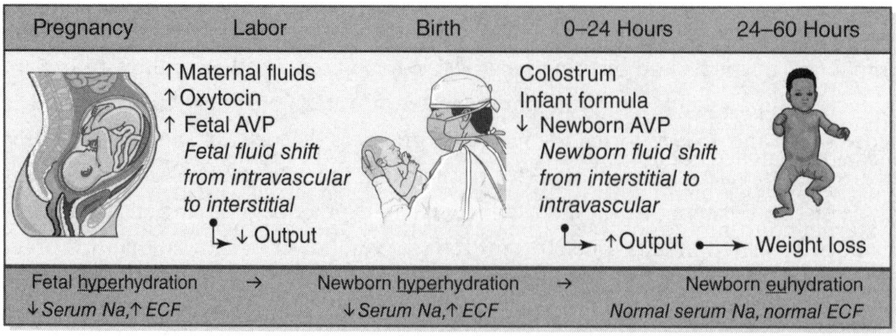

Figure 1-2 Healthy newborn hydration model.

Modified from Mulder, P. J. & Gardner, S. E. (2015). The healthy newborn hydration model: A new model for understanding newborn hydration immediately after birth. *Biological Research for Nursing, 17*, 94–99. First published on April 15, 2014 doi:10.1177/1099800414529362

exposure to high maternal fluid intake during labor may need to lose more than 7% of their birth weight to achieve normal body water content. In contrast, infants with low fluid reserves at birth may encounter under-hydration (even with less than a 7% weight loss), suggesting a better indicator than just percentage of weight loss is needed to determine newborn hydration status.

Mulder and Gardner (2015) suggest using serum sodium measurement along with daily weight loss as a more accurate means of determining hydration status and avoiding the use of supplements when they are not necessary. Serum sodium would be measured in cord blood to establish the baseline hydration status; it would be measured again at 24 hours following birth, with a serum sodium sample being obtained from the heel stick for the metabolic screen. Weight loss patterns should show a greater weight loss in the first 24 hours after birth, followed by a continued weight loss in the second 24 hours, with the lowest point being reached at 3 days. After this time the infant should be gaining weight due to the occurrence of lactogenesis II.

Flaherman and colleagues (2015) analyzed hourly weight-loss patterns of 108,907 healthy, term, exclusively breastfed newborns from 6 to 72 hours of age for vaginally delivered infants and from 6 to 96 hours for those born via cesarean section. Almost 5% of vaginally delivered newborns and almost 10% of those delivered by cesarean section had lost more than 10% of their birth weight by 48 hours after birth. The researchers used their data to create a weight-loss nomogram to help inform clinical care; it is available at http://www.newbornweight.org. However, they did not take the influence of maternal IV fluids during labor into account. Diuresis of large amounts of fluid or large meconium stooling can also result in large weight losses. Other parameters must be considered as well, such as amount of colostrum transferred and number and weight of voids and stools, before a supplementation intervention is undertaken.

Healthcare providers must clearly understand the unwanted outcomes of excessive water supplementation and adequately convey these concerns to parents. An approach to help eliminate water supplementation is as follows:

- Teach and assess proper positioning, latch, and milk transfer.
- Document swallowing and ensure that the mother knows when her baby is swallowing milk.
- Avoid using sterile water or dextrose water. If a breastfed infant requires supplementation, use expressed colostrum/milk.
- Educate the parents and extended family regarding the hazard of giving young breastfed babies bottles of water or other fluids, even in hot weather.
- Avoid placing water bottles in the infant's bassinet in the hospital.
- Remind mothers that babies also nurse at the breast for thirst, frequently coming off the breast after only a few minutes of nursing.
- If a baby is latched but not swallowing adequately, have the mother use alternate massage (massage and compress the breast during pauses between sucking bursts) to sustain sucking and swallowing.
- Maternal consumption of water in excess of thirst does not increase milk production and can cause the mother to produce less milk (Dusdieker, Booth, Stumbo, & Eichenberger, 1985).

Lipids

Milk lipids (among other components) have generated intense interest from numerous studies showing that formula-fed infants and children demonstrate less advanced cognitive development and poorer psychomotor development compared with breastfed children (**Box 1-1**). Guxens and colleagues (2011) found that duration of exclusive breastfeeding was associated with an increase of 0.37 points on mental development scores per month of exclusive breastfeeding. Higher levels of docosahexaenoic acid (DHA) and n-3 polyunsaturated fatty acids and higher ratios between n-3/n-6 polyunsaturated fatty acids in colostrum and breastmilk were associated with higher infant mental scores. Infants whose mothers had high levels of total n-3 polyunsaturated fatty acids such as DHA and a longer duration of breastfeeding had significantly higher mental scores than infants whose mothers had lower amounts of these fatty acids and shorter durations of breastfeeding. Each month of breastfeeding has been associated with an increase of 0.16 IQ points (Kanazawa, 2015). Gustafsson, Duchen, Birberg, and Karlsson (2004) found that colostrum levels of long-chain polyunsaturated fatty acids (LCPUFAs) were significantly associated with cognitive development at 6.5 years. A number of components found in human milk that are absent from unsupplemented formulas are thought to contribute to cognitive deficits seen in non-breastfed infants, including particular LCPUFAs.

Box 1-1 Artificially Fed Infants Demonstrate Different Neurodevelopment and Cognitive Outcomes

- A different brain composition than breastfed infants (Uauy, 1990)
- Reduced concentrations of brain sialic acid, leading to potential deficits in neurodevelopment and cognition (Wang, McVeagh, Petocz, & Brand-Miller, 2003)
- Poorer neurobehavioral organization at 1 week of age (Hart, Boylan, Carroll, Musick, & Lampe, 2003)
- Less mature brain development within the first 2 months of life (Herba et al., 2012)
- Lower neurodevelopmental response at 4 months of age (Agostoni, Trojan, Bellu, Riva, & Giovannini, 1995)
- Lower cognitive development observed from 6 months through 16 years (Anderson, Johnstone, & Remley, 1999)
- Lower mental development and psychomotor development scores at 12 months (Agostoni, Marangoni, Giovannini, Galli, & Riva, 2001)
- Lower probability of scoring in the upper quartile for the Mental Development Index and psychomotor Index on the Bayley Scales of Infant Development (Andres et al., 2012)
- Less mature nervous systems at 1 year of age and attainment of near-adult values of central and peripheral conduction later than breastfed infants (Khedr, Farghaly, El-Din Amry, & Osman, 2004)
- Lower mental development scores at 18 months (Florey, Leech, & Blackhall, 1995)
- Poorer developmental outcome of very-low-birth-weight infants at 18 months of age (Vohr et al., 2006)
- Lower mental development scores at 2 years of age (Morrow-Tlucak, Haude, & Ernhart, 1988)
- Lower cognitive development at 3 years of age (Bauer, Ewald, Hoffman, & Dubanoski, 1991; Johnson & Swank, 1996)
- Lower cognitive function of very-low-birth-weight infants at 5 years of age (Tanaka, Kon, Ohkawa, Yoshikawa, & Shimizu, 2009)
- Less likely to have achieved a good level of overall educational achievement at age 5 years (Heikkila, Kelly, Renfrew, Sacker, & Quigley, 2014)

- Lower IQ scores over the entire preschool period of time (Jedrychowski et al., 2012)
- Lower IQ scores at 6.5 years (Kramer et al., 2008)
- Lower IQ scores at 7 years (Lucas, Morley, Cole, Lister, & Leeson-Payne, 1992)
- Twice the rate of minor neurological dysfunction at 9 years (Lanting, Fidler, Huisman, Touwen, & Boersma, 1994)
- Significantly lower test scores in reading and mathematics in 9-year-old children (McCrory & Layte, 2011)
- Lower IQ scores at 11–16 years (Greene, Lucas, Livingstone, Harland, & Baker, 1995)
- Lower IQ scores and lower attainment in school at 18 years (Horwood & Fergusson, 1998)
- Lower IQ scores, educational attainment, and income at age 30 years (Victora et al., 2015)
- Lower cognitive development when born small for gestational age (Rao, Hediger, Levine, Naficy, & Vik, 2002; Slykerman et al., 2005)
- Increased risk for specific language impairment (Tomblin, Smith, & Zhang, 1997)
- Half the DHA as in the brain of a breastfed infant (Cunnane, Francescutti, Brenna, & Crawford, 2000)
- Significantly lower DHA in the gray and white matter of the cerebellum (coordinates movement and balance) (Jamieson et al., 1999)
- Slower brainstem maturation in preterm infants (Amin, Merle, Orlando, Dalzell, & Guillet, 2000)
- Increased abnormalities in neurobehaviors of preterm infants (Brown, Doyle, Bear, & Inder, 2006)
- Poorer stereoacuity at 3.5 years and at 6 years of age (Singhal et al., 2007; Williams, Birch, Emmett, Northstone, & Avon Longitudinal Study of Pregnancy and Childhood Study Team, 2001)
- Suboptimal quality of general movements that correlate with poorer neurobehavioral condition of children at school age (Bouwstra et al., 2003)
- Increased gross motor delay (Sacker, Quigley, & Kelly, 2006)
- Poorer speech processing with the potential for less optimal linguistic and cognitive development (Ferguson & Molfese, 2007)
- Lower IQ scores in young adults (Mortensen, Michaelsen, Sanders, & Reinisch, 2002)
- Lower general intelligence and cortical thickness in adolescents who had been formula fed (Kafouri et al., 2012)
- Lower child development test scores; subsequent schooling and other experiences during adolescence did not eliminate the breastfeeding gap that appeared in very early childhood (Huang, Peters, Vaughn, & Witko, 2014)

Many classes of lipids and thousands of subclasses exist. The fat content of human milk varies widely, ranging from 3.5% to 4.5% (2–9 g of lipids per 100 mL). It is influenced by a number of factors (**Table 1-2**).

Lipids provide a well-tolerated energy source, contributing approximately 50% of the calories in milk. They provide essential fatty acids, lipid-soluble vitamins, and cholesterol. The milk fat is formed from circulating lipids that are derived from the maternal diet and from maternal body stores. Maternal body fat stores with a relatively slow turnover contribute greatly to the formation of human milk lipids. Short-term variations in dietary fat composition and consumption are somewhat buffered metabolically by maternal fat stores, resulting in a fairly constant LCPUFA content in the milk (Koletzko et al., 2001).

Table 1-2 Factors Influencing Human Milk Fat Content and Composition

Factor	Influence
During a feeding	Rises over the course of a feeding. This was further explained when the fat content of the milk was measured before and after every feed for 24 hours. Rather than fat content being related to the presence of foremilk or hindmilk, the fat content was related to the degree of fullness of the breast. As the breast is progressively drained, the fat content in the milk increases (Daly, Di Rosso, Owens, & Hartmann, 1993).
Volume	Lower milk fat content with higher volumes of milk.
Number of days postpartum	Phospholipid and cholesterol levels are highest in early lactation.
Diurnal rhythm	Varies.
Length of gestation	LCPUFA secretion increases with shortening length of gestation.
Parity	Endogenous fatty acid synthesis decreases with increased parity.
Maternal diet	Can change the LCPUFA profile as well as medium-chain fatty acids (increases with a low-fat diet).
Length of time between feeds	The shorter the interval, the higher the fat concentration.
Maternal energy status	A high weight gain in pregnancy is associated with increased milk fat.
Maternal age	Fat content in colostrum is higher in mothers older than 35 years of age (Lubetzky, Sever, Mimouni, & Mandel, 2015).
Method of milk expression	Manually expressed milk has a higher fat content than milk expressed by an electric pump during the first 72 hours postpartum (Mangel et al., 2015).
Smoking	Active maternal smoking decreases the fat content. Passive smoking (second-hand smoke) exposure reduces milk-lipid profiles (Baheiraei et al., 2014).

Data from Picciano, M. F. (2001). Nutrient composition of human milk. *Pediatric Clinics of North America, 48*, 53–67.

The long-term diet of the mother thus influences milk fat composition. Milk phospholipids contribute to the lipid composition of human milk. Among the several classes of sphingo- and glycolipids are gangliosides, which contribute to the host defense by binding bacterial toxins. Triacylglycerols account for more than 98% of the lipids in milk. The composition of triacylglycerols is usually shown in terms of the kinds and amounts of fatty acids. A shorthand notation is commonly used when discussing fatty acids. The chemical formula is abbreviated by stating the number of carbons to the left of the colon and the number of double bonds to the right of the colon:

- 16:0 palmitic acid
- 18:2 linoleic acid
- 20:4 arachidonic acid (AA)
- 22:6 docosahexanoic acid (DHA)

Unlike breastmilk, unsupplemented infant formula does not contain the LCPUFAs DHA and AA. These two fatty acids are found in abundance as structural lipids in the infant's brain, retina, and central nervous system. Because the animal butterfat of cow's milk formula is replaced with plant oils, human milk and formula have quite different fatty acid profiles. Infant formulas typically contain soy oil, corn oil, sunflower oil, and tropical oils such as palm and coconut oils; these oils may be well absorbed but are not used by the brain in the same way LCPUFAs are from human milk.

Concentrations of DHA and AA in human milk are highly variable and depend on the amount of these preformed fatty acids in the mother's diet and their biosynthesis from precursors (Brenna et al., 2007). Higher DHA values have been identified in preterm mothers' milk compared with those found in term human milk, underscoring the importance of using the mother's own milk to feed her preterm infant (Bokor, Koletzko, & Decsi, 2007). Because there appears to be a higher concentration of DHA in preterm milk, preterm infant formula supplemented with DHA may not contain high enough levels compared with preterm human milk. Parity has an influence on milk lipid concentration, with milk lipid content increasing with subsequent infants at least up to the third delivery (Bachour, Yafawi, Jaber, Choueiri, & Abdel-Razzak, 2012). Genetic polymorphisms (natural variations in a gene, DNA sequence, or chromosome) influence the activity of enzymes involved in the metabolism of polyunsaturated fatty acids (PUFAs) in both the mother and the infant (Glaser, Heinrich, & Koletzko, 2010). For example, the genes FADS1 and FADS2 play an important role in determining the PUFA levels in breastmilk or in the infant's ability to convert precursor fatty acids into their long chain derivatives (Moltó-Puigmartí et al., 2010; Xie & Innis, 2008). This may partially explain the differences in PUFA levels among mothers and the amounts of PUFA ultimately available to their infants. Differences in the fatty acid composition of breastmilk have also been noted in women with eczema and/or respiratory allergy. Johansson, Wold, and Sandberg (2011) reported that lower levels of several PUFAs, including DHA, were seen in the milk of mothers with eczema and/or respiratory allergies, in spite of high amounts of maternal fish intake in the diet. This finding could be the result of dysfunction in the enzymes associated with converting shorter chain fatty acids into longer chain PUFAs. Lower levels of the n-3 fatty acids in allergic women could also be due to the body's enhanced consumption of PUFAs during allergic inflammation within the allergic process.

LCPUFAs have been added to term and preterm formulas in an attempt to provide infants with an exogenous source of these fully formed fatty acids. Infant formulas are supplemented with differing amounts of DHA and AA that are typically based on the average amount found in term human milk. The source of the DHA and AA varies. Infant formulas in the United States use DHA from fermented microalgae (*Crypthecodiunium cohnii*) and AA from soil fungus (*Mortierelle alpina*). These ingredients are new to the food chain and in animal studies showed side effects such as fat loss through stool, oily soft stools (steatorrhea) in acute toxicity tests, higher liver weights in male rats, and increased fetal and neonatal undeveloped renal papilla and dilated renal pelvises (Life Sciences Research Office Report, 1998). Little evidence exists showing that supplementing formula with LCPUFAs confers any significant long-term benefit to term or preterm infants (Life Sciences Research Office Report, 1998; Simmer, 2002a, 2002b). The results of most of the well-conducted, randomized, controlled trials have not shown beneficial effects of LCPUFA supplementation of infant formula on the physical, visual, and neurodevelopmental outcomes of term or preterm infants. Routine supplementation of infant formula with LCPUFA to improve the physical, neurodevelopmental, or visual outcomes of term or preterm infants cannot be recommended based on the current evidence (Simmer, Patole, & Rao, 2008; Simmer, Schulzke, & Patole, 2008).

Because of concerns regarding the safety and effectiveness of the DHA/AA additive, the U.S. Food and Drug Administration (FDA) and Health Canada commissioned the Institute of Medicine to evaluate the process used to determine the safety of new ingredients added to infant formulas. The Institute of Medicine's subsequent report noted a number of shortcomings, including the absence of a structured approach to monitoring side effects after the new formula had been introduced to the market (see the additional reading list at the end of this chapter for information on the full report).

The bioactive fatty acids DHA and AA, when consumed in human milk, are part of a complex matrix of other fatty acids. Important physiological considerations related to this matrix are not accounted for by the simple addition of nonhuman LCPUFAs to infant formula. Many concerns have been raised about these additives (Heird, 1999):

- Supplementation with highly unsaturated oils increases the susceptibility of membranes to oxidant damage and disrupts the antioxidant system. Damage from oxygen radicals can provoke diseases thought to be related to oxidant damage, such as NEC, bronchopulmonary dysplasia, and retrolental fibroplasia (Song, Fujimoto, & Miyazawa, 2000; Song & Miyazawa, 2001). LCPUFA administration has effects on retinol and alpha-tocopherol metabolism (Decsi & Koletzko, 1995).
- Oxidation of PUFAs is enhanced by storage time, temperature, and light exposure. End products of PUFA oxidation occur in large amounts in infant formula, including malondialdehyde (MDA), 4-hydroxyhexanal (4-HHE) specific to the oxidation of DHA, and 4-hydroxynonenal (4-HNE) specific to the oxidation of AA (Genot & Michalski, 2010). Even a few minutes after powdered formula is prepared, substantial amounts of MDA, 4-HHE, and 4-HNE are present, especially in formula enriched with added PUFAs. Human milk is remarkably stable against oxidation. Even though 7 times the amount of vitamin E is found in breastmilk as an antioxidant, infant formula shows extremely high levels of these oxidative end products, especially after open storage (Michalski, Calzada, Makino, Michaud, & Guichardant, 2008). In animal studies, these oxidative end products have been associated with accumulation in the liver and the development of chronic intestinal disorders or cancers. Both 4-HHE and 4-HNE are capable of altering insulin signaling. The question remains as to whether chronic exposure to 4-HHE and 4-HNE from oxidized lipids in infant formula might cause deleterious effects on infant metabolism (Michalski, 2013). Higher levels of PUFAs in muscle cell membranes have been related to increased insulin sensitivity (Pan, Hylbert, & Storlien, 1994).
- There is a possible effect on gene transcription (Clarke & Jump, 1996).
- High-fat supplementation of formula and commercial jarred baby foods has raised the concern that these additives may contribute to the obesity epidemic (Massiera et al., 2003).
- Increasing DHA fortification of commercial baby food adds to the concerns about excessive intake and/or imbalanced ratios of n-6 and n-3 fatty acids.
- Imbalanced ratios of fatty acids can result in altered growth patterns (Carlson, Cooke, Werkman, & Tolley, 1992; Carlson, Werkman, Peeples, Cooke, & Tolley, 1993).
- Many studies have insufficient sample sizes to determine any functional benefit or safety profile; comparison of research results is confounded by the use of different sources of DHA and AA,

different amounts and ratios of these fatty acids, different compositions of the base formulas, and different lengths of time the study formulas were consumed (Koo, 2003).

- Most studies compare supplemented versus unsupplemented formulas to each other but lack a control group of exclusively breastfed infants; many have high attrition rates.
- The accuracy and reliability of the tests used to determine visual and cognitive effects of LCPUFAs during the first 2 years are controversial.
- Enrollment criteria for most studies typically excluded sick infants, twins and higher order multiples, and most infants with any type of problem. This population choice may leave doubts about the suitability of fatty acid–supplemented formula for these infants, regardless of the source of the LCPUFAs. Many of these studies did not include newborn infants or infants during the early days and weeks following birth.
- Meta-analysis of randomized trials suggests that any functional benefit in visual development or neurodevelopment from LCPUFA supplementation of infant formula is likely to be of minor clinical significance, at least for the term infant (Koo, 2003).
- Little evidence indicates that LCPUFA-containing infant formula provides clinically significant improvements in vision and intelligence in healthy term infants. The 25% higher cost can place a significant burden on a family's budget and on public nutrition programs.
- Human milk contains LCPUFAs other than DHA and AA that can be converted to DHA and AA and affects the conversion of alpha-linolenic and linoleic acid to DHA and AA. Their presence may partially explain the apparent need for greater amounts of DHA and AA in formula to achieve the same plasma lipid content of these fatty acids observed in human milk–fed infants (Clandinin et al., 1997).
- Breastmilk contains lipases that enhance fat digestion in breastfed infants; it is a complex matrix, containing numerous bioactive components, hormones, and live cells not found in infant formula. Important physiological considerations relative to the matrix are not accounted for by the simple addition of LCPUFAs to infant formula (Office of Food Additive Safety, 2001).

Clinical Implications

The provision of breastmilk during the period of brain development is important for several reasons:

- IQ studies are remarkably consistent in their demonstration of higher IQ scores that are dose dependent relative to the number of months a child has been breastfed.
- The brain composition of formula-fed infants is measurably and chemically different; namely, DHA levels remain static in formula-fed infants but rise in breastfed infants (Farquharson, Cockburn, Patrick, Jamieson, & Logan, 1992).
- Unsupplemented formula contains no DHA or AA, just their precursors, linolenic and linoleic acid. Infants must rely on an immature liver to synthesize enough of these LCPUFAs to meet the needs of the developing brain.
- Supplemented formulas have unknown side effects:
    1. Fermented microalgae and soil fungus could contain contaminants from the fermentation and oil extraction process, such as hexane residue.

2. Positional distributions of plant-based LCPUFAs on triacylglycerols are different from those of human milk triglycerides. Triacylglycerols or triglycerides are the form in which the body stores fat. They consist of a glycerol spine with three attached fatty acids. The location of the fatty acid on the glycerol spine is identified by stereospecific numbering (sn). Fatty acids are not randomly distributed among the three positions but selectively placed, with human fatty acids having preferences for binding at certain positions. Most saturated fatty acid in human milk is palmitic acid, which is about 20–25% of the total fatty acids in human milk. Palmitic acid is predominantly found in the sn-2 position (Lopez-Lopez, Lopez-Sabater, Campoy-Folgoso, Rivero-Urgell, & Castellote-Bargallo, 2002; Straarup, Lauritzen, Faerk, Høy, & Michaelsen, 2006; Valentine et al., 2010). Palmitic acid in infant formulas, where vegetable oils are the main constituents of infant formula fat, is predominantly found in the sn-1 and sn-3 positions. When palmitic acid is in the sn-2 position, it is well absorbed, but in the sn-1 or sn-3 position, it is released as free fatty acids and forms insoluble soaps that can produce harder stools and constipation in infants.
    a. Infant formula strives to match the overall fatty acid composition of human milk, but it cannot duplicate the triacylglycerol structure that alters lipid metabolism in infants not fed human milk (Nelson & Innis, 1999). Even though the formula is supplemented with DHA and AA, the shape of the molecule is different from that of the DHA and AA found in human milk.
    b. AA and DHA in human milk are present in the sn-1 or sn-2 positions but can be present in all three positions in the single-cell oils (Myher, Kuksis, Geher, Park, & Diersen-Schade, 1996). In human milk, 55% of DHA is found in the sn-2 position.
    c. Human milk triglycerides usually contain no more than one molecule of DHA or AA, whereas some single-cell triglycerides contain two or even three such molecules. Most of the LCPUFAs in formula are located in the outer positions of the triacylglycerol molecule, placing them at potential risk for slow and low absorption (Straarup et al., 2006).
    d. DHA and AA added to infant formula can act differently in the body from human DHA and AA, depending on where and in what proportion they are found on the triglyceride molecule. It is unknown how these differences in molecular shape and triglyceride positioning could affect their metabolism and functioning.

- Fungal sources of AA pose a risk of introducing mycotoxins that could act as opportunistic pathogens in an immunocompromised host.
- Fungal and microalgal oil supplements have been shown to cause a dose-dependent increase in excess gas and belching in adults (Innis & Hansen, 1996).
- The National Alliance for Breastfeeding Advocacy has received numerous complaints of infants experiencing watery explosive diarrhea, diaper rash, excessive foul-smelling gas, and abdominal cramping from ingesting infant formula with the highest levels of LCPUFA supplementation. Also reported was obesity in 6-month-old infants who initially breastfed but had DHA/AA-supplemented formula added to their diet as a supplement, followed by infant cereal at 4 months of age.
- The FDA has received approximately 100 reports from healthcare providers and parents describing adverse reactions to DHA/AA-supplemented formulas. Reports state that numerous

side effects such as vomiting and diarrhea disappeared as soon as the infant was switched to a formula without these additives (Vallaeys, 2008). Some infants may have more difficulty digesting triglycerides, with multiple DHA molecules occupying two or three places on the glycerol spine. Also, a possible contributor to variations in how infants handle these oils is the fact that they contain 40–50% DHA and AA, with the remaining components being high-oleic sunflower oil, diglycerides, and nonsaponifiable materials.

- Studies on LCPUFA-supplemented formula have shown no consistent beneficial outcomes (Follett, Ishii, & Heinig, 2003).
- Neural maturation of formula-fed preterm infants shows a deficit compared with those fed human milk.
- Delayed maturation in visual acuity can occur in both term and preterm formula-fed infants. This delay may affect other mental and physical functions linked to vision in later development (Birch et al., 1993).

The sterol content of human milk ranges from 10 to 20 mg/dL, rising over the course of the lactation, with cholesterol as the major component. Cholesterol is an essential part of all membranes and is required for normal growth and functioning. Breastfed infants' serum cholesterol levels are higher than those of formula-fed infants. This difference may have a long-term effect on the ability of the adult to metabolize cholesterol. Cholesterol is part of and necessary for the laying down of the myelin sheath that is involved in nerve conduction in the brain. Formula contains little to no cholesterol. Information for parents pertinent to the fat component of human milk includes the following:

- Inform parents of the developmental and cognitive differences between infants fed formula versus breastmilk. The average 8-point IQ score elevation in breastfed infants can be the difference between optimal and suboptimal functioning, especially in disadvantaged environments. Eight points is one-half of a standard deviation and is thought to provide a buffer to the neonatal brain from such detrimental factors as maternal smoking, maternal polychlorinated biphenol (PCB) ingestion, and lead ingestion in infancy. One IQ point has been estimated to be worth $14,500 in economic benefits from improved worker productivity (Grosse, Matte, Schwartz, & Jackson, 2002).
- The fatty acid composition of breastmilk can be altered by the maternal diet. Lowering the amounts of trans-fatty acids from hydrogenated fats and increasing the amounts of omega-3 fatty acids from eggs and fish are both beneficial.
- Teach mothers to allow the baby to finish the first side before switching to the second breast. This allows the baby to self-regulate his or her intake, receive the maximum amount of calories (from fat levels that rise at the end of a feeding), and avoid low-calorie, high-lactose feedings that result from placing time limits on the first breast "so the baby will take the second side."
- For infants experiencing slow weight gain, mothers can be guided to finish the first side by using alternate massage before offering the second side and to shorten the intervals between daytime feeds to increase the fat content of the milk.
- It was previously thought that the highest fat content in breastmilk occurred in breastmilk obtained immediately after the feeding begins. Following the initial increase in milk fat content

at the end of a feeding or pumping session, research has shown that the highest levels of both milk fat and live cells in breastmilk appear at 30 minutes after the feeding ends (Hassiotou et al., 2013). Maximum fat levels at 30 minutes post-feed were 1.5- to 8-fold higher compared to prefeeding values. These findings have implications for when milk should be expressed or feedings at breast should occur in the presence of low milk production or infant weight gain issues. It would seem prudent that, with preterm infants or any infants requiring a higher fat content milk for improved weight gain, mothers be instructed to feed again or pump at 30 minutes post feed to maximize milk fat content and improve milk production.

- When breastmilk is stored in the refrigerator or freezer, the fat rises to the top of the container. This can be skimmed off and given to a slow-gaining or preterm infant for extra calories. This milk can be quite calorie dense at 26–28 calories per ounce.
- The prevalence of smoking among pregnant women is between 15% and 20% (Mackay, Eriksen, & Shafey, 2006) and is of importance, as smoking decreases the fat content of breastmilk. Smoking has been associated with earlier weaning (Andersen et al., 1982), decreased milk production, and a lower fat content and lower long-chain fatty acid content in the first 6 months of lactation (Agostoni et al., 2003). Agostoni and colleagues (2003) also showed that smoking in early pregnancy was associated with lower milk fat content later during the first months of lactation. This delayed effect (at least 5 months) may be related to toxicants from smoking being stored in maternal fat tissues (particularly the breasts), which when mobilized during lactation find their way into the milk. Hopkinson, Schanler, Fraley, and Garza (1992) reported that milk fat content was 19% lower in mothers who smoked. Vio, Salazar, and Infante (1991) described milk volume, fat content, and infants' average weight gain over a 14-day study of maternal smokers and nonsmokers. Mean milk volume of nonsmokers was 961 ± 120 g/day, whereas the mean volume of maternal smokers was 693 ± 110 g/day. Fat concentration of nonsmokers' milk was 4.05%, whereas that of smokers was 3.25%. Infants' average weight increase over the 14-day study period was 550 ± 130 g (19.6 oz) for children of nonsmokers and 340 ± 170 g (12.1 oz) for children of smokers. Bachour and colleagues (2012) reported that smoking was associated with a 26% decrease in milk lipids, a 12% decrease in milk protein, and a slower infant growth rate. Infants whose mothers smoke need careful follow-up and frequent weight checks. These infants may need more frequent feeding.

Protein

Human milk proteins, like so many other milk components, exert multiple physiological activities, including enhancement of the immune system; defensive duties against pathogenic bacteria, viruses, and yeast; and the development of the gut. New research now shows that human milk contains at least 761 distinct proteins, including low-abundance and minor protein fractions (D'Alessandro, Scaloni, & Zolla, 2013). The protein concentration of human milk is high during the colostrum period, leveling off to about 0.8–1.0% in mature milk. It is also higher in preterm milk initially than in term milk. Infant formula can have as much as 40% more protein than human milk due to the reduction in digestibility, bioavailability, and efficiency of utilization of cow's milk proteins. Higher concentrations of serum insulin are seen in formula-fed infants, possibly due to elevated levels of insulinogenic amino acids such as valine, leucine, and isoleucine. The long-term consequences of this early hyperinsulinemia are unknown, but the condition might increase the risk of diabetes and obesity in formula-fed infants (Lonnerdal, 2014). Mothers who smoke have been shown to have a 12% decrease in milk proteins (Bachour et al., 2012). Smoking decreases the basal prolactin levels at birth and during lactation, which might partially explain the lower protein levels in smokers' milk because prolactin induces the expression of milk protein–encoding genes. Milk proteins have classically been divided into casein and whey proteins. A third group of proteins, called mucins, surrounds the lipid globules in milk and contributes only a small percentage of the total protein content.

Caseins of human milk constitute 10–50% of the total protein, with this percentage rising over the course of the lactation. Colostrum and preterm milk either do not contain or are very low in casein. Casein gives milk its characteristic white appearance. This easily digested protein provides amino acids and aids in calcium and phosphorus absorption in the newborn. Bovine casein is less easily digested in human infants and may not exert the same effect that human milk casein does. The casein protein that predominates in cow's milk forms a tough rubbery curd in the stomach of an infant and requires a longer time to break down and digest. The whey-to-casein ratio in human milk changes over the course of lactation from 90:10 in the early milk, to 60:40 in mature milk, and to 50:50 in late lactation, and as a consequence of the continually changing ratio, there is really no fixed ratio of casein to whey in human milk (Lonnerdal, 2003). By comparison, these ratios do not change in infant formula and can, in fact, be directly opposite that of human milk.

Maternal dietary intake of protein can influence differing protein fractions in human milk (Lopez Alvarez, 2007). In a well-nourished population of mothers with widely varying differences in protein and energy intake, the nitrogen component as well as the protein fraction in their breastmilk remained unaffected (Boniglia, Carratu, Chiarotti, Giammarioli, & Manzini, 2003). However, in a malnourished sample of Colombian mothers, those who did not receive sufficient protein intake experienced a two-thirds reduction in protein content of early milk and diminished C4 complement, IgA, and IgG (Picciano, 1998). In a study that sought to improve the quality of breastmilk through protein supplementation, Chao et al. (2004) supplemented mothers with a protein-rich chicken extract from the 37th week of gestation until 3 days postpartum. Total protein in colostrum did not significantly change; however, dietary supplementation resulted in up to a 35% increase in breastmilk lactoferrin, a 62% increase in epidermal growth factor, and a 196% increase in TGF-beta 2.

Whey proteins are very diverse. Alpha-lactalbumin and lactoferrin are the chief fractions. Human alpha-lactalbumin has a high nutritional value and has been shown to have antitumor activity (Hákansson, Zhivotovsky, Orrenius, Sabharwal, & Svanborg, 1995). Alpha-lactalbumin can appear as a large complex in human milk and is modified in the infant's stomach into a molecular complex called HAMLET (human alpha-lactalbumin made lethal to tumor cells) and in this form has been shown to kill transformed cells (Gustafsson et al., 2005; Newburg, 2005) as well as 40 different carcinoma and lymphoma cell lines (Svensson, Hákansson, Mossberg, Linse, & Svanborg, 2000). HAMLET has been suggested as a possible reason why breastfeeding results in lower rates of childhood leukemia and a reduced incidence of breast cancer (Hanson, 2004). Lactoferrin is an iron-binding protein. Colostrum contains 5–7 g/L of lactoferrin, which gradually decreases over time. A 1-month-old infant consumes about 260 mg/kg/day of lactoferrin and at 4 months about 125 mg/kg/day (Butte et al., 1984). Lactoferrin promotes the growth of intestinal epithelium and has been thought to exert its bacteriocidal effect through withholding iron from iron-requiring pathogens. This type of inhibition can be reversed by the addition of iron in excess of the binding capacity of lactoferrin. It may, however, have a more important effect, which is to alter the properties of the bacterial cell membrane, making it more vulnerable to the killing effects of lysozyme. Immunoglobulins are part of the whey protein fraction, as are enzymes.

A minor portion of the proteins in human milk reside in the lipid fraction, as an integral part of the membrane surrounding the fat globules. The milk fat globule membrane (MFGM) contains sphingomyelin, gangliosides, sialic acid, and cholesterol, all of which are involved in brain myelination and function. The MFGM is lacking in most formulas because this fraction is lost during the dairy's processing of cow's milk.

S100B protein, brain-derived neurotrophic factor (BDNF) and glial cell line-derived neurotrophic factor (GDNF) are little known proteins with interesting effects. These factors are critical molecules that support the process of neuronal growth, development, protection, and repair, and the modulation of learning and memory. BDNF plays an important role in the development of the enteric nervous system, defense against intestinal infection, and modulation of GI motility. GDNF has been shown to support the development of human enteric nervous system and intestinal epithelial barrier integrity (Li, Xia, Zhang, & Wu, 2011).

Immunoglobulins are members of the defense agent team in breastmilk. The predominant immunoglobulin in human milk is immunoglobulin A (IgA). Concentrations of IgA are highest in colostrum and gradually decline to a plateau of about 1 mg/mL for the duration of lactation. The infant's approximate mean intake of IgA is 125 mg/kg/day at 1 month and 75 mg/kg/day by 4 months (Butte et al., 1984). Breastfeeding actively stimulates and directs the immune response of the breastfed infant. Vaccine responses to oral polio virus vaccine and parenteral tetanus and diphtheria toxoid vaccines are enhanced by breastfeeding, with formula-fed infants sometimes showing lower antibody levels to their immunizations (Hahn-Zoric et al., 1990; Pickering et al., 1998). Intestinal dysbiosis may play a role in the infant's response to oral and parenteral vaccines. High abundance of gut *Bifidobacterium*, as seen in breastfed infants, has been associated with higher responses to oral and parenteral vaccines and a larger thymus. High abundance of *Clostridia*, *Enterobacteriales*, and *Pseumonadales*, as seen in the guts of formula-fed infants, has been associated with neutrophilia (increased white cells associated with inflammation and infection) and lower vaccine responses (Huda et al., 2014).

Human milk also contains numerous enzymes. Some function in the mammary gland, some act in the infant, and some have unknown functions. Many are involved in the digestive process, whereas others function in defense against disease. For example, lysozyme is active against the human immunodeficiency virus and plays a role in the antibacterial activity of human milk, showing the most effect against Gram-positive bacteria. High concentrations are present throughout lactation, whereas concentrations are several orders of magnitude lower in bovine milk. Whereas secretory IgA and lactoferrin levels decrease after the early period of lactation, lysozyme levels remain higher during the 6-month to 2-year period of lactation than they were during the first month of breastfeeding.

Platelet-activating factor acetylhydrolase (PAF-AH) plays an important role in the prevention of NEC, an often fatal bowel disease in preterm infants. PAF is a potent ulcerative agent in the GI tract. NEC can be induced within hours after administration of PAF in experimental animals. PAF-AH hydrolyzes

PAF to produce an inactive form, thereby helping to prevent the development of NEC in infants receiving breastmilk (Furukawa, Lee, & Johnston, 1993). It is interesting to note that among the species studied, the only one devoid of milk PAF-AH was bovine milk; thus, cow's milk products cannot substitute for human milk (Park, Bulkley, & Granger, 1983).

There is also a connection between the breastmilk protein known as neuregulin-4 (NRG4) and protection against NEC. NRG4 promotes epithelial cell survival, with NRG4 receptors being present in the developing human intestine. NEC is known to be characterized by the loss of specialized intestinal cells known as Paneth cells, which help protect the gut from damage from pathological organisms and maintain healthy populations of intestinal stem cells. Such stem cells are essential to facilitate the intestine's ongoing ability to regenerate cells lost to damage and disease. Both animal studies and studies on human cell lines have shown that when fed or exposed to infant formula, Paneth cells are lost; in contrast, when fed or exposed to human milk, Paneth cells are maintained. Given that NRG4 is found only in breastmilk and not in infant formula, infants fed formula are missing out on a protective mechanism for the immature gut. Thus, when a formula-fed infant encounters a NEC trigger such as intestinal infection or injury, he or she may be at an increased risk for acquiring NEC (McElroy et al., 2014).

The nonprotein nitrogen fraction of human milk accounts for 20–25% of the total nitrogen found in human milk. It is made up of peptides, urea, uric acid, ammonia, free amino acids, creatine, creatinine, nucleic acids, nucleotides, polyamines, carnitine, choline, amino alcohols of phospholipids, amino sugars, peptide hormones, and growth factors. Nucleotides have received increased attention because some infant formulas have been supplemented with them. Human milk has a specific content of free nucleotides that differs from the mix found in cow's milk. Nucleotides are involved in the modulation of the immune system, the intestinal microenvironment, and the absorption and metabolism of nutrients. The total nucleotide content of human milk, if nucleic acid content is included, greatly exceeds the levels found in formula supplemented with nucleotides. Although nucleotide-supplemented formula is marketed as "being closer to breastmilk," it remains unproven whether this contributes to decreased morbidity, or only increased revenues.

Clinical Implications

Cow's milk serves as the base of most infant formulas. The prevalence of cow's milk allergy has been placed at between 2% and 5% of infants (Host, Jacobsen, Halken, & Holmenlund, 1995). Risk factors include a family history of atopy and early dietary exposure to cow's milk. The age at onset is directly correlated with the time of introduction of infant formula (Oski, DeAngeles, Feigin, & McMillan, 1994). Even exclusively breastfed infants can develop symptoms of cow's milk protein intolerance that may respond to elimination of the offending agent from the mother's diet.

Because of the high cross-reactivity to soy protein, the potential for soy allergy is 10–14%; thus, soy protein is not used for infants with documented cow's milk allergy. Soy formula neither reduces allergic symptoms nor delays allergies (Chandra & Hamed, 1991). Soy formula has no advantage as a supplement to breastmilk, has no proven value in the prevention or management of infant colic or fussiness, and is indicated only for infants with galactosemia or hereditary lactase deficiency (extremely rare), or when the family prefers a vegetarian diet (Bhatia & Greer, 2008). Although cow's milk protein–based lactose-free formulas are available, they have not been shown to have any clinical impact on colic, growth, or development, and they are not recommended for infants with diarrhea (Heyman, 2006). Breastfed infants should be continued on human milk during episodes of diarrhea. Human milk proteins play a critical role in directing the construction of the immune system. Infants fed soy formula have the lowest antibody titers to their vaccines, and those fed cow's milk–based formula are still below breastfed infants both in antibody titers and incidence of illness (Zoppi et al., 1983). Some soy formula–fed infants have had to be reimmunized after soy formula feeding. Compared with girls fed non–soy-based infant formula or milk (early formula), early soy-fed girls were at a 25% higher risk of earlier menarche (Adgent et al., 2012). It is recommended that the clinician take the following steps:

- Prenatally, help parents understand the importance of exclusive breastfeeding for about 6 months, especially those with a family history of allergies and diabetes.
- Avoid giving bottles of formula (cow's milk based or soy based) in the hospital. Even one bottle can sensitize a susceptible infant and provoke an allergy later when challenged again.
- Encourage frequent breastfeeding, 8–12 times every 24 hours right from the start. Colostrum contains large amounts of protein, especially the sIgA that helps protect the infant against disease. These protein levels in colostrum also serve to prevent hypoglycemia.

Carbohydrates

The principal carbohydrate in human milk is lactose (galactose + glucose), with other carbohydrates occurring in smaller amounts, such as oligosaccharides, monosaccharides, and peptide-bound and protein-bound carbohydrates. Lactose is the most abundant component of human milk (70 g/L). It is thought to have several functions:

- Lactose favors the colonization of the infant's intestine with microflora that competes with and excludes pathogens.
- Infants undergo rapid brain development during the nursing period, with the natural period of exclusive breastfeeding coinciding with the most rapid period of brain development. Myelination requires large amounts of galactosylceramide (galactocerebrosides) and other galactolipids that are major components of this growth. The infant liver may be unable to synthesize all the galactolipids needed at this time. Milk galactose is most likely present to ensure an adequate supply of galactocerebrosides for optimal brain development. Brain growth and development during this time are known to be vulnerable to many types of nutrient deficiencies. This vulnerability has important ramifications for infants on artificial diets, especially when lactose is removed from their sole source of nutrition, as with soy formula or cow's milk–based formula that has had the lactose removed.
- Lactose enhances calcium absorption. Infants fed cow's milk–based formula with the lactose removed show reduced calcium absorption (Abrams, Griffin, & Davila, 2002). Lactose levels are quite stable, showing little or no change in response to a wide variety of environmental or dietary challenges. Infants are well suited to use lactose because lactase, a brush border intestinal enzyme that digests lactose, is present by 24 weeks of fetal life. Lactase levels increase

throughout the last trimester of fetal life, reaching concentrations at term that are two to four times the levels seen at 2–11 months of age. One hypothesis suggests that a relationship exists between the relative size of the brain and the level of lactose in a species' milk. Humans, with their large brains, have very high lactose levels in their milk compared with other species.

Oligosaccharides are biologically active carbohydrates. More than 200 neutral and acidic oligosaccharides have been identified to date at levels of approximately 12–14 g/L (1.2–1.4 g/dL), which represents 1% of human milk and 10% of its caloric content. This makes these carbohydrates collectively the third largest solid component of human milk. Oligosaccharides are essentially indigestible by the infant's gut mucosa and are not utilized as a macronutrient. Instead, they are delivered to the gut intact, where they nourish the infant's gut microbiota, thereby acting as the infant's first prebiotic. An individual mother's milk can contain anywhere from a few dozen to more than a hundred different oligosaccharides. The concentration of oligosaccharides in cow's milk is about 20-fold lower than that found in human milk (Veh et al., 1981). Oligosaccharides have water-soluble cell surface analogs that can inhibit enteropathogen binding to host cell receptors. Oligosaccharides can inhibit the binding to their intestinal cell receptors of such bacteria as *Streptococcus pneumoniae*, *Haemophilus influenzae*, *E. coli*, and *Campylobacter jejuni*. They essentially act as decoys through their ability to mimic intestinal cell receptors, preventing bacteria from attaching to their respective receptors in the host cells.

Milk oligosaccharides also contain human blood group antigens, with women from different blood group types exhibiting distinct patterns.

Lactating mothers differ genetically in their ability to produce protective oligosaccharides and thus may influence their breastfed infant's susceptibility to enteric disease (Morrow et al., 2004; Uauy & Araya, 2004). Newborns fed breastmilk from mothers who exhibit higher levels of certain oligosaccharides may be better protected against certain pathogens such as *E. coli* than infants whose mother's milk contains a genetically programmed lower amount of such disease fighters (Thurl et al., 2010). This distinction is thought to be related to the Lewis blood group to which a mother belongs. Four human milk groups have been identified based on the Lewis blood group system. Each of these groups produces different amounts and kinds of oligosaccharides that appear in the respective mother's breastmilk (Zivkovic, German, Lebrilla, & Mills, 2011).

Oligosaccharide composition also depends on the mother's secretor status. Mothers whose milk-making cells turn "on" the FUT2 gene produce a different set of milk sugars that are more protective than those produced in the absence of a functioning FUT2 gene. Those mothers with a functional FUT2 gene are called "secretors." In contrast, "nonsecretors" have a disabling mutation in the FUT2 (α-1,2-fucosyltransferase) gene, such that they produce sugars with different linkages in their milk. Approximately 20% of mothers are nonsecretors. Both secretors and nonsecretors produce the lactose and fucose molecules, but an important difference is how the fucose attaches to the lactose. If the fucose attaches via an α-1,2 linkage, the sugar is called 2′-FL and has a variety of protective actions; if the fucose links via an α-1,3 linkage, the sugar is called 3′-FL and loses some of its defensive ability, rendering it less protective for the infant. Researchers have shown that bifidobacteria are established earlier and more often in infants fed by secretor mothers than in infants fed by nonsecretor mothers (Lewis et al., 2015). In Lewis et al.'s (2015) study, infants fed by nonsecretor mothers had 10 times fewer bifidobacteria and were delayed in the establishment of bifidobacteria-laden microbiota, possibly due to difficulties in the infant acquiring a species of *Bifidobacterium* that is able to consume the specific milk oligosaccharides provided by the mother.

This finding is true for the milk of preterm mothers as well. Preterm human milk tends to have a lower lactose content than term milk. High concentrations of oligosaccharides exist in the milk of certain Lewis blood group preterm mothers. The use of donor-pooled milk is of benefit rather than single donor milk because the pooled milk is likely to average out the large interindividual variations in oligosaccharide amounts and composition (Gabrielli et al., 2011).

Infant formulas have an oligosaccharide-bound sialic acid content that is 10 to 27 times lower than that of human milk because the manufacturing process for infant formulas has virtually eliminated this component from the finished product (Martin-Sosa, Martin, Garcia-Pardo, & Hueso, 2003). Formula-fed infants have a reduced intake and number of oligosaccharides than human milk–fed infants in their stool and urine, which also differ in composition from those of breastfed infants (Hanson, 2004). Many infant formulas have been supplemented with plant-based oligosaccharides in an effort to mimic the function and outcome seen in breastfed infants, such as inducing softer stools and creating gut flora patterns similar to those of breastfed infants. One potential side effect of this type of supplementation is the possibility of bacterial translocation. The term bacterial translocation is used to describe the passage of viable resident bacteria from the GI tract to normally sterile tissues such as the mesenteric lymph nodes and other internal organs. Barrat et al. (2008) reported that in a study of rats fed a formula with added oligosaccharides and inulin, an increase in bacterial translocation occurred in the immature gut. This side effect may pose a potential infectious risk and requires further study. Oligosaccharides currently added to infant formulas are structurally different from human milk oligosaccharides (HMOs) and most likely are not functionally equivalent (Jantscher-Krenn & Bode, 2012). Xia and colleagues (2012) measured the abundance of commensal and beneficial bacteria (*Bacteroides*, *Bifidobacterium*, and *Lactobacillus*) and pathogenic bacteria (*Clostridium difficile* and *E. coli*) in breastfed infants and infants fed formula supplemented with various amounts of fructo-oligosaccharides. Results showed that formula-fed infants harbored a greater abundance of *C. difficile* and *E. coli* and similar amounts of beneficial bacteria as breastfed infants. The addition of nonhuman oligosaccharides had no significant prebiotic effect with respect to increasing beneficial bacteria or decreasing pathogenic bacteria in formula-fed infants. Some commercially available prebiotics (FOS and GOS) have been shown to stimulate the growth of pathogenic microorganisms such as *Clostridia* (Bunesova et al., 2012), which raises a question about the desirability of supplementing infant formula with these substances.

HMOs are an important source of sialic acid for the infant. Sialic acid is an integral part of the plasma membranes of nerve cells concentrated in the region of nerve endings and dendrites in the brain. The brains of breastfed infants have higher amounts of sialic acid than those of formula-fed infants (Wang et al., 2003). Formula-fed infants derive less than 25% of the amount of sialic acid that is supplied to breastfed infants through mature human milk. Formula-fed infants have a lower dietary source of sialic acid and are unable to synthesize the difference (McVeagh & Miller, 1997). Soy formulas have almost undetectable amounts of sialic acid (Wang, Brand-Miller, McVeagh, & Petocz, 2001). In animal models, an exogenous source of sialic acid increased learning performance as well as the concentration of sialic acid in the frontal cortex of the brain (Wang et al., 2007). Because breastmilk is such a rich source of sialic acid, this suggests that the rapid formation of brain gangliosides during the infant's first month depends on the steady and abundant supply of this brain growth factor. Concentrations of several of the oligosaccharides are higher in colostrum than in mature milk, suggesting that the early days of brain growth are enhanced by the presence of particular factors in breastmilk that are vital for the proper development of the rapidly growing brain (Asakuma et al., 2007). Large amounts of sialylated oligosaccharides may be one mechanism by which breastfeeding promotes higher cognitive performance in children. Infant formula does not have sufficient amounts of Neu5Ac sialic acid (the predominant sialic acid form in healthy humans). It does, however, contain Neu5Gc, which is normally absent in humans and which has often been associated with human inflammatory diseases (Wang, Hu, & Yu, 2006).

Because oligosaccharides present in human milk are able to modulate the microbiota of breastfed infants, it might be possible that HMOs could also modulate the bacterial communities in the breast itself. While milk of secretor women is rich in 2′-fucosyllactose and other α-1,2-fucosylated HMOs, nonsecretor women lack a functional FTU2 enzyme, resulting in milk that does not contain α-1,2-fucosylated HMOs. Interestingly, some strains of *Staphylococcus*—the major bacterial contributor to mastitis—bind to 2′-fucosyllactose (Lane, Mehra, Carrington, & Hickey, 2011). Thus, susceptibility to acquire mastitis might be determined not only by the bacterial composition of the milk, but also by the blood group and corresponding type of HMOs contained in each individual mother's milk (Jeurink et al., 2013). In essence, some mothers can be protected from mastitis by their own HMOs.

Clinical Implications

Human milk provides several tiers of protection from pathogens, and those tiers have the potential to work synergistically. The processing of infant formulas based on cow's milk utilizes procedures that exclude from the final product colostrum, MFGM, and fractions that contain DNA. Milk oligosaccharides from other species confer protection to the young of that species. Random additions of a few synthesized, structurally different oligosaccharides to infant formula would not be expected to generate a tier of disease protection because those oligosaccharides in breastmilk are unique to human milk and have not been replicated synthetically. Reassure parents that it is uncommon for infant fussiness to be related to lactose intolerance. Primary lactose intolerance (lactase deficiency) is extremely rare. Weaning a breastfed infant to a lactose-free formula removes all layers of disease protection and changes the nature of the nutrient supply to the brain. There is a 10-fold difference in sialic concentrations among different types of formulas, with none containing more than 25% of the brain builders found in human milk. The oligosaccharides contained in some infant formulas are synthesized by bacterial enzymes or isolated from plants and lack fucose and sialic acid. These components are essential to realize the beneficial effects of HMOs. The oligosaccharides in formula are unable to mimic the structure-specific effects of the HMOs and may leave formula-fed infants without essential brain nutrients.

Vitamins

The water-soluble vitamins in human milk are ascorbic acid (vitamin C), thiamin (vitamin B_1), riboflavin (vitamin B_2), niacin, pyridoxine (vitamin B_6), folate, pantothenate, biotin, and vitamin B_{12}. The concentration of water-soluble vitamins in human milk shows variations reflecting the stage of lactation, maternal intake, and delivery before term. The breast cannot synthesize water-soluble vitamins, so their origins lie in the maternal plasma, derived from the maternal diet. Concentrations are generally lower in the early days of breastfeeding compared with those found in mature milk. In mothers who are adequately nourished, maternal supplementation in higher than physiological doses either has no effect or is transient. Maternal vitamin supplementation generally shows benefits only when the mother herself is malnourished.

Storage and handling of expressed human milk can alter some of the vitamin components in it. Total ascorbic acid (vitamin C) levels decreased on average by one-third after 24 hours of storage at 4°C (39.2°F), with wide variations between individual mothers (Buss, McGill, Darlow, & Winterbourn, 2001). Francis, Rogers, Brewer, Dickton, and Pardini (2008) found that various bottle systems showed measurable decreases in the mean concentration of ascorbic acid over a 20-minute sampling period (the approximate time of a feeding). Those bottles with the largest milk-to-air interface had the greatest decreases in mean concentration of ascorbic acid over time. The air moving through the milk and the formation of bubbles on the surface of the milk could be factors in the observed decreases of ascorbic acid concentration. Ascorbic acid is also degraded by exposure to light, suggesting that tinted bottles for expressing, storing, and feeding human milk might be appropriate. Those infants who are solely dependent on bottle-feeds for their total ascorbic acid intake by formula or breastmilk, especially high-risk or preterm infants, may need their ascorbic acid status evaluated. Caregivers (parents and health professionals) should avoid shaking the bottle, may wish to use bottle systems with lower milk-to-air surface interfaces, and may wish to consider using tinted bottles for expressing, storing, and feeding purposes.

Micronutrients such as vitamins C and E are essential to the health of the infant's antioxidant defense system. Mothers who were supplemented with 500 mg of vitamin C and 100 mg of vitamin E showed a significant increase in the antioxidant capacity of their breastmilk (Zarban et al., 2015), While a healthy balanced diet may outweigh single supplements, mothers with a diet deficient in vitamins C and E may benefit from supplementation to help enrich their milk with these antioxidants.

Vitamin B_{12} is needed by the infant's developing nervous system. This vitamin occurs exclusively in animal tissue, is bound to protein, and is minimal to absent in vegetable protein. A mother consuming a vegan diet, without meat or dairy products, may have milk deficient in vitamin B_{12}. Infants who present with infections, pallor, hypotonia, neurodevelopmental delays, refusal to suck, failure to thrive, hematological issues, or fatigue may benefit from a check of their vitamin B_{12} levels. Mothers should be asked if they are consuming a vegetarian diet and should also have their vitamin B_{12} status evaluated (Akcaboy et al., 2015).

The fat-soluble vitamins are A, D, E, and K. Vitamin A and its precursors, known as carotenoids (beta-carotene), occur at twice the levels in colostrum as in mature human milk. The level of vitamin A in the milk of well-nourished mothers delivering prematurely is even higher. This vitamin is important in infant growth and development. An inverse relationship exists between the risk of morbidity and mortality and vitamin A status. Even after breastfeeding is discontinued, it appears to confer a protective effect due to some of the vitamin A provided by breastmilk being stored in the child's liver.

Vitamin D comprises a group of related fat-soluble compounds with antirachitic (rickets) activity. Vitamin D is not actually a vitamin or a nutrient but a precursor of a steroid hormone formed when the skin is directly exposed to ultraviolet B radiation in sunlight. It is essential for the normal absorption of calcium from the gut. There are two forms of vitamin D, D_2 (ergocalciferol, which is synthesized by plants) and D_3 (cholecalciferol, which is synthesized by mammals). The main source of vitamin D for humans is through its synthesis in the skin when exposed to ultraviolet B radiation in the range of 290–315 nm, with less than 10% derived from dietary sources. The most common food source of vitamin D is the plant steroid ergosterol, the liver and oils of some fatty fish, and foods fortified with vitamin D such as milk, orange juice, margarine, and cereals. Although vitamin D is synthesized in the skin upon exposure to

Box 1-2 Details on Vitamin D

- Breastmilk contains an average vitamin D content of 26 IU/L (range, 5–136 IU) in a vitamin D-sufficient mother (Institute of Medicine, Food and Nutrition Board, & Standing Committee on the Evaluation of Dietary Reference Intakes, 1997).
- Infant formula contains 400 IU (10 mg) per liter (Life Sciences Research Office Report, 1998).
- If an infant consumes an average of 750 mL/day of breastmilk, exclusive breastfeeding without sun exposure would provide a range of 11–38 IU/day of vitamin D, which is below the recommended minimum intake of 400 IU/day (Wagner, Greer, American Academy of Pediatrics Section on Breastfeeding, & American Academy of Pediatrics Committee on Nutrition, 2008).
- An adequate intake level of vitamin D for infants with some sunlight exposure has not been established, but breastfed infants with limited sunlight exposure have not been shown to develop rickets.
- The cost of averting a single case of rickets by universally dosing infants with vitamin D could be between $252,614 and $958,293 per case (Vitamin D Expert Panel, & Centers for Disease Control and Prevention, 2001).
- The cost to breastfeeding initiation and duration rates has not been accounted for, nor has the concern that formula manufacturers will promote their products in such a way as to imply that breastmilk is inadequate and that their products should be used to prevent a condition caused by the use of "deficient" breastmilk (Heinig, 2003).

sunlight, many people derive much of their vitamin D from foods that are supplemented or enriched with it. Levels of this vitamin vary in breastmilk and are often reported as being inadequate (**Box 1-2**).

Human milk is not necessarily deficient in vitamin D. Approximately 20% of maternal circulating vitamin D is transferred to the infant through the mother's milk. Infants suffering from vitamin D deficiency and rickets do so from a deficit of exposure of the skin to sunlight or may be born deficient if their mother was also deficient during the pregnancy. Vitamin D content in human milk is sufficient when the mother's levels are sufficient (Henderson, 2005). Attaining sufficient and safe sunlight exposure for infants has been complicated by the recommendation from the AAP to keep infants less than 6 months of age out of direct sunlight and to use sunscreen on older infants and children (AAP & Committee on Environmental Health, 1999). Rickets and poor bone mineralization are rare in breastfed infants but do occur. Vitamin D insufficiency and actual deficiency can occur in breastfed infants who are not supplemented with extra vitamin D (Merewood et al., 2012). Incidents of vitamin D deficiency in its extreme form, rickets, are still reported. Rickets is primarily associated with dark-skinned children on vegetarian diets, dark-skinned infants exclusively breastfed beyond 3 to 6 months of age, premature infants, and infants born to mothers who are vitamin D deficient themselves (Misra, Pacaud, Petryk, Collett-Solberg, & Kappy, 2008). Greer and associates (1982) randomized infants into a group receiving a placebo and a group receiving a supplement of 10 mg of vitamin D daily. The bone-mineral content of the placebo group was significantly lower in the first few months after birth but at the end of the first year was actually higher than that in the supplemented group.

Exclusive breastfeeding results in normal infant bone-mineral content when maternal vitamin D status is adequate (Greer & Marshall, 1989), when neonatal stores are normal, and when the infant is regularly exposed to sunlight. Specker, Valanis, Hertzberg, Edwards, and Tsang (1985) reported that

30 minutes of sun exposure per week for infants wearing only a diaper and 2 hours of sun exposure per week for fully clothed infants without a hat maintained vitamin D levels of greater than 27.5 nmol/L. Merewood and colleagues (2012) showed that as little as 10 minutes outside once per week is protective against vitamin D deficiency. However, the duration of sun exposure that is necessary for differing categories of infants (e.g., dark skinned, living at differing latitudes, clothed or just diapered) to maintain vitamin D levels at greater than 50 nmol/L, the currently accepted level for vitamin D sufficiency in children, is undetermined. Darkly pigmented infants require a greater exposure to sunshine to initiate the synthesis of vitamin D in the skin (Clemens, Adams, Henderson, & Holick, 1982). It has been shown that 400 IU/day of vitamin D maintains serum concentrations at greater than 50 nmol/L in exclusively breastfed infants (Wagner, Hulsey, Fanning, Ebeling, & Hollis, 2006). Reports in the literature of confirmed rickets in breastfed infants (Kreiter et al., 2000; Shah, Salhab, Patterson, & Seikaly, 2000) have led to a recommendation by the AAP that all breastfed infants be supplemented with 400 IU of vitamin D per day beginning in the first few days of life (Wagner et al., 2008). Controversy has been generated by this recommendation and the concomitant urging by the AAP that people limit their exposure to sunlight to reduce the incidence of skin cancer. Vitamin D status in infants also depends on numerous factors:

- Is the infant being exclusively breastfed? Is he or she being given medications, other foods, or drinks that could interfere with absorption of nutrients such as calcium? Chronic calcium deficiency increases vitamin D metabolism with secondary vitamin D deficiency (Clements, Johnson, & Fraser, 1987).
- What was the vitamin D status of the mother during her pregnancy? Maternal vitamin D concentrations largely determine the vitamin D status of the fetus and newborn infant. A mother deficient in vitamin D during her pregnancy will give birth to a vitamin D–deficient infant or an infant who will reach vitamin D deficiency more quickly than an infant born to a vitamin D–sufficient mother. Was the infant preterm? Preterm infants lack the necessary time to accumulate vitamin D stores. What is the mother's current vitamin D intake and exposure to sunlight?
- Is the infant's skin deeply pigmented? Approximately 90% of all reported cases of nutritional rickets have occurred in African American children, identifying a population of infants at higher risk for rickets and for whom maternal supplementation or direct supplementation of vitamin D may be more important (Hirsch, 2007). Is the infant from a poor socioeconomic background? Is he or she malnourished or does the infant have fat malabsorption? How old is the infant? Overt rickets is more common in children older than 6 months of age (Pugliese, Blumberg, Hludzinski, & Kay, 1998; Sills, Skuza, Horlick, Schwartz, & Rapaport, 1994).

A number of environmental, genetic, hormonal, nutritional, and cultural factors interact and/or overlap, putting some susceptible children at risk for rickets (Mojab, 2002):

- Maternal deficiency (prenatal and postpartum)
- Daylight hours spent indoors
- Living conditions such as residence in high latitudes and urban areas with buildings or pollution that block sunlight
- Cultural practices such as restricting postpartum women from outdoor exposure during the first month postpartum

- Dark skin pigmentation
- Use of sunscreen
- Covering the body when outside (cold climate, fear of skin cancer, cultural dress customs)

The antirachitic activity in human milk varies by season, maternal vitamin D intake, sun exposure, and race. Various levels of maternal vitamin D supplementation have been studied in an attempt to delineate how much is necessary to increase an infant's vitamin D levels to a midrange of normal through the consumption of breastmilk. Researchers have supplemented lactating mothers with 2,000–4,000 IU of vitamin D per day for 3 months, causing a significant rise in maternal vitamin D levels as well as improving vitamin D levels in breastmilk and in the recipient infants (Basile, Taylor, Wagner, Horst, & Hollis, 2006; Hollis & Wagner, 2004). Such a dose is much higher than the current Dietary Reference Intake for lactating mothers (400 IU/day). Concern has been raised regarding the safety of this practice; however, Vieth, Chan, and MacFarlane (2001) and Heaney, Davies, Chen, Holick, and Barger-Lux (2003) show that vitamin D intakes of 10,000 IU/day (250 mg) or more are safe for periods up to 5 months. Further research is necessary to determine optimal vitamin D intakes for pregnant and lactating women from both sunlight and supplements.

Delineating high-risk groups of infants suitable for supplementation such as dark-skinned, exclusively breastfed infants who spend much time indoors has been suggested as a means of providing supplemental vitamin D appropriately, while avoiding the implication that breastmilk is deficient in this substance (Weisberg, Scanlon, Li, & Cogswell, 2004). Ponnapakkam, Bradford, and Gensure (2010) performed a prospective clinical trial comparing vitamin D supplementation of breastfeeding infants with a placebo as control in southern Louisiana. Those infants in the placebo group showed borderline deficiency at the 2- and 4-month points, but by 6 months, the 25-OHD levels were comparable with those of the treated group. The authors state that there appears to be a critical time period for developing vitamin D insufficiency in infants, which is between 2 and 4 months of age. There was no measurable consequence to this transient vitamin D insufficiency, but it may indicate a period that is more critical for infants who are at a higher risk for developing rickets. They saw no evidence of a benefit of universal vitamin D supplementation for breastfed infants to prevent rickets. High-dose vitamin D supplementation (6,400 IU daily) in nursing mothers may be a workable strategy for improving the vitamin D status of both the mothers and their exclusively breastfeeding infants (Haggerty, 2011). Welch, Bergstrom, and Tsang (2000) recommend viewing vitamin D supplementation as a mechanism to ensure an adequate substrate for a hormone whose normal production has been adversely affected by the realities of modern living conditions—not as a treatment for nutritional inadequacy of human milk. Research has shown that adequate vitamin D maternal supplementation (6400 IU per day) significantly increases the antirachitic activity in breastmilk and is as effective in increasing the infant's vitamin D levels as actually supplementing the infant with 400 IU of vitamin D daily (Hollis et al., 2015; Wagner et al., 2006). Supplementing the mother also reduces the risk of any side effects from supplementing the infant directly. Katikaneni, Ponnapakkam, Ponnapakkam, and Gensure (2009) found that supplementation of infants with standard vitamin D preparations (400 IU/day) was associated with a 76% increased risk of urinary tract infections.

Vitamin E (alpha-tocopherol) functions as an antioxidant. It protects cell membranes and is required for muscle integrity. This vitamin's concentration in colostrum is higher than in mature milk because vitamin E levels are low in the newborn and absorption is inefficient. Human milk supplies more than adequate amounts of vitamin E to the infant.

Vitamin K is essential for the formation of several proteins required for blood clotting. It is produced by the intestinal flora but takes several days in the previously sterile neonatal gut to be effective. Vitamin K stores at birth are very low, so newborns are immediately dependent on an external source for the vitamin. A deficiency of vitamin K increases the risk of a syndrome called hemorrhagic disease of the newborn. The early-onset form occurs at 2–10 days of age in 1 of every 200 to 400 newborns who do not receive additional vitamin K. The late-onset form occurs around 1 month of age in 1 of every 1,000 to 2,000 unsupplemented newborns. The most dependable method of preventing hemorrhagic disease of the newborn is an injected or oral dose of vitamin K at birth (Kleinman, 2004). Vitamin K levels in human milk respond to maternal supplements, but this response is variable and has not been well studied. Vitamin K is localized in the milk-fat globule, with hindmilk containing twofold higher vitamin K concentrations than milk collected from a full breast pumping.

Minerals and Trace Elements

The most prevalent monovalent ions in human milk are sodium, potassium, and chloride; the most prevalent divalent ions are calcium, magnesium, citrate, phosphate, and sulfate. Numerous factors affect the levels of these minerals in human milk. During pregnancy, involution, and mastitis, the junctions between the alveolar cells remain open, allowing sodium and chloride to enter the milk space, drawing water along with them. Lactose and potassium are also thought to move from the milk space to the blood. The net result is that under these conditions, milk has greatly increased concentrations of sodium and chloride and decreased concentrations of lactose and potassium. The presence of high sodium concentrations in human milk is diagnostic of either mastitis or low milk-volume secretion. Colostrum has much higher concentrations of sodium and chloride than does mature milk because the gland is undergoing the transition between pregnancy, when the junctions are open, and full lactation, when they are closed. Preterm milk shows lower concentrations of sodium and chloride, which rise to normal levels approximately 30 days postpartum.

The concentrations in milk of the major divalent ions are species specific. The calcium level increases markedly during the first few days postpartum but then decreases gradually over the course of the lactation. Citrate and phosphate concentrations rise in parallel with the sharp increase in milk volume between 2 to 4 days postpartum. The calcium-to-phosphorus ratio is lower in cow's milk (1:4) than in human milk (2:2). Lactation also affects the mother's calcium movement. Calcium uptake in the maternal duodenum is enhanced during lactation. After weaning, women who have lactated show significantly more bone in the lumbar spine than women who have not lactated (Kalkwarf, Specker, Heubi, Vieira, & Yergey, 1996).

Microminerals

Microminerals (trace minerals or trace elements) can be classified into four categories:

1. Essential: required in the diet, such as iron, zinc, copper, manganese, molybdenum, cobalt, selenium, iodine, and fluorine.
2. Possibly essential: chromium, nickel, silicon, tin, and vanadium.
3. Toxic in excess: aluminum, arsenic, cadmium, lead, and mercury. Soy-based infant formulas, hypoallergenic formulas, and formulas for premature infants have aluminum levels far in excess

of human milk (50 ng/g). Aluminum levels in cow's milk–based formulas have been measured in ranges from 10 to 3,400 ng/g; in soy-based formula, aluminum levels range from 230 to 1,100 ng/g; and in formula for preterm infants, aluminum ranges from 365 to 909 ng/g (Dabeka, Fouquet, Belisle, & Turcotte, 2011). The high aluminum content seen in infant formulas originates from both the myriad ingredients used to produce the product and aluminum from the packaging (Chuchu, Patel, Sebastian, & Exley, 2013). The immature physiologies of infants' GI tract, kidneys, and blood–brain barrier may predispose them to aluminum toxicity.

4. All other elements.

Because infants typically receive their entire nutrition from a single type of food, it is important that the proper trace elements are present and occur in the appropriate concentrations.

The iron concentration in human milk is highest during the first few days after birth and diminishes with the progression of lactation. Compared with the calculated requirements for the growing infant (8–10 mg/day), human milk appears to be relatively low in iron, at a concentration of 0.2–0.8 mg/L. In reality, the full-term infant is born with large physiological stores in the liver and hemoglobin, which, along with the iron in breastmilk, are sufficient to meet requirements for about 6 months if infants are exclusively breastfed. Approximately 50% of the iron from human milk is absorbed by the infant, compared with 2–19% from iron-fortified formula and 4% from fortified infant cereals. Iron concentrations increase during the weaning period and when women produce less than 300 mL/day after 7 months (Dewey, Finley, & Lonnerdal, 1984). The iron concentration in milk is not influenced by the maternal iron status. The infant who is exclusively breastfed for the first 6 months of life is not at risk for iron-deficiency anemia (Duncan, Schifman, Corrigan, & Schaefer, 1985). Caution has been advised with supraphysiological iron supplementation, however, because it can cause as much as a 40-fold increase in iron retention (Schulz-Lell, Buss, Oldigs, Dorner, & Schaub, 1987). Lactose, which promotes iron absorption, is present in higher concentrations in breastmilk, especially compared with commercial formulas, some of which contain no lactose at all. Breastfed infants do not suffer microhemorrhages of the bowel as some formula-fed infants do, so they will not have iron depletion through blood loss. Pisacane and coworkers (1995) studied the iron status of infants breastfed for 1 year who were never given cow's milk, supplemental iron, or iron-enriched formula. None who were exclusively breastfed for 7 months were anemic. Those breastfed exclusively for 6.5 months versus 5.5 months were less likely to be anemic. Iron supplementation of normal, healthy, full-term infants in the first 6 months therefore appears unnecessary and, in fact, increases the risk of disease by saturating lactoferrin. Supplementary foods reduce the intake of human milk and may impair iron absorption. Early introduction of highly bioavailable iron supplements, before 6 months of age, may be beneficial in a high-risk population, such as preterm infants who lack their full complement of iron stores. However, some studies have reported detrimental effects such as decreased growth and increased morbidity (Dewey et al., 2002), decreased zinc absorption (Lind et al., 2004), and altered vitamin A metabolism (Wieringa et al., 2003) when iron supplements are provided to infants who do not need them. It is possible that young infants may lack the capacity to downregulate iron absorption, either due to immaturity or to other micronutrient deficiencies, and that iron given to such infants may cause adverse effects (Hicks, Zavaleta, Chen, Abrams, & Lonnerdal, 2006). Deleterious effects of iron supplementation appear to affect infants who have adequate iron stores to begin with. Ziegler, Nelson, and Jeter (2009) conducted a study to assess the effect of universal early iron supplementation (all breastfed infants) versus selective supplementation (only at-risk infants) from ages 1 month to 5.5 months of age. While 7 mg/day of iron caused some preservation of the infants' iron stores, the effect was modest and did not extend beyond the period of supplementation. Iron supplementation in this study significantly decreased the weight gain (but not length) of female infants. The authors concluded that iron supplementation of breastfed infants from an early age was feasible but only temporarily affected the iron status of the infants. Because of the low prevalence of iron deficiency, selective treatment of only those infants at risk for iron deficiency would be a more suitable approach to prevention of iron deficiency than universal supplementation of all breastfed infants.

Zinc is an essential component of more than 200 enzymes that have both catalytic and structural roles. This nutrient appears to play a critical role in gene expression. Many DNA-binding proteins are zinc complexes. Zinc concentration in colostrum ranges from 8 to 12 mg/mL and in mature milk from 1 to 3 mg/mL. The zinc in human milk is more efficiently utilized by infants than the zinc in cow's milk or formulas. Zinc bioavailability from soy formulas is considerably lower than that from milk-based formulas due to the phytate content of soy protein isolates. The full-term breastfed infant is at little risk for zinc deficiency. Only in rare cases have breastfed infants experienced such a deficiency, usually because of defective zinc uptake by the mammary gland. Transient zinc deficiency due to increased zinc requirements in breastfed mainly preterm infants is a condition similar to acrodermatitis enteropathica, an autosomal recessive disorder of enteric zinc absorption affecting almost exclusively nonbreastfed infants. Early recognition of the disorder and introduction of zinc supplementation rapidly reverses transient zinc deficiency. The term acrodermatitis enteropathica (AE) is used for all patients with acral dermatitis related to zinc deficiency, although it should be strictly confined to hereditary forms. Hypozincemia in infancy is divided into three types. Type I is characterized by an inherent defect in the absorption of zinc from the gut. Type II occurs because of defective secretion of zinc in mother's milk. Type III develops in preterm infants who are put on prolonged parenteral alimentation deficient in zinc.

Copper, selenium, chromium, iodide, manganese, nickel, fluorine, molybdenum, and cobalt all appear in adequate amounts in human milk. Healthy, full-term, breastfed infants require no supplementation of any of these minerals, including fluoride. However, the iodine content of the breastmilk of mothers who smoke cigarettes is lower than that of nonsmokers. Mothers who smoke have been reported to have higher levels of thiocyanate, which may reduce iodide transport into breastmilk. Infants of mothers who smoke may need to have their iodine levels monitored and to be given iodine supplements if appropriate (Laurberg, Nohr, Pedersen, & Fuglsang, 2004).

Clinical Implications

Continued research has revealed the highly complex nature of human milk. Many of the ingredients in breastmilk participate in multiple functions (**Table 1-3**). The interrelationships among the various components may be more significant than the amounts present or their levels of uptake. The ability of human milk and the act of breastfeeding to promote affiliative behavior, protect infant health, and support normal growth and development is unmatched by any other feeding system. Normal, healthy, full-term infants who are exclusively breastfed typically do not need vitamin or mineral supplements, with the exception of some high-risk infants who may need additional vitamin D or iron.

Table 1-3 Multiple Functions of the Major Nutrients of Human Milk in the Infant

Nutrients	Amount	Function
Protein		
sIgA	50–100 mg/dL	Immune protection
IgM	2 mg/dL	Immune protection
IgG	1 mg/dL	Immune protection
Lactoferrin	100–300 mg/dL	Anti-infective, iron carrier
Lysozyme	5–25 mg/dL	Anti-infective
Alpha-lactalbumin	200–300 mg/dL	Ion carrier (Ca^{2+}), part of lactose synthase
Casein	200–300 mg/dL	Ion carrier, inhibits microbial adhesion to mucosal membranes
Carbohydrate		
Lactose	6.5–7.3 g/L	Energy source
Oligosaccharides	1.0–1.5 g/L	Microbial ligands
Glycoconjugates	—	Microbial and viral ligands
Fat		
Triglyceride	3.0–4.5 g/L	Energy source
LCPUFA	—	Essential for brain and retinal development and for infant growth
FFA	—	Anti-infective

FFA, free fatty acids, produced from triglycerides during fat digestion in the stomach and intestine.

Reprinted from Hamosh, M. (2001). Bioactive factors in human milk. *Pediatric Clinics of North America, 48*(1), 69–86. With permission from Elsevier, Inc.

Lactating mothers rarely need supplemental vitamins and minerals because most supplements do not appreciably affect milk nutrient concentrations. However, vegetarian mothers may need either a vitamin B_{12} supplement or consultation regarding acceptable food sources of this vitamin in their diet. Mothers who have undergone gastric bypass surgery will also need a source for vitamin B_{12} supplementation. Celiker and Chawla (2009) reported on the infant of a mother who had undergone gastric bypass surgery 6 years previous to the birth. The infant was born with congenital B_{12} deficiency. It is important that clinicians are aware that B_{12} deficiency may be congenital as well as occur as a result of being fed breastmilk deficient in vitamin B_{12}.

Although diet can affect the composition of fatty acids in the mother's milk, no definitive data support the practice of supplementing the mother with additional DHA to raise DHA levels in her milk or indicate that doing so results in any long-term benefits to her infant (Follett et al., 2003). The association between maternal supplementation with DHA and infant status is a saturable curve (Gibson, Neumann, & Makrides, 1997). As Follett and colleagues (2003) state, "Increasing supplementation of mothers is not associated with increased infant erythrocyte DHA if a level of 0.8% has been reached. Therefore, higher levels of DHA do not result in higher stores or improved function in the infant." In a review of 8 radomized controlled trials that included 1,567 women, LCPUFA supplementation of breastfeeding mothers did not appear to improve children's neurodevelopment, visual acuity, or growth (Delgado-Noguera, Calvache, Bonfill Cosp, Kotanidou, & Galli-Tsinopoulou, 2015). Mitoulas (2000) advises that maternal supplementation of particular medium- or long-chain fatty acids may adversely affect other fatty acids such that the proportions of various fatty acids may become unbalanced, decreasing the proportion of some when others are increased. It is unknown what effect altered fatty acid profiles have on other human milk components or the recipient infant. Cheatham, Nerhammer, Asserhøj, Michaelsen, and Lauritzen (2011) examined whether fish oil supplementation during lactation affects processing speed, working memory, inhibitory control, and socioemotional development of children at 7 years of age. Early fish oil supplementation of breastfeeding mothers may actually have a negative effect on later infant cognitive abilities. The speed of cognitive processing scores were predicted by maternal n-3 LCPUFA intake during the study intervention period, which showed a negative relation (lower scores in the supplemented group). Stroop scores indicative of working memory and inhibitory control were predicted by infant erythrocyte DHA status at 4 months of age, again with a negative relation.

Fluoride supplementation is no longer recommended for infants younger than 6 months of age and only thereafter for infants living in communities with suboptimally fluoridated water supplies. Adding solid foods or infant formula before about 6 months of age may interfere with iron uptake in the breastfed infant and saturate the iron-binding capacity of lactoferrin, increasing the infant's risk of GI disease. Some commercially available bottled baby water contains added fluoride. Parents should be advised that breastfed infants do not require additional water or fluoride and should be told to check with their primary healthcare provider about the safety of such products advertised for young infants.

DEFENSE AGENTS

The immune system of human milk is a complex interplay between milk factors, the matrix of human milk, synergistic activities of defense components, differences in resident gut microflora of the infant, and individual differences in mothers and infants. Defensive characteristics of human milk are potent inhibitors of numerous diseases. As little as 2 weeks of exclusive breastfeeding reduces enterovirus infections in infants for up to 1 year (Sadeharju et al., 2007). Although breastmilk is often referred to as the infant's first immunization, it has been shown that breastfed infants also show a better developed response to a number of vaccines such as *H. influenzae* and pneumococcal (Silfverdal, Ekholm, & Bodin, 2007). Human milk provides the recipient infant with several tiers of protection against pathogens, resulting in the reduced incidence of a number of acute and chronic diseases and conditions long after breastfeeding has ceased (Hanson et al., 2002). These include the following:

- Nutrients that facilitate optimal development of the infant, including the immune system and intestinal mucosa (**Table 1-4**)
- Antibodies in the milk to specific environmental pathogens
- Broad-spectrum protective agents such as lactoferrin and fatty acids that provide a third layer of defense (see **Table 1-3**)
- Glycoconjugates and oligosaccharides
- Live cells
- Anti-inflammatory agents (**Table 1-5**)
- Immunostimulating agents

Table 1-4 Protective Components in Human Milk

Immune Protection	Function
sIgA, G, M, D, E	Specific antigen-targeted anti-infective activity
Nonspecific protection	Antibacterial, antiviral, and antimicrobial-toxin, enhancing newborn's immune system maturation
Major and minor nutrients	See Table 1-3
Nucleotides	Enhance T-cell maturation, natural killer cell activity, antibody response to certain vaccines, intestinal maturation, and repair after diarrhea
Vitamins	
A (beta-carotene)	Anti-inflammatory (scavenging of oxygen radicals)
C (ascorbic acid)	Anti-inflammatory (scavenging of oxygen radicals)
E (alpha-tocopherol)	Anti-inflammatory (scavenging of oxygen radicals)
Enzymes	
Bile salt–dependent lipase	Production of FFA with antiprotozoan and antibacterial activity
Catalase	Anti-inflammatory (degrades H_2O_2)
Glutathione peroxidase	Anti-inflammatory (prevents lipid peroxidation)
PAF acetylhydrolase	Protects against NEC (hydrolysis of PAF)
Hormones	
Prolactin	Enhances the development of B and T lymphocytes, affects differentiation of intestinal lymphoid tissue
Cortisol, thyroxine, insulin, and growth factors	Promote maturation of the newborn's intestine and development of intestinal host-defense mechanism
Cells	
Macrophages, PMNs, and cytokines	Microbial phagocytosis, production of lymphokines and lymphocytes, interaction with and enhancement of other protective agents
Cytokines	Modulate functions and maturation of the immune system

PAF, platelet-activating factor; PMN, polymorphonuclear.
Reprinted from Hamosh, M. (2001). Bioactive factors in human milk. *Pediatric Clinics of North America, 48*(1), 69–86. With permission from Elsevier, Inc.

Jensen (1995) described common features of the biochemically diverse defense agents in human milk:

- An inverse relationship often exists between the production of these factors in the breast and their production by the infant over time.
- As lactation progresses, the concentrations of many of these factors in human milk decline. At the same time, the production at the mucosal sites of those very factors increases in the developing infant.
- Most components of the immunological system in human milk are produced throughout lactation and during gradual weaning.
- The factors are usually common to other mucosal sites.

Table 1-5 Anti-inflammatory Components of Human Milk

Component	Function
Vitamins	
A	Scavenges oxygen radicals
C	Scavenges oxygen radicals
E	Scavenges oxygen radicals
Enzymes	
Catalase	Degrades H_2O_2
Glutathione peroxidase	Prevents lipid peroxidation
PAF-acetylhydrolase	Degrades PAF, a potent ulcerogen
Antienzymes	
$Alpha_1$-antitrypsin	Inhibits inflammatory proteases
$Alpha_1$-antichymotrypsin	Inhibits inflammatory proteases
Prostaglandins	
PGE_1	Cytoprotective
PGE_2	Cytoprotective
Growth Factors	
EGF	Promotes gut growth and functional maturation
TGF-alpha	Promotes epithelial cell growth
TGF-beta	Suppresses lymphocyte function
Cytokines	
IL-10	Suppresses function of macrophages and natural killer and T cells
Cytokine Receptors	
TGF-alpha; RI, RII	Bind to and inhibit TGF-alpha

EGF, epidermal growth factor; IL, interleukin; PAF, platelet-activating factor; PGE, prostaglandin E; TGF, transforming growth factor.

Reprinted from Hamosh, M. (2001). Bioactive factors in human milk. *Pediatric Clinics of North America, 48*(1), 69–86. With permission from Elsevier, Inc.

- They are adapted to resist digestion in the GI tract of the recipient infant.
- They offer protection via noninflammatory mechanisms.
- The agents act synergistically with one another or with defense agents produced by the body.

Types of Defense Agents

Human milk contains a potent mixture of agents that work synergistically to form an innate immune system that allows the nursing mother to protect her infant from a host of diseases.

Direct-Acting Antimicrobial Agents

- Oligosaccharides and glycoconjugates: These agents inhibit toxin binding from *Vibrio cholerae* and *E. coli* and interfere with the attachment of *H. influenzae*, *S. pneumoniae*, and *C. jejuni*.

- Proteins: Many of the whey proteins have direct antimicrobial actions. Lactoferrin competes with bacteria for ferric iron and disrupts their proliferation. A concentration of approximately 5–6 mg/mL is found in colostrum, with the concentration decreasing to 2 mg/mL at 4 weeks and to 1 mg/mL in milk thereafter. Lysozyme lyses susceptible bacteria. The approximate mean intake of milk lysozyme per day in healthy full-term infants is about 3–4 mg/kg/day at 1 month and 6 mg/kg/day at 4 months. Fibronectin facilitates the actions of mononuclear phagocytic cells. Complement components are present as well. Immunoglobulins represent important defensive agents. The predominant immunoglobulin in human milk is sIgA. IgE, the principal type of antibody responsible for immediate hypersensitivity reactions, is absent from human milk. Mucins defend against *E. coli* and rotavirus. Nucleotides are thought to enhance the growth of beneficial bacteria in the gut.
- Bifidus growth promoter.
- Defense agents: These are created from partially digested substrates from human milk. Fatty acids and monoglycerides are able to disrupt enveloped viruses (Isaacs, 2005), with lipid-induced active antiviral activity apparent in the infant's stomach within 1 hour of feeding (Isaacs, Kashyap, Heird, & Thormar, 1990).
- Leukocytes: These are living white cells present in human milk in highest concentrations during the first 2–4 days of lactation. The leukocyte component of human milk is made up of lymphocytes, macrophages, and polymorphonuclear leukocytes (neutrophils and eosinophils). Neutrophils and macrophages are the most abundant in human milk. Lymphocytes are found in human milk, with 80% of them appearing as T cells. They synthesize IgA antibody. Milk lymphocytes manufacture several chemicals, including gamma-interferon, migration inhibition factor, and monocyte chemotactic factor, all of which augment the body's own immune response.
- Anti-inflammatory agents:
  1. Factors that promote the growth of epithelium
     a. Cortisol
     b. Epithelial growth factor
     c. Polyamines
     d. Lactoferrin
  2. Antioxidants
     a. Ascorbate-like compound.
     b. Uric acid.
     c. Beta-carotene.
     d. Carotenoids such as lutein can also act as antioxidants. In the eye, certain other carotenoids (lutein and zeaxanthin) apparently act directly to absorb damaging blue and near-ultraviolet light, in order to protect the macula lutea. Because humans cannot synthesize lutein, this carotenoid must be supplied by dietary sources. Exclusively breastfed infants have six times the mean serum lutein concentration compared with infants consuming formula that is not supplemented with lutein, with four times more lutein needed in formula to achieve similar concentrations seen in breastfed neonates (Bettler, Zimmer, Neuringer, & DeRusso, 2010). With some formulas being supplemented with

these high levels of lutein, it remains unknown what side effects, if any, this might have on recipient infants.

3. Prostaglandins
4. PAF-AH
5. Immunomodulators
   a. Alpha-tocopherol.
   b. Cytokines regulate many epithelial cell functions and are at their highest in human milk when they are at their lowest in the recipient infant. Most of the cytokines that are known to be deficient in the neonate are found in significant amounts in breastmilk. Cytokines have been shown to be higher in milk samples from Asian mothers compared with African mothers and may vary according to race (Chirico, Marzollo, Cortinovis, Fonte, & Gasparoni, 2008). Some of these cytokines are IL-1B, IL-6, IL-8, and IL-10.
   c. Granulocyte-colony stimulating factor.
   d. Macrophage-colony stimulating factor.
   e. TNF-alpha, interferon, epithelial growth factor, TGF-alpha, and TGF-beta2.

CAN BREASTMILK TELL TIME?

The pineal hormone melatonin has been shown to exhibit a circadian rhythm when measured in body fluids. It has a hypnotic effect as well as a relaxing effect on the smooth muscle of the GI tract. Illnerova, Buresova, and Presl (1993) measured melatonin in human milk samples and found that it displayed a circadian rhythm. Melatonin in breastmilk that was expressed during the day was beyond the limits of detection, but breastmilk melatonin during the night was measured at 99 $\pm$ 26 pmol/L. Does breastmilk communicate time of day information to breastfed infants? Cohen Engler, Hadash, Shehadeh, and Pillar (2011) assessed the differences in the prevalence and severity of colic and nocturnal sleep between breastfed and formula-fed 2- to 4-month-old infants. They also characterized the melatonin secretion profile in human milk and formula. Their results showed that breastfed infants had a significantly lower incidence of colic attacks, lower severity of irritability attacks, and a trend for longer nocturnal sleep duration. Melatonin in human milk showed a clear circadian rhythm (higher at night) and was not measurable in infant formula.

The circadian rhythm of melatonin in breastmilk could contribute to the consolidation of infants' sleep–wake cycle until maturation of their own circadian system occurs. It might be useful to breastfeed in the dark for nighttime feedings, as exposure to light causes melatonin suppression in breastmilk. Milk banks might consider having donor mothers label day- and nighttime-expressed milk so that recipient infants can be fed with the milk that corresponds to day or night feeds (Sanchez-Barcelo, Mediavilla, & Reiter, 2011).

People with atopic eczema frequently complain of sleep disturbance, and their levels of blood melatonin are decreased in comparison to healthy subjects. Melatonin levels in breastmilk have only been reported in healthy mothers. Knowing that laughter increases natural killer cell activity in blood and free radical-scavenging capacity in saliva in healthy subjects, Kimata (2007) studied the effects of laughter on the levels of melatonin in the breastmilk of mothers with atopic eczema. Also studied was the effect of feeding with breastmilk after laughter on allergic responses in the infants of the allergic mothers. All infants had allergic eczema and were allergic to latex and house dust mites. Mothers viewed a humorous 87-minute DVD or an 87-minute DVD on the weather. Laughter increased the levels of breastmilk melatonin in both allergic and healthy mothers. Feeding infants with milk that contained increased levels of melatonin reduced allergic responses in the infants. While laughter is often called the best medicine, it seems to have a clear place in influencing melatonin levels in breastmilk and positively affecting allergic, irritable, and colicky infants.

HUMAN MILK FORTIFICATION

Whereas the immunological factors in breastmilk are important for all infants, they are essential to preterm or ill infants whose immune systems may be immature or challenged by other health conditions. Nutrient fortification of preterm mothers' milk is seen in NICUs when an infant's needs exceed the capacity of breastmilk to provide selected nutrients in amounts that support a particular growth velocity.

Most NICUs do not use single-nutrient fortification but rely on multinutrient commercial fortifiers of differing composition. Preterm mothers' milk inhibits the growth of many bacteria, including *E. coli*, *Staphylococcus*, *Enterobacter sakazakii*, and group B *Streptococcus*; however, the addition of a cow's milk protein–based powdered human milk fortifier high in iron can neutralize the ability of human milk to kill these bacterial species (Chan, 2003). The addition to human milk of an older formulation of the same product decreased the IgA levels to *E. coli* and resulted in a 19% decrease in lysozymal activity in human milk, a measure of bacterial lysis (Jocson, Mason, & Schanler, 1997). The addition of a relatively large amount of iron directly into human milk may interfere with the ability of lactoferrin to bind iron and lyse bacterial cell walls. Quan et al. (1994) reported significant decreases in lysozyme content and IgA specific for *E. coli* when commercial fortifiers were added to fresh frozen milk. Chan, Lee, and Rechtman (2007) compared the antibacterial activity of preterm milk that had a commercial cow's milk–based high iron fortifier added to it or a human milk–based fortifier that was lower in iron. The commercial fortifier sample was shown to almost completely eliminate the bacterial inhibitory actions of the milk compared with the human milk fortifier sample, which retained its bacteriocidal activity. Fortifiers can be added to expressed hindmilk when the rate of weight gain is low. Some fortifiers can increase the osmolality of the milk, increasing the risk for GI irritation and feeding intolerance (Fenton & Belik, 2002; Rochow, Landau-Crangle, & Fusch, 2015; Srinivasan, Bokiniec, King, Weaver, & Edwards, 2004). They may also contain cow's milk protein and soy, which presents allergy as a potential side effect. The addition of human milk fortifier may temporarily delay gastric emptying and cause a short-term increase in gastric residuals and emesis.

Commercially available human milk fortifiers may add needed nutrients to mothers' expressed breastmilk but contain casein and whey proteins derived from bovine milk, lipids from both plants and microbial sources, and carbohydrates derived from plants. Although the addition of non–human milk-derived components to human milk is beneficial for promoting the growth of the preterm infant, bovine milk proteins have a different amino acid composition and are not as efficiently digested as human milk proteins. In addition, infants fed fortified human milk may exhibit higher rates of feeding intolerance and NEC. Sullivan and colleagues (2010) showed that NEC was reduced by 76% in preterm infants whose mother's milk was fortified with a human milk-based fortifier compared with a bovine milk-based fortifier. The addition of a bovine fortifier to breastmilk is associated with an acute increase in GI tract inflammation (Panczuk et al., 2016). An alternative to fortifying human milk with commercially available human milk fortifiers is to use human milk products that are derived from donated human milk (Czank, Simmer, & Hartmann, 2010). Ganapathy, Hay, and Kim (2012) conducted a cost-effectiveness analysis of using a human milk–based fortifier compared with a bovine milk–based fortifier on the cost of NEC. They showed that an exclusively human milk–based feeding strategy saved $8,167 per infant who received a diet of exclusive human milk (expressed breastmilk plus a human milk–based fortifier). One study was done to determine the in vitro effect(s) of a bovine-based human breastmilk fortifier (HMF) on human intestinal cells. HMF increased the expression of BCL2/adenovirus E1B 19 kDa protein-interacting protein (Bnip3) and cell death. The outcome supported the hypothesis that HMF increases intestinal Bnip3 in vitro, and that the gene product triggers intestinal cell death (Diehl-Jones et al., 2015). This would raise the prospect of using caution when fortifying human milk with a nonhuman milk fortifier.

Lessaris, Forsythe, and Wagner (2000) showed that human milk fortifier differentially altered the biochemical profile of human milk with regard to TGF-alpha (a gut peptide that exerts a maturational effect on the neonatal gut) concentration and molecular mass profile. What effect this alteration in human milk biochemistry has on neonatal gut function remains unknown. The addition of iron and vitamin C to preterm human milk was shown to increase oxidative stress and reduce the content of mono- and polyunsaturated fatty acids (Friel, Diehl-Jones, Suh, Tsopmo, & Shirwadkar, 2007).

Caution should be exercised when adding a preparation to human milk, such as a fortifier, that neutralizes the milk's ability to destroy harmful bacteria, especially if the potential for bacterial contamination is contained in the fortifier itself. Fortified human milk can be stored in a refrigerator at 2–4°C (35–40°F) for no longer than 24 hours. Once fortified human milk is prepared, it can remain at room temperature for 4 hours (Telang et al., 2005). The American Dietetic Association recommends a hang time for fortified breastmilk of no longer than 4 hours at room temperature (25°C/77°F) (Robbins & Meyers, 2011). Fortified human milk should not be used if it is unrefrigerated for more than a total of 2 hours. After a bottle-feeding begins, it must be used within 1 hour or discarded.

Powdered infant formula is not sterile, including powdered human milk fortifiers. Some samples of powdered infant formula have been found to harbor *E. sakazakii* (*Chronobacter sakazaki*) (Baker, 2002). The FDA discourages the use of powdered forms in the NICU secondary to contamination risk (Himelright et al., 2002). The FDA also advises that "alternatives to powdered forms should be chosen when possible." However, in a study on the use of a new acidified liquid human milk fortifier, a number of poor infant outcomes were seen, such as poor growth, increased acidosis, increased incidence of NEC, metabolic acidosis, feeding intolerance, and diaper dermatitis (Thoene et al., 2014).

One way to avoid the unwanted side effects from use of a cow's milk–based liquid or powered fortifier is to use a donor human milk–derived fortifier, which would result in an exclusively human milk–based diet. In one study, a feeding protocol with early and rapid advancement using a human milk–based fortifier resulted in adequate growth and a low rate of extrauterine growth restriction (Hair, Hawthorne, Chetta, & Abrams, 2013).

Protein is often the limiting factor in breastmilk-fed to very preterm infants. While protein is higher during the early days of lactation, protein concentrations in mother's milk decreases quickly to the point that it may not be sufficient for the needs of a very premature infant. Protein levels vary in maternal and banked donor milk, presenting the problem of how much protein is actually provided to an individual infant. Studies on increasing the amount of protein in fortifiers have shown better weight gain and fewer infants who remain in less than the 10th percentile for length (Miller et al., 2012). Rather than using a shotgun approach to fortification as in standard commercial fortifiers, there are two individualized methods of fortification that may provide a better outcome—adjustable fortification and targeted fortification (Arslanoglu, Moro, Ziegler, & The WAPM Working Group on Nutrition, 2010). Targeted fortification is a method that analyzes the expressed milk for the amounts of particular nutrients—in this case, protein. The amount of fortifier added to the milk is targeted such that the particular nutrient in question reaches a certain level in the milk. Adjustable fortification looks at the individual infant's metabolic response to the contents of the milk. There is no assumption of the infant's protein needs, as periodic sampling of the blood urea nitrogen levels determines adjustments needed in the level of protein intake. Adjustment in protein levels is based on the metabolic response of the infant to avoid under- or overfortification of protein (Arslanoglu, Moro, & Ziegler, 2006).

A best practice concept for the provision of human milk in the NICU is use of a centralized facility or a human milk management center that allows staff to analyze human milk, perform creamatocrits, conduct nutrient analysis, fortify milk under aseptic conditions, make skim milk, and tailor the milk to meet each infant's needs (Spatz, Schmidt, & Kinzler, 2014). One study reported use of a mobile milk cart for the preparation and fortification of breastmilk in a hospital that lacked a central space for the management of human milk nutrition for its preterm patients (Barbas, 2013). Technology for human milk analysis exists in the form of several human milk analyzers that a number of NICUs already utilize to augment their overall nutritional support plans. Given the large variability between inter-woman and intra-woman milk samples, the expressed milk of many mothers of preterm infants as well as pasteurized banked donor human milk may not contain the average 20 kcal/oz and 1.5 g/dL of protein (Adamkin & Radmacher, 2014). Precise analysis and individualized fortification give preterm infants an enhanced ability to have their nutritional needs adequately met.

MILK TREATMENT AND STORAGE

The antioxidant activity of human milk is diminished by both refrigeration and freezing, and over the course of time; however, it remains significantly higher than infant formula in antioxidant capacity despite how it is stored or when it is collected or ingested by the infant (Ezaki, Ito, Suzuki, & Tamura, 2008; Hanna et al., 2004). This is extremely important to preterm infants who are born before their antioxidant defense system is fully developed and functional (Baydas et al., 2002; Georgeson et al., 2002).

Preterm infants can experience oxidative stress from conditions such as infection and chronic lung disease and from interventions such as mechanical ventilation, oxygen therapy, IV nutrition, and blood transfusions. Some of the conditions and diseases common to preterm infants, such as NEC and retinopathy of prematurity, are often attributed to a profusion of oxidative stress and a deficiency in the oxidative defense system. Ingesting human milk rapidly increases antioxidant concentrations (Ostrea, Balun, Winkler, & Porter, 1986; Sommerburg, Meissner, Nelle, Lenhartz, & Leichsenring, 2000; Zoeren-Grobben, Moison, Ester, & Berger, 1993), partially explaining the reduced incidence of NEC and retinopathy of prematurity in infants protected by the consumption of human milk (Hylander, Strobino,

Pezzullo, & Dhanireddy, 2001). Preterm infants with a birth weight below 1,000 grams and a gestational age below 30 weeks may be at high risk of acquiring a symptomatic cytomegalovirus (CMV) infection through their mother's milk if she is CMV positive. Refrigeration and freezing of milk from preterm mothers may reduce the risk of transferring CMV to the infant but does not eliminate it (Hamprecht, Maschmann, Jahn, Poets, & Goelz, 2008). Most preterm infants remain asymptomatic when infected with CMV through breastmilk (Omarsdottir et al., 2015). One study showed that transmission of CMV from seropositive mothers via breastmilk to preterm infants did not appear to have major adverse effects on clinical outcomes, growth, neurodevelopmental status, or hearing function at 12 and 24 months corrected age (Jim et al., 2015). Inactivation of CMV can be accomplished by Holder pasteurization (heating to 62.5°C/144.5°F for 30 minutes) but can decrease the immunological components in breastmilk. Rapid high-temperature treatment of human milk (72°C/161.6°F for 5 or 15 seconds) has been shown to eliminate CMV infectivity without destroying many of the anti-infective capabilities of the milk (Lawrence, 2006). Ehlinger and colleagues (2011) studied methods to reduce CMV virus shedding into mother's milk as a method to lower the potential of postnatal CMV transmission to preterm infants. Rather than treat the milk, antibody-based maternal vaccines might prove more useful for protection against symptomatic postnatal CMV.

The goal of milk treatment and storage is to preserve the nutrient and protective properties of the milk. Heat treatment includes the following processes:

- Microwaving. Refrigerated or frozen breastmilk is sometimes microwaved by parents to quickly thaw or heat it, but microwaving for 50 seconds destroys 30.5% of the milk's IgA. Quan and coworkers (1992) found that microwaving breastmilk at 72–98°C (162–208°F) decreases the activity of lysozyme by 96% and that of total IgA by 98%. Treatment at low temperatures, 20–53°C (68–127°F), did not affect total IgA but decreased lysozyme by 19%. Subsequent *E. coli* growth 3.5 hours after treatment was 5.2 times greater than in the control at low microwave temperatures and 18 times greater at the high temperatures, showing dramatic loss of anti-infective factors. Microwaving bottles of expressed breastmilk also poses a risk of injury to the infant from hot spots in the milk, which could burn the tongue, mouth, and throat as well as cause scalding and full-thickness burn injuries to the body from exploding bottles and nipples. In spite of these microwaving hazards, one study showed that 10% of mothers heated their expressed breastmilk in a microwave (Labiner-Wolfe & Fein, 2013). Advise parents to place the bottle of expressed breastmilk under warm running water or in a bowl of warm water. Human milk is delivered to the baby at body temperature, leaving little reason to heat milk beyond 36.9°C (98.4°F).
- Pasteurization.
  - Human milk is most often pasteurized by milk banks for use as donor milk for preterm or ill infants, in special situations where the unique defense properties in human milk would be therapeutic, when infants cannot tolerate artificial baby milks, and so forth. Banked donor human milk can be obtained by prescription from any of the human milk banks listed in Appendix 1-2. Heat treatment can reduce the effectiveness of some of the defense factors in milk such as the B- and T-cell components of milk, lactoferrin, and IgA. The Human

Milk Banking Association of North America (2008) requires the use of Holder pasteurization (62.5°C/144.5°F for 30 minutes) to eliminate viral contaminants such as human immunodeficiency virus, human T-cell lymphotropic virus-1, and CMV as well as common bacterial contaminants. High-temperature, short-time processing can also be done with human milk at 70°C (158°F) or 75°C (167°F) for 15 seconds. Silvestre, Ruiz, Martinez-Costa, Plaza, and Lopez (2008) noted that the temperature applied is more important than the duration of application for preserving the bactericidal capacity of pasteurized human milk. They found that when comparing untreated milk, milk pasteurized at 63°C (145.4°F) for 30 minutes, and milk pasteurized at 75°C (167°F) for 15 seconds, growth of *E. coli* was reduced by 70.10%, 52.27%, and 36.9%, respectively. The lower milk processing temperature was preferable for preserving more bactericidal capacity. Refrigeration of this pasteurized milk did not further reduce its antibacterial properties.

- Baro and colleagues (2011) compared Holder pasteurization with high-temperature, short-time pasteurization regarding the effects on bile salt–stimulated lipase, lactoferrin, and components of the immune system. Holder pasteurization decreased the amount of bile salt–stimulated lipase and lactoferrin while the high-temperature, short-time method did not alter the activity of bile salt–stimulated lipase, lactoferrin, and IgA. Ley, Hanley, Stone, and O'Connor (2011) reported a reduction in adiponectin (32.8%) and insulin (46.1%) after Holder pasteurization of 17 different batches of donor human milk. Holder pasteurization also preserves the effects of HMOs (Bertino et al., 2008). Pasteurization can reduce the antioxidant capacity of expressed breastmilk (Silvestre, Miranda, et al., 2008). Vieira, Soares, Pimenta, Abranches, & Moreira (2011) reported a 5.5% reduction in fat and a 3.9% reduction in protein after milk was pasteurized. Valentine and colleagues (2010) showed that there was a reduction in DHA levels in pasteurized milk as well as lower concentrations of a number of amino acids. A newer high-temperature, short-time form of pasteurization has been developed that better maintains the immunological quality of the milk (Chen & Allen, 2001). The high-temperature, short-time method of milk pasteurization may hold more promise for reducing alterations of many human milk components.
- Pasteurized donor human milk is a precious resource whose supply is limited. The current standard protocol is that once pasteurized donor human milk is thawed, any remaining milk should be discarded after 24 hours to avoid microbial contamination (Jones, 2011). However, it has been shown that there is no evidence of microbial growth in pasteurized donor human milk when defrosted and stored at 4°C (39.2°F) for up to 9 days (Vickers, Starks-Solis, Hill, & Newburg, 2015). Longer storage times of defrosted donor milk could reduce waste of this valuable resource and increase the availability of human milk for vulnerable infants.
- Boiling human milk is probably the most damaging to its components (Ballard & Morrow, 2013).

- Evaporation. In an effort to engineer human milk as an appropriate fortifier for preterm milk, Braga and Palhares (2007) evaporated pasteurized human milk samples by removing 30% of the water. The pasteurized evaporated human milk met the recommended requirements of sodium, potassium, magnesium, protein, fat, and lactose but not calcium and phosphorus requirements. Further studies are needed to see if this type of human milk manipulation is appropriate for preterm infants, especially if calcium and phosphorus were added.

- Refrigeration and freezing. Human milk can be safely stored under appropriate conditions to ensure infants receive their mother's or banked milk under a variety of conditions (Lawrence, 1999; Ogundele, 2000). Recommendations for storage times and temperatures vary among sources. The Academy of Breastfeeding Medicine recommends storage at room temperature, 16–29°C (60–85°F), for 3–4 hours as optimal; storage for 6–8 hours is acceptable under very clean conditions. Storage in the refrigerator at < 4°C (39°F) for 72 hours is recommended as optimal, with a longer period of 5–8 days being acceptable under very clean conditions. In the freezer < −17°C (0°F) for 6 months is recommended as optimal, with 12 months being acceptable (Academy of Breastfeeding Medicine Protocol Committee, & Eglash, 2010). According to the Human Milk Banking Association of North America (2011), freshly expressed milk can be stored at room temperature for < 6 hours, in the refrigerator for < 5 days for a term infant and for < 8 days for an older child, and in the freezer ideally for 3 months, optimally for < 6 months, although 12 months is acceptable if in a deep freezer (−20°C/−4°F). Previously frozen milk that has been thawed in the refrigerator but not warmed can be stored at room temperature for < 4 hours and in the refrigerator for < 24 hours, but should not be refrozen.

With previously frozen milk that has been brought to room temperature, the feeding should be completed within 1 hour at room temperature, then any remaining milk should be discarded. It can stay up to 4 hours in the refrigerator but should not be refrozen. If the infant has started feeding, the feeding should be completed and the milk can be placed in the refrigerator for up to 4 hours but should not be refrozen.

Storage of milk overnight results in formation of a cream layer on top containing about 20% fat and a skim layer below it containing about 1% fat. These layers are generally mixed before being fed to the infant. However, in special situations, such as a slow-gaining or preterm infant, the top high-fat layer can be skimmed off and given to infants as physiological high-calorie supplements.

Few data are available on storage times and conditions for fortified preterm human milk. Refrigerated fortified human milk should generally be used within 24 hours of when it was prepared (Jocson et al., 1997). Martínez-Costa et al. (2007) showed that refrigeration for 48 hours did not cause significant modifications in antibacterial properties of human milk, but storage beyond 72 hours significantly lowered the degree of bacteriolysis versus fresh milk.

Ogundele (2002) reported that although the bactericidal activities of refrigerated samples diminished rapidly, up to two-thirds of the original activity level was maintained by freezing for up to 3 months. The ability of MFGM to adhere to suspended bacteria was gradually lost in frozen milk samples, whereas it was greatly enhanced during the first few days in refrigerated samples, before declining sharply. This study shows that loss of bactericidal activity in refrigerated milk is well compensated for by enhanced bacteria sequestration activity.

Takci and colleagues (2012) reported that freezing at −20°C (−4°F) for 1 month did not cause statistically significant alteration in the bactericidal activity of expressed milk, but storage for 2 months at this temperature significantly lowered the degree of bactericidal activity against *E. coli*. Bactericidal activity was protected when the milk samples were stored at −80°C (−112°F). There was no statistically significant difference in bactericidal activity of human milk against *E. coli* between freezing at −20°C and −80°C for 1 month; however, when milk was stored for 3 months, storage at −80°C was significantly more protective. Freezing at −20°C and −80°C for 1 and 3 months did not cause any significant change for bactericidal activity against *Pseudomonas aeruginosa*. Tacken and colleagues (2009) found that triglyceride (fat) and carotenoid concentrations in human milk remained stable after refrigeration and freezing as well as low-temperature microwave heating, except for lutein, which decreased after refrigeration and freezing.

Xavier, Rai, and Hegde (2011) showed that when expressed transitional and mature milk were refrigerated or frozen, the total antioxidant capacity of the milk was reduced by 10–20% for 48 hours of storage and by 15–30% for 1 week of storage. This emphasizes the importance of using fresh expressed breastmilk for preterm infants or milk that has been stored only for short periods of time to ensure that a robust antioxidant system is retained in the milk, as preterm infants are highly subject to conditions related to oxidative stress. Slutzah, Codipilly, Potak, Clark, and Schanler (2010) demonstrated that fresh mother's milk may be stored at refrigerator temperature (4°C/39.2°F) for as long as 96 hours with minimal changes and with the overall integrity of the milk during refrigerator storage being preserved.

Prolonged refrigeration of human milk for 96 hours has also been shown to maintain the milk's overall lipid composition. Bile salt–dependent lipase activity, LCPUFAs, and medium-chain saturated fatty acid concentrations were unaffected during the 96 hours of refrigerator storage in one study, as was the milk's overall oxidative status (Bertino et al., 2013).

Human milk also contains bacteria that represent an important factor in the initiation and development of the normal and proper neonatal gut microbiota (Collado, Delgado, Maldonado, & Rodriguez, 2009). While concern about the growth of pathological bacteria in stored human milk is valid, consideration needs to be given to whether cold storage affects the natural bacterial composition of human milk. Marin et al. (2009) found that cold storage of human milk at −20°C (−4°F) for 6 weeks did not significantly affect either the quantitative or the qualitative natural bacterial composition of the milk. However, it was interesting that bacterial counts in milk expressed with a mechanical breast pump were higher than in samples obtained by manual expression. Thawing and warming of previously frozen human milk changes the integrity of the milk, but does not lead to any adverse effects (Handa et al., 2014).

Human milk contains two lipases (enzymes that digest fat) that do not change the lipid structure during refrigeration. However, when milk is frozen, lipolysis can occur. As this process continues, soaps form that can change the taste and smell of the milk. It is speculated that some mothers have more lipase activity than others, which can lead to a more rancid milk that some infants reject. If this occurs, these mothers can be advised to heat their milk to a scald (not boiling) after expressing it, then immediately cool and freeze it to stop the fat from being broken down (Jones, 2011). Hamosh, Ellis, Pollock, Henderson, and Hamosh (1996) studied the stability of protein and lipids as well as bacterial growth in expressed milk of employed mothers and generated the recommendations for short-term milk storage included in **Box 1-3**.

Box 1-3 Storage of Breastmilk for Healthy Infants

38°C (100°F) room air: Safe storage for less than 4 hours
25°C (77°F) room air: Safe storage for as long as 4 hours
15°C (59°F): Safe storage for 24 hours (equivalent to a Styrofoam box with blue ice)
4°C (39°F): In a refrigerator 72 hours and probably longer
Previously thawed milk in a refrigerator: 24 hours
Freezer inside refrigerator compartment: 2 weeks
−20°C (−4°F) freezer separate from refrigerator: 3 to 6 months, or up to 12 months (Milk should not be stored in shelves on the door but in the back of the freezer. Storage containers should be placed on a rack above the floor of the freezer to avoid warming during the automatic defrost cycle in freezers above the refrigerator compartment.)
−70°C (−94°F) deep freezer: Longer than 12 months

Modified from Hamosh, M., Ellis, L. A., Pollock, D. R., Henderson, T. R., & Hamosh, P. (1996). Breastfeeding and the working mother: Effect of time and temperature of short-term storage on proteolysis, lipolysis, and bacterial growth in milk. *Pediatrics, 97*(4), 492–498; Williams-Arnold, L. D. (2000). *Human milk storage for healthy infants and children.* Sandwich, MA: Health Education Associates.

STORAGE

Breastmilk can be stored in a number of ways (**Table 1-6**) (Arnold, 1995; Manohar, Williamson, & Koppikar, 1997; Tully, 2000; Williamson & Murti, 1996). Because human milk is a live fluid, capable of engaging in biological processes, it is important to understand that it remains active during storage. The defense agents in human milk allow it to be stored under a number of conditions and in a variety of containers. When discussing storage conditions and containers, it is also important to differentiate between the needs and tolerances of a healthy full-term infant and those of a sick or preterm infant (Jones, 2011).

Parents may wish to use glass or polypropylene bottles for feeding and storage of breastmilk (Environmental Working Group, 2007). Polycarbonate bottles have been shown to contain bisphenol A (BPA), a plasticizer that mimics estrogen. BPA has been shown to be a developmental, neural, and reproductive toxicant that can interfere with healthy growth and body function (Gibson, 2007). The amount of BPA that leaches from heated baby bottles is within the range shown to cause harm in animal studies (Workgroup for Safe Markets, 2008). Patients should avoid clear, hard plastic bottles marked with a 7 or "PC." Infant formula itself can be contaminated with BPA. Liquid formula packaged in metal cans often contains BPA from the BPA-based epoxy resin coating that lines the formula cans (Cao et al., 2008).

Polyethylene bags are a popular container for storing expressed breastmilk, as they take up less space than bottles and can be connected directly to a breast pump. A recent study showed that the bactericidal activity against *E. coli* in refrigerated human milk stored in polyethylene bags decreased significantly compared with that in expressed milk stored in Pyrex bottles at 24 and 48 hours (Takci, Gulmez, Yigit, Dogan, & Hascelik, 2013). This effect could be due to selective binding of antibodies to the container's walls or surface. Fat loss from breastmilk stored in 9 different containers was reported to range from 8.2% to 9.4%, with the highest loss from a bag with an outer layer of polyester and an inner layer of polyethylene (Chang, Chen, & Lin, 2012). This fat loss was most likely due to the adherence of milk to

Table 1-6 Selected Characteristics of Various Breastmilk Storage Containers

Container Type	Description	Advantages	Disadvantages	Effect on Milk	Healthy Full Term	Child in Day Care	Preterm, Ill, Hospitalized
Polyethylene bags	Thin bottle liner, freezer bags, bags for storage, doubled bags	Inexpensive, do not require washing	Fragile, compromised by expansion of milk during freezing, easily punctured, leak, hard to pour, need support, volume marks inaccurate	Fat loss, easily contaminated, photodegradation of nutrients, loss of sIgA	OK	No	No
Hard plastic (bottles, urine specimen cups, graduated feeders, centri-fuge tubes)	Polypropyl-ene (cloudy, semi-flexible)	Good for short-term storage of colostrum in a refrigerator (retains good cell count and viability)	Can become scratched if frequently reused, increasing chance of bacterial buildup in scratches in stored milk	Small loss of cellular components	OK	OK	OK with tight-fitting lids, short storage times
	Polycarbonate (clear, hard plastic)	More durable, less prone to scratching					
Glass	Bottles, canning jars, sterile water bottles	Best for preserving immune compo-nents of milk	Can break or chip	Possible photodeg-radation, cellular components adhere to walls of container but drop back into the milk sooner than with plastic	OK	OK	OK with tight-fitting lids, better for longer storage, less loss of immune components
Stainless steel	Not typically used in the United States						
Other containers	Ice cube trays, popsicle molds	Handy items found around the house		No data	OK	No	No

Data from Arnold, L. D. W. (1995). Storage containers for human milk: An issue revisited. *Journal of Human Lactation, 11*, 325–328; Human Milk Banking Association of North America. (2006). *Best practice for expressing, storing and handling of mother's own milk in hospital and at home.* Raleigh, NC: Author; Manohar, A. A., Williamson, M., & Koppikar, G. V. (1997). Effect of storage of colostrum in various containers. *Indian Pediatrics, 34,* 293–295; Tully, M. R. (2000). Recommendations for handling of mother's own milk. *Journal of Human Lactation, 16,* 149–151; Williamson, M. T., & Murti, P. K. (1996). Effects of storage, time, temperature, and composition of containers on biologic components of human milk. *Journal of Human Lactation, 12,* 31–35.

the container wall, and less likely due to lipolysis, or lipid peroxidation. It is unknown what the clinical impact of this loss would be on an infant (up to 2.7 kcal/dl).

Many hospital neonatal care units use polypropylene sterile specimen containers to store expressed breastmilk. Such containers are used for collecting tissues or body fluids, not food. Most of these containers are made of polypropylene but may have polyethylene caps. They have many of the characteristics recommended in clinical guidelines, but there are few data on their chemical safety or the potential effect on the milk or infants' health from the use of such containers (Blouin, Coulombe, & Rhainds, 2014).

Clinical Implications

Raw cow's milk contains numerous antimicrobial agents, primarily in colostrum, that are beneficial to the calf. These, however, are of little significance to the human infant consumer of a cow's milk product. Bovine colostrum is not used in the milk supply, and the effectiveness of any defense agent is neutralized by the removal of all cells, pasteurization, and homogenization. Bovine milk is intended to be consumed unaltered by the calf and conveys no disease defense to the human infant. In contrast, the immunological composition of human milk has evolved and adapted to offset the postnatal delays in the development of the human immune system. The thymus is the central organ of the immune system in an infant. Within this organ, T lymphocytes mature and multiply, including killer cells that are important for defense and regulatory T cells that are important for the prevention of autoimmune diseases (Wing, Ekmark, Karlsson, Rudin, & Suri-Payer, 2002). The thymus of a fully breastfed infant is twice the size of a formula-fed infant's thymus (Ngom et al., 2004). The thymic index has been correlated to the percentage of CD8+ cells, with a higher CD8 percentage seen in breastfed compared with formula-fed infants at 8 months of age (Jeppesen, Hasselbalch, Lisse, Ersboll, & Engelmann, 2004). The infant is exposed to microbial immunogens while receiving protective agents in human milk. This process creates an attenuated immunization, in that the pathogenicity of the microbial agent is reduced by the accompanying immune factors. Human milk also prepares the recipient infant to resist certain immune-mediated diseases and a host of other acute and chronic diseases and conditions.

Because formula-fed infants have higher rates of illness, artificial feeding results in higher costs to the healthcare system. Ball and Wright (1999) calculated the costs to the healthcare system associated with three common childhood diseases: otitis media, lower respiratory tract illness (bronchiolitis, croup, bronchitis, pneumonia), and GI illness. The excess total direct medical costs incurred by never-breastfed infants during the first year of life for these three illnesses alone ranged between $331 and $475 per infant, more than the costs incurred by breastfed infants. The authors reported 2,033 excess office visits, 212 excess days of hospitalization, and 609 excess prescriptions for these illnesses per 1,000 never-breastfed infants compared with 1,000 infants exclusively breastfed for at least 3 months. If 90% of U.S. families could comply with medical recommendations to breastfeed exclusively for 6 months, the United States would save $13 billion per year and prevent an excess 911 deaths, nearly all of which would be in infants (or $10.5 billion and 741 deaths at 80% compliance) (Bartick & Reinhold, 2010). The state of Louisiana would save $216,103,368 if 90% of newborns in that state were exclusively breastfed for the first 6 months of life, and 18 infant deaths would be prevented (Ma, Brewer-Asling, & Magnus, 2013). At 80% compliance, Louisiana would save $186,371,125 and prevent 16 infant deaths. The family of a formula-fed infant incurs direct costs for care if uninsured or for copayments if insured, as well as nonmedical costs such as family care and transportation to and from the physician's office and/or hospital. Missed days of work are costly to both employee and employer. If a parent misses 2 hours of work for the excess illnesses attributable to formula feeding, then more than 2,000 hours, the equivalent of 1 year of employment, are lost per 1,000 never-breastfed infants.

It is recommended that clinicians take the following steps to help ensure optimal breastfeeding outcomes:

1. Ensure that infants receive colostrum and human milk as the preferred food and first immunization.
2. Educate mothers/caregivers to avoid actions that dilute the anti-infective properties of human milk such as maternal smoking, mixing human milk with formula in the same container, and microwaving expressed milk.
3. Become familiar with data on the effects of heat treatment, refrigeration, freezing, and storage containers on the defense agents in human milk, and share this information with caregivers (**Table 1-7**).

Table 1-7 Results of Various Treatments on Human Milk

Treatment	Results
Refrigerated Storage	
4°C (39°F), 72 hours	Creaming, decrease in bacterial growth, possible lipolysis
−20°C (−4°F), 12 months	Lipolysis, possible demulsification and protein denaturation when thawed
−70°C (−94°F), indefinite	Possible demulsification and protein denaturation when thawed
Pasteurization	
56°C (132.8°F), 30 minutes	Inactivation of enzymes and antimicrobial proteins, partial loss of some vitamins, destruction of microorganisms
62.5°C (149.36°F), 30 minutes	Inactivation of enzymes and antimicrobial proteins, partial loss of some vitamins, destruction of microorganisms
70°C (158°F), 15 seconds	Inactivation of enzymes and antimicrobial proteins, partial loss of some vitamins, destruction of microorganisms
Microwave treatment	Decrease in IgA and lysozyme, substantial increase in coliforms
Sonication	Homogenization of milk-fat globules
Shaking vs. stirring	Vigorous shaking of breastmilk breaks the MFGM allowing fat to flow together into clumps irreversibly separating the fat from the milk. Stored breastmilk should be gently swirled to distribute the fat layer that has risen to the top of the container.
Selection/fractionization	Selection of high-protein milks, use of high-fat hindmilk
Supplementation	Addition of nutrients for preterm infants
Processing	Treatment of milk to isolate fats, proteins, and other components; fractions then added to milk
Centrifuge	Production of skim (fat-free) milk for infant with chylothorax; performance of creamatocrit
Manipulation of mother's diet	Change the fatty acid profile
Freeze-drying	Increases shelf life of human milk

Data from Jensen, R. G., & Jensen, G. L. (1992). Specialty lipids for infant nutrition. I. Milks and formulas. *Journal of Pediatric Gastroenterology & Nutrition*, 15, 232–245.

SUMMARY: THE DESIGN IN NATURE

Lactation is an ancient physiological process, dating back almost 200 million years. Human lactation and human milk have evolved to meet the needs and address the vulnerabilities of the human young. Milk intended for a four-legged, cud-chewing, nonverbal species may cause human infants to grow, but their growth and development will take a different trajectory than that of their breastfed counterparts. Infant formula and human milk components are not interchangeable. Artificial diets are not the same as human milk. The immuno-nutrition provided by human milk has no equal.

REFERENCES

Aaltonen, J., Ojala, T., Laitinen, K., Poussa, T., Ozanne, S., & Isolauri, E. (2011). Impact of maternal diet during pregnancy and breastfeeding on infant metabolic programming: A prospective randomized controlled study. *European Journal of Clinical Nutrition, 65*, 10–19.

Abrams, S. A., Griffin, I. J., & Davila, P. M. (2002). Calcium and zinc absorption from lactose-containing and lactose-free infant formulas. *American Journal of Clinical Nutrition, 76*, 442–446.

Academy of Breastfeeding Medicine Protocol Committee, & Eglash, A. (2010). ABM clinical protocol #8: Human milk storage information for home use for full-term infants (original protocol March 2004; revision #1 March 2010). *Breastfeeding Medicine, 5*, 127–130.

Adamkin, D. H., & Radmacher, P.G. (2014). Fortification of human milk in very low birth weight infants (VLBW $<$ 1500g birth weight). *Clinics in Perinatology, 41*, 405–421.

Adgent, M. A., Daniels, J. L., Rogan, W. J., Adair, L., Edwards, L. J., Westreich, D., . . . Marcus, M. (2012). Early-life soy exposure and age at menarche. *Paediatric and Perinatal Epidemiology, 26*, 163–175.

Adlerberth, I., & Wold, A. E. (2009). Establishment of the gut microbiota in Western infants. *Acta Paediatrica, 98*, 229–238.

Agostoni, C., Marangoni, F., Giovannini, M., Galli, C., & Riva, E. (2001). Prolonged breastfeeding (six months or more) and milk fat content at six months are associated with higher developmental scores at one year of age within a breastfed population. *Advances in Experimental Medicine and Biology, 501*, 137–141.

Agostoni, C., Marangoni, F., Grandi, F., Lammardo, A. M., Giovannini, M., Riva, E., & Galli, C. (2003). Earlier smoking habits are associated with higher serum lipids and lower milk fat and polyunsaturated fatty acid content in the first 6 months of lactation. *European Journal of Clinical Nutrition, 57*, 1466–1472.

Agostoni, C., Trojan, S., Bellu, R., Riva, E., & Giovannini, M. (1995). Neurodevelopmental quotient of healthy term infants at 4 months and feeding practice: The role of long-chain polyunsaturated fatty acids. *Pediatric Research, 38*, 262–265.

Akcaboy, M., Malbora, B., Zorlu P., Altinel, E., Oquz, M. M., & Sevel, S. (2015). Vitamin B_{12} deficiency in infants. *Indian Journal of Pediatrics, 82*(7), 619–624. doi:10.1007/s12098-015-1725-3

Almroth, S., & Bidinger, P. D. (1990). No need for water supplementation for exclusively breast-fed infants under hot and arid conditions. *Transactions of the Royal Society of Tropical Medicine and Hygiene,84*, 602–604.

American Academy of Pediatrics, Committee on Environmental Health. (1999). Ultraviolet light: A hazard to children. *Pediatrics, 104*, 328–333.

American Academy of Pediatrics, Committee on Nutrition. (2000). Hypoallergenic formulas. *Pediatrics, 106*, 346–349.

American Academy of Pediatrics, Work Group on Cow's Milk Protein and Diabetes Mellitus. (1994). Infant feeding practices and their possible relationship to the etiology of diabetes mellitus. *Pediatrics, 94*, 752–754.

Amin, S. B., Merle, K. S., Orlando, M. S., Dalzell, L. E., & Guillet, R. (2000). Brainstem maturation in premature infants as a function of enteral feeding type. *Pediatrics, 106*, 318–322.

Andersen, A. N., Lund-Andersen, C., Larsen, J. F., Christensen, N. J., Legros, J. J., Louis, F., . . . Molin, J. (1982). Suppressed prolactin but normal neurophysin levels in cigarette smoking breastfeeding women. *Clinical Endocrinology, 17,* 363–368.

Anderson, J. W., Johnstone, B. M., & Remley, D. T. (1999). Breastfeeding and cognitive development: A meta-analysis. *American Journal of Clinical Nutrition, 70,* 525–535.

Andres, A., Cleves, M. A., Bellando, J. B., Pivik, R. T., Casey, P. H., & Badger, T. M. (2012). Developmental status of 1-year-old infants fed breast milk, cow's milk formula, or soy formula. *Pediatrics, 129,* 1134–1140.

Arnold, L. D. W. (1995). Storage containers for human milk: An issue revisited. *Journal of Human Lactation, 11,* 325–328.

Arslanoglu, S., Moro, G. E., & Ziegler, E. E. (2006). Adjustable fortification of human milk fed to preterm infants: Does it make a difference? *Journal of Perinatology, 26,* 614–621.

Arslanoglu, S., Moro, G. E., Ziegler, E. E., & The WAPM Working Group on Nutrition. (2010). Optimization of human milk fortification for preterm infants: New concepts and recommendations. *Journal of Perinatal Medicine, 38,* 233–238.

Asakuma, S., Akahori, M., Kimura, K., Watanabe, Y., Nakamura, T., Tsunemi, M., . . . Urashima, T. (2007). Sialyl oligosaccharides of human colostrum: Changes in concentration during the first three days of lactation. *Bioscience, Biotechnology, and Biochemistry, 7,* 1447–1451.

Ashraf, R. N., Jalil, F., Aperia, A., & Lindblad, B. F. (1993). Additional water is not needed for healthy breastfed babies in a hot climate. *Acta Paediatrica Scandinavica, 82,* 1007–1011.

Bachour, P., Yafawi, R., Jaber, F., Choueiri, E., & Abdel-Razzak, Z. (2012). Effects of smoking, mother's age, body mass index, and parity number on lipid, protein and secretory immunoglobulin A concentrations of human milk. *Breastfeeding Medicine, 7(3),* 179–188.

Backhed, F., Ding, H., Wang, T., Hooper, L. V., Koh, G. Y., Nagy, A., . . . Gordon, J. I. (2004). The gut microbiota as an environmental factor that regulates fat storage. *Proceedings of the National Academy of Sciences of Sciences of the United States of America, 101,* 15718–15723.

Baheiraei, A., Shamsi, A., Khaghani, S., Shams, S., Chamari, M., Boushehri, H., & Khedri, A. (2014). The effects of maternal passive smoking on maternal milk lipid. *Acta Medica Iranica, 52,* 280–285.

Baker, R. D. (2002). Infant formula safety. *Pediatrics, 110,* 833–835.

Ball, T. M., & Wright, A. L. (1999). Health care costs of formula-feeding in the first year of life. *Pediatrics, 103,* 870–876.

Ballard, O., & Morrow, A. L. (2013). Human milk composition: Nutrients and bioactive factors. *Pediatric Clinics of North America, 60,* 49–74.

Barbas, K. H. (2013). Mother's milk technicians: A new standard of care. *Journal of Human Lactation, 29,* 323–327.

Baro, C., Giribaldi, M., Arslanoglu, S., Giuffrida, M. G., Dellavalle, G., Conti, A., . . . Bertino, E. (2011). Effect of two pasteurization methods on the protein content of human milk. *Frontiers in Bioscience (Elite Ed), 3,* 818–829.

Barrat, E., Michel, C., Poupeau, G., David-Sochard, A., Rival, M., Pagniez, A., . . . Darmaun, D. (2008). Supplementation with galactooligosaccharides and insulin increases bacterial translocation in artificially reared newborn rats. *Pediatric Research, 64,* 34–39.

Bartick, M., & Reinhold, A. (2010). The burden of suboptimal breastfeeding in the United States: A pediatric cost analysis. *Pediatrics, 125,* e1048–e1056.

Basile, L. A., Taylor, S. N., Wagner, C. L., Horst, R. L., & Hollis, B. W. (2006). The effect of high-dose vitamin D supplementation on serum vitamin D levels and milk calcium concentration in lactating women and their infants. *Breastfeeding Medicine, 1,* 27–35.

Bauer, G., Ewald, S., Hoffman, J., & Dubanoski, R. (1991). Breastfeeding and cognitive development of three-year-old children. *Psychological Reports, 68,* 1218.

Baydas, G., Karatas, F., Gursu, M. F., Bozkurt, H. A., Ilhan, N., Yasar, A., & Canatan, H. (2002). Antioxidant vitamin levels in term and preterm infants and their relation to maternal vitamin status. *Archives of Medical Research, 33,* 276–280.

Belderbos, M. E., Houben, M. L., van Bleek, G. M., Schuijff, L., van Uden, N. O. P., Bloemen-Carlier, E. M., . . . Bont, L. J. (2012). Breastfeeding modulates neonatal innate immune responses: A prospective birth cohort study. *Pediatric Allergy and Immunology, 23,* 65–74.

Bertino, E., Coppa, G. V., Giuliani, F., Coscia, A., Gabrielli, O., Sabatino, G, . . . Fabris, C. (2008). Effects of Holder pasteurization on human milk oligosaccharides. *International Journal of Immunopathology and Pharmacology, 21,* 381–385.

Bertino, E., Giribaldi, M., Baro, C., Giancotti, V., Pazzi, M., Peila, C., . . . Gastaldi, D. (2013). Effect of prolonged refrigeration on the lipid profile, lipase activity, and oxidative status of human milk. *Journal of Pediatric Gastroenterology and Nutrition, 56,* 390–396.

Bettler, J., Zimmer, J. P., Neuringer, M., & DeRusso, P. A. (2010). Serum lutein concentrations in healthy term infants fed human milk or infant formula with lutein. *European Journal of Nutrition, 49,* 45–51.

Bhatia, J., & Greer, F. (2008). Committee on Nutrition. Use of soy protein–based formulas in infant feeding. *Pediatrics, 212,* 1062–1068.

Birch, E. E., Birch, D. G., Hoffman, D. R., Hale, L., Everett, M., & Uauy, R. (1993). Breastfeeding and optimal visual development. *Journal of Pediatric Ophthalmology and Strabismus, 30,* 33–38.

Blouin, M., Coulombe, M., & Rhainds, M. (2014). Specimen plastic containers used to store expressed breast milk in neonatal care units: A case of precautionary principle. *Canadian Journal of Public Health, 105,* e218–e220.

Blyth, R., Creedy, D. K., Dennis, C. L., Moyle, W., Pratt, J., & DeVries, S. (2002). Effect of maternal confidence on breastfeeding duration: An application of breastfeeding self-efficacy theory. *Birth, 29,* 278–284.

Bokor, S., Koletzko, B., & Decsi, T. (2007). Systematic review of fatty acid composition of human milk from mothers of preterm compared to full-term infants. *Annals of Nutrition and Metabolism, 51,* 550–556.

Boniglia, C., Carratu, B., Chiarotti, F., Giammarioli, S., & Manzini, E. (2003). Influence of maternal protein intake on nitrogen fractions of human milk. *International Journal for Vitamin and Nutrition Research, 73,* 447–452.

Bouwstra, H., Boersma, E. R., Boehm, G., Dijck-Brouwer, D. A. J., Muskiet, F. A. J., & Hadders-Algra, M. (2003). Exclusive breastfeeding of healthy term infants for at least 6 weeks improves neurological condition. *Journal of Nutrition, 133,* 4243–4245.

Braga, L. P. M., & Palhares, D. B. (2007). Effect of evaporation and pasteurization in the biochemical and immunological composition of human milk. *Jornal de Pediatria (Rio J), 83,* 59–63.

Brandtzaeg, P. (2003). Mucosal immunity: Integration between mother and the breastfed infant. *Vaccine, 21,* 3382–3388.

Brenna, J. T., Varamini, B., Jensen, R. G., Diersen-Schade, D. A., Boettcher, J. A., & Arterburn, L. M. (2007). Docosahexaenoic and arachidonic acid concentrations in human breast milk worldwide. *American Journal of Clinical Nutrition, 85,* 1457–1464.

Brill, H. (2008). Approach to milk protein allergy in infants. *Canadian Family Physician, 54,* 1258–1264.

Brown, E. W., & Bosworth, A. W. (1922). Studies of infant feeding SVI. A bacteriological study of the feces and the food of normal babies receiving breastmilk. *American Journal of Diseases of Children, 23,* 243.

Brown, N. C., Doyle, L. W., Bear, M. J., & Inder, T. E. (2006). Alterations in neurobehavior at term reflect differing exposures in very preterm infants. *Pediatrics, 118,* 2461–2471.

Bullen, C. L., Tearle, P. V., & Stewart, M. G. (1977). The effect of humanized milks and supplemented breast feeding on the faecal flora of infants. *Journal of Medical Microbiology, 10,* 403–413.

Bunesova, V., Vlkova, E., Rada, V., Knazovicka, V., Rockova, S., Geigerova, M., & Bozik, M. (2012). Growth of infant fecal bacteria on commercial prebiotics. *Folia Microbiologica, 57,* 273–275.

Buss, I. H., McGill, F., Darlow, B. A., & Winterbourn, C. C. (2001). Vitamin C is reduced in human milk after storage. *Acta Paediatrica, 90,* 813–815.

Butte, N. F., Goldblum, R. M., Fehl, L. M., Loftin, K., Smith, E. O., Garza, C., & Goldman, A. S. (1984). Daily ingestion of immunologic components in human milk during the first four months of life. *Acta Paediatrica Scandinavica, 73,* 296–301.

Cabrera-Rubio, R., Collado, M. C., Laitinen, K., Salminen, S., Isolauri, E., & Mira, A. (2012). The human milk microbiome changes over lactation and is shaped by maternal weight and mode of delivery. *American Journal of Clinical Nutrition, 88,* 894–899.

Cantani, A., & Micera, M. (2005). Neonatal cow milk sensitization in 143 case-reports: Role of early exposure to cow's milk formula. *European Review for Medical and Pharmacological Sciences, 9,* 227–230.

Cao, X. L., Dufresne, G., Belisle, S., Clement, G., Falicki, M., Beraldin, F., & Rulibikiye, A. (2008). Levels of bisphenol A in canned liquid infant formula products in Canada and dietary intake estimates. *Journal of Agricultural and Food Chemistry, 56,* 7919–7924.

Cardwell, C. R., Stene, L. C., Joner, G., Cinek, O., Svensson, J., Goldacre, M. J., . . . Patterson, C. C. (2008). Caesarean section is associated with an increased risk of childhood-onset type 1 diabetes mellitus: A meta-analysis of observational studies. *Diabetologia, 51,* 726–735.

Carlson, S. E., Cooke, R. J., Werkman, S. H., & Tolley, E. A. (1992). First year growth of preterm infants fed standard compared to marine oil n-3 supplemented formula. *Lipids, 27,* 901–907.

Carlson, S. E., Werkman, S. H., Peeples, J. M., Cooke, R. J., & Tolley, E. A. (1993). Arachidonic acid status correlates with first year growth in preterm infants. *Proceedings of the National Academy of Sciences of the United States of America, 90,* 1073–1077.

Castellote, C., Casillas, R., Ramirez-Santana, C., Pérez-Cano, F. J., Castell, M., Moretones, M. G., . . . Franch, A. (2011). Premature delivery influences the immunological composition of colostrum and transitional and mature human milk. *Journal of Nutrition, 141,* 1181–1187.

Catassi, C., Bonucci, A., Coppa, G. V., Carlucci, A., & Giorgi, P. L. (1995). Intestinal permeability changes during the first month: Effect of natural versus artificial feeding. *Journal of Pediatric Gastroenterology and Nutrition, 21,* 383–386.

Celiker, M. Y., & Chawla, A. (2009). Congenital B_{12} deficiency following maternal gastric bypass. *Journal of Perinatology, 29,* 640–642.

Centers for Disease Control and Prevention. (1993). Hyponatremic seizures among infants fed with commercial bottled drinking water: Wisconsin, 1993. *Morbidity and Mortality Weekly Report, 43,* 641–643.

Centers for Disease Control and Prevention. (2007). Breastfeeding-related maternity practices at hospitals and birth centers—United States, 2007. *Morbidity and Mortality Weekly Report 57(23),* 621–625.

Centers for Disease Control and Prevention. (2010). HealthStyles survey: Breastfeeding practices: 2010. Retrieved from http://www.cdc.gov/breastfeeding/data/healthstyles_survey/survey_2010.htmf2010

Centers for Disease Control and Prevention. (2014a). HealthyStyles survey: Public beliefs and attitudes about breastfeeding: 2014. Retrieved from http://www.cdc.gov/breastfeeding/data/healthstyles_survey/index.htm

Centers for Disease Control and Prevention. (2014b). mPINC results tables. Retrieved from http://www.cdc.gov/breastfeeding/data/mpinc/results-tables.htm.

Chan, G. (2003). Effects of powdered human milk fortifiers on the antimicrobial actions of human milk. *Journal of Perinatology, 23,* 620–623.

Chan, G. M., Lee, M. L., & Rechtman, D. J. (2007). Effects of a human milk–derived human milk fortifier on the antibacterial actions of human milk. *Breastfeeding Medicine, 2,* 205–208.

Chandra, R. K. (2000). Food allergy and nutrition in early life: Implications for later health. *Proceedings of the Nutrition Society, 59,* 273–277.

Chandra, R. K., & Hamed, A. (1991). Cumulative incidence of atopic disorders in high risk infants fed whey hydrolysate, soy, and conventional cow milk formulas. *Annals of Allergy, 67*, 129–132.

Chang, Y-C., Chen, C-H., & Lin, M-C. (2012). The macronutrients in human milk change after storage in various containers. *Pediatrics and Neonatology, 53*, 205–209.

Chantry, C., Nommsen-Rivers, L., Peerson, J., Cohen, R., & Dewey, K. (2011). Excess weight loss in first-born breastfed newborns relates to maternal intrapartum fluid balance. *Pediatrics, 127*, e171–e179.

Chao, J. C. J., Tseng, H. P., Chang, C. W., Chien, Y. Y., Au, H. K., Chen, J. R., & Chen, C. F. (2004). Chicken extract affects colostrum protein composition in lactating women. *Journal of Nutritional Biochemistry, 15*, 37–44.

Cheatham, C. L., Nerhammer, A. S., Asserhøj, M., Michaelsen, K. F., & Lauritzen, L. (2011). Fish oil supplementation during lactation: Effects on cognition and behavior at 7 years of age. *Lipids, 46*, 637–645.

Chen, H.-Y., & Allen, J. C. (2001). Human milk antibacterial factors: The effect of temperature on defense systems. *Advances in Experimental Medicine and Biology, 501*, 341–348.

Chirico, G., Marzollo, R., Cortinovis, S., Fonte, C., & Gasparoni, A. (2008). Antiinfective properties of human milk. *Journal of Nutrition, 138*, 1801S–1806S.

Chuchu, N., Patel, B., Sebastian, B., & Exley, C. (2013). The aluminum content of infant formulas remains too high. *BMC Pediatrics, 13*, 162.

Clandinin, M. T., van Aerde, J. E., Parrot, A., Field, C. J., Euler, A. R., & Lien, E. L. (1997). Assessment of the efficacious dose of arachidonic and docosahexaenoic acids in preterm infant formulas: Fatty acid composition of erythrocyte membrane lipids. *Pediatric Research, 42*, 819–825.

Clarke, S. D., & Jump, D. B. (1996). Polyunsaturated fatty acid regulation of hepatic gene transcription. *Journal of Nutrition, 126*(Suppl), 1105–1109.

Claud, E. C., & Walker, W. A. (2001). Hypothesis: Inappropriate colonization of the premature intestine can cause neonatal necrotizing enterocolitis. *FASEB Journal, 15*, 1398–1403.

Clemens, T. L., Adams, J. S., Henderson, S. L., & Holick, M. F. (1982). Increased skin pigment reduces capacity of skin to synthesize vitamin D_3. *Lancet, 1*, 74–76.

Clements, M. R., Johnson L., & Fraser, D. R. (1987). A new mechanism for induced vitamin D deficiency in calcium deprivation. *Nature, 325*, 62–65.

Cohen, R. J., Brown, K. H., Rivera, L. L., & Dewey, K. G. (2000). Exclusively breastfed, low birthweight infants do not need supplemental water. *Acta Paediatrica, 89*, 550–552.

Cohen Engler, A., Hadash, A., Shehadeh, N., & Pillar, G. (2011). Breastfeeding may improve nocturnal sleep and reduce infantile colic: Potential role of breastmilk melatonin. *European Journal of Pediatrics, 171*(4), 729–732.

Collado, M. C., Delgado, S., Maldonado, A., & Rodriguez, J. M. (2009). Assessment of the bacterial diversity of breast milk of healthy women by quantitative real-time PCR. *Letters in Applied Microbiology, 48*, 523–528.

Collado, M. C., Isolauri, E., Laitinen, K., & Salminen, S. (2010). Effect of mother's weight on infant's microbiota acquisition, composition, and activity during early infancy: A prospective follow-up study initiated in early pregnancy. *American Journal of Clinical Nutrition, 92*, 1023–1030.

Cunnane, S. C., Francescutti, V., Brenna, J. T., & Crawford, M. A. (2000). Breastfed infants achieve a higher rate of brain and whole body docosahexaenoate accumulation than formula-fed infants not consuming dietary docosahexaenoate. *Lipids, 35*, 105–111.

Czank, C., Simmer, K., & Hartmann, P. E. (2010). Design and characterization of a human milk product for the preterm infant. *Breastfeeding Medicine, 5*, 59–66.

Dabard, J., Bridonneau, C., Phillipe, C., Anglade, P., Molle, D., Nardi, M., . . . Fons, M. (2001). A new antibiotic produced by a *Ruminococcus gnavus* strain isolated from human feces. *Applied and Environmental Microbiology, 67*, 4111–4118.

Dabeka, R., Fouquet, A., Belisle, S., & Turcotte, S. (2011). Lead, cadmium and aluminum in Canadian infant formulae, oral electrolytes and glucose solutions. Food Additives and Contaminants. *Part A, Chemistry, Analysis, Control, Exposure and Risk Assessment, 28,* 744–753.

Dai, D., & Walker, W. A. (1999). Protective nutrients and bacterial colonization in the immature human gut. *Advances in Pediatrics, 46,* 353–382.

D'Alessandro, A., Scaloni, A., & Zolla, L. (2013). Human milk proteins: Strides in proteomics and benefits in nutrition research. In A. Zibadi, R. R. Watson, & V. R. Preedy (Eds.), *Handbook of dietary and nutritional aspects of human breast milk* (pp. 249–291). Wageningen, Netherlands: Wageningen Academic Publishers.

Daly, S. E. J., Di Rosso, A., Owens, R. A., & Hartmann, P. E. (1993). Degree of breast emptying explains changes in the fat content, but not fatty acid composition, of human milk. *Experimental Physiology, 78,* 741–755.

DeCarvalho, M., Klaus, M. H., & Merkatz, R. B. (1982). Frequency of breastfeeding and serum bilirubin concentration. *American Journal of Diseases of Children, 136,* 737–738.

Decker, E., Engelmann, G., Findeisen, A., Gerner, P., Laass, M., Ney, D., . . . Hornef, M. W. (2010). Cesarean delivery is associated with celiac disease but not inflammatory bowel disease in children. *Pediatrics, 125,* 1433–1440.

Decker, E., Hornef, M., & Stockinger, S. (2011). Cesarean delivery is associated with celiac disease but not inflammatory bowel disease in children. *Gut Microbes, 2,* 91–98.

Decsi, T., & Koletzko, B. (1995). Growth, fatty acid composition of plasma lipid classes, and plasma retinol and alpha-tocopherol concentrations in full-term infants fed formula enriched with n-6 and n-3 long-chain polyunsaturated fatty acids. *Acta Paediatrica Scandinavica, 84,* 725–732.

Delgado-Noguera, M. F., Calvache, J. A., Bonfill Cosp, X., Kotanidou, E. P., & Galli-Tsinopoulou, A. (2015). Supplementation with long chain polyunsaturated fatty acids (LCPUFA) to breastfeeding mothers for improving child growth and development. *Cochrane Database of Systematic Reviews.* Issue 7. Art. No.:CD007901. doi:10.1002/14651858.CD007901.pub3

Dewey, K. (2003). Is breastfeeding protective against childhood obesity? *Journal of Human Lactation, 19,* 9–18.

Dewey, K. G., Domellof, M., Cohen, R. J., Landa Rivera, L., Hernell, O., & Lonnerdal, B. (2002). Iron supplementation affects growth and morbidity of breast-fed infants: Results of a randomized trial in Sweden and Honduras. Journal of *Nutrition, 132,* 3249–55.

Dewey, K. G., Finley, D. A., & Lonnerdal, B. (1984). Breastmilk volume and composition during late lactation (7–20 months). *Journal of Pediatric Gastroenterology and Nutrition, 3,* 713–720.

Diehl-Jones, W., Arcgibald, A., Gordon, J. W., Mughal, W., Hossain, Z., & Friel, J. K. (2015). Human milk fortification increases Bnip3 expression associated with intestinal cell death in vitro. *Journal of Pediatric Gastroenterology and Nutrition, 61,* 583–590.

Dogaru, C. M., Strippoli, M-P. F., Spycher, B. D., Frey, U., Beardsmore, C. S., Silverman, M., & Kuehni, C. E. (2012). Breastfeeding and lung function at school-age: Does maternal asthma modify the effect? *American Journal of Respiratory and Critical Care Medicine, 185*(8), 874–880.

Duncan, B., Schifman, R. B., Corrigan, J. J., & Schaefer C. (1985). Iron and the exclusively breastfed infant from birth to six months. *Journal of Pediatric Gastroenterology and Nutrition, 4,* 421.

Dusdieker, L. B., Booth, B. M., Stumbo, P. J., & Eichenberger, J. M. (1985). Effect of supplemental fluids on human milk production. *Journal of Pediatrics, 106,* 207.

Edwards, C. A., & Parrett, A. M. (2002). Intestinal flora during the first months of life: New perspectives. *British Journal of Nutrition, 88*(Suppl 1), S11–S18.

Ehlinger, E. P., Webster, E. M., Kang, H. H., Cangialose, A., Simmons, A. C., Barbas, K. H., . . . Permar, S. R. (2011). Maternal cytomegalovirus-specific immune responses and symptomatic postnatal cytomegalovirus transmission in very low birth weight preterm infants. *Journal of Infectious Diseases, 204,* 1672–1682.

Environmental Working Group. (2007). EWG's guide to infant formula and baby bottles. Retrieved from http://www.ewg.org/book/export/html/25570

Evans, K. C., Evans, R. G., Royal, R., Esterman, A. J., & James, S. L. (2003). Effect of cesarean section on breastmilk transfer to the normal term newborn over the first week of life. *Archives of Disease in Childhood—Fetal and Neonatal Edition, 88,* F380–F382.

Ezaki, S., Ito, T., Suzuki, K., & Tamura, M. (2008). Association between total antioxidant capacity in breastmilk and postnatal age in days in premature infants. *Journal of Clinical Biochemistry and Nutrition, 42,* 133–137.

Fantuzzi, G. (2005). Adipose tissue, adipokines, and inflammation. *Journal of Allergy and Clinical Immunology, 115,* 911–919.

Farquharson, J., Cockburn, F., Patrick, W. A., Jamieson, E. C., & Logan, R. W. (1992). Infant cerebral cortex phospholipid fatty-acid composition and diet. *Lancet, 340,* 810.

Favier, C. F., Vaughan, E. E., De Vos, W. M., & Akkermans, A. D. L. (2002). Molecular monitoring of succession of bacterial communities in human neonates. *Applied and Environmental Microbiology, 68,* 219–226.

Fenton, T. R., & Belik, J. (2002). Routine handling of milk fed to preterm infants can significantly increase osmolality. *Journal of Pediatric Gastroenterology and Nutrition, 35,* 298–302.

Ferguson, M., & Molfese, P. J. (2007). Breastfed infants process speech differently from bottle-fed infants: Evidence from neuroelectrophysiology. *Developmental Neuropsychology, 31,* 337–347.

Field, C. J. (2005). The immunological components of human milk and their effect on immune development in infants. *Journal of Nutrition, 135,* 1–4.

Flaherman, V. J., Schaefer, E. W., Kuzniewicz, M. W., Li, S. X., Walsh, E. M., & Paul, I. M. (2015). Early weight loss nomograms for exclusively breastfed newborns. *Pediatrics, 135,* e16–e23.

Florey, C., du, V., Leech, A. M., & Blackhall, A. (1995). Infant feeding and mental and motor development at 18 months of age in first born singletons. *International Journal of Epidemiology, 24*(Suppl 1), S21–S26.

Follett, J., Ishii, K. D., & Heinig, M. J. (2003). The role of long-chain fatty acids in infant health: Helping families make informed decisions about DHA. In *Independent Study Workbook 50301.* Davis, CA: UC Davis Human Lactation Center. Retrieved from http://lactation.ucdavis.edu

Francis, J., Rogers, K., Brewer, P., Dickton, D., & Pardini, R. (2008). Comparative analysis of ascorbic acid in human milk and infant formula using varied milk delivery systems. *International Breastfeeding Journal, 3,* 19. Retrieved from http://www.internationalbreastfeedingjournal.com/content/3/1/19

Friel, J. K., Diehl-Jones, W. L., Suh, M., Tsopmo, A., & Shirwadkar, V. P. (2007). Impact of iron and vitamin C–containing supplements on preterm human milk: In vitro. *Free Radical Biology and Medicine, 42,* 1591–1598.

Furukawa, M., Lee, E. L., & Johnston, J. M. (1993). Platelet-activating factor–induced ischemic bowel necrosis: The effect of platelet-activating factor acetylhydrolase. *Pediatric Research, 34,* 237–241.

Gabrielli, O., Zampini, L., Galeazzi, T., Padella, L., Santoro, L., Peila, C., . . . Coppa, G. V. (2011). Preterm milk oligosaccharides during the first month of lactation. *Pediatrics, 128,* e1520–e1531.

Ganapathy, V., Hay, J. W., & Kim, J. H. (2012). Costs of necrotizing enterocolitis and cost-effectiveness of exclusively human milk–based products in feeding extremely premature infants. *Breastfeeding Medicine, 7,* 29–37.

Genot, C., & Michalski, M. C. (2010). [Metabolic impact of lipid structure and oxidation in foods]. *Innovations Agronomiques, 10,* 43–67.

Georgeson, G. D., Szony, B. J., Streitman, K., Varga, I. S., Kovacs, A., Kovacs, L, & Laszlo, A. (2002). Antioxidant enzyme activities are decreased in preterm infants and in neonates born via cesarean section. *European Journal of Obstetrics and Gynecology and Reproductive Biology, 103,* 136–139.

Gerstley, J. R., Howell, K. M., & Nagel, B. R. (1932). Some factors influencing the fecal flora of infants. *American Journal of Diseases of Children, 43,* 555.

Gibson, L. (2007). Toxic baby bottles. Environment California Research & Policy Center. Retrieved from http://www.environmentcalifornia.org/reports/environmental-health/environmental-health-reports/toxic-baby-bottles

Gibson, R. A., Neumann, M. A., & Makrides, M. (1997). Effect of increasing breastmilk docosahexaenoic acid on plasma and erythrocyte phospholipid fatty acids and neural indices of exclusively breastfed infants. *European Journal of Clinical Nutrition, 51,* 578–584.

Giugliani, E. R. J., Santo, L. C. D. E., de Oliveira, L. D., & Aerts, D. (2008). Intake of water, herbal teas and non-breast milks during the first month of life: Associated factors and impact on breastfeeding duration. *Early Human Development, 84,* 305–310.

Glaser, C. Heinrich, J., & Koletzko, B. (2010). Role of FADS1 and FADS2 polymorphisms in polyunsaturated fatty acid metabolism. *Metabolism, 59,* 993–999.

Glover J, & Sandilands M. (1990). Supplementation of breastfeeding infants and weight loss in hospital. *Journal of Human Lactation, 6,* 163–166.

Grapov, D., Lemay, D. G., Weber, D., Phinney, B. S., Azulay Chertok, I. R., Gho, D. S., . . . Smilowitz, J. T. (2015). The human colostrum whey proteome is altered in gestational diabetes mellitus. *Journal of Proteome Research, 14,* 512–520.

Greene, L. C., Lucas, A., Livingstone, M. B., Harland, P. S., & Baker, B. A. (1995). Relationship between early diet and subsequent cognitive performance during adolescence. *Biochemical Society Transactions, 23,* 376S.

Greer, F. R., & Marshall, S. (1989). Bone mineral content, serum vitamin D metabolite concentrations and ultraviolet B light exposure in infants fed human milk with and without vitamin D_2 supplements. *Journal of Pediatrics, 114,* 204–212.

Greer, F. R., Searcy, J. E., Levin, R. S., Steichen, J. J., Asch, P. S., & Tsang, R. C. (1982). Bone mineral content and serum 25-hydroxyvitamin D concentrations in breastfed infants with and without supplemental vitamin D: One year follow-up. *Journal of Pediatrics, 100,* 919–922.

Greer, F. R., Sicherer, S. H., & Burks, A. W. (2008). Committee on Nutrition and Section on Allergy and Immunology. Effects of early nutritional interventions on the development of atopic disease in infants and children: The role of maternal dietary restriction, breastfeeding, timing of introduction of complementary foods, and hydrolyzed formulas. *Pediatrics, 121,* 183–191.

Gronlund, M. M., Arvilommi, H., Kero, P., Lehtonen, O. P., & Isolauri, E. (2000). Importance of intestinal colonization in the maturation of humoral immunity in early infancy: A prospective follow up study of healthy infants 0–6 months. *Archives of Disease in Childhood Fetal and Neonatal Edition, 83,* F186–F192.

Gronlund, M. M., Gueimonde, M., Laittinen, K., Kociubinski, G., Gronroos, T., Salminen, S., & Isolauri, E. (2007). Maternal breastmilk and intestinal bifidobacteria guide the compositional development of the *Bifidobacterium* microbiota in infants at risk of allergic disease. *Clinical and Experimental Allergy, 3Z,* 1764–1772.

Gronlund, M. M., Lehtonen, O. P., Eerola, E., & Kero, P. (1999). Fecal microflora in healthy infants born by different methods of delivery: Permanent changes in intestinal flora after cesarean delivery. *Journal of Pediatric Gastroenterology and Nutrition, 28,* 19–25.

Grosse, S. D., Matte, T. D., Schwartz, J., & Jackson, R. J. (2002). Economic gains resulting from the reduction in children's exposure to lead in the United States. *Environmental Health Perspectives, 110,* 563–569.

Grummer-Strawn, L. M., Scanlon, K. S., & Fein, S. B. (2008). Infant feeding and feeding transitions during the first year of life. *Pediatrics, 122,* S36–S42.

Gustafsson, L., Hallgren, O., Mossberg, A.-K., Pettersson, J., Fischer, W., Aronsson, A., & Svanborg, C. (2005). HAMLET kills tumor cells by apoptosis: Structure, cellular mechanisms, and therapy. *Journal of Nutrition, 135,* 1299–1303.

Gustafsson, P. A., Duchen, K., Birberg, U., & Karlsson, T. (2004). Breastfeeding, very long polyunsaturated fatty acids (PUFA) and IQ at 6H years of age. *Acta Paediatrica, 93,* 1280–1287.

Guxens, M., Mendez, M. A., Moltó-Puigmartí, C., Julvez, J., Garcia-Esteban, R., Forns, J., . . . Sunyer, J. (2011). Breastfeeding, long-chain polyunsaturated fatty acids in colostrum, and infant mental development. *Pediatrics, 128*, e880–e889.

Haggerty, L. L. (2011). Maternal supplementation for prevention and treatment of vitamin D deficiency in exclusively breastfed infants. *Breastfeeding Medicine, 6*, 137–144.

Hahn-Zoric, M., Fulconis, F., Minoli, I., Moro, G., Carlsson, B., Bottiger, M., . . . Hanson, L. A. (1990). Antibody responses to parenteral and oral vaccines are impaired by conventional and low protein formulas as compared to breastfeeding. *Acta Paediatrica Scandinavica, 79*, 1137–1142.

Hair, A. B., Hawthorne, K. M., Chetta, K. E., & Abrams, S. A. (2013). Human milk feeding supports adequate growth in infants ≤ 1250 grams birth weight. *BMC Research Notes, 6*, 459.

Hákansson, A., Zhivotovsky, B., Orrenius, S., Sabharwal, H., & Svanborg, C. (1995). Apoptosis induced by a human milk protein. *Proceedings of the National Academy of Sciences of the United States of America, 92*, 8064–8068.

Hamosh, M. (2001). Bioactive factors in human milk. *Pediatric Clinics of North America, 48*(1), 69–86.

Hamosh, M., Ellis, L. A., Pollock, D. R., Henderson, T. R., & Hamosh, P. (1996). Breastfeeding and the working mother: Effect of time and temperature of short-term storage on proteolysis, lipolysis, and bacterial growth in milk. *Pediatrics, 97*(4), 492–498.

Hamprecht, K., Maschmann, J., Jahn, G., Poets, C. F., & Goelz, R. (2008). Cytomegalovirus transmission to preterm infants during lactation. *Journal of Clinical Virology, 41*, 198–205.

Handa, D., Ahrabi, A. F., Codipilly, C. N., Shah, S., Ruff, S., Potak, D., . . . Schanler, R. J. (2014). Do thawing and warming affect the integrity of human milk? *Journal of Perinatology, 34*, 863–866.

Hanna, N., Ahmed, K., Anwar, M., Petrova, A., Hiatt, M., & Hegyi, T. (2004). Effect of storage on breastmilk antioxidant activity. *Archives of Disease in Childhood—Fetal and Neonatal Edition, 89*, F518–F520.

Hanson, L. A. (2004). *Immunobiology of human milk: How breastfeeding protects babies.* Amarillo, TX: Pharmasoft Publishing.

Hanson, L. A., Korotkova, M., Haversen, L., Mattsby-Baltzer, I., Hahn-Zoric, M., Silfverdal, S. A., . . . Telemo, E. (2002). Breastfeeding, a complex support system for the offspring. *Pediatrics International, 44*, 347–352.

Hart, S., Boylan, L. M., Carroll, S., Musick, Y. A., & Lampe, R. M. (2003). Brief report: Breast-fed one-week-olds demonstrate superior neurobehavioral organization. *Journal of Pediatric Psychology, 28*, 529–534.

Hassiotou, F., & Hartmann, P. E. (2014). At the dawn of a new discovery: The potential of breast milk stem cells. *Advances in Nutrition, 5*, 770–778.

Hassiotou, F., Hepworth, A. R., Williams, T. M., Twigger, A-J., Perrella, S., Lai, C. T., . . . Hartmann, P. E. (2013). Breastmilk cell and fat contents respond similarly to removal of breastmilk by the infant. *PLoS One, 8*, e78232.

Heaney, R. P., Davies, K. M., Chen, T. C., Holick, M. F., & Barger-Lux, M. J. (2003). Human serum 25-hydroxycholecalciferol response to extended oral dosing with cholecalciferol. *American Journal of Clinical Nutrition, 77*, 204–210.

Heikella, M. P., & Saris, P. E. J. (2003). Inhibition of *Staphylococcus aureus* by the commensal bacteria of human milk. *Journal of Applied Microbiology, 158*, 471–478.

Heikkila, K., Kelly, Y., Renfrew, M. J., Sacker, A., & Quigley, M. A. (2014). Breastfeeding and educational achievement at age 5. *Maternal and Child Nutrition, 10*, 92–101.

Heinig, M. J. (2003). Vitamin D and the breastfed infant: Controversies and concerns. *Journal of Human Lactation, 19*, 247–249.

Heird, W. C. (1999). Biological effects and safety issues related to long-chain polyunsaturated fatty acids in infants. *Lipids, 34*, 103–224.

Henderson, A. (2005). Vitamin D and the breastfed infant. *Journal of Obstetric, Gynecologic, and Neonatal Nursing, 34*, 367–372.

Herba, C. M., Roza, S., Govaert, P., Hofman, A., Jaddoe, V., Verhulst, F. C., & Tiemeier, H. (2013). Breastfeeding and early brain development: The Generation R study. *Maternal and Child Nutrition, 9*, 332–349.

Heyman, M. B. (2006). Lactose intolerance in infants, children, and adolescents. *Pediatrics, 118*, 1279–1286.

Hicks, P. D., Zavaleta, N., Chen, Z., Abrams, S. A., & Lonnerdal, B. (2006). Iron deficiency, but not anemia, upregulates iron absorption in breast-fed Peruvian infants. *Journal of Nutrition, 136*, 2435–2438.

Himelright, I., Harris, E., Lorch, V., Anderson, M., Jones, T., Craig, A., . . . Jernigan, D. (2002). *Enterobacter sakazakii* infections associated with the use of powdered infant formula—Tennessee, 2001. *Morbidity and Mortality Weekly Report, 51*, 297–300.

Hirsch, D. S. (2007). Vitamin D and the breastfed infant. In T. W. Hale & P. E. Hartmann (Eds.), *Textbook of human lactation* (pp. 425–461). Amarillo, TX: Hale Publishing.

Hollis, B. W., & Wagner, C. L. (2004). Assessment of dietary vitamin D requirements during pregnancy and lactation. *American Journal of Clinical Nutrition, 79*, 717–726.

Hollis, B. W., Wagner, C. L., Howard, C. R., Ebeling, M., Shary, J. R., Smith, P. G., . . . Hulsey, T. C. (2015). Maternal versus infant vitamin D supplementation during lactation: A randomized controlled trial. *Pediatrics, 136*, 625–634.

Holmberg, H., Wahlberg, J., Vaarala, O., Ludvigsson, J., & ABIS Study Group. (2007). Short duration of breast-feeding as a risk-factor for beta-cell autoantibodies in 5-year-old children from the general population. *British Journal of Nutrition, 97*, 111–116.

Hopkins, M. J., Macfarlane, G. T., Furrie, E., Fite, A., & Macfarlane, S. (2005). Characterisation of intestinal bacteria in infant stools using real-time PCR and northern hybridization analyses. *FEMS Microbiology Ecology, 54*, 77–85.

Hopkinson, J. M., Schanler, R. J., Fraley, J. K., & Garza, C. (1992). Milk production by mothers of premature infants: Influence of cigarette smoking. *Pediatrics, 90*, 934–938.

Horwood, L. J., & Fergusson, D. M. (1998). Breastfeeding and later cognitive and academic outcomes. *Pediatrics, 101*(1), e9. Retrieved from http://www.pediatrics.org/cgi/content/full/101/1/e9

Host, A. (1991). Importance of the first meal on the development of cow's milk allergy and intolerance. *Allergy Proceedings, 10*, 227–232.

Host, A., & Halken, S. (2005). Primary prevention of food allergy in infants who are at risk. *Current Opinion in Allergy and Immunology, 5*, 255–259.

Host, A., Husby, S., & Osterballe, O. (1988). A prospective study of cow's milk allergy in exclusively breastfed infants. *Acta Paediatrica Scandinavica, 77*, 663–670.

Host, A., Jacobsen, H. P., Halken, S., & Holmenlund, D. (1995). The natural history of cow's milk protein allergy/intolerance. *European Journal of Clinical Nutrition, 49*(Suppl 1), S13–S18.

Huang, J., Peters, K. E., Vaughn, M. G., & Witko, C. (2014). Breastfeeding and trajectories of children's cognitive development. *Developmental Science, 17*, 452–461.

Huda, M. N., Lewis, Z., Kalanetra, K. M., Rashid, M., Ahmad, S. M., Raqib, R., . . . Stephensen, C. B. (2014). Stool microbiota and vaccine responses of infants. *Pediatrics,134*, e362–e372.

Human Milk Banking Association of North America. (2006). *Best practice for expressing, storing and handling of mother's own milk in hospital and at home*. Raleigh, NC: Author.

Human Milk Banking Association of North America. (2008). In M. R. Tully (Ed.), *Guidelines for the establishment and operation of a donor human milk bank*. Raleigh, NC: Author.

Human Milk Banking Association of North America. (2011). *Best practice for expressing, storing and handling human milk in hospitals, homes and child care settings* (3rd ed.). Raleigh, NC: Author.

Hunt, K. M., Foster, J. A., Forney, L. J., Schutte U. M. E., Beck, D. L., . . . McGuire, M. A. (2011). Characterization of the diversity and temporal stability of bacterial communities in human milk. *PLoS One, 6*, e21313.

Hylander, M. A., Strobino, D. M., Pezzullo, J. C., & Dhanireddy, R. (2001). Association of human milk feedings with a reduction in retinopathy of prematurity among very low birthweight infants. *Journal of Perinatology, 21*, 356–362.

Hypponen, E., Sovio, U., Wjst, M., Patel, S., Pekkanen, J., Hartikainen, A. L., & Jarvelinb, M. R. (2004). Infant vitamin D supplementation and allergic conditions in adulthood: Northern Finland birth cohort 1966. *Annals of the New York Academy of Sciences, 1037,* 84–95.

Illnerova, H., Buresova, M., & Presl, J. (1993). Melatonin rhythm in human milk. *Journal of Clinical Endocrinology and Metabolism, 77,* 838–841.

Innis, S. M., & Hansen, J. W. (1996). Plasma fatty acid responses, metabolic effects, and safety of microalgal and fungal oils rich in arachidonic and docosahexaenoic acids in healthy adults. *American Journal of Clinical Nutrition, 64,* 159–167.

Institute of Medicine, Food and Nutrition Board, & Standing Committee on the Evaluation of Dietary Reference Intakes. (1997). Vitamin D. In *Dietary reference intakes for calcium, phosphorus, magnesium, vitamin D and fluoride* (pp. 250–287). Washington, DC: National Academy Press.

Isaacs, C. E. (2005). Human milk inactivates pathogens individually, additively and synergistically. *Journal of Nutrition, 135,* 1286–1288.

Isaacs, C. E., Kashyap, S., Heird, W. C., & Thormar, H. (1990). Antiviral and antibacterial lipids in human milk and infant formula feeds. *Archives of Disease in Childhood, 65,* 861–864.

Jamieson, E. C., Farquharson, J., Logan, R. W., Howatson, A. G., Patrick, W. J., Weaver, L. T., & Cockburn, F. (1999). Infant cerebellar gray and white matter fatty acids in relation to age and diet. *Lipids, 34,* 1065–1071.

Jantscher-Krenn, E., & Bode, L. (2012). Human milk oligosaccharides and their potential benefits for the breastfed neonate. *Minerva Pediatrica, 64,* 83–99.

Jedrychowski, W., Perera, F., Jankowski, J., Butscher, M., Mroz, E., Flak, E., . . . Sowa, A. (2012). Effect of exclusive breastfeeding on the development of children's cognitive function in the Krakow prospective birth cohort study. *European Journal of Pediatrics, 171,* 151–158.

Jensen, R. G. (Ed.). (1995). *Handbook of milk composition.* San Diego, CA: Academic Press.

Jensen, R. G., & Jensen, G. L. (1992). Specialty lipids for infant nutrition. I. Milks and formulas. *Journal of Pediatric Gastroenterology & Nutrition,* 15, 232–245.

Jeppesen, D. L., Hasselbalch, H., Lisse, I. M., Ersboll, A. K., & Engelmann, M. D. (2004). T-lymphocyte subsets, thymic size and breastfeeding in infancy. *Pediatric Allergy and Immunology, 15,* 127–132.

Jeurink, P. V., van Bergenhenegouwen, J., Jimenez, E., Knippels, L. M. J., Fernandez, L., Garssen, J., . . . Martin, R. (2013). Human milk: A source of more life than we imagine. *Beneficial Microbes, 4,* 17–30.

Jim, W. T., Chiu, N. C., Ho, C. S., Shu, C. H., Chang, J. H., Hung, H. Y., . . . Chuu, C. P. (2015). Outcome of preterm infants with postnatal cytomegalovirus infection via breastmilk: A two-year prospective follow-up study. *Medicine (Baltimore), 94,* e1835.

Jimenez, E., Marin, M. L., Martin, R., Odriozola, J. M., Olivares, M., Xaus, J., . . . & Rodriguez, J. M. (2008). Is meconium from healthy newborns actually sterile? *Research in Microbiology, 159,* 187–193.

Jocson, M. A. L., Mason, E. O., & Schanler, R. J. (1997). The effects of nutrient fortification and varying storage conditions on host defense properties of human milk. *Pediatrics, 100,* 240–243.

Johansson, S., Lindow, S., Kapadia, H., & Norman, M. (2002). Perinatal water intoxication due to excessive oral intake during labour. *Acta Paediatrica, 91,* 811–814.

Johansson, S., Wold, A. E., & Sandberg, A-S. (2011). Low breast milk levels of long-chain n-3 fatty acids in allergic women, despite frequent fish intake. *Clinical and Experimental Allergy, 41,* 505–515.

Johnson, D. L., & Swank, P. R. (1996). Breastfeeding and children's intelligence. *Psychological Reports, 79,* 1179–1185.

Jones, F. (2011). *Best practice for expressing, storing and handling human milk* (3rd ed.). Fort Worth, TX: Human Milk Banking Association of North America.

Kafouri, S., Kramer, M., Leonard, G., Perron, M., Pike, B., Richer, L., . . . Paus, T. (2013). Breastfeeding and brain structure in adolescence. *International Journal of Epidemiology, 42,* 150–159.

Kainonen, E., Rautava, S., & Isolauri, E. (2013). Immunological programming by breast milk creates an anti-inflammatory cytokine milieu in breastfed infants compared to formula-fed infants. *British Journal of Nutrition, 109*, 1962–1970.

Kalkwarf, H. J., Specker, B. L., Heubi, J. E., Vieira, N. E., & Yergey, A. L. (1996). Intestinal calcium absorption of women during lactation and after weaning. *American Journal of Clinical Nutrition, 63*, 526.

Kalliomaki, M., Collado, M. C., Salminen, S., & Isolauri, E. (2008). Early differences in fecal microbiota composition in children may predict overweight. *American Journal of Clinical Nutrition, 87*, 534–538.

Kalliomaki, M., Kirjavainen, P., Eerola, E., Kero, P., Salminen, S., & Isolauri, E. (2001). Distinct patterns of neo-natal gut microflora in infants developing or not developing atopy. *Journal of Allergy and Clinical Immunology, 107*, 129–134.

Kanazawa, S. (2015). Breastfeeding is positively associated with child intelligence even net of parental IQ. *Developmental Psychology, 51*, 1683–1689.

Karjalainen, J., Martin, J. M., Knip, M., Ilonen, J., Robinson, B. H., Savilahti, E., . . . Dosch, H. M. (1992). A bovine albumin peptide as a possible trigger of insulin-dependent diabetes mellitus. *New England Journal of Medicine, 327*, 302–307.

Katikaneni, R., Ponnapakkam, T., Ponnapakkam, A., & Gensure, R. (2009). Breastfeeding does not protect against urinary tract infection in the first 3 months of life, but vitamin D supplementation increases the risk by 76%. *Clinical Pediatrics (Philadelphia), 48*, 750–755.

Keating, J. P., Shears, G. J., & Dodge, P. R. (1991). Oral water intoxication in infants, an American epidemic. *American Journal of Diseases of Children, 145*, 985–990.

Kelleher, S. L., & Lonnerdal, B. (2001). Immunological activities associated with milk. *Advances in Nutrition Research, 10*, 39–65.

Khedr, E. M. H., Farghaly, W. M. A., El-Din Amry, S., & Osman, A. A. A. (2004). Neural maturation of breastfed and formula-fed infants. *Acta Paediatrica, 93*, 734–738.

Kimata, H. (2007). Laughter elevates the levels of breast-milk melatonin. *Journal of Psychosomatic Research, 62*, 699–702.

Kimpimaki, T., Erkkola, M., Korhonen, S., Kupila, A., Virtanen, S. M., Ilonen, J., . . . Knip, M. (2001). Short-term exclusive breastfeeding predisposes young children with increased genetic risk of type 1 diabetes to progressive beta-cell autoimmunity. *Diabetologia, 44*, 63–69.

Kleinman, R. E. (Ed.). (2004). *Pediatric nutrition handbook* (5th ed.). Elk Grove Village, IL: American Academy of Pediatrics.

Koletzko, B., Rodriguez-Palmero, M., Demmelmair, H., Fidler, N., Jensen, R., & Sauerwald, T. (2001). Physiological aspects of human milk lipids. *Early Human Development, 65*(Suppl), S3–S18.

Koo, W. W. K. (2003). Efficacy and safety of docosahexaenoic acid and arachidonic acid addition to infant formulas: Can one buy better vision and intelligence? *Journal of the American College of Nutrition, 22*, 101–107.

Kostraba, J. N., Cruickshanks, K. J., Lawler-Heavner, J., Jobim, L. F., Rewers, M. J., Gay, E. C., . . . Hamman, R. F. (1993). Early exposure to cow's milk and solid foods in infancy, genetic predisposition, and risk of IDDM. *Diabetes, 42*, 288–295.

Kramer, M. S., Aboud, F., Mironova, E., Vanilovich, I., Platt, R. W., Matush, L., . . . Promotion of Breastfeeding Intervention Trial (PROBIT) Study Group. (2008). Breastfeeding and child cognitive development: New evidence from a large randomized trial. *Archives of General Psychiatry, 65*, 578–584.

Kreiter, S. R., Schwartz, R. P., Kirkman, H. N. Jr, Charlton, P. A., Calikoglu, A. S., & Davenport, M. L. (2000). Nutritional rickets in African American breast-fed infants. *Journal of Pediatrics, 137*, 153–157.

Labiner-Wolfe, J., & Fein, S. B. (2013). How US mothers store and handle their expressed breast milk. *Journal of Human Lactation, 29*, 54–58.

Lane, J. A., Mehra, R. K., Carrington, S. D., & Hickey, R. M. (2011). Development of biosensor-based assays to identify anti-infective oligosaccharides. *Analytical Biochemistry, 410,* 200–205.

Lanting, C. I., Fidler, V., Huisman, M., Touwen, B. C., & Boersma, E. R. (1994). Neurological differences between 9 year old children fed breastmilk or formula milk as babies. *Lancet, 344,* 1319–1322.

Laurberg, P., Nohr, S. B., Pedersen, K. M., & Fuglsang, E. (2004). Iodine nutrition in breast-fed infants is impaired by maternal smoking. *Journal of Clinical Endocrinology and Metabolism, 89,* 181–187.

Lawrence, R. A. (1999). Storage of human milk and the influence of procedures on immunological components of human milk. *Acta Paediatrica, 88*(Suppl), 14–18.

Lawrence, R. M. (2006). Cytomegalovirus in human breastmilk: Risk to the premature infant. *Breastfeeding Medicine, 1,* 99–107.

Lee, Y. K., & Puong, K. Y. (2002). Competition for adhesion between probiotics and human gastrointestinal pathogens in the presence of carbohydrate. *British Journal of Nutrition, 88*(Suppl 1), S101–S108.

Le Huerou-Luron, I., Blat, S., & Boudry, G. (2010). Breast- v. formula-feeding: Impacts on the digestive tract and immediate and long-term health effects. *Nutrition Research Reviews, 23,* 23–36.

Lessaris, K. J., Forsythe, D. W., & Wagner, C. L. (2000). Effect of human milk fortifier on the immunodetection and molecular mass profile of transforming growth factor-alpha. *Biology of the Neonate, 77,* 156–161.

Leung, A. K., McArthur, R. G., McMillan, D. D., Ko, D., Deacon, J. S., Parboosingh, J. T., & Lederis, K. P. (1980). Circulating antidiuretic hormone during labour and in the newborn. *Acta Paediatrica Scandinavica, 69,* 505–510.

Lewis, Z. T., Totten, S. M., Smilowitz, J. T., Popovic, M., Parker, E., Lemay, D.G., . . . Mills, D. A. (2015). Maternal fucosyltransferase 2 status affects the gut bifidobacterial communities of breastfed infants. *Microbiome, 3,* 13.

Ley, R., Backhed, F., Turnbaugh, P., Lozupone, C., Knight, R., & Gordon, J. (2005). Obesity alters gut microbial ecology. *Proceedings of the National Academy of Sciences of the United States of America, 102,* 11070–11075.

Ley, S. H., Hanley, A. J., Stone, D., & O'Connor, D. L. (2011). Effects of pasteurization on adiponectin and insulin concentrations in donor human milk. *Pediatric Research, 70,* 278–281.

Li, R., Rock, V. J., & Grummer-Strawn, L. (2007). Changes in public attitudes toward breastfeeding in the United States, 1999–2003. *Journal of the American Dietetic Association, 107,* 122–127.

Li, R., Xia, W., Zhang, Z., & Wu, K. (2011). S100B Protein, brain-derived neurotrophic factor, and glial cell line–derived neurotrophic factor in human milk. *PLoS One, 6,* e21663.

Life Sciences Research Office Report. (1998). Executive summary for the report: Assessment of nutrient requirements for infant formulas. *Journal of Nutrition, 128*(11 Suppl), 2059S–2293S.

Lind, T., Lonnerdal, B., Stenlund, H., Gamayanti, I. L., Ismail, D., Seswandhana, R., & Persson, L. (2004). A community-based randomized controlled trial of iron and zinc supplementation in Indonesian infants: Effects on growth and development. *American Journal of Clinical Nutrition, 80,* 729–736.

Lonnerdal, B. (2014). Infant formula and infant nutrition: Bioactive proteins of human milk and implications for composition of infant formulas. *American Journal of Clinical Nutrition, 99*(Suppl), 712S–717S.

Lonnerdal, B. (2003). Nutritional and physiologic significance of human milk proteins. *American Journal of Clinical Nutrition, 77,* 1537S–1543S.

Lopez Alvarez, M. J. (2007). Proteins in human milk. *Breastfeeding Review, 15,* 5–16.

Lopez-Lopez, A., Lopez-Sabater, M. C., Campoy-Folgoso, C., Rivero-Urgell, M., & Castellote-Bargallo, A. I. (2002). Fatty acid and sn-2 fatty acid composition in human milk from Granada (Spain) and in infant formulas. *European Journal of Clinical Nutrition, 56,* 1242–1254.

Lubetzky, R., Sever, O., Mimouni, F. B., & Mandel, D. (2015). Human milk macronutrients content: Effect of advanced maternal age. *Breastfeeding Medicine, 10,* 433–436.

Lucas, A., Morley, R., Cole, T. J., Lister, G., & Leeson-Payne, C. (1992). Breastmilk and subsequent intelligence quotient in children born preterm. *Lancet, 339,* 261–264.

Lund-Blix, N. A., Stene, L. C., Rasmussen, T., Torjesen, P. A., Andersen, L. F., & Ronningen, K. S. (2015). Infant feeding in relation to islet autoimmunity and type I diabetes in genetically susceptible children: The MIDIA study. *Diabetes Care, 38,* 257–263.

Ma, P., Brewer-Asling, M., & Magnus, J. H. (2013). A case study on the economic impact of optimal breastfeeding. *Maternal and Child Health Journal, 17,* 9–13.

Mackay, J., Eriksen, M., & Shafey, O. (2006). *The tobacco atlas*. Atlanta, GA: American Cancer Society.

Mackie, R. I., Sghir, A., & Gaskins, H. R. (1999). Developmental microbial ecology of the neonatal gastrointestinal tract. *American Journal of Clinical Nutrition, 69*(Suppl), 1035S–1045S.

Madan, J. C., Hoen, A. G., Lundgren, S. N., Farzan, S. F., Cottingham, K. L., Morrison, H. G., . . . Karagas, M. R. (2016). Association of cesarean delivery and formula supplementation with the intestinal microbiome of 6-week-old infants. *JAMA Pediatrics, 11.* doi:10.1001/jamapediatrics.2015.3732

Mangel, L., Ovental, A., Batscha, N., Arnon, M., Yarkoni, I., & Dollberg, S. (2015). Higher fat content in breastmilk expressed manually: A randomized trial. *Breastfeeding Medicine, 10,* 352–354.

Manohar, A. A., Williamson, M., & Koppikar, G. V. (1997). Effect of storage of colostrum in various containers. *Indian Pediatrics, 34,* 293–295.

Marchbank, T., Weaver, G., Nilsen-Hamilton, M., & Playford, R. J. (2009). Pancreatic secretory trypsin inhibitor is a major motogenic and protective factor in human breast milk. *American Journal of Physiology—Gastrointestinal and Liver Physiology, 296,* G697–G703.

Marin, M. L., Arroyo, R., Jimenez, E., Gomez, A., Fernandez, L., & Rodriguez, J. M. (2009). Cold storage of human milk: Effect on its bacterial composition. *Journal of Pediatric Gastroenterology and Nutrition, 49,* 343–348.

Martelli, A., De Chiara, A., Corvo, M., Restani, P., & Fiocchi, A. (2002). Beef allergy in children with cow's milk allergy: Cow's milk allergy in children with beef allergy. *Annals of Allergy, Asthma & Immunology, 89*(6 Suppl 1), 38–43.

Martínez-Costa, C., Silvestre, M. D., López, M. C., Plaza, A., Miranda, M., & Guijarro, R. (2007). Effects of refrigeration on the bactericidal activity of human milk: A preliminary study. *Journal of Pediatric Gastroenterology and Nutrition, 45,* 275–277

Martin-Sosa, S., Martin, M. J., Garcia-Pardo, L. A., & Hueso, P. (2003). Sialyloligosaccharides in human milk and in infant formulas: Variations with the progression of lactation. *Journal of Dairy Science, 86,* 52–59.

Massiera, F., Saint-Marc, P., Seydoux, J., Murata, T., Kobayashi, T., Narumiya, S., . . . Ailhaud, G. (2003). Arachidonic acid and prostacyclin signaling promote adipose tissue development: A human health concern? *Journal of Lipid Research, 44,* 271–279.

Mathur, N. B., Dwarkadas, A. M., Sharma, V. K., Saha, K., & Jain, N. (1990). Anti-infective factors in preterm human colostrum. *Acta Paediatrica Scandinavica, 79,* 1039–1044.

Mayer, E. J., Hamman, R. F., Gay, E. C., Lezotte, D. C., Savitz, D. A., & Klingensmith, G. J. (1988). Reduced risk of IDDM among breastfed children. The Colorado IDDM Registry. *Diabetes, 37,* 1625–1632.

McCrory, C., & Layte, R. (2011). The effect of breastfeeding on children's educational test scores at nine years of age: Results of an Irish cohort study. *Social Science in Medicine, 72,* 1515–1521.

McElroy, S. J., Castle, S. L., Bernard, J. K., Almohazey, D., Hunter, C. J., Bell, B. A., . . . Frey, M. R. (2014). The ErbB4 ligand neuregulin-4 protects against experimental necrotizing enterocolitis. *American Journal of Pathology, 184,* 2768–2778.

McVeagh, P., & Miller, J. B. (1997). Human milk oligosaccharides: Only the breast. *Journal of Paediatrics and Child Health, 33,* 281–286.

Merewood, A., Mehta, S. D., Grossman, X., Chen, T. C., Mathieu, J., Holick, M. F., & Bauchner, H. (2012). Vitamin D status among 4 month old infants in New England: A prospective cohort study. *Journal of Human Lactation, 28,* 159–166.

Michalski, M. C. (2013). Lipids and milk fat globule properties in human milk. In S. Zibadi, R. R. Watson, & V. R. Preedy (Eds.), *Handbook of dietary and nutritional aspects of human breast milk* (pp. 315–334). Wageningen, Netherlands: Wageningen Academic Publishers.

Michalski, M. C., Calzada, C., Makino, A., Michaud, S., & Guichardant, M. (2008). Oxidation products of polyunsaturated fatty acids in infant formulas compared to human milk: A preliminary study. *Molecular Nutrition Food Research, 52,* 1478–1485.

Miller, J., Makrides, M., Gibson, R. A., McPhee, A. J., Stanford, T. E., Morris, S., . . . Collins, C. T. (2012). Effect of increasing protein content of human milk fortifier on growth in preterm infants born at <31 wk gestation: A randomized controlled trial. *American Journal of Clinical Nutrition, 95,* 648–655.

Milner, J. D., & Gergen, P. J. (2005). Transient environmental exposures on the developing immune system: Implications for allergy and asthma. *Current Opinion in Allergy and Immunology, 5,* 235–240.

Miniello, V. L., Francavilla, R., Brunetti, L., Franco, C., Lauria, B., Lieggi, M. S., . . . Armenio, L. (2008). Primary allergy prevention: Partially or extensively hydrolyzed infant formulas? *Minerva Pediatrica, 60,* 1437–1443.

Misra, M., Pacaud, D., Petryk, A., Collett-Solberg, P. F., & Kappy, M. (2008). Vitamin D deficiency in children and its management: Review of current knowledge and recommendations. *Pediatrics, 122,* 398–417.

Mitoulas, L. R. (2000). *Short- and long-term variation in the production and content and composition of human milk fat* (Unpublished PhD dissertation). Perth: University of Western Australia.

Mojab, C. G. (2002). Sunlight deficiency and breastfeeding. *Breastfeeding Abstracts, 22,* 3–4.

Moltó-Puigmartí, C., Plat, J., Mensink, R. P., Müller, A., Jansen, E., Zeegers, M. P., & Thijs, C. (2010). FADS1 FADS2 gene variants modify the association between fish intake and the docosahexaenoic acid proportions in human milk. *American Journal of Clinical Nutrition, 91,* 1368–1376.

Moodley-Govender, E., Mulol, H., Stauber, J., Manary, M., & Coutsoudis, A. (2015). Increased exclusivity of breastfeeding associated with reduced gut inflammation in infants. *Breastfeeding Medicine, 10,* 488–492.

Morceli, G., Franca, E. L., Magalhaes, V. B., Damasceno, D. C., Calderon, I. M., & Honorio-França, A. C. (2011). Diabetes induced immunological and biochemical changes in human colostrum. *Acta Paediatrica, 100,* 550–556.

Morelli, L. (2008). Postnatal development of intestinal microflora as influenced by infant nutrition. *Journal of Nutrition, 138,* 1791S–1795S.

Morrow, A. L., Ruiz-Palacios, G. M., Altaye, M., Jiang, X., Guerrero, M. L., Meinzen-Derr, J. K., . . . Newburg, D. S. (2004). Human milk oligosaccharides are associated with protection against diarrhea in breastfed infants. *Journal of Pediatrics, 145,* 297–303.

Morrow-Tlucak, M., Haude, R. H., & Ernhart, C. B. (1988). Breastfeeding and cognitive development in the first 2 years of life. *Social Science and Medicine, 26,* 635–639.

Mortensen, E. L., Michaelsen, K. F., Sanders, S. A., & Reinisch, J. M. (2002). The association between duration of breastfeeding and adult intelligence. *Journal of the American Medical Association, 287,* 2365–2371.

Mosconi, E., Rekima, A., Seitz-Polski, B., Kanda, A., Fleury, S., Tissandie, E., . . . & Verhasselt, V. (2010). Breast milk immune complexes are potent inducers of oral tolerance in neonates and prevent asthma development. *Mucosal Immunology, 3,* 461–474.

Mountzouris, K. C., McCartney, A. L., & Gibson, G. R. (2002). Intestinal microflora of human infants and current trends for its nutritional modulation. *British Journal of Nutrition, 87,* 405–420.

Mulder, P., Johnson, T., & Baker, L. (2010). Excessive weight loss in breastfed infants during the postpartum hospitalization. *Journal of Obstetric, Gynecologic and Neonatal Nursing, 39,* 15–26.

Mulder, P. J., & Gardner, S. E. (2015). The healthy newborn hydration model: A new model for understanding newborn hydration immediately after birth. *Biological Research for Nursing, 17,* 94–99.

Musumeci, M., & Musumeci, S. (2013). Biologic substances present in human colostrums. In S. Zibadi, R. R. Watson, & V. R. Preedy (Eds.), *Handbook of dietary and nutritional aspects of human breast milk.* Human Health Handbooks no. 5 (pp. 217–233).Wageningen, Netherlands: Wageningen Academic Publishers.

Myher, J. J., Kuksis, A., Geher, K., Park, P. W., & Diersen-Schade, D. A. (1996). Stereospecific analysis of triacylglycerols rich in long-chain polyunsaturated fatty acids. *Lipids, 31*, 207–215.

Nelson, C. M., & Innis, S. M. (1999). Plasma lipoprotein fatty acids are altered by the positional distribution of fatty acids in infant formula triacylglycerols and human milk. *American Journal of Clinical Nutrition, 70*, 62–69.

Neu, J., & Walker, W. A. (2011). Necrotizing enterocolitis. *New England Journal of Medicine, 364*, 255–264.

Newburg, D. S. (2005). Innate immunity and human milk. *Journal of Nutrition, 135*, 1308–1312.

Newburg, D. S., & Walker, W. A. (2007). Protection of the neonate by the innate immune system of developing gut and of human milk. *Pediatric Research, 61*, 2–8.

Ngom, P. T., Collinson, A. C., Pido-Lopez, J., Henson, S. M., Prentice, A. M., & Aspinall, R. (2004). Improved thymic function in exclusively breastfed infants is associated with higher interleukin 7 concentrations in their mothers' breastmilk. *American Journal of Clinical Nutrition, 80*, 722–728.

Nicoll, A., Ginsburg, R., & Tripp, J. H. (1982). Supplementary feeding and jaundice in newborns. *Acta Paediatrica Scandinavica, 71*, 759–761.

Norris, J., Barriga, K., Klingensmith, G., Hoffman, M., Eisenbarth, G. S., Erlich, H. A., & Rewers, M. (2003). Timing of initial cereal exposure in infancy and risk of islet autoimmunity. *Journal of the American Medical Association, 290*, 1713–1720.

Office of Food Additive Safety. (2001). *GRAS Notice No. GRN 000041 (May 17, 2001).* Washington, DC: U.S. Food and Drug Administration.

Oftedal, O. T. (2002). The origin of lactation as a water source for parchment-shelled eggs. *Journal of Mammary Gland Biology and Neoplasia, 7*, 253–266.

Ogundele, M. O. (2000). Techniques for the storage of human breastmilk: Implications for anti-microbial functions and safety of stored milk. *European Journal of Pediatrics, 159*, 793–797.

Ogundele, M. O. (2002). Effects of storage on the physicochemical and antibacterial properties of human milk. *British Journal of Biomedical Science, 59*, 205–211.

Omarsdottir, S., Casper, C., Naver, L., Legnevall, L., Gustafsson, F., Grillner, L., . . . Vanpee, M. (2015). Cytomegalovirus infection and neonatal outcome in extremely preterm infants after freezing of maternal milk. *Pediatric Infectious Disease Journal, 34*, 482–489.

Osborn, D. A., & Sinn, J. (2006). Soy formula for the prevention of allergy and food intolerance in infants. *Cochrane Database of Systematic Reviews, 18*(4), CD003741.

Oski, F. A., DeAngeles, C. D., Feigin, R. D., & McMillan, J. A. (1994). *Principles and practice of pediatrics.* Philadelphia, PA: Lippincott.

Ostrea, E. M. Jr., Balun, J. E., Winkler, R., & Porter, T. (1986). Influence of breastfeeding on the restoration of the low serum concentration of vitamin E and beta-carotene in the newborn infant. *American Journal of Obstetrics and Gynecology, 154*, 1014–1017.

Pan, D. A., Hylbert, A. J., & Storlien, L. H. (1994). Dietary fats, membrane phospholipids and obesity. *Journal of Nutrition, 124*, 1555–1565.

Panczuk, J. K., Unger, S., Francis, J., Bando, N., Kiss, A., & O'Connor, D. L. (2016). Introduction of bovine-based nutrient fortifier and gastrointestinal inflammation in very low birth weight infants as measured by fecal calprotectin. *Breastfeeding Medicine, 11*, 2–5.

Park, D. A., Bulkley, G. B., & Granger, D. N. (1983). Role of oxygen-derived free radicals in digestive tract disease. *Surgery, 94*, 415–422.

Penn, A. H., Altshuler, A. E., Small, J. W., Taylor, S. F., Dobkins, K. R., & Schmid-Schonbein, G. W. (2012). Digested formula but not digested fresh human milk causes death of intestinal cells in vitro: Implications for necrotizing enterocolitis. *Pediatric Research, 72*, 560–567.

Perrier, C., & Corthesy, B. (2011). Gut permeability and food allergies. *Clinical and Experimental Allergy, 41*, 20–28.

Picciano, M. F. (1998). Human milk: Nutritional aspects of a dynamic food. *Biology of the Neonate, 74*, 84–93.

Picciano, M. F. (2001). Nutrient composition of human milk. *Pediatric Clinics of North America, 48*, 53–67.

Pickering, L. K., Granoff, D. M., Erickson, J. R., Masor, M. L., Cordle, C. T., Schaller, J. P., . . . Hilty, M. D. (1998). Modulation of the immune system by human milk and infant formula containing nucleotides. *Pediatrics, 101*, 242–249.

Pisacane, A., DeVizia, B., Valíante, A., Vaccaro, F., Russo, M., Grillo, G., & Giustardi, A. (1995). Iron status in breastfed infants. *Journal of Pediatrics, 127*, 429.

Piskin, E., Karavar, N., Arasli, M., & Ermis, B. (2012). Effect of maternal smoking on colostrum and breast milk cytokines. *European Cytokine Network, 23*, 187–190.

Ponnapakkam, T., Bradford, E., & Gensure, R. (2010). A treatment trial of vitamin D supplementation in breastfed infants: Universal supplementation is not necessary for rickets prevention in southern Louisiana. *Clinical Pediatrics, 49*, 1053–1060.

Prescott, S., & Nowak-Wegrzyn, A. (2011). Strategies to prevent or reduce allergic disease. *Annals of Nutrition and Metabolism, 59*(Suppl 1), 28–42.

Pugliese, M. F., Blumberg, D. L., Hludzinski, J., & Kay, S. (1998). Nutritional rickets in suburbia. *Journal of the American College of Nutrition, 17*, 637–641.

Quan, R., Yang, C., Rubinstein, S., Lewiston, N. J., Stevenson, D. K., & Kerner, J. A. Jr. (1994). The effect of nutritional additives on anti-infective factors in human milk. *Clinical Pediatrics (Philadelphia), 33*, 325–328.

Quan, R., Yang, C., Rubinstein, S., Lewiston, N. J., Sunshine, P., Stevenson, D. K., & Kerner, J. A. Jr. (1992). Effects of microwave radiation on anti-infective factors in human milk. *Pediatrics, 89*, 667

Rao, M. R., Hediger, M. L., Levine, R. J., Naficy, A. B., & Vik, T. (2002). Effect of breastfeeding on cognitive development of infants born small for gestational age. *Acta Paediatrica, 91*, 267–274.

Ratner, B. (1935). The treatment of milk allergy and its basic principles. *Journal of the American Medical Association, 105*, 934–939.

Robbins, S. T., & Meyers, R. (Eds.); Pediatric Nutrition Practice Group. (2011). *Infant feedings: Guidelines for preparation of human milk and formula in health care facilities* (2nd ed.). Chicago, IL: American Dietetic Association.

Rochow, N., Landau-Crangle, E., & Fusch, C. (2015). Challenges in breast milk fortification for preterm infants. *Current Opinion in Clinical Nutrition and Metabolic Care, 18*, 276–284.

Rozenfeld, P., Docena, G. H., Añón, M. C., & Fossati, C. A. (2002). Detection and identification of a soy protein component that cross-reacts with caseins from cow's milk. *Clinical and Experimental Immunology, 130*, 49–58.

Rubaltelli, F. F., Biadaioli, R., Pecile, P., & Nicoletti, P. (1998). Intestinal flora in breast and bottle-fed infants. *Journal of Perinatal Medicine, 26*, 186–191.

Ruth-Sanchez, V., & Greene, C. V. (1997). Water intoxication in a three day old: A case presentation. *Mother and Baby Journal, 2*, 5–11.

Sachdev, H. P. S., Krishna, J., Puri, R. K., Satyanarayana, L., & Kumar, S. (1991). Water supplementation in exclusively breastfed infants during summer in the tropics. *Lancet, 337*, 929–933.

Sacker, A., Quigley, M. A., & Kelly, Y. J. (2006). Breastfeeding and developmental delay: Findings from the Millennium Cohort study. *Pediatrics, 118*, e682–e689.

Sadeharju, K., Knip, M., Virtanen, S. M., Savilahti, E., Tauriainen, S., Koskela, P., . . . Finnish TRIGR Study Group. (2007). Maternal antibodies in breastmilk protect the child from enterovirus infections. *Pediatrics, 119*, 941–946.

Salminen, S. J., Gueimonde, J., & Isolauri, E. (2005). Probiotics that modify disease risk. *Journal of Nutrition, 135*, 1294–1298.

Sanchez-Barcelo, E. J., Mediavilla, M. D., & Reiter, R. J. (2011). Clinical uses of melatonin in pediatrics. *International Journal of Pediatrics, 2011,* 892624.

Savilahti, E., Tuomilehto, J., Saukkonen, T. T., Virtala, E. T., & Akerblom, H. K. (1993). Increased levels of cow's milk and beta-lactoglobulin antibodies in young children with newly diagnosed IDDM. *Diabetes Care, 16,* 984–989.

Scariati, P. D., Grummer-Strawn, L. M., & Fein, S. (1997). Water supplementation of infants in the first month of life. *Archives of Pediatrics and Adolescent Medicine, 151,* 830–832.

Schulz-Lell, G., Buss, R., Oldigs, H. D., Dorner, K., & Schaub, J. (1987). Iron balances in infant nutrition. *Acta Paediatrica Scandinavica, 76,* 585.

Scott, J. A., Binns, C. W., & Oddy, W. H. (2007). Predictors of delayed onset of lactation. *Maternal and Child Nutrition, 3,* 186–193.

Sevelsted, A., Stokholm, J., Bennelykke, K., & Bisgaard, H. (2015). Cesarean section and chronic immune disorders. *Pediatrics, 135,* e92–e98.

Shah, M., Salhab, N., Patterson, D., & Seikaly, M. G. (2000). Nutritional rickets still afflict children in North Texas. *Texas Medicine, 96,* 64–68.

Silfverdal, S. A., Ekholm, L., & Bodin, L. (2007). Breastfeeding enhances the antibody response to Hib and pneumococcal serotype 6B and 14 after vaccination with conjugate vaccines. *Vaccine, 25,* 1497–1502.

Sills, I. N., Skuza, K. A., Horlick, M. N., Schwartz, M. S., & Rapaport, R. (1994). Vitamin D deficiency rickets. Reports of its demise are exaggerated. *Clinical Pediatrics (Philadelphia), 33,* 491–493.

Silvers, K. M., Frampton, C. M., Wickens, K., Pattemore, P. K., Ingham, T., Fishwick, D., . . . Epton, M. J. (2012). Breastfeeding protects against current asthma up to 6 years of age. *Journal of Pediatrics, 160,* 991–996.

Silvestre, D., Miranda, M., Muriach, M., Almansa, I., Jareño, E., & Romero, F. J. (2008). Antioxidant capacity of human milk: Effect of thermal conditions for the pasteurization. *Acta Paediatrica, 97,* 1070–1074.

Silvestre, D., Ruiz, P., Martinez-Costa, C., Plaza, A., & Lopez, M. C. (2008). Effect of pasteurization on the bactericidal capacity of human milk. *Journal of Human Lactation, 24,* 371–376.

Simmer, K. (2002a). Longchain polyunsaturated fatty acid supplementation in infants born at term (Cochrane Review). In *The Cochrane Library, 1.* Oxford, UK: Update Software.

Simmer, K. (2002b). Longchain polyunsaturated fatty acid supplementation in preterm infants (Cochrane Review). In *The Cochrane Library, 1.* Oxford, UK: Update Software.

Simmer, K., Patole, S. K., & Rao, S. C. (2008, January 23). Longchain polyunsaturated fatty acid supplementation in infants born at term. *Cochrane Database of Systematic Reviews, 1,* CD000376.

Simmer, K., Schulzke, S. M., & Patole, S. (2008, January 23). Longchain polyunsaturated fatty acid supplementation in preterm infants. *Cochrane Database of Systematic Reviews, 1,* CD000375.

Simsek, Y., Karabiyik, P., Polat, K., Duran, Z., & Polat, A. (2014). Mode of delivery changes oxidative and antioxidative properties of human milk: A prospective controlled clinical investigation. *Journal of Maternal, Fetal and Neonatal Medicine, 28,* 734–738.

Singhal, A., Morley, R., Cole, T. J., Kennedy, K., Sonksen, P., Isaacs, E., . . . Lucas, A. (2007). Infant nutrition and stereoacuity at age 4–6 y. *American Journal of Clinical Nutrition 85,* 152–159.

Singhi, S., Chookang, E., Hall, J. S., & Kalghangi, S. (1985). Iatrogenic neonatal and maternal hyponatremia following oxytocin and aqueous glucose infusion during labour. *British Journal of Obstetrics and Gynecology, 92,* 356–363.

Slutzah, M., Codipilly, C. N., Potak, D., Clark, R. M., & Schanler, R. J. (2010). Refrigerator storage of expressed human milk in the neonatal intensive care unit. *Journal of Pediatrics, 156,* 26–28.

Slykerman, R. F., Thompson, J. M. D., Becroft, D. M. D., Robinson, E., Pryor, J. E., Clark, P. M., . . . Mitchell, E. A. (2005). Breastfeeding and intelligence of preschool children. *Acta Paediatrica, 94,* 832–837.

Sommerburg, O., Meissner, K., Nelle, M., Lenhartz, H., & Leichsenring, M. (2000). Carotenoid supply in breastfed and formula-fed neonates. *European Journal of Pediatrics, 159,* 86–90.

Song, J. H., Fujimoto, K., & Miyazawa, T. (2000). Polyunsaturated (n-3) fatty acids susceptible to peroxidation are increased in plasma and tissue lipids of rats fed docosahexaenoic acid–containing oils. *Journal of Pediatrics, 130,* 3028–3033.

Song, J. H., & Miyazawa, T. (2001). Enhanced level of n-3 fatty acid in membrane phospholipids induces lipid peroxidation in rats fed dietary docosahexaenoic acid oil. *Atherosclerosis, 155,* 9–18.

Spatz, D. L., Schmidt, K. J., & Kinzler, S. (2014). Implementation of a human milk management center. *Advances in Neonatal Care, 14,* 253–261.

Specker, B. L., Valanis, B., Hertzberg, V., Edwards, N., & Tsang, R. C. (1985). Sunshine exposure and serum 25-hydroxyvitamin D concentrations in exclusively breastfed infants. *Journal of Pediatrics, 107,* 372–376.

Srinivasan, L., Bokiniec, R., King, C., Weaver, G., & Edwards, A. D. (2004). Increased osmolality of breastmilk with therapeutic additives. *Archives of Disease in Childhood—Fetal and Neonatal Edition, 89,* F514–F517.

Stewart, J. A., Chadwick, V. S., & Murray, A. (2006). Carriage, quantification, and predominance of methanogens and sulfate-reducing bacteria in fecal samples. *Letters in Applied Microbiology, 43,* 58–63.

Straarup, E. M., Lauritzen, L., Faerk, J., Høy, C. E., & Michaelsen, K. F. (2006). The stereospecific triacylglycerol structures and fatty acid profiles of human milk and infant formulas. *Journal of Pediatric Gastroenterology and Nutrition, 42,* 293–299.

Sullivan, S., Schanler, R. J., Kim, J. H., Patel, A. L., Trawoger, R., Kiechl-Kohlendorfer, U., . . . Lucas, A. (2010). An exclusively human milk–based diet is associated with a lower rate of necrotizing enterocolitis than a diet of human milk and bovine milk–based products. *Journal of Pediatrics, 156,* 562–567.

Svensson, M., Hákansson, A., Mossberg, A. K., Linse, S., & Svanborg, C. (2000). Conversion of alpha-lactalbumin to a protein inducing apoptosis. *Proceedings of the National Academy of Sciences of the United States of America, 97,* 4221–4226.

Tacken, K. J., Vogelsang, A., van Lingen, R. A., Slootstra, J., Dikkeschei, B. D., & van Zoeren-Grobben, D. (2009). Loss of triglycerides and carotenoids in human milk after processing. *Archives of Disease in Childhood—Fetal and Neonatal Edition, 94,* F447–F450.

Takci, S., Gulmez, D., Yigit, S., Dogan, O., Dik, K., & Hascelik, G. (2012). Effects of freezing on the bactericidal activity of human milk. *Journal of Pediatric Gastroenterology and Nutrition, 55*(2), 146–149.

Takci, S., Gulmez, D., Yigit, S., Dogan, O., & Hascelik, G. (2013). Container type and bactericidal activity of human milk during refrigerated storage. *Journal of Human Lactation, 29,* 406–411.

Tanaka, K., Kon, N., Ohkawa, N., Yoshikawa, N., & Shimizu, T. (2009). Does breastfeeding in the neonatal period influence the cognitive function of very-low-birth-weight infants at 5 years of age? *Brain Development, 31,* 288–293.

Tanaka, S., Kobayashi, T., Songjinda, P., Tateyama, A., Tsubouchi, M., Kiyohara, C., . . . Nakayama, J. (2009). Influence of antibiotic exposure in the early postnatal period on the development of intestinal microbiota. *FEMS Immunology and Medical Microbiology, 56,* 80–87.

Tarnow-Mordi, W. O., Shaw, J. C., Liu, D., Gardner, D. A., & Flynn, F. V. (1981). Iatrogenic hyponatremia of the newborn due to maternal fluid overload: A prospective study. *British Medical Journal—Clinical Research Edition, 283,* 639–642.

Telang, S., Berseth, C. L., Ferguson, P. W., Kinder, J. M., DeRoin, M., & Petschow, B. W. (2005). Fortifying fresh human milk with commercial powdered human milk fortifiers does not affect bacterial growth during 6 hours at room temperature. *Journal of the American Dietetic Association, 105,* 1567–1572.

Thavagnanam, S., Fleming, J., Bromley, A., Shields, M. D., & Cardwell, C. R. (2008). A meta-analysis of the association between caesarean section and childhood asthma. *Clinical and Experimental Allergy, 38,* 629–633.

Thoene, M., Hanson, C., Lyden, E., Dugick, L., Ruybal, L., & Ansercon-Berry, A. (2014). Comparison of the effect of two human milk fortifiers on clinical outcomes in premature infants. *Nutrients, 6,* 261–275.

Thomas, E., Zeps, N., Cregan, M., Hartmann, P., & Martin, T. (2011). 14-3-3σ (sigma) regulates proliferation and differentiation of multipotent p63-positive cells isolated from human breastmilk. *Cell Cycle, 10,* 278–284.

Thurl, S., Munzert, M., Henker, J., Boehm, G., Muller-Werner, B., Jelinek, J., & Stahl, B. (2010). Variation of human milk oligosaccharides in relation to milk groups and lactational periods. *British Journal of Nutrition, 104,* 1261–1271.

Tomblin, J. B., Smith, E., & Zhang, X. (1997). Epidemiology of specific language impairment: Prenatal and perinatal risk factors. *Journal of Communicable Disorders, 30,* 325–344.

Tullus, K., & Burman, L. G. (1989). Ecological impact of ampicillin and cefuroxime in neonatal units. *Lancet, 1,* 1405–1407.

Tully, M. R. (2000). Recommendations for handling of mother's own milk. *Journal of Human Lactation, 16,* 149–151.

Uauy, R. (1990). Are omega-3 fatty acids required for normal eye and brain development in the human? *Journal of Pediatric Gastroenterology and Nutrition, 11,* 296–302.

Uauy, R., & Araya, M. (2004). Novel oligosaccharides in human milk: Understanding mechanisms may lead to better prevention of enteric and other infections. *Journal of Pediatrics, 145,* 283–285.

Vaarala, O., Paronen, J., Otonkoski, T., & Akerblom, H. K. (1998). Cow milk feeding induces antibodies to insulin in children: A link between cow milk and insulin-dependent mellitus? *Scandinavian Journal of Immunology, 47,* 131–135.

Valentine, C. J., Morrow, G., Fernandez, S., Gulati, P., Bartholomew, D., Long, D., . . . Rogers, L. K. (2010). Docosahexaenoic acid and amino acid contents in pasteurized donor milk are low for preterm infants. *Journal of Pediatrics, 157,* 906–910.

Vallaeys, C. (2008). *Replacing mother-imitating human breastmilk in the laboratory. Novel oils in infant formula and organic foods: Safe and valuable functional food or risky marketing gimmick?* Cornucopia, WI: Cornucopia Institute. Retrieved from http://www.cornucopia.org/2008/01/replacing-mother-infant-formula-report

Vandenplas, Y., Brueton, M., Dupont, C., Hill, D., Oranje, A. P., Brueton, M., . . . Dupont, C. (2007). Guidelines for the diagnosis and management of cow's milk protein allergy in infants. *Archives of Disease in Childhood, 92,* 902–908.

van Odijk, J., Kull, I., Borres, M. P., Brandtzaeg, P., Edberg, U., Hanson, L. A., . . . Wille, S. (2003). Breastfeeding and allergic disease: A multidisciplinary review of the literature (1996–2001) on the mode of early feeding in infancy and its impact on later atopic manifestations. *Allergy, 58,* 833–843.

Veh, R. W., Michalski, J. C., Corfiend, A. P., Sander-Wewer, M., Gies, D., & Schauer, R. (1981). New chromatographic system for the rapid analysis and preparation of colostrum sialyl oligosaccharides. *Journal of Chromatography, 212,* 313–322.

Vickers, A. M., Starks-Solis, S., Hill, D. R., & Newburg, D. S. (2015). Pasteurized donor human milk maintains microbiological purity for 4 days at 4°C. *Journal of Human Lactation, 31,* 401–405.

Victora, C. G., Horta, B. L., Loret de Mola, C., Quevedo, L., Pinheiro, R. T., Gigante, D. P., . . . Barros, F.C. (2015). Association between breastfeeding and intelligence, educational attainment, and income at 30 years of age: A prospective birth cohort study from Brazil. *Lancet Global Health, 3,* e199–e205.

Vieira, A. A., Soares, F. V., Pimenta, H. P., Abranches, A. D., & Moreira, M. E. (2011). Analysis of the influence of pasteurization, freezing/thawing, and other processes on human milk's macronutrient concentrations. *Early Human Development, 87,* 577–580.

Vieth, R., Chan, P. C. R., & MacFarlane, G. D. (2001). Efficiency and safety of vitamin D_3 intake exceeding the lowest observed adverse effect level (LOAEL). *American Journal of Clinical Nutrition, 73,* 288–294.

Vio, F., Salazar, G., & Infante, C. (1991). Smoking during pregnancy and lactation and its effects on breast-milk volume. *American Journal of Clinical Nutrition, 54,* 1011–1016.

Vitamin D Expert Panel, Centers for Disease Control and Prevention. (2001). Final report. Retrieved from http://www.cdc.gov/nccdphp/dnpa/nutrition/pdf/Vitamin_D_Expert_Panel _Meeting.pdf

Vohr, B. R., Poindexter, B. B., Dusick, A. M., McKinley, L. T., Wright, L. L., Langer, J. C., . . . NICHD Neonatal Research Network. (2006). Beneficial effects of breastmilk in the neonatal intensive care unit on the developmental outcome of extremely low birth weight infants at 18 months of age. *Pediatrics, 118,* e115–e123.

Von Berg, A., Koletzko, S., Grubl, A., Filipiak-Pittroff, B., Wichmann, H. E., Bauer, C. P., . . . German Infant Nutritional Intervention Study Group. (2003). The effect of hydrolyzed cow's milk formula for allergy prevention in the first year of life: The German Infant Nutritional Intervention Study, a randomized double-blind trial. *Journal of Allergy and Clinical Immunology, 111,* 533–540.

Vorbach, C., Capecchi, M. R., & Penninger, J. M. (2006). Evolution of the mammary gland from the innate immune system? *BioEssays, 28,* 606–616.

Wagner, C. L., Greer, F. R., American Academy of Pediatrics Section on Breastfeeding, & American Academy of Pediatrics Committee on Nutrition. (2008). Prevention of rickets and vitamin D deficiency in infants, children, and adolescents. *Pediatrics, 122,* 1142–1152.

Wagner, C. L., Hulsey, T. C., Fanning, D., Ebeling, M., & Hollis, B. W. (2006). High-dose vitamin D_3 supplementation in a cohort of breastfeeding mothers and their infants: A six-month follow-up pilot study. *Breastfeeding Medicine, 1,* 59–70.

Wang, B., Brand-Miller, J., McVeagh, & Petocz, P. (2001). Concentration and distribution of sialic acid in human milk and infant formulas. *American Journal of Clinical Nutrition, 74,* 510–515.

Wang, B., Hu, H., & Yu, B. (2006). Molecular characterization of pig ST8SiaIV: A critical gene for the formation of neural cell adhesion molecule and its response to sialic acid supplement in piglets. *Nutritional Neuroscience, 9,* 3–4.

Wang, B., McVeagh, P., Petocz, P., & Brand-Miller, J. (2003). Brain ganglioside and glycoprotein sialic acid in breastfed compared with formula-fed infants. *American Journal of Clinical Nutrition, 78,* 1024–1029.

Wang, B., Yu, B., Karim, M., Hu, H., Sun, Y., McGreevy, P., . . . Brand-Miller, J. (2007). Dietary sialic acid supplementation improves learning and memory in piglets. *American Journal of Clinical Nutrition, 85,* 561–569.

Weisberg, P., Scanlon, K. S., Li, R., & Cogswell, M. E. (2004). Nutritional rickets among children in the United States: Review of cases reported between 1986 and 2003. *American Journal of Clinical Nutrition, 80*(Suppl), 1697S–1705S.

Welch, T. R., Bergstrom, W. H., & Tsang, R. C. (2000). Vitamin D–deficient rickets: The reemergence of a once-conquered disease. *Journal of Pediatrics, 137,* 143–145.

West, P. A., Hewitt, J. H., & Murphy, O. M. (1979). The influence of methods of collection and storage on the bacteriology of human milk. *Journal of Applied Bacteriology, 46,* 269–277.

Wieringa, F. T., Dijkhuizen, M. A., West, C. E., Thurnham, D. I., Muhilal, & Van der Meer, J. W. (2003). Redistribution of vitamin A after iron supplementation in Indonesian infants. *American Journal of Clinical Nutrition, 77,* 651–657.

Williams, C., Birch, E. E., Emmett, P. M., Northstone, K., & Avon Longitudinal Study of Pregnancy and Childhood Study Team. (2001). Stereoacuity at age 3.5 years in children born full-term is associated with prenatal and postnatal dietary factors: A report from a population-based cohort study. *American Journal of Clinical Nutrition, 73,* 316–322.

Williams, H. G. (2006). "And not a drop to drink": Why water is harmful for newborns. *Breastfeeding Review, 14,* 5–9.

Williams-Arnold, L. D. (2000). *Human milk storage for healthy infants and children.* Sandwich, MA: Health Education Associates.

Williamson, M. T., & Murti, P. K. (1996). Effects of storage, time, temperature, and composition of containers on biologic components of human milk. *Journal of Human Lactation, 12,* 31–35.

Wing, K., Ekmark, A., Karlsson, H., Rudin, A., & Suri-Payer, E. (2002). Characterization of human CD25+ CD4+ T cells in thymus, cord and adult blood. *Immunology, 106,* 190–199.

Wojcicki, J. M., Holbrook, K., Lustig, R. H., Caughey, A. B., Munoz, R. F., & Heyman, M. B. (2011). Infant formula, tea, and water supplementation of Latino infants at 4–6 weeks postpartum. *Journal of Human Lactation, 27,* 122–130.

Workgroup for Safe Markets. (2008). Baby's toxic bottle: Bisphenol A leaching from popular baby bottle. Retrieved from http://www.greentogrow.com/BabysToxicBottleFinal.pdf

Xavier, A. M., Rai, K., & Hegde, A. M. (2011). Total antioxidant concentrations of breastmilk: An eyeopener to the negligent. *Journal of Health, Population and Nutrition, 29,* 605–611.

Xia, Q., Williams, T., Hustead, D., Price, P., Morrison, M., & Yu, Z. (2012). Quantitative analysis of intestinal bacterial populations from term infants fed formula supplemented with fructo-oligosaccharides. *Journal of Pediatric Gastroenterology and Nutrition, 55*(3), 314–320

Xie, L., & Innis, S. M. (2008). Genetic variants of the FADS1 FADS2 gene cluster are associated with altered (n-6) and (n-3) essential fatty acids in plasma and erythrocyte phospholipids in women during pregnancy and in breast milk during lactation. *Journal of Nutrition, 138,* 2222–2228.

Yamauchi, Y., & Yamanouchi, H. (1990). Breastfeeding frequency during the first 24 hours after birth in full-term neonates. *Pediatrics, 86,* 171–175.

Young, T. K., Martens, P. J., Taback, S. P., Sellers, E. A., Dean, H. J., Cheang, M., & Flett, B. (2002). Type 2 diabetes mellitus in children. *Archives of Pediatrics and Adolescent Medicine, 156,* 651–655.

Zagierski, M., Szlagatys-Sidorkiewicz, A., Jankowska, A., Krzykowski, G., Korzon, M., & Kaminska, B. (2011). Maternal smoking decreases antioxidative status of human breast milk. *Journal of Perinatology, 32,* 593–597.

Zarban, A., Toroghi, M. M., Asli, M., Jafari, M., Vejdan, M., & Sharifzadeh, G. (2015). Effect of vitamin C and E supplementation on total antioxidant content of human breastmilk and infant urine. *Breastfeeding Medicine, 10,* 214–217.

Zeiger, R. (1999). Prevention of food allergy in infants and children. *Immunology And Allergy Clinics of North America, 19,* 619–646.

Zetterstrom, R., Bennet, R., & Nord, K. E. (1994). Early infant feeding and micro-ecology of the gut. *Acta Paediatrica Japan, 36,* 562–571.

Ziegler, A., Schmid, S., Huber, D., Hummel, M., & Bonifacio, E. (2003). Early infant feeding and risk of developing type I diabetes–associated antibodies. *Journal of the American Medical Association, 290,* 1721–1728.

Ziegler, E. E., Nelson, S. E., & Jeter, J. M. (2009). Iron supplementation of breastfed infants from an early age. *American Journal of Clinical Nutrition, 89,* 525–532.

Zivkovic, A. M., German, J. B., Lebrilla, C. B., & Mills, D. A. (2011). Human milk glycobiome and its impact on the infant gastrointestinal microbiota. *Proceedings of the National Academy of Sciences, 108*(Suppl 1), 4653–4658.

Zoeren-Grobben, D., Moison, R. M., Ester, W. M., & Berger, H. M. (1993). Lipid peroxidation in human milk and infant formula: Effect of storage, tube feeding and exposure to phototherapy. *Acta Paediatrica, 82,* 645–649.

Zoppi, G., Gasparini, R., Mantovanelli, F., Gobio-Casali, L., Astolfi, R., & Crovari, P. (1983). Diet and antibody response to vaccinations in healthy infants. *Lancet, 2,* 11–14.

ADDITIONAL READING AND RESOURCES

Guo, M. (Ed.). (2014). *Human milk biochemistry and infant formula manufacturing technology.* Cambridge, UK: Woodhead Publishing.

Hanson, L. A. (2004). *Immunobiology of human milk: How breastfeeding protects babies.* Amarillo, TX: Hale Publishing.

Health Policy Advocacy. (2012). At what cost: When profits are put before mothers and babies [Online video]. Retrieved from http://vimeo.com/54697462

Institute of Medicine. (2004). *Infant formula: Evaluating the safety of new ingredients.* Washington, D.C.: The National Academies Text. Available from http://books.nap.edu/catalog/10935.html or http://www.nap.edu

Kent, G. (2011). *Regulating infant formula.* Amarillo, TX: Hale Publishing.

Wagner, C. L., Taylor, S. N., & Hollis, B. W. (2010). *New insights into vitamin D during pregnancy, lactation and early infancy.* Amarillo, TX: Hale Publishing.

Zibadi, S., Watson, R. R., & Preedy, V. R. (Eds.). (2013). *Handbook of dietary and nutritional aspects of human breast milk.* Wageningen, Netherlands: Wageningen Academic Publishers.

Appendix 1-1

Summary Interventions Based on the Biospecificity of Breastmilk

1. Promote breastfeeding as the normal and best way to feed an infant.
   - Educate parents regarding:
     - The components of breastmilk and formula. Remind them that the two are not the same and that health and developmental outcomes can be different.
     - Defense factors in breastmilk. Explain that these factors protect the infant from acute and chronic diseases, resulting in fewer days of missed work. Formula cannot duplicate the health-protective factors in human milk and increases the risk of acute and chronic disease, autoimmune disease, and conditions such as overweight, obesity, asthma, and diabetes.
   - Inform parents of the developmental and cognitive differences when infants are fed formula, such as lower IQ scores and poorer school performance.
   - Assist parents to critically evaluate infant formula marketing by helping them understand that formula is not equivalent to human milk.
2. Keep mother and baby together during their hospital stay.
   - If separated, have the mother spend time in the baby's environment (nursery, special care).
3. Avoid giving the baby infant formula in the hospital or before gut closure occurs.
   - In breastfed infants at risk, hypoallergenic formulas can be used to supplement breastfeeding if medically necessary and mother's own milk or banked donor milk is not available.
4. Ensure 8–12 feedings each 24 hours, starting in the hospital.
5. Teach and assess proper positioning, latch, and milk transfer.
   - Document swallowing and ensure that the mother knows when her baby is swallowing milk.
   - If a baby is latched but not swallowing adequately, have the mother use alternate massage (massage and compress the breast during pauses between sucking bursts) to sustain sucking and swallowing.
6. Avoid using sterile water or dextrose water. If used, chart the amount and reason for use.
   - Educate the parents and extended family regarding the hazard of giving young breastfed infants bottles of water, even in hot weather.

- Avoid placing water bottles in the infant's bassinet in the hospital.
- Remind mothers that babies also nurse at the breast for thirst, frequently coming off the breast after only a few minutes of nursing.

7. Mothers do not need excessive amounts of water and simply need to drink to quench thirst.
    - Maternal consumption of water in excess of thirst does not increase milk supply and can decrease milk production.
8. Teach mothers to allow the baby to finish the first side before switching to the second breast.
    - For infants experiencing slow weight gain, mothers can be guided to finish the first side using alternate massage before offering the second side and to shorten the intervals between daytime feeds to increase the fat content of the milk.
    - When breastmilk is stored in the refrigerator or freezer, the fat rises to the top of the container; it can be skimmed off and given to slow gaining or preterm infants for extra calories.
    - Avoid vigorously shaking stored breastmilk to redistribute the fat layer. Doing so can damage some of the cellular components and inject air into the milk.
    - Infants whose mothers smoke need to be carefully monitored and to have frequent weight checks.
9. Prenatally, help parents understand the importance of exclusive breastfeeding for about 6 months, especially those with a family history of allergies and diabetes.
10. Reassure parents that it is uncommon for infant fussiness to be related to lactose intolerance. Primary lactose intolerance (lactase deficiency) is extremely rare.
11. Lactating mothers rarely need supplemental vitamins and minerals.
    - Fluoride supplementation is no longer recommended for infants younger than 6 months of age and only thereafter for infants living in communities with suboptimally fluoridated water supplies.
    - Mothers can maintain good vitamin D status by consuming vitamin D–fortified food and through exposure to sunlight. If mothers are vitamin D deficient, vitamin D supplements can be taken to raise their levels and the vitamin D levels in their milk.
    - Child care providers should be instructed to take infants outside for short periods each day.
        - Breastfed infants require 30 minutes of exposure to sunlight each week if wearing only a diaper or 2 hours per week if fully clothed without a hat to maintain normal vitamin D levels. Darkly pigmented infants require a greater exposure to sunshine to initiate the synthesis of vitamin D in the skin. Some infants may require additional vitamin D supplements, especially if they are dark skinned, experience reduced sunlight exposure, or demonstrate signs of suboptimal vitamin D intake.
        - Vegetarian mothers may either need a vitamin B_{12} supplement or consultation regarding acceptable food sources of this vitamin in their diet.
12. Adding solid foods or infant formula before about 6 months of age may interfere with iron uptake in the breastfed infant and saturate the iron-binding capacity of lactoferrin, increasing the risk of GI disease.

13. Some commercially available bottled baby water contains added fluoride. Parents should be advised that breastfed infants do not require additional water or fluoride and to check with their primary healthcare provider about the safety of products advertised for young infants.
14. Microwaving bottles of expressed breastmilk can interfere with the disease-protective factors in breastmilk and poses an injury hazard to the infant. Advise parents to place the bottle of expressed breastmilk under warm running water or in a bowl of warm water.
15. Human milk can be safely stored under appropriate conditions.

Appendix 1-2

Human Milk Banks in North America

UNITED STATES

Alabama
Mother's Milk Bank of Alabama
107 Walter Davis Dr.
Birmingham, AL 35209
Phone: (205) 942-8911
Website: http://www.mmbal.org

California
Mothers' Milk Bank
751 South Bascom Ave.
San Jose, CA 95128
Phone: (408) 998-4550
Fax: (408) 297-9208
Website: http://www.mothersmilk.org
Email: donate@mothersmilk.org

Colorado
Mothers' Milk Bank, a program of Rocky Mountain Children's Health Foundation
394 Marshall St, Suite 400
Arvada, CO 80002
Phone: (303) 869-1888
Website: http://rmchildren.org/mothers-milk-bank
Email: mothersmilkbank@rmchildren.org

Florida
Mothers' Milk Bank of Florida
8669 Commodity Circle
Suite 490
Orlando, FL 32819
Phone: (407) 248-5050
Email: info@milkbankofflorida.org

Illinois
Mothers' Milk Bank of the Western Great Lakes
1691 Elmhurst Road
Elk Grove Village, IL 60007
Phone: (847) 262-5134
Website: http://www.milkbankwgl.org
Email: info@milkbankwgl.org

Indiana
The Milk Bank
5060 E. 62nd Street, Suite 128
Indianapolis, IN 46220
Phone: (317) 536-1670
Toll-free: (877) 829-7470
Fax: (317) 536-1676
Website: http://www.themilkbank.org
Email: info@themilkbank.org

Iowa
Mother's Milk Bank of Iowa
Department of Food and Nutrition Services
University of Iowa Hospitals and Clinics
University of Iowa at Liberty Square

119 2nd Street, Suite 400
Coralville, IA 52241
Phone: (319) 384-9929
Website: http://www.uichildrens.org/mothers-milk-bank
Email: jean-drulis@uiowa.edu

Michigan
Bronson Mothers' Milk Bank
601 John Street, Suite N1300
Kalamazoo, MI 49007
Phone: (269) 341-6146
Fax: (269) 341-8365
Website: http://www.bronsonhealth.com
Email: Duffc@bronsonhg.org

Mississippi
Mothers' Milk Bank of Mississippi
2001 Airport Road, Suite 204
Flowood, MS 39232
Phone: (601) 939-6555
Website: http://www.msmilkbank.org

Missouri
Heart of America Mothers' Milk Bank at
St. Luke's Hospital
4401 Wornail Rd.
Kansas City, MO 64111
Phone: (816) 932-4888
Website: http://www.stlukeshealthsystem.org
Email: kcmilkbank@saint-lukes.org

Montana
Mothers' Milk Bank of Montana
734 Kensington Ave.
Missoula, MT 59801
Phone: (406) 529-2749
Email: mothersmilkbankofmt@yahoo.com

New England
Mothers' Milk Bank of Northeast
377 Elliot St.
Newton Upper Falls, MA 02464
Phone: (617) 527-6263
Website: http://www.milkbankne.org
Email: info@milkbankne.org

North Carolina
WakeMed Mothers' Milk Bank and
Lactation Center
3000 New Bern Ave.
Raleigh, NC 27610
Phone: (919) 350-8599
Website: http://www.wakemed.org/
Email: mothersmilkbank@wakemed.org

Ohio
Ohio Health Mothers' Milk Bank
4850 E. Main St.
Columbus, OH 43213
Phone: (614) 566-0630
Website: http://www.ohiohealth.com
Email: helen.harding@ohiohealth.com

Oklahoma
Oklahoma Mothers' Milk Bank Inc.
901 N. Lincoln Blvd., Suite #330
Oklahoma City, OK 73104
Phone: (405) 297-LOVE
Website: http://www.okmilkbank.org
Email: becky@okmilkbank.org

Oregon
Northwest Mothers Milk Bank
417 SW 117th Ave, Suite #105
Portland, OR 97225
Phone: (503) 469-0955
Email: joanne@nwmmb.org

Pennsylvania
CHOP Mothers' Milk Bank
34th and Civic Center Blvd.
Philadelphia, PA 19104
Email: CHOPmmb@email.chop.edu

South Carolina
Mothers' Milk Bank of South Carolina
Charleston, South Carolina
To find a depot site near you, please contact:
Ann Harvey Shrum, Milk Bank Coordinator
Director Email: Frampton@musc.edu
Phone: (843) 792-5415
Email: scmilkbank@musc.edu

Texas
Mothers' Milk Bank at Austin
2911 Medical Arts St., Suite 12
Austin, TX 78705
Phone: (512) 494-0800
Toll-free: (877) 813-MILK (6455)
Website: http://www.milkbank.org
Email: info@milkbank.org

Mothers' Milk Bank of North Texas
600 West Magnolia Ave
Ft. Worth, TX 76104
Phone: (817) 810-0071
Toll-free: (866) 810-0071
Website: http://www.texasmilkbank.org
Email: info@TexasMilkBank.org

Virginia
The King's Daughters Milk Bank
The Children's Hospital of the King's Daughters
400 Gresham Dr., Suite 410
Norfolk, VA 23507
Phone: (757) 668-6455
Email: Kdmilkbank@chkd.org

CANADA

Alberta
NorthernStar Mothers Milk Bank
103-10333 Southport Rd. S.W.
Calgary, Alberta T2W 3X6
Phone: (403) 475-6455
Fax: (888) 334-4372
Website: http://northernstarmilkbank.ca/
Email: contact@northernstarmilkbank.ca

British Columbia
BC Women's Provincial Milk Bank
BCW Lactation Services
1U 50-4450 Oak St.
Vancouver, BC V6H 3N1
Phone: (604) 875-2282
Website: http://www.bcwomensmilkbank.ca
Email: fjones@cw.bc.ca

Ontario
Rogers Hixon Ontario Human Milk Bank
Mount Sinai Hospital
600 University Avenue
Toronto, Ontario, Canada M5G 1X5
Phone: (416) 586-4800 x 3053
Website: http://www.milkbankontario.ca
Email: info@milkbankontario.ca

Chapter 2

Influence of the Maternal Anatomy and Physiology on Lactation

INTRODUCTION

The mammary gland, or breast, and its ability to produce milk for the young of a species are one of the common links among all mammals. The breast grows and develops over time, as it is not a fully functional organ at birth. It reaches its full functional capacity during pregnancy and childbirth. The breast performs through an elegant interplay occurring among all of the body's systems, and changes its composition, function, and architecture over time with mediation from marked changes in gene expression. There is a typical progression of growth and development, sometimes with deviations that may affect either the breast's ability to synthesize milk or the infant's ability to remove it. Breast development first occurs in several stages during the embryonic and fetal periods. Prenatal breast developmental stages can be described using gestational week or the 10 stages relative to embryonic and fetal length (**Table 2-1**).

Small amounts of milk secretion (colostrum) are present in the breasts of the newborn under the influence of circulating maternal hormones. This secretion, which is referred to as "witch's milk," ceases once the maternal hormones have cleared the infant's system, usually within 3–4 weeks. The lactiferous ducts communicate with a small depression known as the mammary pit. This depression later elevates, forming the nipple and areola. A true inverted nipple occurs because of the failure of the pit to elevate.

Usually, one pair of glands develops along each milk line; when fully developed they lie between the second and sixth rib arches. However, accessory or supernumerary nipples and breast tissue can develop anywhere along the milk lines (**Figure 2-1**). The prevalence of accessory nipples is approximately 2–10%, with white Europeans and black Americans having frequencies of 0.2% and 1.6%, respectively, and Jewish women, 2.5% (Mathes, Seyfer, & Miranda, 2006). Approximately 20% of ectopic breast tissue occurs in the axillae (Surajit, Basanti, & Basanti, 2007) and results when the mammary ridge fails to resolve during embryonic development. These extra nipples and breast tissue occasionally swell and secrete milk during lactogenesis II. Although the enlargement and activity of accessory breast tissue and nipples have no physiological significance, they do have the potential to significantly grow during pregnancy and lactation and become painful or make breastfeeding awkward. No special management is necessary, but if axillary tissue becomes significantly enlarged and painful, warm compresses may provide symptomatic relief. Some ectopic tissue may be differentiated enough to actually secrete milk. Faridi and Dewan (2008)

Table 2-1 Stages of Fetal Breast Development

Stage by Fetal Length	Stage by Gestational Age
1: Ridge stage—embryo less than 5 mm	5–6 wk; milk line appears (ectodermal ridge)
2: Milk hill stage-embryo more than 5.5 mm	7–8 wk; mammary disc appears; primitive blood vessels form
3: Mammary disc stage—embryo 10–11 mm	10–12 wk; epithelial buds form
4: Lobule-type stage—embryo 11.0–25.0 mm	12–16 wk; smooth musculature of areola and nipple are formed
5: Cone stage—embryo 25–30 mm	16 wk; vascular system completely formed
6: Budding stage—embryo 30–68 mm	13–20 wk; parenchymal branching
7: Indentation stage—embryo 68 mm to 10 cm	20 wk; 15–20 ductal structures formed
8: Branching stage—fetus 10 cm	32 wk; canalization forms primary milk ducts
9: Canalization stage—20–32 wk gestation	32 wk to term; lobulo-alveolar development; increased periductal stroma; lobules show single layer of epithelium
10: End-vesicle stage with vesicles composed of a single layer of epithelium and containing colostrum	

Data from Russo, J., & Russo, I. H. (2004). Development of the human breast. *Maturitas, 49*, 2–15; Geddes, D. T. (2007). Gross anatomy of the lactating breast. In T. W. Hale & P. E. Hartmann (Eds.), *Textbook of human lactation* (Ch. 2, pp. 19–34). Amarillo, TX: Hale Publishing.

reported a mother who chose to express milk from ectopic tissue in the axilla, but most mothers simply allow the tissue to involute and do not remove milk. Breast development during childhood is a quiescent period of time with mammary growth simply reflecting general body growth.

Puberty

Hormones such as estrogen and growth hormone stimulate the growth of mammary ducts, whereas progesterone secreted by the ovary results in modest lobular–alveolar development. About 11 alveolar buds form in clusters around each terminal duct to create a lobule. The areola enlarges and darkens, and the breasts increase to the adult size, mostly through the deposition of adipose tissue. Each ovulatory or menstrual cycle facilitates a little more mammary development that continues until about age 35.

Pregnancy

The breast completes the majority of its growth and maturation during pregnancy under the influence of a number of hormones such as progesterone, prolactin, human placental lactogen, growth hormone, and insulin-like growth factor. By 16–20 weeks of gestation, the breast is capable of secreting its first milk: colostrum. Lactose appears in the blood and urine, heralding the stage called lactogenesis I. Preterm delivery (< 28 weeks of gestation) interrupts the development of the breast but does not preclude breastfeeding. Mothers delivering very preterm infants may see a delay in lactogenesis II, the onset of copious milk production, and experience diminished amounts of milk in the early week or two postpartum. Note that breast growth and accompanying change in the size of the breasts varies greatly from woman to woman. The greatest rate of breast growth usually occurs during the first 5 months of pregnancy, but such growth can also occur gradually throughout the entire pregnancy. The increase in breast volume can range from 12 to 227 mL. Some women, however, experience minimal breast enlargement during pregnancy, defined by Neifert et al. (1990) as an increase of less than one cup size. Breast size achieved during pregnancy does not reliably indicate lactation potential, as it does not account for the volume of active secretory tissue present in the breast.

No relationship has been found between breast growth in pregnancy and milk production at 1 month in mothers breastfeeding as frequently as desired or needed (Cox, Kent, Casey, Owens, & Hartmann, 1999). Indeed, the human mammary glands may have the ability to increase secretory tissue during lactation in response to increased demand for milk. Hytten (1954) reported that the breast volume of one mother who reported no breast growth during pregnancy rose 160% by the 7th day postpartum. Irrespective of the size of their breasts before pregnancy, an increase in size of up to 200 mL or one bra cup size during pregnancy or the first month postpartum usually indicates sufficient secretory tissue proliferation for ample milk production (Czank, Henderson, Kent, Lai, & Hartmann, 2007). Russo and Russo (2004) discussed the effects that breast changes during pregnancy have on increasing the protectiveness against breast cancer. They postulate that the mammary gland's differentiation activates specific genes that imprint the breast epithelia to subsequent hormonal milieu, providing protection against neoplastic changes. It has been suggested that longer breastfeeding duration facilitates the depletion of stem/progenitor populations, with proliferative capacity reducing the risk for developing aggressive forms of breast cancer (Hassiotou & Geddes, 2013).

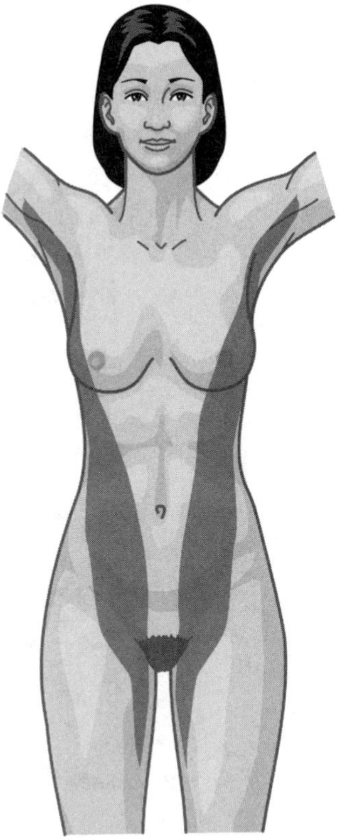

Figure 2-1 Areas for possible accessory breast/nipple tissue growth.

It is not unusual for a woman to have breasts that are slightly different in size and shape from each other. About one in five women have breasts that differ in volume by more than 25% (Loughry et al., 1989).

Breast size is generally not related to overall milk-making capacity. Nevertheless, breasts that are significantly asymmetrical, tubular, or cone shaped may be at a higher risk for producing insufficient milk. Breast abnormalities that could be predictive of insufficient milk-making capacity include those in the hypoplastic (underdevelopment) categories described by Heimburg, Exner, Kruft, and Lemperle (1996) and adapted by Huggins, Petok, and Mireles (2000) into four breast types of concern (**Figure 2-2**):

- Type 1: round breasts, no hypoplasia in the lower medial or lateral quadrants
- Type 2: hypoplasia of the lower medial quadrant
- Type 3: hypoplasia of both the lower medial and the lateral quadrants
- Type 4: severe constriction with a minimal breast base

Other aspects of concern include breasts with exceptionally large areolas relative to the size of the breast, herniation of breast tissue into the nipple–areolar complex, marked asymmetry of the breast, hypoplastic breasts that point down and sideways, and an intramammary distance of more than 1.5 inches (indicating medial breast hypoplasia). The aesthetic and plastic surgery literature describes

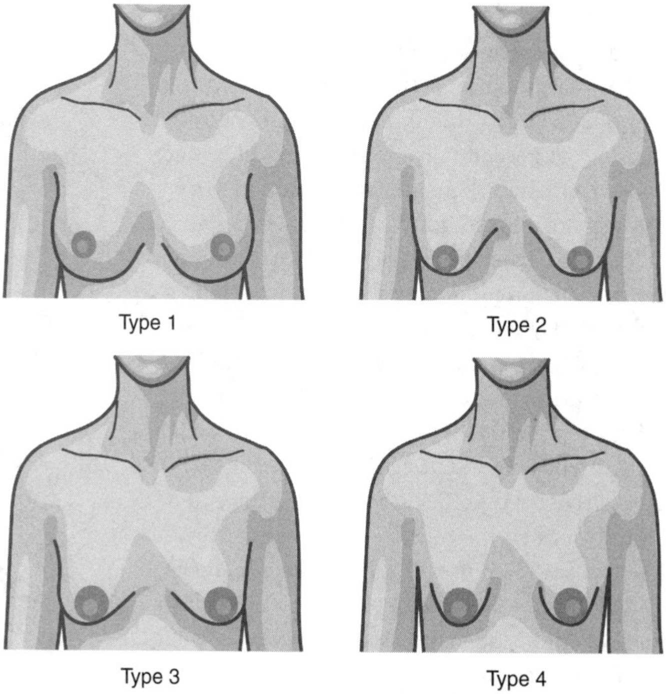

Figure 2-2 Breast classifications.

four classifications of tuberous breasts (**Table 2-2**), which range from mild hypoplasia of the inferior medial quadrant of the breast to major hypoplasia of all four quadrants, with varying degrees of tissue herniation into the areola, areolar enlargement, and breast asymmetry. Costagliola, Atiyeh, and Rampillon (2013) propose an explanation for these differences, whereby hormonal influences on the breast result in thrusting forces with both horizontal (estrogen) and vertical (progesterone) vectors that fall out of balance and result in a tuberous breast anomaly. The anomaly consists of a dermal (skin) weakness of the nipple–areolar complex. The main anomaly in a tuberous breast is the underlying abnormality in the quality of the skin of the areola, with a deficiency of areolar fascial support being noted. Enlarging breast tissue at puberty pushes through the area of weakness and causes stretching of the areolar skin. If the gland grows rapidly, it does not have time to spread radially and instead develops anteriorly, further expanding the areolar skin and herniating into the areola.

In a study of 34 women with varying types of hypoplastic breasts, most women produced less than 50% of the milk necessary for their infants during the first week postpartum. Many reported little to no growth during pregnancy, with a finding that the more severe the hypoplasia, the poorer the milk production in the first week postpartum (Huggins et al., 2000).Women with mammary hypoplasia may have normal hormonal levels and innervation but are lacking sufficient glandular tissue, increasing their risk of insufficient milk supply (Arbour & Kessler, 2013). It is important that clinicians identify this condition by visual and tactile examination of the breasts, either prenatally or immediately following delivery, so as to initiate suitable interventions early in the course of lactation (Duran & Spatz, 2011).

Table 2-2 Classification of Tuberous Breasts

Von Heimburg	Grolleau		Costagliola et al.
		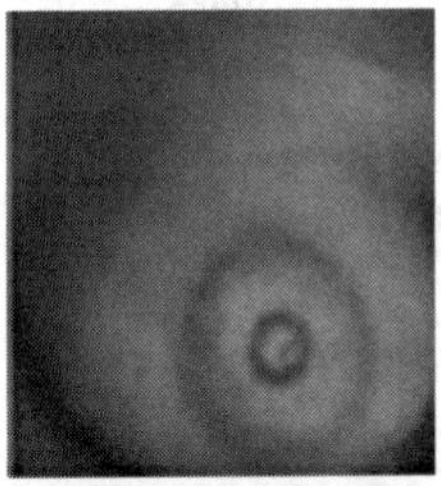 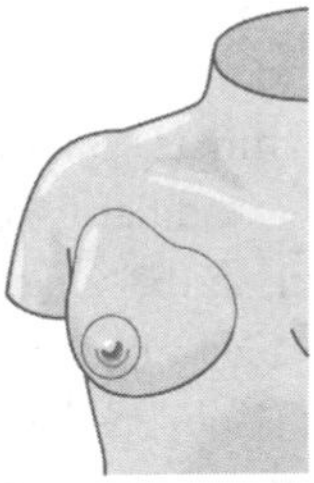	Type 0: normal mammary base; isolated areolar complex herniation sometimes intermittent
Type I: hypoplasia of the lower medial quadrant	Type I: defect of inferior medial part of mammary base; S italics aspect	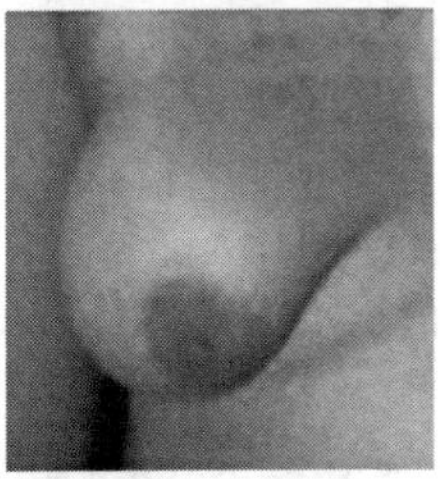 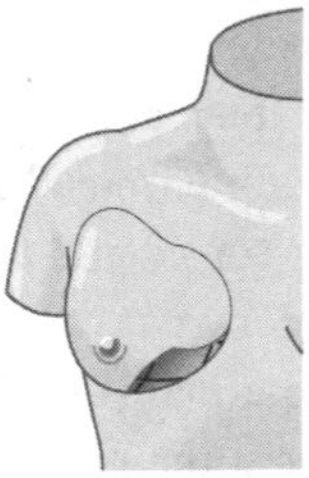	Type I: defect of inferior medial part of mammary base. S italics aspect
Type II: hypoplasia of the lower medial and lateral quadrants, sufficient skin in the subareolar region Type III: hypoplasia of the lower medial and lateral quadrants, deficiency of skin in the subareolar	Type II: defect of lower pole	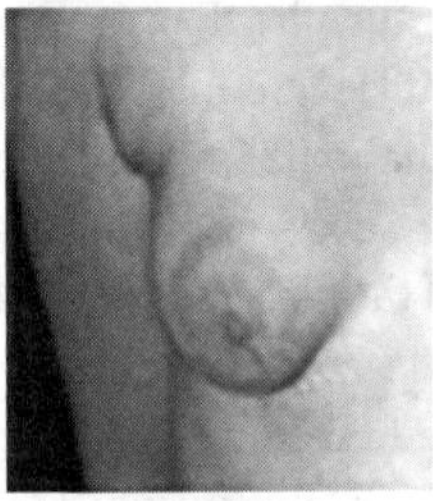 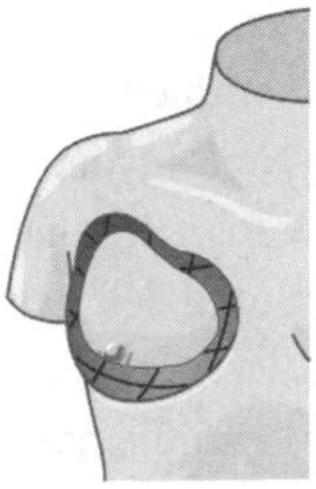	Type II: defect of lower pole
Type IV: severe breast constriction, minimal breast base	Type III: defect of total base. Extremely narrow-based breast. Tubular Snoopy deformity.	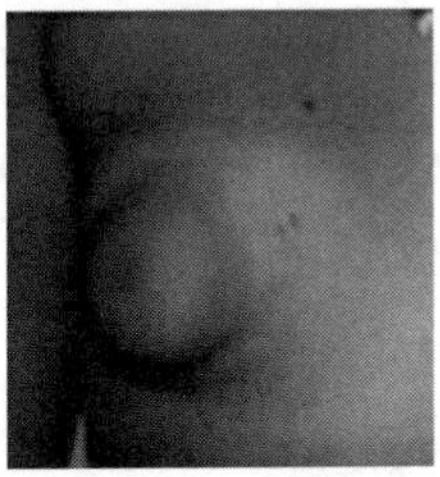 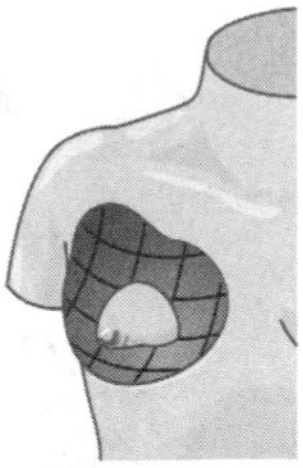	Type III: defect of total base, extremely narrow-based breast. Tubular Snoopy deformity.

Reproduced from Costagliola, M., Atiyeh, B., & Rampillon, F. (2013). Tuberous breast: Revised classification and a new hypothesis for its development. *Aesthetic Plastic Surgery, 37*, 896–903.

FUNCTIONAL ANATOMY OF THE BREAST

Breast imaging modalities have improved over recent years and are providing new insights and data on the inner workings of the mammary glands (Geddes, 2009). The breast is composed of glandular tissue, embedded in fatty tissue (the fatty patterns in the breast vary from woman to woman), and is supported by fibrous connective tissue and suspensory ligaments (Cooper's ligaments) (**Figure 2-3**). Some mammary glandular tissue projects into the axilla (tail of Spence) and is connected to the normal duct system. A large proportion of the glandular tissue is located at a 30-mm (1.18-inch) radius from the base of the nipple, with the breast being considered as a tree-shaped mass transfer structure (Mortazavi, Geddes, Hassioutou, & Hassanipour, 2014). Approximately 5–10 or so main ducts branch and extend from the nipple in a complex and intertwined pattern. Lobules extend from these ducts; they are composed of branching ductules that terminate in alveolar clusters. The alveolus, the milk-secreting unit, is lined with alveolar milk-secreting epithelial cells surrounded by supporting structures, a rich vascular supply, and myoepithelial cells. Although the size and number of alveolar units increase during pregnancy, the high circulating levels of estrogen and progesterone during pregnancy suppress most alveolar function until delivery of the placenta. Relatively large gaps exist between the milk-secreting cells during the first 4 days postpartum, enhancing the passage into milk of components such as immunoglobulins, cells such as lymphocytes and macrophages, and most drugs (**Figure 2-4**). After this time, the alveolar cells swell under the influence of prolactin, which closes these gaps. As a consequence, drug entry into milk may occur more readily during the early days until these gaps close.

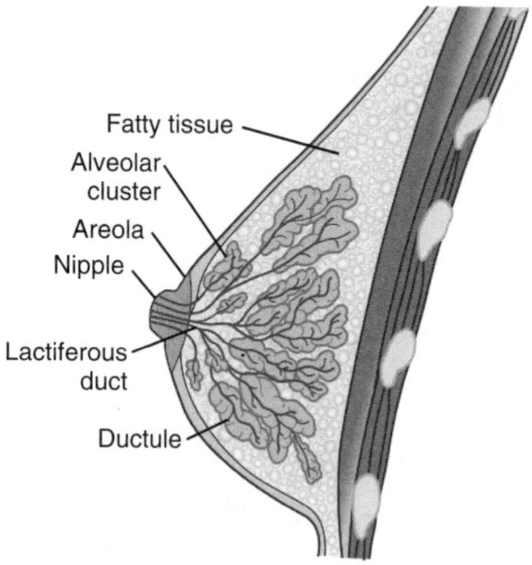

Figure 2-3 Side view of lactating breast.

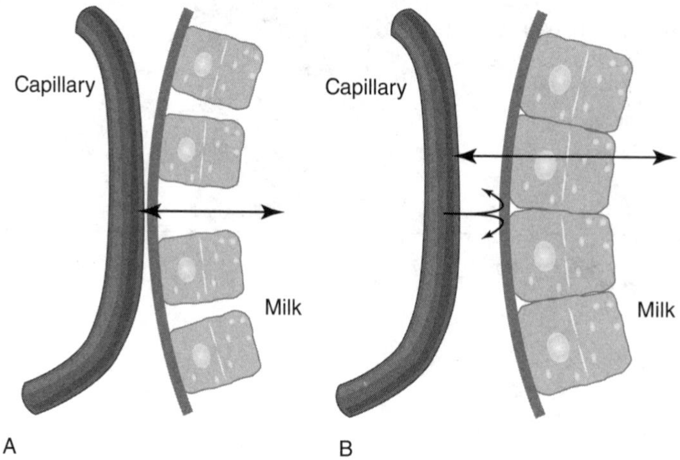

Figure 2-4 Alveolar cell gaps as a function of days postpartum.

Myoepithelial cells are smooth muscle contractile cells responsible for ejecting milk into the ductules under the influence of the hormone oxytocin (known as the milk ejection reflex or the letdown reflex). Ducts can be as small as 2 mm or less in diameter, tend to be superficial, and are easily compressed (Geddes, 2007b). Under ultrasound, an average 79% increase in duct diameter can be shown when milk ejection occurs, usually within 54 seconds after the infant goes to breast (Hartmann, 2000).

The nipple sits in the center of the areola and contains many nerve fiber endings, 5–10 main milk ducts and 10–15 other pores, smooth muscle fibers, and a rich blood supply. Most investigations have shown between 17 and 27 ducts within the nipple and 5 to 9 orifices or actual openings at the tip (Going & Moffat, 2004; Taneri et al., 2006). Although older textbooks describe 15–25 ductal openings on the nipple, direct observation, three-dimensional modeling, ultrasound, ductography, and actual dissections of the nipple have helped clarify its internal structure (Geddes, 2007a). Five to 10 true mammary or lactiferous ducts transport milk from the lobules they drain (Going & Moffat, 2004; Love & Barsky, 2004; Ramsay, Kent, Hartmann, & Hartmann, 2005) to the nipple tip, even though there are many more ducts within the nipple. This finding is in agreement with the classic work on breast anatomy conducted by Sir Astley Cooper in 1840 (Cooper, 1840) showing 7–12 patent nipple ducts in cadaver dissections (**Figure 2-5**). Rusby, Brachtel, Michaelson, Koerner, and Smith (2007) found a mean of 24 ducts within sectioned nipples with a range of 5–50 ducts. Although Ramsay et al. (2005) found approximately nine ducts in the nipple, it must be remembered that ultrasound cannot identify ducts of less than 0.5 mm.

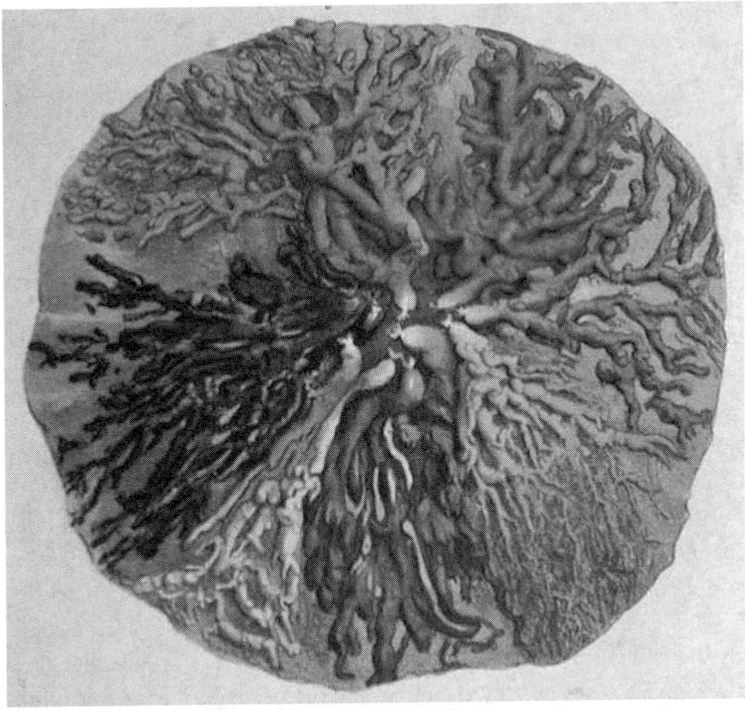

Figure 2-5 Wax-injected ductal system in cadaver dissection.

Cooper, A. P. (1840). *Anatomy of the breast*. London, UK: Longman, Orme, Green, Browne, and Longmans.

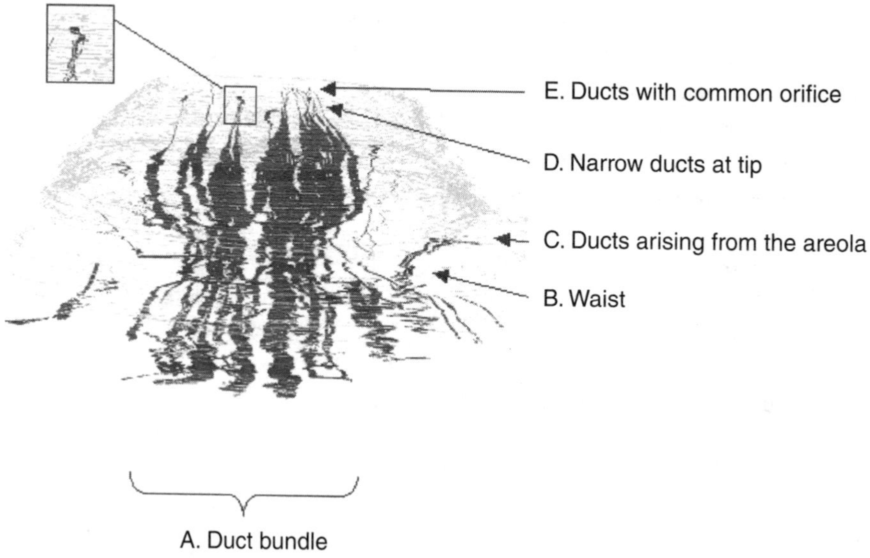

Figure 2-6 Pattern of ducts within the nipple. The ducts are arranged in a central bundle. The bundle narrows to a waist just beneath the skin. Some ducts originate on the areola or part way up the nipple. Most ducts narrow as they approach the tip of the nipple. Many of the ducts originate from a few clefts.
Rusby, J. E., Brachtel, E. F., Michaelson, J. S., Koerner, F. C., & Smith, B. L. (2007). Breast duct anatomy in the human nipple: Three-dimensional patterns and clinical applications. *Breast Cancer Research and Treatment, 106*, 171–179.

Jutte, Hohoff, Sauerland, Wiechmann, and Stamm (2014) designed a study intended to provide clinical identification of milk duct orifices under direct observation during manual milk expression. During manual expression, an average of 3.9 ductal orifices per nipple were identified by milk exiting the orifices. A mean of 4.2 ductal orifices were seen in the right nipple of mothers of boys, compared with a mean of 3.5 ductal orifices in the right nipple of mothers of girls. The study did not determine whether the same ductal orifices were active each time milk was expressed or whether other ductal orifices had milk exiting them at differing times.

Several ducts can arise from the same cleft in the nipple tip, accounting for the discrepancy between the number of ducts in the nipple and the number of openings that can be counted externally. The shared opening of multiple ducts on the surface of the nipple tip can be seen in **Figure 2-6**. There is usually a group of central orifices with peripheral ductal openings surrounding the central openings in a somewhat concentric pattern. Rusby et al. (2007) described the spatial arrangement of ducts within the nipple. Most ducts are arranged in a central bundle that narrows to a "waist" approximately 2 mm beneath the skin (**Figure 2-7**). This central bundle occupies 21–67% of the cross-sectional area of the nipple. Multiple ducts may branch and end within the nipple, whereas others end as lobular tissue or as a blind-ending sinus. Other ducts originate at the base of the nipple and on the areola and are morphologically different from the ducts within the central bundle. At 1 and 1.5 mm beneath the tip of the nipple, the average duct

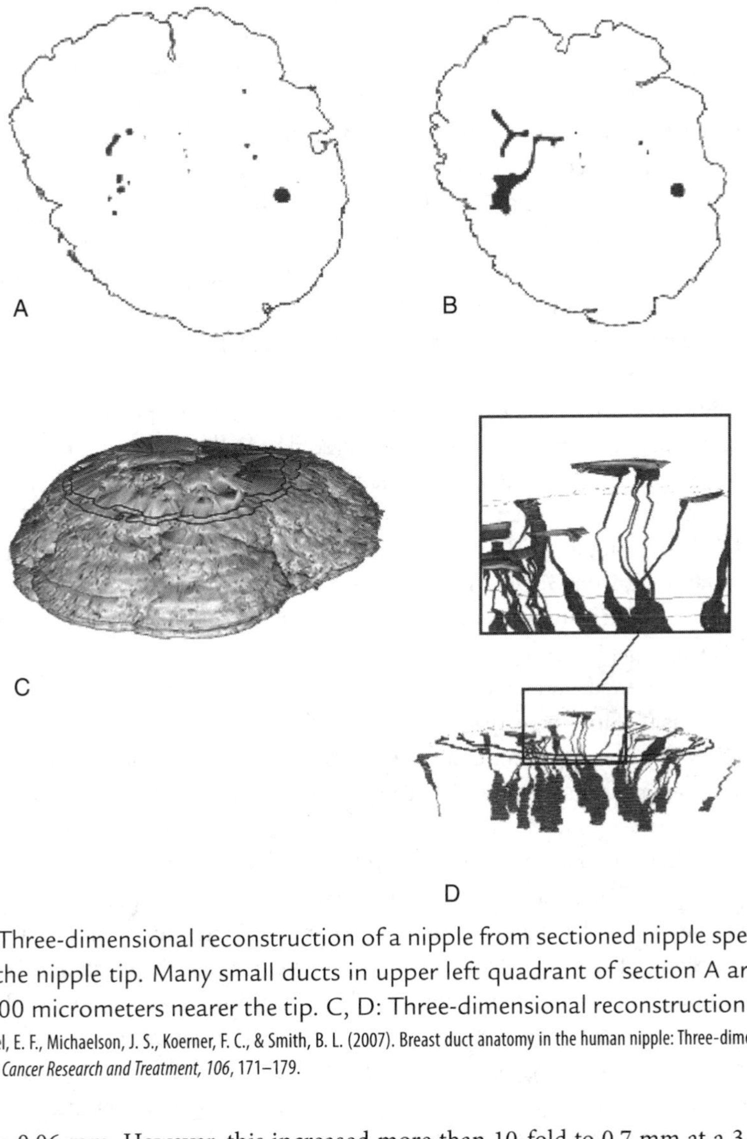

Figure 2-7 Three-dimensional reconstruction of a nipple from sectioned nipple specimens. A, B: Two sections of the nipple tip. Many small ducts in upper left quadrant of section A arise from a cleft in section B, 100 micrometers nearer the tip. C, D: Three-dimensional reconstruction of a nipple tip.
Rusby, J. E., Brachtel, E. F., Michaelson, J. S., Koerner, F. C., & Smith, B. L. (2007). Breast duct anatomy in the human nipple: Three-dimensional patterns and clinical applications. *Breast Cancer Research and Treatment, 106*, 171–179.

diameter was 0.06 mm. However, this increased more than 10-fold to 0.7 mm at a 3-mm depth. There was no relationship between the size of the duct and whether it ended within the nipple or passed deeper into the breast. The other types often disappear into a skin appendage and are most likely tubercles, tubes, sebaceous (oil-secreting) gland orifices, and sweat gland openings that lie superficial to the areola but do not communicate with the milk-secreting and transporting apparatus. Duct diameters greater than 2–3 mm are considered enlarged and may indicate ductal ectasia or mastalgia, but ductal diameters can range from 0.6 to 4.4 mm with no evidence of pathology (Ballesio et al., 2007; Peters, Diemer, Mecks, & Behnken, 2003; Tedeschi, Ahari, & Byrne, 1963).

Milk ducts at the base of the nipple are very superficial and easily compressed. Their depth ranges from 0.7 to 7.9 mm. This anatomic feature may be of importance, as excessive compression or compression applied incorrectly may occlude these ducts, impeding the flow of milk out of the nipple. Proper latch and sucking become important for clinicians to monitor, as does the fit of the shield or flange on a breast pump to avoid excessive pressure on the superficial ductwork of the nipple. Ducts are not always arranged symmetrically and their course is often erratic.

Under ultrasound examination, Ramsay et al. (2005) were unable to visualize the commonly described lactiferous sinus or dilated sac under the areola. Because the internal workings of the breast are dynamic, the frequently drawn "lactiferous sinus" could possibly be attributed to graphic renderings of a dilated duct immediately below the areola after a milk ejection or the convergence and branching of two ducts. Using three-dimensional ultrasound scanning, Gooding, Finlay, Shipley, Halliwell, and Duck (2010) confirmed the absence of "milk sinuses" or any sac-like features behind the areola. Their scans showed no sacs, but the widening of a duct in the nipple generally occurring after the first branching point.

In one study, nipple length and diameter were measured during the course of pregnancy in 56 Thai mothers. Mothers with a nipple length of greater than or equal to 7 mm were eligible for the study. From early gestation until term, the mean nipple length increased significantly from 9.3 ± 1.5 mm to 11.2 ± 1.8 mm and the mean nipple width increases from 13.6 ± 1.8 mm to 15.9 ± 2.3 mm. The areolar width increased substantially, from 37.9 ± 8.9 mm to 50.1 ± 10.9 mm. This areolar expansion assists with the property of elasticity that supports the formation of a graspable teat for the infant to latch onto (Thanaboonyawat, Chanprapaph, Lattalapkul, & Rongluen, 2013).

In another study, nipple length and its relation to successful breastfeeding as measured by the LATCH assessment tool were measured in 449 postpartum women on day 1 postpartum. The results showed that a 7-mm nipple length was the cut-off point that gave a 97% success rate of proper latch-on by the infant (Puapornpong, Raungrongmorakot, Paritakul, Ketsuwan, & Wongin, 2013). When latch is successful there is a greater tendency to see a successful breastfeeding experience. In an earlier study of 114 mothers, those with a nipple length of 7 mm or more were 4.38 times more likely to achieve successful breastfeeding, as measured by a score of 7 or greater on the LATCH assessment tool, compared with mothers whose nipples were shorter than 7 mm (Thanaboonyawat, Chanprapaph, Puriyapan, & Lattalapkul, 2012).

Separate ductal systems of varying extent and differing lobe sizes may be present in the same breast quadrant with or without being connected. Ohtake et al. (2001) showed that different lobular systems could be connected to each other (anastomoses between ducts of different lobes) and demonstrated connections within the same lobular system. Going and Moffat (2004) described an autopsied breast through the use of 2-mm sections that showed that one main collecting duct and its branches drained up to 23% of the total breast volume, the largest three systems drained 50%, and the largest six systems drained 75% of the breast. They likened the human breast to not one gland but many, with the lobes or ductal systems as separate domains. Some preliminary data indicate that hormone levels differ in different ductal systems, possibly representing diverse microenvironments among various lobes in the same breast (Elia et al., 2002).

Murase and colleagues (2009) showed that milk synthesis differs in each mammary lobe, even within the same breast. The degree of fullness in each mammary lobe seems to play the most important role in determining the fat content of the milk synthesized in each lobe. The protein content in the milk from each mammary lobe is also different and presumably determined by the feedback inhibitor of lactation, accumulated in the corresponding mammary lobe.

The areola is a circular pigmented area that generally enlarges and darkens during pregnancy. The pigments in the nipple and areola are brown eumelanin and to a greater extent pheomelanin (a red pigment). The amount of melanin in the areola and nipple skin, which gives the nipple/areola its darker color, is more than twice that found in surrounding breast skin (Dean et al., 2005). Melanin has many functions, one of which includes helping the skin resist abrasion. There is a wide variation in the size of the nipple–areolar complex among mothers. The mean diameter of the areola is 4 cm (range, 2.0–7.0 cm) (Mathes et al., 2006). In Korean, Chinese, and Japanese women, the diameter of the areola was measured to be between 3.32 cm to 4 cm (Park, Kim, Jo, Lee, & Kim, 2014); in Caucasian women, it was found to be somewhat larger, at 5 cm. The skin of the areola does not contain fat, but does contain smooth muscle and elastic tissues in radial and circular arrangements. Between 1 and 15 Montgomery tubercles or glands become prominent during pregnancy and can secrete substances, including a small amount of milk. The tubercles vary in size and number, with sebaceous glands often emptying near or into the Montgomery gland ducts. Because the glands have a secretory apparatus, they can become inflamed, infected, or obstructed. If mothers present with a red raised bump or fluid-filled blister on the areola, the clinician should check to see if pump flanges, breast shells, topical preparations, or nipple shields are irritating or blocking the glands of Montgomery. These glands are functional during lactation, serving as a communication conduit with the infant through odor, providing protective properties to the areola, and enhancing infant sucking.

Doucet, Soussignan, Sagot, and Schaal (2007) showed that infants behaved differently when presented with a breast covered in a plastic film versus a breast with either the nipple, areola, or whole breast revealed. When exposed to volatile compounds originating in areolar secretions or milk itself, infants demonstrated a delayed onset of crying, stimulation of eye opening, and mouthing behaviors. Infants exposed to the breast covered in a plastic film cried earlier and longer and opened their eyes less. Doucet, Soussignan, Sagot, and Schaal (2009) compared newborn infant responses to odor substrates collected directly from Montgomery glands to infant responses to other substrates, including human milk, vanilla, infant formula, and cow's milk. Presenting odor substrates from Montgomery glands directly under the newborns' noses elicited significantly increased amounts of head turning, lip pursing, and tongue protrusion as well as greater reactivity than any of the other substrates presented in the same manner. The Montgomery gland odor resulted in immediate motor and respiratory responses of high amplitude during the time it was presented compared with all of the other odors, which showed a lower magnitude of responses that were also slower to appear. The volatile compounds from the Montgomery glands readily activated behavioral and autonomic responses in newborns that were similar to behaviors seen when an infant is put to the breast for a feeding. Increased numbers of Montgomery glands have been associated with increased infant weight gain during the first 3 days, improved latching and sucking activity, and a quicker onset of lactation in primiparous women (Schaal, Doucet, Sagot, Hertling, & Soussignan, 2006).

Doucet, Soussignan, Sagot, and Schaal (2012) assessed the areolae of 121 breastfeeding mothers during the first 3 days postpartum. They found that 97% of mothers had identifiable areolar glands, 80.2% had 1–20 glands per areola, and 33% were secreting a visible fluid. Infants of mothers with lower numbers of areolar glands had a lower weight gain than infants of mothers with higher amounts of areolar glands. The onset of copious milk production took longer in mothers with lower counts of areolar glands.

In addition to the important olfactory properties associated with the areola, Schaal and colleagues discussed other attributes of the areola, such as its higher surface temperature compared to the nipple and surrounding breast tissue. This feature is thought to aid in the evaporation of the areolar odorants, enhancing their effectiveness as a chemical attractant to the infant. Areolar temperature elevation is triggered by infant crying, which results in a maximal amount of odor being released when the infant approaches the breast (Vuorenkoski, Wasz-Hockert, Koivisto, & Lind, 1969). The higher temperature of the areola has also been shown to be accompanied by a higher pH and lower elasticity (Zanardo & Straface, 2015). Sebum is a fatty secretion from sebaceous glands and Montgomery tubercles that is thought to act as an odor fixative to stabilize the olfactory mixture of substances formed on the surface of the areola. It may also function as a lubricant to reduce mechanical stress on the nipple/areola and to protect the areolar skin from factors in the infant's saliva that may break down tissue. The increased activity of the areolar glands during pregnancy and lactation may help protect the nipple/areolar epidermis and ductal openings from pathogens.

These studies point to the importance of keeping mothers and infants together skin to skin immediately after birth and during the early days of breastfeeding. This contact allows these odor stimuli to enhance the intake of colostrum and strengthen the maternal/infant bond. When an infant is held skin to skin between the breasts and in close proximity to the nipple–areolar complex, important olfactory feeding and orienting cues are presented to the infant in the early days that would otherwise be missed if the infant were placed in a bassinet. Breast olfactory signals activate oral activity by the infant directed to the nipple and start a cascade of behavioral responses that include neural, neuroendocrine, and endocrine functions in both the infant and the mother.

It is important that these areolar secretions are not washed, wiped off, or masked by topical preparations applied to the nipple/areola in the first few days following birth. Routine application of creams or ointments to the nipples in the early days should be avoided. Such practices may eliminate an important olfactory stimulus necessary to facilitate an optimal start to breastfeeding. Full contact nipple shields might also mask olfactory cues during the early days of infant learning. If a shield is absolutely required during the first few days postpartum, perhaps the cutout version of shield would still allow areolar odors to reach the infant.

When the nipple is stimulated, the muscular fibroelastic system in the nipple and areola contracts, decreasing the surface area of the areola and producing nipple erection. The areola is rich in horizontal muscle fibers and wrinkles during its erection, which reduces its surface area. This response results in the nipple becoming smaller, firmer, and more prominent. Sphincter-like smooth muscles present in the distal ducts prevent milk leakage between feedings (Tezer, Bakkaloglu, Erguven, Bilir, & Kadioglu, 2011).

Nipples vary in size and shape, with some variations carrying the potential for a difficult latch such as those that are flat, inverted, dimpled, bulbous, bifurcated, exceptionally large, or double (**Table 2-3**). In a study of 300 Japanese women (600 breasts), Sanuki, Fukama, and Uchida (2008) classified nipples as type I when the nipple height was greater than the diameter, type II when the nipple height was shorter than the diameter, type III when the nipple was inverted, and type IV when the nipple was of other shapes such as multiple or divided. They also subclassified types I and II according to the location of strictures (**Figure 2-8**). The mean diameter of the nipple was 1.3 cm (range, 0.6–2.3 cm), and the mean height of the

Table 2-3 The Five Basic Types of Nipples

Type of Nipple	Before Stimulation	After Stimulation
The majority of mothers have a **common nipple**. It protrudes slightly when at rest and becomes erect and more graspable when stimulated. A baby has no trouble finding and grasping this nipple to pull in a large amount of breast tissue and stretch it to the roof of his or her mouth.	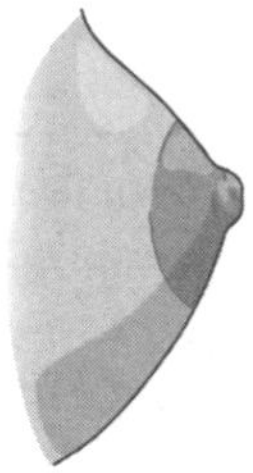	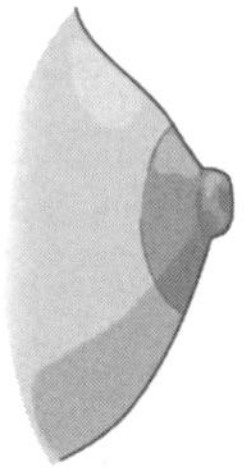
The **flat nipple** has a very short shank that makes it less easy for the baby to find and grasp. In response to stimulation, slight movement inward or outward may be present, but not enough to aid the baby in finding and initially grasping the breast on center.	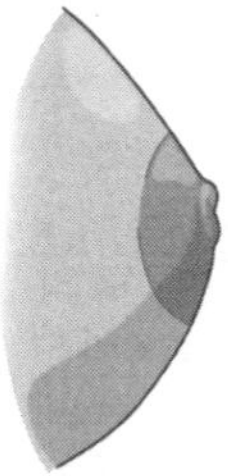	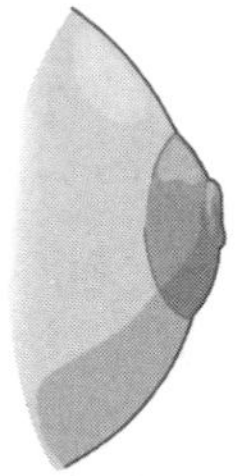
An **inverted-appearing nipple** may appear inverted but becomes erect and easily graspable after stimulation.	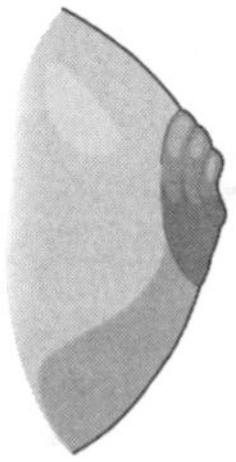	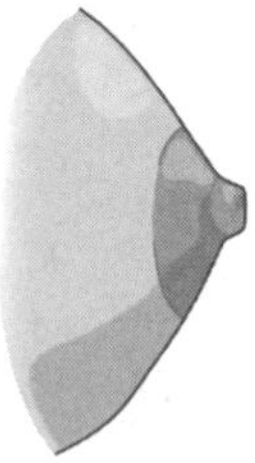
The **retracted nipple** is the most common type of inverted nipple. On stimulation it retracts, making attachment difficult.	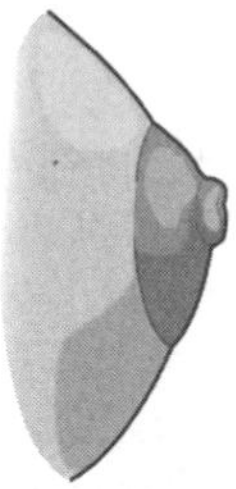	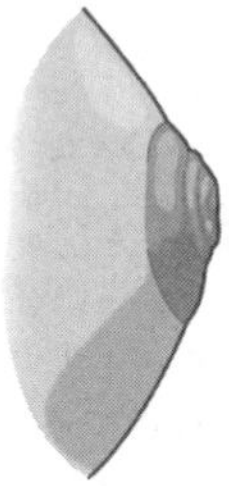
The truly **inverted nipple** is retracted both at rest and when stimulated. Such a nipple is very uncommon and more difficult for the baby to grasp.	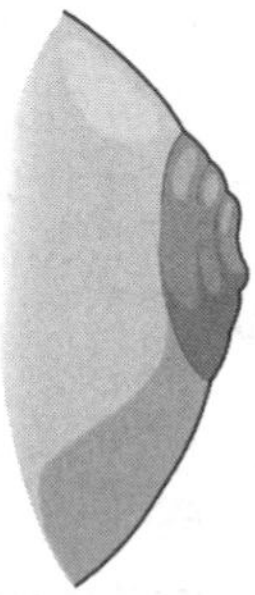	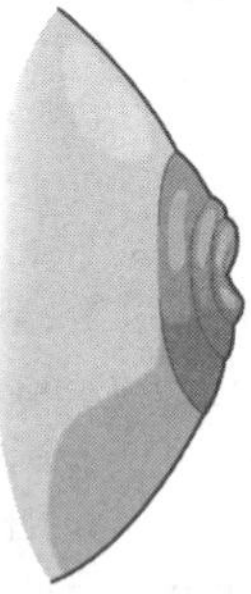

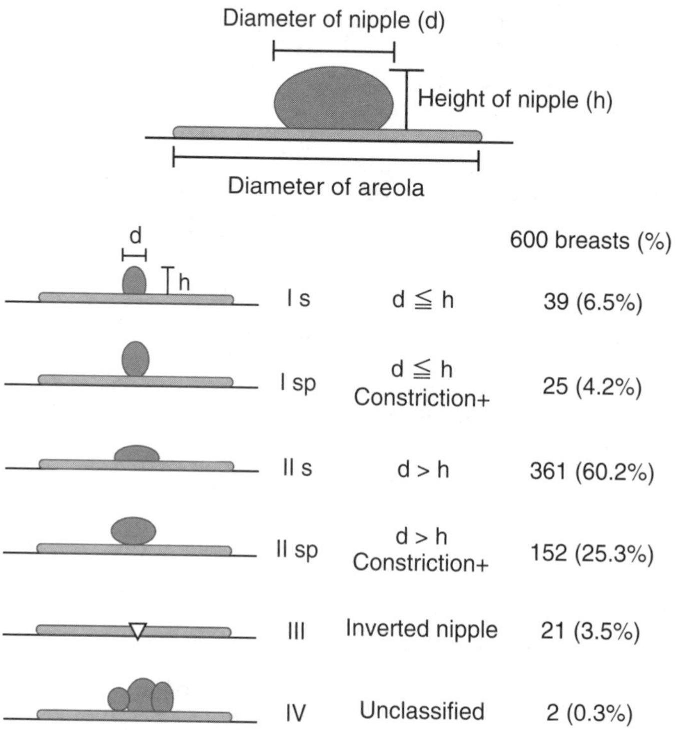

Figure 2-8 Nipple classification system by type.

Reproduced from Sanuki, J., Fukama, E., & Uchida, Y. (2008). Morphologic study of nipple–areola complex in 600 breasts. *Aesthetic Plastic Surgery, 33*, 295–297. doi: 10.1007/s00266-008-9194-y

nipple was 0.9 cm (range, 0–2.0 cm). Type II without constriction was the most common type of nipple (60.2%) followed by type II with constriction (25.3%). Inverted nipples were found in 3.5% of the breasts.

The breast is highly vascular, with 60% of the blood supply carried by the internal mammary artery and about 30% supplied by the lateral thoracic artery. During pregnancy, mammary blood flow increases to double the prepregnancy levels by 24 weeks and remains constant thereafter (Thoresen & Wesche, 1988; Vorherr, 1974). The 24-hour mammary blood flow necessary to produce 1 L of milk is about 400:1. Mammary blood flow, however, is markedly reduced in a breast that is synthesizing relatively small amounts of milk compared with one producing a normal volume (Geddes et al., 2012). Sucking causes an increase in mammary blood flow. Blood flow to the breast decreases by 40–50% just before milk ejection, increasing in the next 1–2 minutes (Janbu, Koss, Thoresen, & Wesche, 1985). The lymphatic system of the breast is quite extensive—collecting excess fluid, bacteria, and cast-off cell parts—with the main drainage channeled to the axillary nodes. The breast is innervated mainly from branches of the fourth, fifth, and sixth intercostal nerves. The fourth intercostal nerve becomes more superficial as it approaches the areola, where it divides into five branches. The lowermost branch penetrates the areola at the 5 o'clock position on the left breast and the 7 o'clock position on the right breast. If this lowermost branch experiences trauma or is severed (during surgery), loss of sensation to the nipple and areola could result.

Sucking by the infant is detected by touch receptors within the nipple. These touch receptors are afferents that are part of the third, fourth, and fifth intercostal nerves. Impulses from the touch receptors are relayed to the spinal cord and on to projections in the median eminence of the hypothalamus, where prolactin and oxytocin are subsequently released (Koyama, Wu, Easwaran, Thopady, & Foley, 2013).

Clinical Implications

Lactation can be sustained within wide variations of breast size, shape, and appearance because the basic anatomic structure and physiological functioning are remarkably adept at performing under diverse conditions. A number of breast changes are commonly experienced during pregnancy, including breast enlargement, increased tenderness, darkening and/or enlargement of the areola, small amounts of colostrum leakage, increased visibility of veining on the chest, prominence of the glands of Montgomery, protrusion of the nipple, and appearance of stretch marks on the breasts. Absence of such changes may cause concern in both mothers and healthcare providers and may signal a need for closer follow-up after birth. Even so, mothers should still be encouraged to breastfeed.

NIPPLE PREPARATION

Prenatal nipple preparation techniques, such as pulling on or manipulating the nipple, have generally fallen out of favor today. Earlier studies showed no improvement in flat nipples produced by wearing breast shells under the bra during pregnancy (Alexander, Grant, & Campbell, 1992; MAIN Trial Collaborative Group, 1994). However, a newer study of 90 Thai mothers whose nipples measured less than 7 mm showed significant elongation after wearing breast shells 8 hours per day starting at 18–20 weeks' gestation (Chanprapaph, Luttarapakul, Siribariruck, & Boonyawanichkul, 2013). Women with inverted nipples were not included in the study. Perhaps women with a nipple length longer than 7 mm derive no benefit from wearing breast shells prenatally.

The nipple (including its attachment to the areola) is an elastic structure, capable of stretching two to three times its resting length (Smith, Erenberg, & Nowak, 1988). Infant suckling and/or mechanical pumping after birth usually cause a protrusive response in flat nipples. Accessory nipples may secrete milk, generally do not interfere with breastfeeding, and may be associated with urinary tract anomalies. Some mothers are not aware that what looks like a mole to them is actually a nipple and may be surprised if it secretes drops of milk. Because there is usually little underlying ductal or glandular tissue, these nipples tend to cease secreting milk soon after lactogenesis II. However, some mothers report continuous milk secretion from accessory nipples that are much more developed.

Hypoplastic breasts require close follow-up and monitoring of infant weight postpartum. Every effort should be made to help such breasts maximize their milk production within the early days and weeks of lactation. Insufficient glandular tissue may present as a flaccid breast with only patchy areas of glandular tissue evident upon palpation. Subsequent transillumination of the breast or ultrasound imaging may confirm the reduced amount of functional tissue (Neifert, Seacat, & Jobe, 1985). Endocrine pathologies such as polycystic ovary syndrome may also contribute to insufficient mammary tissue, increasing the risk of delayed or failed lactogenesis II, reduced weight gain in infants, and the need for intense lactation support (Marasco, Marmet, & Shell, 2000).

BREAST AUGMENTATION

Breast augmentation has been the most common cosmetic surgical procedure in the United States since 2006. Approximately 290,000 breast augmentation procedures were performed in 2013. Silicone implants were used in 72% of these procedures and saline implants in 28% of all breast augmentation procedures in 2013 (American Society of Plastic Surgeons, 2013).

Surgical procedures to the breasts such as augmentation mammaplasty or reduction mammaplasty can potentially affect lactation and milk production. Andrade, Coca, and Abrao (2010) reported that the probability of an infant being exclusively breastfed at the end of the first month of life was 29% in women with reduction surgery, 54% in those with augmentation surgery, and 80% in women who had no breast surgery. The risk of an infant being nonexclusively breastfed was 5 times greater in women with reduction surgery compared to women with no surgery, and 2.6 times greater with augmentation surgery compared with no surgery. Otherwise, there is scant literature on the impact of breast augmentation on breastfeeding outcomes. A systematic review suggested that breast augmentation was associated with a 40% decrease in the likelihood of exclusive breastfeeding among women who breastfed (Schiff, Algert, Ampt, Sywak, & Roberts, 2014). Infants of mothers who have had breast augmentation are less likely to receive breastmilk at hospital discharge than infants of women without such augmentation. Women who underwent augmentation surgery between births have also been found to be less likely to breastfeed the subsequent infant (Roberts, Ampt, Algert, Sywak, & Chen, 2015).

Augmentation is accomplished with the insertion of an implant that consists of a silicone outer shell and a filler (most commonly silicone gel or saline), either under the chest muscle (submuscular) or on top of the muscle and under the glandular tissue (subglandular) (**Figure 2-9**). The implants may be inserted in a number of ways, including through an axillary incision (under the arm), inframammary incision (under the breast), or periareolar incision (along the edge of the areola) (**Figure 2-10**). Currently, five silicone gel-filled implants are approved by the FDA for use in such

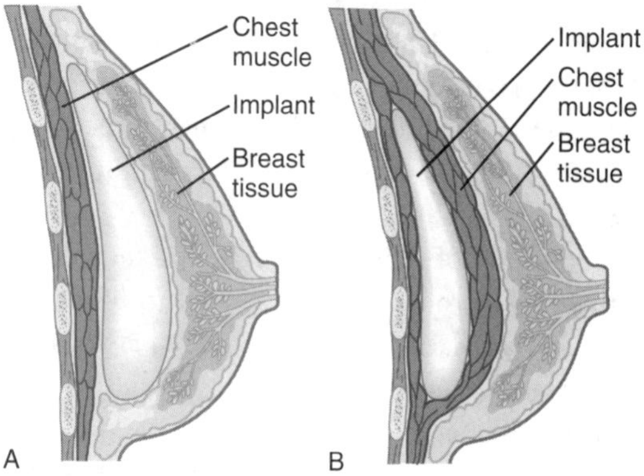

Figure 2-9 Location of breast implants: (A) Implant between breast and muscle. (B) Implant under muscle.

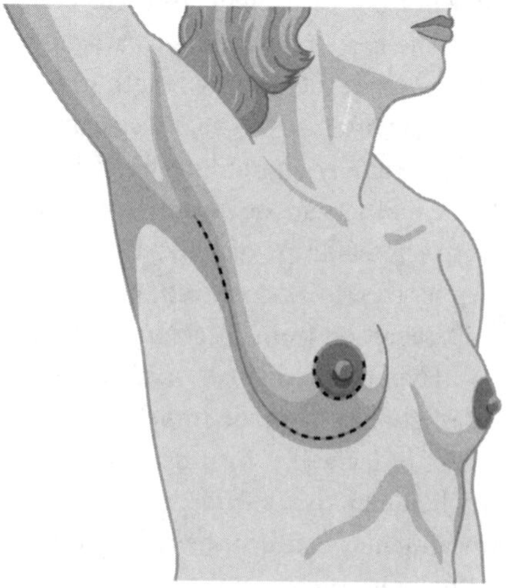

Figure 2-10 Breast augmentation incisions: through the armpit, under the areola, under the breast.

surgery in the United States. As conditions of approval, the FDA required each manufacturer to conduct postapproval studies to characterize the long-term performance and safety of the devices. In June 2011, the FDA issued an Update on the Safety of Silicone Gel-Filled Breast Implants (Center for Devices and Radiological Health, U.S. Food and Drug Administration, 2011).

A number of complications can occur from breast augmentation and potentially impact the normal functioning of the breasts (Center for Devices and Radiological Health, U.S. Food and Drug Administration, 2014):

- Capsular contracture occurs when the scar tissue or capsule that normally forms around the implant tightens and squeezes the implant. With greater degrees of contracture, the breast may present as hard and painful and appear visibly distorted. Surgery is usually required to remedy this problem. Engorged breasts are also hard, painful, and swollen and may exacerbate the capsular contracture.
- Deflation or rupture of the implant may occur due to capsular contracture, mammography, physical manipulation, trauma, or normal aging of the implant. Affected women may notice decreased breast size, pain, tingling, swelling, numbness, burning, or changes in sensation. With silicone implants, silicone gel may migrate away from the implant, causing hard knots in the breast and lumps (granulomas) in the chest wall, armpit, arm, or abdomen. In such cases the implant needs to be surgically removed. The FDA recommends that women with silicone gel-filled breast implants obtain MRI screenings for silent ruptures 3 years after they receive the implants and every 2 years after that.
- Pain may occur at any time with implants.
- Breast infections may occur at any time and are more difficult to treat because the bacteria may not respond to common antibiotics.
- Galactoceles are relatively uncommon complications after breast augmentation surgery but should be considered in the differential of an enlarged breast (Tung & Carr, 2011).
- Women with breast implants may have a very small but increased likelihood of being diagnosed with anaplastic large cell lymphoma.
- Necrosis (formation of dead tissue around the implant) may occur and require surgical correction or removal.
- Tissue atrophy occurs when pressure from the implant causes the breast tissue to thin and shrink. It has also been speculated that pressure from the implant on milk-secreting cells may diminish milk secretion (Hurst, 1996).
- The periareolar incision site is associated with the highest risk of inability to breastfeed. In a retrospective study that compared lactation outcomes between augmented and nonaugmented women, 64% of 42 augmented women experienced insufficient lactation compared with less than 7% of 42 nonaugmented women (Hurst, 1996). Strom, Baldwin, Sigurdson, and Schusterman (1997) reported on breastfeeding outcomes of 28 women from a study of 292 cosmetic saline implant patients, 46 of whom had children after the procedure. Of the 28 women who breastfed, 11 reported problems and 8 reported breastfeeding problems they perceived as being related to the implants. Seven of the 8 women had implants placed through a periareolar incision. Nerves innervating the nipple and areola are best protected if resections at the base of the breast and skin incisions at the medial areolar border are avoided (Schlenz, Kuzbari, Gruber, & Holle, 2000).

- Ranges of sensation in the nipple and breast vary after surgery from increased intensity to elimination of all feeling. Such changes can be temporary or permanent. If the primary nerve that innervates the nipple–areolar complex is stretched, cut, or cauterized during breast augmentation surgery, then nipple sensation might be affected. Sensation generally returns to the nipple/areolar complex with no problems if the nerve is just stretched. If the nerve is cut, nipple sensation is unlikely to return. If the nerve is cauterized, there is a chance that nipple sensation will return, depending on the extent of the cauterization. The risk of permanent nipple numbness from augmentation surgery is about 15%. Using an implant whose diameter is larger than the breast's diameter increases the risk of nipple numbness. Women who choose very large implants relative to their breast skin envelopes are at an increased risk of losing nipple sensation (Mofid, Klatsky, Singh, & Nahabedian, 2006). Sensation in some nipples can take up to 2 years to return following augmentation surgery. The periareolar incision site is often associated with the highest risk of interference with breastfeeding.
- Concern has been expressed over the possibility of silicone leaking into tissues and milk from ruptured silicone implants. No data exist that contraindicate breastfeeding with silicone implants, nor do mothers need to have these devices removed before lactating or have milk levels checked during lactation. When silicon was used as a proxy measure for silicone, Semple, Lugowski, Baines, Smith, & McHugh (1998) found that silicon levels were significantly higher in infant formula than in either the blood or breastmilk of mothers with implants.
- Breast implants are not lifetime devices and will not last forever. Revisions are done frequently to address breast ptosis (drooping), change the desired size, repair saline implants that have deflated, repair capsular contraction, and revise scarring. The average time from initial implant to the need for a revision is 7 years (Spear, Low, & Ducic, 2003). If implants are removed and not replaced, the breasts may become excessively droopy and have a dimpled and/or puckered appearance. Revisions to the initial breast augmentation procedure, especially for capsular contracture, can further damage nerves and functional breast tissue, increasing the risk of insufficient milk production (Michalopoulos, 2007).
- Mothers may not be informed that their breasts could actually be hypoplastic, with only small amounts of functional tissue, or that augmentation mammaplasty has the potential to reduce lactation ability. Cruz and Korchin (2010) compared two groups of mothers, one group with and one group without a saline breast implant, relative to breastfeeding success and the need to supplement feedings. Successful breastfeeding occurred in 88% of the control group without implants and 63% of the group with implants. The need to supplement breastfeeding was seen in 27% of the control group and 46% of the mothers with implants. The authors did not see a significant difference in the breastfeeding experience between those mothers with a periareolar incision or the inframammary approach. Loss of nipple sensation was reported by 2% in both the periareolar and inframammary subgroups. The success of breastfeeding decreased approximately 25% and the need to supplement breastfeeding increased 19% after augmentation mammaplasty.

Breast implants are regulated by the FDA as medical devices. Brown, Todd, Cope, & Sachs (2006) accessed 339 adverse event reports on breast implants between 1968 and 2002 from the FDA database on adverse event reports of medical devices. Almost half (46%) mentioned problems with breastfeeding, such as inadequate milk supply, pain from the implant, rupture or contracture of the implant, silicone measured or seen in the mother's milk, and unspecified breastfeeding problems. Seroma is a complication that involves a collection of serous clear fluid in a surgically dissected area where there has been a creation of a cavity or a dead space. Asymmetric breast enlargement may be seen and may need to be drained. Engorgement is generally bilateral, and seroma should be ruled out when it presents as a unilateral breast enlargement. Seroma can occur in the immediate postoperative period or many weeks later. One case study reported a massive seroma in an augmented breast associated with the use of a breast pump. Small repetitive traumas may have provoked the seroma formation through both mechanical and inflammatory mechanisms (Meggiorini et al., 2013).

Most reports also mentioned anxiety regarding the health of the infant and the safety of breastfeeding with silicone implants. Anxiety on the part of the mother regarding the integrity of the implant, whether breastfeeding will ruin the implant, and safety issues of breastfeeding with implants need to be discussed with mothers to prevent the avoidance of breastfeeding.

BREAST REDUCTION

Indications for breast reduction surgery include musculoskeletal stress from large, heavy breasts, pain, poor body image, and restrictions on physical activities. Older surgical techniques that involved the "free nipple graft" technique or the complete removal of the nipple–areolar complex and reattachment often resulted in impaired or impossible lactation. Nipple sensation is usually greatly diminished in these women but not necessarily absent (Ahmed & Kolhe, 2000). A number of newer surgical techniques are able to preserve the attachment of the nipple–areola to underlying tissue as well as improve the vascular supply to the nipple with less disruption of sensory nerves (Gonzalez, Brown, Gold, Walton, & Shafer, 1993; Hallock, 1992; Nahabedian & Mofid, 2002). Certain types of reduction mammaplasty may result in much less of a compromise to lactation (Mottura, 2002; Ramirez, 2002), making it important to inform women before reduction surgery about the procedure's potential effect on lactation. Because of the intermixing of adipose tissue and glandular tissue and the adhesion of one to the other, breast reduction surgery cannot be accomplished by a simple removal of "fat deposits" (Nickell & Skelton, 2005). Preserving the glandular tissue within the first 30 mm of the nipple and using a surgical technique that keeps the pedicle supporting the nipple–areolar complex as thick as possible may maximize the potential for optimal milk production (Nickell & Skelton, 2005; Ramsay et al., 2005). If a woman has only five or six main milk ducts, removal or destruction of just a few of those central ducts could permanently impair the milk production potential of that breast (Ramsay et al., 2005).

Mothers who have had reduction surgery should be encouraged to breastfeed with proper infant follow-up. The breastfeeding practices of a series of postpartum women who had undergone prior reduction mammaplasty by means of an inferior pedicle approach were reported in a retrospective study by Brzozowski, Niessen, Evans, and Hurst (2000), who also examined the factors that influenced the decision to breastfeed postoperatively. Successful breastfeeding was defined as the ability to feed for a duration equal to or greater than 2 weeks. Seventy-eight patients had children after their breast reduction surgery. Fifteen of the 78 patients (19.2%) breastfed exclusively, 8 (10.3%) breastfed with formula supplementation, 14 (17.9%) had an unsuccessful breastfeeding attempt, and 41 (52.6%) did not attempt breastfeeding. Of the 41 patients not attempting to breastfeed, 9 patients did so as a direct consequence of discouragement by a healthcare professional. Of the 78 women who had children postoperatively, a total of 27 were discouraged from breastfeeding by medical professionals, with only 8 of the 27 (29.6%) subsequently attempting to do so despite this recommendation. In comparison, 26 patients were encouraged to breastfeed; 19 (73.1%) of them did subsequently attempt breastfeeding. Postpartum breast engorgement and lactation was experienced by 31 of the 41 patients not attempting to breastfeed. Of these 31 patients, 19 believed they would have been able to breastfeed due to the extent of breast engorgement and lactation experienced. In a study of 99 young women who underwent reduction mammaplasty, 67.2% reported decreased nipple sensitivity, and 65.2% reported breastfeeding difficulties, including reduced milk production, unilateral milk production, and latching problems because of an inverted nipple (Nguyen, Palladino, Sonnema, & Petty, 2013).

Studies examining successful lactation outcomes after breast reduction surgery show varying results, with approximately 50% reported as successfully breastfeeding depending on the type of surgery performed. The studies typically define successful breastfeeding as breastfeeding (with or without supplementation) for 2–3 weeks (**Table 2-4**). Using such a definition of "successful breastfeeding" can be misleading to clinicians and mothers. "Successful" breastfeeding could be accomplished for 2 weeks when infant intake may be small. After that time, supplementation may be necessary for some infants if milk production reaches a maximum that is still insufficient for the infant's needs. The loss or reduction of nipple sensation can potentially interrupt feedback from the nipple to the pituitary gland, resulting in the possibility of milk production problems. A mother who cannot feel her nipple may be at an increased risk of damage and trauma to the nipples, infection, and incorrect infant latch. Mothers and infants require close follow-up in the early weeks, with frequent infant weight checks. **Box 2-1** presents a sample feeding plan for mothers who have experienced a breast augmentation or breast reduction procedure.

Table 2-4 Successful Breastfeeding After Breast Reduction Mammaplasty

Study	Comments
Hefter, Lindholm, & Elvenes (2003)	Showed a 54% rate of successful breastfeeding (without supplementation)
Cruz-Korchin & Korchin (2004)	Reported a 60% successful breastfeeding rate where a medial pedicle reduction was performed
Cherchel, Azzam, & De Mey (2007)	Found a 44% successful breastfeeding rate (2 weeks with or without supplementation) with a superior pedicle reduction mammaplasty
Chiummariello et al. (2008)	Examined multiple techniques, finding successful lactation rates of 60% after superior pedicle, 55.1% after lateral pedicle, 48% after medial pedicle, and 43.5% after inferior pedicle, as defined by breastfeeding for 3 weeks without supplementation
Cruz & Korchin (2007)	Compared successful lactation outcomes of superior, inferior, and medial pedicle reduction with each other and with matched control subjects. A 60% success rate was found in each group, which was defined as breastfeeding for 2 weeks with or without supplementation

Box 2-1 Sample Feeding Plan for Mothers with Breast Augmentation or Reduction

Mothers and infants should be followed closely in the early days and weeks after hospital discharge to ensure that infant weight gain is adequate, milk production is sufficient, and damage to nipples is minimized. Mothers should be provided with a specific written feeding plan for use after leaving the hospital. Mothers need the contact information of someone who will be following breastfeeding progress once home.

- Advise mothers that reduction or augmentation surgery has the potential to disrupt breastfeeding.
- Assess latch and correct if necessary.
- Use methods to evert the nipple prior to feedings if nipple inversion from breast surgery is present.
- Feed 8–12 times per 24 hours.
- Hand express or pump milk if infant does not latch or feeds poorly. Some clinicians advise to pump after all daytime feedings to maximize milk production.
- Ensure milk transfer.
  - Use alternate massage on each breast at each feeding to optimize milk intake (alternate massage involves massaging and compressing the breast during each pause between sucking bursts).
  - If the mother's breasts have been augmented, she can compress the breast from above rather than squeezing from below the breast. The sides of the breast should be compressed such that pressure is avoided on the implant to prevent implant rupture.
  - If needed, perform pre- and postfeed weights to quantify milk intake and determine if supplementation is necessary.
- Pump after feedings following discharge if needed.
  - Enhance milk output with power pumping, as follows: With double collection kit, pump for 5–8 minutes until milk flow slows with first letdown, remove pump and start pumping again 20 minutes later, and repeat a third time; another power pumping session can be done in the evening.
- Weigh infant every 3 days until adequate weight gain pattern is established.
  - Weigh infant the day after discharge to prevent excessive weight loss and high bilirubin levels. This is especially important if the infant is a late preterm infant, the mother has delivered by cesarean section, the mother is diabetic, or the mother is a primipara. These situations place the mother at an increased risk for a delay in the milk coming in and further increase the potential for insufficient milk intake.
- Use expressed milk if supplement is needed; expressed milk can be delivered through a tube feeding device at the breast to maximize breast stimulation. If sufficient breastmilk is not available, supplement with banked donor human milk or infant formula.
- Check nipples for pain or trauma with corrective actions taken.

Data from Walker, M. (2010). *The nipple and areola in breastfeeding and lactation.* Amarillo, TX: Hale Publishing.

Some mothers who have undergone surgical procedures on their breasts may complain of breast pain during lactation. This may be due to the formation of scar tissue. Clinicians will need to rule out other causes of breast pain, such as infection or improper latch. West and Hirsch (2008) noted that post-surgical mothers often experience nipple blanching or vasospasm of the nipple. Blanching may be due to a blood supply interruption or nerve trauma to the nipple–areola during the surgery, although the true cause is unknown. Mothers may find some relief from this painful condition by compressing the areola and mechanically squeezing blood back into the nipple (West & Hirsch, 2008). Clinicians can refer mothers to the additional readings and resources at the end of this chapter.

Other types of surgery, such as placement of chest drains during infancy, can also affect the development and functioning of the breasts. Skin incisions for chest drains can be misplaced, resulting in breast deformity from dermal adhesions and underdevelopment of the breast. This situation should be corrected when breast development begins at adolescence to allow unrestricted growth of the entire breast. Severe, uncorrected cases may result in the inability to breastfeed (Rainer et al., 2003). A number of aspects of the breast and nipple anatomy of lactating mothers may need closer observation and follow-up when present or absent.

BREAST ANOMALIES

When assisting breastfeeding mothers, visually assess the conformation of both breasts, checking for size, symmetry, distortions, scars, accessory breast tissue in the axilla, edema, and erythema (redness).

Ask whether the breasts underwent changes during pregnancy. Check the origin of all scars.

- Mothers with breasts that are significantly hypoplastic, that have a wide intramammary space, or that have been augmented or reduced need intense lactation support. Infants should be breastfed 8–12 times each 24 hours, or pumping should be commenced in the absence of a vigorously suckling infant. Infant weights should be closely monitored (as frequently as every 2–3 days in the beginning) to ensure adequate intake. Mothers who have undergone a significant breast reduction may need to be advised that supplementation could be necessary if the breasts are unable to increase their production to meet the growing needs of the infant. Some mothers produce adequate amounts of colostrum in the hospital and early days but do not report lactogenesis II. Some mothers' breasts may be unable to produce an abundant amount of milk to meet the infant's increasing needs. Skin incisions on the medial borders of the areola or under the breast may result in diminished sensation to the nipple–areolar complex, with mothers being unable to feel whether the infant is latched correctly. This factor increases the risk for not only insufficient milk production but also nipple and areolar damage.
- Mothers who have had breast augmentation should be asked whether the intent was to cosmetically enhance the breasts or to compensate for a lack of development of normal breast tissues during adolescence. Augmentation will obviously not improve milk production if insufficient glandular tissue was present initially. Breast augmentation, as well as the underlying reason for the procedure, has the potential to alter breastfeeding outcomes through a number of factors: use of a periareolar incision, severing of milk ducts, altered nipple sensation, lack of functional breast tissue, little or no breast changes during pregnancy, and minimal postpartum engorgement

(Hill, Wilhelm, Aldag, & Chatterton, 2004). Mothers should be asked whether they experienced any previous hormonal aberrations that would have affected normal breast development.

- Medications to enhance milk production are usually ineffective if breast tissue is absent or significantly underdeveloped.
- Some mothers may not self-report augmentation or reduction mammaplasty. This information should be ascertained during telephone contacts if mothers call for help with insufficient milk or slow infant weight gain or weight loss.
- Mothers with anatomic breast problems can be offered the option of using a tube-feeding device at the breast to optimize breastmilk production, deliver a supplement if necessary, and enjoy the close contact and pleasure of feeding at the breast.
- Breasts that are edematous may be engorged—a normal event, but one that is managed by frequent breastfeeding (or pumping/hand expression if necessary) to prevent overfullness, reduced milk production, nipple trauma, and insufficient milk later on. Accessory breast tissue in the tail of Spence can swell and become engorged during lactogenesis II. Cold compresses may help reduce the edema. Care should be taken that a tight brassiere or underwires do not curtail drainage from this area.
- Red patches on the breast usually indicate areas of inflammation where milk is not draining adequately. Proper positioning, latch, suck, and swallow need to be ensured, with alternate massage being added to help the affected areas drain more efficiently. Alternate massage involves massaging and compressing the breast during the pause between the infant's sucking bursts to encourage the infant to sustain sucking and manually increase the internal pressure in the breast to improve milk transfer (Bowles, Stutte, & Hensley, 1987; Stutte, Bowles, & Morman, 1988). Some mothers also benefit from taking anti-inflammatory medication.

NIPPLE ANOMALIES

Accessory breast tissue or extra nipples may look like moles or may be more developed with the appearance of small nipples and/or areolae. Occasionally, a mother may have an ectopic duct that drains milk to the skin surface but is located on the areola or even farther back on the breast tissue. Some nipples are not symmetrical and may have the appearance of a raspberry or even look like two nipples are present on the areola. Extra nipples and ectopic ducts may leak milk upon letdown but usually cause no problems during breastfeeding.

Flat, retracted, or "inverted" nipples are not unusual. A true inverted nipple—that is, one that fails to elevate from the mammary pit—may be visibly assessed. In contrast, flat or retracted nipples are typically discovered either when the infant has difficulty latching on or prenatally if the mother or healthcare provider compresses the tissue behind the nipple to see whether it protrudes (somewhat comparable with the infant latching on). The nipple should protrude, not retract, when this manipulation is performed. In older texts, this is referred to as the "pinch test." To successfully transfer milk, the infant must be able to grasp the nipple and one-half inch or so of the areola and pull it back almost to the junction of the hard and soft palates. The nipple–areolar complex stretches to two or three times its resting length during this maneuver. A nipple that pulls back from the infant when he or she grasps the breast may make latch-on more difficult for some infants and damage the nipple. Engorgement may cause the areola and nipple to flatten out and lose their elasticity. If the infant cannot latch in this situation, a mother can apply a cold compress and hand express or pump some milk to soften the areola.

Some mothers given large amounts of intravenous fluids during labor and/or whose labors have been induced or augmented with Pitocin have been anecdotally reported to experience edematous areolae that envelop the nipple, causing latch problems and pain. These nipples are not flat, just difficult to access. Cold compresses, cabbage leaves, and foods with a diuretic effect (watermelon) have all been anecdotally recommended to help decrease the swelling. Placing a breast pump and applying vacuum to an edematous areola may exacerbate the problem because nipples typically swell after pumping (Wilson-Clay & Hoover, 2013). Areolar compression that shifts excess fluid away from the areola should be considered before placing a pump on an areola already distended with fluid (Miller & Riordan, 2004). A technique called "reverse pressure softening" mechanically displaces areolar interstitial fluid inward, temporarily increasing elasticity and permitting an easier latch (Cotterman, 2004).

Double or bifurcated nipples are occasionally seen when two nipples appear on an areola that may be completely separate from each other or may be joined by a ridge of areolar tissue. Each nipple may have its own ductal system, with the areola being enlarged on the affected side. Some arrangements may present as a cluster of small nipples resembling a mulberry. An infant with a small mouth may experience difficulty taking the whole structure into his or her mouth. If the mother is using a pump, the nipple arrangement must fit properly into the pump flange to avoid tissue damage.

HORMONES OF LACTATION

A remarkable procession of hormones, summarized in **Table 2-5**, is involved in facilitating the process of lactation.

Prolactin

Prolactin is a single-chain protein hormone secreted in the anterior pituitary and several other sites. This multifunctional hormone has more than 300 separate biological activities. Its receptors are found not just in the breast but also at many other sites throughout the body, including the ovaries, central nervous system (CNS), immune system, and a wide range of peripheral organs. Prolactin's effects have been linked to maternal behavior (Grattan et al., 2001), and the hormone even plays a role in the immune response. Most notable is the role that prolactin plays in the regulation of the humoral and cellular immune responses in normal physiological states as well as pathological conditions such as autoimmune diseases (Neidhart, 1998). Prolactin facilitates lobuloalveolar growth during pregnancy and promotes lactogenesis by acting together with cortisol and insulin to stimulate the transcription of the genes that encode for milk proteins.

The hypothalamus is the regulator of prolactin secretion, acting as a limiting agent on its expression until the restraint is removed. Dopamine is a major prolactin-inhibiting factor (i.e., brake on prolactin secretion). Agents, stimuli, or drugs that interfere with dopamine secretion or receptor binding lead to enhanced secretion of prolactin. Drugs can also inhibit release of prolactin from the pituitary, such as ergot alkaloids. Prolactin is positively regulated by a number of other hormones, including thyroid-releasing hormone, gonadotropin-releasing hormone, and vasoactive intestinal polypeptide. Prolactin

1:02 pm

404 - 707 - 7410

313-343-3146

ZC.

Zatonya Padgett,

7/20/1988 Donovan returned her call.

Table 2-5 Hormonal Regulation of Breast Development and Function

Phase/Stage	Hormones	Function	Local Control
Pregnancy	Progesterone	Lobular formation	
	Prolactin	Completes lobular/alveolar development; stimulates glandular production of colostrum	
	Placental lactogen	Increases prolactin	
	Estrogen	Ductular sprouting	
Birth (lactogenesis II)	Removal of progesterone	Allows prolactin to exert its effect	
	Prolactin		
	Removal of progesterone	Lactogenic trigger	
	Glucocorticoids	Supportive and/or permissive	
	Insulin	Assists in milk production	
	Cortisol	Supports milk production	
Maintenance of lactation (lactogenesis III)	Prolactin	Along with cortisol and insulin, acts to stimulate transcription of genes that encode milk proteins	Feedback inhibitor of lactation ([FIL], a whey protein)
	Oxytocin	Facilitates milk transfer	Stretch
	Thyroid hormone	Increases responsiveness of mammary cells to prolactin	Back pressure
	Parathyroid hormone		Degree of drainage
	Growth hormone		Frequency of feeds
			Infant appetite
			Milk storage capacity of breasts
Suckling	Prolactin	Stimulates milk synthesis	
	Oxytocin	Responsible for milk ejection and mothering behavior	
	Prolactin-inhibiting factor	Depressed by suckling; controls release of prolactin from the hypothalamus	

is released when the nipple is stimulated during nursing due to a spinal reflex arc that causes release of prolactin-stimulating hormones from the hypothalamus (**Figure 2-11**).

Prolactin levels rise during pregnancy from about 10 ng/mL in the nonpregnant state to approximately 200 ng/mL at term. Baseline levels do not drop back to normal in a lactating woman but average about 100 ng/mL at 3 months and 50 ng/mL at 6 months. Prolactin levels can double with the stimulus of suckling. After about 6 months of breastfeeding, the prolactin rise with suckling amounts to only 5–10 ng/mL. This diminished level reflects the increased prolactin-binding capacity or sensitivity of the mammary tissue, which allows full lactation in the face of falling prolactin levels over time. It is interesting to note that the level of inhibition of prolactin that is necessary to suppress lactation is over 80%, meaning that the typical levels of prolactin seen in mothers in Western countries with term infants is considerably in excess of the levels required to maintain lactation. The high levels of prolactin seen during

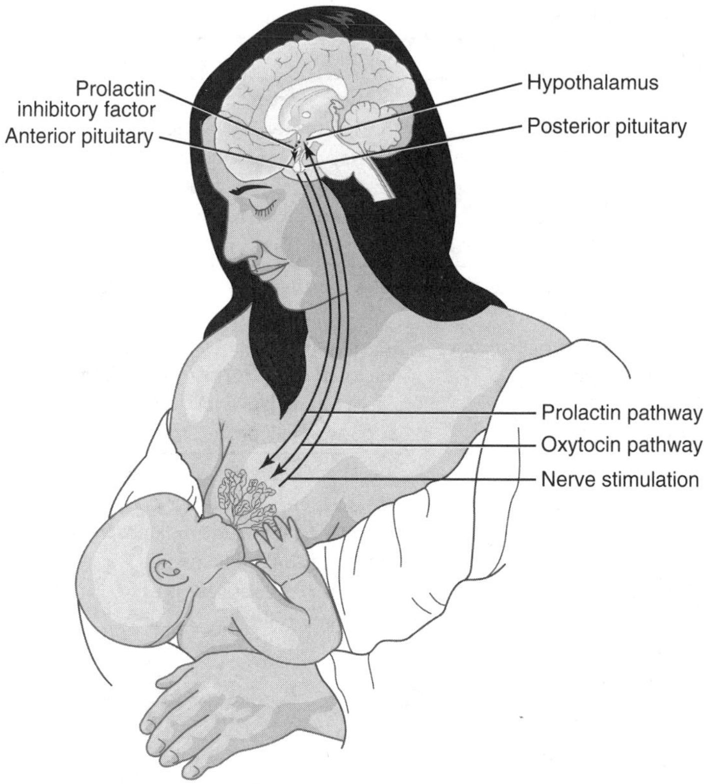

Figure 2-11 Hormone pathways during suckling.

pregnancy and early lactation may also serve to increase the number of prolactin receptors and depend on tactile input for stimulation and release. Despite its importance to the initiation of lactation, prolactin does not directly regulate the short-term or long-term rate of milk synthesis (Cox, Owens, & Hartmann, 1996). Once lactation is well established, prolactin is still required for milk synthesis to occur, but its role is permissive rather than regulatory (Cregan, De Mello, & Hartmann, 2000).

Prolactin concentration in the plasma is highest during sleep and lowest during the waking hours; it operates as a true circadian rhythm (Stern & Reichlin, 1990). The prolactin response is superimposed on the circadian rhythm of prolactin secretion, meaning that the same intensity of suckling stimulus can elevate prolactin levels more effectively at certain times of the day when the circadian input enhances the effect of the suckling stimulus (Freeman, Kanyicska, Lerant, & Nagy, 2000).

Prolactin is seen in the maternal cerebrospinal fluid from which it diffuses into various regions of the brain, with the hypothalamus itself showing increases in prolactin receptors. Prolactin influences numerous brain functions, including maternal behavior, feeding and appetite, and oxytocin secretion. Given the high circulating levels of prolactin during pregnancy and lactation and the increased expression of prolactin receptors in the hypothalamus, prolactin stands as a key player in the coordination of neuroendocrine and behavioral adaptations in the maternal brain (Grattan, 2001). Oxytocin is required for the secretion of prolactin, with the finding that there are nerves containing oxytocin in the anterior pituitary. Prolactin secretion is affected by stress as well as a number of hormones, including oxytocin and vasopressin (the antidiuretic hormone). The most common disease related to vasopressin is diabetes insipidus, a condition that results from a deficiency in secretion of vasopressin from the posterior pituitary or the inability of the kidney to respond to the hormone. Although the major sign of diabetes insipidus is excessive urine output, this magnitude of disturbance in water and electrolyte regulation can impede suckling-induced prolactin release. A number of other factors can also affect prolactin:

- Hill and colleagues (2009) studied the differences in prolactin and oxytocin levels between term and preterm mothers (who were completely pump dependent). Preterm mothers had significantly lower prolactin levels than term mothers. However, with simultaneous breast pumping, preterm mothers achieved similar prolactin levels as term mothers, though their milk yield was still lower. There was a notable interaction between pumping frequency and prolactin in the preterm mothers. More frequent breast stimulation in preterm mothers exposed the breasts to higher than basal levels of prolactin, reinforcing the position of clinicians that very frequent breast pumping is (hormonally) necessary for mothers of preterm infants.
- Certain drugs administered during and after labor may interfere with prolactin secretion. Prostaglandins administered for the induction of labor are dopamine agonists that reduce prolactin secretion. Ergometrine to reduce postbirth bleeding is also a dopamine agonist that suppresses prolactin secretion. Jordan and colleagues (2009) found that in an analysis of a large obstetric database, oxytocin and ergometrine in the third stage of labor and prostaglandins for the induction of labor were associated with a significant reduction in breastfeeding. Routine prevention of postpartum hemorrhage with oxytocin, either alone or combined with ergometrine, was associated with a 6–8% reduction in breastfeeding at 48 hours.
- Mothers who have delivered by cesarean section have lower prolactin levels than mothers who deliver vaginally.
- Mennella and Pepino (2008) studied the relationship between alcohol ingestion, prolactin, and milk yield in 13 lactating women. They found that prolactin levels were higher at the start of a pumping session and for at least the next hour when less time had elapsed between pumping sessions. Alcohol ingestion modified the prolactin response to breast pumping but depended on when the pumping occurred along the blood alcohol concentration curve. As blood alcohol concentration rose, pumping during that time enhanced the prolactin response, but pumping during the descending phase as blood alcohol levels decreased resulted in a blunted prolactin response. However, during the immediate hours after lactating women drank a moderate dose of alcohol, their infants consumed less milk at the breast (Mennella, 2001). One reason for this is that mothers produce less milk within the immediate hours after drinking. In contrast to prolactin, oxytocin levels decrease significantly during the hours immediately following alcohol ingestion and the diminished oxytocin responses are significantly related to deficits in milk yield and delay in milk ejection (Mennella, Pepino, & Teff, 2005). These studies refute the folklore that alcohol acts as a galactagogue. Alcohol should not be recommended as an intervention to improve milk production.

- Mennella and Pepino (2010) found that having a family history of alcoholism in a first-degree relative is a determinant of hormonal and behavioral responses to breast stimulation and alcohol consumption in lactating women. The women with a family history of alcoholism who are not alcoholics themselves exhibited smaller prolactin responses to sucking with an alcohol challenge than women without such a family history. Women who had no family history of alcoholism exhibited an increase in peak prolactin response to breast stimulation after an alcohol challenge compared to women with such a history. Regardless of the prolactin response, alcohol consumption did not result in greater milk production during the 16-minute pumping periods of the study. A blunted prolactin response does not mean that a woman cannot successfully breastfeed. A prolactin-promoting intervention would include more frequent breastfeeding during the afternoon and evening hours when prolactin levels are normally lowest due to the circadian rhythms of prolactin secretion. Women with blunted prolactin responses may need more opportunities to expose their breasts to prolactin.
- A wide range of prolactin values are compatible with exclusive breastfeeding. Baseline prolactin levels at 8 weeks postpartum may vary depending on the frequency of feedings, being higher with increased feeding frequency (Stuebe, Meltzer-Brody, Pearson, Pedersen, & Grewen, 2015).

Oxytocin

Oxytocin is a nine-amino-acid peptide that is synthesized in the hypothalamus and then transported to the posterior pituitary, from which it is released into the blood. It is simultaneously released through a closed system into the brain. Oxytocin differs from vasopressin by just two of the nine amino acids from which it is composed. Actions of oxytocin cause contraction of the smooth muscle myoepithelial cells surrounding the mammary alveoli, moving milk into the collecting ducts, which dilates these ducts and propels milk toward the nipple. The resulting increase in intraductal pressure and duct dilatation increases the milk flow rate. Even though oxytocin reaches the alveoli at approximately the same time, the myoepithelial cells' contraction may vary in response to this hormone. There can be a 2- to 8-second difference in the timing of duct dilatation and milk flow in the main milk ducts draining different lobes in the same breast (Gardner, Kent, Hartmann, & Geddes, 2015). Milk that is not removed flows in a retrograde fashion and is redistributed through the breast.

Multiple milk ejections typically occur during both breastfeeding and milk expression (Mitoulas, Lai, Gurrin, Larsson, & Hartmann, 2002), with many mothers able to feel the first milk ejection but not subsequent ones. The amount of milk ingested by the infant is related to the number of milk ejections per feeding and is independent of the amount of time spent at the breast (Ramsay, Kent, Owens, & Hartmann, 2004). Successful lactation depends on the milk ejection reflex, as only small volumes of milk (1–10 mL) can be either expressed (Kent, Ramsay, Doherty, Larsson, & Hartmann, 2003) or removed by the breastfeeding infant (Ramsay et al., 2004) before milk ejection.

Oxytocin also exerts effects on neuroendocrine reflexes, produces analgesic effects, reduces the stress and anxiety response, causes contractions of the uterus, and contributes to the establishment of social and bonding behaviors related to caring for offspring (Gimpl & Fahrenholz, 2001). Breastfeeding within an hour of birth, when oxytocin levels are very high, supports a close maternal–infant bond. Upon nipple stimulation, oxytocin is released in a pulsatile nature consisting of brief 3- to 4-second bursts of oxytocin into the bloodstream at 90-second intervals, resulting in milk ejection from the breast (Uvnas-Moberg, 2015). Oxytocin cells fire in bursts so that oxytocin is secreted in pulses. The breast responds to oxytocin only at relatively high concentrations, and it rapidly desensitizes in response to continued exposure, so pulsatile delivery of oxytocin is essential for efficient milk ejection. This pulse shortens and widens the lactiferous ducts, increasing the pressure inside the breast, and is essential for maximum removal of milk from the breast (Neville, 2001). Mothers who deliver by cesarean section may lack a significant rise in prolactin levels 20–30 minutes after the onset of breastfeeding and experience fewer oxytocin pulses than mothers who have a vaginal delivery.

Administration of oxytocin to women who labor with epidural analgesia may interfere with the release of endogenous oxytocin (Wiklund, Norman, Uvnas-Moberg, Ransjo-Arvidson, & Andolf, 2009). Plasma levels of oxytocin are reduced in mothers who receive epidural analgesia (Rahm, Hallgren, Hogberg, Hurtig, & Odlind, 2002) and may play a role in the delayed onset of breastfeeding in the postpartum period. Correlations between oxytocin pulsatility on day 2 and the duration of exclusive breastfeeding suggest that the development of an early pulsatile oxytocin pattern is of importance for sustained exclusive breastfeeding (Nissen, Uvnas-Moberg, Svensson, Stock, Widstrom, & Winberg, 1996). Jonas and colleagues (2009) compared oxytocin and prolactin release in response to breastfeeding during the second day postpartum in two groups of women: (1) women who had received oxytocin either intravenously for stimulation of labor or intramuscularly for prevention of postpartum hemorrhage and/or epidural analgesia and (2) women receiving no such treatment during labor. The median oxytocin level was lower in the group of mothers who received epidural analgesia combined with oxytocin. The higher the dose of oxytocin infusion that women received during labor, the lower the women's endogenous oxytocin levels were during a breastfeeding episode on day 2. A feedback inhibition of oxytocin release seems to have been induced as a reaction to the high and unphysiological oxytocin levels during labor resulting from the oxytocin infusions. This inhibition may occur because the administration of epidural analgesia inhibits transmission of nerve fibers mediating the sense of pain in the spinal cord, and nerve fibers mediating oxytocin release might also be affected by epidural analgesia. Oxytocin can also be released before the infant is placed at breast and is not solely dependent on tactile stimulation for release.

Both drugs and a mother's emotional state can affect oxytocin secretion. Morphine administration to breastfeeding women can lower the oxytocin response to sucking (Lindow, Hendricks, Nugent, Dunne, & van der Spuy, 1999). Wright (1985) showed experimentally that the administration of morphine into the lumbar subarachnoid space inhibited the milk ejection reflex. In addition, ethyl alcohol is an inhibitor of oxytocin release that can act in a dose-dependent manner (Cobo, 1973). Pain and psychological stress can inhibit the milk ejection reflex by reducing the number of oxytocin pulses during suckling episodes (Ueda, Yokoyama, Irahara, & Aono, 1994). Opiate and beta-endorphin release during stress can block stimulus-related oxytocin secretion (Lawrence & Lawrence, 2010).

Lactation performance is influenced by stress surrounding labor and delivery, and it is different in women who underwent elective cesarean delivery compared with spontaneous vaginal delivery. Zanardo and colleagues (2012) assessed the relationship between cortisol and prolactin following elective cesarean delivery and lactation performance, from the delivery to the sixth month of life. Basal stress, lactogenic hormones, cortisol, and prolactin were comparable on day 3 postpartum in all of the mothers.

Multivariate analysis indicated that elective cesarean delivery has a negative impact (OR; 95% CI) on breastfeeding prevalence on the seventh day (0.14; 0.0–0.44, $p = .008$) and at the third month postpartum (0.19; 0.05–0.71, $p = .05$) in comparison to vaginal delivery. In addition, prolactin levels proved to have a statistically significant role in early breastfeeding (1.01; 1–1.01, $p = .002$). The authors concluded that elective cesarean delivery is a risk factor for successful lactation performance.

Significant elevations of oxytocin occur 15, 30, and 45 minutes after delivery and are thought to enhance mother–child interactions by shaping maternal behavior (Nissen, Lilja, Widstrom, & Uvnas-Moberg, 1995). Not only does a systemic release of oxytocin into the bloodstream occur with infant suckling, but a closed system exists within the brain whereby oxytocin is also secreted into areas of the brain responsible for affiliative behavior. This secretion may be functionally related to the initiation of maternal behavior after birth (Nelson & Panksepp, 1998). Lactation, through its oxytocin mediation within the maternal brain, reduces responses to stressful situations, may protect some women from mental disorders (Cowley & Roy-Byrne, 1989; Klein, Skrobala, & Garfinkel, 1995), and aids in the mother's ability to deal with the demands of child rearing. The effects of oxytocin and vasopressin indicate that lactation is associated with a reduction in anxiety, obsessiveness, and stress reactivity that may create an adaptive state that favors the interests of the infant over those of the mother (Carter, Altemus, & Chrousos, 2001). Bottle-feeding mothers experience a greater cardiovascular response to psychological stressors, have higher incidences of psychiatric and cardiovascular disorders (Mezzacappa, Kelsey, & Katlin, 1999), and have higher blood pressure (Light et al., 2000) than do breastfeeding mothers. Oxytocin release during stress is higher in lactating mothers, leading to suppressed stress responsivity in these women (Uvnas-Moberg & Eriksson, 1996). Research suggests that the hormonal milieu of lactation may diminish the physiological stress response as well as the psychological perceptions of stress (Groer & Davis, 2002). High levels of cortisol are related to stress and low levels to relaxation. Cortisol levels are in turn regulated by adrenocorticotropic hormone (ACTH). Handlin and colleagues (2009) explored the relationship among circulating oxytocin, ACTH, and cortisol levels during breastfeeding. Mothers who received oxytocin infusions during labor had higher cortisol levels than did controls. Both cortisol and ACTH levels decreased in response to breastfeeding. Skin-to-skin contact prior to breastfeeding also decreased cortisol levels. The increased cortisol levels in mothers who received oxytocin infusions during labor may be an expression of an increased sensitivity to some types of stress as a result of the lowered function in their oxytocinergic system, both within the brain and in the circulation. Some data suggest reason for concern regarding the effects of epidural analgesia on the blocking of oxytocin release at delivery (Goodfellow, Hull, Swaab, Dogterom, & Buijs, 1983). Exogenous oxytocin thus has the potential to interrupt the initiation of lactation by (1) disrupting the endogenous pulsatile secretion of oxytocin; (2) augmenting the stress response, which replaces pulsatile secretion of oxytocin with continuous secretion and inhibits lactation; and (3) desensitizing and downregulating the myoepithelial receptors of oxytocin.

Prefeeding cues are oral–motor neurobehaviors that communicate feeding readiness, and the ability to self-comfort and regulate behavioral state. Infants exposed to synthetic oxytocin during labor demonstrate fewer prefeeding cues and a low level of prefeeding organization, with the exposed infants having 11.5 times the odds of demonstrating low prefeeding cues compared to non-exposed infants (Bell, White-Traut, & Rankin, 2013). Primitive neonatal reflexes comprise a group of reflexive spontaneous behaviors and reactions to stimuli that are seen in all normal healthy newborns; one of the rhythmic primitive neonatal reflexes is sucking. When administered in high doses, synthetic oxytocin crosses the infant's blood–brain barrier and can disrupt the neuroendocrine environment of the fetal nervous system (Gabriel et al., 2015). One consequence of this intervention is interference with the expression of primitive neonatal reflexes.

A negative association has been observed between intrapartum doses of synthetic oxytocin, newborn sucking, and increased early risk of unwanted breastfeeding discontinuation. In one study, higher doses of intrapartum oxytocin had an inhibitory effect on newborn sucking and mothers who had received a higher dose of oxytocin were highly unlikely to be exclusively breastfeeding at 3 months postpartum (Fernandez et al., 2012). In another study, synthetic oxytocin administered during labor increased the risk of bottle-feeding in exposed newborns and multiplied the risk of abandoning breastfeeding at 3 months by 2.29 times (Garcia-Fortea et al., 2014).

The hormonal environment of lactation can be further disrupted by the ingestion of alcohol. Some mothers are still advised by their healthcare providers or cultural surroundings that alcohol will serve as a lactation aid or help calm a fussy baby. Consuming alcohol at a level of 0.4 g/kg resulted in a rise in prolactin and a depressed oxytocin release such that there was a delay in milk ejection and lower milk yields when pumping (Mennella et al., 2005). Prolactin and oxytocin normally behave in tandem, but consumption of alcoholic beverages disrupts this synchrony. Infants have been shown to consume 20% less milk after their mothers' consumption of alcohol (Mennella & Beauchamp, 1991). Chien, Huang, Hsu, Chao, and Liu (2008) studied Chinese lactating mothers who were given a traditional soup that contained rice wine. Milk ejection was delayed in these mothers, milk composition was altered, prolactin levels were raised, and milk yields were reduced. Although an occasional alcoholic beverage may have little effect on the overall lactation process, regular alcohol consumption may be problematic in terms of milk composition and infant weight gain.

Effects of Other Hormones Influenced by Suckling

Not only are prolactin and oxytocin released during infant suckling, but a simultaneous activation of 19 different maternal and infant gastrointestinal (GI) hormones also enhances the mother's and baby's digestive capacity as a mechanism against energy loss and as a way to ensure adequate energy supply for milk production and infant growth (Uvnas-Moberg, Widstrom, Marchini, & Winberg, 1987) (**Table 2-6**). Bone mineral density is enhanced after weaning in lactating women (Polatti, Capuzzo, Viazzo, Colleoni, & Klersy, 1999).

Clinical Implications

Alterations in prolactin secretion can affect lactogenesis II and III.

- Retained placental fragments can inhibit the withdrawal of progesterone and the subsequent prolactin release (Neifert, McDonough, & Neville, 1981). Other more uncommon conditions of the placenta that prolong the elevation of pregnancy hormones, such as placenta increta (invasion of the myometrium by the chorionic villi), may also interfere with lactogenesis II (Anderson, 2001).
- Sheehan syndrome is caused by such a severe postpartum hemorrhage that it leads to pituitary infarction, hypoperfusion, or other vascular injury to the pituitary. The pituitary gland is very vascular and becomes more sensitive to a decreased blood flow at the end of a pregnancy.

Table 2-6 Selected GI Hormones Associated with Suckling

Hormone	Action	Effect from Suckling
Gastrin: released in response to protein intake	Stimulates acid secretion in the stomach and growth of gastric mucosa; trophic; promotes glucose-induced insulin release	Rise in maternal levels within 30 seconds of onset of breastfeeding
Cholecystokinin: released in response to fat intake	Stimulates contraction and growth of the gallbladder; promotes glucose-induced insulin release; induces satiety and post-prandial sedation and sleep	Released in response to suckling in both mother and baby
Somatostatin: 90% released from stomach	Inhibits GI secretions, motility, blood flow, most GI hormones; released during stress; higher in sick infants	Decreases 1 hour after the onset of breastfeeding
Insulin	Metabolic regulator	Rises in response to suckling in both mother and baby; stabilizes blood sugar levels; promotes storage of ingested nutrients in infants

GI, gastrointestinal.

- Other conditions that affect prolactin secretion, such as hypothyroidism, diabetes insipidus, and polycystic ovary syndrome, may become evident during early lactation.
- Surgical interruption of sensory nerves to the nipple–areola may remove the tactile stimulation, leading to altered prolactin secretion.
- Pituitary surgery has the potential for diminishing total prolactin secretion as well as the normal prolactin surge during suckling. However, evidence has also shown that with early frequent suckling, adequate breast drainage, and close follow-up, lactation can successfully take place (DeCoopman, 1993).
- Certain medications may suppress prolactin secretion, usually dopamine agonists such as ergot alkaloids (cabergoline, ergotamine) and early use of oral contraceptives containing estrogens (Hale & Ilett, 2002).

Because prolactin concentrations are highest during sleep, recommendations to breastfeed at night become important in the early days and weeks when lactation is becoming established. Separating mother and baby in the hospital should be avoided, as should recommendations to stretch out feedings at night or have the father give a bottle at night so the mother can sleep.

Oxytocin is important to both mothering behavior and the delivery of milk to the infant. It also functions to contract the uterus so as to minimize bleeding from the placental attachment site. Mothers, especially multiparous mothers, feel this as uterine cramping (afterpains) during the milk ejection reflex. Oxytocin has a calming effect, lowers maternal blood pressure, and decreases anxiety. Women receiving magnesium sulfate and/or who are placed on seizure precautions due to pregnancy-induced hypertension may find that breastfeeding is therapeutic. Some mothers also report feeling a tingling or heavy sensation in the breasts upon letdown (albeit infrequently in the early days after birth), feeling thirsty, experiencing a warm or flushed feeling, sensing increased heat from the breasts, feeling sleepy (Mulford, 1990), or encountering headaches or nausea when the milk lets down. Many of these seemingly random feelings are generated in response to the complex interplay of oxytocin and a variety of metabolic hormones that are simultaneously released each time the infant goes to the breast. Mothers who experience nausea when breastfeeding often find that eating a cracker before nursing lessens this problem. Other mothers have found relief by wearing "sea bands," cuffs worn around the wrists that either place pressure on the nausea acupressure points, deliver adjustable vibrations over acupressure points, or deliver small electrical charges to these areas.

Synthetic oxytocin has historically been recommended for mothers who experience difficulty with their letdown reflex. Use of oxytocin nasal spray to enhance letdown has been reported (Newton & Egli, 1958), as well as use to help establish breastfeeding and improve milk output in puerperal women (Huntingford, 1961). When oxytocin nasal spray was used by a group of infrequently pumping preterm mothers, a 3.5 times increase in volume of milk pumped by those using oxytocin nasal spray before each pumping session was observed (Ruis, Holland, Doesburg, Broeders, & Corbey, 1981). A review in the Cochrane Database (Renfrew, Lang, & Woolridge, 2000) reported that sublingual or buccal preparations of oxytocin were also associated with increased milk production, although most of these early studies suffer from methodology problems and samples of mothers with very restricted breastfeeding "schedules." Fewtrell, Loh, Blake, Ridout, and Hawdon (2006) did not find significant differences in milk output of preterm pumping mothers when using oxytocin nasal spray. Because oxytocin nasal spray is not generally used to increase milk production but to aid in the milk ejection, this is not surprising. However, it was noted that many mothers in this study complained that their milk production decreased after they ceased using the spray. Using the spray may be beneficial in helping mothers through the early difficult days of breastfeeding or pumping milk for a preterm infant because milk output was increased during the first couple of days in the group using the spray. This finding may encourage some mothers to continue pumping. Use of oxytocin nasal spray may give mothers a boost of confidence as they see milk issuing from their breasts. Since the commercial preparation of intranasal oxytocin was removed from the market, its use has diminished. However, the preparation can be created by a compounding pharmacy, and some mothers may benefit from its judicious use.

The hormonal milieu of lactation is usually taken for granted until a problem arises. In general, breastfeeding management guidelines should reflect the nature of and work with the process of lactation.

The optimal functioning of the hormones involved in lactation starts with the earliest contact between mother and infant after birth.

- Newborn infants placed in uninterrupted skin-to-skin contact on their mother's chest immediately after birth engage in a prefeeding sequence of behaviors designed to locate and latch to the nipple. This process takes about an hour in infants from unmedicated labors (Widstrom et al., 1987). One behavior demonstrated by newborns is the stimulation and massage of the mother's breast before latch-on. Oxytocin levels rise in response to this massage, causing nipple erection and stimulating the milk ejection reflex before it has become conditioned to the sucking stimulus (Matthiesen, Ransjo-Arvidson, Nissen, & Uvnas-Moberg, 2001). These high levels of oxytocin persist when the infant suckles and flood the mothering center in the maternal brain, thereby enhancing maternal behavior (Widstrom et al., 1990). Early and extended contact has long been known to result in prolonged breastfeeding (Salariya, Easton, & Cater, 1978). Newborns should be placed and left on the mother's chest to engage in this behavior immediately after birth.

- Mothers should be encouraged to breastfeed frequently according to infant behavioral feeding cues, helping to increase the number and sensitivity of prolactin receptors.
- Mothers should be encouraged to breastfeed at night when prolactin levels are highest and when suckling enhances prolactin's effects. Mothers with risk factors for impaired prolactin secretion should be encouraged to breastfeed frequently during the late afternoon and early evening when prolactin levels are low to expose the breasts to a prolactin-enhancing environment.
- Any medical history or observation of elements known to affect lactation should be charted and the mother encouraged to breastfeed. Close follow-up is needed in special situations.

LACTOGENESIS II

Lactogenesis II is described as the onset of copious milk production occurring between 32 and 96 hours postpartum. The timing of this event varies among mothers. Some women experience delayed lactogenesis II. Delayed lactogenesis II has been defined as milk transfer of less than 9.2 g per feeding at 60 hours after birth and maternal perception of the lack of breast fullness, edema, and leaking at 72 or more hours postpartum (Chapman & Perez-Escamilla, 2000a). Its incidence in the United States ranges from 23% to 44% in various populations. Delayed onset of lactation is associated with the cessation of any and exclusive breastfeeding at 4 weeks postpartum and is a marker for the need for additional professional lactation support (Brownell, Howard, Lawrence, & Dozier, 2012).

The rapid drop in maternal progesterone levels after expulsion of the placenta, in combination with the secretion of prolactin and other permissive hormones such as cortisol and insulin, triggers lactogenesis II. Milk synthesis occurs during the first 3 days postpartum even in the absence of infant suckling or milk expression, with similar prolactin levels found in both lactating and nonlactating mothers. The composition of colostrum has been shown to be similar between breastfeeding and nonbreastfeeding women during the first 3 days after birth, but prolactin levels begin dropping in nonlactating mothers on day 3. Beginning on day 4, however, nonbreastfeeding women's milk reverts to the composition of colostrum, whereas the chemical composition of breastfeeding women's milk changes to that of more mature milk. This change illustrates that efficient milk removal is essential for continued lactation (Kulski & Hartmann, 1981).

Biochemical markers that are associated with lactogenesis II include an increase in concentration of breastmilk lactose, glucose, and citrate, with parallel decreases occurring in levels of protein, nitrogen, sodium, chloride, and magnesium that are mostly complete by 72 hours postpartum (Neville et al., 1991). These changes result from the closure of the gaps between the milk-secreting cells and generally precede the onset of the large increase in milk volume by about 24 hours (Neville, Morton, & Umemora, 2001).

Maternal perception of lactogenesis II follows the biochemical changes and varies widely, with mothers reporting breast fullness, heaviness, hardness, swelling, and leaking from 1 to 148 hours after birth (Chapman & Perez-Escamilla, 1999). No single indicator for lactogenesis II exists. Misunderstanding of this process can lead mothers and healthcare providers to unnecessarily use formula supplements and further compromise the process (Chapman & Perez-Escamilla, 2000b).

Within the first 24 hours after birth, 100 mL or less of colostrum is available to the infant. This amount increases approximately 36 hours after birth and reaches an average of 500 mL at 4 days (Neville et al., 1991). The large increase in volume between 36 and 96 hours postpartum is usually perceived by the mother as the milk coming in and is a reliable indicator for this event (Pérez-Escamilla & Chapman, 2001). Women with delayed onset of lactogenesis II tend toward a lower level of milk output, and their infants lose more weight during the early postpartum period. Edema further increases the feeling of fullness and swelling.

Factors Related to Delayed Lactogenesis II

Whereas delayed lactogenesis II refers to a longer than usual time to the onset of copious milk production, failed lactogenesis II describes either a primary inability to produce adequate milk volumes or secondary conditions that impede full milk production (Hurst, 2007). The prevalence of delayed onset of lactation in primíparas is common and ranges from 33% to 44%, alerting clinicians that first-time mothers need close follow-up during the first 2 weeks postpartum. The odds of any breastfeeding at 6 weeks postpartum are nearly fivefold higher in women with a timely onset of lactation compared with those who have a delayed onset of lactation (Nommsen-Rivers, Mastergeorge, Hansen, Cullum, & Dewey, 2009).

A variety of factors have been identified that can delay or otherwise affect lactogenesis II (Neville & Morton, 2001):

- Preglandular: hormonal causes such as:
  - Retained placenta—that is, the failure of progesterone withdrawal or reduced prolactin release or other placental abnormalities such as placenta increta (Anderson, 2001; Betzold, Hoover, & Snyder, 2004; Neifert et al., 1981)
  - Gestational ovarian theca lutein cysts that elevate testosterone levels, thereby suppressing milk production (Hoover, Barbalinardo, & Platia, 2002)
- Glandular (Neifert et al., 1985): surgical procedures, insufficient mammary tissue.
- Postglandular: ineffective or infrequent milk removal, ineffective breastfeeding, cesarean delivery, primiparity (Scott, Binns, & Oddy, 2007), peripartum complications, and formula supplementation (Sievers, Haase, Oldigs, & Schaub, 2003).

Other factors that can influence lactogenesis II include preterm delivery, insulin-dependent diabetes mellitus (IDDM), gestational diabetes, metabolic status/health, obesity, older maternal age, and stress. Not all mechanisms involved are well understood. The breast is unique in that it is probably the only organ in the body that does not have a specific diagnostic test to measure its adequacy (Hartmann & Cregan, 2001). Because there is no test to determine whether or not the breast will lactate adequately, the clinician must use indirect or secondary measures to determine lactation sufficiency (Hurst, 2007).

Metabolic Status/Health

Nommsen-Rivers, Dolan, and Huang (2012) discuss factors that contribute to delayed lactogenesis II relative to maternal metabolic status. They describe three risk factors for delayed lactogenesis—higher body mass index (BMI; overweight/obesity), increased maternal age, and larger infant birth weight—as known correlates with carbohydrate intolerance and systemic inflammation. The primary predictors of the onset of lactation in this study of normal glycemic primiparous mothers was serum concentrations for insulin and for glucose, and insulin-to-glucose ratio (I:G)—a measure of 1-hour insulin relative to 1-hour glucose concentration. They found that a woman at the median for I:G ratio will experience the onset of lactation at approximately 66 hours. If her I:G ratio is in the bottom 25% of this ratio, her onset of lactation will be approximately 21–30 hours later, well beyond the 72-hour cutoff for normal onset of lactation. Thus, a lower serum insulin secretion relative to the serum glucose level after a glucose challenge during pregnancy is associated with subsequent delayed onset of lactation. This finding is cause for concern because among exclusively breastfeeding mothers who experience a delayed onset of lactation, 40% of their infants will lose more than 10% of their birth weight by the fourth day of life (Chantry, Nommsen-Rivers, Peerson, Cohen, & Dewey, 2011; Nommsen-Rivers, Heinig, Cohen, & Dewey, 2008).

Prematurity

Lactogenesis II and subsequent milk volumes can be compromised in mothers delivering prematurely (Cregan & Hartmann, 1999) for any number of reasons, including delayed initiation of pumping (Hopkinson, Schanler, & Garza, 1988) and ineffectiveness of pumps in removing milk (Hartmann, Mitoulas, & Gurrin, 2000). Chemical markers of lactogenesis II in milk samples of preterm mothers show delayed changes in concentrations relative to milk samples of full-term mothers, resulting in lower milk production (Cregan et al., 2000). Preterm mothers with chemical markers outside the range of markers observed in full-term mothers produced significantly lower amounts of milk than did preterm mothers with markers within the range for full-term women. Some speculation has been put forward that antenatal corticosteroid therapy given in high-risk pregnancies could unintentionally stimulate the breast, causing lactogenesis II to occur before delivery (Hartmann & Cregan, 2001). Henderson, Hartmann, Newnham, and Simmer (2008) showed that delivery at gestational ages less than 28 weeks caused a significant delay in the onset of lactogenesis II. The volume of milk was even more suppressed when antenatal corticosteroids were administered between 28 and 34 weeks of gestation and delivery occurred 3–9 days later. Mothers of premature infants who pumped less than six times a day also experienced a delay in lactogenesis II.

Insulin-Dependent Diabetes Mellitus

Lactogenesis II can be delayed in both mothers with IDDM and mothers with gestational diabetes. When milk levels of lactose and citrate were used as markers of lactogenesis II, Arthur, Smith, and Hartmann (1989) found a 15- to 28-hour delay in mothers with IDDM as well as a decrease in milk volume in the first 3 days postpartum. When the milk markers of lactose and total nitrogen were used, a delay of approximately 24 hours was confirmed (Neubauer et al., 1993). During the first postpartum week, serum prolactin levels were lower in mothers with IDDM and were related to elevated serum glucose concentrations (Ostrom & Ferris, 1993). Mothers with poor glycemic control should be encouraged to breastfeed very frequently during the early days of lactation. The breast contains insulin-sensitive tissue and requires insulin to initiate milk production. This delay in lactogenesis II may illustrate how the mother's body competes with the breasts for the available insulin. Less optimal breastfeeding management may also contribute to the physiological delay in lactogenesis II in diabetic women. Mothers with IDDM have been observed to start breastfeeding an average of 24 hours later than nondiabetic women (Ferris et al., 1988). An increased number of breastfeeding episodes within the first 12 hours postpartum have been shown to be critical in stimulating lactogenesis II in mothers with IDDM (Ferris et al., 1993). A possible contributor to delayed lactogenesis in diabetic mothers may be the reduced amount of circulating human placental lactogen, which is positively correlated with breast growth in pregnancy (Hartmann & Cregan, 2001).

Delayed onset of lactation has been shown to be common in women with recent gestational diabetes mellitus, with one third of subjects reporting a delayed arrival of milk in a study of 883 new mothers with gestational diabetes (Matias, Dewey, Quesenberry, & Gunderson, 2014). In this investigation, the researchers identified maternal obesity, insulin treatment during pregnancy (an indicator of greater severity of gestational diabetes mellitus), and suboptimal in-hospital breastfeeding management as key risk factors for delayed lactogenesis II. Insulin treatment during pregnancy should be considered an indicator of the need for immediate skilled lactation support following delivery. Older maternal age is a risk factor for gestational diabetes and is associated with increased odds of delayed onset of lactation, with a 5-year increase in maternal age being associated with a 26% increase in risk of experiencing delayed lactogenesis II (Matias et al., 2014). Marked disturbances in insulin and glucose metabolism during pregnancy may interfere with the hormonal pathways for initiation of lactogenesis.

A recent study looked at gene expression profiles at different stages of lactation and suggested that decreased insulin sensitivity may delay milk production as a result of overexpression of protein tyrosine phosphatase, receptor type F, in the breast (Lemay et al., 2013).

Obesity

Overweight (BMI of 26–29 kg/m^2) and obesity (BMI greater than 29 kg/m^2) have been shown to be risk factors for avoidance of breastfeeding, delayed onset of lactation and shorter duration of breastfeeding. Mothers with a heavy or obese build have been identified as experiencing delayed onset of lactogenesis and demonstrating reduced milk transfer at 60 hours postpartum (Chapman & Perez-Escamilla, 1999, 2000b). Women who are overweight or obese are also less likely to be breastfeeding at hospital discharge (Hilson, Rasmussen, & Kjolhede, 1997). Mothers with delayed lactogenesis (72 hours or later postpartum) were significantly more likely to have a higher prepregnant BMI than mothers with earlier onset of lactogenesis II (Hilson, 2000; Rasmussen, Hilson, & Kjolhede, 2001). Obese mothers demonstrate a lower prolactin response to suckling, especially during the early days of lactation when this response is more important than in later lactation (Rasmussen & Kjolhede, 2004). Nommsen-Rivers, Chantry, Peerson, Cohen, and Dewey (2010) found a dose–response relationship between BMI and delayed onset of lactation. The incidence of delayed onset of lactation was 1.84 times higher in overweight mothers and 2.21 times higher in obese mothers compared with mothers in the normal BMI range.

A relationship between postpartum BMI and duration of breastfeeding has been established as well. When comparing BMI and breastfeeding duration, an inverse relationship is seen whereby breastfeeding duration decreases as BMI increases (Donath & Amir, 2000). In this dose–response pattern, overweight women have an increased risk of unsuccessful initiation and continuation of breastfeeding compared with normal weight mothers. Obese mothers have a further elevated risk. Rutishauser and Carlin (1992) reported that 18% of women with a BMI between 26 and 30 discontinued breastfeeding between 14 and 60 days postpartum, whereas 37% of women with a BMI greater than 30 ceased breastfeeding during this period. Forty-one percent of the failure in breastfeeding initiation in this study population was attributable to prepregnant overweight and obesity.

Data from a study involving 151 women showed that a 1-unit (1 kg/m^2) increase in prepregnant BMI was associated with a 0.5-hour delay in lactogenesis II (Hilson et al., 2004). The clinical implications of this calculation become apparent when comparing the difference in the onset of lactation between a mother with a BMI of 40 kg/m^2 and a mother with a BMI of 20 kg/m^2. A 10-hour delay in lactogenesis II for an obese mother can contribute to supplementation of the infant because the concerned mother becomes anxious about the delayed milk arrival (Hilson et al., 2004). Dewey, Nommsen-Rivers, Heinig, and Cohen (2003) found that women with a BMI greater than 27 kg/m^2 were 2.5 times more likely to experience a delayed onset of lactation and their infants were 3 times more likely to demonstrate suboptimal breastfeeding on day 7. With as many as 35.8% of American women being obese and given the increasing obesity trend among African American and Hispanic women (Flegal, Carroll, Kit, & Ogden, 2012), higher BMIs may present continuing and increasing challenges to both the initiation and the duration of breastfeeding in this population.

Other factors, such as the role of race/ethnicity, gestational weight gain, and other comorbidities, may contribute to the adverse effects of higher BMI on breastfeeding (Wojcicki, 2011). Additional possible contributors to the adverse breastfeeding outcomes seen in overweight and obese mothers include the following:

- Obese women have a higher risk of cesarean delivery and of bearing a large infant:
    - This may result in a delay of the infant going to breast as well as discomfort or illness in the mother.
    - The infant may suffer birth trauma and/or unstable blood glucose values, resulting in formula supplementation and possible delay in early and frequent suckling.
- Gestational diabetes mellitus is more prevalent in obese women than in overweight women and may delay lactogenesis II.
- Mechanical difficulties may exist in positioning and latching an infant onto a large breast.
- Maternal obesity may be associated with metabolic or steroidal hormonal alterations that affect the breasts' ability to initiate and produce sufficient quantities of milk or particular nutrients. Rasmussen and Kjolhede (2004) demonstrated that obese women had a lower prolactin response to suckling. A blunted prolactin response to suckling in the early days when lactation is becoming established may not only delay lactogenesis II but may also establish low levels of milk production, leading to early supplementation and premature weaning.

Stress

A relationship between stress experienced during labor and delivery and delayed lactogenesis II has been observed in mothers experiencing long stage II durations and urgent cesarean sections. Chen, Nommsen-Rivers, Dewey, and Lonnerdal (1998) demonstrated that a number of markers of maternal and fetal distress during labor and delivery were associated with delayed breast fullness, smaller milk volume on day 5, and/or delayed casein appearance. Chapman and Perez-Escamilla (1999) reported that, among other risk factors, unscheduled cesarean section and prolonged stage II of labor were associated with delayed onset of breast fullness (more than 72 hours postpartum). Dewey, Nommsen-Rivers, Heinig, and Cohen (2002) described delayed lactogenesis II as being more common if there was a long duration of labor (more than 14 hours), the mother had an urgent cesarean section, and the infant had a low sucking score on day 3. All these conditions are strongly related to the amount of stress experienced by both the mother and the infant during labor and delivery, can have a marked impact on lactogenesis II, and may be partially predictive of the magnitude of infant weight loss by day 3.

Complex interrelationships exist among the various factors that may affect lactogenesis, making it difficult to separate the effects of stress from those of other variables. When lactogenesis II is impaired, leading to delayed onset of milk production, insufficient milk volume, and/or infant weight loss, this problem can also be due to the combined result of stress with one or more maternal, infant, or environmental factors (Dewey, 2001). Chatterton et al. (2000) found a relationship between salivary amylase (a measure of stress) and decreased prolactin levels at 6 weeks postpartum in preterm mothers who were pumping their milk. This degree of suppression of prolactin levels could represent a declining responsiveness that results in inadequate milk production in mothers of some preterm infants.

Timing of First Breast Stimulation Following Delivery

Parker, Sullivan, Krueger, Kelechi, and Mueller (2012) studied the effects of early initiation of milk expression on the onset of lactogenesis II and milk volume in mothers of very-low-birth-weight infants. Twenty women were randomized to initiate milk expression either within 60 minutes of birth (group 1) or 1 to 6 hours following delivery (group 2). Milk volume and timing of lactogenesis II was compared between the two groups. Group 1 produced significantly more milk than group 2 during the first 7 days and at week 3. Group 1 also demonstrated a significantly earlier onset of lactogenesis II. The common recommendation to initiate milk expression during the first 6 hours following birth was shown to be ineffective in inducing earlier lactogenesis II and increased milk production unless milk expression was begun within 1 hour of birth (Parker, Sullivan, Krueger, & Meuller, 2015). Clinicians may wish to recommend that mothers of preterm or ill infants start milk expression within an hour of birth if possible when the infant cannot be put to breast during that time.

Disruption of Circadian Systems

Given the metabolic/hormonal influences may act to delay lactogenesis II, it is interesting to note that the circadian and metabolic systems are closely linked. It has been suggested that disruption of the circadian timing system during pregnancy and the peripartum could negatively affect lactogenesis II (Fu et al., 2015). Circadian rhythms are generated at the molecular level by circadian clocks, with the master circadian clock being located in the suprachiasmatic nuclei of the hypothalamus. In addition, peripheral clocks are distributed in every body organ. Depression, light, activity (especially at night, such as night-shift work), excessive weight, stress, and sleep disturbances are all factors that can disrupt circadian rhythms. Changes in glucose and lipid metabolism, abnormally high levels of cortisol at night, changes in melatonin and thyroid levels, and development of type 2 diabetes may also disrupt circadian rhythms.

Prolactin, milk synthesis, and milk composition show circadian variations in lactating mothers. In fact, almost 7% of the genes expressed in the lactating breast show circadian oscillation. It has been proposed that interventions might potentially be able to prevent circadian misalignment so as to ameliorate the altered timing of lactogenesis II among many mothers at risk for delayed onset of lactation (Fu et al., 2015). Such interventions might include lighting environments that are more closely aligned with the natural light–dark cycles of the earth. Ideally, infants should be exposed to a natural light–dark cycle after birth, not 24-hour bright lights as are found in a nursery. Optical filters could be placed on lights for nighttime lighting when it is necessary to perform procedures that require nighttime exposure to light. Mothers should experience a natural light–dark cycle while in the hospital, along with limited visiting hours, to reduce their levels of stress.

Suckling and Suckling Frequency

The function of infant suckling (or mechanical milk removal) varies between lactogenesis II, the onset of copious milk production, and lactogenesis III, the maintenance of abundant milk production. Lactogenesis II occurs in the absence of milk removal over the first 3 days postpartum, but changes in milk composition and volume will not proceed along the continuum to maximum milk production and mature milk composition in the absence of frequent milk removal after that time. Although suckling (or mechanical milk removal) may not be a prerequisite for lactogenesis II, poor sucking can delay it and sucking is critical for lactogenesis III. Delayed suckling by the infant, whether due to premature delivery (Cregan et al., 2000), cesarean delivery (Sozmen, 1992), or other factors that necessitate mechanical milk removal, may affect the timing or delay the onset of lactogenesis II. Nommsen-Rivers and colleagues (2010) reported that delayed onset of lactation was associated with infants who were described as not breastfeeding well twice during the first 24 hours. Delayed onset of lactation was also more common with higher amounts ($>$ 60 mL) of formula supplementation during the first 48 hours. Breastfeeding frequency was not associated with delayed onset of lactation, but poor quality of breastfeeding was. Lower LATCH scores during the first 24 hours (reflecting suboptimal breastfeeding during the hospital stay) have been associated with increased odds of experiencing delayed onset of lactation (Matias et al., 2014). Additional breast pumping after a couple of breastfeeds before the onset of lactogenesis II has not been shown to hasten the event or result in increased milk transfer to the baby at 72 hours (Chapman, Young, Ferris, & Perez-Escamilla, 2001). However, direct suckling at the breast during the first 24 hours postpartum interacts with maternal obesity status to determine milk transfer at 60 hours postpartum. Mothers who exclusively formula feed their infants perceive the onset of lactation as being significantly later than those who breastfeed (Chapman & Perez-Escamilla, 1999).

Direct, early, and frequent suckling at the breast during the early days of lactation has the following effects:

- It prevents a delayed onset of lactogenesis II or conversely facilitates the normal timing for the onset of lactogenesis II.
- It properly hydrates the infant.
- It provides sufficient calories for infant growth.
- It prevents excessive infant weight loss.
- It stabilizes infant blood glucose levels.
- It moderates infant bilirubin levels.
- It may prime the breasts by increasing the number and sensitivity of prolactin receptors in milk-secreting cells, setting the stage for abundant milk synthesis following lactogenesis II.

Clinical Implications

The early breastfeeding experience contributes to the timing of the onset of lactation. Maternity care practices in hospitals during the early days postpartum should be consistent with those contained in the Baby-Friendly Hospital Initiative. These practices increase the likelihood of effective breastfeeding within the first 24 hours and reduce practices that result in delayed onset of lactation.

Woolridge (1995) provided a practical identification of six separate stages in the lactation process:

1. Priming (changes of pregnancy).
2. Initiation (birth and the management of early breastfeeding).
3. Calibration (the concept that milk production gets under way without the breasts actually "knowing" how much milk to make in the beginning). Over the first 3 to 5 weeks after birth, milk output is progressively calibrated to the infant's needs, usually building up (upregulating) but occasionally down-regulating to meet the infant's needs.
4. Maintenance (the period of exclusive breastfeeding).
5. Decline (the period after complementary foods or supplements are added).
6. Involution (weaning).

The second, third, and fourth time periods are crucial to ensuring abundant milk production and optimal weight gain in the infant. Dewey et al. (2003) identified a number of factors that can negatively affect lactogenesis II, infant breastfeeding behaviors, and excessive weight loss: primiparity, urgent cesarean section, long/stressful labor, labor pain medications, high maternal BMI, flat or inverted nipples, non-breastmilk fluid supplementation in the first 48 hours, and pacifier use. Close attention must be given to any of the previously mentioned alterations that could affect the breasts' ability to calibrate their milk output to the needs of the infant.

Medications

Medications for lactation have mostly centered around preparations that are used to increase faltering milk volumes. Because prolactin is necessary for the initiation of lactation, a new treatment using recombinant human prolactin may be helpful in those mothers with prolactin deficiency or blunted prolactin responses (Page-Wilson, Smith, & Welt, 2007). Powe and colleagues (2011) conducted a study to determine the impact of recombinant human prolactin (r-hPRL) on the nutritional and immunological composition of breastmilk. One group of prolactin-deficient, preterm mothers in the study was noted to still be producing only small amounts of milk at entry into the study (< 8 mL/day) at a mean time of 12.4 weeks following delivery. After administration of recombinant human prolactin, baseline and peak prolactin levels adjusted to normal ranges and milk production increased significantly. Essentially, these women had failed to experience lactogenesis II but did so when provided with a source of prolactin. The prolactin administration was associated with compositional changes in the milk that mirrored those in women undergoing normal lactogenesis in the first 2–10 days following birth. There was an increase in lactose concentrations and a decrease in milk sodium concentrations with the recombinant prolactin treatment. These changes are consistent with closure of the tight junctions between mammary epithelial cells in the breast, which prohibits sodium entry from the interstitium into milk and traps lactose in the ducts. When tight junctions open, milk production decreases because osmotically active milk components cannot be retained in the duct. Increased milk sodium is known to be associated with events such as mastitis, weaning, insufficient milk, and breastfeeding failure. This study demonstrated the role of prolactin in human lactogenesis through direct administration of prolactin to mothers with prolactin deficiency. R-hPRL was used successfully in a breastfeeding mother with no detectable prolactin due to prolactin deficiency associated with autoantibodies against prolactin-secreting cells (Iwama, Welt, Romero, Radovick, & Caturegli, 2013). Future studies with recombinant human prolactin are looking at its use in mothers with Sheehan syndrome, in adoptive mothers, and as an aid to induce lactation. Thyroid hormones are important for milk production and in animals are necessary for the mammary glands to be responsive to prolactin during lactation (Hapon, Simoncini, Via, & Jahn, 2003). Insufficient lactation in women has been treated with nasal administration of thyrotropin-releasing hormone, which has been shown to increase prolactin levels and daily milk volume (Peters, Schulze-Tollert, & Schuth, 1991).

LACTOGENESIS III

The maintenance of milk production is influenced by three levels of controls: endocrine, autocrine (local), and metabolic. The endocrine system is thought to set each individual woman's maximum potential to produce milk, but it is the local control mechanisms acting in concert that actually regulate the short-term synthesis of milk (Hartmann, Sherriff, & Mitoulas, 1998).

Autocrine or Local Control of Milk Synthesis

Local control of milk synthesis is governed by a number of factors:

1. Degree of breast fullness
    - Computerized breast measurements (Daly et al., 1992) have shown that the degree of fullness of the breast and the short-term rate of milk synthesis (between feeds) are inversely related; that is, the emptier the breast, the higher the rate of milk synthesis.
    - Milk synthesis is a continuous process governed in part by a mechanism that is sensitive to the degree of fullness in the breast (Lai, Hale, Simmer, & Hartmann, 2010).
    - There is a wide variability in the rate of milk synthesis, ranging from 11 to 58 mL/h; however, the infant does not drain the breasts to the same degree at consecutive feedings. The amount of milk available in the breasts does not necessarily determine the amount of milk the infant removes at each feeding.
    - On average over a 24-hour period, infants remove approximately 76% of the available milk at a feeding (Daly, Kent, Owens, & Hartmann, 1996). The breast can rapidly change the rate of milk synthesis from one feeding interval to the next.
    - There is an inverse relationship between the breast volume and the fat content of the milk. At the maximum breast volume when the breast is full of milk, minimum fat content is seen in the milk. When the breast is well drained and at minimum volume, the milk is seen with maximum fat content (Kent et al., 2006).
    - As milk accumulates in the breast, the binding of prolactin to its membrane receptors is reduced, an event that occurs independently within each breast, facilitating an inhibitory

effect on milk secretion rates (Cox et al., 1996). Prolactin uptake from the blood by the lactocytes (milk-secreting cells) depends on the fullness of the breast, such that prolactin uptake may be inhibited in full alveoli (Cregan, Mitoulas, & Hartmann, 2002).

- Each breast can control the rate of milk synthesis independently of the other, even though both are exposed to the same hormonal stimuli. Thus one breast may produce more milk than the other (Daly, Owens, & Hartmann, 1993). In 7 of 10 mothers, the right breast is more productive, with no association between handedness or preferential offering to the infant (Kent et al., 2006). The differences between milk output appear early in the postpartum period and remain relatively constant throughout the day and over many weeks of lactation (Engstrom, Meier, Jegier, Motykowski, & Zuleger, 2007). Milk production in each mammary lobe may be controlled separately, as each can contain milk of a different composition. The creamatocrit value of hindmilk obtained from separate ducts represents the degree of emptying of each mammary lobe that is drained (Mizuno et al., 2008). Moreover, the quality of the infant's latch (deep or shallow) affects the degree of drainage of the respective mammary lobes (Mizuno et al., 2008). Although the difference in output between breasts is normal, it is still important to recognize when reduced output in a breast signals a problem (blocked milk duct, mastitis, tight breast pump flange, or, more rarely, neoplastic changes). This recognition is especially important if the onset of reduced production is sudden or appears as a significant discrepancy from previous milk production. Although the reasons for milk output differences are unknown, it has been speculated that the right breast receives more blood flow than the left breast, giving it an advantage in the mechanics of milk production (Aljazaf, 2004).

2. Infant appetite
    - Maternal milk supply is balanced to the infant's demand for or intake of milk because the average mother's potential for milk production exceeds the average infant's appetite (Daly & Hartmann, 1995a).
    - Approximately 29% of infants whose mothers have a high milk storage capacity choose to take smaller feeds even though more milk is available, whereas 40% of infants whose mothers have a low milk storage capacity choose to take larger feeds and drain the breast more thoroughly at each feeding (Kent, 2007).
    - If an infant's demand or need for milk increases, the infant may choose to feed at the same frequency but increase the amount of milk ingested at the feed. Thus the degree to which the breast is emptied may be the factor driving overall milk synthesis.
    - Frequency of breastfeeding may be critical in some mothers, especially those expressing milk in the absence of an infant at breast.
3. Storage capacity of the breasts
    - The size of the breast typically has no relationship to the overall amount of milk it is capable of synthesizing. However, larger breasts (that may contain more glandular tissue) may be able to store more milk between feedings, partially determining how the infant's demand for milk is met by the mother. Mothers with smaller storage capacities make similar amounts of milk over 24-hour periods but may need to feed their infant more frequently than mothers with larger breastmilk storage capacity (Daly & Hartmann, 1995b).

4. Feedback inhibitor of lactation
   - Feedback inhibitor of lactation (FIL) is an active whey protein that inhibits milk secretion as alveoli become distended and milk is not removed (Prentice, Addey, & Wilde, 1989). Its concentration increases with longer periods of milk accumulation, downregulating milk production in a chemical feedback loop.
   - The inhibition of milk secretion is reversible and depends on concentration; it does not affect the composition of the milk because it affects the secretion of all milk components simultaneously.
   - Short feedings from both breasts remove the FIL, as its volume is highest in the foremilk. If one breast is not used for many feedings or not drained very well, then its milk production could be reduced. This knowledge is used in efforts to reduce overproduction by limiting sucking at the breast.
5. Breastfeeding method
   - Feeding methods may also influence milk synthesis. Little information is available on the physiology of the length of feeding times as they relate to milk production. Prolonged feeds (greater than 30 minutes) may demonstrate diminishing returns relative to milk synthesis (and milk intake). In a study looking at milk volume, breastfeeding frequency, and duration in mothers with nipple pain, McClellan and colleagues (2012) found that clinically, the only predictor of lower milk production was meal durations lasting longer than 33 minutes in the women with persistent nipple pain.
   - Walshaw (2010) noted three factors that may act to reduce milk supply during long feedings:
     - Sensory input from the nipple depends on nerve receptors on the tip of the nipple that are the quick-adapting type and sensitive to stretching. As milk flow rates slow toward the end of a feeding and pauses increase in length, continued feeding over a prolonged period of time with little milk flow and long applications of vacuum to the nipple may result in only a weak signal passed to the hypothalamus.
     - Continuous nipple stimulation over a long period may result in a continuous low output of oxytocin rather than the normal pulsatile release seen with shorter, more vigorous feedings. The continuous low output of oxytocin may result in tetanic asynchronous contractions of the myoepithelial cells, which may not cause an effective vigorous release of milk. The baby may need to be eventually removed from the breast in order to let the oxytocin levels fall.
     - Downregulation of oxytocin receptors within the breast may take place during prolonged feedings. Some of these receptors may downregulate after a relatively short exposure to oxytocin, with a long exposure resulting in abnormal milk flow and possible decreased milk production (Walshaw, Owens, Scally & Walshaw, 2008). Shorter feedings with gaps between feeds may help to maintain optimal function of the oxytocin receptors.

Volume of Milk Production over Time

Milk production varies widely among breastfeeding mothers, and a number of factors may influence a woman's lactation capacity. The range of milk volumes varies among mothers from 500 mL/day to

1,200 mL/day, with calculations of breastmilk transfer to the infant gradually increasing from approximately 650 mL/day at 1 month, to 770 mL/day at 3 months, to 800 mL/day at 6 months, when it seems to level off (Neville et al., 1988). As solid foods are introduced around 6 months, milk production decreases to between 95 and 315 mL/day at 15 to 30 months (Hennart, Delogne-Desnoeck, Vis, & Robyn, 1981; Kent, Mitoulas, Cox, Owens, & Hartmann, 1999; Neville et al., 1991). The milk composition changes with decreases in the concentration of glucose, citrate, phosphate, and calcium and increases in the concentrations of fat, protein, lactose, and sodium. The amount of breast tissues remains constant between 1 and 6 months of lactation and decreases significantly between 6 and 9 months, with only a small drop in milk production. The breasts return to their preconception size by 15 months of lactation (Kent et al., 1999). Mothers may become concerned during this time that their milk production is insufficient because of the change in breast size. Clinicians can assure mothers that this is part of the normal process of breast involution. Involution of the breast occurs in two stages. First the lactocytes (milk-producing cells) are removed by apoptosis (programmed cell death), and then the surrounding stroma (supporting tissue) is remodeled (Watson, 2006).

THE NEWBORN STOMACH

During the first few days after birth, the breasts secrete colostrum in amounts that seem small compared with what a formula-fed infant can be compelled to consume. The amounts and composition of colostrum and milk are synchronized to the newborn infant's anatomy, physiology, needs, and stores (**Table 2-7**). Misunderstanding of this unique matchup can lead to unnecessary supplementation.

Table 2-7 Volume of Milk Production and Intake

Time Postpartum	Volume/Day Average (Range)	Volume/Feed Average	Notes	References
Day 1 (0–24 h)	37 mL (7–123 mL) 6 mL/kg (vaginal) 4 mL/kg (cesarean)	7 mL	Matches the physiological capacity of the newborn stomach	Casey, Neifert, Seacat, & Neville, 1986; Evans, Evans, Royal, Esterman, & James, 2003; Houston, Howie, & McNeilly, 1983; Roderuck, Williams, & Macy, 1946; Saint, Smith, & Hartmann, 1984
Day 2 (24–48 h)	84 mL (44–335 mL) 25 mL/kg (vaginal) 13 mL/kg (cesarean)	14 mL		Evans et al., 2003; Houston et al., 1983
24 hours 30 hours 36 hours 48 hours 60 hours 72 hours		4.2 mL ± 10.6 3.1 mL ± 6.6 3.1 mL ± 4.9 6.4 mL ± 6.8 14.0 mL ± 13.5 26.1 mL ± 26.6	Nonpumping cesarean mothers; multiparous mothers had increased milk volumes	Chapman et al., 2001

(*continues*)

Table 2-7 Volume of Milk Production and Intake (*Continued*)

Time Postpartum	Volume/Day Average (Range)	Volume/Feed Average	Notes	References
Day 3 (48–72 h)	408 mL (98–775) 66 mL/kg (vaginal) 44 mL/kg (cesarean)	38 mL	Lactogenesis II occurs in this time period	Casey et al., 1986; Evans et al., 2003; Houston et al., 1983; Neville et al., 1988; Saint et al., 1984
Day 4 (72–96 h)	625 mL (378–876) 106 mL/kg (vaginal) 82 mL/kg (cesarean)	58 mL	Delayed lactogenesis II results in decreased milk volumes	Houston et al., 1983; Saint et al., 1984; Evans et al., 2003
Day 5	200–900 g 123 mL/kg (vaginal) 111 mL/kg (cesarean)		Milk output is calibrated to meet infant needs over 3–5 weeks	Woolridge, 1995; Evans et al., 2003
Day 6	138 mL/kg (vaginal) 129 mL/kg (cesarean)			Evans et al., 2003
Day 7	576 mL (mean) (200–1,013)	65 mL	Multiparous women produced an average of 142 mL more milk each 24 h	Ingram, Woolridge, Greenwood, & McGrath, 1999
4 weeks	750 mL (mean) (328–1,127) 675 mL (600–950)	94 mL		Ingram et al., 1999
2–6 months 2.5 months	1,680–3,000 mL 3080 mL		Milk yields in mothers of twins; mothers of triplets	Saint, Maggiore, & Hartmann, 1986
3 months	750 mL (609–837) 720 mL (550–880)			Butte, Garza, O'Brien Smith, & Nichols, 1984
5 months	770 mL (630–950)			
6 months	800 mL			Neville et al., 1988
1–6 months	750 mL ± 200 mL	71.8 mL ± 26.3 mL	All infants were fully breastfed on demand; includes both multiparous and primiparous mothers	Mitoulas et al., 2002
9 months	740 mL			Kent et al., 1999
12 months	520 mL			
18 months	218 mL			
24 months	114 mL			

Modified from Royal College of Midwives. (2002). *Successful breastfeeding* (3rd ed.). London, UK: Churchill Livingstone, p. 26.

Table 2-8 Factors Related to Feed Size/Frequency in the Early Hours and Days After Birth

Factor	Comment
Physiological diuresis of excess fluid	Lack of hunger or thirst (CNS depression, changing hormonal concentrations)
Immaturity of gastric function	Noncompliant, nonrelaxing stomach
Stomach capacity	Size related to birth weight
Physiological vs. anatomic capacity	The volume that fits comfortably as a feed vs. the amount that can be held to the point of discomfort and pain
Gastric emptying time	Generally delayed in the first 12 hours of life; faster for breastmilk than for formula
Increasing age and number of feedings	Encourages the stomach to relax and stretch to better accommodate increasing volumes of milk

The volume of a feeding in the early hours and days after birth is quite small. A number of factors contribute to this normal state (**Table 2-8**).

Clinical Implications

A newborn infant may show a delayed interest in feeding if the mother has been heavily medicated during labor and/or has received large quantities of fluid during labor, adding to the excess extracellular fluid burden that accompanies the transition to postnatal life. The newborn stomach is rather noncompliant and does not easily relax to accommodate a feeding during the early hours after birth. Over the next 3 days of life, a reduction in the gastric tone and an increase in compliance allow the stomach to accept increasing volumes of milk per feeding (Zangen et al., 2001). Clinically, this change is seen as infants ingesting very small volumes of milk (5 mL = 1 teaspoon) and regurgitating milk or formula if they are persuaded to accept more than their stomachs can physiologically accommodate.

There is a difference between the physiological and anatomic capacity of the newborn stomach (**Table 2-9** and **Table 2-10**). The physiological capacity is what an infant can comfortably ingest at a feeding (feeding volume as determined by pre- and post-feed weights), whereas the anatomic capacity is what the stomach will hold at its maximum fullness (as determined on autopsy). Physiological capacity (Scammon & Doyle, 1920) is considerably less than anatomic capacity during the early days. Physiological and anatomic stomach capacities begin to approximate each other around 4 days of age. The actual size of the newborn stomach has received little attention, especially in regard to the volume of what a "normal" feeding should be. Widstrom et al. (1988) studied gastric aspirates in newborns immediately after birth, showing gastric contents of 0–11 mL. They suggested that the fetus typically drinks about 10-mL portions of amniotic fluid, which are gradually emptied from the stomach.

Using real-time ultrasound imaging, Nagata, Koyanagi, Fukushima, Akazawa, and Nakano (1994) calculated fetal stomach volume at 38 weeks to be approximately 9.9 mL, whereas Sase et al. (2005) using ultrasound calculated newborn stomach volumes at approximately 10 mL. Naveed, Manjunath, and Sreenivas (1992) calculated the anatomic stomach capacity at autopsy of 100 perinatal stillbirths and 37 deaths

Table 2-9 Average Physiological Capacity of the Stomach in the First 10 Days of Life

Physiological stomach capacity birth weights 2.0–4.0+ kg (4.4–8.8 lb), 14,571 feeding records of 323 breastfed newborns

Day of Life	mL	mL/kg
1	7	2
2	13	4
3	27	8
4	46	14
5	57	17
6	64	19
7	68	21
8	71	22
9	76	23
10	81	24

Scammon, R. E., & Doyle, L. O. (1920). Observations on the capacity of the stomach in the first ten days of postnatal life. *American Journal of Diseases in Children, 20*, 516–538.

Table 2-10 Average Anatomic Capacity of the Stomach in Newborns

Physiological stomach capacity birth weights 2.0–4.0+ kg (4.4–8.8 lb), 14,571 feeding records of 323 breastfed newborns

Age/Weight	Average Capacity (mL)
Newborn 1.5–2.0 kg	22
Newborn 2.0–2.5 kg	30
Newborn 2.5–3.0 kg	30
Newborn 3.0–3.5 kg	35
Newborn 3.5–4.0 kg	35
Newborn 4.0+ kg	38
1 week, all weights	45
2 weeks, all weights	75

Scammon, R. E., & Doyle, L. O. (1920). Observations on the capacity of the stomach in the first ten days of postnatal life. *American Journal of Diseases in Children, 20*, 516–538.

occurring in the first week. They found that the larger the infant, the greater the anatomic capacity of the stomach. An infant over 5.5 lb (2,500 g) was shown to have an anatomic capacity of 18–21 mL. Hata and colleagues (2010) used three-dimensional ultrasound to study the volume of the fetal stomach. The fetal gastric volume calculated by two-dimensional ultrasound is about one-third smaller than the maximum volume using three-dimensional ultrasound. These authors found that at 36 weeks, the maximum volume of the fetal stomach was almost 14 mL. The functional capacity was somewhat less. Bergman (2013) suggested that the anatomic capacity of the stomach at birth is approximately 20 mL, and that when sleep cycles and gastric emptying times are taken into account, the feeding frequency of one hour more closely matches the physiology and capacities of the newborn. Hourly breastfeedings would avoid the stress to newborns from large feeding volumes, state disorganization, reflux, hypoglycemia, and spitting up—all outcomes to which unphysiological feeding volumes and long intervals between feeds can contribute.

Communicating the concept of the small stomach size and the need for small feedings and avoidance of large formula supplements during the early days led to the concept of a visual aid to illustrate the small size of the newborn stomach (Spangler, Randenberg, Brenner, & Howett, 2008). Objects such as marbles, ping pong balls, and eggs illustrate the approximate breastmilk intake of infants at various ages and help parents and clinicians understand that encouraging infants to take volumes beyond their physiological capacity may be detrimental. The anatomic and physiological capacities of the newborn stomach vary widely and depend on gestational age and feeding history. There is really no single visual aid such as a walnut that accurately reflects the exact volume a specific infant can safely consume. Many clinicians use a teaspoon to represent an average feeding volume on day 1 because 5 mL is within the range of intakes of normal term breastfed infants.

Human milk is easily and rapidly digested. The mean gastric half-emptying time for formula is 65 minutes (range, 27–98 minutes), whereas the mean gastric half-emptying time for breastmilk is 47 minutes (range, 16–86 minutes) (Lambrecht, Robberecht, Deschynkel, & Afschrift, 1988; Van den Driessche et al., 1999). Thus breastfed infants can be hungry sooner than 2 or 3 hours after a feeding. Routine or capricious supplementation of a breastfed infant with water or formula after nursing is not supported by the data.

SUMMARY: THE DESIGN IN NATURE

Lactation is a robust process that is organized to meet the nutritional, emotional, developmental, and health needs of the infant and young child. Breastfeeding is a dynamic coordination between the changing needs, stores, and capacities of a child and the delivery of appropriate nutrients, immune factors, and physical contact necessary to support the normal growth and development of a new person. Breastfeeding and lactation can occur within a wide range of anatomic and physiological parameters in both the infant and the mother. It is the clinician's responsibility to ensure that both happen (**Appendix 2-1**).

REFERENCES

Ahmed, O. A., & Kolhe, P. S. (2000). Comparison of nipple and areolar sensation after breast reduction by free nipple graft and inferior pedicle techniques. *British Journal of Plastic Surgery, 53,* 126–129.

Alexander, J., Grant, A., & Campbell, M. J. (1992). Randomized controlled trial of breast shells and Hoffman's exercises for inverted and non-protractile nipples. *British Medical Journal, 304,* 1030–1032.

Aljazaf, K. M. (2004). *Ultrasound imaging in the analysis of the blood supply and blood flow in the human lactating breast* (Dissertation). Medical Imaging Science, Curtin University of Technology, Perth, Australia.

American Society of Plastic Surgeons. (2013). 2013 plastic surgery statistics report. Retrieved from http://www.plasticsurgery.org/Documents/news-resources/statistics/2013-statistics/plastic-surgery-statistics-full-report-2013.pdf

Anderson, A. M. (2001). Disruption of lactogenesis by retained placental fragments. *Journal of Human Lactation, 17,* 142–144.

Andrade, R. A., Coca, K. P., & Abrao, A. C. (2010). Breastfeeding pattern in the first month of life in women submitted to breast reduction and augmentation. *Journal de Pediatría (Rio J), 86,* 239–244.

Arbour, M. W., & Kessler, J. L. (2013). Mammary hypoplasia: Not every breast can produce sufficient milk. *Journal of Midwifery & Women's Health, 58,* 457–461.

Arthur, P. G., Smith, M., & Hartmann, P. E. (1989). Milk lactose, citrate, and glucose as markers of lactogenesis in normal and diabetic women. *Journal of Pediatric Gastroenterology and Nutrition, 9,* 488–496.

Ballesio, L., Maggi, C., Savelli, S., Angeletti, M., Rabuffi, P., Manganaro, L., & Porfiri, L. M. (2007). Adjunctive diagnostic value of ultrasonography evaluation in patients with suspected ductal breast disease. *La Radiologia Medica, 112,* 354–365.

Bell, A. F., White-Traut, R., & Rankin, K. (2013). Fetal exposure to synthetic oxytocin and the relationship with prefeeding cues within one hour postbirth. *Early Human Development, 89,* 137–143.

Bergman, N. J. (2013). Neonatal stomach volume and physiology suggest feeding a 1-h intervals. *Acta Paediatrica, 102,* 773–777.

Betzold, C. M., Hoover, K. L., & Snyder, C. L. (2004). Delayed lactogenesis II: A comparison of four cases. *Journal of Midwifery and Women's Health, 49,* 132–137.

Bowles, B. C., Stutte, P. C., & Hensley, J. H. (1987). New benefits from an old technique: Alternate massage in breastfeeding. *Genesis, 9,* 5–9, 17.

Brown, S. L., Todd, J. F., Cope, J. U., & Sachs, H. C. (2006). Breast implant surveillance reports to the US Food and Drug Administration: Maternal–child health problems. *Journal of Long-Term Effects of Medical Implants, 16,* 281–290.

Brownell, E., Howard, C. R., Lawrence, R. A., & Dozier, A. M. (2012). Does delayed onset lactogenesis II predict the cessation of any or exclusive breastfeeding? *Journal of Pediatrics, 161,* 608–614.

Brzozowski, D., Niessen, M., Evans, H. B., & Hurst, L. N. (2000). Breastfeeding after inferior pedicle reduction mammaplasty. *Plastic and Reconstructive Surgery, 105,* 530–534.

Butte, N., Garza, C., O'Brien Smith, E., & Nichols, B. L. (1984). Human milk intake and growth in exclusively breastfed infants. *Journal of Pediatrics, 104,* 187–195.

Carter, C. S., Altemus, M., & Chrousos, G. P. (2001). Neuroendocrine and emotional changes in the postpartum period. *Progress in Brain Research, 133,* 241–249.

Casey, C., Neifert, M., Seacat, J., & Neville, M. (1986). Nutrient intake by breastfed infants during the first five days after birth. *American Journal of Diseases of Children, 140,* 933–936.

Center for Devices and Radiological Health, U.S. Food and Drug Administration. (2011). FDA Update on the Safety of Silicone Gel-Filled Breast Implants. Retrieved from http://www.fda.gov/downloads/MedicalDevices/ProductsandMedicalProcedures/ImplantsandProsthetics/BreastImplants/UCM260090.pdf

Center for Devices and Radiological Health, U.S. Food and Drug Administration (2014). Breast implant complications booklet. Retrieved from http://www.fda.gov/MedicalDevices/ProductsandMedicalProcedures/ImplantsandProsthetics/BreastImplants/ucm259296.htm

Chanprapaph, P., Luttarapakul, J., Siribariruck, S., & Boonyawanichkul, S. (2013). Outcome of non-protractile nipple correction with breast cups in pregnant women: a randomized controlled trial. *Breastfeeding Medicine, 8,* 408–412.

Chantry, C. J., Nommsen-Rivers, L. A., Peerson, J. M., Cohen, R. J., & Dewey, K. G. (2011). Excess weight loss in first-born breastfed newborns relates to maternal intrapartum fluid balance. *Pediatrics, 127,* e171–e179.

Chapman, D., & Perez-Escamilla, R. (1999). Identification of risk factors for delayed onset of lactation. *Journal of the American Dietetic Association, 99,* 450–454.

Chapman, D. J., & Perez-Escamilla, R. (2000a). Lactogenesis stage II: Hormonal regulation, determinants, and public health consequences. *Recent Research Developments in Nutrition, 3,* 43–63.

Chapman, D. J., & Perez-Escamilla, R. (2000b). Maternal perception of the onset of lactation is a valid, public health indicator of lactogenesis state II. *Journal of Nutrition, 130,* 2972–2980.

Chapman, D. J., Young, S., Ferris, A. M., & Perez-Escamilla, R. (2001). Impact of breast pumping on lactogenesis stage II after cesarean delivery: A randomized clinical trial. *Pediatrics, 107,* e94.

Chatterton, R. T., Hill, P. D., Aldag, J. C., Hodges, K. R., Belknap, S. M., & Zinaman, M. J. (2000). Relation of plasma oxytocin and prolactin concentrations to milk production in mothers of preterm infants: Influence of stress. *Journal of Clinical Endocrinology and Metabolism, 85,* 3661–3668.

Chen, D., Nommsen-Rivers, L., Dewey, K. G., & Lonnerdal, B. (1998). Stress during labor and delivery and early lactation performance. *American Journal of Clinical Nutrition, 68,* 335–344.

Cherchel, A., Azzam, C., & De Mey, A. (2007). Breastfeeding after vertical reduction mammaplasty using a superior pedicle. *Journal of Plastic, Reconstructive, and Aesthetic Surgery, 60,* 465–70.

Chien, Y. C., Huang, Y. J., Hsu, C. S., Chao, J. C., & Liu, J. F. (2008). Maternal lactation characteristics after consumption of an alcoholic soup during the postpartum "doing the month" ritual. *Public Health Nutrition, 22,* 1–7.

Chiummariello, S., Cigna, E., Buccheri, E. M., Dessy, L. A., Alfano, C., & Scuderi, N. (2008). Breastfeeding after reduction mammaplasty using different techniques. *Aesthetic Plastic Surgery, 32,* 294–297.

Cobo, E. (1973). Effect of different doses of ethanol on the milk-ejecting reflex in lactating women. *American Journal of Obstetrics and Gynecology, 115,* 817–821.

Cooper, A. P. (1840). *Anatomy of the breast.* London, UK: Longman, Orme, Green, Browne, and Longmans.

Costagliola, M., Atiyeh, B., & Rampillon, F. (2013). Tuberous breast: Revised classification and a new hypothesis for its development. *Aesthetic Plastic Surgery, 37,* 896–903.

Cotterman, K. J. (2004). Reverse pressure softening: A simple tool to prepare areola for easier latching during engorgement. *Journal of Nutrition, 20,* 227–237.

Cowley, D. S., & Roy-Byrne, P. P. (1989). Panic disorder during pregnancy. *Journal of Psychosomatic Obstetrics and Gynaecology, 10,* 193–210.

Cox, D. B., Kent, J. C., Casey, T. M., Owens, R. A., & Hartmann, P. E. (1999). Breast growth and the urinary excretion of lactose during human pregnancy and early lactation: Endocrine relationships. *Experimental Physiology, 84,* 421–434.

Cox, D. B., Owens, R. A., & Hartmann, P. E. (1996). Blood and milk prolactin and the rate of milk synthesis in women. *Experimental Physiology, 81,* 1007–1020.

Cregan, M. D., De Mello, T. R., & Hartmann, P. E. (2000). Pre-term delivery and breast expression: Consequences for initiating lactation. *Advances in Experimental Medicine and Biology, 478,* 427–428.

Cregan, M. D., & Hartmann, P. E. (1999). Computerized breast measurement from conception to weaning: Clinical implications. *Journal of Human Lactation, 15,* 89–96.

Cregan, M. D., Mitoulas, L. R., & Hartmann, P. E. (2002). Milk prolactin, feed volume and duration between feeds of women breastfeeding their full-term infants over a 24 h period. *Experimental Physiology, 87,* 207–214.

Cruz, N. I., & Korchin, L. (2007). Lactational performance after breast reduction with different pedicles. *Plastic and Reconstructive Surgery, 120,* 35–40.

Cruz, N. I., & Korchin, L. (2010). Breastfeeding after augmentation mammaplasty with saline implants. *Annals of Plastic Surgery, 64,* 530–533.

Cruz-Korchin, N., & Korchin, L. (2004). Breast-feeding after vertical mammaplasty with medial pedicle. *Plastic and Reconstructive Surgery, 114,* 890–894.

Czank, C., Henderson, J. J., Kent, J. C., Lai, C. T., & Hartmann, P. E. (2007). Hormonal control of the lactation cycle. In T. W. Hale & P. E. Hartmann (Eds.), *Textbook of human lactation.* Amarillo, TX: Hale Publishing.

Daly, S. E. J., & Hartmann, P. E. (1995a). Infant demand and milk supply. Part 1: Infant demand and milk production in lactating women. *Journal of Human Lactation, 1,* 21–26.

Daly, S. E. J., & Hartmann, P. E. (1995b). Infant demand and milk supply. Part 2: The short-term control of milk synthesis in lactating women. *Journal of Human Lactation, 11,* 27–37.

Daly, S. E. J., Kent, J. C., Huynh, D. Q., Owens, R. A., Alexander, B. F., Ng, K. C., & Hartmann, P. E. (1992). The determination of short-term breast volume changes and the rate of synthesis of human milk using computerized breast measurement. *Experimental Physiology, 77,* 79–87.

Daly, S. E. J., Kent, J. C., Owens, R. A., & Hartmann, P. E. (1996). Frequency and degree of milk removal and the short-term control of human milk synthesis. *Experimental Physiology, 81,* 861–875.

Daly, S. E. J., Owens, R. A., & Hartmann, P. E. (1993). The short-term synthesis and infant-regulated removal of milk in lactating women. *Experimental Physiology, 78,* 209–220.

Dean, N., Haynes, J., Brennan, J., Neild, T., Goddard, C., Dearman, B., & Cooter, R. (2005). Nipple–areolar pigmentation: Histology and potential for reconstitution in breast reconstruction. *British Journal of Plastic Surgery, 58,* 202–208.

DeCoopman, J. (1993). Breastfeeding after pituitary resection: Support for a theory of autocrine control of milk supply? *Journal of Human Lactation, 9,* 35–40.

Dewey, K. G. (2001). Maternal and fetal stress are associated with impaired lactogenesis in humans. *Journal of Nutrition, 131,* 3012S–3015S.

Dewey, K. G., Nommsen-Rivers, L., Heinig, M. J., & Cohen, R. J. (2002). Lactogenesis and infant weight change in the first weeks of life. *Advances in Experimental Medicine and Biology, 503,* 159–166.

Dewey, K. G., Nommsen-Rivers, L., Heinig, M. J., & Cohen, R. J. (2003). Risk factors for suboptimal infant breastfeeding behavior, delayed onset of lactation, and excess neonatal weight loss. *Pediatrics, 112,* 607–619.

Donath, S. M., & Amir, L. H. (2000). Does maternal obesity adversely affect breastfeeding initiation and duration? *Journal of Paediatrics and Child Health, 36,* 482–486.

Doucet, S., Soussignan, R., Sagot, P., & Schaal, B. (2007). The "smellscape" of mother's breast: Effects of odor masking and selective unmasking on neonatal arousal, oral, and visual responses. *Developmental Psychobiology, 49,* 129–138.

Doucet, S., Soussignan, R., Sagot, P., & Schaal, B. (2009). The secretion of areolar (Montgomery's) glands from lactating women elicits selective, unconditional responses in neonates. *PLoS One,* 4(10), e7579. Retrieved from http://www.plosone.org/article/info:doi%2F10.1371%2Fjournal.pone.0007579

Doucet, S., Soussignan, R., Sagot, P., & Schaal, B. (2012). An overlooked aspect of the human breast: Areolar glands in relation with breastfeeding pattern, neonatal weight gain, and the dynamics of lactation. *Early Human Development, 88,* 119–128.

Duran, M. S., & Spatz, D. L. (2011). A mother with glandular hypoplasia and a late preterm infant. *Journal of Human Lactation, 27,* 394–397.

Elia, M., Handpour, S., Terranova, P., Anderson, J., Klemp, J. R., & Fabian, C. (2002). Marked variation in nipple aspirate fluid (NAF), estrogen concentration and NAF/serum ratios between ducts in high risk women [abstract]. *Proceedings of the American Association of Cancer Research, 43,* 820: abstract no. 4072.

Engstrom, J. L., Meier, P. P., Jegier, B., Motykowski, J. E., & Zuleger, J. L. (2007). Comparison of milk output from the right and left breasts during simultaneous pumping in mothers of very low birthweight infants. *Breastfeeding Medicine, 2,* 83–91.

Evans, K. C., Evans, R. G., Royal, R., Esterman, A., & James, S. (2003). Effect of caesarean section on breastmilk transfer to the normal term newborn over the first week of life. *Archives of Disease in Childhood—Fetal and Neonatal Edition, 88,* F380–F382.

Faridi, M. M. A., & Dewan, P. (2008). Successful breastfeeding with breast malformations. *Journal of Human Lactation, 24,* 446–450.

Fernandez, I. O., Gabriel, M. M., Martinez, A. M., Morillo, A. F-C., Sanchez, F. L., & Costarelli, V. (2012). Newborn feeding behavior depressed by intrapartum oxytocin: A pilot study. *Acta Paediatrica, 101,* 749–754.

Ferris, A. M., Dalidowitz, C. K., Ingardia, C. M., Reece, E. A., Fumia, F. D., Jensen, R. G., & Allen, L. H. (1988). Lactation outcome in insulin-dependent diabetic women. *Journal of the American Dietetic Association, 88,* 317–322.

Ferris, A. M., Neubauer, S. H., Bendel, R. R., Green, K. W., Ingardia, C. J., & Reece, E. A. (1993). Perinatal lactation protocol and outcome in mothers with and without insulin-dependent diabetes mellitus. *American Journal of Clinical Nutrition, 58,* 43–48.

Fewtrell, M. S., Loh, K. L., Blake, A, Ridout, D. A., & Hawdon, J. (2006). Randomised, double blind trial of oxytocin nasal spray in mothers expressing breast milk for preterm infants. *Archives of Disease in Childhood—Fetal and Neonatal Edition, 91,* F169–F174.

Flegal, K. M., Carroll, M. D., Kit, B. K., & Ogden, C. L. (2012). Prevalence of obesity and trends in the distribution of body mass index among US adults, 1999–2010. *Journal of the American Medical Association, 307*(5), 491–497.

Freeman, M. E., Kanyicska, B., Lerant, A., & Nagy, G. (2000). Prolactin: Structure, function, and regulation of secretion. *Physiological Reviews, 80,* 1523–1631.

Fu, M., Zhang, L., Ahmed, A., Plaut, K., Haas, D. M., Szucs, K., & Casey, T. M. (2015). Does circadian disruption play a role in the metabolic–hormonal link to delayed lactogenesis II? *Frontiers in Nutrition, 2,* 4.

Gabriel, M. A. M., Fernandez, I. O., Martinez, A. M. M., Armengod, C. G., Costarelli, V., Santos, I. M., . . . Murillo, L. G. (2015). Intrapartum synthetic oxytocin reduce the expression of primitive reflexes associated with breastfeeding. *Breastfeeding Medicine, 10,* 209–213.

Garcia-Fortea, P., Gonzalez-Mesa, E., Blasco, M., Cazorla, O., Delgado-Rios, M., & Gonzalez-Valenzuela, M. J. (2014). Oxytocin administered during labor and breastfeeding: A retrospective cohort study. *Journal of Maternal–Fetal & Neonatal Medicine, 27,* 1598–1603.

Gardner, H., Kent, J. C., Hartmann, P. E., & Geddes, D. T. (2015). Asynchronous milk ejection in human lactating breast: Case series. *Journal of Human Lactation, 31,* 254–259.

Geddes, D. T. (2007a). Gross anatomy of the lactating breast. In T. W. Hale & P. E. Hartmann (Eds.), *Textbook of human lactation* (pp. 19–34). Amarillo, TX: Hale Publishing.

Geddes, D. T. (2007b). Inside the lactating breast: The latest anatomy research. *Journal of Midwifery and Women's Health, 52,* 556–563.

Geddes, D. T. (2009). Ultrasound imaging of the lactating breast: Methodology and application. *International Breastfeeding Journal, 4,* 4.

Geddes, D. T., Aljazaf, K. M., Kent, J. C., Prime, D. K., Spatz, D. L., . . . Hartmann, P. E. (2012). Blood flow characteristics of the human lactating breast. *Journal of Human Lactation, 28,* 145–152.

Gimpl, G., & Fahrenholz, F. (2001). The oxytocin receptor system: Structure, function, and regulation. *Physiological Review, 81,* 629–683.

Going, J. J., & Moffat, D. F. (2004). Escaping from flatland: Clinical and biological aspects of human mammary duct anatomy in three dimensions. *Journal of Pathology, 203,* 538–544.

Gonzalez, F., Brown, F. E., Gold, M. E., Walton, R. L., & Shafer, B. (1993). Preoperative and postoperative nipple–areola sensibility in patients undergoing reduction mammaplasty. *Plastic and Reconstructive Surgery, 92,* 809–814.

Goodfellow, C. F., Hull, M. G. R., Swaab, D. F., Dogterom, J., & Buijs, R. M. (1983). Oxytocin deficiency at delivery with epidural analgesia. *British Journal of Obstetrics and Gynecology, 90,* 214–219.

Gooding, M. J., Finlay, J., Shipley, J. A., Halliwell, M., & Duck, F. A. (2010). Three-dimensional ultrasound imaging of mammary ducts in lactating women. *Journal of Ultrasound in Medicine, 29,* 95–103.

Grattan, D. R. (2001). The actions of prolactin in the brain during pregnancy and lactation. *Progress in Brain Research, 133,* 153–171.

Grattan, D. R., Pi, X. J., Andrews, Z. B., Augustine, R. A., Kokay, I. C., Summerfield, M. R., . . . Bunn, S. J. (2001). Prolactin receptors in the brain during pregnancy and lactation: Implications for behavior. *Hormones and Behavior, 40,* 115–124.

Groer, M. W., & Davis, M. W. (2002). Postpartum stress: Current concepts and the possible protective role of breastfeeding. *Journal of Obstetric, Gynecologic, and Neonatal Nursing, 31,* 411–417.

Hale, T. W., & Ilett, K. F. (2002). *Drug therapy and breastfeeding: From theory to clinical practice.* New York: Parthenon.

Hallock, G. G. (1992). Prediction of nipple viability following reduction mammoplasty using laser Doppler flowmetry. *Annals of Plastic Surgery, 29,* 457–460.

Handlin, L., Jonas, W., Petersson, M., Ejdeback, M., Ranjo-Arvidson, A-B., Nissen, E., & Uvnas-Moberg, K. (2009). Effects of sucking and skin-to-skin contact on maternal ACTH and cortisol levels during the second day postpartum: Influence of epidural analgesia and oxytocin in the perinatal period. *Breastfeeding Medicine, 4,* 207–220.

Hapon, M. B., Simoncini, M., Via, G., & Jahn, G. A. (2003). Effect of hypothyroidism on hormone profiles in virgin, pregnant and lactating rats, and on lactation. *Reproduction, 126,* 371–382.

Hartmann, P. (2000). *Human lactation: Current research and clinical implications.* Presented at ALCA 2000: 5th Biennial Conference of the Australian Lactation Consultants' Association, Melbourne, Australia.

Hartmann, P., & Cregan, M. (2001). Lactogenesis and the effects of insulin-dependent diabetes mellitus and prematurity. *Journal of Nutrition, 131,* 3016S–3020S.

Hartmann, P. E., Mitoulas, L. R., & Gurrin, L. C. (2000). Physiology of breast milk expression using an electric breast pump. *Proceedings of the 10th International Conference of the Research on Human Milk and Lactation (ISRHML),* Tucson, AZ.

Hartmann, P. E., Sherriff, J. L., & Mitoulas, L. R. (1998). Homeostatic mechanisms that regulate lactation during energetic stress. *Journal of Nutrition, 128,* 394S–399S.

Hassiotou, F., & Geddes, D. (2013). Anatomy of the human mammary gland: Current status of knowledge. *Clinical Anatomy, 26,* 29–48.

Hata, T., Tanaka, H., Noguchi, J., Inubashiri, E., Yanagihara, T., & Kondoh, S. (2010). Three-dimensional sonographic volume measurement of the fetal stomach. *Ultrasound in Medicine and Biology, 36,* 1808–1812.

Hefter, W., Lindholm, P., & Elvenes, O. P. (2003). Lactation and breast-feeding ability following lateral pedicle mammaplasty. *British Journal of Plastic Surgery, 56,* 746–751.

Heimburg, D., Exner, K., Kruft, S., & Lemperle, G. (1996). The tuberous breast deformity: Classification and treatment. *British Journal of Plastic Surgery, 49,* 339–345.

Henderson, J. J., Hartmann, P. E., Newnham, J. P., & Simmer, K. (2008). Effect of preterm birth and antenatal corticosteroid treatment on lactogenesis II in women. *Pediatrics, 121,* e92–e100.

Hennart, P., Delogne-Desnoeck, J., Vis, H., & Robyn, C. (1981). Serum levels of prolactin and milk production in women during a lactation period of thirty months. *Clinical Endocrinology, 14,* 349–353.

Hill, P. D., Aldag, J. C., Demirtas, H., Naeem, V., Parker, N. P., Zinaman, M. J., & Chatterton, R. T. (2009). Association of serum prolactin and oxytocin with milk production in mothers of preterm and term infants. *Biological Research for Nursing, 10,* 340–349.

Hill, P. D., Wilhelm, P. A., Aldag, J. C., & Chatterton, R. T. (2004). Breast augmentation and lactation outcome: A case report. *American Journal of Maternal Child Nursing, 29,* 238–242.

Hilson, J. A. (2000). *Maternal obesity and breastfeeding success* (PhD thesis). Cornell University, Ithaca, NY.

Hilson, J. A., Rasmussen, K. M., & Kjolhede, C. L. (1997). Maternal obesity and breastfeeding success in a rural population of white women. *American Journal of Clinical Nutrition, 66,* 1371–1378.

Hilson, J. A., Rasmussen, K. M., & Kjolhede, C. L. (2004). High prepregnant body mass index is associated with poor lactation outcomes among white, rural women independent of psychosocial and demographic correlates. *Journal of Human Lactation, 20,* 18–29.

Hoover, K. L., Barbalinardo, L. H., & Platia, M. P. (2002). Delayed lactogenesis II secondary to gestational ovarian theca lutein cysts in two normal singleton pregnancies. *Journal of Human Lactation, 18,* 264–268.

Hopkinson, J. M., Schanler, R. J., & Garza, C. (1988). Milk production by mothers of premature infants. *Pediatrics, 81,* 815–820.

Houston, M. J., Howie, P., & McNeilly, A. S. (1983). Factors affecting the duration of breastfeeding: 1. Measurement of breastmilk intake in the first week of life. *Early Human Development, 8,* 49–54.

Huggins, K. E., Petok, E. S., & Mireles, O. (2000). Markers of lactation insufficiency: A study of 34 mothers. In *Current issues in clinical lactation* (pp. 25–35). Sudbury, MA: Jones and Bartlett.

Huntingford, P. J. H. (1961). Intranasal use of synthetic oxytocin in management of breast-feeding. *British Medical Journal, 243,* 709–711.

Hurst, N. M. (1996). Lactation after augmentation mammoplasty. *Obstetrics and Gynecology, 87,* 30–34.

Hurst, N. M. (2007). Recognizing and treating delayed or failed lactogenesis II. *Journal of Midwifery and Women's Health, 52,* 588–594.

Hytten, F. E. (1954). Clinical and chemical studies in human lactation: VI The functional capacity of the breast. *British Medical Journal, 1*(4867), 912–915.

Ingram, J. C., Woolridge, M. W., Greenwood, R. J., & McGrath, L. (1999). Maternal predictors of early breast milk output. *Acta Paediatrica, 88,* 493–499.

Iwama, S., Welt, C. K., Romero, C. J., Radovick, S., & Caturegli, P. (2013). Isolated prolactin deficiency associated with serum autoantibodies against prolactin-secreting cells. *Journal of Clinical Endocrinology and Metabolism, 98,* 3920–3925.

Janbu, T., Koss, K. S., Thoresen, M., & Wesche, J. (1985). Blood velocities in the female breast during lactation and following oxytocin injections. *Journal of Developmental Physiology, 7,* 373–380.

Jonas, W., Johansson, L. M., Nissen, E., Ejdeback, M., Ranjo-Arvidson, A. B., & Uvnas-Moberg, K. (2009). Effects of intrapartum oxytocin administration and epidural analgesia on the concentration of plasma oxytocin and prolactin, in response to suckling during the second day postpartum. *Breastfeed Medicine, 4,* 71–82.

Jordan, S., Emery, S., Watkins, A., Evens, J. D., Storey, M., & Morgan, G. (2009). Associations of drugs routinely given in labour with breastfeeding at 48 hours: Analysis of the Cardiff Births Survey. *British Journal of Gynecology, 116,* 1622–1632.

Jutte, J., Hohoff, A., Sauerland, C., Wiechmann, D., & Stamm, T. (2014). In vivo assessment of number of milk duct orifices in lactating women and association with parameters in the mother and the infant. *BMC Pregnancy and Childbirth, 14,* 124.

Kent, J. C. (2007). How breastfeeding works. *Journal of Midwifery and Women's Health, 52,* 564–570.

Kent, J. C., Mitoulas, L. R., Cox, D. B., Owens, R. A., & Hartmann, P. E. (1999). Breast volume and milk production during extended lactation in women. *Experimental Physiology, 84,* 435–447.

Kent, J. C., Mitoulas, L. R., Cregan, M. D., Ramsay, D. T., Doherty, D. A., & Hartmann, P. E. (2006). Volume and frequency of breastfeeds and fat content of breast milk throughout the day. *Pediatrics, 117,* e387–e395.

Kent, J. C., Ramsay, D. T., Doherty, D., Larsson, M., & Hartmann, P. E. (2003). Response of breasts to different stimulation patterns of an electric breast pump. *Journal of Human Lactation, 19,* 179–187.

Klein, D. F., Skrobala, A. M., & Garfinkel, R. S. (1995). Preliminary look at the effects of pregnancy on the course of panic disorder. *Anxiety, 1,* 227–232.

Koyama, S., Wu, H.-J., Easwaran, T., Thopady, S., & Foley, J. (2013). The nipple: A simple intersection of mammary gland and integument, but focal point of organ function. *Journal of Mammary Gland Biology and Neoplasia, 18,* 121–131.

Kulski, J., & Hartmann, P. (1981). Changes in human milk composition during initiation of lactation. *Australian Journal of Experimental Biology and Medical Science, 59,* 101–114.

Lai, C. T., Hale, T. W., Simmer, K., & Hartmann, P. E. (2010). Measuring milk synthesis in breastfeeding mothers. *Breastfeeding Medicine, 5,* 103–107.

Lambrecht, L., Robberecht, E., Deschynkel, K., & Afschrift, M. (1988). Ultrasonic evaluation of gastric clearing in young infants. *Pediatric Radiology, 18,* 314–318.

Lawrence, R. A., & Lawrence, R. M. (2010). *Breastfeeding: A guide for the medical profession* (7th ed.). Philadelphia, PA: Elsevier Mosby.

Lemay, D. G., Ballard, O. A., Hughes, M. A., Morrow, A. L., Horseman, N. D., & Nommsen-Rivers, L. A. (2013). RNA sequencing of the human milk fat layer transcriptome reveals distinct gene expression profiles at three stages of lactation. *PLoS One, 8,* e67531.

Light, K., Smith, T., Johns, J., Brownley, K. A., Hofheimer, J. A., & Amico, J. A. (2000). Oxytocin responsivity in mothers of infants: A preliminary study of relationships with blood pressure during laboratory stress and normal ambulatory activity. *Health Psychology, 19,* 560–567.

Lindow, S. W., Hendricks, M. S., Nugent, F. A., Dunne, T. T., & van der Spuy, Z. M. (1999). Morphine suppresses the oxytocin response in breastfeeding women. *Gynecologic and Obstetric Investigation, 48,* 33–37.

Loughry, C. W., Sheffer, D. B., Price, T. E., Einsporn, R. L., Bartfai, R. G., Morek, W. M., & Meli, N. M. (1989). Breast volume measurement of 598 women using biostereometric analysis. *Annals of Plastic Surgery, 22,* 380–385.

Love, S. M., & Barsky, S. H. (2004). Anatomy of the nipple and breast ducts revisited. *Cancer, 101,* 1947–1957.

MAIN Trial Collaborative Group. (1994). Preparing for breastfeeding: Treatment of inverted and non-protractile nipples in pregnancy. *Midwifery, 10,* 200–214.

Marasco, L., Marmet, C., & Shell, E. (2000). Polycystic ovary syndrome: A connection to insufficient milk supply? *Journal of Human Lactation, 16,* 143–148.

Mathes, S. J., Seyfer, A. E., & Miranda, E. P. (2006). Congenital anomalies of the chest wall. In S. J. Mathes & V. R. Hentz (Eds.). *Plastic surgery VI* (pp. 457–537). Philadelphia, PA: Elsevier.

Matias, S. L., Dewey, K. G., Quesenberry, C. P., Jr., & Gunderson, E. P. (2014). Maternal prepregnancy obesity and insulin treatment during pregnancy are independently associated with delayed lactogenesis in women with recent gestational diabetes mellitus. *American Journal of Clinical Nutrition, 99,* 115–121.

Matthiesen, A.-S., Ransjo-Arvidson, A.-B., Nissen, E., & Uvnas-Moberg, K. (2001). Postpartum maternal oxytocin release by newborns: Effects of infant hand massage and sucking. *Birth, 28,* 13–19.

McClellan, H. L., Hepworth, A. R., Kent, J. C., Garbin, C. P., Williams, T. M., Hartmann, P. E., & Geddes, D. T. (2012). Breastfeeding frequency, milk volume, and duration in mother–infant dyads with persistent nipple pain. *Breastfeed Medicine, 2,* 275–281.

Meggiorini, M. L., Maruccia, M., Carella, S., Sanese, G., De Felice, C., & Onesti, M. G. (2013). Late massive breast implant seroma in postpartum. *Aesthetic Plastic Surgery, 37,* 931–935.

Mennella, J. A. (2001). Regulation of milk intake after exposure to alcohol in mothers' milk. *Alcoholism: Clinical and Experimental Research, 25,* 590–593.

Mennella, J. A., & Beauchamp, G. K. (1991). The transfer of alcohol to human milk: Effects on flavor and the infant's behavior. *New England Journal of Medicine, 325,* 981–985.

Mennella, J. A., & Pepino, M. Y. (2008). Biphasic effects of moderate drinking on prolactin during lactation. *Alcoholism: Clinical and Experimental Research, 32,* 1899–1908.

Mennella J. A., & Pepino, M. Y. (2010). Breastfeeding and prolactin levels in lactating women with a family history of alcoholism. *Pediatrics, 125,* e1162–e1170.

Mennella, J. A., Pepino, M. Y., & Teff, K. L. (2005). Acute alcohol consumption disrupts hormonal milieu of lactating women. *Journal of Clinical Endocrinology and Metabolism, 90,* 1979–1985.

Mezzacappa, E., Kelsey, R., & Katlin, E. (1999). *A preliminary study of maternal cardiovascular function and breastfeeding in the first year.* Poster session at annual meeting, American Psychosomatic Society, Vancouver, BC, Canada.

Michalopoulos, K. (2007). The effects of breast augmentation surgery on future ability to lactate. *Breast Journal, 13,* 62–67.

Miller, V., & Riordan, J. (2004). Treating postpartum breast edema with areolar compression. *Journal of Human Lactation, 20,* 223–226.

Mitoulas, L. R., Lai, C. T., Gurrin, L. C., Larsson, M., & Hartmann, P. E. (2002). Efficacy of breast milk expression using an electric breast pump. *Journal of Human Lactation, 18,* 344–352.

Mizuno, K., Nishida, Y., Mizuno, N., Taki, M., Murase, M., & Itabashi, K. (2008). The important role of deep attachment in the uniform drainage of breastmilk from mammary lobe. *Acta Paediatrica, 97,* 1200–1204.

Mofid, M. M., Klatsky, S. A., Singh, N. K., & Nahabedian, M. Y. (2006). Nipple–areola complex sensitivity after primary breast augmentation: A comparison of periareolar and inframammary incision approaches. *Plastic and Reconstructive Surgery, 117,* 1694–1698.

Mortazavi, S. N., Geddes, D., Hassioutou, F., & Hassanipour, F. (2014). Mathematical analysis of mammary ducts in lactating human breast. *Conference Proceedings of IEEE Engineering in Medicine and Biology Society, 2014,* 5687–5690.

Mottura, A. A. (2002). Circumvertical reduction mammaplasty. *Clinics in Plastic Surgery, 29,* 393–399.

Mulford, C. (1990). Subtle signs and symptoms of the milk ejection reflex. *Journal of Human Lactation, 5,* 177–178.

Murase, M., Mizuno, K., Nishida, Y., Mizuno, N., Taki, M., Yoshizawa, M., . . . Mukai, Y. (2009). Comparison of creamatocrit and protein concentration in each mammary lobe of the same breast: Does the milk composition of each mammary lobe differ in the same breast? *Breastfeed Medicine, 4,* 189–195.

Nagata, S., Koyanagi, T., Fukushima, S., Akazawa, K., & Nakano, H. (1994). Change in the three-dimensional shape of the stomach in the developing human fetus. *Early Human Development, 37,* 27–38.

Nahabedian, M. Y., & Mofid, M. M. (2002). Viability and sensation of the nipple–areolar complex after reduction mammaplasty. *Annals of Plastic Surgery, 49,* 24–31.

Naveed, M., Manjunath, C., & Sreenivas, V. (1992). An autopsy study of relationship between perinatal stomach capacity and birth weight. *Indian Journal of Gastroenterology, 11,* 156–158.

Neidhart, M. (1998). Prolactin in autoimmune disease. *Proceedings of the Society of Experimental Biology and Medicine, 217,* 408–419.

Neifert, M., DeMarzo, S., Seacat, J., Young, D., Leff, M., & Orleans, M. (1990). The influence of breast surgery, breast appearance, and pregnancy-induced breast changes on lactation sufficiency as measured by infant weight gain. *Birth, 17,* 31–38.

Neifert, M. R., McDonough, S. L., & Neville, M. C. (1981). Failure of lactogenesis associated with placental retention. *American Journal of Obstetrics and Gynecology, 140,* 477–478.

Neifert, M. R., Seacat, J. M., & Jobe, W. E. (1985). Lactation failure due to insufficient glandular development of the breast. *Pediatrics, 76,* 823–828.

Nelson, E. E., & Panksepp, J. (1998). Brain substrates of infant–mother attachment: Contributions of opioids, oxytocin, and norepinephrine. *Neuroscience and Biobehavioral Reviews, 22,* 437–452.

Neubauer, S. H., Ferris, A. M., Chase, C. G., Fanelli, J., Thompson, C. A., Lammi-Keefe, C. J., . . . Green, K. W. (1993). Delayed lactogenesis in women with insulin-dependent diabetes mellitus. *American Journal of Clinical Nutrition, 58,* 54–60.

Neville, M. C. (2001). Anatomy and physiology of lactation. *Pediatric Clinics of North America, 48,* 13–34.

Neville, M. C., Allen, J. C., Archer, P., Casey, C. E., Seacat, J., Keller, R. P., . . . Neifert, M. (1991). Studies in human lactation: Milk volume and nutrient composition during weaning and lactogenesis. *American Journal of Clinical Nutrition, 54,* 81–93.

Neville, M., Keller, R., Seacat, J., Lutes, V., Neifert, M., Casey, C., . . . Archer, P. (1988). Studies in human lactation: Milk volumes in lactating women during the onset of lactation and full lactation. *American Journal of Clinical Nutrition, 48,* 1375–1386.

Neville, M. C., & Morton, J. (2001). Physiology and endocrine changes underlying human lactogenesis II. *Journal of Nutrition, 131,* 3005S–3008S.

Neville, M. C., Morton, J. A., & Umemora, S. (2001). Lactogenesis: The transition between pregnancy and lactation. *Pediatric Clinics of North America, 48,* 35–52.

Newton, M., & Egli, G. E. (1958). The effect of intranasal administration of oxytocin on the let-down of milk in lactating women. *American Journal of Obstetrics and Gynecology, 76,* 103–107.

Nguyen, J. T., Palladino, H., Sonnema, A. J., & Petty, P. M. (2013). Long-term satisfaction of reduction mammoplasty for bilateral symptomatic macrosomia in younger patients. *Journal of Adolescent Health, 53,* 112–117.

Nickell, W. B., & Skelton, J. (2005). Breast fat and fallacies: More than 100 years of anatomical fantasy. *Journal of Human Lactation, 21,* 126–130.

Nissen, E., Lilja, G., Widstrom, A.-M., & Uvnas-Moberg, K. (1995). Elevation of oxytocin levels early postpartum in women. *Acta Obstetricia et Gynecologica Scandinavica, 74,* 530–533.

Nissen, E., Uvnas-Moberg, K., Svensson, K., Stock, S., Widstrom, A. M., & Winberg, J. (1996). Different patterns of oxytocin, prolactin but not cortisol release during breastfeeding in women delivered by cesarean section or by the vaginal route. *Early Human Development, 45,* 103–118.

Nommsen-Rivers, L. A., Chantry, C. J., Peerson, J. M., Cohen, R. J., & Dewey, K. G. (2010). Delayed onset of lactogenesis among first-time mothers is related to maternal obesity and factors associated with ineffective breastfeeding. *American Journal of Clinical Nutrition, 92,* 574–584.

Nommsen-Rivers, L. A., Dolan, L. M., & Huang, B. (2012). Timing of stage II lactogenesis is predicted by antenatal metabolic health in a cohort of primiparas. *Breastfeed Medicine, 7,* 43–49.

Nommsen-Rivers, L. A., Heinig, M. J., Cohen, R. J., & Dewey, K. G. (2008). Newborn wet and soiled diaper counts and timing of onset of lactation as indicators of breastfeeding inadequacy. *Journal of Human Lactation, 24,* 27–33.

Nommsen-Rivers, L. A., Mastergeorge, A. M., Hansen, R. L., Cullum, A. S., & Dewey, K. G. (2009). Doula care, early breastfeeding outcomes, and breastfeeding status at 6 weeks postpartum among low-income primiparae. *Journal of Obstetric, Gynecologic, and Neonatal Nursing, 38,* 157–173.

Ohtake, T., Kimijima, I., Fukushima, T., Yasuda, M., Sekikawa, K., Takenoshita, S., & Abe, R. (2001). Computer-assisted complete three-dimensional reconstruction of the mammary ductal/lobular systems. *Cancer, 91,* 2263–2272.

Ostrom, K. M., & Ferris, A. M. (1993). Prolactin concentrations in serum and milk of mothers with and without insulin dependent diabetes mellitus. *American Journal of Clinical Nutrition, 58,* 49–53.

Page-Wilson, G., Smith, P. C., & Welt, C. K. (2007). Short-term prolactin administration causes expressible galactorrhea but does not affect bone turnover: Pilot data for a new lactation agent. *International Breastfeed Journal, 2,* 10.

Park, I. Y., Kim, M. R., Jo, H. H., Lee, M. K., & Kim, M. J. (2014). Association of the nipple–areola complexes with age, parity, and breastfeeding in Korean premenopausal women. *Journal of Human Lactation, 30,* 474–479.

Parker, L. A., Sullivan, S., Krueger, C., Kelechi, T., & Mueller, M. (2012). Effect of early breast milk expression on milk volume and timing of lactogenesis stage II among mothers of very low birth weight infants: A pilot study. *Journal of Perinatology, 32,* 205–209.

Parker, L. A., Sullivan, S., Krueger, C., & Mueller, M. (2015). Association of timing of initiation of breastmilk expression on milk volume and timing of lactogenesis stage II among mothers of very low-birth-weight infants. *Breastfeeding Medicine, 10,* 84–91.

Pérez-Escamilla, R., & Chapman, D. J. (2001). Validity and public health implications of maternal perception of the onset of lactation: An international analytical overview. *Journal of Nutrition, 131,* 3021S–3024S.

Peters, F., Diemer, P., Mecks, O., & Behnken, L. J. (2003). Severity of mastalgia in relation to milk duct dilatation. *Obstetrics and Gynecology 101,* 54–60.

Peters, F., Schulze-Tollert, J., & Schuth, W. (1991). Thyrotropin-releasing hormone: A lactation-promoting agent? *British Journal of Obstetrics and Gynecology, 98,* 880–885.

Polatti, F., Capuzzo, E., Viazzo, F., Colleoni, R., & Klersy, C. (1999). Bone mineral changes during and after lactation. *Obstetrics and Gynecology, 94,* 52–56.

Powe, C. E., Puopolo, K. M., Newburg, D. S., Lonnerdal, B., Chen, C., Allen, M., . . . Welt, C. K. (2011). Effects of recombinant human prolactin on breast milk composition. *Pediatrics, 127,* e359–e366.

Prentice, A., Addey, C. V. P., & Wilde, C. J. (1989). Evidence for local feedback control of human milk secretion. *Biochemical Society Transactions, 17,* 122.

Puapornpong, P., Raungrongmorakot, K., Paritakul, P., Ketsuwan, S., & Wongin, S. (2013). Nipple length and its relation to success in breastfeeding. *Journal of the Medical Association of Thailand, 96*(Suppl 1), S1–S3.

Rahm, V. A., Hallgren, A., Hogberg, H., Hurtig, I., & Odlind, V. (2002). Plasma oxytocin levels in women during labor with or without epidural analgesia: A prospective study. *Acta Obstetricia et Gynecologica Scandinavica, 81,* 1033–1039.

Rainer, C., Gardetto, A., Fruhwirth, M., Trawoger, R., Meirer, R., Fritsch, H., & Piza-Katzer, H. (2003). Breast deformity in adolescence as a result of pneumothorax drainage during neonatal intensive care. *Pediatrics, 111,* 80–86.

Ramirez, O. M. (2002). Reduction mammaplasty with the "owl" incision and no undermining. *Plastic and Reconstructive Surgery 109,* 512–522.

Ramsay, D. T., Kent, J. C., Hartmann, R. A., & Hartmann, P. E. (2005). Anatomy of the lactating breast redefined with ultrasound imaging. *Journal of Anatomy, 206,* 525–534.

Ramsay, D. T., Kent, J. C., Owens, R. A., & Hartmann, P. E. (2004). Ultrasound imaging of milk ejection in the breast of lactating women. *Pediatrics, 113,* 361–367.

Rasmussen, K. M., Hilson, J. A., & Kjolhede, C. L. (2001). Obesity may impair lactogenesis II. *Journal of Nutrition, 131,* 3009S–3011S.

Rasmussen, K. M., & Kjolhede, C. L. (2004). Prepregnant overweight and obesity diminish the prolactin response to suckling in the first week postpartum. *Pediatrics, 113,* e465–e471.

Renfrew, M. J., Lang, S., & Woolridge, M. (2000). Oxytocin for promoting successful lactation (Cochrane Review). In *The Cochrane Library, 3.* Oxford, UK: Update Software.

Roberts, C. L., Ampt, A. J., Algert, C. S., Sywak, M. S., & Chen, J. S. C. (2015). Reduced breast milk feeding subsequent to cosmetic breast augmentation surgery. *Medical Journal of Australia, 202,* 324–329.

Roderuck, C., Williams, H. H., & Macy, I. G. (1946). Metabolism of women during the reproductive years. *Journal of Nutrition, 32,* 267–283.

Royal College of Midwives. (2002). *Successful breastfeeding* (3rd ed.). London, UK: Churchill Livingstone, p. 26.

Ruis, H., Rolland, R., Doesburg, W., Broeders, G., & Corbey, R. (1981). Oxytocin enhances onset of lactation among mothers delivering prematurely. *British Medical Journal (Clinical Research Edition), 283,* 340–342.

Rusby, J. E., Brachtel, E. F., Michaelson, J. S., Koerner, F. C., & Smith, B. L. (2007). Breast duct anatomy in the human nipple: Three-dimensional patterns and clinical applications. *Breast Cancer Research and Treatment, 106,* 171–179.

Russo, J., & Russo, I. H. (2004). Development of the human breast. *Maturitas, 49,* 2–15.

Rutishauser, I. H. E., & Carlin. J. B. (1992). Body mass index and duration of breastfeeding: A survival analysis during the first six months of life. *Journal of Epidemiology and Community Health, 46,* 559–565.

Saint, L., Maggiore, P., & Hartmann, P. E. (1986). Yield and nutrient content of milk in eight women breastfeeding twins and one woman breastfeeding triplets. *British Journal of Nutrition, 56,* 49–58.

Saint, L., Smith, M., & Hartmann, P. (1984). The yield and nutrient content of colostrum and milk from giving birth to one month postpartum. *British Journal of Nutrition, 52,* 87–95.

Salariya, E. M., Easton, P. M., & Cater, J. I. (1978). Infant feeding: Duration of breast-feeding after early initiation and frequent feeding. *Lancet, 2,* 1141–1143.

Sanuki, J., Fukama, E., & Uchida, Y. (2008). Morphologic study of nipple–areola complex in 600 breasts. *Aesthetic Plastic Surgery, 33,* 295–297.

Sase, M., Miwa, I., Sumie, M., Nakata, M., Sugino, N., Okada, K., . . . Ross, M. G. (2005). Gastric emptying cycles in the human fetus. *American Journal of Obstetrics and Gynecology, 193,* 1000–1004.

Scammon, R. E., & Doyle, L. O. (1920). Observations on the capacity of the stomach in the first ten days of postnatal life. *American Journal of Diseases of Children, 20,* 516–538.

Schaal, B., Doucet, S., Sagot, P., Hertling, E., & Soussignan, R. (2006). Human breast areolae as scent organs: Morphological data and possible involvement in maternal–neonatal adaptation. *Developmental Psychobiology, 48,* 100–110.

Schiff, M., Algert, C. S., Ampt, A., Sywak, M. S., & Roberts, C. L. (2014). The impact of cosmetic breast implants on breastfeeding: A systematic review and meta-analysis. *International Breastfeeding Journal, 9,* 17.

Schlenz, I., Kuzbari, R., Gruber, H., & Holle, J. (2000). The sensitivity of the nipple–areola complex: An anatomic study. *Plastic and Reconstructive Surgery, 105,* 905–909.

Scott, J. A., Binns, C. W., & Oddy, W. H. (2007). Predictors of delayed onset of lactation. *Maternal and Child Nutrition, 3,* 186–193.

Semple, J. L., Lugowski, S. J., Baines, C. J., Smith, D. C., & McHugh, A. (1998). Breast milk contamination and silicone implant: Preliminary results using silicon as a proxy measurement for silicone. *Plastic and Reconstructive Surgery, 102,* 528–533.

Sievers, E., Haase, S., Oldigs, H. D., & Schaub, J. (2003). The impact of peripartum factors on the onset and duration of lactation. *Biology of the Neonate, 83,* 246–252.

Smith, W., Erenberg, A., & Nowak, A. (1988). Imaging evaluation of the human nipple during breastfeeding. *American Journal of Diseases of Children, 142,* 76–78.

Sozmen, M. (1992). Effects of early suckling of cesarean-born babies on lactation. *Biology of the Neonate, 62,* 67–68.

Spangler, A. K., Randenberg, A. L., Brenner, M. G., & Howett, M. (2008). Belly models as teaching tools: What is their utility? *Journal of Human Lactation, 24,* 199–205.

Spear, S. L., Low, M., & Ducic, I. (2003). Revision augmentation mastopexy: Indications, operations, and outcomes. *Annals of Plastic Surgery, 51,* 540–546.

Stern, J. M., & Reichlin, S. (1990). Prolactin circadian rhythm persists throughout lactation in women. *Neuroendocrinology, 51,* 31–37.

Strom, S. S., Baldwin, B. J., Sigurdson, A. J., & Schusterman, M. A. (1997). Cosmetic saline breast implants: A survey of satisfaction, breastfeeding experience, cancer screening, and health. *Plastic Reconstructive Surgery, 100,* 1553–1557.

Stuebe, A. M., Meltzer-Brody, S., Pearson, B., Pedersen, C., & Grewen, K. (2015). Maternal neuroendocrine serum levels in exclusively breastfeeding mothers. *Breastfeeding Medicine, 10,* 197–202.

Stutte, P. C., Bowles, B. C., & Morman, G. Y. (1988). The effects of breast massage on volume and fat content of human milk. *Genesis, 10,* 22–25.

Surajit, N., Basanti, A., & Basanti, D. (2007). Polymastia of the axillae. *Indian Journal of Dermatology, 52,* 118–120.

Taneri, F., Kurukahvecioglu, O., Akyurek, N., Tekin, E. H., Ilhan, M. N., Cifter, C., . . . Onuk, E. (2006). Microanatomy of milk ducts in the nipple. *European Surgical Research, 38,* 545–549.

Tedeschi, L., Ahari, S., & Byrne, J. (1963). Involutional mammary duct ectasia and periductal mastitis. *American Journal of Surgery, 106,* 517–521.

Tezer, M., Bakkaloglu, H., Erguven, M., Bilir, A., & Kadioglu, A. (2011). Smooth muscle morphology in the nipple–areola complex. *Journal of Morphological Science, 28,* 171–175.

Thanaboonyawat, I., Chanprapaph, P., Lattalapkul, J., & Rongluen, S. (2013). Pilot study of normal development of nipples during pregnancy. *Journal of Human Lactation, 29,* 480–483.

Thanaboonyawat, I., Chanprapaph, P., Puriyapan, A., & Lattalapkul, J. (2012). Association between breastfeeding success rate and nipple length and diameter in Thai pregnant women. *Siriraj Medical Journal, 64,* 18–21.

Thoresen, M., & Wesche, J. (1988). Doppler measurements of changes in human mammary and uterine blood flow during pregnancy and lactation. *Acta Obstetricia et Gynecologica Scandinavica, 67,* 741–745.

Tung, A., & Carr, N. (2011). Postaugmentation galactocele: A case report and review of literature. *Annals of Plastic Surgery, 67,* 668–670.

Ueda, T., Yokoyama, Y., Irahara, M., & Aono, T. (1994). Influence of psychological stress on suckling-induced pulsatile oxytocin release. *Obstetrics and Gynecology, 84,* 259–262.

Uvnas-Moberg, K. (2015). *Oxytocin: The biological guide to motherhood.* Plano, TX: Hale Publishing.

Uvnas-Moberg, K., & Eriksson, M. (1996). Breastfeeding: Physiological, endocrine and behavioral adaptations caused by oxytocin and local neurogenic activity in the nipple and mammary gland. *Acta Paediatrica, 85,* 525–530.

Uvnas-Moberg, K., Widstrom, A. M., Marchini, G., & Winberg, J. (1987). Release of GI hormones in mother and infant by sensory stimulation. *Acta Paediatrica Scandinavica, 76,* 851–860.

Van den Driessche, M., Peeters, K., Marien, P., Ghoos, Y., Devlieger, H., & Veereman-Wauters, G. (1999). Gastric emptying in formula-fed and breastfed infants measured with the 13C-octanoic acid breath test. *Journal of Pediatric Gastroenterology and Nutrition, 29,* 46–51.

Vorherr, H. (1974). *The breast: Morphology, physiology and lactation.* London, UK: Academic Press.

Vuorenkoski, V., Wasz-Hockert, O., Koivisto, E., & Lind, J. (1969). The effect of cry stimulus on the temperature of the lactating breast of primipara. *Experientia, 25,* 1286–1287.

Walker, M. (2010). *The nipple and areola in breastfeeding and lactation.* Amarillo, TX: Hale Publishing.

Walshaw, C. A. (2010). Are we getting the best from breastfeeding? *Acta Paediatrica, 99,* 1292–1297.

Walshaw, C. A., Owens, J. M., Scally A. J., & Walshaw, M. J. (2008). Does breastfeeding method influence weight gain? *Archives of Disease in Childhood, 93,* 292–296.

Watson, C. J. (2006). Involution: Apoptosis and tissue remodeling that convert the mammary gland from milk factory to a quiescent organ. *Breast Cancer Research, 8,* 203.

West, D., & Hirsch, E. M. (2008). *Breastfeeding after breast and nipple procedures: A guide for healthcare professionals.* Amarillo, TX: Hale Publishing.

Widstrom, A. M., Christensson, K., Ransjo-Arvidson, A. B., Matthiesen, A. S., Winberg, J., & Uvnas-Moberg, K. (1988). Gastric aspirates of newborn infants: pH, volume and levels of gastrin- and somatostatin-like immunoreactivity. *Acta Paediatrica Scandinavica, 77,* 502–508.

Widstrom, A.-M., Ransjo-Arvidson, A.-B., Christensson, K., Matthiesen, A. S., Winberg, J., & Uvnas-Moberg, K. (1987). Gastric suction in healthy newborn infants: Effects on circulation and developing feeding behavior. *Acta Paediatrica, 76,* 566–572.

Widstrom, A.-M., Wahlberg, V., Matthiesen, A. S., Eneroth, P., Uvnas-Moberg, K., Werner, S., & Winberg, J. (1990). Short term effects of early suckling and touch of the nipple on maternal behavior. *Early Human Development, 21,* 153–163.

Wiklund, I., Norman, M., Uvnas-Moberg, K., Ransjo-Arvidson, A.-B, & Andolf, E. (2009). Epidural analgesia: Breastfeeding success and related factors. *Midwifery, 25,* e31–e38.

Wilson-Clay, B., & Hoover, K. (2013). *The breastfeeding atlas* (5th ed.). Austin, TX: LactNews Press.

Wojcicki, J. M. (2011). Maternal prepregnancy body mass index and initiation and duration of breastfeeding: A review of the literature. *Journal of Women's Health, 20,* 341–347.

Woolridge, M. W. (1995). Breastfeeding: Physiology into practice. In D. P., Davies (Ed.). *Nutrition in child health* (pp. 13–31). Proceedings of conference jointly organized by the Royal College of Physicians of London and the British Paediatric Association. UK: RCPL Press.

Wright, D. M. (1985). Evidence for a spinal site at which opioids may act to inhibit the milk ejection reflex. *Journal of Endocrinology, 106,* 401–407.

Zanardo, V., Savona, V., Cavallin, F., D'Antona, D., Giustardi, A., & Trevisanuto, D. (2012). Impaired lactation performance following elective delivery at term: Role of maternal levels of cortisol and prolactin. *Journal of Maternal and Fetal Neonatal Medicine, 25,* 1595–1598.

Zanardo, V., & Straface, G. (2015). The higher temperature in the areola supports the natural progression of the birth to breastfeeding continuum. *PLoS One, 10,* e0118774.

Zangen, S., Di Lorenzo, C., Zangen, T., Mertz, H., Schwankovsky, L., & Hyman, P. E. (2001). Rapid maturation of gastric relaxation in newborn infants. *Pediatric Research, 50,* 629–632.

ADDITIONAL READING AND RESOURCES

Breastfeeding After Breast and Nipple Surgeries website: http://www.bfar.org

Cassar-Uhl, D. (2014). *Finding sufficiency.* Amarillo, TX. Praeclarus Press.

FDA consumer website regarding breast implants: http://www.fda.gov/MedicalDevices/ProductsandMedicalProcedures/ImplantsandProsthetics/BreastImplants/

Hale, T. W., & Hartmann, P. E. (2007). *Textbook of human lactation.* Amarillo, TX: Hale Publishing.

Low Milk Supply website: http://www.lowmilksupply.org

Mothers Overcoming Breastfeeding Issues website: http://www.mobimotherhood.org

West, D. (2001). *Defining your own success: Breastfeeding after breast reduction surgery.* Schaumburg, IL: La Leche League International.

West, D., & Marasco, L. (2008). *The breastfeeding mother's guide to making more milk.* New York, NY: McGraw-Hill.

Appendix 2-1

Summary Interventions Based on the Maternal Anatomy and Physiology of Lactation

1. Breastfeeding can and should be recommended, even when alterations in breast appearance and function may be present. Precise management instructions are needed plus very close follow-up of infant weight gain.
   - Early, frequent feeds plus pumping after feedings should be performed during the early days to maximize output from whatever secretory tissue is present.
   - Infant weight checks should be performed approximately every 3 days after discharge until weight gain stabilizes.
   - Pumped breastmilk can be given as a supplement through a tube-feeding device at breast. If maximal milk production has been reached and is still insufficient for normal infant growth, supplemental infant formula can be provided through a tube-feeding device at breast.
   - Alternate breast massage can be performed by the mother on each breast at each feeding to maximize breast drainage and promote as much milk synthesis as possible (Bowles, Stutte, & Hensley, 1987; Stutte, Bowles, & Morman, 1988).
   - Endocrine pathologies that result in marginal breast growth or milk output should be followed up by the primary healthcare provider and/or specialist.
2. Mothers with breast augmentation/reduction should be encouraged to breastfeed. Ascertain the location of the incisions. Ask the mother whether her breasts before augmentation were hypoplastic, had a wide intramammary gap, were asymmetrical, or herniated into the areola. These types of breasts may be at risk for insufficient milk production. Lack of sensation in the areola and nipple also puts mothers at a significant risk for damage to the nipple because they may be unable to feel incorrect latch or sucking.
   - Precise position, latch, suck, and swallow observations are necessary as well as frequent infant weight checks. Mothers should be able to state when the baby is swallowing milk and should be instructed to always check that the baby's mouth is wide open and properly latched to the breast.
   - Breastmilk or formula supplements can be delivered to the baby at the breast through a tube-feeding device.

3. Assist mothers with achieving an optimal latch. Assess whether nipples are anomalous, flat, inverted, enveloped by an edematous areola, or supernumerary. Select an appropriate intervention if necessary.
    - Ensure that the infant has a wide gape with at least a 150-degree angle of opening at the corner of his or her mouth, especially if the nipple is bulbous or unusually shaped.
    - Flat nipples can be gently pulled out and rolled before latch-on to help them become erect. Mothers can use a modified syringe to evert flat or inverted nipples. Reverse pressure softening can be applied for an edematous areola.
4. Risk factors for delayed lactogenesis II should be identified as early as possible (Dewey, Nommsen-Rivers, Heinig, & Cohen, 2003).
    - Mothers with IDDM should be encouraged to breastfeed their infant as many times as possible as soon after delivery as possible, especially during the first 12–24 hours.
    - Obese mothers may need extra help in positioning their infant at breast and require close follow-up regarding milk production and infant weight gain. A rolled-up towel or receiving blanket can be placed under the breast to support it and avoid the baby pulling down on the nipple or a heavy breast resting on the baby's chest if in a clutch or football hold.
    - Mothers with long stage II labors or urgent cesarean sections should be encouraged to breastfeed frequently in the hospital and called or seen on day 3 or 4 to ensure adequate infant weight gain.
    - Infants who fail to suck correctly or frequently enough will need a referral immediately upon discharge from the hospital with frequent weight checks.
    - Infants should be breastfed 8–12 times each 24 hours during the early weeks of breastmilk calibration.
    - Nighttime feedings are important during the early days and weeks when milk production is being calibrated to take advantage of sucking that is superimposed over higher nocturnal prolactin levels.
    - Avoid supplementing the breastfed infant unless medically indicated.

Chapter 3

Influence of the Infant's Anatomy and Physiology

INTRODUCTION

The newborn infant brings a unique set of anatomic structures, physiological activities, reflexive behaviors, and nutritional needs and stores to the breastfeeding relationship. The mechanical acts of latching, suckling, swallowing, and breathing must all occur in a synchronized interplay among anatomic structures, physiological parameters, and the infant's immediate environment. After birth, the fetus must transition to extrauterine life and undergo extraordinary changes in an amazingly short time. Some of these changes affect and are affected by breastfeeding. This chapter views breastfeeding from the perspective of the infant and the structures and functions that he or she brings to the breastfeeding process.

FUNCTIONAL INFANT ANATOMY AND PHYSIOLOGY ASSOCIATED WITH BREASTFEEDING

To breastfeed effectively, an infant must engage in and coordinate the three basic processes of suck, swallow, and breathe. Anatomic structures contributing to these processes are usually in close proximity to one another and may overlap in function (**Figure 3-1**). This topic is covered in depth by Wolf and Glass (1992) and Morris and Klein (2000). Knowledge of these structures, their functions, and their interrelatedness allows the clinician to assess the feeding process and to recognize anatomic or physiological deviations and how they affect the ability to breastfeed effectively (**Box 3-1**).

Oral Cavity

The oral cavity or the mouth consists of the lips, upper jaw (maxilla), lower jaw (mandible), cheeks, tongue, floor of the mouth, gum ridges, hard and soft palates, and uvula.

Lips and Cheeks

- The lips help locate the nipple and bring it into the mouth (not necessary with bottle-feeding).
- The lips stabilize the position of the nipple–areolar complex within the mouth.
  - The lips help form the anterior seal around the nipple–areolar complex.
  - The cheeks provide stability and maintain the shape of the mouth.

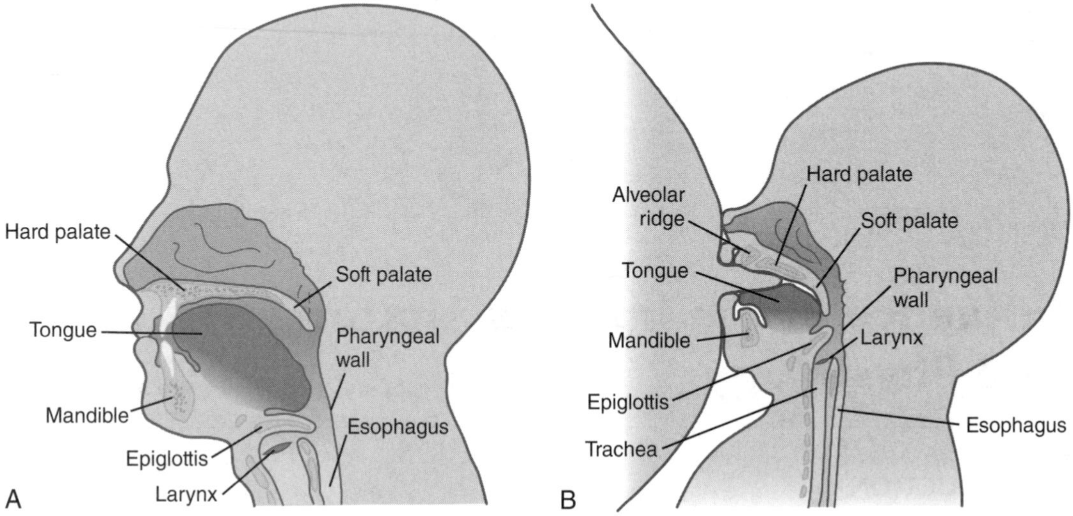

Figure 3-1 Swallowing anatomy: Midsagittal sections of the cranial and oral anatomy of an adult (A) and an infant (B) swallowing.

Box 3-1 Evaluation of Oral Structures

Tongue

Key Functions

- Assists in sealing oral cavity anteriorly and posteriorly
- Changes configuration to provide compression to nipple to increase volume of oral cavity for suction
- Bolus formation

Normal Position and Movement

- Position: Soft, with well-defined shape that is thin and flat with a rounded tip.
- Rests in the bottom of the mouth, and not seen when the lips are closed.
- Movement: Actively cups around the finger, forming a central groove.
- Movements should be rhythmic, wavelike, and in small excursions.
- Compression and suction should be present.

Abnormalities of Position and Movement

- Position: Protruding out of the mouth, retracting into the mouth, or humped/bunched with a thick feeling. Tip should not be elevated against the palate.
- Movement: Protrusion or thrusting during sucking, lack of central grooving, arrhythmic movements.

Jaw

Key Functions

- Provides a stable base for movements of the tongue
- Helps create negative pressure by slight downward movement

Normal Position and Movement

- Position: Upper and lower alveolar ridges are aligned, with loose opposition.
- Movement: Smooth, rhythmic movement in small excursions.

Abnormalities of Position and Movement

- Position: Hanging open, clenched tightly, or lower jaw retracted (micrognathia).
- Movement: Wide or excessive jaw excursion, clenching or biting during sucking.

Lips

Key Functions

- Assist in forming anterior seal
- Assist in stabilizing nipple position

Normal Position and Movement

- Lips are soft, shape to the nipple, and provide slight pressure at corners.

Abnormal Position and Movement

- Loose and floppy with poor seal around nipple, or tight and pursed.

Cheeks

Key Functions

- Provide stability to oral cavity
- Aid in bolus formation

Normal Position and Movement

- Fat pads visible, soft profile, with little movement during sucking.

Abnormalities of Position and Movement

- Floppy or stiff, pulling in during sucking.

Palate

Key Functions

- Hard palate: Helps compress nipple, maintains nipple position
- Soft palate: Assists in creating posterior seal, elevates during swallow

Normal Position and Movement

- Hard and soft palates should be intact with smooth contours.

Abnormalities of Position and Movement

- Clefts of any portion of the palate, high-arched hard palate, bifid uvula, decreased movement of soft palate.

Glass, R. P., & Wolf, L. S. (1994). A global perspective on feeding assessment in the neonatal intensive care unit. *American Journal of Occupational Therapy, 48*(6), 514–526.

- In young infants, the fat pads passively provide the majority of positional stability.
- As the infant grows, the fat pads diminish and the cheek muscles provide active stability.
- The cheeks provide lateral boundaries for food on the tongue and help in bolus formation.
- The fat pads are visible through 6–8 months of age.
- Fat pads are considerably diminished in preterm infants.

The labial or maxillary frenum (the terms "frenum" and "frenulum" are used interchangeably) attaches the upper lip to the upper gum. It has been defined as a vertical band of lip tissue extending from the inside portion of the upper lip and attaching to the alveolar mucosa of the maxillary arch (Kotlow, 2011a). A tight labial frenum or "lip-tie" may create difficulty flanging the upper lip and maintaining a seal on the breast (Wiessinger & Miller, 1995), possibly resulting in sore nipples, decreased milk intake, and engorgement, and later contributing to dental caries and creating a gap between the child's front teeth. A maxillary lip-tie has also been associated with reflux and colic-like symptoms in infants from swallowing excessive amounts of air due to the inability to form a tight seal around the breast while sucking (Kotlow, 2011b).

Mandible (Lower Jaw) and Maxilla (Upper Jaw)

- The jaw is innervated by cranial nerve V, the trigeminal (motor).
- It provides a base for movements of the tongue, lips, and cheeks.
- Downward movement during sucking expands the size of the sealed oral cavity to create suction.
- A receding jaw positions the tongue posteriorly, where it can lead to obstruction of the airway.
- A receding jaw can contribute to sore nipples unless the chin is brought closer to the breast.
- Breastfeeding creates beneficial forces on the development of the jaws during a period of very rapid growth. The forward forces of suckling (as in breastfeeding) oppose the backward forces of sucking (as in bottle-feeding) (Page, 2001). Breastfeeding helps correct physiological mandibular retrognathism (the normal slightly retracted mandible that usually self-corrects during growth, due to the jaws increasing in size). Bottle-feeding causes the buccinator muscle (used for obtaining milk from a bottle) to become hypertrophic (enlarged or overgrown), which can alter the growth trajectory of the mandible and maxilla (Carrascoza, Possobon, Tomita, & de Moraes, 2006). Breastfeeding allows the masseter muscle (the principal muscle of breastfeeding), which elevates the mandible, to strengthen and grow appropriately for facilitating normal craniofacial growth. This development also allows for the ideal positioning of the mandible for tooth eruption (Gomes, Thomson, & Cardoso, 2009).
- Sanchez-Molins, Carbo, Gaig, and Torrent (2010) found that breastfeeding had a very positive influence on the growth of the orofacial structures compared to bottle-feeding. Craniofacial features were compared in breastfed and bottle-fed 6- to 11-year-old children. Bottle-fed children showed a more retrusive mandible, with facial growth described as dolichocephalic (or long face). Breastfed children had a mandibular arch that determined a more brachycephalic growth (or short face).
- Medeiros, Ferreira, and de Felicio (2009) reported that 6- to 12-year-old children who had been breastfed had better mobility of the tongue and jaw than children who had been bottle-fed. The enhanced orofacial structures showed breastfed children performing better in tests of speech

repetition, chewing and swallowing, and lip, tongue, and mandible mobility, compared with children who had been bottle-fed as infants.

Tongue

- The tongue is innervated by:
  - Cranial nerve VII, facial (sensory)
  - Cranial nerve IX, glossopharyngeal (taste)
  - Cranial nerve XII, hypoglossal (motor muscles of the tongue)
- During breastfeeding the tongue actively brings the nipple into the mouth, shapes the nipple and areola into a teat, and stabilizes the teat's position.
- During bottle-feeding the tongue is not needed to draw the artificial nipple into the mouth, but the tongue still helps stabilize the position of the nipple.
- The tongue helps seal the oral cavity (the anterior portion along with the lower lip seal against the nipple–areolar complex, while the posterior portion seals against the soft palate until the soft palate lifts for swallowing).
- By changing configuration, the tongue is the primary means of increasing the volume of the oral cavity to create negative pressure/suction.
- The tongue provides compression against the nipple–areolar complex or teat (Bosma, Hepburn, Josell, & Baker, 1990).
- The tongue forms a central groove to channel liquid toward the pharynx, and the lateral portions of the tongue elevate and curl to provide the framework or a cylindrical pathway for the movement of milk (Tamura, Horikawa, & Yoshida, 1996).
- The neonatal tongue differs morphologically from the adult tongue in that it is specialized for suckling, especially in the adaptation that allows the curling of the lateral edges of the tongue (Iskander & Sanders, 2003).
- The tongue helps form a bolus and holds it in the oral cavity until swallowing is triggered.
- When muscle force (strength) of the tongue and posterior tongue thickness were compared in full-term and preterm infants, researchers found that full-term infants had stronger tongue muscle force and increased posterior tongue thickness compared with preterm infants (Capilouto et al., 2014). Posterior tongue thickness was measured in this study, as it was considered to be the aspect of the infant tongue most responsible for propelling a bolus to the back of the throat. Preterm infants often engage in non-nutritive sucking, but may lack sufficient tongue muscle force to extract milk and propel it to the posterior pharyngeal wall to initiate the swallow. This reduced muscle force could disrupt the sequence and timing of the suck–swallow–breathe cycle, leading to a reduced transfer of milk during nutritive sucking. Interventions for strengthening tongue strength might be a valuable approach to improving milk transfer rates in preterm infants. Non-nutritive sucking may not improve tongue muscle strength in preterm infants as much as functional resistance exercises do.
- The lingual frenulum is a fold of mucous membrane that extends from the floor of the mouth to the midline of the undersurface of the tongue, anchoring the tongue to the base of the mouth. Tongue functioning can be impaired if the frenulum is tight or short.

Carrascoza and colleagues (2006) studied the effects of the use of feeding bottles on the oral facial development of children who were breastfed and those who were bottle-fed. They reported the following:

- The tongue of bottle-fed infants tended to rest in the mandibular arch, indicating somewhat hypotonic tongue muscles compared with the resting position of the tongue of breastfed infants. The tongue of breastfed infants normally rests in the maxillary arch.
- Sucking movements of breastfeeding place the tongue in the palatal region of the central incisors, preventing air from passing through the mouth, which favors nose breathing. While this type of breathing heats, humidifies, and filters air prior to reaching the lungs, it is also considered the functional matrix for growth of the maxilla. The passage of air through the nose exerts pressure on the palate, resulting in the lowering and expanding of the structure, which allows the face bones to accompany general body growth.
- In bottle-fed infants, the tongue rests in an unphysiological position that promotes mouth breathing and discourages nose breathing. The result can be maxillary atresia (narrowing of the maxilla and a V-shaped palate rather than a U-shaped palate), compromise of the aesthetic appearance and function of the nose, and alteration of the shape of the face.

Hard Palate

Wolf and Glass (1992) describe the hard palate's functions as assisting with the positioning and stability of the nipple when drawn into the mouth and working in conjunction with the tongue in the compression of the nipple–areolar complex. The contour of the palate is shaped in utero and after birth by the continuous pressure of the tongue against the palate when the mouth is closed. A palate with a high arch or one that is very narrow may be an indication of an abnormality or a restriction of tongue movement.

Palmer (1998) described the palate as being almost as malleable as softened wax while in the early stages of oral cavity development. It can therefore be subject to alterations, depending on what is placed in the mouth (artificial nipples, intubation, pacifiers). Pressure from objects can easily mold the shape of the palate. The soft human breast in the infant's mouth contributes to a rounded U-shaped palatal configuration because the flexible and supple breast flattens and broadens in response to the infant's tongue action. An appropriately shaped palate aligns the teeth properly and does not infringe upward, thus avoiding a contributing factor to reducing the size of the nasal cavity.

Snyder (1995) describes size parameters of the reference palate as being 0.75 inch (2 cm) in width (as measured from the lateral aspects of the alveolar ridges midway to the junction of the hard and soft palates) and approximately 1 inch (2.5 cm) from the anterior superior alveolar ridge to the hard and soft palates' junction. Wilson-Clay and Hoover (2002) measured the palates of 98 infants ranging in age from 35 weeks of gestation to age 3 months by inserting a gloved finger to a depth that triggered sucking. The length from lip closure to the hard and soft palates' juncture ranged from 0.75 to 1.26 inches (1.9–3.2 cm). Palatal variations have been described as narrow, grooved or channeled, high, flat, V-shaped, short, long, and bubble.

Hohoff, Rabe, Ehmer, and Harms (2005) describe the hard palate of the newborn as already exhibiting rugae (ridges or folds), which are also present on the adult hard palate. These rugae or ridges are thought to help anchor the breast in the mouth so it does not slip or slide out of position during sucking (Crelin, 1976). The maxilla of the newborn is further characterized by a system of grooves (**Figure 3-2**). By the age of 5 years, the lateral palatine ridges are no longer apparent and the palate becomes similar to that of the

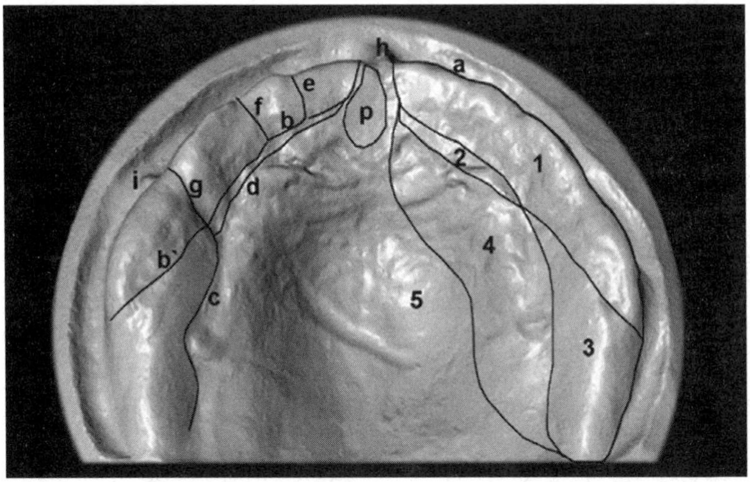

Nomenclature of Palatal Structures

a	outer alveolar groove	h	frenum labii
b	alveo-palatinal sulcus	i	frenulum of cheek
b′	postero-lateral sulcus	p	papilla insicive
b + b′	tooth germ groove	1	alveolar wall
c	transitory palatal fold	2	tektal wall
d	anterior palatal groove	3	dental molar wall
e	anterior sulcus	4	lateral palatine ridge
f	antero-lateral sulcus	5	palatal vault
g	lateral sulcus		

Figure 3-2 Newborn palate.

Hohoff, A., Rabe, H., Ehmer, U., & Harms, E. (2005). Palatal development of preterm and low birthweight infants compared to term infants: What do we know? Part 1: The palate of the term newborn. *Head and Face Medicine, 1*, 8. Retrieved from http://www.ncbi.nlm.nih.gov/pmc/articles/PMC1308841/?tool=pubmed

adult. Epstein's pearls are white or yellow inclusion cysts that may be present on the palate and are remnants of epithelial tissue trapped during palatal fusion. These cysts generally disappear within a few weeks of birth.

Soft Palate (Velum)

The soft palate is continuous and extends directly posterior to the hard palate. It does not have a bony core but rather a layer of fibrous tissue called the palatine aponeurosis, to which all soft palate musculature is attached. The soft palate makes up the posterior third of the palate, is fleshy and moveable, and raises during swallowing so that food passes into the esophagus and not up into the nasal cavity. The boundary between the hard and soft palates has traditionally indicated how far back into the mouth the nipple should extend at maximum suction. However, Jacobs, Dickinson, Hart, Doherty, and Faulkner (2007) demonstrated under ultrasound that only about 25% of infants in their study positioned the nipple at exactly the junction of the hard and soft palates. The mean distance from the tip of the nipple to the junction of the hard and soft palates was 5 mm in breastfeeding couples with no nipple pain or milk transfer issues, which illustrated that most infants did not draw the nipple–areola as far into the mouth as once thought. The nipple was not stationary during feedings, with a movement of 4.0 ± 1.3 mm. Hanging from the posterior edge of the soft palate is the uvula, which contains some muscle fibers.

Nasal Cavity

Inspired air passes through the nasal cavity, where the palatine bone or hard palate separates the oral cavity from the nasal cavity. The opening to the eustachian tube is present in this area (nasopharynx). The nasal cavity is sealed off from the oropharynx and oral cavity when the soft palate is fully elevated.

Pharynx

The pharynx, a soft tube involved in swallowing, is divided into three regions: the nasopharynx; the oropharynx, which is the space between the elevated soft palate and the epiglottis; and the hypopharynx or laryngeal pharynx, which is the area and the structures between the epiglottis and the sphincter at the top of the esophagus. Changes in head position (flexion, extension, sideways movement) influence the diameter of the pharynx, which is thought to be related to protection of the airway.

Larynx

The larynx is composed primarily of cartilage and contains structures necessary for producing sounds and protecting the airway during swallowing. The epiglottis is a structure that rests at the base of the tongue and folds down during swallowing to close and seal off the inlet to the larynx and trachea, thereby preventing liquid and food from entering the airway. At rest, it is elevated and allows air to flow freely through the larynx into the trachea.

Trachea

The trachea is a semirigid tube composed of semicircular rings of cartilage connected to each other and to the larynx. As it descends, it branches into the two primary bronchi that go to each lung.

Hyoid Bone

The hyoid is a small, free-floating bone that is the nexus of connections between the structures involved in the anatomy and physiology of sucking, swallowing, and breathing as well as in head and neck control. The hyoid is held in position by seven connections: to the scapula, sternum, cervical vertebrae, laryngeal cartilage, tongue, mandible, and temporal bone. When the hyoid moves up and forward during swallowing, the appropriate connections help open the entry to the esophagus. The muscles attached to the hyoid are involved in the bulk of mechanical breastfeeding behaviors, and their ability to function optimally depends on the position of the head and neck. Movement of the hyoid bone is a direct indication of swallowing. Abnormal movement of the hyoid is considered an indication of a sensory-deficit or abnormal motor response (Sonies, Wang, & Sapper, 1996).

Esophagus

The esophagus is the tube through which food passes on its way to the stomach, propelled by smooth and striated muscles that create peristalsis. It terminates at the stomach at the lower esophageal sphincter, which relaxes during peristalsis to allow food or fluid to enter the stomach. The lower esophageal sphincter remains closed at rest and provides protection from the upward flow or reflux of stomach contents into the esophagus. The oral, pharyngeal, and laryngeal structures are in close proximity during the early months of life. Because these structures and functions are interrelated, structural defects or disorganized functional problems in one area may adversely affect other areas.

Muscles

More than 40 muscles participate in the complex process of coordinating the movement of food and air through the oral cavity. Muscles act in synchrony and function to effect lip movement, allow graded jaw movements, influence the shape and action of the tongue and cheeks, elevate the soft palate to seal the nasopharynx, protect the airway, and move and clear a bolus of food. Orofacial muscles that are recruited for breastfeeding include the submental muscles—especially the mylohyoideus, which depresses the mandible; the masseter and temporal muscles on the side of the face, which move the jaw; the orbicularis oris complex of muscles, which encircles the mouth and is responsible for lip closure; the buccinator muscles at the side of the face, which are responsible for check compression and air expulsion; and the tongue. Surface electromyography has shown differences in facial muscles' activity between breastfeeding and bottle-feeding (Gomes, Trezza, Murade, & Padovani, 2006).

The masseter muscle is heavily involved during feeding at the breast; its activity is used as a measurement standard when comparing alternative feeding methods. This muscle is much more active during breastfeeding than bottle-feeding and has been shown to demonstrate higher electrical activity during breastfeeding than during bottle-feeding or cup feeding when measured by electromyography (Franca, Sousa, Aragao, & Costa, 2014). During bottle-feeding, the masseter, temporalis, pterygoid, tongue, and lips operate suboptimally or in hypofunction, while the mentalis and buccinators are overfunctioning or in hyperactivity. The increased activity of the buccinators restricts jaw movement, facilitates tongue retraction, and can change the functioning of the tongue.

Activity of the masseter muscle during cup feeding is higher than during bottle-feeding. Cup feeding may provide more of an opportunity to develop better oral muscle function for breastfeeding or, conversely, to avoid weakening of the muscles used for breastfeeding (Franca et al., 2014).

A study that analyzed the relative roles of three groups of muscles used in breastfeeding (submental group, orbicularis oris, and sternocleidomastoid) found that all three muscle groups were active during breastfeeding (Ratnovsky et al., 2013). The sternocleidomastoid muscle is an accessory inspiratory muscle located along each side of the neck and is thought to contribute to the development of intraoral vacuum generation.

Neural Control

Just as the anatomic structures and functions of suck, swallow, and breathe overlap, so too do the nerves that innervate these structures and functions. Six cranial nerves overlap in neural function to enable the suck, swallow, and breathe functions (**Table 3-1**).

Reflexes

Full-term infants come equipped with a number of well-developed reflexes that aid in securing food in a safe and efficient manner.

- Swallowing is seen in the fetus as early as 12 weeks of gestation. Infants are born with considerable experience in swallowing from the routine ingestion of amniotic fluid before birth.
- Sucking is present by 24 weeks of gestation, with the fetus being capable of turning his or her head toward oral stimulation. Sucking is initiated by stimulation in the infant's mouth that causes the infant to extend his or her tongue over the lower gum, raise the mandible, draw the

Table 3-1 Cranial Nerves Associated with Suck, Swallow, and Breathe

Cranial Nerve	Function
I—Olfactory nerve (sensory)	Responsible for the sense of smell, which also affects the perception of taste.
V—Trigeminal (sensory and motor) • Maxillary branch • Mandibular branch • Ophthalmic branch (purely sensory and not involved with sucking, swallowing, or breathing)	Channels sensory information from the mouth (suck), soft palate (swallow), nose (breathe). Gathers sensory input from the cheeks, nose, upper lip, teeth. Gathers sensory input from the skin over the lower jaw, the lower lip, and lower teeth. Motor aspect of the nerve innervates muscles that control chewing.
VII—Facial (sensory and motor)	Sensory fibers on the anterior two-thirds of the tongue for sweet, salty, and sour tastes. The motor fibers are involved with the muscles of facial expressions and the salivary glands.
IX—Glossopharyngeal (sensory and motor)	Sensory fibers on the posterior third of the tongue for bitter taste. Motor fibers go to the muscles used in swallowing, and to the salivary glands, and innervate the gag reflex.
X—Vagus (sensory, somatic, and autonomic)	Sensory information from the palate, uvula, pharynx, larynx, esophagus, visceral organs. Motor connections to the pharynx, larynx, and heart. Autonomic nervous system functions are involved in heart rate, smooth muscle activity in the gut, glands that alter gastric motility, respiration, and blood pressure.
XII—Hypoglossal (motor)	Contraction of the muscles of the tongue. Involved in the peristaltic action in bolus preparation, sucking, and swallowing.

nipple–areola into his or her mouth, and initiate the sequence of sucking behaviors. Sucking is a reflex at birth, with the infant "obligated" to suck on anything placed in the mouth. By about 3 months, sucking changes from reflexive or automatic to voluntary. Some parents see this transition as a breastfeeding infant who refuses to suck on artificial nipples (even if they have been given in combination with breastfeeding since early after birth).

- The gag reflex is apparent at 26 weeks of gestation and is quite strong in a newborn. At first it can be stimulated when the posterior two-thirds of the tongue is touched. It gradually changes such that the gag reflex is elicited farther back on the posterior one-third of the tongue.
- The phasic bite and transverse tongue reflexes appear at around 28 weeks of gestation. The phasic bite reflex is seen as the rhythmic opening and closing of the jaw when the gums are stimulated. The transverse tongue reflex is seen as the tongue gravitating toward a stimulus, elicited by tracing the lower gum ridge and brushing the lateral edge of the tongue with the examiner's finger.
- The rooting reflex is seen at 32 weeks of gestation and occurs in response to stroking of the skin around the mouth. This mouth-orienting reflex is strongest around 40 weeks and fades after 3 months.

Sucking Mechanisms

Components of sucking, swallowing, and breathing, along with the coordination between the three activities, mature at different times and rates depending on the gestational age of the infant. For example, expression (positive pressure) matures before suction. These activities also need to occur sequentially from the oral phase to the pharyngeal (swallowing) phase to the pulmonary or breathing phase while ensuring that the swallow takes place during a safe phase of the respiratory cycle (Amaizu, Shulman, Schanler, & Lau, 2008). Sucking at the breast involves a complex series of behaviors that have been studied for a number of years by various means. Changing research modalities have allowed researchers and clinicians to refine their understanding of how this process unfolds. There are numerous interpretations of suck mechanisms:

- Ardran, Kemp, and Lind (1958) were among the first researchers to visualize the breast inside the infant's mouth. In their study the breast was coated with a barium sulfate paste, and radiographic films were made while the infant nursed. Infants were positioned on a couch with the mother leaning over the baby, which may have prevented a deep latch and partially accounted for observations that have since been refined with newer imaging techniques. Notable was the confirmation that the nipple and areola were drawn into the mouth to the junction of the hard and soft palates and that the nipple widened and extended to about three times its resting length, forming the nipple–areolar complex or a teat. These authors also described the action of the infant forming the nipple–areola into a teat and drawing it far back into the mouth, with the tongue playing a major part in the sucking process and the breast being soft and pliable enough to allow this activity. According to these authors, "Any factor which causes edema or congestion [of the breast] will probably interfere with suckling." Their study was confined to the lateral plane and could not visualize other tongue actions. It also relied on X-rays, the hazards of which halted the use of this type of research.
- The use of real-time ultrasound refined the interpretation of the sucking process at breast. Smith, Erenberg, Nowak, and Franken (1985) and Smith, Erenberg, and Nowak (1988) noted the following points:
  1. Failure of the lips to form a complete seal is manifested on a scan by air leaking into the oral cavity.
  2. Tongue and jaw movements compress the nipple, which is highly elastic, elongating it along with 2 cm of areola to twice its resting length and to 70% of its original diameter.
  3. During the peristaltic action of the tongue, the teat is compressed 60% more in the vertical direction and widens by 20% in the lateral direction.
  4. The buccal mucosa and musculature (sucking pads, buccinator muscle) move inward as the tongue is depressed. This maintains a tight seal on the nipple–areola, conducts the milk toward the central depression in the posterior portion of the tongue, and allows the milk to be propelled toward the oropharynx.
- Weber, Woolridge, and Baum (1986) described both feeding movements and the coordination of sucking, swallowing, and breathing:
  1. The action of the tongue in a breastfed infant was described as a rolling or peristaltic undulation in an anterior to posterior direction, whereas in bottle-fed infants the tongue

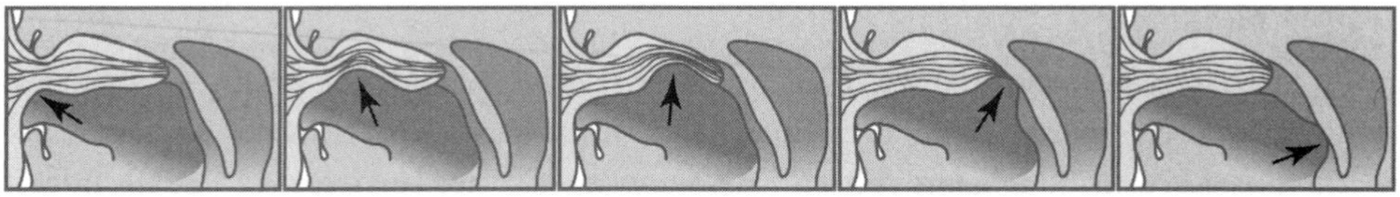

Figure 3-3 Complete suck cycle on breast.

worked in an up-and-down piston-type motion; when not sucking, the breastfed infants maintained their grasp on the nipple, with the teat still moderately indented by the tongue.

2. The lateral margins of the tongue cupped around the nipple, forming a central groove.
3. One- to 3-day-old infants showed distinct interruptions of their breathing movements when a swallow occurred, whereas in infants 4 days and older, the breathing trace appeared as a smooth uninterrupted movement with swallows occurring at the natural boundary between expiration and inspiration.

Figure 3-3, a graphic rendering of ultrasound studies, summarizes the dynamics of a complete suck cycle that was postulated from this study (Woolridge, 1986).

Woolridge and Drewett (1986) also noted the importance of taking into account both positive and negative pressures. Fluid movement during breastfeeding occurs from an area of high pressure inside the breast—created by fluid volume and the milk ejection reflex—to an area of low pressure inside the infant's mouth, where suction or vacuum is created by sealing the oral cavity and enlarging it when the jaw and tongue drop. During bottle-feeding, either suction or compression can be the predominant determinant of efficient fluid flow, depending on the type of nipple and opening in the nipple. Preterm infants are able to express milk from a bottle without applying vacuum (Lau, Sheena, Shulman, & Schanler, 1997), and although they may effectively feed from a bottle, they can demonstrate difficulty in removing milk from the breast. This finding suggests that the mechanics of milk removal from a bottle versus from the breast are different (Meier, 2003). Although infants can receive some milk by compressing an artificial nipple, in the absence of negative pressure (i.e., in infants who cannot develop sufficient suction), adequate amounts of milk may be lacking unless modifications are made to the nipple.

Current, more sensitive ultrasound studies describe the infant sucking dynamic (**Figures 3-4** and **3-5**) as follows (Geddes, Kent, Mitoulas, & Hartmann, 2008; Jacobs et al., 2007):

- Negative pressure draws the nipple–areola into the mouth, usually several millimeters anterior to the junction of the hard and soft palates, forms a teat, and holds it in place with a baseline vacuum of –60 mm Hg over the entire breastfeeding.
- The motion of the tongue during a suck cycle does not show a peristaltic action (as in bottle-feeding), but rather the tongue is up and in apposition with the hard palate, with the anterior tongue not indenting the nipple.
- Vacuum is generated as the tongue and jaw move down, which allows milk flow from the nipple. When the posterior part of the tongue lowers, milk ducts in the nipple open and milk flows into the infant's mouth. Peak vacuum coincides with the tongue at its lowermost position.

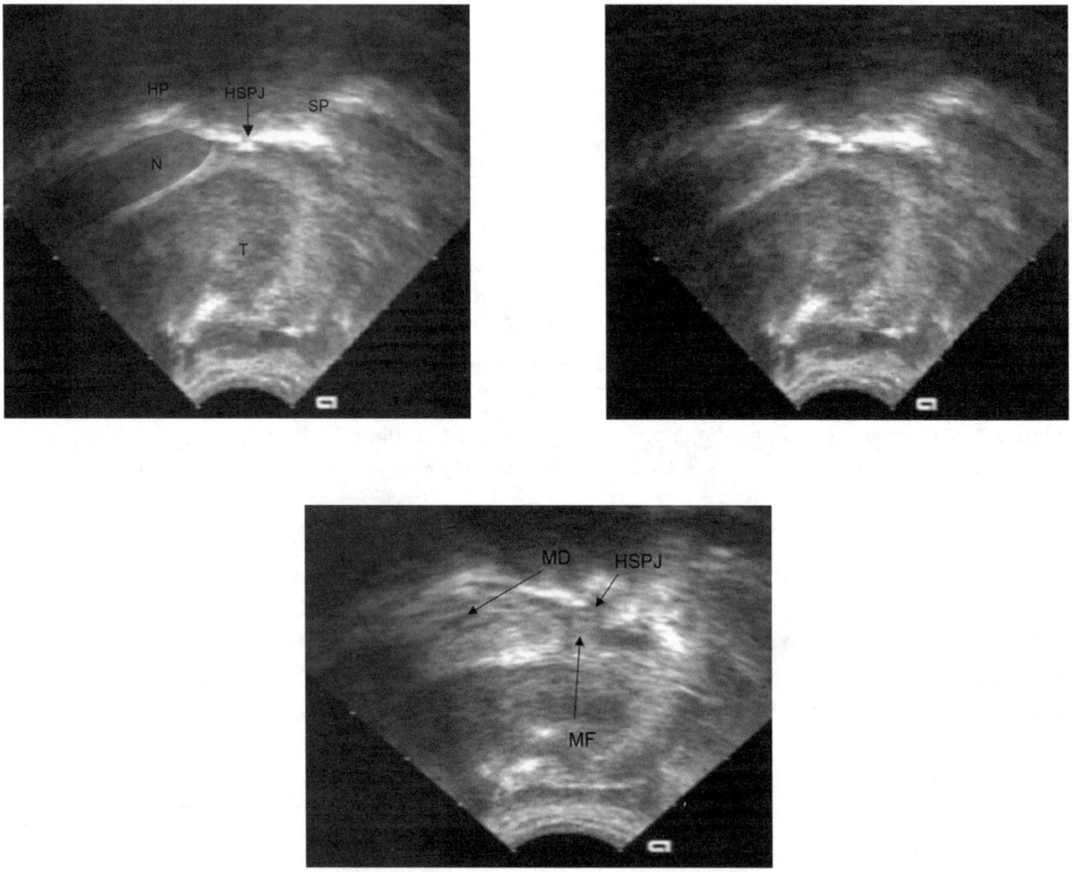

Figure 3-4 Ultrasound images of intra-oral cavity during breastfeeding.

Reprinted from Geddes, D. T., Kent, J. C., Mitoulas, L. R., & Hartmann, P. E. (2008). Tongue movement and intra-oral vacuum in breastfeeding infants. *Early Human Development, 84*, 7.

- As the tongue moves back up, vacuum decreases and milk flow ceases. Milk ducts within the nipple and milk flow cannot be seen on ultrasound. The tongue captures the milk that has flowed into the nipple, holding it in place until the tongue and jaw lower again, with the milk subsequently flowing into the oral cavity. This mechanism ensures that milk is not constantly flowing into the oral cavity but is apportioned into manageable boluses so that excessive swallowing does not interfere with breathing and oxygenation.

McClellan, Sakalidis, Hepworth, Hartmann, and Geddes (2010) investigated infant sucking using ultrasound and measured the nipple diameter and placement of the nipple within the infant oral cavity during breastfeeding. They found that the nipple diameter does not remain consistent along the length of the nipple during sucking, and changes in nipple diameter associated with tongue movement were also

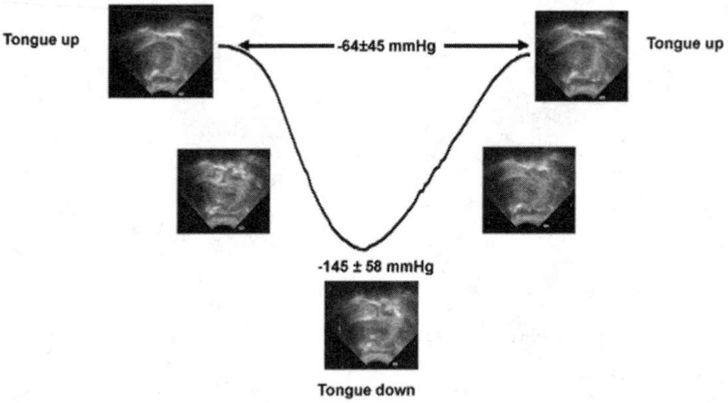

Figure 3-5 Changes in infant tongue position during one complete suck cycle.

Reprinted from Geddes, D. T., Kent, J. C., Mitoulas, L. R., & Hartmann, P. E. (2008). Tongue movement and intra-oral vacuum in breastfeeding infants. *Early Human Development, 84*, 7.

significantly different. All nipple diameter measurements significantly increased between the tongue-up and tongue-down movements, which the authors concluded was not consistent with a peristaltic tongue action. Sakalidis, Williams, and colleagues (2013) found that there was a difference in tongue movement between nutritive and non-nutritive sucking at the breast. During nutritive sucking, the infant's midtongue lowered farther and the sucking was significantly slower compared to non-nutritive sucking.

In contrast, using ultrasound videos to describe the sucking sequence, Monaci and Woolridge (2011) reported that during non-nutritive sucking prior to eliciting the milk ejection reflex, the infant's tongue engaged in a peristaltic motion. After the milk ejection reflex, a swallow was seen corresponding to each suck and a more pronounced vacuum action (tongue depression) was seen, similar to the previously discussed description of Geddes and Jacobs. Therefore it is thought that infants may use both a peristaltic tongue action to move the milk into the oropharynx and a tongue depression to generate vacuum, which allows milk from the breast to enter the oral cavity of the infant (Woolridge, 2011). Woolridge (2012) identified both propulsive or peristaltic movements of the tongue as well as extractive or vacuum application during feedings at the breast. Alteration of vacuum and compression may allow compression to regulate milk flow by stopping it to allow swallowing and the refilling of the nipple ducts while vacuum draws the milk from the nipple into the oral cavity. While each of the two types of tongue movements may be capable of removing milk independently, they are more likely to complement each other and act synergistically to accomplish the most efficient method of removing milk from the breast (Sakalidis & Geddes, 2015).

In a study using three-dimensional (3D) ultrasound rather than two-dimensional (2D) ultrasound, researchers found evidence of both peristaltic and up-and-down movements in the tongue during breastfeeding, but cautioned that visualization of these parameters varied depending on which plane was examined during the scan (Burton, Deng, McDonald, & Fewtrell, 2013). Differing scan planes could yield differing results, as the authors found that positioning the scan probe on the mid-sagittal plane (not just along the mid-sagittal line) was most important. When the probe was placed slightly off the mid-sagittal plane, fewer peristaltic tongue patterns were observed.

In an analysis of mid-sagittal submental 3D ultrasound video clips, the anterior portion of the tongue was found to move as a rigid body with the cycling motion of the mandible. The posterior section of the tongue undulates in a peristaltic wave, which facilitates swallowing of the milk bolus (Elad et al., 2014). The anterior tongue, while moving with the mandible, also moves slightly anteriorly (outside the mouth) as the mandible moves down. This anterior motility illustrates the infant's tongue thrust reflex and may be of concern if it is absent due to a tongue-tie.

Thus sucking seems to be a dynamic process, shifting between peristaltic movements and vacuum-generating movements, possibly in response to the varying rate of milk release from the breast. Vacuum-generating movements of the tongue may be superimposed on the peristaltic movements of the tongue and are generated as part of the same suck cycle. Mothers can remove milk by positive pressure only, as with manual expression and the milk ejection reflex, or by negative pressure, as with a breast pump. However, unless milk ejection occurs (positive pressure) when using a pump, mothers may not express very much milk. Vacuum seems to be the driving force working in concert with an intact milk ejection reflex to ensure maximum milk expression when using a breast pump. Mothers using a breast pump experience maximum milk yield in the shortest time when using the highest comfortable vacuum. Most of the milk is collected during the first two milk ejections, occurring on average within the first 8 minutes after the start of the first milk ejection (Kent et al., 2008). Whereas too little vacuum may be problematic in removing milk from the breast, too much vacuum has also been shown to present potential problems. McClellan and colleagues (2008) studied two groups of mothers: those experiencing nipple pain during or after feedings and a control group with no complaints of pain. In spite of ongoing professional help by International Board Certified Lactation Consultants, infants of mothers with persistent nipple pain applied significantly stronger vacuums and transferred less milk than infants not causing pain. All components of the suck cycle were stronger, with the baseline vacuum or seal on the breast 61% stronger and the peak vacuum being 31% stronger in the infants causing the persistent nipple pain. These infants also applied more vacuum than an electric breast pump at the mothers' maximum comfort vacuum values. Mothers maintained their milk supply through expressing breastmilk if their nipples were too painful for direct breastfeeding.

Quantifying the Sucking Episode

A number of infant sucking and breast functioning parameters have been measured that are of interest in the understanding of sucking as well as in the assessment of what is in the range of normal and what may constitute a deviation or alteration from the norm (**Table 3-2**).

Sucking patterns change over the course of a feed. Older studies have described a typical 1:1 ratio of sucking to swallowing with changes by the end of a feed to a ratio of 2:1 or 3:1 sucks per swallow (Weber et al., 1986). Newer ultrasound studies revealed that the suck-swallow-breathe ratios were highly variable during a breastfeeding with ratios ranging from 1:1:1 to 12:1:4 during nutritive sucking and 2:0:1 to 23:1:23 during non-nutritive sucking (Sakalidis, Kent, et al., 2013). The amount of milk transferred tends be higher from the first breast suckled and lower from the second breast. Prieto and colleagues (1996) showed a 58% decrease in amount of milk transferred from the second breast compared with the first: 63 ± 9 g from the first breast and 27 ± 8 g from the second breast in infants aged 21–240 days. Drewett

Table 3-2 Infant Sucking and Breast Functioning Parameters

Parameter	Value	Reference
Infant negative-pressure ranges		
Mean pressure	−50 ± 0.7 mm Hg	Prieto et al., 1996
Average range of pressure	−50 to −155 mm Hg	
Maximum pressure range	−197 ± 1 to −241 mm Hg	
Basal resting pressure to keep nipple in mouth	−70 to −200 mm Hg	
Infant positive-pressure ranges		
Baby's tongue	73–3.6 mm Hg	
Baby's jaw	200–300 g	Kron & Litt, 1971
Full breast	28 mm Hg	Egnell, 1956
Additional pressure of milk ejection reflex	10–20 mm Hg	
Infant mechanics		
Cycles (sucks)	36–126 (mean 74) per minute	Bowen-Jones, Thompson, & Drewett, 1982
Duration of a suck	0.77 s	Chetwynd, Diggle, Drewett, & Young, 1998
Duration of rest	0.7 s	
Sucks per second	1.28	Ramsay & Gisel, 1996
Intersuck interval	0.5–0.6 s with no milk flow	Woolridge, How, Drewett, Rolfe, & Baum,
	0.9–1.0 s at a flow rate of 0.5 g/suck	1982; Bowen-Jones et al., 1982
Volume of milk per suck	0.14–0.21 mL at beginning of a feed	
	0.01–0.04 mL at the end of a feed	Chetwynd et al., 1998
Number of sucks per burst at beginning of feed	11 (with considerable variation)	Chetwynd et al., 1998
Number of sucks per burst at end of feed	5 (with considerable variation)	Shawker, Sonies, Stone, & Baum, 1983
Velocity of peristaltic wave motion of the tongue	15 cm/s	
Breast function parameters		
Mean diameter of lactiferous ducts before milk ejection	2.83 mm (range 1.1–5.9 mm)	Kent, Ramsay, Doherty, Larsson, & Hartmann, 2003
Increase in cross-sectional area of ducts following milk ejection	6.45 mm ± 0.98 mm	Kent et al., 2003
Length of time ducts remain dilated per each milk ejection	86 s	Ramsay, Kent, Owens, & Hartmann, 2001
Average yield for each milk ejection	35 g	Ramsay, Ramsay, Doherty, Larsson, &
Milk flow rate from breast	24.4 g/min	Hartmann, 2001
Time from beginning of sucking to milk ejection	56 s	Ramsay et al., 2001
Time to milk ejection with pump	121 ± 11 s to 149 ± 12 s	Kent et al., 2003
		Kent et al., 2003

and Woolridge (1981) measured 38.5 g from the first breast and 21.8 g from the second breast in 5- to 7-day-old infants. The volume of milk per suck also changes, with more than a 50% reduction from peak volume seen at the end of the feed on the second breast. The intake of the infants in these studies was not limited by the milk supply available but rather by the behavior of the infant in regulating his or her own intake.

Infants suck in bursts separated by rests, typically defined as a sequence of sucks with intersuck intervals of less than 2 seconds (Woolridge & Drewett, 1986). The sucking rate on the breast varies as a function of milk flow rate (Bowen-Jones, Thompson, & Drewett, 1982); the higher the milk flow rate, the slower the sucking rate. The intersuck intervals (within bursts) range from 0.5 to 1.3 seconds depending on milk flow rates, leading these researchers to conclude that there was not a distinct separation of nutritive and non-nutritive sucking at breast (as with bottle-feeding) but rather a graded distribution between the two. Ramsay and Gisel (1996) measured a higher sucking rate in breastfed infants compared with bottle-fed infants and showed that infants spent 50% more time sucking when they were alert than when they were asleep. Also noted was that infants identified in this study as having feeding difficulties demonstrated shorter continuous sucking bursts and shorter sucking times than infants who had no problems feeding. Infants who later showed some feeding difficulties were already exhibiting poorer feeding ability shortly after birth.

Bromiker and colleagues (2006) demonstrated that full-term infants of insulin-managed mothers with diabetes had poorer sucking patterns. These infants averaged 5.2 fewer sucking bursts and 42 fewer sucks per 5-minute interval. This finding is consistent with descriptions by Pressler, Hepworth, LaMontagne, Sevcik, and Hesselink (1999) of significantly poorer performance for motor processes and reflex functioning in infants of insulin-managed mothers with diabetes. These infants may be less neurologically mature, which would help explain the decrease seen in the number of sucks and number of bursts per 5-minute interval. Thus clinicians may wish to monitor these infants more closely, especially during the early days when breastfeeding is being established.

Moral and colleagues (2010) found that in 3- to 4-week-old infants who were exclusively bottle-fed, the mechanics of sucking showed fewer suck movements and the same number of pauses but of longer duration when compared to exclusively breastfed infants. In infants who were mixed fed (by both bottle and breast) there were 8.7% fewer suction movements compared to exclusively breastfed infants. Aizawa, Mizuno, and Tamura (2010) found that jaw and throat region movements differ between breastfed and bottle-fed infants. Jaw and throat region movements were significantly smaller during breastfeeding than during bottle-feeding. The angle of the mouth during breastfeeding was larger than during bottle-feeding. These differences were partly due to the difference in the angle of the mouth demonstrated during each type of feeding. These studies refute some of the marketing claims of artificial nipples being advertised as equivalent to feeding at the breast.

Ramsay, Kent, Owens, and Hartmann (2001) found that milk intake was related to the number of milk ejections experienced by the mother rather than the total time an infant spent at the breast. Each milk ejection makes a certain amount of milk available to the infant, whereas the vacuum applied by the infant affects how fast this milk is removed.

While the suck–swallow–breathe pattern in full-term newborn infants is intact and capable of transferring sufficient amounts of milk to enable the child to grow appropriately, infants clearly become more efficient at breastfeeding as they grow older. During the first 4 months after birth, infants increase their sucking burst durations and reduce their pause durations while transferring a similar amount of milk from the breast in a shorter period of time (Sakalidis, Kent, et al., 2013). Elevated heart rates and lower oxygenation are present in these younger infants owing to their need to pause more during milk removal to maintain adequate oxygen levels. These parameters, however, change over time. Older infants become more efficient through adaptation, conditioning, or "practice." Older infants with short sucking bursts and long pauses between bursts may be signaling fatigue, insufficient milk transfer, or poorer cardiovascular regulation.

Swallowing

More than two dozen muscles are involved in the process of swallowing. Coordination of swallowing with suck and breathing is fundamental to effective and safe feeding. There are three phases of swallowing: oral, pharyngeal, and esophageal. The pharyngeal swallow is thought to achieve rhythmic stability as early as 32–34 weeks of gestation (Gewolb, Vice, Schweitzer-Kenney, Taciak, & Bosma, 2001). Swallowing in the infant is initiated when the milk bolus accumulates either in the space between the soft palate and the tongue or in the space between the soft palate and the epiglottis. To enable them to work in tandem, swallowing, sucking, and esophageal motility are linked together within a control center originating in a central pattern generator in the brainstem (Jean, 2001). Central pattern generators are adaptive networks of interneurons that activate groups of motor neurons to engage in specific motor patterns of behavior. Interneurons in the brainstem can generate a basic swallow pattern. Swallowing is seen in the fetus by 11 weeks' gestation as a means to regulate amniotic fluid volume.

Swallowing is not a simple reflex, but rather a complex coordinated process generated by multiple levels of neural control. The swallowing network is adaptive and can be modified by experience. In healthy term infants, nutritive swallows occur predominantly at the cusp of inspiration and expiration; in contrast, in preterm infants, the swallow occurs predominantly during respiratory pauses (Barlow, 2009a).

The development of a rhythmic pattern of sucking, swallowing, and breathing is often interrupted by interventions in preterm infants that provide abnormal stimulation to sensitive oral structures. Placement of tubes and tape around the nostrils, mouth, and lower face, for example, may restrict the range of oral movements during a critical period of time when disruption of the trigeminal sensory field may delay the attainment of oromotor feeding skills (Barlow, 2009b).

There are differences between an infant's and an adult's anatomy relative to the act of swallowing. In the infant, the hyoid and larynx are located higher in the neck and the pharynx is smaller. As the infant grows and matures, the hyoid and larynx migrate downward, the epiglottis and soft palate are no longer in direct approximation after 3 to 4 months of age, and more mature protection of the airway allows the infant to cease relying on specialized anatomic structures and configurations to support sucking, swallowing, and breathing.

Respiration ceases for a short period during swallowing. Geddes, Chadwick, Kent, Garbin, and Hartmann (2010a) found a significant correlation between swallow apnea and the movement of milk through the pharyngeal area, as detected by ultrasound.

Figures 3-6 and **3-7** show the progression of a milk bolus as it traverses the three phases of swallowing in a breastfed infant. The respiratory phase at which swallowing is timed differs between 2 weeks and

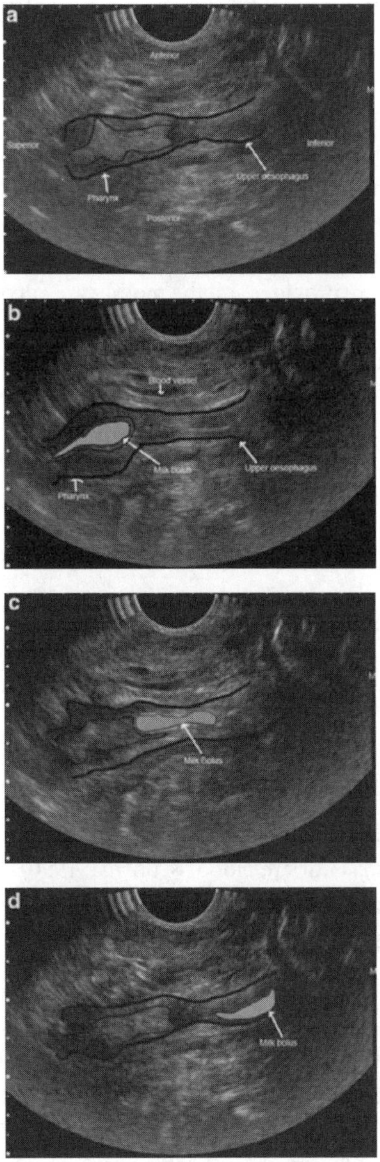

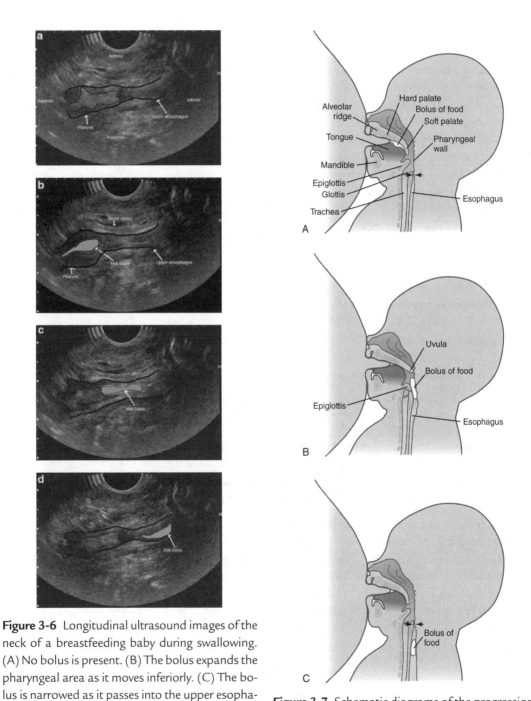

Figure 3-6 Longitudinal ultrasound images of the neck of a breastfeeding baby during swallowing. (A) No bolus is present. (B) The bolus expands the pharyngeal area as it moves inferiorly. (C) The bolus is narrowed as it passes into the upper esophageal region. (D) The bolus is almost cleared.

Geddes, D. T., Chadwick, L. M., Kent, J. C., Garbin, C. P., & Hartmann, P. E. (2010). Ultrasound imaging of infant swallowing during breastfeeding. *Dysphagia, 25*, 183–191.

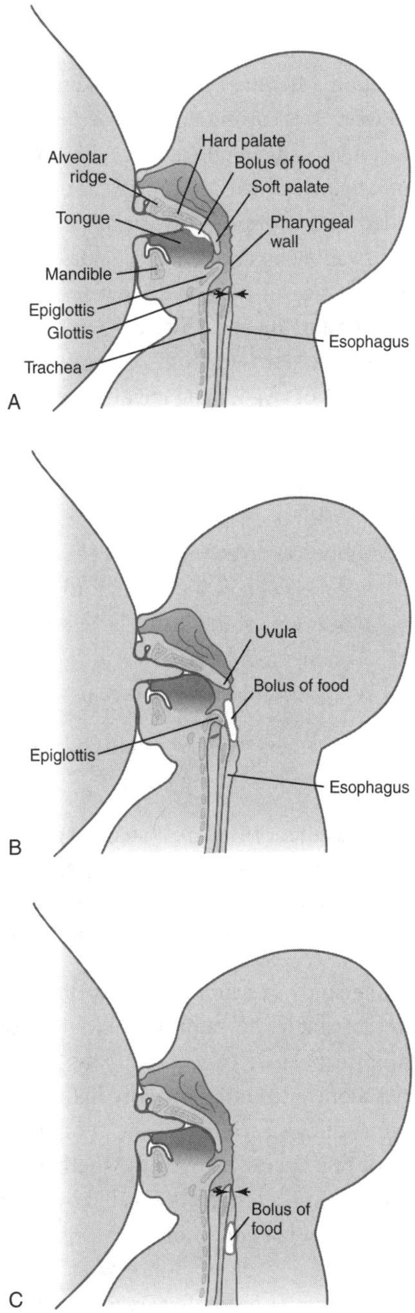

Figure 3-7 Schematic diagrams of the progression of the milk bolus in a breastfed infant.

Geddes, D. T., Chadwick, L. M., Kent, J. C., Garbin, C. P., & Hartmann, P. E. (2010). Ultrasound imaging of infant swallowing during breastfeeding. *Dysphagia, 25*, 183–191.

2 months of age and has been attributed to a critical window of neural development occurring during that time (Kelly, Huckabee, Jones, & Frampton, 2007). Swallowing in breastfed infants is typically followed by expiration. Mizuno, Ueda, and Takeuchi (2002) studied the effects of different fluids on the coordination between swallowing and breathing during bottle-feedings. When receiving breastmilk, compared with formula or distilled water in the bottle, the infants showed a significantly higher breathing rate. Swallows followed by inspiration were demonstrated less often with breastmilk in the bottle. The authors concluded that expressed breastmilk is more suitable for neonates because of the better coordination between swallowing and breathing, making subclinical aspiration less likely.

Swallowing can and should be assessed. Both the healthcare provider and the mother are encouraged to assess swallowing at each feeding in the early days to ensure milk transfer has occurred. Although an infant's jaw may move up and down, mimicking breastfeeding, jaw movement is not indicative of milk transfer. Signs of swallowing include the following:

- Deep jaw excursion (as opposed to shallow, biting, or chewing-like movements)
- Audible sound of swallowing
- Visualization of the throat during a swallow
- Vibration on the occipital region of the infant (a hand placed on the back of the baby's head may feel the swallow as a vibration)
- Movement of the throat felt by a finger over the trachea
- A small sound made by a puff of air from the nose
- A "ca" sound from the throat

Clinicians can assess swallow sounds by cervical auscultation with a stethoscope if they are uncertain that swallowing of milk is taking place.

- Placement of a small stethoscope adjacent to the lateral aspect of the larynx provides access to the sounds of the pharyngeal swallow (Vice, Heinz, Giuriati, Hood, & Bosma, 1990).
- In the absence of definitive evidence of swallowing, pre- and postfeed weights could be taken, if necessary, to validate whether milk transfer took place.

In one study, researchers found that swallow counts alone in infants who were 9 to 75 hours old were not a reliable indicator of milk intake or adequacy of a feeding (Cote-Arsenault & McCoy, 2012). A significant positive relationship was noted between number of swallows and breastmilk intake, but swallows alone accounted for only half of the variance in milk intake. Most likely, other factors in addition to swallows account for the volume of milk intake. These other predictive factors might include volume of milk per swallow and whether lactogenesis II has occurred—after this point, more milk is available and milk transfer is assisted by the milk ejection reflex. It is possible to visualize the swallowing process in a breastfed infant through a fiberoptic endoscopic evaluation. If feeding difficulties are suspected to be a result of problematic swallowing or swallowing is affected by structural, neurological, metabolic, or cardiorespiratory issues, such an exam helps pinpoint the origin of the problem and allows a more individualized feeding plan to be created. In one study, noisy breathing (with or without feeding), cyanosis, and "feeding difficulty" were the three most common presenting symptoms that prompted a fiberoptic study of swallowing (Willette, Molinaro, Thompson, & Schroeder, 2015).

Breathing

Breathing must also be coordinated while feeding. The airway is protected during sucking and swallowing and must remain stable (resist collapse) during feeding because sucking and swallowing occur in a rapid sequence. The patency of the airway can be affected by the sleep state, structural abnormalities, position of the neck, rate of milk flow, maturation (preterm vs. full term), illness, or central nervous system involvement. Increasing neck flexion causes the airway to become more prone to collapse; conversely, increasing neck extension helps increase the resistance to collapse. Some infants who suffer respiratory distress or who are premature may adopt an extended head and neck position because this posture makes it easier for them to breathe.

Breathing always takes precedence over feeding. Feeding difficulties can sometimes be an indicator of breathing problems, either from faulty positioning or an anatomic or physiological aberration in the infant. Positioning such infants at the breast may include subtle adjustments in the position of the head and proper shoulder girdle support to allow infants to remain well ventilated while they feed. Although infants prefer to breathe through their noses, they are not obligate nose breathers. Infants can breathe through their mouths for short periods of time, but it is accomplished at the expense of respiratory efficiency (Miller et al., 1985).

The bulk of research looking at suck–swallow–breathe synchrony has been conducted during bottle-feeding (Mathew, 1991a; Mathew & Bhatia, 1989; Meier, 1988, 1996). Repeated airway closure during swallowing has been shown to interrupt breathing. The more rapid milk flow from soft artificial nipples with large holes results in more frequent swallowing, less frequent opportunities for breathing, and significantly increased interruption in ventilation (Duara, 1989; Mathew, 1991b). These breathing alterations are more pronounced in preterm infants but also occur in full-term infants (Mathew, 1988; Mathew & Bhatia, 1989). Sucking during bottle-feeding interrupts breathing more frequently and for more sustained durations than sucking during breastfeeding (Meier, Lysakowski, Engstrom, Kavanaugh, & Mangurten, 1990). During bottle-feedings, infants alternate clusters of sucks and breaths. During breastfeeding, breathing is integrated into the sucking bursts. The suck–breathe pattern during breastfeeding suggests that infants may manipulate sucking parameters to control milk flow and accommodate breathing in such a way that apnea, bradycardia, and fatigue do not occur (Meier, 2001).

Differing bottle systems can affect oxygenation and how swallows are distributed during feedings. Goldfield, Richardson, Lee, and Margetts (2006) demonstrated that swallowing during breastfeeding was distributed nonrandomly and occurred at the peaks of intraoral sucking pressures. A group of infants in this study using a Playtex bottle system displayed a pattern of sucking, swallowing, and breathing that was more similar to the physiological norm of breastfeeding than the pattern observed in a group of infants using an Avent bottle system. If infants need to be supplemented and a bottle is chosen to provide extra milk, clinicians may wish to choose those bottles that disrupt breastfeeding the least (Peterson & Harmer, 2010).

Entrainment

Entrainment is the synchronization and control of a physiological rhythm by an external stimulus, influencing the body's ability to regulate. Sucking is a rhythmic behavior controlled primarily by the suck central pattern generator. Centrally generated patterns produced by the suck central pattern generator can be entrained in infants by the application of a rhythmic stimulus to the perioral and intraoral tissues (Barlow & Estep, 2006).

In one example, researchers adapted a pacifier to become a pulsating nipple that delivered the temporal pattern of a well-formed non-nutritive sucking burst to 31 tube-fed preterm infants with no functional suck. Repeated exposure to this type of stimulus over 7–10 days provided the infants with a neural entrainment experience that strengthened the central pathways that regulate suck, as evidenced by the rapid emergence of non-nutritive sucking and increased oral intake at feedings (Barlow, Finan, Lee, & Chu, 2008).

Music therapy has also been shown to improve sucking in preterm infants, especially live music when a lullaby is sung by a parent or when the infant is exposed to entrained rhythms from a Gato box that simulates the heartbeat sound that the infant would hear in utero (Loewy, Stewart, Dassier, Telsey, & Homel, 2013). Live, organized, entrained, rhythmic sounds are able to improve sustained sucking patterns. This noninvasive therapy can help turn the chaotic acoustical environment of a neonatal intensive care unit into a more organized and therapeutic environment. Akca and Aytekin (2014) studied the effects of soothing noise on the sucking outcomes of full-term infants as measured on the LATCH breastfeeding assessment tool. Sixty-four infants in the experimental group were exposed to the song "Don't Let Your Baby Cry-2" from the album *Colic* (released by Othan Osman of the On Music Production Company) and compared to 63 infants in the control group who were not exposed to the music. The music was played during the first breastfeeding after birth and again 24 hours later. The LATCH scores in the experimental group (8.61 ± 1.37) who were exposed to the music were found to be significantly higher than those in the control group (6.52 ± 1.79). Music therapy interventions may be a low-cost, noninvasive method of improving sucking and overall feeding outcomes.

Clinical Implications

Alterations in an infant's functional anatomy and physiology related to feeding may affect milk intake to a greater or lesser extent. During breastfeeding evaluations and especially if an infant presents with feeding problems, it is important to include an assessment of the infant's anatomic structures related to breastfeeding and their functioning.

Assessment of the Lips. The lips should present with the following characteristics:

- The lips should appear soft at rest, remain closed when awake and asleep, have a bow-shaped upper lip, and have a well-defined philtrum (the median groove between the upper lip and the nose).
- Both the upper and the lower lip should flange or flare outward when attached to the nipple/areola.
- When properly latched to the breast, the infant's lips should be parted at a wide angle when measured from the corner of the mouth. Aizawa and colleagues (2010) measured oral angles of breastfeeding and bottle-feeding infants, showing that the angle of the opened mouth of breastfed infants while nursing was approximately double that of infants sucking on standard artificial nipples. The angle at the corner of the mouth of infants feeding at the breast ranged from

112 degrees to 152 degrees, while infants sucking on a standard artificial nipple had an oral angle ranging from 55 degrees to 72 degrees.

- The lips should exert slight pressure to maintain a seal.

Alterations may include the following:

- Cleft lip: There is a great variation in cleft lip presentation, ranging from a small notch in the upper lip, either unilateral or bilateral, to a complete cleft through the lip into the nostril and through the upper alveolar ridge. A cleft in the lip compromises the seal needed to create negative pressure in the oral cavity. Many mothers fill the gap in the lip by manipulating the areola, their thumb, and the breast tissue to cover the defect. Infants with clefts of the lip are capable of generating suction, especially if the cleft is small (Reid, Reilly, & Kilpatrick, 2007). "Kissing" sounds heard during the feeding indicate that the anterior seal is being broken intermittently, which may compromise milk intake with each suck (Glass & Wolf, 1999).
- Loose, floppy, or asymmetrical lips: This problem can be associated with generalized hypotonia, partial paralysis or underdevelopment of the facial nerve (cranial nerve VII), facial asymmetry, and mouth droop or immobility. Any of these conditions may result in failure to form a seal for the oral cavity, causing periodic breaks in suction, inability to generate suction, smacking sounds, and/or milk leaking from the corners of the mouth. Asymmetrical lips may be seen if there is nerve damage or muscle weakness on either side of the face, causing one side of the mouth to droop and become slack on the weaker side.
- Retracted (forming a tight horizontal line over the mouth), pursed, or hypertonic lips: Increased tone may impair latch-on and active suckling, damage the nipple, and result in poor milk transfer. Pursed lips may result from feeding with artificial nipples that encourage mouth and lip closure. Lip retraction may also result from poor positioning where the neck or shoulder girdle is in extension.
- Tight (or short, inelastic) labial frenulum: This alteration may impede the flanging of the upper lip over the areola, as a restriction in the range of motion of the upper lip interferes with the upward and outward movement of the lip. An indication of a tight labial frenulum or "lip-tie" is an infant who purses the lips rather than flaring out the upper lip, resulting in a shallower, ineffective latch. This could result in nipple abrasion, painful or improper sucking, difficulty achieving a proper latch, or awkward positioning attempts by the infant (Wiessinger & Miller, 1995). The lip-tie may appear as a small, string-like to wide fan-like band of connective tissue extending from the inside of the upper lip and attaching to the alveolar mucosa of the maxillary arch. If a small crease appears in the upper lip between the nose and the lip, it is a sign that the lip is being tethered to the maxillary gum tissue, impeding the ability of the lip to extend upward (Kotlow, 2013). The lips should normally extend 1–1.5 inches (2.5–3.8 cm) beyond the base of the nipple when the infant is latched to the breast. Lip-tie may further contribute to reduced milk transfer, slow weight gain, fussiness from excessive air intake, colic-like symptoms, reflux, poor drainage in areas of the breast, reduced milk supply, and persistence of these problems after normal interventions have been tried. Kotlow (2004a; 2004b; 2011a) developed a classification

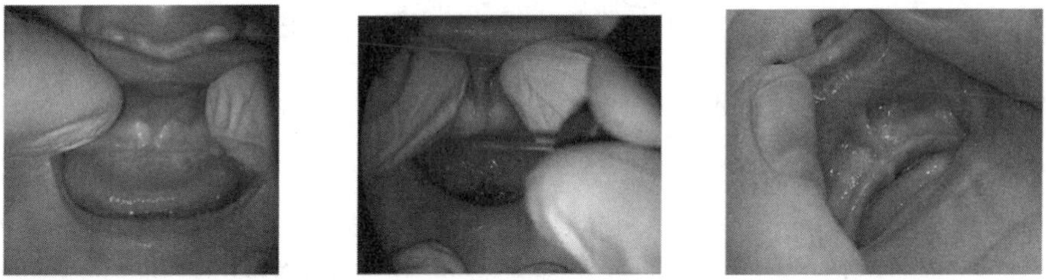

Class II
Attaches mostly into the gingival tissue

Class III
Attaches just in front of the anterior papilla*

Class IV
Attaches into the papilla* extending into the hard palate

*The papilla is the small bump of tissue just behind the area where the upper front teeth will erupt.

Figure 3-8 Kotlow classification of infant maxillary frenum attachment.

Used with permission from Kotlow, L. (2010a). Why can't my baby breastfeed: The effects of an abnormal maxillary frenum attachment. Retrieved from http://www.kiddsteeth.com/maxillaryfrenum_and_nursingfinal.pdf

of maxillary frenum attachments to aid in the clinical diagnosis of this condition (**Figure 3-8**). Class I is a normal attachment and requires no intervention. Class II attaches mostly into the gingival tissue. Class III attaches just in front of the anterior papilla, and class IV attaches into the papilla and extends into the hard palate. The papilla is the small bump of tissue just behind the area where the upper front teeth will erupt. Clinicians may wish to check for lip-tie when tongue-tie (ankyloglossia) is present and when normal interventions for common problems are ineffective. Lip-tie can be revised by clipping or by using a dental laser.

- Lip-ties that have not been revised in older infants can create a pocket for milk retention around the central incisors. This may facilitate the pooling of milk in the pockets created by the lip-tie when infants feed at night and contribute to the development of dental caries on the anterior surface of the two front teeth (Kotlow, 2010b).
- Corresponding alterations in cheek functioning: Lips and cheeks work together. Deviations or alterations in function in one affect the efficiency and functioning in the other.

Assessment of the Jaw. The lower jaw or mandible is typically in a neutral position at rest, with the lips touching. It moves in a smooth manner, correctly graded to engage in coordinated small excursions with a rhythmic quality. Several alterations in the structure of the jaw are possible.

Assessment of the Cheeks. The cheeks should appear soft, be symmetrical, have well-defined sucking pads, and maintain good tone during sucking. Cheeks with low tone or that are unstable may be pulled inward during the generation of vacuum, appearing as dimpled cheeks. In addition, they may contribute to reduced suction overall. Damage to cranial nerves VII (facial) and V (trigeminal) (either prenatally or from mechanical forces during delivery) could produce weakness or low tone in the cheeks, rendering them less able to sustain sucking during feeding. A tongue that is retracted or that lodges behind the lower gum line during sucking also produces dimpled cheeks. Dimpled cheeks indicate incorrect latch and/or suckling. Preterm infants have diminished sucking pads, such that the buccal surfaces of the cheeks may not come in contact with the mother's nipple–areola. This contributes to reduced stability and weaker structural support during feedings. Clinicians can advise mothers to use the Dancer hand position, which allows the mother's fingers to compress the infant's cheeks, placing the inner cheeks in contact with the nipple/areola. Preterm infants may have difficulty both in opening their mouths wide enough and in closing their mouths over the areola.

- In a recessed or retracted jaw structure (not caused by muscle tension or the normal slight recess of the newborn's jaw), the lower gum ridge is posterior to the upper gum ridge. The tongue is usually of normal size but is positioned farther back in the mouth. In utero, micrognathia can interfere with the normal positioning of the tongue, contributing to lack of fusion of the palatal shelves, and potentially lead to a cleft palate. Because of its posterior positioning, the tongue may be unable to move forward enough to engage in normal movements. The infant may also have difficulty opening the mouth wide enough to latch to the breast. Micrognathia frequently appears as part of various syndromes such as the following:
  - Pierre Robin syndrome, which also includes a small tongue and usually a wide, U-shaped cleft palate. Infants have a great deal of difficulty breastfeeding, usually because of the cleft. They also need to be placed in a prone position for feeding due to the tendency of the tongue to fall back into the throat, obstructing the airway.
  - Hemifacial microsomia. In this condition, one side of the child's face is underdeveloped, affecting mainly the ear, mouth, and jaw. It is the second most common congenital facial anomaly after cleft lip/palate, occurring in 1 in every 3,000–5,600 live births. Involvement may range from mild, with just minor jaw asymmetry, to severe, with additional eye, vertebral, and cardiac involvement, which is known as Goldenhar syndrome. There may be unequal cheek fullness due to underdevelopment of the fat pad and muscles. If the central nervous system is affected, then there may be asymmetry in facial movements. Underdevelopment of the jaw necessitates careful and creative positioning and close monitoring of milk transfer and weight gain.
- Asymmetrical jaw or deviations to one side may be the result of asymmetrical muscle tone, a structural defect, positioning in utero, or torticollis. Torticollis may be caused by fibrosis (replacement with connective tissue) of the SCM muscle, resulting in rotation of the head to the opposite side. Physical features of torticollis include variable degrees of the following: plagiocephaly, misalignment of the eyes, asymmetry of the ears, a depression of the side of the neck under the ear, flattening of the mandible, upward tilting of the lower jaw and gum line, elevation of the temporomandibular joint (TMJ), limited neck movement, and occasional asymmetries of the back, chest, hips, and feet. Flattening of the lower jaw may be visible. On the same side as the torticollis, the mandible may be flattened and the TMJ is elevated. Because of the pressure of the shoulder, the mandible is tilted up and the lower alveolar ridge is not parallel to the upper ("jaw tilt"). The typical right-sided head position preference when supine, cranial flattening, and long periods in the supine position with the head turned to the right may contribute to a shortening of the SCM. Infants with localized head flattening (plagiocephaly) at birth have an increased risk for other deformational anomalies, such as mandibular hypoplasia (underdeveloped lower jaw) (Peitsch, Keefer, LaBrie, & Mulliken, 2002).

Boere-Boonekamp and van der Linden-Kuiper (2001) examined 7,609 infants from a general population and found that 10% of infants less than 2 months of age had a preference for holding the head to one side and typically breastfed better on one side. The infant with torticollis has spent many weeks in utero with the head turned to one side while pushing on the opposite shoulder. Breastfed infants may have difficulty achieving a comfortable breastfeeding position with the shortened SCM muscle (Stellwagen, Hubbard, & Vaux, 2004). Wall and Glass (2006) reported that mothers of infants with mandibular asymmetry may experience sore nipples, difficult latch, and reduced milk transfer. Chin support and use of a nipple shield may be necessary. The infant's shortened SCM muscle may not be able to provide the power needed for the proper jaw excursions during active breastfeeding, leading to a weaker suck. Mothers may find it helpful to use breast compressions to facilitate milk transfer. A gap at the corner of the infant's mouth should be closed by pressing into the cheek, and sublingual pressure (a fingertip pressing gently under the soft area behind the chin) can be applied to make sure that the tongue is properly positioned and supported (Genna, 2015).

The most expeditious intervention during the early days when an infant demonstrates torticollis/asymmetrical jaw is to position the infant at the breast with the head turned to the preferred side. Rather than switching positions to feed on the second breast, the infant is slid over in the same position to feed from the other breast. The straddle position or a ventral position may also be helpful. Stretching exercises may be prescribed or referral to an occupational or physical therapist may be necessary to improve the condition.

- Alterations in jaw functioning may show up as exaggerated jaw movements, jaw clenching, wide jaw excursions, clamping or biting down to achieve stability and hold onto the nipple, and low tone or poor control of the TMJ. The TMJ may be affected by birth forces or instrument deliveries and may have an altered or limited range of movement. This joint moves in rather intricate ways: up and down like a hinge and gliding forward and down. A limited opening of the mouth caused by the inability of the TMJ to move in a full cycle of opening and closing may contribute to incremental latch-on in which an infant bites or nibbles his or her way onto the nipple rather than opening to a more optimal 160-degree angle. Wide jaw excursions beyond a 150- to 160-degree angle may be heard as smacking sounds as the tongue loses contact with the nipple–areola. Jaw instability is common in preterm infants and those with low orofacial tone, resulting in an unstable base for tongue movements. Sucking can be inefficient, and if the lips are unable to close, milk will leak from the corners of the mouth.

Assessment of the Tongue. The tongue should appear soft at rest, lying in the bottom of the mouth with a well-defined bowl shape. It should appear thin and flat, with a rounded tip and cupped sides. The tongue should neither protrude over the lips nor be seen when the mouth is closed. It should have sufficient tone and mobility to lift, extend, groove, and lateralize in a smooth and symmetrical manner. When a finger is placed in the infant's mouth, the tongue should cup around the finger, forming a distinct groove, and move in a rhythmic manner either in and out or up and down. Sucking pressure should be felt equally over the entire surface of the inserted finger. Besides playing a major role in sucking and swallowing, the tongue is an important oral structure that affects the shape of the palate, is involved in speech, contributes to the position of the teeth, and affects the development of the face.

Alterations of the tongue may include the following conditions:

- In tongue-tip elevation, the tip of the tongue is in opposition to the upper gum ridge, making it difficult for an infant to latch to the breast.
- Bunched (compressed in a lateral direction), retracted, or humped (in an anterior–posterior direction) tongue may be part of an infant's high tone. The tongue is unable to form a central groove in any of these positions.
- A tongue with low tone may demonstrate little to no shape, may feel excessively soft, may protrude over the lower gum ridge, or may appear excessively wide or large for the mouth.
- Tongue thrust (an in-and-out pattern of movement with a strong protrusion or push out of the mouth) during active sucking may be associated with high tone and result in difficulty generating negative pressure.
- Tongue alterations may be a sign of oral defensiveness or, with tongue protrusion, may be a result of respiratory problems where the infant positions the tongue forward to increase respiratory capacity.
- Tongue movement anomalies may be seen in cesarean-born infants from traction forces placed on the cranial base during delivery. The hypoglossal canal, through which the hypoglossal nerve passes, can be disrupted as the head is lifted through the cesarean incision (Smith, 2004).
- The action of the tongue can be altered by the use of artificial nipples. Whereas the shape of the human nipple–areola conforms to the inner boundaries of the infant's mouth, the infant's tongue and oral cavity are obligated to conform to the parameters presented to them by the shape and rigidity of an artificial nipple. The artificial nipple positions the tongue behind the lower gum (**Figure 3-9**). If a breastfed infant were to do this at the breast, both the upper and lower gum would be in opposition to each other and the infant would actually bite the nipple. Such a scenario could result in extreme pain for the mother along with nipple damage and little milk transfer. High-flow artificial nipples may result in decreased oxygen levels due

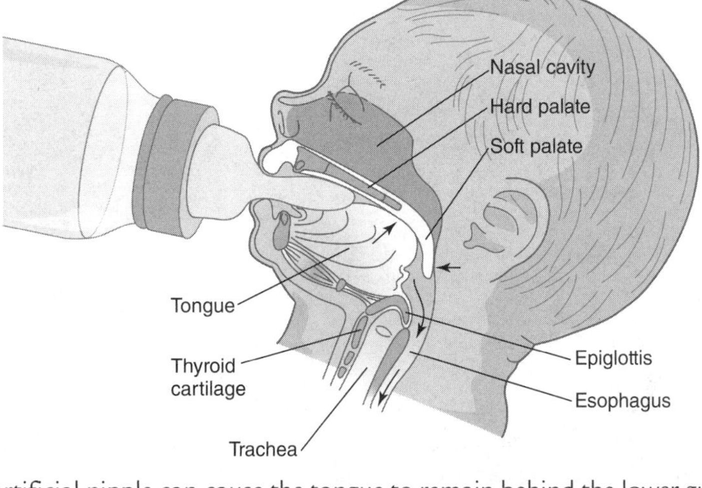

Figure 3-9 The artificial nipple can cause the tongue to remain behind the lower gum.

to rapid swallowing and limited intervals for breathing (**Figure 3-10A**). The artificial nipple (**Figure 3-10B**) does not fill the oral cavity, alters the labial seal, may obliterate the central grooving of the tongue, and may result in forces that impinge on the alveolar ridges and press them inward. Even so-called orthodontic improvements made to artificial nipples still force the normal shape and physiological action of the tongue to change (**Figure 3-10C**).

- Recent research on the sucking action of infants on artificial nipples has been conducted in an effort to manufacture artificial nipples that can claim to elicit similar sucking actions as on the breast. Segami, Mizuno, Taki, and Itabashi (2013) studied an experimental artificial nipple with a wide base, a firm shaft, and a valve at the base such that milk flowed only when the infant exerted vacuum. They concluded that there were no significant differences in perioral movements between breastfeeding and feeding on this experimental nipple. However, one important difference was noted: The vacuum generated during sucking on the experimental nipple was significantly smaller than that observed during feeding on the breast. This would be of concern if an infant transferred a lower vacuum to the breast and such a weaker sucking pressure was unable to transfer milk efficiently from the breast. The same observation of reduced vacuum application was seen in a study conducted by Geddes and colleagues (2012) on the development

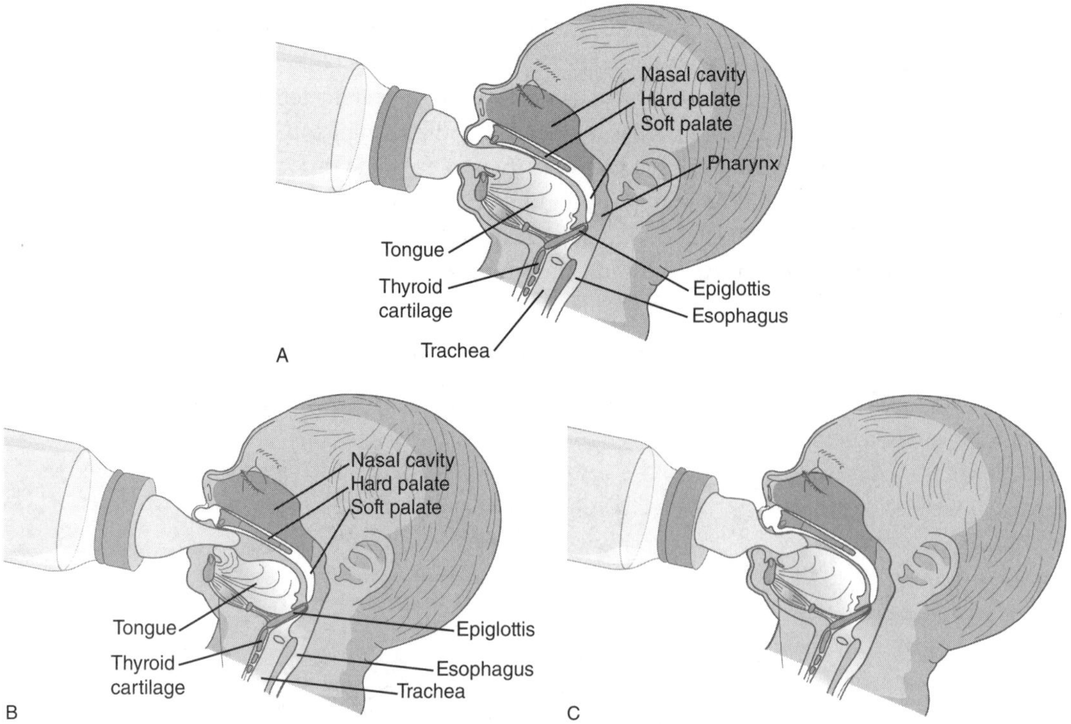

Figure 3-10 (A) Throat conformation for swallowing within the bottle suck cycle. (B) Traditional artificial nipple does not fill the oral cavity. (C) Altered "orthodontic" artificial nipple alters tongue position, compromising physiologic tongue action.

of a new artificial nipple that relies solely on vacuum to transfer milk from the bottle. Baseline (–12 mm Hg vs. –31 mm Hg) and peak vacuum (–67 mm Hg vs. –122 mm Hg) generation on the experimental artificial nipple was significantly lower than that applied at the breast. During the development of this same artificial nipple, Sakalidis and colleagues (2012) again demonstrated that sucking pressures on the artificial nipple were lower than at the breast. Use of artificial nipples that lower vacuum generation could have negative implications when used by infants who already have a weak suck, reinforcing diminished vacuum application at the breast. Woolridge (2012) found that under ultrasound, peristaltic movements of the tongue could be visualized when infants were sucking on a different artificial nipple, with both vacuum and peristaltic tongue movements present during the same feeding.

Tongue-tie, or ankyloglossia, is one of the most common tongue alterations and can affect infant milk intake and the integrity of the mother's nipples. The exact incidence of tongue-tie is unknown, but studies report a 4.2–4.8% incidence in general populations of newborns (Ballard, Auer, & Khoury, 2002; Messner, Lalakea, Aby, Macmahon, & Bair, 2000). Definitions and descriptions vary. Fernando (1998) described the condition based on both visual and functional aspects of the frenum: "Tongue-tie is a congenital condition, recognized by an unusually thickened, tightened, or shortened frenum [frenulum], which limits movement of the tongue in activities connected with feeding and which has an adverse impact on both dental health and speech." Hazelbaker (1993) defined tongue-tie as "impaired tongue function resulting from a tight and/or short lingual frenulum which may or may not involve fibers of the genioglossus muscle. Complete ankyloglossia can be defined as a 'fusing' of the tongue to the floor of the mouth."

Ankyloglossia limits the range of motion of the tongue and affects not only sucking but also speech, the position of the teeth, periodontal tissue (the tongue cannot clear residual fluid and food from the buccal cavities), jaw development, and swallowing. It has been associated with deviation of the epiglottis and larynx, harsh breath sounds, and mild oxygen desaturation during sucking (Mukai, Mukai, & Asaoka, 1991).

Tongue-tie is sometimes visualized during the newborn exam before hospital discharge. Mothers may complain of nipple pain and sore nipples, difficult latch, unsustained sucking, or the infant "popping" on and off the breast. Inability to transfer milk because of a mechanical difficulty can also lead to and present with insufficient milk, slow weight gain, engorgement, and plugged ducts. Observations of the breastfeeding may reveal milk leaking from the sides of the mouth, slow feeding, a clicking or smacking sound as the tongue loses contact with the nipple–areolar complex, sucking blisters on the infant's lips, and distorted appearance of the nipple when released from the infant's mouth. Tongue-tie has been described and assessed by the appearance of the tongue, the functioning of the tongue, or a combination of both parameters. The affected tongue has variously been described as heart shaped (**Figure 3-11**), notched, unable to protrude beyond the lower gum or elevate to the roof of the mouth, unable to cup and form a central groove, having a short and/or tight frenulum, having a thick or thin frenulum, having

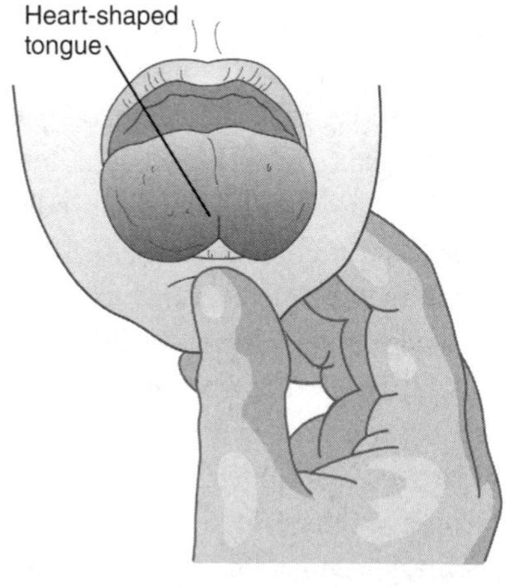

Figure 3-11 Heart-shaped tongue.

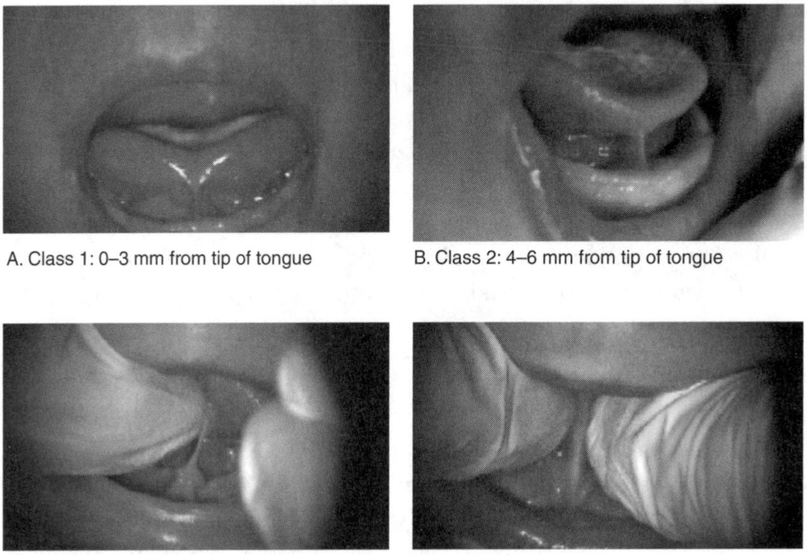

A. Class 1: 0–3 mm from tip of tongue

B. Class 2: 4–6 mm from tip of tongue

C. Class 3: 7–9 mm from tip of tongue

D. Class 4: 10–12 mm from tip of tongue

Figure 3-12 Kotlow classification of infant tongue-tie.

Kotlow, L. (2011b). Infant reflux and aerophagia associated with the maxillary lip-tie and ankyloglossia (tongue-tie). *Clinical Lactation, 2*, 25–29.

a frenulum attached anywhere along the underside of the tongue, and being anchored in various places, from the lower alveolar ridge or farther back along the floor of the mouth. A tight or short frenulum may be less than 1 cm in length and feel tight when a finger is placed under the midline of the tongue (Notestine, 1990). During a digital assessment of the tongue, it may be felt to snap back to the mandibular floor because it may be unable to elevate or maintain extension for very long (Marmet, Shell, & Marmet, 1990).

Consistent definitions and assessment tools are scarce. Kotlow (2004a) classifies tongue-ties based on the distance of the insertion of the lingual frenum to the tip of the tongue. A normal distance is 16 mm. Class IV is defined as a distance of 10–12 mm from the tip of the tongue; class III is a moderate tongue-tie, with a distance of 7–9 mm from the tip of the tongue; class II is severe, with a distance of 4–6 mm from the tip of the tongue; and class I is complete, with a distance of 0–3 mm from the tip of the tongue (**Figure 3-12**). If this distance is less than 8 mm, Kotlow (2004c) recommends that the frenum be revised.

Edmunds, Miles, and Fulbrook (2011) analyzed the evidence regarding tongue-tie to determine if tongue-tie could have a significant impact on breastfeeding and if frenotomy was a viable option. They found that for most infants, frenotomy offered the best chance of improved and continued breastfeeding and that the procedure did not lead to complications for the infant or the mother. Kumar and Kalke (2011) analyzed prospective cohort studies and randomized controlled trials regarding whether breastfeeding was adversely affected by tongue-tie and if frenotomy was helpful in rectifying the associated breastfeeding problems. They found a strong association between the presence of tongue-tie and breastfeeding problems in neonates. Their analysis revealed that neonates with tongue-tie are at increased risk for breastfeeding difficulties and that those with breastfeeding difficulties should be immediately referred to a lactation consultant with experience in handling this situation. They also stated that the presence of tongue-tie along with breastfeeding difficulties in an infant should constitute a valid indication for a referral for frenotomy. The data confirmed that frenotomy usually results in very rapid improvement in the symptoms associated with tongue-tie.

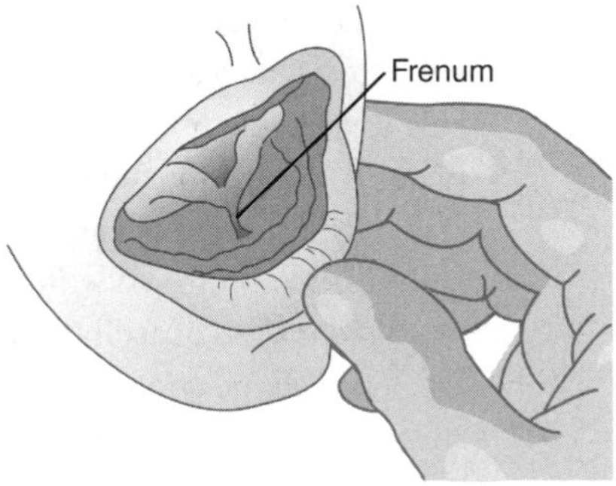

Figure 3-13 Tight frenum causes problems elevating tongue.

A prospective longitudinal study was conducted to observe changes in breastfeeding parameters following lingual frenotomy that included number of sucks, length of pauses between sucking bursts, and complaints from mothers (Martinelli, Marchesan, Gusmao, Honorio, & Berretin-Felix, 2015). Following frenotomy, the number of sucks increased, the length of pauses decreased, feedings were of shorter duration, infants no longer slipped off the nipple, and nipple pain was eliminated. The provision of frenotomy seems to be time sensitive, in that a delay in this procedure beyond 4 weeks from referral to assessment of tongue-tie is more likely to be associated with abandonment of breastfeeding (Donati-Bourne, Batool, Hendrickse, & Bowley, 2015).

Some mothers present with excoriated nipples caused by the infant's altered tongue movements. The compression between the gums and the up-and-down movements of the tongue may result in abrasions on the upper aspect of the nipple as it rubs against the upper gum ridge or rugae of the hard palate or on the underside of the nipple as it experiences friction over the uncovered lower gum. If the frenulum is attached at the very tip of the tongue, the tongue can actually curl under. Tongue-tie restricts the tongue to a limited range of movements (**Figure 3-13**), making it problematic if the tongue tip remains unable to elevate as the jaw drops and/or interferes with the posterior tongue's movements in swallowing. Infants often engage in a number of compensatory movements to facilitate milk intake, such as reliance on negative pressure to obtain milk, fluttering action of the tongue as it seeks the nipple, chewing motions, biting actions to hold onto the nipple in place, and head movements to help with swallowing.

Tongue-tie is usually an isolated condition, but it can be seen as part of congenital syndromes. It is more common in boys than in girls, and is often familial. If the mother has a small breast, if the breast is highly elastic, and if the infant can draw in enough of the areola, breastfeeding may not become compromised. In a small study of five breastfed infants with tongue-tie, Geddes and colleagues (2010b) found that in these mothers, nipple pain, milk intake by the infant, and milk production were not impacted by the tongue-tie. This finding suggests that some mothers may have certain breast, nipple, milk supply, or milk ejection characteristics that allow infants with tongue-tie to breastfeed successfully. However, failure to correct the tongue-tie at this stage may simply postpone the procedure until problems with eating, dentition, and speech require it at an older age.

Assessment of the Hard Palate. The hard palate should be intact, smoothly contoured, and appear as if the tongue would comfortably fit within its contours. There are a number of alterations to the hard palate.

- Cleft lip and cleft palate constitute the fourth most common congenital disability, affecting 1 in 700 children in the United States. A cleft of the palate can include the hard and/or soft palate, with or without involvement of the lip; can be unilateral or bilateral; and may exhibit varying degrees of severity and involvement. Clefting may occur as an isolated event or may be part of a syndrome such as Pierre Robin syndrome or Turner syndrome. A submucous cleft of the hard palate can sometimes be felt as a notch or depression in the bony palate when palpated with a finger. Although tongue movements during sucking may be normal, compression can be generated only if there is adequate hard palate surface to compress against; sealing of the oral cavity is always compromised with both hard and soft palate clefts (Glass & Wolf, 1999). Feedings are long, and if signs of aspiration, such as frequent coughing, choking, sputtering, or color change, are observed, position changes may be required or assistive devices may be needed to ensure adequate intake (Edmondson & Reinhartsen, 1998). Usually, no airway obstruction or swallowing abnormalities are present, but with clefts of the palate, air is vented through the cleft, making it difficult to impossible to achieve vacuum, depending on how much of the palate is involved. Infants born with a cleft lip only usually have fewer problems breastfeeding than those with palatal defects.

- Breastfeeding infants with clefts (or supplying pumped breastmilk) provides the same disease protection as for any other infant. Indeed, breastmilk is especially important in reducing the otitis media that infants with cleft palate are so prone to develop. Breastfeeding encourages the proper use of the oral and facial musculature, promotes better speech development, and, when the infant is at breast, helps normalize maternal–infant interactions.
- Infants with cleft lip/palate are at an increased risk for insufficient milk intake. Weight gain, number of feedings, intake at each feeding, and diaper counts must be monitored to determine the need for supplemental breastmilk or other foods (Dowling, Danner, & Coffey, 1997).
- Poor feeding skills may sometimes be seen in newborns with cleft palate or cleft lip/cleft palate, and are even more commonly seen in infants with Pierre Robin syndrome, along with other syndromes. Many infants with isolated cleft lip and/or palate have normal feeding skills and experience problems only with vacuum generation, slow feedings, and nasal regurgitation. Actual oral motor dysfunction seen in infants with various syndromes can include minimal jaw excursions and absence of normal jaw and tongue movements for long periods. Reid, Kilpatrick, and Reilly (2006) found that babies with smaller clefts such as cleft lips and minor soft palate clefts were more likely to generate normal levels of suction on a bottle than infants with larger clefts, but not always for a long time. Infants with cleft lip and palate were also reported to have lower compression readings on the artificial nipple. This decreased compression could be due to the absence of palatal tissue against which to press the nipple or it could be a learned behavior from feeding with compressible bottles/nipples, which deliver milk regardless of whether suction or compression is generated.

Masarei and colleagues (2007) looked at bottle sucking patterns of infants with unilateral cleft lip and palate and of infants with a cleft of the soft palate and at least two-thirds of the hard palate. They found two patterns of feeding—one in which the infants did not produce an identifiable sucking burst, but used a continuous disorganized pattern, and one in which the infants generated a short rhythmic sucking burst/pause pattern that was sustained for only 2 to 3 minutes followed by sucking disorganization. Sucking rates of these infants were more rapid than in infants with no cleft—109.26 sucks per minute in infants with clefts compared with

75.05 sucks per minute in infants without clefts. Infants with clefts generated compression or positive pressure for 71% of the feeding, while infants without clefts generated positive pressure for 26% of the feeding. Infants with clefts demonstrated an inconsistent range of tongue and jaw movements, arrhythmic tongue and jaw movements, and an altered rate of sucking. Many of these sucking alterations appear to be attempts by the infants to compensate for the anatomic abnormalities. Lacking enough vacuum for milk removal, infants compensated with faster and more compressions or positive pressure generation to remove milk by using a mechanical ability that they possessed. While this study only looked at feeding patterns on a bottle, it is likely that infants with cleft defects will also attempt to compensate in a similar manner at the breast. Clinicians might wish to visualize the entire mouth (including the hard and soft palate) of an infant who is demonstrating the feeding patterns just described. Feeding inefficiency is predictive of poor feeding in young infants. Neonates transferring less than 2.2 mL/minute of milk and infants transferring less than 3.3 mL/minute of milk are highly predictive of poor feeding skills (Reid et al., 2006). The more severe the cleft, the more likely associated disorders or syndromes are to be present (de Vries et al., 2014). During early assessment, clinicians will need to explore the possibility of other disorders or syndromes in infants with clefts, especially if there is severe clefting.

- If the infant is unable to withdraw sufficient milk from the breast, expressed breastmilk can be provided through a supplemental tube feeding device at breast or through a special bottle-feeder. Mothers will need an electric breast pump and a pumping plan to provide breastmilk and maintain an adequate supply. They may use alternate massage when the infant is at breast or hand express milk directly into the infant's mouth, but the infant may be unable to adequately drain the mother's breasts, increasing the risk of insufficient milk supply, engorgement, plugged ducts, and mastitis unless the breasts are more thoroughly drained at each feeding (Biancuzzo, 1998).
- Some infants may be fitted with a palatal obturator (a prosthesis molded to fill the cleft and provide an "artificial" palate). This device is designed to provide a solid surface against which to compress the nipple and seal the oral cavity to facilitate achieving negative pressure for milk withdrawal. It may also help to decrease the amount of time it takes for each feeding, reducing the fatigue for both infant and parents.
- Managing the infant with a cleft defect is typically accomplished by a team of healthcare professionals, with surgeries, treatment, and therapy that can continue for many years. Because most orofacial clefts are immediately apparent after birth, it is important that healthcare providers experienced with feeding cleft-involved infants be readily available to parents. Parents are especially concerned about feeding issues, and nurses caring for mothers of newborns with orofacial clefts should quickly refer mothers to lactation specialists/consultants experienced with the associated feeding complications (Byrnes, Berk, Cooper, & Marazita, 2003).
- Other palatal variations such as a bubble palate (**Figure 3-14**) may also impede breastfeeding. A bubble palate is defined as a "concavity in the hard palate, usually about 3/8 to 3/4 in (1–2 cm) in diameter and 1/4 in (1/2 cm) deep" (Marmet & Shell, 1993). Because of the position of the mother's nipple relative to the bubble, the nipples can become abraded, inflamed, and sore if the nipple rubs against the anterior ridge of the bubble. Weight gain problems may also ensue if the infant is unable to transfer sufficient milk (Snyder, 1997).

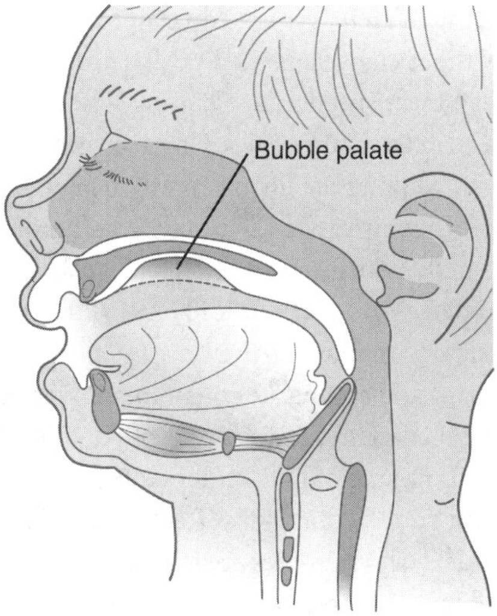

Figure 3-14 Bubble palate.

Assessment of the Soft Palate. The soft palate generally has thinner mucosa than the hard palate and may be somewhat darker in color. It is firm but spongy, the uvula should be in the midline and intact, and the soft palate should not sag to either side. The following notes relate to alterations of the soft palate:

- Cleft of the soft palate and uvula is always midline. Submucous clefts are a subgroup of clefts with intact mucosa lining the roof of the mouth that can make it difficult to see when looking into the mouth. The underlying muscle and bone are at least partially divided, indicating insufficient median fusion of the muscles of the soft palate. A submucous cleft may be identified by the presence of a bifid uvula, a very thin translucent strip of mucosa in the middle of the roof of the mouth, and a notch at the back edge of the hard palate that can be felt with the fingertip. Reiter and colleagues (2012) found a potential role of maternal smoking during pregnancy in the formation of a submucous cleft palate, especially if the infants had particular genetic variants that predisposed for orofacial clefts. Infants may experience swallowing difficulties and persistent middle-ear disease. Damage to the glossopharyngeal nerve (cranial nerve IX) and the vagus nerve (cranial nerve X) may cause a paralysis of the soft palates, which will sag on the affected side. Babies with this type of cleft suck rhythmically but generate only weak suction and may feed for prolonged periods but transfer little milk, resulting in inadequate weight gain. They may have nasal snorting, frequent sneezing, or regurgitation through the nares. Clefts of the soft palate will not be detected on digital exam. The examiner needs to visualize the soft palate by using a light and a tongue depressor on the posterior tongue.
- A congenital short palate can result in velopharyngeal insufficiency, as can insufficient tissue repair of a cleft palate (Morris & Klein, 2000).
- The soft palate is typically involved when the hard palate has a cleft. This can result in an open nasopharynx during swallowing and reflux of milk into the nasal cavity, swallowing of air into the stomach, and, if ear tubes are present, milk sometimes leaking through the tubes and out the ear.

Some clefts can be identified on fetal ultrasound as early as 14–16 weeks' gestation, especially if the cleft palate is severe and occurs along with a cleft lip. Not all clefts are identified at birth or on day 1, with delayed detection of clefts experienced by some families. Habel, Elhadi, Sommerlad, and Powell (2006) found that isolated cleft palates that were U shaped were more often detected on day 1 than were narrow V-shaped clefts (**Figure 3-15**). A delay in detection is more likely in the case of small narrow clefts in the soft palate. Digital examination of the infant's mouth can miss small clefts, and in the presence of symptoms (e.g., feeding difficulties, nasal regurgitation), a visual examination of the mouth

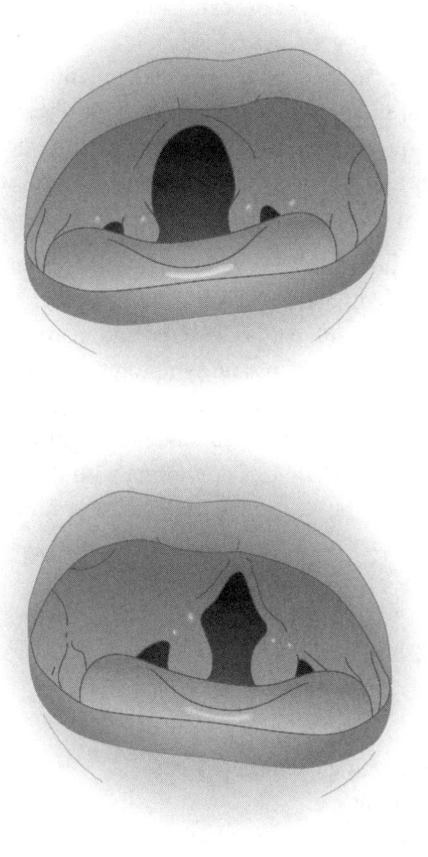

Figure 3-15 Clefting that might be missed without direct visualization of the palates. (A) Broad U-shaped cleft palate extending one-third way into the hard palate. (B) Narrow V-shaped cleft palate at the junction of the soft and hard palates.
Habel, A., Elhadi, N., Sommerlad, B., & Powell, J. (2006). Delayed detection of cleft palate: An audit of newborn examination. *Archives of Disease in Childhood, 91*, 238–240.

should be performed. The tongue needs to be sufficiently depressed to visualize the back of the mouth with a flashlight.

Assessment of the Nasal Cavity, Pharynx, Larynx, and Trachea. These structures can be assessed with varying tests and instruments when significant deviations from normal are suspected. Alterations in swallowing and breathing or problems with the coordination of suck, swallow, breathe may alert the clinician to an anatomic or structural defect, such as the following:

- Choanal atresia—occlusion of the passage between the nose and pharynx by a bony or membranous structure.
- Vocal cord anomalies or paralysis.

- Edema from trauma such as intubation, extubation, or suctioning.
- Structural narrowing such as subglottic stenosis.
- Instability of a structure, such as tracheomalacia (softening of the tracheal cartilage) or laryngomalacia (softening of the tissues of the larynx, typically when the epiglottis bends over and partially obstructs the opening to the larynx). Infants with tracheomalacia, laryngomalacia, and laryngotracheomalacia also have a higher incidence of gastroesophageal reflux (Bibi et al., 2001).
- Spasms of a structure, such as laryngospasm.

Because these structures are not readily visible, the clinical presentation, feeding and health history, and behavioral observation of a feeding are necessary to gather data for a feeding plan and/or referral. Infants may present with one or a combination of signs and symptoms. The underlying cause of the problems may be unclear because similar signs and symptoms may reflect different etiologies. Complex medical diseases and conditions (e.g., bronchopulmonary dysplasia, cardiac problems, cerebral palsy, genetic syndromes) may also produce some of the following signs and symptoms even if they are not related to structural or anatomic defects. Infants presenting with these symptoms should be checked by their primary care provider and may be referred to a specialist or undergo testing (Arvedson & Lefton-Greif, 1998) to determine the primary problem:

- Noisy breathing
- Chronic congestion
- Inadequate weight gain
- Refusal to feed
- Apnea/bradycardia
- Coughing, choking, or gagging during a feeding
- Cyanosis, pallor, or sweating
- Wheezing, stridor, or suprasternal retractions
- Excessive drooling

Depending on the type and extent of interference with feeding at the breast, modifications may be warranted in such elements as total body positioning, flexion or extension of the head, use of a nipple shield, expression of milk, and use of alternate feeding devices.

Assessment of the Esophagus. The most common disorder related to the esophagus in an infant is gastroesophageal reflux (GER), although other esophageal disorders can interfere with swallowing (e.g., upper or lower esophageal sphincter dysfunction, esophageal dysmotility, extrinsic compression, or mechanical obstruction) (Arvedson & Lefton-Greif, 1998). GER entails the passive backflow of stomach contents into the esophagus and implies a functional or physiological process in a healthy infant with no underlying systematic abnormalities. This disorder is associated with a transient relaxation of the lower esophageal sphincter due to fundal stimulation, which allows gastric contents to wash back into the lower esophagus and often be regurgitated. GER (spitting up) generally peaks between 1 and 4 months of age and is seen in 40–65% of healthy infants. The supine position and the slumped seated position can exacerbate reflux during the times that the lower esophageal sphincter relaxes (Jung, 2001). Some infants with frequent GER have an inflamed throat and a hoarse cry. Infants may arch their neck and back when feeding, may gag or cough, and engage in chewing motions (rumination or "cud chewing"). Infants with an unexplained chronic cough should be evaluated for GER (Borrelli et al., 2011). Jadcherla and colleagues (2012) looked at how GER might be influenced by certain feeding mechanics and found that at least in preterm infants, feeding duration and feeding flow rate modifications could significantly reduce GER events. In bottle- and gavage-fed infants, slowing down the feeding and decreasing the milk flow rate significantly reduced the total number of GER events. The authors speculated that a large volume of swallowed milk and air over a short period of time could contribute to the gastric distention and fundal stimulation that precipitate GER events. Applying this finding to the breastfeeding situation might suggest that in infants with GER, mothers might wish to elicit the milk ejection reflex before putting the baby to breast to reduce the volume and speed of milk intake. Mothers might also consider extending the feeding time by allowing some periods of rest to prolong the feeding.

Gastroesophageal reflux disease (GERD) is a pathological process characterized by clinical features such as regurgitation with poor weight gain, irritability, pain in the lower chest, possible apnea and cyanosis, wheezing, laryngospasm, and possibly aspiration, chronic cough, and stridor. An infant with GERD may have more than five episodes of reflux per day, regurgitate approximately 28 g per episode, and refuse or show irritability during feedings (Arguin & Swartz, 2004). Some infants with GERD do not respond to medication. In infants with more severe GERD, an abnormal hyperextension of the neck with torticollis (Sandifer syndrome) may be seen.

Infants with GER or GERD may demonstrate feeding resistance, arching at the breast, limited feeding time at the breast, and discomfort when fed in the cradle position. These infants feed better when breastfed in an elevated position of 45 degrees or more (Boekel, 2000; Wolf & Glass, 1992). After each feeding, infants should be kept upright, as in a front pack carrier or wrap, rather than slumped down in an infant seat or immediately put in a supine position. Care must be taken when using a sling so as not to increase intra-abdominal pressure. Proton-pump inhibitors are frequently prescribed for GER symptoms, but crying infants less than 3–4 months of age with vomiting, back-arching, and aversive feeding behaviors very rarely have macroscopic esophageal lesions on endoscopy. Gastric acid is buffered for 2 hours after feedings, so gastric reflux contents during this time period do not irritate the esophageal mucosa (Douglas, 2013). Other physical/medical conditions should be ruled out and breastfeeding properly assessed and managed before medications for GER or GERD are prescribed.

Kotlow (2011b) describes tongue-tie and maxillary lip-tie as potential contributors to symptoms typically associated with reflux and colic. The association is the large amount of air that can be swallowed and the inability of the lips to form a complete seal on the breast. Once a maxillary lip-tie and/or a tongue-tie is released, the lips can form a more complete seal and the tongue remains in contact with the nipple/areola, reducing the intake of air. Alcantara and Anderson (2008) report that chiropractic and cranial–sacral therapy may provide relief for some infants suffering from GER.

PUTTING IT ALL TOGETHER

The infant's feeding anatomy and associated physiology come together at feeding times in a complex series of actions that must occur in synchrony to ensure transfer of sufficient milk from the mother's breast into the infant. Guidelines for assessing the breastfeeding mother and infant have emphasized the importance of the visual assessment conducted in a coordinated manner (Walker, 1989). Assessment is the foundation of professional practice. Breastfeeding assessment is part of the community standard of care for hospital maternity units. The Committee on Fetus and Newborn of the American Academy of Pediatrics (2010) recommends that a number of criteria be met before any newborn discharge, including items specific to breastfeeding:

1. The infant has completed at least two successful feedings, with documentation that the infant is able to coordinate sucking, swallowing, and breathing while feeding.
2. The mother's knowledge, ability, and confidence to provide adequate care for her baby are documented by the fact that she has received training and demonstrated competency regarding the importance and benefits of breastfeeding. The breastfeeding mother and baby should be assessed by trained staff regarding breastfeeding position, latch-on, and adequacy of swallowing.

Tools

Tools have been developed to predict future problems or to help identify mothers who are at risk for early weaning. Assessing breastfeeding activities using a systematic approach can be undertaken in a number of ways. Some clinicians use (or adapt) one of a number of short clinical assessment tools that have been developed for the following purposes:

- Organize the breastfeeding assessment
- Identify both normal and abnormal patterns at the breast
- Determine whether milk transfer has occurred
- Document and chart breastfeeding behaviors
- Direct professional intervention and patient education to areas where it is needed
- Serve as a communication vehicle among professional caregivers
- Establish evaluation and teaching standards
- Reduce inappropriate supplementation
- Predict which infants are at risk for early weaning
- Recognize mother–baby pairs in need of referrals and follow-up

Using a clinical assessment tool helps objectively document feedings and may be expedient in the hospital or clinic setting. Some of the tools assign a score with cut-off points that serve as a basis for making referrals. Several have been shown to be predictive of risk for early weaning and are also used to justify the need for more intensive breastfeeding assistance. Not all tools have been shown to be valid (i.e., the tool measures what it states it measures) and/or clinically reliable (i.e., it consistently measures the intended behavior). However, the tools that assess feedings at the breast depend on the clinician's observation of a feeding and do not rely on subjective descriptions of "good, fair, poor" or number of minutes at each breast, descriptions that are inappropriate, inaccurate, and of little clinical relevance.

Infant Breastfeeding Assessment Tool

Matthews (1988) noted that Infant Breastfeeding Assessment Tool (IBFAT) scores (**Table 3-3**) were not predictive of abandonment of breastfeeding but rather illustrated that sucking behaviors improved over time. There was a significant difference in breastfeeding competence between infants of first-time

Table 3-3 Infant Breastfeeding Assessment Tool

Component	**3**	**2**	**1**	**0**
Readiness to feed	Started to feed readily without effort	Needed mild stimulation to start feeding	Needed vigorous stimulation to feed	Cannot be roused
Rooting	Rooted effectively at once	Needed coaxing to root	Rooted poorly, even with coaxing	Did not try to root
Fixing (latch-on)	Started to feed at once	Took 3–10 minutes to start feeding	Took > 10 minutes to start feeding	Did not feed
Sucking pattern	Sucked well on one or both breasts	Sucked off and on, but needed encouragement	Some sucking efforts for short periods	Did not suck

Maximum score: 12
Score of 10–12 = Effective vigorous feeding
Score of 7–9 = Moderately effective feeders
Score 0–6 = Effective sucking rhythm not established
Data from Matthews, M. K. (1988). Developing an instrument to assess infant breastfeeding behaviour in the early neonatal period. *Midwifery, 4,* 154–165.

mothers, who took a mean of 35 hours to establish effective breastfeeding, compared with infants of multiparous mothers, who took a mean of 21.2 hours to establish effective breastfeeding. A longer period to establish effective breastfeeding was also associated with the timing of drug administration in labor, as 83.4% of primiparous mothers received alphaprodine (Nisentil) within 1–4 hours before delivery compared with 45% of multiparous mothers.

The IBFAT does not assess swallowing, which can be a drawback in its use unless swallowing is included in the "sucking pattern" measurement score. Matthews (1991) also observed that mothers can use the IBFAT to assess their infants' feeding progress, with infants who score the highest having mothers who are more pleased with the feeding. Primiparous mothers had a significantly higher percentage of feedings at which they were dissatisfied, with low scores tending to occur predominantly during the first 48 hours after birth. Mothers' satisfaction or positive feedback is important in the maternal decision to continue breastfeeding and persevere during breastfeeding difficulties. Mothers who experience dissatisfaction during the early time after birth will need more intensive support to curtail the negative feedback generated when an infant struggles to breastfeed. An infant who does not achieve a score in the 10 to 12 range of the IBFAT upon discharge from the hospital should be referred for follow-up (Matthews, 1993).

Latch Assessment Documentation Tool

This latch assessment tool (**Table 3-4**) was developed to serve as a quick and easy method for documenting a mother's ability to attach her baby properly to the breast and to observe the infant's sucking. Each component was defined and a plus or minus used to indicate whether the behavior was present or absent, respectively. If any component of the latch assessment is charted as insufficient, the nurse writes a progress note to detail the deviation or variance as well as to chart what corrective action was taken. Use of this form served to visually remind nurses to follow up with mothers who needed assistance to latch their infants successfully (Jenks, 1991). Swallowing was not evaluated as a separate component but was mentioned as part of the adequate suction measurement (e.g., "suck/swallow ratio is 1–2/second").

Table 3-4 Latch Assessment Documentation Tool

Parameter	Code + (Normal and Sufficient) − (Insufficient)
Baby's gum line placed over mother's lactiferous sinuses	
Both lips are flanged	
Complete jawbone movement	
Tongue is positioned under the areola	
Adequate suction	

Data from Jenks, M. (1991). Latch assessment documentation in the hospital. *Journal of Human Lactation, 7*, 19–20.

No numerical score is assigned to the feeding effort; however, this tool is designed to identify breastfeeding problems so that a plan of care can be initiated as early as possible.

Breastfeeding Assessment Tool

Inaccurate, inadequate, or subjective/qualitative descriptions of breastfeeding in the hospital perpetuate inconsistencies in care and sometimes the communication of useless information. In an effort to improve breastfeeding assessment, the Breastfeeding Assessment Tool was developed to improve documentation of objective observations of breastfeeding status (Bono, 1992). Although nurses resisted filling out another form, practices supportive of breastfeeding increased with the improved awareness of the necessity of such documentation. Tools such as the Breastfeeding Assessment Tool, which includes audible swallowing as a component to be assessed, help prevent hospital staff from minimizing the importance of ongoing assessment of the breastfeeding couple.

Systematic Assessment of the Infant at Breast

It is recommended that each component of the Systematic Assessment of the Infant at the Breast (SAIB; **Box 3-2**) be evaluated as part of an initial breastfeeding assessment and completed at least once before the mother and baby are discharged home. The SAIB delineates the essential components of a breastfeeding episode that are central to effective breastfeeding and milk transfer. It emphasizes the importance of assessing for and documenting that swallowing has occurred. Without an assessment of swallowing,

Box 3-2 Systematic Assessment of the Infant at Breast

Alignment

- Infant is in flexed position, relaxed with no muscular rigidity.
- Infant's head and body are at breast level.
- Infant's head is aligned with trunk and is not turned laterally, hyperextended, or hyperflexed.
- Correct alignment of infant's body is confirmed by an imaginary line from ear to shoulder to iliac crest.
- Mother's breast is supported with cupped hand during first 2 weeks of breastfeeding.

Areolar Grasp

- Mouth is open widely; lips are not pursed.
- Lips are visible and flanged outward.
- Complete seal and strong vacuum are formed by infant's mouth.
- Approximately ½ inch of areolar tissue behind the nipple is centered in the infant's mouth.
- Tongue covers lower alveolar ridge.
- Tongue is troughed (curved) around and below areola.
- No clicking or smacking sounds are heard during sucking.
- No drawing in (dimpling) of cheek pad is observed during sucking.

Areolar Compression

- Mandible moves in a rhythmic motion.
- If indicated, a digital suck assessment reveals a wavelike motion of the tongue from the anterior mouth toward the oropharynx (a digital suck assessment is not routinely performed).

Audible Swallowing

- Quiet sound of swallowing is heard.
- Sound may be preceded by several sucking motions.
- Sound may increase in frequency and consistency after milk ejection reflex occurs.

Data from Shrago, L., & Bocar, D. (1990). The infant's contribution to breastfeeding. *Journal of Obstetric, Gynecologic, and Neonatal Nursing, 19*, 209–215.

it cannot be assumed that the infant has received any milk. A continuing pattern of no audible swallowing signals the need for careful investigation into the cause (Shrago & Bocar, 1990).

Mother–Baby Assessment Tool

The Mother–Baby Assessment (MBA) Tool (**Table 3-5**) focuses on the mother's and baby's efforts in learning to breastfeed and tracks the progress of both partners (Mulford, 1992). The total number of pluses yields a numerical score that indicates the effectiveness of the breastfeeding session:

- A score of 3 or lower indicates that one partner (mother or baby) tried to initiate breastfeeding but the other was not ready.
- A score of 4 or 5 indicates that the infant was put to the breast but did not latch.
- A score of 6 indicates possible milk transfer.
- A score of 7 or 8 gives clearer evidence of milk transfer.
- A score of 9 or 10 scored consistently over a number of feedings indicates the need for only minimal follow-up.

The higher the MBA score, the more effective the breastfeeding episode. A low score indicates the need for assistance from a skilled lactation specialist or consultant.

Table 3-5 Mother–Baby Assessment Tool

Steps/Points	What to Look For/Criteria
#1 Signaling	
1	Mother watches and listens for baby's cues. She may hold, stroke, rock, talk to baby. She stimulates baby if he is sleepy, calms baby if he is fussy.
1	Baby gives readiness cues: stirring, alertness, rooting, sucking, hand-to-mouth, vocal cues, cry.
#2 Positioning	
1	Mother holds baby in good alignment within latch-on range of the nipple. Baby's body is slightly flexed, entire ventral surface facing mother's body. Baby's head and shoulders are supported.
1	Baby roots well at breast, opens mouth wide, tongue cupped and covering lower gum.
#3 Mixing	
1	Mother holds her breast to assist baby as needed, brings baby in close when his mouth is wide open. She may express drops of milk.
1	Baby latches on, takes all of nipple and about 2 cm (1 inch) of areola into mouth, then suckles, demonstrating a recurrent burst-pause sucking pattern.
#4 Milk Transfer	
1	Mother reports feeling any of the following: thirst, uterine cramps, increased lochia, breast ache or tingling, relaxation, sleepiness. Milk leaks from opposite breast.
1	Baby swallows audibly; milk is observed in baby's mouth; baby may spit up milk when burping. Rapid "call-up sucking" rate (two sucks/second) changes to "nutritive sucking" rate of about 1 suck/second.
#5 Ending	
1	Mother's breasts are comfortable; she lets baby suckle until he is finished. After nursing, her breasts feel softer; she has no lumps, engorgement, or nipple soreness.
1	Baby releases breast spontaneously, appears satiated. Baby does not root when stimulated. Baby's face, arms, and hands are relaxed; baby may fall asleep.

The MBA is an assessment method for rating the progress of a mother and baby who are learning to breastfeed. For every step, both mother and baby should receive a + before either one can be scored on the following step. If the observer does not observe any of the designated indicators, score 0 for that person on that step. If help is needed at any step for either the mother or the baby, check "Help" for that step. This notation will not change the total score for mothers and babies.
Data from Mulford, C. (1992). The mother–baby assessment (MBA): An "Apgar score" for breastfeeding. *Journal of Human Lactation, 8*, 79–82.

Via Christi Breastfeeding Assessment Tool

The Via Christi Breastfeeding Assessment Tool (Riordan & Riordan, 2000) (**Table 3-6**) assigns a score of 1 or 2 to five factors. Scores range from 0 to 10.

- Immediate high risk: All mothers who have had breast surgery; all infants who have lost more than 10% of their birth weight
- 0 to 2 = High risk: Close, immediate postdischarge follow-up needed; phone call and visit to healthcare provider within 24 hours

Table 3-6 Via Christi Breastfeeding Assessment Tool

Assessment Factors	0 Points	1 Point	2 Points	Score
Latch-on	No latch-on achieved	Latch-on after repeated attempts Eagerly grasped breast to latch on		
Length of time before latch-on and suckle	Over 10 minutes	4–6 minutes	0–3 minutes	
Suckling	Did not suckle	Suckled but needed encouragement	Suckled rhythmically and lips flanged	
Audible swallowing	None	Only if stimulated	Under 48 hours, intermittent; over 48 hours, frequent	
Mom's evaluation	Not pleased	Somewhat pleased	Pleased	
Total Score:				

Data from Riordan, J. (1999). *Via Christi breastfeeding assessment tool* (Unpublished).

- 3 to 6 = Medium risk: Postdischarge phone call within 2 days; visit to healthcare provider within 3 days
- 7 to 10 = Low risk: Information given to mother and routine phone call

This tool was developed as an expedient way to assess excessively sleepy infants whose mothers received high doses of labor analgesia and are at risk for breastfeeding problems. This research-based assessment tool scores early breastfeedings to establish a risk category for assigning appropriate follow-up.

Latch-on Assessment Tool

The Lactation Assessment Tool (**Box 3-3**) is a guided assessment form emphasizing comprehensive assessment from prefeeding behaviors through latch-on and during the actual feeding process. When used

Box 3-3 Latch-on Assessment Tool/Lactation Assessment Tool

The Latching Process

- Rooting
- Gape
- Suck
- Seal

Angle of Infant's Mouth Opening

- 160 degrees
- 100 degrees
- 90 degrees
- 60 degrees

Infant's Lip Position

- Top and bottom lips flanged
- Top lip turned in
- Bottom lip turned in
- Top and bottom lips turned in

Infant's Head Position

- Nose and chin
- Chin away
- Nose away
- Chin and nose away

Infant's Cheek Line

- Smooth
- Broken
- Dimpled

Height at the Breast

- Nose opposite nipple
- Too high
- Too low

Body Rotation

- Chest to mother's breast
- Head only turned to breast

Body Relationship

- Horizontal
- Angle

Breastfeeding Dynamic

- Bursts 2:1 or 1:1
- Occasional 8+:1
- Sucks, no swallows

Rhythm of Mother's Breast While Breastfeeding

- Breast moves rhythmically
- Breast stays stationary

Data from *Healthy Children Project 2000*. Healthy Children Project.

to study the elements of the feeding process that are thought to be related to nipple pain and damage, positioning errors were found to be related to pain, but no one element was shown to be the sole cause of sore nipples. Rather, many aspects of the breastfeeding episode, especially the latching process, contribute to elevating or reducing the mother's level of pain (Blair, Cadwell, Turner-Maffei, & Brimdyr, 2003).

LATCH Scoring System

Mothers who use the LATCH criteria after discharge have reported increased confidence in the assessment of their infants' breastfeeding and knowledge about when to seek help for breastfeeding problems (Hamelin & McLennan, 2000). Audible swallowing is an integral part of this tool, which evaluates the amount of help a mother needs to physically breastfeed. A composite score ranging from 0 to 10 is possible in the LATCH scoring system (**Table 3-7**), facilitating the identification of needed interventions and improving charting (Jensen, Wallace, & Kelsay, 1994). Breastfeeding behavioral changes can be followed over time, and the tool can also be used by mothers as a means of continuing assessment.

Table 3-7 LATCH Criteria

	0	1	2
L			
Latch	Too sleepy or reluctant No latch achieved	Repeated attempts Hold nipple in mouth Stimulate to suck	Grasps breast Tongue down Lips flanged Rhythmic sucking
A			
Audible swallowing	None	A few with stimulation	Spontaneous and intermittent $<$ 24 hours Spontaneous and frequent $>$ 24 hours
T			
Type of nipple	Inverted	Flat	Everted (after stimulation)
C			
Comfort (breast/nipple)	Engorged Cracked, bleeding, large blisters, or bruises Severe discomfort	Filling Reddened/small blisters or bruises Mild/moderate discomfort	Soft Tender
H			
Hold (positioning)	Full assist (staff holds infant at breast)	Minimal assist (i.e., elevate head of bed; place pillows for support) Teach one side; mother does the other Staff holds and then mother takes over	No assist from staff Mother able to position/hold infant

Data from Jensen, D., Wallace, S., & Kelsay, P. (1994). LATCH: A breastfeeding charting system and documentation tool. *Journal of Obstetric, Gynecologic, and Neonatal Nursing, 23,* 27–32.

A recent study looked at whether the LATCH scoring system could help determine whether term and preterm infants were taking in enough breastmilk according to their postnatal age and weight (Altuntas, Kocak, Akkurt, Razi, & Kislal, 2015). Milk intake and LATCH scores were found to be lower in preterm infants compared to full-term infants. In this study, 93.8% of preterm infants and 100% of term infants with a LATCH score of 7 and higher received more than 50% of milk volume according to calculations for their age and weight. However, LATCH scores cannot substitute for test weights in preterm infants because of the variability in minimum and maximum milk intake per LATCH score.

Breastfeeding Assessment Score

The Breastfeeding Assessment Score (**Table 3-8**) is designed to be administered before hospital discharge to identify infants at risk for breastfeeding cessation in the first 7–10 days of life (Hall et al., 2002). Hall and colleagues (2002) demonstrated that approximately 10.5% of mothers from the study sample of 1, 075 women had completely weaned by 7–10 days postpartum. Scoring with the tool ranges from 0 to 2, representing low, moderate, or high risk of early weaning. The highest overall score is 10, with 2 points being subtracted for each of the three variables of previous breast surgery, maternal hypertension, and vacuum extraction at delivery, creating a score range of –6 to +10. Results from the study were as follows:

Score	No. of Mothers	Cessation Rate at 7–10 Days Postpartum
≥8	705 of 1,075	5% (37 of 705)
≤ 8	370 of 1,075	21% (77 of 370)

The Breastfeeding Assessment Score identifies those mothers most in need of additional follow-up. The 370 women scoring lower than 8 on this screening tool represented about one-third of the study population, pointing out the significant need for continued professional lactation support (Nommsen-Rivers, 2003). The mean age of breastfeeding cessation was 5.4 days (± 2.2), suggesting a strong association between events occurring during the first 3–5 days of life and the early abandonment of breastfeeding.

Table 3-8 Breastfeeding Assessment Score

Variable	0	1	2
Maternal age (y)	< 21	21-24	> 24
Previous breastfeeding experience	Failure	None	Success
Latching difficulty	Every feeding	Half the feedings	< 3 feedings
Breastfeeding interval (hours between feedings)	> 6	3-6	> 3
Number of bottles of formula before enrollment (Babies were enrolled into the study if they were at least 20 hours old)	> 2	1	0

Two points each should be subtracted for the presence of previous breast surgery, maternal hypertension during pregnancy, and/or vacuum vaginal delivery.

Data from Hall, R. T., Mercer, A. M., Teasley, S. L., McPherson, D. M., Simon, S. D., Santos, S. R., . . . Hipsh, N. E. (2002). A breastfeeding assessment score to evaluate the risk for cessation of breastfeeding by 7 to 10 days of age. *Journal of Pediatrics, 141*, 659–664.

Maternal Breastfeeding Evaluation Scale

The Maternal Breastfeeding Evaluation Scale (MBFES) (Leff, Jeffries, & Gagne, 1994) consists of 30 items divided into three categories identified as maternal perceptions of successful breastfeeding: (1) maternal enjoyment/role attainment, (2) infant satisfaction/growth, and (3) lifestyle/body image. The MBFES is designed to measure the positive and negative aspects of breastfeeding that mothers deem important in defining successful breastfeeding.

Potential Early Breastfeeding Problem Tool

The Potential Early Breastfeeding Problem Tool (PEBPT) was developed to determine which breastfeeding problems rated highest among breastfeeding mothers (Kearney, Cronenwett, & Barrett, 1990). This tool uses 23 questions with a 4-point Likert scale questionnaire, giving a possible total score of 88. Higher scores indicate that more breastfeeding problems have occurred.

H & H Lactation Scale

The H & H Lactation Scale and its three subscales (maternal confidence/commitment to breastfeeding, perceived infant breastfeeding satiety, and maternal/infant breastfeeding satisfaction) are designed to measure a mother's perception of insufficient milk supply, a leading cause of premature weaning from the breast (Hill & Humenick, 1996). This tool can be used prospectively with both full-term and preterm mothers.

Breastfeeding Self-Efficacy Scale

The Breastfeeding Self-Efficacy Scale (BSES) (Dennis & Faux, 1999) is a 33-item self-report tool that assesses breastfeeding self-efficacy expectations in new mothers. Self-efficacy is the mother's perception regarding her ability to perform a specific behavior—in this case, breastfeeding. The scale is designed to identify mothers with low breastfeeding confidence and to provide assessment information to assist the healthcare provider in creating care plans specific to the items identified as problematic (Dennis, 1999). The BSES was modified to a shortened version (BSES-SF) that keeps 14 items and deletes 18 items that were shown to be redundant, making it easier and quicker to administer (Dennis, 2003).

Breastfeeding Attrition Prediction Tool

The Breastfeeding Attrition Prediction Tool (BAPT) (Janke, 1992) uses four subscales to measure the theory of planned behavior: positive breastfeeding sentiment (18 items), negative breastfeeding sentiment (9 items), social and professional support (10 items), and control (12 items). The original tool used 49 items to help predict breastfeeding status at 8 weeks postpartum.

Neonatal Oral–Motor Assessment Scale

This scale assesses 28 characteristics of sucking and is used to diagnose both disorganized and dysfunctional sucking (Palmer, Crawley, & Blanco, 1993). This differentiation is often subtle, necessitating that users of the Neonatal Oral–Motor Assessment Scale be certified in the administration and scoring of the tool. Deviations in sucking include a disorganized suck that is defined as a lack of rhythm of the total sucking activity (Crook, 1979), with the infant demonstrating difficulty in coordinating sucking and swallowing with breathing. Clinical signs of disorganized sucking include labored breathing, color changes, apnea, bradycardia, and nasal flaring (Palmer, 1993), often seen with premature infants. Dysfunctional sucking is characterized by abnormality in orofacial tone that may present as minimal jaw excursions, excessively wide jaw excursions, tongue retraction, and/or flaccid tongue (Palmer, 2002). Such situations usually require specialized referrals and follow-up because dysfunctional sucking in the neonate has been correlated with developmental delay at 24 months of age (Hawdon, Beauregard, & Kennedy, 2000; Palmer & Heyman, 1999).

Newborn Individualized Developmental Care and Assessment Program

The Newborn Individualized Developmental Care and Assessment Program (NIDCAP) is an infant behavior assessment system (Als, 1995) originally developed for preterm infants that assesses behavior in the autonomic system (heart rate, respiration, skin color, startles, twitches, gastrointestinal signs), motor system (muscle tone, posture, active movements), state system (level of wakefulness, clarity of state, pattern of state transitions), and attention or interaction (availability, responsiveness). The observation is designed to provide data for descriptions of an infant's strengths and weaknesses, current developmental goals, and recommendations for caregiving, including feeding. NIDCAP observations have been used to guide modifications to the infant's environment and to provide recommendations to facilitate optimal breastfeeding experiences for compromised infants (Nyqvist, Ewald, & Sjoden, 1996). Most users of the NIDCAP tool are certified in its administration and interpretation.

Preterm Infant Breastfeeding Behavior Scale

The Preterm Infant Breastfeeding Behavior Scale was developed to describe the maturational steps and developmental stages in preterm infant breastfeeding behavior through operational definitions ranging from immature to mature behavior (Nyqvist, Sjoden, & Ewald, 1999). It is also used to reduce the delays in going to breast that commonly occur with preterm infants by quantifying the appearance of parameters necessary for full breastfeeding (Nyqvist et al., 1999; Nyqvist, Rubertsson, Ewald, & Sjoden, 1996). Maturational steps in preterm infants' breastfeeding behavior are scored for rooting, areolar grasp, latching, sucking, longest sucking burst, and swallowing.

Mother–Infant Breastfeeding Progress Tool

This tool was developed in recognition that both the mother and the infant contribute to the development and success of breastfeeding (Johnson, Mulder, & Strube, 2007). The Mother–Infant Breastfeeding Progress Tool is designed to evaluate the presence of maternal and infant behaviors that are necessary for the mother to independently latch her infant to the breast. The tool is used during breastfeeding and consists of eight items (**Table 3-9**). Rather than using a single score to identify or predict problems and guide interventions, the checklist is not scored but is used over time to assess whether progress toward effective breastfeeding is being made. It is unclear whether swallowing is included under nutritive sucking. If swallowing does not happen, then no milk transfer occurs and the infant is left undernourished even though he or she may be latched to the breast and the mother can independently breastfeed her infant.

Beginning Breastfeeding Survey

The Beginning Breastfeeding Survey (BBS) is designed to measure the mother's perception of her ability to breastfeed effectively during the first few days postpartum (Mulder & Johnson, 2010). It is designed as a measure of breastfeeding effectiveness for a single breastfeeding episode that has already occurred.

Table 3-9 Mother-Infant Breastfeeding Progress Tool

Mother responds to infant feeding cues	Infant eagerly roots and latches
Mother goes no longer than 3 h between feeding attempts	Infant grasps areolar tissue with mouth open wide, lips visible and flanged outward Nutritive sucking bursts noted
Mother independently positions self for feeding	Does not require assistance, including position pillows
Mother can independently latch infant onto breast	Does not require any assistance to position herself or infant for latch
No nipple trauma is present	Includes redness, blistering, bruising, bleeding, or scabbing
No negative comments about breastfeeding	No comments that reflect insecurity about ability to breast-feed or satisfy her infant

Data from Johnson, T. S., Mulder, P. J., & Strube, K. (2007). Mother–infant breastfeeding progress tool: A guide for education and support of the breastfeeding dyad. *Journal of Obstetric, Gynecologic, and Neonatal Nursing, 36,* 319–327.

Each item in the BBS is indicative of an infant or maternal need that is met or unmet. There are 26 items in the tool, 16 maternal need items and 10 infant need items. This tool potentially provides a quick and easy screening method that can be completed during the hospitalization to determine which mothers would benefit from further breastfeeding support in the hospital and following discharge.

Bristol Breastfeeding Assessment Tool

The Bristol Breastfeeding Assessment Tool (BBAT) (**Table 3-10**) was developed to be used consistently by healthcare providers as a simple tool to measure breastfeeding proficiency both in research studies and in clinical practice. This tool was also designed to measure breastfeeding efficiency before and after a procedure such as a frenotomy and to evaluate breastfeeding dyads over time. Good internal reliability has been reported for the BBAT (Ingram, Johnson, Copeland, Churchill, & Taylor, 2015).

Validity and Reliability

The validity and reliability of breastfeeding assessment tools vary depending on a number of issues, including the outcome criteria under study. Some tools were constructed for charting and descriptive purposes, not necessarily for their predictive value. Efforts have been made to scrutinize a number of breastfeeding assessment tools to discover their usefulness in the clinical setting as well as in areas of policy and research. Howe, Lin, Fu, Su, and Hsieh (2008) reviewed seven clinical feeding assessment tools, five of which related to breastfed infants (IBFAT, LATCH, MBS, Preterm Infant Breastfeeding Behavior Scale, and SAIB). They reported that none was satisfactory in terms of being empirically validated. Mixed results of reliability and validity were noted for the LATCH and IBFAT, and limited evidence of psychometric properties was seen for the MBA and SAIB.

LATCH, IBFAT, and MBA

Riordan and Koehn (1997) assessed three tools, LATCH, IBFAT, and MBA, to ascertain whether any or all were accurate predictors of adequate infant intake, especially after discharge. Each tool uses different components to assess effective breastfeeding. Interrater agreement among the tools was low on some of

Table 3-10 Bristol Breastfeeding Assessment Tool

	0 (Poor)	1 (Moderate)	2 (Good)	Score
Positioning				
Baby well supported: tucked against mother's body; lying on side/neck not twisted; nose to nipple; mother confident handling baby	No or few elements achieved Needs to be talked through positioning	Achieving some elements Some positioning advice still needed	Achieving all elements No positioning advice needed	
Attachment				
Positive rooting; wide-open mouth; baby achieving quick latch with a good amount of breast tissue in mouth; baby stays attached with a good latch throughout feed	Baby unable to latch onto breast or achieves poor latch No/few elements achieved Needs to be talked through attachment	Achieving some elements Some advice on attachment needed	Achieving all elements No advice on attachment needed	
Sucking				
Able to establish effective sucking pattern on both breasts (initial rapid sucks, then slower sucks with pauses); baby ends feed	No effective sucking; no sucking pattern	Some effective sucking; no satisfactory sucking pattern; on and off the breast	Effective sucking pattern achieved	
Swallowing				
Audible, regular soft swallowing; no clicking	No swallowing heard; clicking noises	Occasional swallowing heard; some swallows noisy or clicking	Regular, audible, quiet swallowing	

the components. Agreement reached 0.90 (a number on which clinical decisions can be made) on two items in the LATCH tool (audible swallowing and type of nipple), two items in the MBA (readiness to feed and positioning), and no items in the IBFAT. The study concluded that none of these tools was reliable or valid in the clinical setting. No tools used any type of swallow count or weight measurements to determine actual intake at a feeding; nor did the study use these techniques to test validity of the tools. Raters were maternity nurses who viewed videotapes of feedings and were not present in the clinical setting where the feedings occurred. In contrast, a more recent study demonstrated that the LATCH, IBFAT, and MBA tools were both compatible and reliable for assessing breastfeeding (Altuntas et al., 2014). Positive and significant correlations were found between raters' scores for 46 observations. These tools were not time consuming to use.

Comparisons among existing tools as a way to test validity may be difficult because they measure feedings at the breast in different ways. Thus the results may not be highly correlated to one another (Riordan, 1998).

Hamelim and McLennan (2000) assessed the relationship between the use of the LATCH tool and breastfeeding outcomes, determining that even after the tool went into use in the hospital setting, breastfeeding outcomes did not improve. The authors concluded that the LATCH tool lacked predictive ability. This result could have been related to hospital practices that delayed the first breastfeed for an average of 2 hours and to the fact that 30% of all infants in the study were supplemented with formula during their hospital stay. Individual LATCH scores of breastfeeding sessions in the hospital setting were not collected.

Adams and Hewell (1997) compared maternally derived LATCH scores and professional LATCH scores to see whether relationships existed between these measures and maternal reports of satisfaction with breastfeeding. Their results showed moderate correlations overall but significant discrepancies in specific areas. The weakest correlations between mother and professional assessments were in the areas of audible swallowing and positioning, where the maternal assessments were less accurate. These areas involve assessing the infant's contribution to breastfeeding rather than the mother's contribution. As the maternal scores increased on the LATCH, mothers ranked themselves as being more satisfied with breastfeeding. The interrater agreement between the researcher and the clinic lactation consultants for total LATCH scores was 94.4%. The interrater agreement was greater than 85% (range, 85.7–100%) for each of the five LATCH components, supporting the reliability of the LATCH as an effective tool for professional assessment of breastfeeding and for the communication of those findings. This conclusion contradicts the findings of Riordan and Koehn, possibly because the Riordan study used maternity nurses who evaluated videotaped breastfeeding sessions, whereas this study used lactation consultants who were physically present to evaluate each feeding.

Kumar, Mooney, Wieser, and Havstad (2006) determined whether LATCH scores assessed by professional staff during in-hospital stays were predictive of breastfeeding at 6 weeks. A score of 9 or above at 16 to 24 hours was the most discriminate of the five time periods examined. Women who met this criterion were 1.7 times more likely to be breastfeeding at 6 weeks compared with women with lower scores. LATCH scores lower than 9 at 16 to 24 hours after birth should be an indicator that more intensive breastfeeding support is needed.

Tornese and colleagues (2012) analyzed the relationship between the LATCH score assessed in the first 24 hours after delivery and non-exclusive breastfeeding at discharge. Their goal was to identify a cutoff for the LATCH score for the purpose of identifying women with higher risk of non-exclusive breastfeeding who may need additional lactation support. The rate of non-exclusive breastfeeding was inversely related to the LATCH score, with non-exclusively breastfeeding infants scoring less (6.9) than infants exclusively breastfed at discharge (7.6). The authors were unable to identify a single LATCH cutoff score that could consistently predict non-exclusive breastfeeding at discharge. However, three subgroups and their cutoff scores for exclusive breastfeeding at discharge were identified. Cesarean delivery was considered a major risk factor for non-exclusive breastfeeding, and phototherapy and primiparity were considered minor factors. In the high-risk group (either presenting with the major risk factor or both minor risk factors), extra support should be provided regardless of the LATCH score. In the presence of both minor risk factors, extra breastfeeding support should be provided to all mothers with a LATCH score of 9 or below. In the moderate-risk group (presence of one minor risk factor), the LATCH score is predictive for non-exclusive breastfeeding and the need for extra support when it is equal to or below 6 when the risk factor is phototherapy and 4 when the risk factor is primiparity.

LATCH/IBFAT and MBFES/PEBPT

The LATCH and IBFAT tools and the MBFES and PEBPT tools were assessed to see whether a relationship existed between scores on the LATCH/IBFAT breastfeeding assessment and maternal satisfaction (MBFES) and breastfeeding problems (PEBPT) experienced at 1 week postpartum (Schlomer, Kemmerer, & Twiss, 1999). A moderate association was seen: As the scores on both the LATCH and IBFAT increased, maternal satisfaction scores increased and breastfeeding problem scores tended to decrease.

The LATCH tool was assessed for its validity in predicting breastfeeding status at 6 weeks postpartum. Mothers who scored lower on the comfort domain (engorged, cracked, or bleeding nipples) were less likely to be breastfeeding at 6 weeks, despite their intention to feed at least that long (Riordan, Bibb, Miller, & Rawlins, 2001). The LATCH tool proved useful in identifying the need for follow-up with breastfeeding mothers at risk for early weaning because of sore nipples. The authors recommend that mothers who score 2 or lower on the comfort measure be closely followed after discharge.

Riordan, Woodley, and Heaton (1994) tested the validity and reliability of the MBFES as a way to directly measure maternal satisfaction with breastfeeding. The MBFES scale and subscales were positively correlated with the length of time the mother intended to breastfeed as well as the length of time she actually breastfed. Maternal satisfaction with breastfeeding was also positively linked to the length of time mothers intended to breastfeed. The MBFES was found to be a valid and reliable tool and was useful for measuring outcomes of interventions such as breastfeeding classes or breastfeeding rounds.

Low breastfeeding satisfaction as measured by the MBFES appeared to be the most important predictor of weaning at survey ages of 6 weeks and 3 months, even after adjusting for other breastfeeding experiences (Cooke, Sheehan, & Schmied, 2003). Most breastfeeding problems were not predictive of weaning. Mothers with low breastfeeding satisfaction scores were 3–15 times more likely to wean during the 2-week, 6-week, and 3-month survey periods in the Cooke study.

H & H Lactation Scale

The H & H Lactation Scale and its three subscales were found to have a high degree of reliability as well as concurrent and predictive validity when used prospectively with breastfeeding mothers of both full-term and preterm infants (Hill & Humenick, 1996). The tool's predictive ability suggested that a mother's perception of insufficient milk supply was most closely tied to her perception of infant satiety.

BSES

Predictive validity for the BSES was demonstrated with positive correlations between BSES scores and infant feeding patterns at 6 weeks postpartum. The BSES was found to be valid and reliable in predicting which women would still be breastfeeding at 6 weeks (Dennis & Faux, 1999). In other words, the higher the BSES score, the more likely the mother would be exclusively breastfeeding at 6 weeks postpartum. The BSES was also shown to be significantly related to breastfeeding duration and intensity (exclusivity).

Low antenatal breastfeeding self-efficacy scores were positively related to bottle-feeding at 1 week postpartum. High self-efficacy scores at 1 week postpartum were related to mothers being more likely to continue to breastfeed until 4 months postpartum and to do so exclusively (Blyth et al., 2002). The BSES has been translated into Spanish and replicated in a sample of 100 Puerto Rican women. It was found to be a valid and reliable measure of breastfeeding confidence among Puerto Rican mothers (Torres, Torres,

Rodriguez, & Dennis, 2003). This tool has also been translated into Mandarin Chinese and shown to be a reliable and valid instrument when administered to 186 Chinese mothers (Dai & Dennis, 2003). The short form, BSES-SF, proved both valid and reliable in identifying mothers who needed additional interventions as well as pointing out that mothers who delivered via cesarean had lower self-efficacy in breastfeeding than those who delivered vaginally (Dennis, 2003).

BAPT

Janke (1994) established construct validity of the BAPT by factor analysis. The original BAPT was able to predict breastfeeding status at 8 weeks in 73% of the mother studies (Janke, 1994). Shortening the instrument increased its reliability scores while maintaining adequate prediction of early attrition. The modified BAPT was an effective predictor of 78% of women who stopped breastfeeding before 8 weeks and 68% of those who were still breastfeeding at that time (Dick et al., 2002). These results were consistent with Wambach's results that showed a mother's attitude and sense of control were the strongest predictors of breastfeeding behavior (Wambach, 1997). Evans, Dick, Lewallen, and Jeffrey (2004) determined that the BAPT was not an effective predictor of early breastfeeding attrition at either the prenatal or postpartum administration of the tool.

BBS

The BBS demonstrated more than adequate internal consistency reliability for a new scale. The BBS was positively correlated with breastfeeding self-efficacy. The group of mothers who were exclusively breastfeeding scored higher than either of the groups of partial breastfeeding or full formula feeding.

BAS

While the BAS is designed to predict the risk for early breastfeeding cessation, a meta-analysis showed that it does so with only moderate accuracy (Raskovalova et al., 2015). The authors strongly recommended locally calibrating the BAS prior to its implementation.

Review of Assessment Tools

Ho and McGrath (2010) conducted a review of seven tools used to assess women's attitudes, experiences, satisfaction, and confidence toward breastfeeding; the Gender-Role Attitudes toward Breastfeeding Scale (GRABS) developed by Kelley, Kviz, Richman, Kim, and Short (1993) used to measure new mother's attitudes and behaviors toward breastfeeding; the Iowa Infant Feeding Attitudes Scale (IIFAS) developed by De la Mora and Russell (1999) to measure attitudes toward infant feeding and to identify factors that influence women's decisions related to infant feeding methods; the MBFES; the BSES; the H & H Lactation Scale; the Breastfeeding Personal Efficacy Beliefs Inventory (BPEBI) developed by Cleveland and McCrone (2005); and the BAPT. Overall, Ho and McGrath (2010) found that these tools were valid, reliable, and feasible self-report measures of attitudes, satisfaction, experiences, or confidence associated with breastfeeding. Clinicians should understand that modifying any of these tools or testing the tools in populations different than the ones in the studies may alter the psychometric properties of the tool and may require testing of the modifications and new populations.

A study was conducted using three International Board Certified Lactation Consultants to assess videotaped breastfeeding sessions of overweight or obese women using 4 assessment tools (IBFAT, a modified Via Christi tool, a modified LATCH tool, and Riordan's Tool). Day 2 scores were significantly different between raters for all of the tools. Day 2 modified LATCH scores had the lowest interrater reliability, and swallowing assessments were unreliable (Chapman, Doughty, Mullin, & Perez-Escamilla, 2015). The low levels of absolute agreement between raters are worrisome and may indicate that these tools are particularly problematic for swallowing assessments throughout the first week postpartum. Clinicians using these tools with overweight or obese mothers should be aware of the psychometric differences among the various tools.

SUMMARY: THE DESIGN IN NATURE

The human infant, although born immature in many regards, is uniquely adapted to secure food and nurturance from the maternal breast right from the start. Alterations in the infant's anatomy and physiology may temporarily (or rarely permanently) affect his or her ability to feed at the breast, but breastmilk can almost always be fed to the infant. Prompt recognition of deviations and appropriate referrals and follow-up often permit breastfeeding or the provision of breastmilk in even the most extreme situations. All infants benefit from human milk, especially in the presence of anatomic or physiological compromise.

REFERENCES

Adams, D., & Hewell, S. (1997). Maternal and professional assessment of breastfeeding. *Journal of Human Lactation, 13,* 279–283.

Aizawa, M., Mizuno, K., & Tamura, M. (2010). Neonatal sucking behavior: Comparison of perioral movement during breastfeeding and bottle feeding. *Pediatrics International, 52,* 104–108.

Akca, K., & Aytekin, A. (2014). Effect of soothing noise on sucking success of newborns. *Breastfeeding Medicine, 9,* 538–542.

Alcantara, J., & Anderson, R. (2008). Chiropractic care of a pediatric patient with symptoms associated with gastroesophageal reflux disease, fuss–cry–irritability with sleep disorder syndrome and irritable infant syndrome of musculoskeletal origin. *Journal of the Canadian Chiropractic Association, 52,* 248–255.

Als, H. (1995). *Manual for the naturalistic observation of newborn behavior.* Boston: Harvard Medical School.

Altuntas, N., Kocak, M., Akkurt, S., Razi, H. C., & Kislal, M. F. (2015). LATCH scores and milk intake in preterm and term infants: A prospective comparative study. *Breastfeeding Medicine, 10,* 96–101.

Altuntas, N., Turkyilmaz, C., Yildiz, H., Kulali, F., Hirfanoglu, I., Onal, E., ... Atalay, Y. (2014). Validity and reliability of the infant breastfeeding assessment tool, the Mother Baby Assessment Tool, and the LATCH scoring system. *Breastfeeding Medicine, 9,* 191–195.

Amaizu, N., Shulman, R. J., Schanler, R. J., & Lau, C. (2008). Maturation of oral feeding skills in preterm infants. *Acta Paediatrica, 97,* 61–67.

American Academy of Pediatrics, Committee on Fetus and Newborn. (2010). Hospital stay for healthy term newborns. *Pediatrics, 125,* 405–409.

Ardran, G. M., Kemp, F. H., & Lind, J. (1958). A cineradiographic study of breast feeding. *British Journal of Radiology, 31,* 156–162.

Arguin, A. L., & Swartz, M. K. (2004). Gastroesophageal reflux in infants: A primary care perspective. *Pediatric Nursing, 30,* 45–71.

Arvedson, J. C., & Lefton-Greif, M. A. (1998). *Pediatric videofluoroscopic swallow studies.* San Antonio, TX: Communication Skill Builders.

Ballard, J. L., Auer, C. E., & Khoury, J. C. (2002). Ankyloglossia: Assessment, incidence, and effect of frenuloplasty on the breastfeeding dyad. *Pediatrics, 110,* e63. Retrieved from http://www.pediatrics.org/cgi/content/full/110/5/e63

Barlow, S. M. (2009a). Central pattern generation involved in oral and respiratory control for feeding in the term infant. *Current Opinions in Otolaryngology Head Neck Surgery, 17,* 187–193.

Barlow, S. M. (2009b). Oral and respiratory control of preterm feeding. *Current Opinions in Otolaryngology Head Neck Surgery, 17,* 179–186.

Barlow, S. M., & Estep, M. (2006). Central pattern generation and the motor infrastructure for suck, respiration and speech. *Journal of Communication Disorders, 39,* 366–380.

Barlow, S. M., Finan, D. S., Lee, J., & Chu, S. (2008). Synthetic orocutaneous stimulation entrains preterm infants with feeding difficulties to suck. *Journal of Perinatology, 28,* 541–548.

Biancuzzo, M. (1998). Yes! Infants with clefts can breastfeed. *AWHONN Lifelines, 2,* 45–49.

Bibi, H., Khvolis, E., Shoseyov, D., Ohaly, M., Ben Dor, D., London, D., & Ater, D. (2001). The prevalence of gastroesophageal reflux in children with tracheomalacia and laryngomalacia. *Chest, 119,* 409–413.

Blair, A., Cadwell, K., Turner-Maffei, C., & Brimdyr, K. (2003). The relationship between positioning, the breastfeeding dynamic, the latching process and pain in breastfeeding mothers with sore nipples. *Breastfeeding Review, 11,* 5–10.

Blyth, R., Creedy, D. K., Dennis, C.-L., Moyle, W., Pratt, J., & Vries, S. M. (2002). Effect of maternal confidence on breastfeeding duration: An application of breastfeeding self-efficacy theory. *Birth, 29,* 278–284.

Boekel, S. (2000*). Gastroesophageal reflux disease (GERD) and the breastfeeding baby.* [Independent Study Module]. Raleigh, NC: International Lactation Consultant Association.

Boere-Boonekamp, M., & van der Linden-Kuiper, L. (2001). Positional preference: Prevalence in infants and follow-up after two years. *Pediatrics, 107,* 339–343.

Bono, B. J. (1992). Assessment and documentation of the breastfeeding couple by health care professionals. *Journal of Human Lactation, 8,* 17–22.

Borrelli, O., Marabotto, C., Mancini, V., Aloi, M., Macri, F., Falconieri, P., . . . Cucchiara, S. (2011). Role of gastroesophageal reflux in children with unexplained chronic cough. *Journal of Pediatric Gastroenterology and Nutrition, 53,* 287–292.

Bosma, J. F., Hepburn, L. G., Josell, S. D., & Baker, K. (1990). Ultrasound demonstration of tongue motions during suckle feeding. *Developmental Medicine and Child Neurology, 32,* 223–229.

Bowen-Jones, A., Thompson, C., & Drewett, R. F. (1982). Milk flow and sucking rate during breastfeeding. *Developmental Medicine and Child Neurology, 24,* 626–633.

Bromiker, R., Rachamim, A., Hammerman, C., Schimmel, M., Kaplan, M., & Medoff-Cooper, B. (2006). Immature sucking patterns in infants of mothers with diabetes. *Journal of Pediatrics, 149,* 640–643.

Burton, P., Deng, J., McDonald, D., & Fewtrell, M. S. (2013). Real-time 3D ultrasound imaging of infant tongue movements during breastfeeding. *Early Human Development, 89,* 635–641.

Byrnes, A. L., Berk, N. W., Cooper, M. E., & Marazita, M. L. (2003). Parental evaluation of informing interviews for cleft lip and/or palate. *Pediatrics, 112,* 308–313.

Capilouto, G. J., Cunningham, T., Frederick, E., Dupont-Versteegden, E., Desai, N., & Butterfield, T. A. (2014). Comparison of tongue muscle characteristics of preterm and full term infants during nutritive and nonnutritive sucking. *Infant Behavior and Development, 37,* 435–445.

Carrascoza, K. C., Possobon, R. de F., Tomita, L. M., & de Moraes, A. B. A. (2006). Consequences of bottle-feeding to the oral facial development of initially breastfed children. *Journal of Pediatrics (Rio J), 82,* 395–397.

Chapman, D. J., Doughty, K., Mullin, E. M., & Perez-Escamilla, R. (2015). Reliability of lactation assessment tools applied to overweight and obese women. *Journal of Human Lactation.* pii: 0890334415597903 [Epub ahead of print].

Chetwynd, A. G., Diggle, P. J., Drewett, R. F., & Young, B. (1998). A mixture model for sucking patterns of breastfed infants. *Statistics in Medicine, 17,* 395–405.

Cleveland, A. P., & McCrone, S. (2005). Development of the breastfeeding personal efficacy beliefs inventory: A measure of women's confidence about breastfeeding. *Journal of Nursing Measurement, 13,* 115–127.

Cooke, M., Sheehan, A., & Schmied, V. (2003). A description of the relationship between breastfeeding experiences, breastfeeding satisfaction, and weaning in the first 3 months after birth. *Journal of Human Lactation, 19,* 145–156.

Cote-Arsenault, D., & McCoy, T. P. (2012). Reliability and validity of swallows as a measure of breastmilk intake in the first days of life. *Journal of Human Lactation, 28,* 483–489.

Crelin, E. (1976). Development of the upper respiratory system. *Ciba Clinical Symposia, 28,* 12.

Crook, C. K. (1979). The organization and control of infant sucking. *Advances in Child Development and Behavior, 14,* 209–252.

Dai, X., & Dennis, C. L. (2003). Translation and validation of the Breastfeeding Self-Efficacy Scale into Chinese. *Journal of Midwifery and Women's Health, 48,* 350–356.

De La Mora, A., & Russell, D. W. (1999). The Iowa Infant Feeding Attitude Scale: Analysis of reliability and validity. *Journal of Applied Social Psychology, 29,* 2362–2380.

De Vries, I. A. C., Breugem, C. C., van der Heul, A. M. B., Eijkemans, M. J. C., Kon, M., & Mink van der Molen, A. B. (2014). Prevalence of feeding disorders in children with cleft palate only: A retrospective study. *Clinical Oral Investigations, 18,* 1507–1515.

Dennis, C.-L. (1999). Theoretical underpinnings of breastfeeding confidence: A self-efficacy framework [Commentary]. *Journal of Human Lactation, 15,* 195–201.

Dennis, C.-L. (2003). The Breastfeeding Self-Efficacy Scale: Psychometric assessment of the short form. *Journal of Obstetric, Gynecologic, and Neonatal Nursing, 32,* 734–744.

Dennis, C.-L., & Faux, S. (1999). Development and psychometric testing of the Breastfeeding Self-Efficacy Scale. *Research in Nursing Health, 22,* 399–409.

Dick, M. J., Evans, M. L., Arthurs, J. B., Barnes, J. K., Caldwell, R. S., Hutchins, S. S., & Johnson, L. K. (2002). Predicting early breastfeeding attrition. *Journal of Human Lactation, 18,* 21–28.

Donati-Bourne, J., Batool, Z., Hendrickse, C., & Bowley, D. (2015). Tongue-tie assessment and division: A time-critical intervention to optimize breastfeeding. *Journal of Neonatal Surgery, 4,* 3.

Douglas, P. S. (2013). Diagnosing gastro-oesophageal reflux disease or lactose intolerance in babies who cry a lot in the first few months overlooks feeding problems. *Journal of Paediatric and Child Health, 49,* E252–E256.

Dowling, D., Danner, S., & Coffey, P. (1997). *Breastfeeding the infant with special needs.* White Plains, NY: March of Dimes.

Drewett, R. F., & Woolridge, M. (1981). Milk taken by human babies from the first and second breast. *Physiology and Behavior, 26,* 327–329.

Duara, S. (1989). Oral feeding containers and their influence on intake and ventilation in preterm infants. *Biology of the Neonate, 56,* 270–276.

Edmondson, R., & Reinhartsen, D. (1998). The young child with cleft lip and palate: Intervention needs in the first three years. *Infants and Young Children, 11,* 12–20.

Edmunds, J., Miles, S. C., & Fulbrook, P. (2011). Tongue-tie and breastfeeding: A review of the literature. *Breastfeeding Review, 19,* 19–26.

Egnell, E. (1956). The mechanism of different methods of emptying the female breast. *Journal of the Swedish Medical Association, 40,* 1–8.

Elad, D., Kozlovsky, P., Blum, O., Laine, A. F., Po, M. J., Botzer, E., . . . Sira, L. B. (2014). Biomechanics of milk extraction during breastfeeding. *Proceedings of the National Academy of Science, 111,* 5230–5235.

Evans, M. L., Dick, M. J., Lewallen, L. P., & Jeffrey, C. (2004). Modified breastfeeding attrition prediction tool: Prenatal and postpartum tests. *Journal of Perinatal Education, 13,* 1–8.

Fernando, C. (1998). *Tongue tie: From confusion to clarity.* Sydney, Australia: Tandem Publications.

Franca, E. C. L., Sousa, C. B., Aragao, L. C., & Costa, L. R. (2014). Electromyographic analysis of masseter muscle in newborns during suction in breast, bottle or cup feeding. *BMC Pregnancy and Childbirth, 14,* 154.

Geddes, D. T., Chadwick, L. M., Kent, J. C., Garbin, C. P., & Hartmann, P. E. (2010a). Ultrasound imaging of infant swallowing during breastfeeding. *Dysphagia, 25,* 183–191.

Geddes, D. T., Kent, J. C., McClellan, H. L., Garbin, C. P., Chadwick, L. M., & Hartmann, P. E. (2010b). Sucking characteristics of successfully breastfeeding infants with ankyloglossia: A case series. *Acta Paediatrica, 99,* 301–303.

Geddes, D. T., Kent, J. C., Mitoulas, L. R., & Hartmann, P. E. (2008). Tongue movement and intra-oral vacuum in breastfeeding infants. *Early Human Development, 84,* 471–477.

Geddes, D. T., Sakalidis, V. S., Hepworth, A. R., McClellan, H. L., Kent, J. C., Lai, C. T., & Hartmann, P. E. (2012). Tongue movement and intra-oral vacuum of term infants during breastfeeding and feeding from an experimental teat that released milk under vacuum only. *Early Human Development, 88,* 443–449.

Genna, C. W. (2015). Breastfeeding infants with congenital torticollis. *Journal of Human Lactation, 31,* 216–220.

Gewolb, I. H., Vice, F. L., Schweitzer-Kenney, E. L., Taciak, V. L., & Bosma, J. F. (2001). Developmental patterns of rhythmic suckle and swallow in preterm infants. *Developmental Medicine and Child Neurology, 43,* 22–27.

Glass, R. P., & Wolf, L. S. (1994). A global perspective on feeding assessment in the neonatal intensive care unit. *American Journal of Occupational Therapy, 48*(6), 514–526.

Glass, R. P., & Wolf, L. S. (1999). Feeding management of infants with cleft lip and palate and micrognathia. *Infants and Young Children, 12,* 70–81.

Goldfield, E. C., Richardson, M. J., Lee, K. G., & Margetts, S. (2006). Coordination of sucking, swallowing, and breathing and oxygen saturation during early infant breastfeeding and bottle-feeding. *Pediatric Research, 59,* 1–7.

Gomes, C. F., Thomson, Z., & Cardoso, J. R. (2009). Utilization of surface electromyography during the feeding of term and preterm infants: A literature review. *Developmental Medicine and Child Neurology, 51,* 936–942.

Gomes, C. F., Trezza, E. M. C., Murade, E. C. M., & Padovani, C. R. (2006). Surface electromyography of facial muscles during natural and artificial feeding of infants. *Journal of Pediatrics (Rio J), 82,* 103–109.

Habel, A., Elhadi, N., Sommerlad, B., & Powell, J. (2006). Delayed detection of cleft palate: An audit of newborn examination. *Archives of Disease in Childhood, 91,* 238–240.

Hall, R. T., Mercer, A. M., Teasley, S. L., McPherson, D. M., Simon, S. D., Santos, S. R., . . . Hipsh, N. E. (2002). A breastfeeding assessment score to evaluate the risk for cessation of breastfeeding by 7 to 10 days of age. *Journal of Pediatrics, 141,* 659–664.

Hamelin, K., & McLennan, J. (2000). Examination of the use of an in-hospital breastfeeding assessment tool. *Mother and Baby Journal, 5,* 29–37.

Hawdon, J. M., Beauregard, N., & Kennedy, G. (2000). Identification of neonates at risk of developing feeding problems in infancy. *Developmental Medicine and Child Neurology, 42,* 235–239.

Hazelbaker, A. K. (1993). *The Assessment Tool for Lingual Frenulum Function (ATLFF): Use in a lactation consultant private practice* [Thesis]. Pasadena, CA: Pacific Oaks College.

Healthy Children Project 2000. (2000). *Latch-on Assessment Tool (LAT).* East Sandwich, MA: Healthy Children Project.

Hill, P., & Humenick, S. (1996). Development of the H & H Lactation Scale. *Nursing Research, 45,* 136–140.

Ho, Y.-J., & McGrath, J. K. (2010). A review of the psychometric properties of breastfeeding assessment tools. *Journal of Obstetric, Gynecologic, and Neonatal Nursing, 39,* 386–400.

Hohoff, A., Rabe, H., Ehmer, U., & Harms, E. (2005). Palatal development of preterm and low birthweight infants compared to term infants—What do we know? Part 1: The palate of the term newborn. *Head and Face Medicine, I,* 8.

Howe, T.-H., Lin, K.-C., Fu, C.-P., Su, C.-T., & Hsieh, C.-L. (2008). A review of psychometric properties of feeding assessment tools used in neonates. *Journal of Obstetric, Gynecologic, and Neonatal Nursing, 37,* 338–349.

Ingram, J., Johnson, D., Copeland, M., Churchill, C., & Taylor, H. (2015). The development of a new breastfeeding assessment tool and the relationship with breastfeeding self-efficacy. *Midwifery, 31,* 132–137.

Iskander, A., & Sanders, I. (2003). Morphological comparison between neonatal and adult human tongues. *Annals of Otology, Rhinology, and Laryngology, 112,* 768–776.

Jacobs, L. A., Dickinson, J. E., Hart, P. D., Doherty, D. A., & Faulkner, S. J. (2007). Normal nipple position in term infants measured on breastfeeding ultrasound. *Journal of Human Lactation, 23,* 52–59.

Jadcherla, S. R., Chan, C. Y., Moore, R., Malkar, M., Timan, C. J., & Valentine, C. J. (2012). Impact of feeding strategies on the frequency and clearance of acid and nonacid gastroesophageal reflux events in dysphagic neonates. *Journal of Parenteral and Enteral Nutrition, 36*(4), 449–455.

Janke, J. R. (1992). Prediction of breastfeeding attrition: Instrument development. *Applied Nursing Research, 5,* 48–53.

Janke, J. R. (1994). Development of the Breastfeeding Attrition Prediction Tool. *Nursing Research, 43,* 100–104.

Jean, A. (2001). Brain stem control of swallowing: Neuronal network and cellular mechanisms. *Physiology Review, 81,* 929–969.

Jenks, M. (1991). Latch assessment documentation in the hospital nursery. *Journal of Human Lactation, 7,* 19–20.

Jensen, D., Wallace, S., & Kelsay, P. (1994). LATCH: A breastfeeding charting system and documentation tool. *Journal of Obstetric, Gynecologic, and Neonatal Nursing, 23,* 27–32.

Johnson, T. S., Mulder, P. J., & Strube, K. (2007). Mother–infant breastfeeding progress tool: A guide for education and support of the breastfeeding dyad. *Journal of Obstetric, Gynecologic, and Neonatal Nursing, 36,* 319–327.

Jung, A. D. (2001). Gastroesophageal reflux in infants and children. *American Family Physician, 64,* 1853–1860.

Kearney, M., Cronenwett, L., & Barrett, J. (1990). Breastfeeding problems in the first week postpartum. *Nursing Research, 39,* 90–95.

Kelley, M. A., Kviz, F., Richman, J. A., Kim, J. H., & Short, C. (1993). Development of a scale to measure gender-role attitudes toward breastfeeding among primiparas. *Women and Health, 20,* 47–68.

Kelly, B. N., Huckabee, M-L., Jones, R. D., & Frampton, C. M. A. (2007). The early impact of feeding on infant breathing–swallowing coordination. *Respiratory Physiology and Neurobiology, 156,* 147–153.

Kent, J. C., Mitoulas, L. R., Cregan, M. D., Geddes, D. T., Larsson, M., Doherty, D. A., & Hartmann, P. E. (2008). Importance of vacuum for breastmilk expression. *Breastfeeding Medicine, 3,* 11–19.

Kent, J. C., Ramsay, D. T., Doherty, D., Larsson, M., & Hartmann, P. E. (2003). Response of breasts to different stimulation patterns of an electric breast pump. *Journal of Human Lactation, 19,* 179–186.

Kotlow, L. (2004a). Oral diagnosis of abnormal frenum attachments in neonates and infants: Evaluation and treatment of the maxillary and lingual frenum using the erbium: YAG laser. *Journal of Pediatric Dental Care, 10,* 11–14.

Kotlow, L. (2004b). Oral diagnosis of abnormal frenum attachments in neonates and infants. *Journal of Pediatric Dental Care, 10,* 26–28.

Kotlow, L. A. (2004c). Using the erbium: YAG laser to correct an abnormal lingual frenum attachment in newborns. *Journal of the Academy of Laser Dentistry, 12,* 22–23.

Kotlow, L. (2010a). *Why can't my baby breastfeed: The effects of an abnormal maxillary frenum attachment.* Retrieved from http://www.kiddsteeth.com/maxillaryfrenum_and_nursingfinal.pdf

Kotlow, L. (2010b). The influence of the maxillary frenum on the development and pattern of dental caries on anterior teeth in breastfeeding infants: Prevention, diagnosis and treatment. *Journal of Human Lactation, 26,* 304–308.

Kotlow, L. (2011a). Diagnosis and treatment of ankyloglossia and tied maxillary fraenum in infants using Er:YAG and 1064 diode lasers. *European Archives in Paediatric Dentistry, 12,* 106–112.

Kotlow, L. (2011b). Infant reflux and aerophagia associated with the maxillary lip-tie and ankyloglossia (tongue-tie). *Clinical Lactation, 2,* 25–29.

Kotlow, L. A. (2013). Diagnosing and understanding the maxillary lip-tie (superior labial, the maxillary labial frenum) as it relates to breastfeeding. *Journal of Human Lactation, 29,* 458–464.

Kron, R. E., & Litt, M. (1971). Fluid mechanics of nutritive sucking behaviour: The suckling infant's oral apparatus analysed as a hydraulic pump. *Medical and Biological Engineering, 9,* 45–60.

Kumar, M., & Kalke, E. (2012). Tongue-tie, breastfeeding difficulties and the role of frenotomy. *Acta Paediatrica, 101,* 687–689.

Kumar, S. P., Mooney, R., Wieser, L. J., & Havstad, S. (2006). The LATCH scoring system and prediction of breastfeeding duration. *Journal of Human Lactation, 22,* 391–397.

Lau, C., Sheena, H. R., Shulman, R. J., & Schanler, R. J. (1997). Oral feeding in low birth weight infants. *Journal of Pediatrics, 130,* 561–569.

Leff, E., Jeffries, S., Gagne, M. (1994). The development of the Maternal Breastfeeding Evaluation Scale. *Journal of Human Lactation, 10,* 105–111.

Loewy, J., Stewart, K., Dassier, A-M., Telsey, A., & Homel, P. (2013). The effects of music therapy on vital signs, feeding, and sleep in premature infants. *Pediatrics, 131,* 902–918.

Marmet, C., & Shell, E. (1993). *Lactation forms: A guide to lactation consultant charting* (pp. 4–7). Encino, CA: Lactation Institute and Breastfeeding Clinic.

Marmet, C., Shell, E., & Marmet, R. (1990). Neonatal frenotomy may be necessary to correct breastfeeding problems. *Journal of Human Lactation, 6,* 117–121.

Martinelli, R. L. de C., Marchesan, I. Q., Gusmao, R. J., Honorio, H. M., & Berretin-Felix, G. (2015). The effects of frenotomy on breastfeeding. *Journal of Applied Oral Science, 23,* 153–157.

Masarei, A. G., Sell, D., Habel, A., Mars, M., Sommerlad, B. C., & Wade, A. (2007). The nature of feeding in infants with unrepaired cleft lip and/or palate compared with healthy noncleft infants. *Cleft Palate–Craniofacial Journal, 44,* 321–328.

Mathew, O. P. (1988). Respiratory control during nipple feeding in preterm infants. *Pediatric Pulmonology, 5,* 220–224.

Mathew, O. P. (1991a). Science of bottle feeding. *Journal of Pediatrics, 119,* 511–519.

Mathew, O. P. (1991b). Breathing patterns of preterm infants during bottle feeding: Role of milk flow. *Journal of Pediatrics, 119,* 960–965.

Mathew, O. P., & Bhatia, J. (1989). Sucking and breathing patterns during breast- and bottle-feeding in term neonates. *American Journal of Diseases in Childhood, 143,* 588–592.

Matthews, M. K. (1988). Developing an instrument to assess infant breastfeeding behaviour in the early neonatal period. *Midwifery, 4,* 154–165.

Matthews, M. K. (1991). Mothers' satisfaction with their neonates' breastfeeding behaviors. *Journal of Obstetric, Gynecologic, and Neonatal Nursing, 20,* 49–55.

Matthews, M. K. (1993). Assessments and suggested interventions to assist newborn breastfeeding behavior. *Journal of Human Lactation, 9,* 243–248.

McClellan, H. L., Geddes, D. T., Kent, J. C., Garbin, C. P., Mitoulas, L. R., & Hartmann, P. E. (2008). Infants of mothers with persistent nipple pain exert strong sucking vacuums. *Acta Paediatrica, 97,* 1205–1209.

McClellan, H. L., Sakalidis, V. S., Hepworth, A. R., Hartmann, P. E., & Geddes, D. T. (2010). Validation of nipple diameter and tongue movement measurements with B-mode ultrasound during breastfeeding. *Ultrasound in Medicine and Biology, 36,* 1197–1807.

Medeiros, A. P. M., Ferreira, J. T. L., & de Felicio, C. M. (2009). Correlation between feeding methods, non-nutritive sucking and orofacial behaviors. *Pro-fono Revista de Atualizacao Cientifica, 21,* 315–319.

Meier, P. P. (1988). Bottle and breastfeeding: Effects on transcutaneous oxygen pressure and temperature in preterm infants. *Nursing Research, 37,* 36–41.

Meier, P. P. (1996). Suck–breathe patterning during bottle and breastfeeding for preterm infants. In J. J. David (Ed.), *Major controversies in infant nutrition* (pp. 9–20). International Congress and Symposium Series 215. London, UK: Royal Society of Medicine Press.

Meier, P. P. (2001). Breastfeeding in the special care nursery: Prematures and infants with medical problems. *Pediatric Clinics of North America, 48,* 425–442.

Meier, P. P. (2003). Supporting lactation in mothers with very low birth weight infants. *Pediatric Annals, 32,* 317–325.

Meier, P. P., Lysakowski, T. Y., Engstrom, J. L., Kavanaugh, K. L., & Mangurten, H. H. (1990). The accuracy of test-weighing for preterm infants. *Journal of Pediatric Gastroenterology and Nutrition, 10,* 62–65.

Messner, A. H., Lalakea, L., Aby, J., Macmahon, J., & Bair, E. (2000). Ankyloglossia: Incidence and associated feeding difficulties. *Archives of Otolaryngology—Head and Neck Surgery, 126,* 36–39.

Miller, M. J., Martin, R. J., Carlo, W. A., Fouke, J. M., Strohl, K. P., & Fanaroff, A. A. (1985). Oral breathing in newborn infants. *Journal of Pediatrics, 107,* 465–469.

Mizuno, K., Ueda, A., & Takeuchi, T. (2002). Effects of different fluids on the relationship between swallowing and breathing during nutritive sucking in neonates. *Biology of the Neonate, 81,* 45–50.

Monaci, G., & Woolridge, M. (2011, September). Ultrasound video analysis for understanding of infant breastfeeding: *International Conference on Signal Processing.* IEEE, Belgium.

Moral, A., Bolibar, I., Seguranyes, G., Ustrell, J. M., Sebastia, G., Martinez-Barba, C., & Rios, J. (2010). Mechanics of sucking: Comparison between bottle feeding and breastfeeding. *BMC Pediatrics, 10,* 6.

Morris, S. E., & Klein, M. D. (2000). *Pre-feeding skills: A comprehensive resource for mealtime development* (2nd ed.). San Antonio, TX: Therapy Skill Builders.

Mukai, S., Mukai, C., & Asaoka, K. (1991). Ankyloglossia with deviation of the epiglottis and larynx. *Annals of Otology, Rhinology, and Laryngology, 100,* 3–20.

Mulder, P. J., & Johnson, T. S. (2010). The Beginning Breastfeeding Survey: Measuring mothers' perceptions of breastfeeding effectiveness during postpartum hospitalization. *Research in Nursing Health, 32,* 329–344.

Mulford, C. (1992). The Mother–Baby Assessment (MBA): An "Apgar score" for breastfeeding. *Journal of Human Lactation, 8,* 79–82.

Nommsen-Rivers, L. (2003). Research Spotlight: Identifying mothers at risk for early abandonment of breastfeeding. *Journal of Human Lactation, 19,* 217–218.

Notestine, G. E. (1990). The importance of the identification of ankyloglossia (short lingual frenulum) as a cause of breastfeeding problems. *Journal of Human Lactation, 6,* 113–115.

Nyqvist, K. H., Ewald, U., & Sjoden, P.-O. (1996). Supporting a preterm infant's behaviour during breastfeeding: A case report. *Journal of Human Lactation, 12,* 221–228.

Nyqvist, K. H., Rubertsson, C., Ewald, U., & Sjoden, P.-O. (1996). Development of the Preterm Infant Breastfeeding Behavior Scale (PIBBS): A study of nurse–mother agreement. *Journal of Human Lactation, 12,* 207–219.

Nyqvist, K. H., Sjoden, P.-O., & Ewald, U. (1999). The development of preterm infants' breastfeeding behavior. *Early Human Development, 55,* 247–264.

Page, D. C. (2001). Breastfeeding and early functional jaw orthopedics (an introduction). *Functional Orthodontist, 18,* 24–27.

Palmer, B. (1998). The influence of breastfeeding on the development of the oral cavity: A commentary. *Journal of Human Lactation, 14,* 93–98.

Palmer, M. M. (1993). Identification and management of the transitional suck pattern in premature infants. *Journal of Perinatal and Neonatal Nursing, 7,* 66–75.

Palmer, M. M. (2002). Recognizing and resolving infant suck difficulties. *Journal of Human Lactation, 18,* 166–167.

Palmer, M. M., Crawley, K., & Blanco, I. (1993). The Neonatal Oral–Motor Assessment Scale: A reliability study. *Journal of Perinatology, 13,* 28–35.

Palmer, M. M., & Heyman, M. B. (1999). Developmental outcome for neonates with dysfunctional and disorganized sucking patterns: Preliminary findings. *Infant–Toddler Intervention: Transdisciplinary Journal, 9,* 299–308.

Peitsch, W. K., Keefer, C. H., LaBrie, R. A., & Mulliken, J. B. (2002). Incidence of cranial asymmetry in healthy newborns. *Pediatrics, 110*(6). Retrieved from http://www.pediatrics.org/cgi/content/full/110/6/e72

Peterson, A., & Harmer, M. (2010). *Balancing breast and bottle: Reaching your breastfeeding goals.* Amarillo, TX: Hale Publishing.

Pressler, J. L., Hepworth, J. T., LaMontagne, L. L., Sevcik, R. H., & Hesselink, L. F. (1999). Behavioral responses of newborns of insulin-dependent and nondiabetic healthy mothers. *Clinical Nursing Research, 8,* 103–118.

Prieto, C. R., Cardenas, H., Salvatierra, A. M., Boza, C., Montes, C. G., & Croxatto, H. B. (1996). Sucking pressure and its relationship to milk transfer during breastfeeding in humans. *Journal of Reproductive Fertility, 108,* 69–74.

Ramsay, D. T., Kent, J. C., Owens, R. A., & Hartmann, P. E. (2001, September). Ultrasound imaging of milk ejection in the human lactating breast (Abstract 30). Paper presented at the Proceedings of the Thirty-Second Annual Conference for the Society for Reproductive Biology, Gold Coast, Queensland.

Ramsay, M., & Gisel, E. G. (1996). Neonatal sucking and maternal feeding practices. *Developmental Medicine and Child Neurology, 38,* 34–47.

Raskovalva, T., Teasley, S. L., Gelbert-Baudino, N., Mauri, P. A., Schelstraete, C., Massoutier, M., . . . Labarere, J. (2015). Breastfeeding Assessment Score: Systematic review and meta-analysis. *Pediatrics, 135*, e1276–e1285.

Ratnovsky, A., Carmeli, Y. N., Elad, D., Zaretsky, U., Dollberg, S., & Mandel, D. (2013). Analysis of facial and inspiratory muscles performance during breastfeeding. *Technology and Health Care, 21,* 511–520.

Reid, J., Kilpatrick, N., & Reilly, S. (2006). A prospective, longitudinal study of feeding skills in a cohort of babies with cleft conditions. *Cleft Palate–Craniofacial Journal, 43,* 702–709.

Reid, J., Reilly, S., & Kilpatrick, N. (2007). Sucking performance of babies with cleft conditions. *Cleft Palate–Craniofacial Journal, 44,* 312–320.

Reiter, R., Brosch, S., Ludeke, M., Fischbein, E., Haase, S., Pickhard, A., . . . Maier, C. (2012). Genetic and environmental risk factors for submucous cleft palate. *European Journal of Oral Science, 120,* 97–103.

Riordan, J. (1998). Predicting breastfeeding problems. *AWHONN Lifelines, 2,* 31–33.

Riordan, J., Bibb, D., Miller, M., & Rawlins, T. (2001). Predicting breastfeeding duration using the LATCH breastfeeding assessment tool. *Journal of Human Lactation, 17,* 20–23.

Riordan, J., & Riordan, S. (2000). *The effect of labor epidurals on breastfeeding. Unit 4/lactation consultant series two.* Schaumburg, IL: La Leche League International.

Riordan, J. M., & Koehn, M. (1997). Reliability and validity testing of three breastfeeding assessment tools. *Journal of Obstetric, Gynecologic, and Neonatal Nursing, 26,* 181–187.

Riordan, J. M., Woodley, G., & Heaton, K. (1994). Testing validity and reliability of an instrument which measures maternal evaluation of breastfeeding. *Journal of Human Lactation, 10,* 231–235.

Sakalidis, V. S., & Geddes, D. T. (2015). Suck-swallow-breathe dynamics in breastfed infants. *Journal of Human Lactation.* pii: 0890334415601093 [Epub ahead of print].

Sakalidis, V. S., Kent, J. C., Garbin, C. P., Hepworth, A. R., Hartmann, P. E., & Geddes, D. T. (2013). Longitudinal changes in suck–swallow–breathe, oxygen saturation, and heart rate patterns in term breastfeeding infants. *Journal of Human Lactation, 29,* 236–245.

Sakalidis, V. S., McClellan, H. L., Hepworth, A. R., Kent, J. C., Lai, C. T., Hartmann, P. E., & Geddes, D. T. (2012). Oxygen saturation and suck–swallow–breathe coordination of term infants during breastfeeding and feeding from a teat releasing milk only with vacuum. *International Journal of Pediatrics, 2012,* Article ID 130769, doi:10.1155/2012/130769.

Sakalidis, V. S., Williams, T. M., Garbin, C. P., Hepworth, A. R., Hartmann, P. E., Paech, M. J., & Geddes, D. T. (2013). Ultrasound imaging of infant sucking dynamics during the establishment of lactation. *Journal of Human Lactation, 29,* 205–213.

Sanchez-Molins, M., Carbo, J. G., Gaig, C. L., & Torrent, J. M. U. (2010). Comparative study of the craniofacial growth depending on the type of lactation received. *European Journal of Paediatric Dentistry, 11,* 87–92.

Schlomer, J. A., Kemmerer, J., & Twiss, J. J. (1999). Evaluating the association of two breastfeeding assessment tools with breastfeeding problems and breastfeeding satisfaction. *Journal of Human Lactation, 15,* 35–39.

Segami, Y., Mizuno, K., Taki, M., & Itabashi, K. (2013). Perioral movements and sucking pattern during bottle feeding with a novel, experimental teat are similar to breastfeeding. *Journal of Perinatology, 33,* 319–323.

Shawker, T. H., Sonies, B., Stone, M., & Baum, B. J. (1983). Real-time ultrasound visualization of tongue movement during swallowing. *Journal of Clinical Ultrasound, 11,* 485–490.

Shrago, L., & Bocar, D. (1990). The infant's contribution to breastfeeding. *Journal of Obstetric, Gynecologic, and Neonatal Nursing, 19,* 209–215.

Smith, L. J. (2004). Physics, forces, and mechanical effects of birth on breastfeeding. In L. J. Smith & M. Kroeger (Eds.), *Impact of birthing practices on breastfeeding* (pp. 119–145). Sudbury, MA: Jones and Bartlett.

Smith, W. L., Erenberg, A., & Nowak, A. (1988). Imaging evaluation of the human nipple during breastfeeding. *American Journal of Diseases in Childhood, 142,* 76–78.

Smith, W. L., Erenberg, A., Nowak, A., & Franken, E. A. (1985). Physiology of sucking in the normal term infant using real-time US. *Radiology, 156,* 379–381.

Snyder, J. B. (1995). *Variation in infant palatal structure and breastfeeding.* (A project submitted in partial fulfillment of the requirements for the degree master of arts in human development specialization in lactation.) Encino, CA: Lactation Institute.

Snyder, J. B. (1997). Bubble palate and failure to thrive: A case report. *Journal of Human Lactation, 13,* 139–143.

Sonies, B. C., Wang, C., & Sapper, D. J. (1996). Evaluation of normal and abnormal hyoid bone movement during swallowing by use of ultrasound duplex–Doppler imaging. *Ultrasound in Medicine and Biology, 22,* 1169–1175.

Stellwagen, L., Hubbard, E., & Vaux, K. (2004). Look for the "stuck baby" to identify congenital torticollis. *Contemporary Pediatrics, 21,* 55.

Tamura, Y., Horikawa, Y., & Yoshida, S. (1996). Coordination of tongue movements and peri-oral muscle activities during nutritive sucking. *Developmental Medicine and Child Neurology, 38,* 503–510.

Tornese, G., Ronfani, L., Pavan, C., Demarini, S., Monasta, L., & Davanzo, R. (2012). Does the LATCH score assessed in the first 24 hours after delivery predict non-exclusive breastfeeding at hospital discharge? *Breastfeeding Medicine, 7,* 423–430.

Torres, M. M., Torres, R. R. D., Rodriguez, A. M. P., & Dennis, C.-L. (2003). Translation and validation of the Breastfeeding Self-Efficacy Scale into Spanish: Data from a Puerto Rican population. *Journal of Human Lactation, 19,* 35–42.

Vice, F. L., Heinz, J. M., Giuriati, G., Hood, M., & Bosma, J. F. (1990). Cervical auscultation of suckle feeding in newborn infants. *Developmental Medicine and Child Neurology, 32,* 760–768.

Walker, M. (1989). Functional assessment of infant breastfeeding patterns. *Birth, 16,* 140–147.

Wall, V., & Glass, R. (2006). Mandibular asymmetry and breastfeeding problems: Experience from 11 cases. *Journal of Human Lactation, 22,* 328–334.

Wambach, K. A. (1997). Breastfeeding intention and outcome: A test of the theory of planned behavior. *Research in Nursing Health, 20,* 51–59.

Weber, F., Woolridge, M. W., & Baum, J. D. (1986). An ultrasonographic study of the organisation of sucking and swallowing by newborn infants. *Developmental Medicine and Child Neurology, 28,* 19–24.

Wiessinger, D., & Miller, M. (1995). Breastfeeding difficulties as a result of tight lingual and labial frena: A case report. *Journal of Human Lactation, 11,* 313–316.

Willette, S., Molinaro, L. H., Thompson, D. M., & Schroeder, J. W., Jr. (2015). Fiberoptic examination of swallowing in the breastfeeding infant. *Laryngoscope.* doi:10.1002/lary.25641 [Epub ahead of print].

Wilson-Clay, B., & Hoover, K. (2002). *The breastfeeding atlas* (2nd ed.). Austin, TX: LactNews Press.

Wolf, L. S., & Glass, R. P. (1992). *Feeding and swallowing disorders in infancy: Assessment and management.* Tucson, AZ: Therapy Skill Builders.

Woolridge, M. (2011). *The mechanisms of breastfeeding revised: New insights into how babies feed provided by a fresh ultrasound studies of breastfeeding* [Abstract]. 5th Europaediatrics Congress.

Woolridge, M. (2012, July). *The mechanics of infant feeding revisited: Fresh ultrasound studies of breastfeeding and bottle-feeding. Do babies extract milk from the breast using peristalsis, suction or a combination of both?* Paper presented at the International Lactation Consultant Association Conference, Orlando, FL.

Woolridge, M., & Drewett, R. (1986). Sucking rates of human babies on the breast: A study using direct observation and intraoral pressure measurements. *Journal of Reproductive and Infant Psychology, 4,* 69–75.

Woolridge, M. W. (1986). The "anatomy" of infant sucking. *Midwifery, 2,* 164–171.

Woolridge, M. W., How, T. V., Drewett, R. F., Rolfe, P., & Baum, J. D. (1982). The continuous measurement of milk intake at a feed in breastfed babies. *Early Human Development, 6,* 365–373.

Chapter 4

Influence of Peripartum Factors, Birthing Practices, and Early Caretaking Behaviors

INTRODUCTION

The environment in which an infant lives before, during, and immediately after birth can affect breastfeeding through a number of mechanisms. Early sucking behaviors can be affected by medications that a mother receives during her pregnancy and during her delivery. Instrument-assisted deliveries can affect the mechanics of breastfeeding. Separation, supplementation, crying, and tight wrapping diminish breastfeeding efforts. This chapter delineates a number of factors in the early environment that can influence the initiation of breastfeeding.

BIRTH INTERVENTIONS AND BREASTFEEDING

"Natural childbirth" is fast becoming an extinct practice. In a 2002 landmark U.S. survey of 1,583 mothers conducted by the Maternity Center Association, no births occurred without some form of medical intervention (Declercq, Sakala, Corry, & Applebaum, 2002). Birth interventions and their side effects have the potential to significantly disrupt early breastfeeding behaviors, especially if more than one intervention is experienced. The Maternity Center Association's Listening to Mothers survey outlined the extent to which childbirth has been transformed into a technologically choreographed event. Similar outcomes were seen in the 1,573 women who participated in the 2006 Listening to Mothers Survey II (**Box 4-1**) conducted by Childbirth Connection (formerly the Maternity Center Association) (Declercq, Sakala, Corry, & Applebaum, 2006). What was once a "normal" progression of labor and delivery has been tinkered with to the point that the absence of birth interventions is rare (Kroeger & Smith, 2004).

For the Listening to Mothers Survey III, 2,400 mothers completed the online survey (Declercq, Sakala, Corry, Applebaum, & Herrlich, 2013). Birth interventions were still common, but many had improved:

- 30% of labors were induced.
- 67% were given epidural or spinal anesthesia.
- 16% were given narcotics such as Demerol or Stadol.
- 62% were given an IV.

Box 4-1 Selected Birth Interventions from Listening to Mothers Survey II

- 41% of women had their labor induced.
- 86% of mothers used one or more types of medication for pain relief.
- 76% of women used epidural or spinal analgesia; 22% were given narcotics such as Demerol or Stadol.
- 80% received intravenous fluids.
- 59% had their membranes broken; 55% received Pitocin to augment the labor.
- 25% had an episiotomy.
- 5% experienced vacuum extraction, and 2% experienced the use of forceps.
- 32% experienced a cesarean delivery.
- 34% of newborn infants were not kept in the mothers' arms.
- 69% of mothers with a vaginal birth experienced rooming-in compared with 49% of cesarean mothers.
- 61% of mothers hoped to breastfeed exclusively; 19% planned to use a combination of breastfeeding and formula; 20% planned to use formula only.
- 34% of mothers perceived that hospital staff expressed no infant feeding preference; 3% encouraged formula feeding.
- Of those mothers intending to breastfeed only, 66% were given free formula samples or offers; 44% of their infants were given pacifiers by staff; 38% were given formula or water supplements.
- One week after giving birth, 51% of the mothers were exclusively breastfeeding; 75% of the mothers intending to breastfeed exclusively were doing so by the end of the first week.

Based on Declercq, E. R., Sakala, C., Corry, M. P., & Applebaum, S. (2002). *Listening to mothers: Report of the first national US survey of women's childbearing experiences.* New York: Maternity Center Association.

- 36% were given Pitocin to augment labor.
- 31% experienced a cesarean delivery.
- 60% experiencing rooming-in.
- 54% planned to exclusively breastfeed.
- 50% of mothers reported exclusive breastfeeding at 1 week.
- 49% of mothers who planned to exclusively breastfeed were given formula samples or offers.
- 29% of mothers intending to exclusively breastfeed were given formula or water to supplement their breastfeeding.

While heartening improvements were seen in a number of areas, many mothers who intended to breastfeed still experienced ill-advised hospital practices that undermine breastfeeding. There was a drop-off of several percentage points in the proportion of mothers who wanted to exclusively breastfeed at the end of pregnancy and the proportion who were doing so 1 week after birth (each percentage point represents approximately 40,000 mother/baby dyads). Just 50% of babies were exclusively breastfed a week after their birth. Among those who were at least 7 months postpartum, just 29% met the international standard of exclusive breastfeeding for 6 months or more.

A predominant characteristic of human birth throughout the evolution of our species has been a nocturnal pattern of delivery. Childbirth without interventions shares a circadian mechanism with non-human primates. Research on the regulation of the timing of birth and contributors to the contractile components of the myometrium (the smooth muscle layer of the uterine wall) have shown that labor is normally the result of increased sensitivity to melatonin, which works synergistically with oxytocin (Sharkey, Puttaramu, Word, & Olcese, 2009). Bernis and Varea (2012) reported that vaginal deliveries without interventions occur with greater frequency during the nighttime hours, and birth with interventions, such as epidural analgesia, predominate during the day. Nocturnal deliveries have the advantage of occurring at the most optimal time for maternal–infant viability and maternal–infant bonding in the less active hours. Nocturnal deliveries tend to be shorter and are the result of ancient evolutionary adaptive patterns. Delivery at night reduces the risk of interventions and better reflects the physiological needs of the mother and infant (labors are shorter, mother–baby bonding is improved, lower risk of interventions that can interfere with the establishment of breastfeeding). These authors recommend an evolutionary approach to birth to reduce unnecessary interventions and improve birthing outcomes.

Abundant physical contact and frequent breastfeeding have been replaced with artificial feeding, minimal contact, early separation, medication, and misinformation. Lozoff, Brittenham, Trause, Kennell, and Klaus (1977) explained that perinatal medical management practices (such as routine postpartum separation) approach the limits beyond which breastfeeding may fail: "the limits of adaptability." For the mother and baby with a problem, breastfeeding success is even more tenuous. Variations in practice abound, with many perinatal interventions claiming to be scientifically based but with large gaps existing between common practices and what the research actually says (Goer, 1995). Interference with the natural process of childbirth should proceed from a sound base of evidence and do more good than harm. Maternity care practices in hospitals and birth centers throughout the intrapartum period, such as ensuring mother–newborn skin-to-skin contact, keeping mother and newborn together, and not giving supplemental feedings to breastfed newborns unless medically indicated, can positively influence breastfeeding behaviors during a period critical to the successful establishment of lactation (Chien, Tai, Chu, Ko, & Chiu, 2007; Dewey, Nommsen-Rivers, Heinig, & Cohen, 2003; DiGirolamo, Grummer-Strawn, & Fein, 2001; Murray, Ricketts, & Dellaport, 2007; Rosenberg, Eastham, & Kasehagen, 2008; World Health Organization [WHO]/United Nations Children's Fund, 1989).

Certain maternity care practices experienced by mothers during their hospital stay have been shown to promote breastfeeding (Cadwell & Turner-Maffei, 2009). Specifically, the Baby-Friendly Hospital Initiative (BFHI), an international initiative introduced in 1991 by the World Health Organization and the United Nations Children's Fund (1989), has been shown to contribute to positive breastfeeding outcomes. Ten evidence-based best practices form BFHI's core of breastfeeding support in the hospital (**Box 4-2**). The Ten Steps address a major factor in the erosion of exclusive and sustained breastfeeding—maternity care practices that interfere with or are ineffective in supporting breastfeeding. Achievement of the components of all 10 steps earns a birthing facility the designation of Baby-Friendly and the assurance to patients that breastfeeding support services engaged in by the hospital are deemed as best practices. During the implementation of the BFHI in one inner city hospital, breastfeeding rates rose from 58–87%. Of note was the increase among U.S.-born African American mothers, whose breastfeeding rates rose from 34–74% (Philipp et al., 2001). Hospitals working on implementing the Ten Steps have seen improvements

Box 4-2 Ten Steps to Successful Breastfeeding

1. Maintain and routinely communicate a written breastfeeding policy to all staff.
2. Train all healthcare staff in skills necessary to implement this policy.
3. Inform all pregnant women about the benefits and management of breastfeeding.
4. Help mothers initiate breastfeeding within 1 hour of birth.
5. Show mothers how to breastfeed and how to maintain lactation, even if they are separated from their infants.
6. Give infants no food or drink other than breastmilk, unless medically indicated.
7. Practice rooming-in, which allows mothers and infants to remain together 24 hours a day.
8. Encourage unrestricted breastfeeding.
9. Give no pacifiers or artificial nipples to breastfeeding infants.
10. Foster the establishment of breastfeeding support groups and refer mothers to them on discharge from the hospital or clinic.

Reprinted from World Health Organization/United Nations Children's Fund. (1989). *Protecting, promoting and supporting breastfeeding: The special role of maternity services.* Geneva, Switzerland: World Health Organization. Used with permission.

in breastfeeding outcomes even before earning the Baby-Friendly designation. DiFrisco and colleagues (2011) reported that mothers who breastfed within the first hour of birth were significantly more likely to be exclusively breastfeeding at 2 to 4 weeks than mothers who did not breastfeed within the first hour of birth. This finding provides further support to the evidence for step 4 of the BFHI, which is to help all mothers initiate breastfeeding within the first hour of birth.

Not only does the number of steps influence breastfeeding duration, but also specific combinations of two steps. Additive effects from various combinations of steps suggest a synergistic relationship exists between particular steps (Nickel, Labbok, Hudgens, & Daniels, 2013). These research findings support a dose–response relationship, with exposure to 6 steps being related to the longest median duration of breastfeeding (48.8 weeks). In the Nickel et al. (2013) study, exposure to 4 or 5 steps resulted in a 9-week reduction in breastfeeding duration compared to exposure to 6 steps. Exposure to 2 or 3 steps showed a 12-week reduction in breastfeeding duration compared to the 6-steps exposure. Mothers who lacked exposure to both step 4 (delayed initiation) and step 9 (pacifier use) demonstrated the largest decrease in breastfeeding duration, 11.8 weeks.

DiGirolamo and colleagues (2001) surveyed 1,085 new mothers in the Infant Feeding Practices Study I regarding the breastfeeding support they received during the hospital stay after the birth of their baby. They studied the presence or absence of 5 of the 10 steps of the BFHI (i.e., initiation of breastfeeding within 1 hour of birth, 24-hour rooming-in, infant receipt of supplements, feeding on cue, and use of pacifiers). All five steps were experienced by only 7% of the mothers surveyed. Mothers experiencing none of the steps were 8 times more likely to have stopped breastfeeding before 6 weeks postpartum. A dose–response relationship was seen, as the more steps a mother experienced, the more likely she was to continue breastfeeding to 6 weeks and beyond. The major risk factors for early abandonment of breastfeeding were late initiation of breastfeeding and supplementation of the infant. A dose–response relationship between the number of steps experienced and the time of breastfeeding discontinuation was replicated in the Infant Feeding Practices Study II (DiGirolamo, Grummer-Strawn, & Fein, 2008). Only 8% of the mothers experienced all six of the steps studied. A consistent association of breastfeeding beyond 6 weeks was seen with initiation of breastfeeding within 1 hour of birth, giving only breastmilk, and avoiding pacifier use. Mothers who experienced none of the practices were 13 times more likely to stop breastfeeding early.

Perrine, Scanlon, Li, Odom, and Grummer-Strawn (2012) found that most mothers who wish to exclusively breastfeed intend to do so for greater than 3 months, but the majority are not meeting their intended duration. Mothers were more likely to achieve their exclusive breastfeeding duration goal when their infant was not supplemented in the hospital. Of the 1,792 mothers who intended to exclusively breastfeed, only 1.1% intended to do so for less than 1 month, but that is how long 41.6% actually exclusively breastfed. Only 32.4% of the mothers in this sample met their own exclusive breastfeeding intention following hospital discharge. The percentage of mothers who met their own exclusive breastfeeding duration goal increased by the number of Baby-Friendly hospital practices they experienced. Mothers experiencing 6 hospital practices were 2.7 times more likely to achieve their exclusive breastfeeding goal compared to mothers who experienced only 1 or no practices. All of the women in this study intended to exclusively breastfeed, but upon discharge from the hospital, 15% had already given up their intention to exclusively breastfeed their infant. The primary hospital practice associated with this outcome was the receipt by the infant of nonbreastmilk feedings.

Using data from the Infant Feeding Practices Study II (DiGirolamo et al., 2008), Nickel (2011) found the following:

- Supplementing breastfed infants during the hospital stay led to a 10.5-week decrease in breastfeeding duration.
- Delaying breastfeeding initiation for more than 1 hour when combined with providing a pacifier during the hospital stay resulted in an 11.8-week decrease in breastfeeding duration.
- Not feeding according to hunger cues when combined with providing a pacifier during the hospital stay resulted in a 6.3-week decrease in breastfeeding duration.
- Separating a mother and infant (not rooming-in) when combined with not feeding according to hunger cues resulted in a 5.6-week decrease in breastfeeding duration.

These studies suggest a cumulative effect of the practices, with no one practice in isolation contributing to enhanced outcomes; rather, the combination of practices is the important goal (Forster & McLachlan, 2007). Hospitals designated as Baby-Friendly have elevated rates of breastfeeding initiation and exclusivity compared with national and state levels, demonstrating the effectiveness of institutional investments in breastfeeding (Merewood, Mehta, Chamberlain, Phillip, & Bauchner, 2005).

One of the most important practices contained in the Ten Steps is that of having a written breastfeeding policy that is routinely communicated to all healthcare staff (Feldman-Winter, Procaccini, & Merewood, 2012). Rosenberg, Stull, Adler, Kasehagen, and Crivelli-Kovach (2008) found that this step was associated with continued breastfeeding at 2 weeks and that if a hospital had to prioritize the Ten Steps, breastfeeding policy development and implementation was an effective place to start. Although there may be concerns or misinformation regarding implementation of the BFHI (Walker, 2007), institutional changes in hospital practices are effective in increasing both initiation and duration of breastfeeding

(Fairbank et al., 2000). Kruse, Denk, Feldman-Winter, and Rotondo (2005) reported that hospital practices are extremely important to breastfeeding outcomes. Although sociodemographic variables predicted about 60% of the variation in hospital-specific rates of exclusive breastfeeding at discharge, other contributions, including hospital practices, predicted the remaining 40%.

In 2007 the Centers for Disease Control and Prevention (CDC) conducted the first national Maternity Practices in Infant Nutrition and Care (mPINC) survey to characterize intrapartum practices in hospitals and birth centers in the United States. Questions regarding maternity practices were grouped into seven categories that served as subscales in the analyses:

1. Labor and delivery
2. Breastfeeding assistance
3. Mother–newborn contact
4. Newborn feeding practices
5. Breastfeeding support after discharge
6. Nurse/birth attendant breastfeeding training and education
7. Structural and organizational factors related to breastfeeding

The findings from the 2,690 hospitals that responded to the survey indicated widespread use of maternity practices that are not evidence-based and that are known to interfere with breastfeeding. For example, 24% of birth facilities reported supplementing more than half of healthy, full-term, breastfed newborns with something other than breastmilk during the postpartum stay, a practice shown to be unnecessary and detrimental to breastfeeding. In addition, 70% of facilities reported giving breastfeeding mothers gift bags containing infant formula samples. Scores on the seven items will help facilities identify specific maternity practices that might be changed to better support breastfeeding (CDC, 2008).

Results from the 2009 mPINC survey found that little progress had been made in improving lactation care in hospitals with maternal and newborn services. Few hospitals were shown to have model breastfeeding policies (14%), limit breastfeeding supplement use (22%), or support mothers postdischarge (27%). From 2007 to 2009, the percentage of hospitals with recommended practices covering at least 9 of 10 indicators increased only slightly, from 2.4–3.5% (CDC, 2011). In 2009, most hospitals reported providing prenatal breastfeeding education (92.8%), teaching women breastfeeding techniques (89.1%), and teaching women how to recognize and respond to infant feeding cues (81.8%). For all other indicators, half or fewer hospitals followed recommended practices. The lowest prevalence of recommended practices related to having a model breastfeeding policy (14.4%); limiting use of formula, water, or glucose supplements for healthy, full-term breastfed infants (21.5%); and providing adequate breastfeeding support to breastfeeding mothers at hospital discharge (26.8%).

The results from the 2011 mPINC survey (CDC, 2012) showed that from 2009 to 2011, the national average mPINC score increased from 65 to 70, with scores increasing by 5 or more points in 26 states and Washington, DC. However, 90% or more infants received breastmilk as their first feeding after a vaginal birth in only 75% of reporting hospitals. In a question looking at formula supplementation, 50% of healthy full-term infants received formula supplementation in up to 49% of hospitals. Use of glucose water or sterile water for breastfed infants was reported in almost 19% of hospitals. mPINC scores are generally higher for hospitals located in more densely populated counties. From 2007 to 2011, the average mPINC score increased from 64 to 71 among hospitals in metropolitan urbanized counties and from 54 to 65 among hospitals in thinly populated counties. This pattern of lower hospital quality scores in more rural areas of the United States was driven by large differences in breastfeeding policies, clinical practice, staff training, and structural and organizational aspects of care (Allen, Perrine, & Scanlon, 2015). These results suggest that a large number of mothers are still not receiving the evidence-based care necessary to meet their breastfeeding intentions.

The 2013 results from the mPINC survey showed that the national average mPINC score increased from 70 to 75. This continuing improvement demonstrates that many hospitals are making great efforts to improve their breastfeeding care and services. Nevertheless, 10–49% of infants in 51.4% of facilities still receive formula supplements. Glucose water/water supplementation was reported in 12% of facilities. Staff competency in breastfeeding management and support was assessed at least once a year in 60.1% of facilities, less than once per year in 12.8 facilities, and not assessed at all in 27.1 facilities—a worrisome finding (CDC, 2014).

Because the mPINC survey questions draw heavily from the Ten Steps to Successful Breastfeeding, the BFHI remains an important goal for hospitals to achieve. At the very least, hospitals should strive to implement the Ten Steps to provide optimal evidence-based breastfeeding support to new mothers. Sources of sample policies and more information on the BFHI can be found in the additional reading and resources list at the end of this chapter.

MATERNITY CARE PRACTICES AND BREASTFEEDING

Prenatal Maternal Medications

Although the possibility always exists that recreational drugs, illicit drugs, or drugs of abuse can affect an infant's feeding behaviors (e.g., maternal prenatal smoking and its association with infantile colic) (Sondergaard, Henriksen, Obel, & Wisborg, 2001), some prescribed medications taken by the mother during the third trimester also have the potential to influence such behaviors. For example, 1.8–2.8% of all pregnant women are prescribed selective serotonin reuptake inhibitors (SSRIs), which are a group of antidepressants used to treat mild to moderate depression. These types of medications easily cross the placental barrier and expose the fetus to increased serotonin levels during a period of rapid growth and development. Of all infants exposed to SSRIs, approximately 30% will develop symptoms of poor neonatal adaptation as they withdraw from the medication. When SSRIs are taken by a mother during the second or third trimester, withdrawal symptoms may be evident in infants during the early days after birth. Generally, most mild symptoms appear between 8 and 48 hours following birth. These symptoms may include irritability, constant crying, shivering, increased tone, feeding and sleeping difficulties, and convulsions, all described as part of the neonatal withdrawal syndrome by Nordeng, Lindemann, Perminov, and Reikvam (2001). Conversely, Laine, Heikkinen, Ekbald, and Kero (2003) suggest that the cluster of symptoms that includes tremor, restlessness, and rigidity, although seen four times more frequently in exposed newborns, is due to central nervous system serotogenic overstimulation (serotonin-using pathways) rather than an actual withdrawal syndrome. Full-term infants exposed to SSRIs have an altered neurobehavioral profile and may demonstrate more signs of central nervous system stress (Salisbury et al., 2011). High doses of prenatal SSRIs may increase the risk of preterm birth (Roca et al., 2011) and all of the attendant problems an early birth presents to breastfeeding. Casper, Gilles, Fleisher, Baran, Enns, and Lazzeroni (2011) reported that a longer SSRI exposure during pregnancy increased the risk of lower Psychomotor Developmental Index and Behavioral Rating Scale scores in infancy. Women taking SSRIs are less likely to initiate breastfeeding compared with unexposed women (Gorman, Kao, & Chambers, 2012). Clinicians should follow these mothers and infants closely postdischarge, making sure to provide written instructions for sufficient feedings during the first week.

Some evidence suggests that symptoms are not always due to toxic or withdrawal actions but that SSRIs may interfere with the physiology of the infant's respiratory system and parasympathetic activity (Gentile, 2007). Symptoms may occur during the early hours after birth and/or may appear after discharge and further include respiratory distress, transient tachypnea, hypoglycemia, bradycardia, and sucking problems, depending on the particular drug and dosage (Fleschler & Peskin, 2008). Some of these symptoms are suggestive of other conditions, such as dehydration or intracranial hemorrhage. Zeskind and Stephens (2004) reported that SSRI-exposed infants showed greater tremulousness, less flexible and dampened state regulation, greater amounts of uninterrupted REM sleep, more startles and arousals, more generalized motor activity, and greater autonomic dysregulation than infants who had not been exposed to these drugs. Clinically these infants may present as underaroused with more tremors and erratic motor movements.

Paroxetine (Paxil) and fluoxetine (Prozac) are most commonly reported as being associated with neonatal side effects (Moses-Kolko et al., 2005). When mothers receive a combination of paroxetine and clonazepam (Klonopin), infants may be at a higher risk of experiencing poor neonatal adaptation (Oberlander et al., 2004). The clinician may need to check the mother's records or ask whether she has taken any of these medications. Education of the parents is important and should include that these symptoms are short-lived (2–4 weeks) and may disrupt feeding, motor tone, sleeping, and consolability of the infant. Although the symptoms may subside during the first 4–7 days or so, extra vigilance and assistance with breastfeeding may be necessary during the hospital stay and the first week home. Suggested interventions include the provision of a dim, quiet environment (visitors should be minimized); frequent small feedings to address increased caloric requirements and feeding difficulties; skin-to-skin contact to improve breastfeeding, behavioral states, and breathing regularity; swaddling; and cue-based feedings.

Extra vigilance is also called for with mothers who have received mood-stabilizing drugs such as lithium for treating bipolar disorders, because a number of undesirable effects have been described in neonates whose mothers received antimanic or maintenance drugs for mood disorders (Iqbal, Gundlapalli, Ryan, Ryals, & Passman, 2001). While most infants show no symptoms, the floppy infant syndrome (characterized by hypotonia, hypothermia, respiratory depression, and decreased sucking reflex) may appear at a low incidence.

Prenatal SSRI use increases the risk for delayed lactogenesis in the mother. Marshall and colleagues (2010) found that mothers taking prenatal SSRIs had a twofold risk of delayed lactogenesis. The median onset of copious milk production was 85.8 hours postpartum in mothers taking SSRIs compared to 69.1 hours in mothers not taking SSRIs. Because of the longer colostral phase, mothers should be advised to feed their infants very frequently, use alternate massage on each breast during each feeding, watch for sufficient diapers, visit the infant's physician for a weight check and jaundice evaluation no later than day 3, and hand express colostrum for feedings if the infant will not latch.

Infants born to mothers who were treated with SSRI medications should be observed for 48 hours after birth in close proximity to their mothers unless significant symptoms are present (such as respiratory distress), which would signal a need for a higher level of monitoring and care (Leibovitch et al., 2013). Breastfeeding should be encouraged if the infant has been exposed to SSRIs, mirtazapine (Remeron), or venlafaxine (Effexor), as this practice probably reduces the risk of poor neonatal adaptation. The small amounts of these medications that are released into breastmilk may lead to a slower decrease in the drug level in the infant and, therefore, fewer symptoms of poor neonatal adaptation (Kieviet, Dolman, & Honig, 2013). As breastfeeding or the provision of human milk can result in a decreased intensity and severity of neonatal abstinence syndrome (Welle-Strand et al., 2013), current recommendations are that when possible, and not otherwise contraindicated, mothers in supervised drug treatment programs should be encouraged to breastfeed (Hudak, Tan, Committee on Drugs, Committee on Fetus and Newborn, & American Academy of Pediatrics, 2012).

Prescription opioid use during pregnancy is common and associated with both poor neonatal adaptation and neonatal abstinence syndrome. In a study of 242 infants with documented neonatal abstinence syndrome, 99.6% of the mothers had used one or more opioids during pregnancy; these drugs included oxycodone, morphine, hydrocodone, hydromorphone, tramadol, meperidine, methadone, and buprenorphine. Reasons for use included illicit (nonmedical) drug abuse treatment, and chronic pain treatment (Lind et al, 2015). In a study of 112,029 pregnant women, 28% filled more than one opioid prescription during their pregnancy (Patrick et al., 2015). This study also demonstrated that cumulative exposure during pregnancy to prescription opioids, tobacco use, and SSRI use increased the risk of the neonatal abstinence syndrome. Clinicians should observe infants with these exposures for feeding difficulties, jaundice, and respiratory distress.

Labor Medications

Pharmacological relief of the pain from labor has a long history. Various drugs, combinations of drugs, and routes of delivery have fallen in and out of favor through the years.

Systemic Agents

Drugs such as opioids provide some pain relief during labor but carry a number of potential side effects. More than 50 years ago, Brazelton (1961) described the central nervous system depressant effects that occurred in newborns of heavily medicated mothers (i.e., those who received scopolamine, barbiturates, spinal block, pudendal block, saddle block, ether, trichloroethylene, Nisentil, or nitrous oxide). Behavioral disorganization, difficulty in the modulation of state control, and difficulties with breastfeeding that included a sleepy, unresponsive infant who was challenging to wake and keep alert were common. Bricker and Lavender (2002) summarized the association of opioid use during labor with neonatal respiratory depression, decreased alertness, inhibition of sucking, lower neurobehavioral scores, and delay in effective feeding. Other side effects in infants exposed to narcotics include a shorter duration of wakefulness, less efficient suckling, depressed visual and auditory attention, longer time to habituate to noise, and decreased social responsiveness. This behavior can be evident for as long as 4 days (Weiner, Hogg, & Rosen, 1977). The drug-to-delivery interval is the time from when the drug was administered to the mother to the time of the infant's birth. It is an important consideration regarding the extent to which the newborn is affected by medications administered to the mother. Effects on newborns are minimized when narcotics have been given within an hour of birth (Rooth, Lysikiewicz, Huch, & Huch, 1983). Maximal accumulation of a drug and its metabolites in fetal tissues occurs when the agent is given more than 3 hours before delivery (Brice, Moreland, & Walker, 1979) or given repeatedly over a longer period of time.

Although older medications may no longer be used during childbirth, drugs used today still exert a number of undesirable effects on the newborn. Demerol (meperidine) replaced morphine as a popular labor medication for many years. It is now being phased out in many institutions due to its unpleasant side effects on laboring mothers, its depressive effects on newborns, its long half-life in neonates (13 hours), and the extremely long half-life of its potent metabolite normeperidine (62 hours in the neonate). Side effects of concern include depressed suckling (Righard & Alade, 1990), decreased tone and reflexes (Coalson & Glosten, 1991), respiratory depression (Hamza et al., 1992), delayed rooting reflex (Nissen, Lilja, Matthiesen, et al., 1995), and delayed neonatal sucking behavior (Nissen et al., 1997).

Nisentil (alphaprodine) is a rapid-acting narcotic analgesic with a short duration of action. Matthews (1989) compared infants from nonmedicated mothers and mothers medicated with Nisentil in terms of time to effective breastfeeding. Also studied was the effect of the drug-to-delivery interval on mean time to effective breastfeeding. Ninety-three percent of the infants of mothers from the nonmedicated group and from a group whose mothers received Nisentil within an hour of delivery were effectively breastfeeding by 24 hours of age. Mean time to effective breastfeeding for this group was 11.86 hours. By comparison, infants of mothers who received Nisentil 1–3 hours before birth experienced a mean time to effective breastfeeding of 21.2 hours. Only 66% of these infants had established effective breastfeeding by 24 hours.

Crowell, Hill, and Humenick (1994) studied Stadol (butorphanol) and Nubain (nalbuphine), comparing the effects on breastfeeding relative to the drug-to-delivery interval and when the first breastfeeding occurred (**Table 4-1**). Their data also identified a subgroup of mothers and infants who were especially at risk of suboptimal breastfeeding, namely primiparous mothers of boys.

In 2005 the U.S. Food and Drug Administration (FDA) approved safety labeling revisions for nalbuphine (Nubain) injection, warning of the risk for serious fetal and neonatal adverse events associated with its use during labor and delivery. Reports to the FDA of fetal and neonatal adverse events have included fetal bradycardia, respiratory depression at birth, apnea, cyanosis, and hypotonia. Some of these events have been life threatening. Although maternal administration of naloxone during labor has sometimes counteracted these effects, severe prolonged fetal bradycardia has occurred and, in some cases, resulted in permanent neurological damage. The FDA advised that nalbuphine be used during

Table 4-1 Comparative Effects on Breastfeeding of DDI and First Breastfeed

IBFAT Scoring System Was Used to Determine the Establishment of Effective Breastfeeding	No Analgesia or Analgesia Administered Less than 1 Hour Prior to Delivery	Analgesia Administered More than 1 Hour Prior to Delivery
Early initiator: Breastfeeding started less than 1 hour after delivery	Mean time to effective breastfeeding: 6.4 hours	Mean time to effective breastfeeding: 50.3 hours
Late initiator: Breastfeeding started more than 1 hour after delivery	Mean time to effective breastfeeding: 49.7 hours	Mean time to effective breastfeeding: 62.5 hours

* DDI: Drug-to-delivery interval.

labor and delivery only if clearly indicated and the potential benefit outweighed the risk to the infant. The FDA recommended that newborns exposed to maternal nalbuphine should be monitored for respiratory depression, apnea, bradycardia, and arrhythmias.

Systemic analgesics can be highly lipid soluble. They rapidly cross the placenta and are quickly absorbed into fetal circulation. Immaturity of the fetal liver and renal system can delay detoxification and clearance of the drug, which prolongs its action, sometimes well past discharge from the hospital. Peak fetal depressant effects can be seen approximately 1.5–2 hours after administration. To reduce the possibility of newborn depression from opioid analgesia, birth should occur within 1 hour of or 4 hours after its administration (Poole, 2003), something over which clinicians have little control.

Remifentanil is a fast-acting synthetic opioid that is administered through the patient-controlled intravenous route at the beginning of a contraction. One study showed that 6.3% of infants exposed to remifentanil during labor experienced breastfeeding difficulties (Evron, Glezerman, Sadan, Boaz, & Ezri, 2005). Remifentanil can also cause respiratory depression in the mother and may not be as effective in pain management as an epidural (Van de Velde, 2015). Additional lactation support may be required for mothers who have received opioids during labor (Anderson, 2011).

Jordan and colleagues (2009) reported lower breastfeeding rates at 48 hours with epidural analgesia, intramuscular opioid analgesia, ergometrine, and oxytocin and prostaglandins for induction of labor. Use of oxytocin either alone or in combination with ergometrine to prevent postpartum hemorrhage decreased breastfeeding at 48 hours by 6–8%. Ergometrine is a prolactin inhibitor, as are prostaglandins. Exogenous oxytocin has the potential to interrupt the initiation of lactation by disrupting the pulsatile secretion of oxytocin with continuous secretion. This disruption may result in a desensitization and downregulation of myoepithelial receptors (Leng, Caquineau, & Sabatier, 2005).

Concerns have surfaced regarding the concept of genetic imprinting at birth for self-destructive behavior and opiate or amphetamine addiction later in life as possible long-term consequences for an infant whose mother received narcotics during labor (Jacobson et al., 1987, 1990; Jacobson, Nyberg, Eklund, Bygdeman, & Rydberg, 1988). The potential for adult drug abuse may be programmed early in life, with obstetric narcotics exposure serving as an early risk factor (Nyberg, Buka, & Lipsitt, 2000). Animal models have demonstrated that the course of behavioral maturation during certain periods of infancy is influenced by both meperidine and bupivacaine administration at birth, possibly by interfering with the programming of brain development or the alteration of early experiences (Golub, 1996).

Regional Analgesia/Anesthesia

These methods include spinal, epidural, intrathecal, and combined spinal and epidural techniques. Use of combined spinal and epidural analgesia is a common intervention in labor, with some states showing over a 75% rate of use (Osterman & Martin, 2011). Practitioners use various types and amounts of drugs and drug combinations and may administer the drugs over short or long periods, before or after the cervix is 3–4 cm dilated, or after laboring women have already been dosed with systemic analgesics. The relationship between epidural use and breastfeeding has yielded conflicting data, with difficulties experienced in comparing studies whose methodologies vary widely and that may not take into account the influence of co-interventions (Camann, 2007). In an analysis of the Infant Feeding Practices Study II that looked at 1,907 mothers who intended to breastfeed for longer than 2 months, mothers who did not receive any pain medication during labor and delivery were more likely to continue breastfeeding beyond 6 weeks. This association remained after controlling for demographic, behavioral, and attitudinal variables (DiGirolamo et al., 2008).

Torvaldsen, Roberts, Simpson, Thompson, and Ellwood (2006) studied 1,295 women to determine any association between epidural analgesia and breastfeeding in the first week postpartum and breastfeeding cessation during the first 6 months. Epidurals were significantly associated with partial breastfeeding during the first week due to difficulty breastfeeding. Women who used no pain medication had the lowest rates of breastfeeding cessation at 6 months; in comparison, mothers who experienced epidurals had the highest rates of abandoning breastfeeding. Although epidural use may not have been causal, breastfeeding difficulties were more frequent during the first week postpartum, formula supplementation occurred early, and breastfeeding cessation was more common in mothers who had been given epidural analgesia. Infants whose mothers received epidural analgesia appear to be at an increased risk for difficulty initiating breastfeeding, being supplemented with formula, and not being breastfed until 6 months of age. These mother–baby pairs will benefit from targeted interventions (Jordan, 2006), and clinicians may wish to place such pairs in a higher risk category for breastfeeding problems and premature weaning.

Early studies failed to examine breastfeeding as an outcome of epidural use and may not have used nonmedicated control groups (Walker, 1997). Nevertheless, epidural analgesia has been associated with neonatal respiratory depression (Kumar & Paes, 2003), a lower rate of spontaneous vaginal delivery, fetal malpositioning, a higher rate of instrumental vaginal delivery, an increased cesarean section rate, longer labors, increased incidence of oxytocin-augmented labor, increased incidence of intrapartum fever (with the infants more likely to be evaluated and treated for suspected sepsis as well as experiencing unexplained neonatal seizures), infant hypotonia, decreased performance on the Neonatal Behavioral Assessment Scale, and increased occurrence of neonatal jaundice (Lieberman & O'Donoghue, 2002).

Co-interventions designed to reduce the common side effects of epidurals have their own side effects (Mayberry, Clemmens, & De, 2002). Epidural drugs and their side effects on the laboring woman, their effects on the labor and delivery, the consequences to the fetus and newborn, plus the co-interventions administered to reduce side effects and their own side effects all make it difficult to pinpoint which intervention affects breastfeeding, how they influence breastfeeding, and how varying combinations of interventions may act synergistically (Riordan & Riordan, 2000). Some studies claim that epidural use does not affect breastfeeding initiation or duration (Halpern et al., 1999) or that epidurals actually promote breastfeeding (Leighton & Halpern, 2002a). Halpern et al. (1999) studied the duration of breastfeeding as a means to evaluate the effect of labor pain medication on successful breastfeeding outcomes. Of the 189 women enrolled in the study, 171 were interviewed at 6–8 weeks postpartum. These mothers had received intravenous (IV) narcotics, epidural analgesia, or no medications for labor pain relief. Although 59% had received epidural anesthesia, there was no discrimination between breastfeeding outcomes among the various labor experiences. Seventy-two percent of the entire sample was breastfeeding exclusively at 6 weeks, 20% were partially breastfeeding, and the rest had weaned. Thirty-six percent reported difficulty in initiating breastfeeding in the hospital, 55 of the mothers visited a free lactation clinic at least once, and intensive breastfeeding support was used during and after the hospital stay. The study did not say whether these problems were associated with analgesia use during labor but concluded that epidurals do not affect breastfeeding. Perhaps breastfeeding succeeded despite the medications, due to the rigorous amount of lactation care and services provided to all the mothers in this study. Wieczorek, Guest, Balki, Shah, and Carvalho (2010) reported that the incidence in their hospital of successful lactation was high in multiparous women who received an epidural with fentanyl. Over 69% of these mothers required some degree of lactation support, with 4.6% needing help with each feeding and 26.4% requiring help at least daily during their hospital stay. The mothers had all breastfed previously. While cessation of breastfeeding at 6 weeks was lower in this sample, these mothers had experience breastfeeding previously and had access to free and sufficient help when it was needed. Not all mothers who receive epidural analgesia will be fortunate enough to have access to the sometimes extensive services of lactation professionals that may be needed to overcome this impediment to breastfeeding. Henderson, Dickinson, Evans, McDonald, & Paech (2003) found that nulliparous women who chose epidural analgesia were significantly more likely to breastfeed for shorter durations.

Handlin and colleagues (2009) found that mothers who received oxytocin infusion during labor had higher cortisol levels than mothers who did not receive oxytocin. High cortisol levels are related to stress. Women who received both oxytocin and an epidural had higher cortisol levels than women who received only an epidural. The more oxytocin a mother received during labor, the lower her oxytocin levels in response to a breastfeed were 2 days later. The administration of epidural analgesia inhibits nerve fiber transmission of pain in the spinal cord, with the possibility that nerve fibers mediating oxytocin release may also be affected by epidural analgesia (Jonas et al., 2009).

Epidural Drugs

All drugs used in epidurals reach the fetus in greater or lesser amounts, including bupivacaine (Kuhnert, Kuhnert, & Gross, 1982), an anesthetic that is measurable in the fetus within 10 minutes of maternal administration (Rosenblatt et al., 1981), and any of the narcotics combined in the epidural, such as fentanyl and sufentanil (Loftus, Hill, & Cohen, 1995). The effects on breastfeeding may be either direct or indirect and can vary from agent to agent. Fentanyl has a half-life of 2–4 hours in an adult but 3–13 hours in neonates (Hale, 2008). If it takes approximately five half-lives to eliminate the drug from the body, a neonate with a sluggish liver could take as long as 65 hours to eliminate the fentanyl that accumulated during the birthing process. The concentration of fentanyl increases as infant pH decreases, placing crying infants and cesarean-delivered infants at an elevated risk for much higher concentrations of fentanyl (Jordan, Emery, Bradshaw, Watkins, & Friswell, 2005). This point is well after discharge from the hospital and may signal the need for closer follow-up in infants whose mothers received fentanyl during labor.

Spontaneous breast-seeking and suckling behaviors soon after delivery are reduced in newborns whose mothers receive analgesics and epidurals (Righard & Alade, 1992; Widstrom et al., 1987). Developing and early discrete breastfeeding movements are also altered or blunted by maternal labor medications. Administration of analgesia and epidurals disturbs the behavioral sequence of prefeeding behaviors immediately after delivery such as hand-to-mouth movements, touching of the areola, suckling movements, and the sucking pattern itself (Ransjo-Arvidson et al., 2001).

Using the Infant Breastfeeding Assessment Tool, Riordan, Gross, Angeron, Krumwiede, and Melin (2000) compared four groups of infants whose mothers received (1) no labor pain medication, (2) only epidural analgesia, (3) only IV narcotics, or (4) both epidural and IV analgesia. On a scale where 12 represented the highest suckling score, infants whose mothers had no labor pain analgesia scored 11.1 ± 0.9.

Infants whose mothers had IV analgesia scored 8.5 ± 3.2, whereas infants whose mothers had an epidural scored 8.5 ± 3.4. Infants whose mothers had both IV analgesia and an epidural had significantly lower suckling scores of 6.4 ± 3.0. Infants with scores less than 10 are in need of significant follow-up, because both IV medications and epidurals diminish neonatal sucking.

Baumgarder, Muehl, Fischer, and Pribbenow (2003) also found that epidural anesthesia had a negative impact on breastfeeding in the first 24 hours of life. The primary outcome of interest in their study was the ability of the infant to accomplish two successful breastfeedings by 24 hours as defined by the LATCH breastfeeding assessment tool. This outcome was achieved by 81% of infants whose mothers did not have an epidural compared with 69.6% of infants whose mothers received epidural analgesia. Another disturbing outcome of this study was the finding that infants exposed to epidural anesthesia were significantly more likely to receive a bottle supplement during hospitalization. Mothers who received an epidural and did not breastfeed within 1 hour of delivery were at extremely high risk for their infants to receive bottle supplementation. Early onset of breastfeeding has been shown to be adversely affected by epidural analgesia (Herrera-Gomez et al., 2015). Clinicians may need to exercise increased vigilance and provide more intense breastfeeding support for mothers who have received an epidural during labor.

Dozier and colleagues (2013) analyzed potential associations between epidural analgesia and overall breastfeeding cessation within 30 days postpartum. While the relationship between epidural use and breastfeeding is complex, this study found that epidural analgesia significantly predicted breastfeeding cessation. Mothers receiving both epidural analgesia and IV oxytocin were the group most likely to abandon breastfeeding within 1 month, while mothers receiving neither of these interventions had the lowest risk of breastfeeding cessation.

Beilin and colleagues (2005) looked at the total dose of epidural opioids relative to breastfeeding impairment. They found that in multiparous women with a history of successful breastfeeding who received > 150 mcg of epidural fentanyl, 19% experienced breastfeeding failure at 6 weeks. This failure rate was significantly higher than in mothers who received < 10 mcg of epidural fentanyl.

Formula supplementation was reported to be more common among infants of mothers who received epidural analgesia containing a bupivacaine concentration of 0.25% (Volmanen, Valanne, & Alahuhta, 2004). Wiklund, Norman, Uvnas-Moberg, Ranjo-Arvidson, and Andolf (2009) reported that compared with infants of mothers not receiving an epidural, fewer infants of mothers with epidurals suckled the breast within the first 4 hours of birth, that they were given formula more often during their hospital stay, and fewer were exclusively breastfed upon discharge.

In an attempt to reduce the negative effects of epidurals on laboring mothers and their newborns, most obstetric services now use an ultra-low dose of drugs in the epidural mixture (0.125% bupivacaine, 50 mcg fentanyl, and 1:600,000 epinephrine as the loading dose and a continuing infusion of 0.044% bupivacaine, 0.000125% fentanyl, and 1:800,000 epinephrine). Radzyminski (2003) concluded that there were no measurable differences between the breastfeeding behaviors of infants of 28 mothers who received this type of epidural and 28 infants whose mothers received no labor medication. However, it is interesting to note that 72% of the medicated mothers received oxytocin to induce or augment their labor compared with 32% of the mothers in the unmedicated group. The subgroup of infants who experienced difficulty in initiating breastfeeding had mothers who experienced more maternal fatigue, anxiety, lack of previous breastfeeding experience, induction of labor, and extremes of the labor curve. One difference between the two groups was the greater amount of swallowing in the unmedicated group, although it was not statistically significant. Bupivacaine in the epidural affected the newborn's passive and active tone and total score on the Neurologic and Adaptive Capacity Score instrument used to measure neurobehavior in this study (Amiel-Tison, Barrier, & Shnider, 1982). This could possibly impede early suckling movements. It remains unknown whether any of these drugs become sequestered in the neonatal central nervous system during the early days after discharge.

It has been shown that the higher the doses of intrapartum fentanyl and synthetic oxytocin, the less the likelihood of the newborn infant achieving successful sucking during the first hour skin to skin after a vaginal birth (Brimdyr et al., 2015). In looking at the varying total amounts of fentanyl given to a laboring mother, this study showed that there was a threshold of the dose that started to degrade infant sucking. Infant sucking started to be affected at a dose of 150 mcg of fentanyl, which correlates with the dose that Beilin et al. (2005) suggested as disturbing to breastfeeding. Brimdyr et al. (2015) also described how as the synthetic oxytocin dose increased, so too did the fentanyl dose. Mothers in this study who received fentanyl without synthetic oxytocin had an average amount of fentanyl of 169.65 mcg (maximum 243.3 mcg, minimum 102.9 mcg). Mothers who received both fentanyl and synthetic oxytocin had an average amount of fentanyl of 264.45 mcg (maximum 613.4 mcg, minimum 15.7 mcg). Clinicians may wish to provide additional breastfeeding monitoring and assistance to mothers whose fentanyl dose exceeded 150 mcg.

In animals, epidural anesthesia can interfere with maternal attachment and the onset of mothering behavior by blocking sensory stimuli for the release of oxytocin (Krehbiel, Pomdron, Levy, & Prud'Homme, 1987). In human mothers, a spontaneous peak of oxytocin release is usually observed about 15 minutes post delivery, with several more peaks of oxytocin occurring up to 60 minutes postpartum (Nissen, Lilja, Winstrom, & Uvnas-Moberg, 1995). Epidural use is associated with a decrease or deficiency in plasma oxytocin levels in mothers after delivery (Goodfellow, Hull, Swaab, Dogterom, & Buijs, 1983; Rahm, Hallgren, Hogberg, Hurtig, & Odlind, 2002). Sepkoski, Lester, Ostheimer, and Brazelton (1992) showed that mothers with bupivacaine (0.5%) epidurals spent less time with their infants while in the hospital (9.7 vs. 13.7 hours) than did a nonmedicated group of mothers. The medicated infants showed clear depression in motor abilities and exhibited poor state control.

Intrapartum fever is associated with epidural use. Whereas maternal fever is a marker for potential infection, most intrapartum fevers originate as a side effect of epidural use (Lieberman et al., 1997). Lieberman and colleagues (1997) analyzed 1,047 laboring women, 63% of whom received epidurals and 37% of whom did not. Of the women who received an epidural, 14.5% developed a fever of more than 38°C (100.4°F) during labor compared with only 1% of women not receiving an epidural. Ninety-six percent of the intrapartum fevers occurred within the group receiving an epidural, resulting in 85.6% of neonatal sepsis workups occurring in the group of infants whose mothers received an epidural. These infants were also four times more likely to be treated with antibiotics.

Gross, Cohen, Lang, Frigoletto, & Lieberman (2002) evaluated the records of 1,233 mothers whose labor analgesia was managed with no medication, epidural medication only, nalbuphine alone, or both epidural and nalbuphine. The incidence of fever was 17% for mothers receiving only epidurals and 1% for the no-medication group. Riley and colleagues (2011) also demonstrated the higher incidence of fever associated with epidural use. Women receiving labor epidural analgesia had fever develop more frequently (22.7%) compared with women not receiving epidural analgesia (6%). These authors also found that epidural fever is associated with an inflammatory state. In a study of 49 laboring mothers who received remifentanil analgesia, 49 mothers who received epidural analgesia, and 49 controls who received no analgesia, it was found that fever greater than 38°C (100.4°F) developed in 10% of the remifentanil mothers, 37% of the epidural mothers, and 7% of the controls (Douma, Stienstra, Middeldorp, Arbous, & Dahan, 2015). Greenwell et al. (2012) found that the proportion of infants experiencing adverse outcomes increased with the degree of epidural-related maternal temperature elevation. Of the 3,209 women in the studied population, 86.8% received epidural analgesia, and 13.2% did not. Over 44% of women with an epidural developed a fever above 37.5°C (99.5°F), compared with 14% not receiving an epidural. Maternal fever above 38°C (100.4°F) developed in 19.2% of women with an epidural compared to 2.4% of women without an epidural. Other interventions were significantly higher in the epidural group, including fetal distress in 13.3% of the epidural group compared with 8% in the nonepidural group, forceps use in 5.7% of the epidural group compared with 0.3% in the nonepidural group, and 12.8% use of vacuum extraction in the epidural groups compared with 3.6% in the nonepidural group. All of these interventions increased as the maternal temperature increased. Adverse neonatal outcomes increased as maternal temperatures increased. The proportion of infants with transient hypotonia increased from 10.8% when maternal temperature was at or below 37.5°C (99.5°F) to 25.2% when fever was above 38.3°C (101°F). Hypotonia can interfere with initial breastfeeding mechanics and disrupt the acquisition of neonatal breastfeeding skills. Infants who are hypotonic require greater body and jaw support when at the breast, may suck with lower amounts of vacuum, may transfer less colostrum and milk per suck and per feeding, and may be at risk for insufficient milk intake.

In a study of 2,520 mothers, those who received labor pain medications had approximately 2 to 3 times higher odds of experiencing delayed onset of lactation compared to mothers who received no labor pain medications and delivered vaginally (Lind, Perrine, & Li, 2014). Given that labor pain medication is a common childbirth intervention, clinicians will need to ensure that these mothers have access to appropriate lactation support services immediately following discharge to avoid neonatal and maternal complications and early abandonment of breastfeeding.

Intrapartum maternal fever is associated with an increased risk of cesarean section and operative vaginal delivery (Lieberman, Cohen, Lang, Frigoletto, & Goetzl, 1999) as well as a number of transient adverse effects in the newborn such as low Apgar score, hypotonia, bag and mask resuscitation, and oxygen therapy in the nursery (Lieberman, Lang, et al., 2000). High maternal fever increases the risk of neurological injury to the fetus independent of infection. It is associated with a 3.4-fold increase in the risk of unexplained neonatal seizures and is a strong predictor of later morbidity and mortality in term infants (Lieberman, Eichenwald, et al., 2000). Even in afebrile mothers, those who receive epidural analgesia have infants who are more likely to be evaluated for sepsis compared with mothers who do not receive such medications (20.4% vs. 8.9%) (Goetzl et al., 2001). Agakidis, Agakidou, Philip Thomas, Murthy, & John Loyd (2011) reported that epidural analgesia is an independent risk factor for fever in term neonates. Fever lasting more than 5 hours would generate the need for a sepsis evaluation. Sepsis workups usually result in separation, invasive procedures, expressing milk rather than having an infant at the breast, and maternal anxiety that contributes to a slow start to breastfeeding.

Delivery and immediate postpartum care practices can affect breastfeeding in mothers who have received an epidural, possibly exacerbating problems that could have been minimized with early frequent contact such as skin to skin (Anderson, Moore, Hepworth, & Bergman, 2003), minimal to no separation

(Leighton & Halpern, 2002b), opportunities for self-attachment to the breast, and frequent feedings. It is possible that with intense lactation care and services both during the hospital stay and after discharge, many of the side effects of epidurals on breastfeeding may be overcome. However, if mothers do not have these services available or lack access to them, then breastfeeding is placed in jeopardy, with mixed feeding and early weaning distinct possibilities.

When an epidural is administered, it is usually accompanied by a cascade of interventions that either individually or in combination can significantly affect breastfeeding:

- IV infusion of regional anesthesia/analgesia can cause hypotension. To reduce the risks of this side effect, a pre-epidural IV infusion of 500–1,000 mL of non-glucose-balanced sodium chloride solution (isotonic saline or lactated Ringer's) is usually administered 15–30 minutes before the procedure. Glucose solutions are contraindicated due to the risk for fetal hyperglycemia and rebound hypoglycemia in the newborn. Large amounts of fluid can be administered over the course of a long labor or if maternal IV medications are used during and after the labor and delivery (1–6 L of fluid are possible). A healthy pregnant woman at term already has approximately 2 L of fluid stored in her extravascular space (Lind, 1983). One adverse outcome of a delay in the expected postpartum fluid shift and diuresis of excess fluid has been observed as areolar edema (Cotterman, 2004). An edematous areola envelops the nipple and increases subareolar tissue resistance, resulting in a difficult, painful latch or an areola that cannot be drawn into the infant's mouth. Fluid retention is further exacerbated by the normally increased vasopressin (antidiuretic hormone) production during childbirth. Hypotension is also managed with IV vasopressor agents, such as ephedrine and phenylephrine (Camann, 2003), adding yet more drugs (which also contribute to fluid retention) into the laboring woman. Although prophylactic ephedrine can prevent maternal hypotension and late fetal decelerations, it is associated with fetal tachycardia (Cleary-Goldman et al., 2005), another unwanted and hazardous side effect. Omitting the fluid preload before epidural administration has been studied, with findings of similar rates of maternal hypotension between no preload and a 1-L preload in low-dose epidurals but with a higher rate of deterioration in fetal heart rates seen where no fluid preload was administered (Kinsella, Pirlet, Mills, Tuckey, & Thomas, 2000). Morbidly obese mothers given an epidural during labor have more hypotension and prolonged fetal heart rate decelerations than women without an epidural (Vricella, Louis, Mercer, & Bolden, 2011). The amount of maternal IV fluid received during labor is significantly associated with maximum weight loss in the newborn. For every 1% increase in average milliliters per hour of IV infusion, the infant maximum weight loss percentage will increase by 0.0077 (Hirth, Weitkamp, & Dwivedi, 2012).
- Oxytocin administration for inducing or augmenting labor can further contribute to edema (as well as dilutional hyponatremia or water intoxication) because it has an antidiuretic effect similar to vasopressin. If oxytocin is administered in a glucose solution, this formulation further potentiates the antidiuretic effects of oxytocin. A few hospitals may still use a dextrose solution for the mainline IV (Ruchala, Metheny, Essenpreis, & Borcherding, 2002). Water overload, dilutional hyponatremia (Omigbodun, Fajimi, & Adeleye, 1991), hyperbilirubinemia (Omigbodun et al., 1993), respiratory distress, and feeding difficulties can be seen in newborns whose mothers are the recipients of excessive or inappropriate fluids during labor (Borcherding & Ruchala, 2002).

More IV fluid may be needed as a treatment for excessive uterine activity from oxytocin augmentation of labor (Simpson, 2011). A fluid bolus of at least 500 mL of lactated Ringer's solution, along with other measures to reduce excessive uterine activity, further adds to the fluid burden experienced by some mothers (Simpson & James, 2008).

- Fetal malposition is strongly and consistently associated with epidural analgesia (Ponkey, Cohen, Heffner, & Lieberman, 2003). Lieberman, Davidson, Lee-Parritz, and Shearer (2005) found that epidurals were associated with a fourfold increase in the risk of occiput posterior birth. Persistent occiput posterior is associated with increased rates of operative vaginal and cesarean deliveries and other peripartum complications such as prolonged first and second stages of labor, oxytocin augmentation, excessive blood loss, third- and fourth-degree perineal lacerations, and chorioamnionitis (Cheng, Shaffer, & Caughey, 2006). Infants of mothers who experienced a cesarean delivery compared with those delivered vaginally were shown to demonstrate poorer scores on the LATCH scoring system at each of their first three feedings (Cakmak & Kuguoglu, 2007), creating the need for more intensive lactation support.
- Instrument delivery by forceps, vacuum extraction, or both are commonly associated with epidural use (Walker & O'Brien, 1999), often due to fetal malposition. Thorp and colleagues (1993) found a fourfold increase in the rate of malposition (19% vs. 4%) in a group of mothers who received epidural analgesia. Epidural analgesia increases the risk for labor dystocia and has been identified as an independent risk factor for vacuum extraction (O'Hana et al., 2008). Vacuum extraction has the potential to disrupt the autonomic balance in infants, increasing their vulnerability to stress (Moehler, Poustka, & Resch 2007; Porges, 1992). Intracranial hemorrhage is higher among infants delivered by forceps or vacuum extraction. Towner, Castro, Eby-Wilkens, and Hilbert (1999) identified one-third of a sample of 583,340 liveborn singleton infants as being born by operative techniques. Intracranial hemorrhage occurred in 1 of 860 infants delivered by vacuum extraction, 1 of 664 infants delivered by forceps, and 1 of 1,900 infants delivered spontaneously. Vacuum extraction causes less maternal trauma but increases the risk of certain types of intracranial hemorrhage such as subarachnoid hemorrhage (Wen et al., 2001). Compared with spontaneous vaginal deliveries, deliveries by sequential use of vacuum and forceps had even higher rates of injuries, with almost four times the rate of intracranial hemorrhage and increased risk of brachial plexus, facial nerve injury, seizures, depressed 5-minute Apgar scores, and maternal perineal lacerations. The relative risk of sequential vacuum and forceps use was greater than the sum of the individual relative risks of each instrument for intracranial hemorrhage, facial nerve injury, seizure, hematoma, and perineal and vaginal lacerations (Gardella, Taylor, Benedetti, Hitti, & Critchlow, 2001).

The FDA became sufficiently concerned about the serious injuries and deaths related to the use of vacuum extraction devices that it issued a public health advisory to healthcare professionals on May 21, 1998 (FDA, 1998). The FDA warned that these devices could cause serious or fatal injuries and noted that those who care for these infants after delivery might not be aware that the devices could produce life-threatening complications. The FDA was also concerned that if healthcare providers were not alerted to an infant who had been vacuum extracted, they might not adequately monitor for signs and symptoms of device-related injuries. Clinicians should be sure to check whether an infant who is having difficulty feeding experienced a vacuum extraction, as lethargy, irritability, and poor feeding are signs and symptoms of intracranial injury. It may also be prudent to remove the infant's little hat to check the fetal scalp for swollen or puffy areas that may indicate damage from the vacuum extraction.

- Infants exposed to vacuum-assisted delivery devices usually have a caput succedaneum—that is, an extracranial hemorrhage-producing edema of the soft tissues of the scalp that resolves spontaneously within the first week of life. Cephalohematomas can lead to hyperbilirubinemia. Clinicians and parents should be aware of the increased risk for jaundice in infants delivered by vacuum extraction. The FDA, however, warned of two major life-threatening complications of vacuum extraction:
    1. Subgaleal hematoma (subaponeurotic hematoma) (Cavlovich, 1994) is an extracranial hemorrhage that represents a significant blood loss to the infant. It occurs when emissary veins are damaged and blood accumulates in the potential space between the galea aponeurotica and the periosteum of the skull. Because this space has no boundaries, blood may accumulate from the orbital ridges above the eyes to the nape of the neck. The signs may be present at delivery or may not become apparent until several hours or days after delivery. Signs include diffuse swelling of the head, pallor, hypotension, tachycardia, lethargy, and increased respiration rate. Significant blood loss can occur with subsequent brain compression, disseminated intravascular coagulation, and shock (Amar, Aryan, Meltzer, & Levy, 2003; Uchil & Arulkumaran, 2003).
    2. Intracranial hemorrhage may include subdural, subarachnoid, intraventricular, and/or intraparenchymal hemorrhage. Signs are not visible from the outside and may include seizure activity, lethargy, apnea, bulging fontanel, poor feeding, increased irritability, bradycardia, and shock. Clinical evidence of neurological damage may develop over time and not become apparent until 4 weeks to 6 months of age (Steinbach, 1999).

The FDA estimated that almost 6% of all deliveries in 1998 used vacuum extraction devices. The rate of delivery by vacuum extraction had increased by 59% between 1990 (3.9%) and 1996–1997 (6.2%) (Martin et al., 2011). The use of vacuum extraction during 2010 births was 4.40%, down from 4.53% in 2009 (Martin, Hamilton, Ventura, Osterman, Wilson, & Mathews, 2012). Use of vacuum extraction continued to decrease to 2.72% of all births in 2013 (Martin, Hamilton, Osterman, Curtin, & Mathews, 2015). This trend may help reduce early breastfeeding problems associated with this delivery practice. Infants delivered by vacuum extraction often start suckling later, are given formula more often, and are breastfed less at night, and their mothers may experience a delay in lactogenesis II (Vestermark, Hogdall, Birch, Plenov, & Toftager-Larsen, 1991). Hall and colleagues (2002) demonstrated that vacuum extraction was a significant contributor to poor scores on the Breastfeeding Assessment Score that was predictive of increased risk of breastfeeding cessation during the first 7–10 days after birth. In some hospitals, vacuum extraction is an indication for a referral to the lactation consultant and a higher level of support and monitoring of breastfeeding.

Cesarean delivery has been identified as a persistent barrier to breastfeeding (Rowe-Murray & Fisher, 2002). With the 2013 cesarean birth rate in the United States at 32.7% (Martin et al., 2015), it is important to offer interventions that can help improve breastfeeding for cesarean mothers. An important intervention is adequate pain control following the surgery, as inadequate pain relief can result in less effective breastfeeding. Woods and colleagues (2012) studied the effects of different maternal pain control modalities on breastfeeding behavior during the first 24 hours following cesarean birth in 621 mothers. Mothers using patient-controlled epidural analgesia reported significantly greater pain relief than mothers using regular patient-controlled analgesia. Women with lower pain scores had significantly more breastfeeding sessions than mothers with high pain scores. Mothers with mild well-controlled pain were 2.4 times more likely to breastfeed 6 or more times in the first 24 hours. Those who put the infant to breast within the first 2 hours following the surgery had 3.5 times the likelihood of breastfeeding 6 or more times in the first 24 hours. Those not receiving any supplemental feedings were 6.9 times as likely to breastfeed 6 or more times within the first 24 hours. However, of concern was the average time to the first feeding, which was 4.2 hours in this sample of mothers. Clinicians may wish to work to provide more effective methods of pain relief to cesarean mothers, assure that the first breastfeeding occurs within an hour or so of birth, facilitate 6 or more feedings within the first 24 hours, and refrain from formula supplementation.

There is increasing interest in making a cesarean delivery a more family-centered and satisfying experience for parents (Smith, Plaat, & Fisk, 2008). Some hospitals have started to modify standard cesarean operative techniques by initiating skin-to-skin contact in the operating room (OR); delivering the infant more slowly to mimic the vaginal squeeze; placing the IV catheter, oximeter, and blood pressure cuff on the same nondominant arm; placing the electrocardiographic leads on the mother's back; using clear surgical drapes so parents can view the birth; and providing for intraoperative breastfeeding (Camann & Trainor, 2012). Skin-to-skin contact in the OR and intraoperative breastfeeding have been shown to significantly decrease formula supplementation during the hospital stay for those infants who experience skin-to-skin contact and breastfeeding in the OR compared to infants who are placed skin to skin 90 minutes following delivery or who do not experience skin-to-skin contact at all (Hung & Berg, 2011). In one study, exclusive breastfeeding rates more than doubled in cesarean-delivered mothers who experienced skin-to-skin interventions in the OR (Brady, Bulpitt, & Chiarelli, 2014).

Separation

When the predominant location for birth moved to the hospital setting in the early 20th century, caretaking routines developed that are still in use today. It is not uncommon to see mothers and their babies separated at birth, infants cared for in a nursery, mothers and babies together only during the day, infant interventions performed not at the bedside but in the nursery, and the expectation that contact between mother and baby will prevent the mother from obtaining sleep. Although there are medical reasons for separation, most occur due to non-evidence-based views; for example, nursery care allows better supervision of the infant, routine monitoring or physician evaluations must be done where better light is available, interventions such as phototherapy must occur in the nursery, or mothers are told that they should allow the nurses to care for the infant (especially at night) so that they can get more rest. Separating mothers and infants reduces the interaction between mother and baby, hinders a mother's opportunity to learn her baby's feeding cues, decreases access to the breast resulting in fewer breastfeeds (Yamauchi & Yamanouchi, 1990b), may increase the occurrence of complementary or supplementary feedings of water or formula, delays lactogenesis II, and produces undesirable physiological side effects in newborns (Anderson, 1989).

Side Effects of Separation

Separation does not result in more sleep for mothers at night if infants are returned to the nursery. Mothers have been shown to receive no more sleep when their infants are sent to the nursery at night than mothers who room-in with their infants (Waldenstrom & Swenson, 1991). Keefe (1988) demonstrated that mothers slept an average of 5.35 hours during an 8-hour night period when their infants were returned to the nursery, whereas mothers who roomed-in with their babies slept an average of 5.55 hours. A strategy to implement close contact during rooming-in in the hospital without the potential risk of bed-sharing was the use of a three-sided bassinet that attached to the maternal bed, keeping the baby within easy reach on the same level as the mother without directly sharing the sleep surface. Ball, Ward-Platt, Heslop, Leech, and Brown (2006) studied the use of such an arrangement and its effect on breastfeeding compared with infants who remained in a bassinet. Infants in the group who were placed in the attached bassinet breastfed more frequently than those in a stand-alone bassinet. This study showed that exclusive breastfeeding at 16 weeks was higher in the group of infants sleeping in the attached bassinet in the hospital (53%) compared with 21% of infants who were still exclusively breastfed at 16 weeks who slept in a stand-alone bassinet (Ball, 2008). The American Academy of Pediatrics (AAP, Section on Breastfeeding, 2012) recommends that mothers sleep in close proximity to their infants to facilitate breastfeeding.

Some mothers believe that giving their infant a bottle of formula before bedtime will make the baby feel fuller and sleep longer, allowing for more maternal sleep at night. A laboratory study has shown that breastfeeding mothers do achieve more deep sleep than formula-feeding mothers (Blyton, Sullivan, & Edwards, 2002). In a study of 120 first-time mothers, nocturnal sleep time at 1 month postpartum was significantly greater for mothers who exclusively breastfed compared to women who used formula at night (Doan, Gay, Kennedy, Newman, & Lee, 2014). The amount of sleep loss in this study between 9:00 pm and 9:00 am experienced by mothers who used formula at night was nearly 3 times the amount of sleep loss experienced by mothers in the exclusively breastfeeding group. The possibility of a little more sleep at night may be another incentive to practice exclusive breastfeeding.

A study that examined the effects on breastfeeding of separation of infants from their mothers for early-onset sepsis evaluation found that this practice was significantly associated with delayed initiation of breastfeeding and increased formula supplementation in the first day of life (Mukhopadhyay, Lieberman, Puopolo, Riley, & Johnson, 2015). The authors suggested that in asymptomatic, well-appearing newborns, frequent, standardized physical examinations might be substituted for laboratory studies to screen infants for group B *Streptococcus* early-onset sepsis. The early-onset sepsis evaluation could be conducted in the mother's delivery room, allowing the first breastfeeding to occur before separation, and/or permitting mother–infant contact during the time required for antibiotic infusion.

Infants cared for in a nursery at night are exposed to greater light and sound levels than those cared for in the mother's room, receive less contact with a caregiver, experience less quiet sleep, and cry more than infants who remain with their mothers. Keefe (1987) reported illumination levels in a nursery as 35-foot candles compared with 3-foot candles in the mother's room. Infants kept in the nursery at night were exposed to noise levels equal to or greater than 80 decibels for approximately one-third of the night. The most persistent and striking noise in the nursery was the sound of infants crying. Infants kept in their mothers' rooms also engaged in more quiet sleep and less crying. The presence of the newborn in the mother's room did not significantly alter maternal sleep but did improve infant sleep.

Infants separated from their mothers cry more, frequently startle, have lower body and skin temperatures, and have lower blood glucose levels than do infants who remain with their mothers after birth. In a study following 50 infants for the first 90 minutes after birth, Christensson and colleagues (1992) found that the maternal body was an efficient heat source for the newborn because the skin-to-skin infants remained warmer. Blood glucose levels in the separated infants at 90 minutes after birth averaged 46.6 mg/dL compared with the skin-to-skin infants, whose blood glucose averaged 57.6 mg/dL. The latter infants also cried significantly less, preserving high blood glucose levels and glycogen stores and contributing to a more rapid metabolic adaptation to extrauterine life. Significantly less hypoglycemia was experienced in infants of diabetic mothers who were kept skin to skin and who were kept with their mothers during rooming-in (Stage, Mathiesen, Emmersen, Greisen, & Damm, 2010). This intervention is especially important for infants of diabetic mothers and late preterm infants to help maintain high blood glucose levels and reduce formula supplementation. Walters, Boggs, Ludington-Hoe, Price, and Morrison (2007) found that skin temperature of newborns rose during skin-to-skin care immediately after delivery. They also reported that blood glucose levels varied between 42 and 85 mg/dL for infants who had not already fed and between 43 and 118 mg/dL for those who had fed when blood glucose levels were measured at 60 minutes after birth. Christidis and colleagues (2003) conducted a thermogram study that showed that the entire infant's body (peripheral and trunk) was heated during skin-to-skin care following delivery rather than just the trunk, as occurs under a radiant warmer. Mothers and infants should be kept together, skin to skin, following delivery to reduce crying, maintain body temperature, prevent low blood glucose levels, and facilitate early breastfeeding. This may be more difficult with a cesarean delivery, but Erlandsson, Dsilna, Fagerberg, and Christensson (2007) showed that when fathers provide the skin-to-skin care following a cesarean delivery, the infants cried less, were calmer, and were comforted better than infants who were placed alone in a bassinet following a cesarean delivery.

The physiological impact of separating newborn infants from their mothers can affect the infant's autonomic nervous system. The physiological stress response is controlled by the autonomic nervous system, with heart rate variability being a marker of autonomic nervous system activity. To investigate the impact of maternal–newborn separation, heart rate variability was measured in infants sleeping in skin-to-skin contact with their mothers and sleeping alone for 1 hour in each place prior to discharge from the hospital. Maternal–newborn separation was associated with a dramatic increase in heart rate variability, with a 176% increase in autonomic activity and an 86% decrease in quiet sleep duration during separation compared with skin-to-skin contact (Morgan, Horn, & Bergman, 2011). Separation at this early time in life may serve as a stressor to the young infant, resulting in dysregulation and epigenetic changes in the infant (Bergman, 2014). Neuroendocrine mechanisms are involved in mother–child attachment during the early sensitive period immediately following delivery and are critically important for the development of attachment behavior (Olza-Fernandez, Gabriel, Gil-Sanchez, Garcia-Segura, & Arevalo, 2014).

Separating mothers and babies during their hospital stay has been associated with a reduced length of breastfeeding (Murray et al., 2007). Rooming-in for 60% or more of the hospital stay is significantly associated with the continuation of full breastfeeding at 4 months of age (Wright, Rice, & Wells, 1996). Rooming-in results in higher milk yields during the first 4 days after birth, most likely due to the high intensity of nonsupplemented breastfeeding (Bystrova et al., 2007). Staff attitudes and support for rooming-in have a significant effect on the practice. Svensson, Matthiesen, and Widstrom (2005) demonstrated that mothers who had not roomed-in with their infants were more likely to perceive that the staff believed their babies should stay in the nursery at night compared with those mothers who roomed-in with their babies. Negative staff attitudes toward night rooming-in may implicitly suggest to mothers that closeness and contact at this time are not important.

Separation has been shown to stress the infant. In animal research, separating the newborn from its mother is a common mechanism to create stress in the neonate in order to study the damaging effects of this practice on the developing newborn brain. Separating human infants from their mothers is a common practice in hospitals, and humans are the only mammals that engage in this practice. Morgan, Horn, and Bergman (2011) investigated the effects that separation of mother and newborn had on the infant's physiological stress response. The physiological stress response is overseen by the autonomic nervous system, and heart rate variability is a means of measuring or quantifying the activity of the autonomic nervous system activity. Heart rate variability is influenced by level of arousal, which can be quantified during sleep. Sleep is essential for early optimal brain development. This study measured heart rate variability in 16 2-day-old full-term infants sleeping in skin-to-skin contact with their mothers and sleeping alone for 1 hour in each place. There was a 176% increase in autonomic activity and an 86% decrease in quiet sleep duration during mother–newborn separation episodes compared with skin-to-skin contact. Separation that is not medically indicated is a practice that unnecessarily stresses the infant, once again demonstrating the importance of skin-to-skin care and keeping the mother and infant together and in contact with each other.

Separation of the mother and infant at birth and the practice of tightly swaddling a newborn was shown to interfere with mother–infant interactions during breastfeeding on day 4. Dumas, Lepage, Bystrova, Matthiesen, Welles-Nystrom, and Widstrom (2013) showed that infants who remained in the newborn nursery during the initial postpartum period were more difficult to wake for feedings and mothers demonstrated rougher techniques when trying to wake a sleepy baby being fed on a schedule. Swaddling and mother–infant separation disturb the normal and expected maternal and infants behaviors during the early hours and days following birth. Gubler, Krahenmann, Roos, Zimmerman, and Ochsenbein-Kolbe (2013) reported that rooming-in for less than 24 hours a day was associated with formula supplementation. This is especially worrisome knowing the importance of avoiding the introduction of foreign proteins into the immature infant gut and the increased emphasis being placed on exclusive breastfeeding in the hospital.

Self-regulation in the newborn is an important task to accomplish in the early hours post birth. Full-term healthy infants, when held skin to skin following birth, engage in 9 instinctive steps as they move toward the first feeding at breast. This inborn biological program to seek out and find the breast involves the birth cry, a relaxation phase, an awakening phase, an active phase, crawling motions, another resting phase, familiarization with the breast, a sucking phase, and finally a sleeping phase (Widstrom et al., 2011). Facilitating these 9 steps optimizes the infant's ability to achieve self-regulation. This point is important, as it has been found that 3-day-old infants with low self-regulation levels are at risk for poorer social and cognitive development as well as regulatory disorders (Lundqvist-Persson, 2001). This relationship highlights the importance of providing the opportunity for the infant to establish early self-regulation by keeping mothers and infants together and not rushing to bathe or separate the infant from the mother unless medically necessary.

CRYING

Adaptation to extrauterine life can be physiologically demanding for an infant. Misconceptions about newborn crying persist, such as the belief that newborns need to cry to expand or exercise their lungs. A full-term newborn's lungs carry an adequate functional reserve after the first breath (Karlberg, 1960) and are as fully expanded at 30 minutes after birth as they are at 24 hours after birth (Klaus, Tooley, Weaver, & Clements, 1963). Crying results in a surprising number of undesirable side effects (Ludington-Hoe, Cong, & Hashemi, 2002), which can render an infant less capable of breastfeeding.

Crying raises the heart rate by at least 19 beats per minute, varying with the intensity and duration of crying, from 170 beats per minute with slight crying to more than 200 beats per minute with hard crying, resulting in tachycardia. Crying causes both systolic and diastolic pressures to increase by 135%, and the all-important pulse pressure is reduced to values less than 1% at rest, impairing circulation to the brain (Dinwiddie, Patel, Kumar, & Fox, 1979). Unoxygenated blood is shunted to the body, reducing arterial oxygen levels by 16.8 mm Hg and resulting in desaturation (Dinwiddie, Pitcher-Wilmott, Schwartz, Shaffer, & Fox, 1979). Decreased oxygen levels and excessive right-sided heart pressures may cause the foramen ovale to open, shunting blood into the left atrium and reestablishing fetal circulation (Brazy, 1988); fluctuations in cerebral blood flow and pressure plus immature vascularization (**Figure 4-1**) can contribute to intraventricular hemorrhage in preterm infants and, if severe, result in developmental delays (Brazy, 1988; Hiraishi et al., 1991).

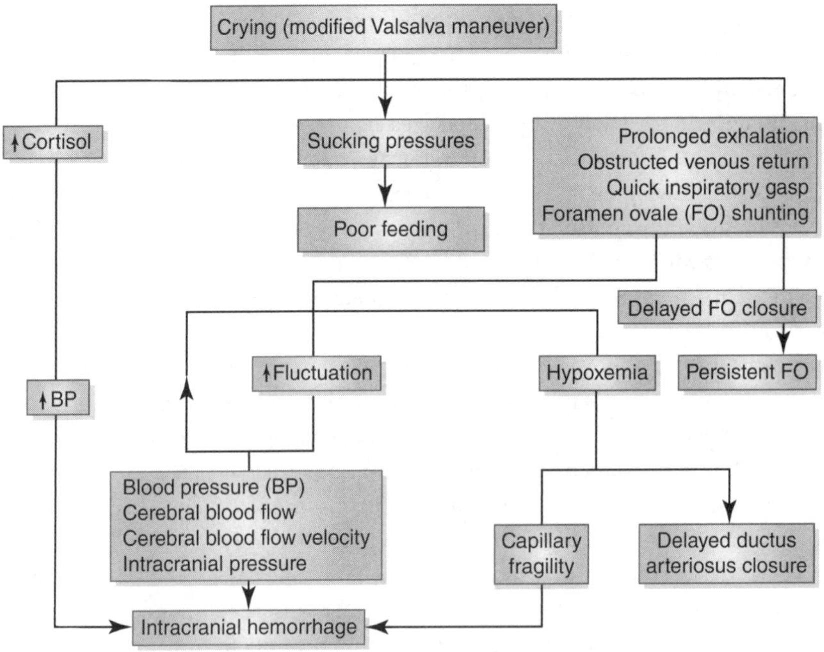

Figure 4-1 Stressor: Crying.

Full-term infants are also vulnerable to intracranial hemorrhage during this transitional time. In a study conducted on 505 asymptomatic, normal, full-term infants in a general nursery, such hemorrhages were documented at 72 hours after birth in 3% of these apparently healthy infants (Hayden et al., 1985).

Salivary cortisol levels increase as the length of crying increases, signaling stress. High levels of cortisol act as an immunosuppressant, weakening the infant's ability to fight infection. Infants can swallow a large amount of air when crying. In a study of 2- to 3-week-old infants, a mean of 360 mL of air was swallowed during crying (Shaker, Schaefer, James, & White, 1973). Distention of the stomach contributes to discomfort, reduced intake of milk, and the possibility of further crying, spitting up, and disruption in the normal feeding and digestive processes. Gastric rupture has been reported with prolonged (30 minutes) hard crying associated with circumcision (Connelly, Shropshire, & Salzberg, 1992); as crying progresses, infant behavior becomes more disorganized (Anderson, 1976) and the exhausted infant may be unable to make eye contact or breastfeed effectively.

Newborns cared for in hospital nurseries rather than in close contact with the mother have often begun crying before they are taken to their mothers. One-hour-old infants were observed displaying many oral cues and signs of stress over a period of 30 minutes before reaching a sustained cry (Gill, White, & Anderson, 1984). In busy hospital nurseries, the sustained cry typically prompts the nurse (or the mother) to determine it is time to feed the infant. A better approach is to take advantage of the infant's feeding readiness cues such as mouthing or hand-to-mouth movements and to feed him or her at that point rather than after crying has begun and the infant experiences stress (**Figure 4-2**).

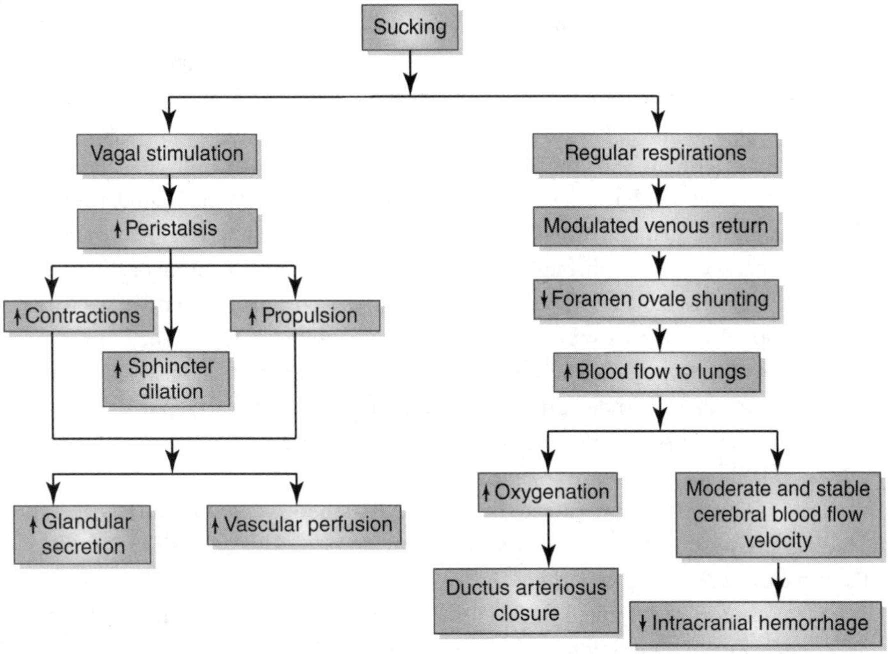

Figure 4-2 Theoretical paradigm: Sucking and crying have opposite effects.

A crying infant is also stressful to the mother, raising a woman's systolic blood pressure by 8–10 mm Hg when she first hears her baby cry (Zeskind, 1980). The cry represents a distress signal and is designed to cause a caregiving response that will meet the needs of the infant at that time (Ludington-Hoe et al., 2002); energy reserves are depleted as a result of vigorous motor movements during crying (Ludington, 1990). When crying is reduced (such as when keeping the mother and baby in close contact), blood glucose levels remain high due to decreased metabolic demand for circulating or stored glucose (Christensson et al., 1992).

Infant crying may be the primary manner in which mothers assess the adequacy of their milk production, the satisfaction or fullness of the infant, and the infant's hunger. Not all crying indicates hunger, but if crying is the primary cue used by mothers to initiate feedings, inappropriate feeding practices may be used to assure satiety, extend the sleep period, and keep the infant full for a longer period of time (Heinig et al., 2006). Giving formula supplements after satiety has been reached to reduce crying may lead to overweight or obesity in the child and early abandonment of breastfeeding. See the Additional Reading and Resources at the end of this chapter for sources to help mothers understand infant crying.

SUPPLEMENTATION

Supplementing or complementing breastmilk with other fluids and foods from an early age has been described since antiquity (Fildes, 1986). Supplementary and complementary feedings have been defined in many ways, and these terms are often used interchangeably in the literature and in clinical practice. Supplementation can refer to a feeding given in place of a breastfeed or as an extra feeding, whereas complementation often describes topping off a breastfeed with formula, water, solid food, or expressed breastmilk. Both mothers and healthcare providers may request or advise that a breastfed infant receive something other than breastmilk for a number of reasons, some of which may not be medically indicated or evidence based. Supplementing breastfed infants both in the hospital and after discharge is a common practice (Kovach, 1997). Abbott Nutritionals (formerly Ross Laboratories and Ross Products Division), an infant formula manufacturer, has collected breastfeeding data through the Mothers Survey since 1955, until the CDC became the primary collector of breastfeeding data. The infant formula manufacturer then conducted its market research through a front called the National Institute of Infant Nutrition. The survey data are no longer available to the public but have shown a disturbing trend of decreasing exclusive breastfeeding in hospital and increasing amounts of supplementation (**Box 4-3**).

Most mothers who want to exclusively breastfeed intend to do so for longer than 3 months, but the majority are not meeting their intended duration. Mothers are more likely to achieve their intended duration when their infant is not supplemented in the hospital. Perrine and colleagues (2012) reported that 40% of the 1,457 infants in their study received supplemental formula feedings in the hospital despite maternal intensions to exclusively breastfeed. In this analysis, there was a substantial gap between exclusive breastfeeding intention and exclusive breastfeeding duration, with only 32.4% of women surveyed achieving their exclusive breastfeeding intention.

Dewey and colleagues (2002) noted that 21% of the 280 infants in their study received water or formula in the hospital. Kurinij and Shiono (1991) reported that 37% of breastfed infants in their sample of 726 mothers were given formula supplementation in the hospital. However, 50% of the infants whose mothers delivered at the public or community hospital were supplemented, compared with 15% of the

Box 4-3 Hospital Formula Supplementation Trends

1971

21% exclusively breastfeeding in hospital
3% additionally supplemented

1982

55% exclusively breastfeeding in hospital
6.9% additionally supplemented

2001

46.3% exclusively breastfeeding in hospital
23% additionally supplemented

2003

44.0% exclusively breastfeeding in hospital
22% additionally supplemented

2006

38.4% exclusively breastfeeding in hospital
25.2% additionally supplemented

2009

36.6% exclusively breastfeeding in hospital
24% additionally supplemented

Based on Ryan, A. S., Wenjun, Z., & Acosta, A. (2002). Breastfeeding continues to increase into the new millennium. *Pediatrics*, 110, 1103–1109; Mothers Survey, Ross Products, Breastfeeding Trends—2003, 2006

newborns delivered at a university hospital. Women giving birth where the supplementation rates were lowest were 3.5 times more likely to be exclusively breastfeeding. The longer a mother waited to initiate breastfeeding, the more likely she was to use formula. Seventeen reasons were cited in the Kurinij and Shiono study for supplementing breastfed infants, with the top three being (1) to give the mother some rest, (2) because the mother was ill, or (3) because the mother did not have enough breastmilk.

Tender and colleagues (2009) reported that 78% of breastfed infants in their study received formula supplementation while hospitalized. Only 13% of these infants received supplementation based on the supplementation guidelines from the Academy of Breastfeeding Medicine (2009). Mothers' reasons for supplementation included the perception that the milk supply was insufficient or that her milk had not "come in" at birth. Providers' reasons for supplementing included that the infant was lactose intolerant, it helped simplify weaning, the mother was taking medications, and it allowed the mother to sleep.

Over 20% of mothers did not know why their infant was supplemented. Within the cohort of women receiving WIC benefits, 80% of breastfed infants were given supplements in the hospital, 87% of which were medically unnecessary. Infants of mothers who did not attend a prenatal breastfeeding class were 4.7 times more likely to receive formula supplementation in hospital. This study demonstrated the importance of improving medical providers' knowledge about breastfeeding and medical indications for supplementation, as well as the necessity of correcting misinformation on the part of the mother.

Crivelli-Kovach and Chung (2011) described current breastfeeding policies and practices among Philadelphia hospitals and changes in their policies and practices over time. Of the 18 participating hospitals, 40% reported that breastfed infants were receiving formula supplementation over 50% of the time, and 68% reported that supplements were given at the mother's request. Most hospitals (89%) reported giving formula supplements, compared with 37% in 1994 and 1999.

Gagnon, Leduc, Waghorn, Yang, and Platt (2005) discovered that the highest risk time of day for an infant to receive supplementation was between 7:00 pm and 9:00 am, regardless of the time of birth. Nurses in this study revealed that "insufficient milk" was a common reason for supplementing. Infant behaviors such as fussiness, sleepiness, or latching difficulties often triggered supplementation even though there are numerous breastfeeding interventions that can address these issues and do not involve supplementation. Highly anxious mothers were a subgroup of women who needed extra support and special interventions to avoid unnecessary supplementation.

Other common reasons for supplementation include a fussy, unsettled infant; a sleepy infant; a certain number of hours have passed without a feeding at the breast; the mother (or nurse) believes she does not have enough milk; and non-evidenced-based assumptions or opinions that supplementation will prevent hypoglycemia, weight loss, dehydration, or hyperbilirubinemia in the breastfed infant. A preponderance of data supports the opposite conclusion (WHO, 1998). Inappropriate supplementation can also negatively affect the immediate and long-term intensity (exclusivity) and duration of breastfeeding (Semenic, Loiselle, & Gottlieb, 2008) and serve as a potential environmental trigger for some acute and chronic diseases and conditions later in life.

Biro, Sutherland, Yelland, Hardy, and Brown (2011) reported that of the 4,085 women who initiated breastfeeding in their study, 23% reported that their infants received formula supplementation. Infants were more likely to be supplemented if the mother was primiparous (perhaps indicating a lack of confidence and/or knowledge), if the mother had a body mass index (BMI) of more than 30 (obesity can delay lactogenesis II), if the mother had a cesarean section (cesareans can delay the time to first breastfeed and the onset of copious milk production), if the infant was low-birth-weight or admitted to the special care nursery (separation and rush to feed formula), or if the infant was born in a hospital without the BFHI accreditation (indicating higher risk of non-evidence-based practice). In a study that characterized the gut microbiome of 102 six-week-old infants (70 vaginally delivered and 32 by cesarean delivery), it was observed that those breastfed infants who were supplemented with formula had intestinal microbial communities similar to those infants who were exclusively formula fed (Madan et al., 2016). Cesarean birth resulted in a significant difference in the gut microbiome compared with vaginally born infants. Alterations in the newborn gut microbiome, whether from mode of delivery or from formula supplementation are known to have lifelong consequences (Thompson, 2012).

Realizing the importance of exclusive breastmilk feeding and the growing problem of inappropriate formula supplementation, The Joint Commission's Pregnancy and Related Conditions core measure set was retired and replaced with the new Perinatal Care core measure set. The new Perinatal Care core measure set became available for selection by hospitals beginning with April 1, 2010, discharges (The Joint Commission, 2011). The Joint Commission has mandated that starting in January 2014, hospitals with more than 1,100 births per year will be mandated to select the Perinatal Care core measure set, which includes the metric of exclusive breastmilk feeding at discharge. Hospitals will be required to measure this as well as being expected to take measures to improve those numbers over time (The Joint Commission, 2012). The Joint Commission assumes that implementation of evidence-based best practices for infant feeding will reduce the number of infants who receive formula supplementation for nonmedical reasons and increase the number of exclusively breastmilk-fed infants at discharge. The Joint Commission has made the distinction between exclusive breastfeeding and exclusive breastmilk feeding to permit infants with breastfeeding difficulties to be supplemented with human milk and still be counted as exclusively breastmilk fed. The Joint Commission realizes that in any hospital there will always be a small number of breastfed infants in whom supplementation is medically indicated, even with exemplary implementation of best practices. The Joint Commission relies on experience with public reporting on exclusive breastfeeding in California, which shows that less than 10% of breastfed infants are supplemented in the top-performing hospitals.

Formula Supplementation Effects on Intensity and Duration of Breastfeeding

Research from as early as the 1970s has shown that the introduction of breastmilk substitutes (water or formula), whether in the hospital or in the first month of life, has a consistently negative effect on the duration of breastfeeding. Blomquist, Jonsbo, Serenius, and Persson (1994) found that breastfed infants who had been given supplements in the hospital were almost four times more likely to have weaned by 3 months of age and were seven times less likely to be breastfed at 3 months if they experienced in-hospital supplementation and experienced a loss of 10% birth weight or more. However, among infants receiving supplements for the specific indications of maternal insulin-dependent diabetes mellitus or gestational diabetes, the duration of breastfeeding was similar to that in the nonsupplemented group. Supplementation without medical reasons significantly reduces the duration of both exclusive and partial breastfeeding; conversely, supplementation for medical reasons does not have this type of dramatic effect on intensity or duration of breastfeeding (Ekstrom, Widstrom, & Nissen, 2003). Even one bottle of formula can affect the duration of breastfeeding. Chezem, Friesen, Montgomery, Fortman, and Clark (1998) looked at the patterns of human milk replacement during hospitalization. In a small sample of 53 mothers, 28% of their infants received at least one oral replacement while in the hospital. Duration of breastfeeding was significantly shorter in women whose infants received any formula during hospitalization (9 weeks) compared with women whose infants were not fed formula (20 weeks). Only 40% of the infants fed formula in the hospital were still breastfeeding at 6 weeks, compared with 88% of those not fed formula.

In a population of low-income women, Bolton, Chow, Benton, and Olson (2009) reported that formula introduction on day 1 postpartum was associated with a significantly shorter breastfeeding duration and that the most dramatic predictor of breastfeeding duration was introduction of formula on day 1. Because early weaning is associated with the early introduction of formula (Hornell, Hofvander, & Kylberg, 2001), delaying formula introduction may be highly effective in lengthening the duration of breastfeeding. Breastfeeding support interventions must address methods to reduce excessive formula supplementation in-hospital.

In a study that examined the relationship between in-hospital formula supplementation and breastfeeding duration among 393 first-time mothers who intended to exclusively breastfeed, it was found that 47% of the infants received formula supplementation in the hospital (Chantry, Dewey, Peerson, Wagner, & Nommsen-Rivers, 2014). Formula supplementation use was associated with almost 2 times the risk of breastfeeding cessation by day 30 and almost 3 times the risk of breastfeeding cessation by day 60. The larger the volume of formula the infant received, the more likely that breastfeeding had ceased by days 30 and 60. When looking at some of the associations between infant formula supplementation and labor and postpartum characteristics, it was found that 70.6% of infants were supplemented if Pitocin was used to induce and augment labor, 69.6% were supplemented if delivered by cesarean section, 91% were supplemented if the mother first held the infant more than 2 hours after delivery, 93% were supplemented if the first breastfeeding occurred more than 4 hours after delivery, and 73.1% were supplemented if the infant breastfed fewer than 8 times in the first 24 hours. Many of the reasons for supplementation (e.g., perceived insufficient milk, concern over infant inadequate intake, poor infant breastfeeding behavior) could have been addressed with early intervention for maternal concerns, maternal education regarding feeding capabilities of newborns, a greater understanding of the physiology of early breastfeeding, and minimizing formula feedings by bottle.

One intervention that reduces formula supplementation in hospitals is to ensure that mothers breastfeed in the labor, delivery, and recovery room (Komara et al., 2007). Newborn medications can be stocked in the labor, delivery, and recovery room so staff can administer the required medications while avoiding the separation of mothers and infants during the early time after birth. Because staff members may perceive infant formula to be free, it is used and given away liberally. Not only is infant formula frequently seen as a fix for breastfeeding problems, but some hospital staffs give large quantities of formula to breastfeeding mothers at discharge from the hospital. One way hospitals have helped restrict formula use in breastfed infants to actual medical indications is to lock up the formula and require staff to log out the formula, noting the formula batch number in case there is a recall, date and time of formula use, patient and staff member's names, and reason for use. Some hospitals manage formula use by placing it in a medication distribution system such as Pyxis. Such protocols help provide information on where additional staff education may be needed and help reduce unnecessary formula supplementation (Cadwell & Turner-Maffei, 2009).

Use of daily human milk replacements is negatively correlated with breastfeeding duration, regardless of the mother's prenatal intentions to exclusively or partially breastfeed (Chezem, Friesen, & Boettcher, 2003). Bottles of formula can be the cause of breastfeeding problems or a symptom of breastfeeding difficulties. Infants who are given non-breastmilk fluids in the first 48 hours or offered pacifiers have been shown to be two to three times more likely to have suboptimal breastfeeding behaviors on days 3 and 7 (Infant Breastfeeding Assessment Tool score < 10), interfering with the establishment of effective breastfeeding (Dewey et al., 2003). Sievers, Haase, Oldigs, and Schaub (2003) studied peripartum indicators for mothers and infants who were most at risk for early lactation failure. Partial feeding of infant formula or an intake of less than 150 g of human milk per day 24–48 hours after lactogenesis II was linked to weaning within 4 weeks.

Supplementation has a marked effect on lactogenesis III, or the calibration and maintenance of a sufficient milk supply (Daly, Owens, & Hartmann, 1993). This interference with the body's ability to accomplish and sustain the production of copious amounts of milk can result in reduced amounts of breastmilk transferred to the infant (Drewett et al., 1989) and a repeating cycle of more formula supplementation until the body receives the signal for breast involution. Breastfeeding frequency and duration decline quickly after the start of regular formula supplementation (one or more bottles of formula per day). Indeed, the younger infants are at the start of regular formula supplementation, the younger they are when they stop breastfeeding (Hornell et al., 2001). The most frequent reason for supplementing young infants is the mother's impression that she does not have enough milk to satisfy the infant. Whether this shortage is real or merely perceived, intervention is needed to prevent the downward spiral toward weaning.

Breastfeeding intensity or degree of exclusivity has been shown to be predictive of duration of breastfeeding up to 1 year of age. Petrova, Hegyi, and Mehta (2007) found that women who exclusively breastfed in the hospital were more likely to be exclusively breastfeeding at 1 month following delivery compared with mothers who introduced formula during the hospital stay. Among mothers who exclusively breastfed in the hospital, 50.9% were exclusively breastfeeding at the end of the first month, compared with 20.3% of mothers who introduced formula during their hospital stay. Hill, Humenick, Brennan, and Woolley (1997) followed 343 mothers for 20 weeks or until weaning, observing the supplementation patterns and subsequent rate of breastfeeding at 5 months postpartum. The breastfeeding rate at 20 weeks was significantly greater for mothers who reported feeding breastmilk exclusively at 2 weeks postpartum (~ 61%) compared with mothers who supplemented with formula (~ 26%). Using data from the 1988 National Maternal–Infant Health Survey, Piper and Parks (1996) reported that exclusive breastfeeding during the first month postpartum was associated with a breastfeeding duration of longer than 6 months. The strongest association with breastfeeding duration of 1 year was a higher breastfeeding intensity during months 4–6 postpartum (Piper & Parks, 2001).

Hispanic infants are at a high risk for being supplemented with not only formula but also tea and water. Wojcicki and colleagues (2011) reported that of 192 Latina mothers in their study, 44.7% of the breastfed infants were supplemented with formula by 4–6 weeks, 9% were fed breastmilk with water or tea, and 37.4% were exclusively breastfed. Including the exclusively formula-fed infants, 25.4% of all of the infants in this study were supplemented with water or teas at 4–6 weeks. Supplementing breastfed infants with water and/or teas increases the risk of micronutrient deficiencies from a diet of reduced breastmilk.

Given that perceived insufficient milk production is a frequent reason for supplementing with formula or abandoning breastfeeding altogether, an intervention that might be helpful in countermanding this perception is weighing the infant before and after each breastfeeding for a full 24-hour period to determine if adequate milk transfer is taking place (Kent, Hepworth, Langton, & Hartmann, 2015). This practice may help confirm if low milk production is present or if the infant is not transferring a sufficient volume of milk. Data from this intervention may direct the clinician to reassure the mother that she has sufficient milk production or alert the clinician that there is a milk transfer problem with the infant.

Distribution of discharge bags from formula companies is another form of supplementation with commercial overtones. These bags represent a marketing tactic (not a gift) designed to cause breastfeeding mothers to supplement and purchase more of the product, thus creating a market where none existed before (Walker, 2007). Women who received these packages were more likely to exclusively breastfeed for fewer than 10 weeks than were women who had not received the packages (Rosenberg, Eastham, & Kasehagen,

2008). The distribution of these bags to new mothers by hospitals is part of a long-standing marketing campaign by infant formula manufacturers and implies hospital and staff endorsement of infant formula. Many hospitals have recognized the ethical problems created by commercial relationships with infant formula manufacturers and have eliminated the distribution of formula company bags. They have created their own bags, marketing their birthing services rather than allowing formula company access to their patients. More than 900 U.S. hospitals have eliminated these bags, often with help from the Ban the Bags campaign (http://www.banthebags.org), which provides materials and assistance with formula company bag elimination. This is reflected in the impressive 41% reduction in hospitals distributing commercial formula gifts, from 72.6% in 2007 to 31.6% in 2013 (Nelson, Li, & Perrine, 2015).

Weight Loss

The AAP states that an acceptable weight loss for breastfed infants during the first 3–5 days of life is up to 7% of the birth weight, with an evaluation for breastfeeding problems if weight loss exceeds 7% (AAP, Section on Breastfeeding, 2012). Concern about the potential for excessive weight loss in an exclusively breastfed infant has been used to justify the prophylactic and "therapeutic" feeding of water, glucose water, and formula. It represents a significant threat to exclusive breastfeeding in the hospital. Lack of understanding regarding the amount of colostrum available and required by newborns has led both parents and healthcare providers to urge breastfed infants to consume sterile water, 5% dextrose water, 10% dextrose water, or formula in an attempt to compensate for "insufficient milk," in an effort to feed the infant "until the milk comes in," or because the infant is "too big" or "too small." Research shows that breastfed infants on average lose about 5–7% of their birth weight in the first few days of life, peaking on day 3 after birth and recovering by day 8 (Crossland, Richmond, Hudson, Smith, & Abu-Harb, 2008; Macdonald, Ross, Grant, & Young, 2003; Rodriguez et al., 2000). Clinicians become watchful and may intervene when this weight loss reaches 7–10%. Weight loss exceeding 10% of birth weight must be addressed. Flaherman, Bokser, and Newman (2010) reported that newborn weight loss in the first 24 hours was a strong predictor of eventual weight loss during the hospital stay. A weight loss greater than 4% by 24 hours was associated with a twofold increase in the odds of eventual in-hospital weight loss equal to or greater than 10%. This study did not take into account the amount of IV fluid received by the mother during labor. Increased weight loss in breastfed infants has also been associated with cesarean delivery (Manganaro, Mami, Marrone, Marseglia, & Gemelli, 2001). Preer, Newby, and Philipp (2012) found that exclusively breastfed infants delivered by cesarean birth in the absence of labor experienced higher than expected weight loss. They speculate that one reason for this heightened weight loss could be that retained lung fluid contributed to a greater percentage of weight loss as the fluid is diuresed during the early hours and days following birth. Slower than normal clearance of lung fluid can result from the absence of labor, which slows the rapid reabsorption of fetal lung fluid seen after a vaginal birth. Clinicians will need to exercise greater vigilance in cesarean-born infants to assure extra breastfeeding support and rapid resolution of any breastfeeding problems. However, Preer and colleagues counsel that if weight loss in these infants is slightly higher than expected, but the infant is latching well, transferring colostrum, and voiding and stooling adequately, then clinical concern may be reduced.

Many mothers receive large amounts of IV fluids during labor. Significant weight loss in the newborn's first days following birth may be related to a fluid shift from the mother to the fetus in the absence of breastfeeding inadequacies or pathology. Because weight loss is often the driver of interventions such as delayed discharge or formula supplementation, it is important that clinicians take into account newborn fluid overload as a contributor to newborn weight loss. Numerous authors have demonstrated a relationship between intrapartum fluid intake and neonatal weight loss:

- Mulder, Johnson, and Baker (2010) studied 53 breastfeeding infants who lost either less than or greater than 7% of the birth weight during the hospital stay. Infants losing greater than 7% of their birth weight were shown to have significantly more total voids and a higher breastfeeding frequency than infants losing less than 7% of their birth weight. In the absence of other indicators of ineffective breastfeeding, infants losing greater than 7% of their birth weight may be experiencing a physiological diuresis not related to their breastfeeding behaviors.
- Lamp and Macke (2010) also showed that a strong predictor of neonatal weight loss within the first 48 hours included the average number of wet diapers.
- Okumus and colleagues (2011) reported that postnatal weight loss was higher in infants whose mothers had a cesarean delivery and epidural analgesia compared with infants whose mothers experienced a vaginal delivery. Postnatal weight losses were correlated with the amount of IV fluid volume infused into the mother during the last 6 hours prior to delivery.
- Chantry, Nommsen-Rivers, Peerson, Cohen, and Dewey (2011) reported that the relative risk of infants losing greater than 10% of their birth weight tripled when women had a positive fluid balance of greater than 200 mL/hour during the intrapartum period.
- Watson, Hodnett, Armson, Davies, and Watt-Watson (2012) showed that weight loss in infants whose mothers received greater than 2,500 mL of IV fluid was significantly higher than in infants whose mothers received lower IV fluid volumes.
- Noel-Weiss, Woodend, Peterson, Gibb, and Groll (2011) demonstrated a correlation between neonatal urine output, the amount of infused maternal IV fluids, and newborn weight loss. For mothers who received 1,200 mL or less of IV fluids, the average percentage of newborn weight loss at 60 hours was 5.51%. The group receiving more than 1,200 mL of total fluids had infants who averaged a 6.93% weight loss. Late onset of lactogenesis II showed a positive correlation to the percentage of newborn weight loss.

These authors suggest that newborns may have an artificially high reference point for newborn weight loss when using birth weight as the reference. Resetting the baseline weight to a point after diuresis has occurred and the weight has stabilized may provide a more accurate way to determine actual weight loss. A frequency analysis of percentage weight loss was conducted to contrast two possible outcomes using a baseline of the actual birth weight compared to weight 24 hours later, after diuresis had occurred in the infants in this study. Using a 24-hour baseline weight, 2.3% of infants lost between 7% and 10% of their birth weight, with none losing more than 10%. However, when using the actual weight at birth as a baseline, 33% of newborns lost between 7% and 10% of their birth weight, and 7.3% lost more than 10%. Perhaps weight at 24 hours is a better reference point at which to start monitoring newborn weight loss, rather than actual weight at birth.

Breastfeeding is not necessarily a risk factor for greater neonatal weight loss if weight loss is monitored, breastfeeding is repeatedly assessed and appropriately supported, and careful supplementation (preferably with expressed colostrum) is judiciously used to treat excess weight loss (Davanzo, Cannioto, Ronfani, Monasta, & Demarini, 2012).

Supplementing breastfed infants in the hospital with water or formula does not necessarily prevent weight loss (Herrera, 1984; Shrago, 1987). Bertini, Dani, Tronchin, and Rubaltelli (2001) also confirmed the relationship between supplementation of breastfed infants with formula and weight loss. Breastfed infants supplemented with formula lost significantly more weight than exclusively breastfed infants or exclusively bottle-fed infants (Bertini et al., 2001). In a chart audit of 74 mothers, breastfed infants who received glucose water demonstrated a larger percentage of birth weight loss (2.43–15.87%) compared with unsupplemented breastfed newborns (2.97–7.48%) (Glover, 1990). Weight loss in infants supplemented with sterile water or 5% glucose water is consistent with the lower caloric density of these fluids compared with colostrum, transitional milk, and mature milk. One ounce of 5% dextrose water contains 5 calories, 1 ounce of 10% dextrose water contains 10 calories, and 1 ounce of colostrum contains 18–20 calories. For each ounce of 5% dextrose water consumed by a breastfed infant, his or her caloric intake is reduced by approximately two-thirds. The risk of excess infant weight loss has been shown to be 7.1 times greater if the mother has delayed onset of milk production (Dewey et al., 2003). Neifert (1998, 1999) recommended that weight loss of 8% or more from birth weight, failure to surpass birth weight by 2 weeks of age, or failure to commence weight gain of approximately 28 g per day by 5 days of age warrants further investigation.

Healthy full-term newborns have an abundance of extracellular and extravascular water. Caution therefore is necessary in the use of water supplementation of newborns. Water intoxication with seizures has been reported in a breastfed infant who was given 675 mL (22.5 oz) of supplementary glucose water during the 24 hours before transfer from the maternity unit to the neonatal intensive care unit (Ruth-Sanchez & Greene, 1997). Supplementation should not be used in place of skilled assessment and prompt and correct lactation care and services. Neonates born to mothers who have received dextrose-containing IV fluids during labor can experience enough of a fluid shift to skew weight loss calculations toward the appearance of a clinical problem of excessive loss of birth weight, when what is really taking place is a diuresis of excess fluid (Keppler, 1988). Dahlenburg, Burnell, and Braybrook (1980) examined the serum sodium levels in newborns whose mothers received IV fluids containing 5% dextrose and oxytocin. The mean sodium levels were significantly lower in the infants whose mothers had IV fluids compared with those who did not. Percentage of weight loss in infants whose mothers received IV fluids was 6.17% ± 3.36% compared with 4.07% ± 2.20% weight loss in infants whose mothers did not receive IV fluids during labor. Both maternal and neonatal serum sodium concentrations are significantly decreased even when dextrose is used only as the diluent (rather than normal saline) for oxytocin infusion in induction or augmentation of labor (Higgins, Gleeson, Holohan, Cooney, & Darling, 1996; Stratton, Stronge, & Boylan, 1995).

Breastfed infants whose mothers received epidurals have been shown to lose more weight in the first 24 hours than infants whose mothers did not have an epidural. Merry and Montgomery (2000) reported that the average weight loss in the first day for infants whose mothers had an epidural was 226 g (8 oz) compared with 142 g (5 oz) in a nonepidural group. It is possible that administration of IV fluids during labor, which is more common in women receiving analgesia or anesthesia, could initially increase the hydration status of the newborn, with a subsequent rapid weight loss mimicking underfeeding. Once started, water supplementation remains prevalent in the first month of life, even in exclusively breastfed infants (Scariati, Grummer-Strawn, & Fein, 1997).

Martens and Romphf (2007) demonstrated that factors significantly increasing the percentage of weight loss in newborn infants included birth weight, female sex, epidural use, and a longer hospital stay. In this study, supplemented breastfed infants lost more weight than exclusively breastfed newborns, as did those whose mothers had epidurals during labor and delivery. Formula-fed infants lost approximately 3% of birth weight, substantially less than a breastfed infant who represents the norm. The authors speculated that formula-fed infants (who were 111 g heavier than breastfed infants during the first 3 days postpartum) may be at risk for overfeeding in the early days and were actually being overfed at a time when early feeding experiences could be critical to metabolic imprinting and future overweight or obesity (de Moura, Lisboa, & Passos, 2008; Lucas, 1998). Unnecessary or unphysiological amounts of formula supplement may predispose infants to later weight problems. Stettler and colleagues (2005) found a 28% increased risk of obesity in adulthood for every 100 g of weight an infant gained in his or her first week of life.

Caglar, Ozer, and Altugan (2006) reported that infants with a weight loss of more than 10% were more likely to be from primiparous mothers, to experience a delay in receiving their first breastfeeding, to pass less than four stools per day, and to have uric acid crystals in their diaper. These findings alert the clinician to the need by first-time mothers for extra vigilance; mothers must know how to tell when the infant is swallowing and ensure that the infant is swallowing milk.

Assessment of effective or ineffective breastfeeding and supplementation interventions must rely on more than just weight loss. Often, the underlying assumption is that weight loss is due to insufficient milk supply or ineffective milk transfer, but other confounding factors may also be present. Birthing practices, hospital routines, maternal IV fluid volume, and birth experiences are also associated with weight loss. Seldom is the amount of stooling and voiding entered into the equation of neonatal weight loss. Weight change patterns help clinicians identify situations of concern, but interventions such as supplementing breastfeeding with formula should not be solely based on maintaining an infant's weight within preestablished norms (Noel-Weiss, Courant, & Woodend, 2008).

Dehydration

Prophylactic or routine administration of water or formula to breastfed infants to prevent dehydration has not been shown to be necessary. Dehydration is unlikely to occur in full-term healthy newborns who are able to successfully transfer colostrum and milk from the breast and who are given ample opportunities to do so when they demonstrate feeding readiness cues. Rodriguez and colleagues (2000) calculated the loss of total body water and body solids during the first 3 days of life. The percentage of total body water actually increased, indicating adequate hydration, whereas the weight of the infant decreased due to the greater loss of body solids (stool), not the loss of total body water. Infants who pass several large meconium stools during the first 24–48 hours may give the appearance of not being adequately fed or hydrated but do not require intervention unless other feeding parameters are not acceptable.

Renal function in the newborn differs from that in older children and adults. The normal neonate has 6–44 mL of urine in the bladder at birth. Approximately 17% of newborns void directly after delivery, 92% by 24 hours, and 99% by 48 hours. Newborns tend to be oliguric (low urinary output) for the first day because of high circulating levels of antidiuretic hormone after birth. If the infant voided at delivery, urine output in the first 24 hours may be misleading (Black, 2001) because another void may not become

Table 4-2 Urine Volume mL/24 h

Full Term	2 Weeks	8 Weeks	1 Year
15–60	250–400	250–400	500–600

Data from Ingelfinger, J. R. (1991). Renal conditions in the newborn period. In J. P. Cloherty & A. R. Stark (Eds.), *Manual of neonatal care* (3rd ed., pp. 477–495). Boston, MA: Little, Brown and Company.

apparent until many hours later. The full-term infant typically creates a urine volume of 15–60 mL per 24 hours. Voiding size is 19.3 mL, with urine formation ranging from 0.5 to 5.0 mg/kg/h at all gestational ages. Normal neonates void 2–6 times per day during the first 48 hours of life and 5–25 times daily thereafter. Voiding during the first 2–3 days reflects the depletion of the infant's extravascular and extracellular reserve and may be reflected in diaper counts of one to two diapers, with amounts increasing as lactogenesis II occurs on days 3–4. Urine output increases rapidly after this time (**Table 4-2**).

Hypernatremic dehydration, however, can represent the extreme spectrum of a deteriorating clinical situation (Neifert, 2001). An infant who is unable to transfer milk and a mother who has a depleted milk supply, delayed lactogenesis II, underproduction, or any number of other risk factors (**Boxes 4-4** and **4-5**) should be evaluated promptly to avoid true infant dehydration. Fever and hypernatremia are often found in neonates with excessive weight loss. In low-risk, full-term infants, fever with no other symptoms during the first days is frequently related to dehydration and problems with breastfeeding. Jaundice and poor sucking may be the major presenting symptoms (Unal, Arhan, Kara, Uncu, & Alliefendioglu, 2007). Hypernatremia can cause disruption in the blood–brain barrier, facilitating the diffusion of bilirubin into the brain. This can lead to a worsening cycle of dehydration, jaundice, and hypernatremia. Often, jaundice is the presenting complaint along with a weight loss of greater than 7% (Uras, Karadag, Dogan, Tonbul, & Tatli, 2007). Hypernatremic dehydration may be difficult to recognize clinically, but weight loss and inadequate stooling are sensitive indicators of dehydration (Moritz, Manole, Bogen, & Ayus, 2005).

Box 4-4 Maternal Risk Factors for Infant Dehydration

- Previous insufficient milk or underweight, breastfed infant
- Flat or inverted nipples affecting infant latch or milk removal
- Breast anomalies such as markedly asymmetrical, tubular, or hypoplastic breasts
- Excessive, prolonged, or unrelieved breast engorgement
- Previous breast surgery (periareolar incisions, abscess)
- Cracked, bleeding nipples or persistent nipple pain
- Perinatal complications (hemorrhage, hypertension, infection)
- Preexisting maternal conditions (overweight, obesity, diabetes, endocrine disorders)
- Lack of previous breastfeeding experience
- Maternal age older than 37 years
- Labor and delivery variations (vacuum extraction, labor medications, prolonged labor)

Box 4-5 Early Infant Breastfeeding Risk Factors for Dehydration

- Gestation age (preterm and near-term 36–37 weeks)
- Small for gestation age, intrauterine growth retardation, low-birth-weight
- Separation from mother for more than 24 hours
- Oral anatomic defects (cleft lip/palate, micrognathia, macroglossia, ankyloglossia, bubble palate)
- Neurological or neuromotor problems (Down syndrome, dysfunctional sucking)
- Sucking variations (nonsustained, non-nutritive, disorganized, weak)
- Hyperbilirubinemia, especially if using phototherapy
- Multiple births
- Systemic illness (increased oxygen requirement, cardiac defect, infection)
- Difficulty latching correctly to one or both breasts
- Sleepy infant with poor or subtle feeding cues
- Irritability, fretfulness, apparent hunger after feeds
- Excessive pacifier use
- Weight loss of more than 7% of birth weight
- Not passing yellow, breastmilk stools by 4 days of age; fewer than four sizable stools per day between 4 days and 4 weeks of age
- Fewer than six clear voids per day by 4 days of age
- Appearance of urate crystals in the diaper after 3 days of age
- Failure to exceed birth weight by 10–14 days of age
- Failure to begin weight gain of approximately 28 g/day after day 4 or 5

Modified from Neifert, M. R. (2001). Prevention of breastfeeding tragedies. *Pediatric Clinics of North America, 48*, 273–297; Walker, M. (1989). Functional assessment of infant breastfeeding patterns. *Birth, 16*, 140–147.

Scant bowel output during the first 5 days after delivery or delayed transition of bowel movements to a yellow color are markers for immediate follow-up (Shrago, Reifsnider, & Insel, 2006).

Konetzny, Bucher, and Arlettaz (2009) found that infants born by cesarean section had a 3.4 times higher risk for hypernatremia than those born vaginally, reminding clinicians that these babies may need closer follow-up both during the hospital stay and after discharge. Weighing infants at 72–96 hours after birth helps in the early recognition of hypernatremic dehydration and reduces the extent of the dehydration and hypernatremia while preserving breastfeeding (Iyer et al., 2008). Mothers should be provided with information (**Figure 4-3**) that addresses feeding adequacy and alerts them to when they should consult a healthcare provider (Livingstone, Willis, Abdel-Wareth, Thiessen, & Lockitch, 2000).

Early signs and symptoms of dehydration include jaundice, decreased bowel movements, decreased urination, dry mucous membranes, sunken fontanel, poor skin turgor, lethargy, fever, and irritability. Charts with standard deviation score (SDS) lines for weight loss in the first month were constructed for 2,359 healthy breastfed newborns and 271 infants with breastfeeding-associated hypernatremic dehydration. Many infants with hypernatremic dehydration and those who eventually developed the condition fell below the −1 SDS line on day 3, the −2 SDS line on day 4, and the −2.5 SDS line on day 5. Even at this early age, the charts demonstrated that weight loss differed between healthy

Breastfeeding Checklist for Newborns

Post on your refrigerator or on the back of your bathroom door.

Baby's birth date and time: ____________________

Your baby will be 4 days old on ____________________

Baby's birth weight: ____________________

Baby's discharge weight: ____________________
(It's normal to lose up to 7% from birth.)

Baby's weight at check-up 2 days after discharge: __________

Baby's second week weight: ____________________
(Baby should have regained his birth weight by 14 days.)

Important Numbers:

Pediatrician: ____________________

OB-GYN Doctor: ____________________

Lactation Consultant: ____________________

Find more support near you at Zipmilk.org – just enter your zip code.

Some signs that breastfeeding is going well:

- ☐ Your baby is breastfeeding at least 8 times every 24 hours.
- ☐ Your baby has at least 4 yellow bowel movements every 24 hours by day 4.
- ☐ You can hear your baby gulping or swallowing at feedings.
- ☐ Once your baby latches on, your nipples do not hurt when your baby nurses.
- ☐ Your baby is receiving only breastmilk.

Check in with your pediatrician's office or lactation consultant if:

- ☐ Your baby is having fewer than 4 poopy diapers per 24 hours by day 4.
- ☐ There are any red stains in the diaper after day 3. (It can be normal in the first 3 days.)
- ☐ Your baby is still having black tarry bowel movements on day 4.
- ☐ Your baby is not breastfeeding at least 8 times every 24 hours.
- ☐ You can't hear your baby gulping or swallowing, or you can't tell.
- ☐ Your nipples hurt during feeding, even after the baby is first latched on.
- ☐ Your baby does not seem satisfied after most feedings.

It is your responsibility to contact your baby's doctor to schedule visits, including a visit 2 days after going home.

Do not wait to call your baby's doctor or the lactation consultant if *you* think breastfeeding is not going well.

Massachusetts Breastfeeding Coalition

www.massbfc.org | zipmilk.org

Figure 4-3 Breastfeeding checklist for newborns.
Massachusetts Breastfeeding Coalition (www.massbfc.org). Used with permission.

term breastfed newborns and those with hypernatremic dehydration (van Dommelen, Boer, Unal, & van Wouwe, 2014). Use of these charts may signal a need for more intense breastfeeding support and help prevent unnecessary formula supplementation.

Hyperbilirubinemia

Prevention of hyperbilirubinemia is a frequently cited reason for recommending supplementation, as is the misconception that bilirubin can be flushed out of the system by increasing water intake. At birth, normal, healthy, full-term infants have a cord total serum bilirubin concentration of about 1.5 mg/dL (25.5 μmol/L). This increases in the early days to a mean peak of approximately 5.5 mg/dL (93.5 |imol/L) by the third day in black and white infants and 10 mg/dL (170 |imol/L) in infants of Asian ethnicity (Halamek & Stevenson, 1996). Breastfed Asian infants (Japanese, Korean, and Chinese) as well as breastfed Navajo Indian and Alaska Native newborns appear to have exaggerated physiological jaundice independent of feeding method (Saland, McNamara, & Cohen, 1974).

Breastfed and formula-fed infants have been shown to have differing bilirubin patterns, with breastfed infants experiencing a more gradual decline in bilirubin levels or with bilirubin concentration reaching a second peak around the 10th day of life (Gartner & Herschel, 2001). Feeding frequency and bilirubin levels are inversely associated in the first 3 days of life. Infants fed eight times or less per 24 hours had significantly higher bilirubin levels on day 3 (9.3 mg/dL) than did infants fed more than eight times per 24 hours (6.5 mg/dL) (De Carvalho, Klaus, & Merkatz, 1982). As the frequency of breastfeeding decreases, the incidence and levels of bilirubin increase over the first week of life. Yamauchi and Yamanouchi (1990a) looked at the frequency of breastfeeding during the first 24 hours and the incidence of bilirubin levels exceeding 15 mg/dL at 6 days. Infants who fed 8–11 times per day had a 0% rate, those feeding 7–8 times per 24 hours had a rate of 11.8%, those feeding 5–6 times per 24 hours yielded a 15.2% rate, those feeding 3–4 times showed a 24.5% rate, and infants fed less frequently than 3 times showed a 28.1% rate of significant jaundice.

- Water supplementation has an inverse relationship with bilirubin levels. The more water given to breastfed infants, the higher their bilirubin levels (Nicoll, Ginsburg, & Tripp, 1982). Supplementary water does not prophylactically prevent or lower bilirubin levels (De Carvalho, Hall, & Harvey, 1981).
- Meconium passage is also related to bilirubin levels. As stooling volume increases, serum bilirubin levels decrease. Early initiation and more frequent breastfeeding avoid delayed fecal bilirubin clearance (De Carvalho, Robertson, & Klaus, 1985).
- High bilirubin levels are related to significant weight loss in the newborn. Lack of calories from inefficient breastfeeding contributes to delayed gastrointestinal motility, increasing the enterohepatic circulation of bilirubin. Salas and colleagues (2009) showed that severe hyperbilirubinemia was significantly related to excessive weight loss in newborns. Chen, Yeh, and Chen (2015) observed that jaundiced neonates showed significantly less body weight gain from hospital discharge to outpatient follow-up. To reduce the incidence of hyperbilirubinemia, discharge instructions were provided to mothers that emphasized frequent breastfeeds. Of the 98 neonates who participated in this study, 63 breastfed fewer than 8 times per day and 35 breastfed 8 or more times per day.

Those infants who breastfed 8 or more times per day exhibited a significantly lower incidence of hyperbilirubinemia. In a study of 343 infants in Taiwan, birth weight loss cutoff values were calculated as a predictive tool for progression to significant hyperbilirubinemia at 72 hours. The results showed that birth weight losses of 4.48% on day 1, 7.60% by day 2, and 8.15% by day 3 were predictive of significant hyperbilirubinemia at 72 hours following birth (Yang et al., 2013). Clinically, this suggests that even in infants with high weight losses on days 1 and 2, optimal interventions may avoid progression to significant hyperbilirubinemia by 72 hours. Such interventions would include 8 or more breastfeedings per 24 hours, documented infant swallowing of colostrum by hospital staff, mother's ability to ascertain when the infant is swallowing, and methods to increase colostrum and milk transfer such as breast compressions while sucking.

Bertini and colleagues (2001) reported a significant correlation between breastfed infants with significant jaundice (bilirubin levels > 12.9 mg/dL; 221 mmol/L) and supplementary feeding. Breastfed infants did not have higher bilirubin levels in the first days of life, except for a subpopulation that showed a greater weight loss than the mean. Jaundice was not associated with breastfeeding per se but rather with an increased weight loss after birth subsequent to fasting, suggesting the important role of caloric intake in the regulation of serum bilirubin. Thus breastfed infants who receive low-calorie supplements in place of colostrum and breastfed infants who are unable to transfer colostrum and subsequently receive supplementation show much higher levels of bilirubin. Among the other conditions favoring jaundice (ABO blood incompatibility, supplementary feeding, weight loss, and Asian ethnicity) was the finding that infants born by vacuum extraction were at a high risk for exaggerated jaundice. Seventeen percent of vacuum-extracted infants had total serum bilirubin values exceeding 12.9 mg/dL. This finding is consistent with the development of scalp or brain bleeding and has been reported in the past (Rubaltelli, 1968).

Once formed, bilirubin cannot be diluted or flushed out by giving additional water. This substance is conjugated by the liver, and almost all of it is excreted via the bile into the stools. Water is not a limiting or facilitating factor in bilirubin metabolism. Giving additional water decreases breastmilk and caloric intake, reduces breast stimulation, increases the risk for insufficient milk, increases bilirubin levels, and is counterproductive to establishing breastfeeding and adequate lactation. Water supplements may result in adequate hydration but create simultaneous caloric deprivation, contributing to the very situation the supplements were supposed to avoid. As Gartner (1994) reminds clinicians, "In the great majority of cases of breastfeeding jaundice, the evidence points to inappropriate or thoughtless policies and procedures regarding breastfeeding advice and management." The AAP (2012) recommends against routine supplementation of nondehydrated breastfed infants with water or dextrose water. Despite the data and recommendations to the contrary, the mPINC survey found that 30% of facilities gave feedings of glucose water and 15% gave water to breastfed infants, practices known to be detrimental to breastfeeding (CDC, 2008). Dextrose/water supplements may prevent clinical interventions necessary to prevent excessive bilirubin levels from developing pre- and postdischarge. Rather than water supplements, clinicians should use a preventive approach to hyperbilirubinemia (Bhutani & Johnson, 2009) that includes optimal breastfeeding support (making sure mothers know when their infant is swallowing milk), referral to an International Board Certified Lactation Consultant in the hospital for breastfeeding problems and following discharge, facilitation of risk assessment for hyperbilirubinemia in the hospital through use of a bilirubin nomogram, more intense monitoring of infants at increased risk (such as late preterm infants), and a follow-up appointment with the infant's physician within 48 hours of discharge.

Hypoglycemia

Hypoglycemia (or the potential for hypoglycemia) represents a frequent reason for supplementing the breastfed newborn. A major physiological challenge for newborns is to establish and regulate their own metabolic processes, including the self-regulation of glucose metabolism when this function is no longer performed by the maternal placental unit. A quarter of a century ago newborns were routinely fed nothing by mouth for 6–12 hours or longer after birth, reflecting a number of non-evidence-based assumptions. Inappropriate supplementation trends persist today due to a lack of consensus on what constitutes hypoglycemia, misunderstanding of neonatal glucose metabolism, and uncertainty about when to intervene. After delivery, the maternal glucose supply is abruptly withdrawn, causing a self-limiting decline in the infant's blood sugar for about the first 3 hours of life (Srinivasan, Pildes, Cattamanchi, Voora, & Lilien, 1986). The infant must then initiate counter-regulatory compensation through three processes, plus start the process for the formation of alternative fuels (Williams, 1997):

1. Glycolysis, the conversion of glucose to lactate and pyruvate
2. Glycogenolysis, the release of glycogen from body stores to form glucose
3. Gluconeogenesis, the production of glucose by the liver and kidneys from substrates such as fatty acids and amino acids

Additional sources of fuel for the brain include ketone bodies derived from a brisk ketogenic response to low blood glucose levels through fatty acid mobilization. Especially at low blood glucose levels, breastfed infants show high concentrations of ketone bodies, a response that is blunted by supplementation with formula (De Rooy & Hawdon, 2002). Early feeding of human milk/colostrum enhances the process of gluconeogenesis by providing amino acid precursors, presents fatty acids that facilitate the formation of an enzyme critical to ketogenesis, and provides lactose that minimizes insulin secretion. Feeding either 5% or 10% glucose water in the immediate period after birth increases insulin secretion (which suppresses gluconeogenesis), decreases secretion of glucagon (a hormone that stimulates the liver to change stored glycogen to glucose and encourages the use of fats and amino acids for energy production), and delays the natural gluconeogenesis and ketogenic processes (Eidelman, 2001). The breastfed term infants who lose the most weight have the highest ketone body concentrations (Hawdon, Ward-Platt, & Aynsley-Green, 1992; Swenne, Sandberg, & Ostenson, 1994), suggesting that ketogenesis is an adaptive response to temporarily low nutrient intake during the time it takes for the infant to successfully establish feeding at the breast (Cornblath et al., 2000).

Lactate is an important cerebral fuel, acting as a glucose generator to support brain metabolism. In fact, it may be more important as an alternative brain fuel than ketones. Plasma concentrations of lactate peak within the first few hours of birth (Hawdon, Ward-Platt, & Aynsley-Green, 1992), exactly when blood glucose concentrations are declining. It has been shown that lactate provides a useful source of cerebral fuel in most hypoglycemic infants, and that those hypoglycemic babies with low plasma lactate concentrations may be at an increased risk for neurological side effects (Harris, Weston, & Harding, 2015).

Table 4-3 Statistical Definition of Hypoglycemia

Author	Age	Serum or Plasma Glucose Concentration
Srinivasan, Pildes, Cattamanchi, Voora, & Lilien (1986)	0–3 hours	< 35 mg/dL (2.0 mmol/L)
	3–24 hours	< 40 mg/dL (2.2 mmol/L)
	24–48 hours	< 45 mg/dL (2.5 mmol/L)
Heck & Erenberg (1987)	0–24 hours	< 30 mg/dL (1.7 mmol/L)
	24–48 hours	< 40 mg/dL (2.2 mmol/L)
Alkalay, Sarnat, Flores-Sarnat, et al. (2006)	1–2 hours	28 mg/dL (1.6 mmol/L)
	3–47 hours	40 mg/dL (2.2 mmol/L)
	48–72 hours	48 mg/dL (2.7 mmol/L)

Formula-fed and breastfed infants demonstrate different patterns of serum glucose concentrations. Hawdon and coworkers (1992) reported a mean of 3.6 mmol/L (58 mg/dL) with a range of 1.5–5.3 mmol/L (27–95 mg/dL) in breastfed infants and a mean of 4.0 mmol/L (72 mg/dL) with a range of 2.5–6.2 mmol/L (45–111 mg/dL) in formula-fed infants. None of the breastfed infants became symptomatic, and all responded with significant increases in ketone bodies. Only the interval between feedings was correlated with glucose concentrations, reinforcing the recommendation for frequent breastfeeding. Considerable controversy exists regarding the actual definition of hypoglycemia, with some current definitions not being applicable to breastfed infants because these infants can tolerate lower plasma glucose levels (Cornblath, Schwartz, Aynsley-Green, & Lloyd, 1990). Statistical rather than functional blood glucose levels have been described for hypoglycemia cutoff points that are the lower limits of normal (**Table 4-3**). These distinctions are based on serum or plasma glucose concentrations, which are 10–15% higher than in whole blood and do not distinguish between breastfed and formula-fed infants.

Symptomatic hypoglycemia is the association of clinical signs (which can be vague and nonspecific) and blood glucose concentrations of less than arbitrary level. Healthy, normal, full-term infants do not develop symptomatic hypoglycemia simply as a result of underfeeding (Williams, 1997) and do not require routine monitoring of blood glucose levels (Eidelman, 2001). The use of bedside screening tests using reagent strips can have as high as a 20% rate of false positives (i.e., normoglycemic infants labeled erroneously as hypoglycemic) (Holtrop, Madison, Kiechle, Karcher, & Batton, 1990; Reynolds & Davies, 1993). Laboratory determinations should confirm the results before supplementing a breastfed infant with formula. Hypoglycemia is minimized in breastfed infants who are fed early, often, and exclusively and who are actually and adequately transferring milk (colostrum), as confirmed by documenting swallowing. Early breastfeeding is not precluded simply because an infant meets the criteria for glucose monitoring (Academy of Breastfeeding Medicine, 2014). Some maternity units supplement normal, healthy, full-term infants as if they were high risk, using specific glucose levels that may inappropriately call for supplementing infants who have no medical need. Maternity units should not use glucose measurements adapted for sick infants, such as in the S.T.A.B.L.E. program (http://www.stableprogram.org/index.php), a program for postresuscitation/pretransport stabilization care of sick infants. Gross overfeeding of breastfed infants with infant formula to prevent or ameliorate low blood sugar levels may unintentionally result in long-term problems. Screening should be restricted to at-risk and symptomatic infants, with symptomatic infants receiving IV glucose therapy, not forced feedings (Wight, 2006).

The AAP provides a practical guide for screening and management of hypoglycemia (Adamkin, Committee on Fetus and Newborn, American Academy of Pediatrics, 2011). It reminds clinicians that any approach to hypoglycemia management should not unnecessarily disrupt breastfeeding.

Maternal Request

Breastfed infants are often supplemented in the hospital at the request of the mother. Cultural factors are frequently attributed to this practice. However, DaMota, Bañuelos, Goldbronn, Vera-Becerra, and Heinig (2012) found in a sample of 97 English- and Spanish-speaking low-income mothers that cultural factors were not mentioned as a reason for supplementation; rather, lack of preparation for what the early postpartum period would be like actually determined mothers' request for the in-hospital use of infant formula. Mothers in this study described an event in the hospital that triggered the request for supplementation. Mothers overestimated the capabilities of a newborn and were not prepared for the frequency of feeding and waking in their newborn. Crying was interpreted as insufficient milk, which called for using a bottle of formula. Unsettled behavior in the infant was thought to occur because the infant was not interested in breastfeeding or desired infant formula. Many mothers thought their milk would come in immediately following delivery, that colostrum was insufficient for their infants, and that their infant would latch on easily and effectively the first time they were put to breast. Some mothers were unaware that they would not have a large amount of milk immediately after birth, concluding they did not have enough milk to satisfy the infant. Mothers did not realize the small amounts of colostrum available during the early days were sufficient for their infants and used bottles of formula to assess how much milk their infants were lacking. Unmet expectations for their infant's behavior, the perception that healthcare providers were unsupportive of breastfeeding, and the unexpected work of new parenting led to the belief that infant formula was necessary. Some mothers who encountered breastfeeding problems requested infant formula rather than asking for help.

Given the unrealistic expectations of many mothers and the lack of understanding of the breastfeeding process, clinicians may be able to help reduce supplementation of breastfeeding that is not medically indicated by doing the following:

- Offering prenatal education and/or education immediately post delivery to improve mothers' expectations about the availability and amount of colostrum and to teach them that not all crying indicates hunger and that many newborns do not feed effectively the first time they are put to breast
- Assuring that mothers are taught techniques to maximize colostrum intake at each feeding, such as correct latch and alternate massage
- Educating mothers regarding the frequency of newborn feeding, how to rest between feedings, and the importance of minimizing the number of visitors and interruptions
- Intervening immediately to correct nipple pain or soreness

- Explaining the capabilities and behavior of a newborn
- Ascertaining how the mother interprets her infant's behavior
- Assuring that mothers learn and can perform the basic skills necessary to recognize hunger cues, latch the infant with no pain, feed enough times each 24 hours, and maximize milk intake at each feeding

"Just One Bottle Won't Hurt" (Or Will It?)

Early supplementation of the breastfed infant with infant formula has significant effects on the recipient infant's gut flora (Brown & Bosworth, 1922; Bullen, Tearle, & Stewart, 1977), can provoke sensitivity and allergy to cow's milk protein (Host, 1991), and has been identified as an environmental triggering event in the development of diabetes in susceptible infants (Karjalainen et al., 1992). Gimeno and deSouza (1997) demonstrated that the introduction to cow's milk products before 8 days of age is a risk factor for insulin-dependent diabetes mellitus. Early introduction of cow's milk proteins results in aberrant humoral immune responses to various cow's milk proteins in children who later progress to type I diabetes (Luopajarvi et al., 2008) and increases the risk of beta-cell autoimmunity and type I diabetes. Exposure to cow's milk is associated with a transient increase in the permeability of the gut (Catassi, Bonucci, Coppa, Carlucci, & Giorgi, 1995) as well as mucosal inflammation, which further increases gut permeability. This allows complex foreign proteins into systemic circulation and increases the levels of antibodies to a number of cow's milk proteins. Early enterovirus infections have been implicated as a strong trigger candidate for beta cell autoimmunity (Knip et al., 2005). Breastfeeding is protective against enterovirus infections, decreasing the risk of enterovirus-triggered beta cell autoimmunity. This protection is partially due to breastmilk's effect on decreasing gut permeability and not allowing these viruses to enter into the circulation.

Careful consideration should be undertaken before supplementing a breastfed infant, including establishing the presence of a history of allergy or diabetes in the infant's family. Liberal or cavalier supplementing of a breastfed infant with standard cow's milk-based formula can have long-lasting negative effects. Exposure of an exclusively breastfed infant to the cow's milk in infant formula during the hospital stay can sensitize the infant to cow's milk protein (Juvonen, Mansson, Kjellman, Bjorkstén, & Jakobsson, 1999), setting up an allergic response when challenged with cow's milk later in the first year of life (Saarinen et al., 1999; Saarinen & Savilahti, 2000). IgA antibodies in colostrum and mature human milk prevent antigen entry at the intestinal surface of a breastfed infant. Infants whose mothers have a low IgA content in their milk may experience defective exclusion of food antigens and be predisposed to the development of food allergies (Jarvinen, Laine, Jarvenpaa, & Suomaiainen, 2000). Only tiny amounts of an allergen are necessary to sensitize a susceptible infant. Just 1 ng of bovine beta-lactalbumin is sufficient to set the stage for an undesired outcome (Businco, Bruno, & Giampietro, 1999). Cantani and Micera (2005) demonstrated that small doses of allergens are more sensitizing than larger ones. Isolated supplementary cow's milk-based formula feedings of breastfed infants should be avoided during the early days. If a formula is needed, a hydrolyzed formula should be used (AAP, Work Group on Cow's Milk Protein and Diabetes Mellitus, 1994). Use of a hydrolyzed formula postpones the introduction of intact cow's milk proteins, which include bovine insulin. Young children who demonstrate early signs of beta cell autoimmunity seem to lack the capacity to develop oral tolerance to bovine insulin during infancy (Vaarala et al., 1999). Thus the initial immune response to bovine insulin may be diverted at a later time into a response that targets human insulin and insulin-producing beta cells in these children (Knip, Virtanen, & Akerblom, 2010). Use of this type of formula may facilitate decreased intestinal permeability. The Nutritional Committees from the AAP and jointly the European Society for Pediatric Allergology and Clinical Immunology and the European Society for Pediatric Gastroenterology, Hepatology, and Nutrition recommend exclusive breastfeeding as the most critical measure for food allergy prevention (Zeiger, 2003).

Indications for Supplementation

According to the World Health Organization, there are a few medical indications in a maternity facility that may require individual infants be given fluids or food in addition to, or in place of, breastmilk (**Box 4-6**).

Box 4-6 Acceptable Medical Reasons for Supplementing Breastfed Infants

It is assumed that severely ill infants, infants in need of surgery, and very low-birth-weight infants will be in a special care unit. Their feeding will be individually decided, given their particular nutritional requirements and functional capabilities, although breastmilk is recommended whenever possible. These infants in special care are likely to include the following groups:

- Infants with very low-birth-weight (less than 1,500 g) or who are born before 32 weeks of gestation
- Infants with severe dysmaturity with potentially severe hypoglycemia or who require therapy for hypoglycemia and who do not improve through increased breastfeeding or by being given breastmilk

For infants who are well enough to be with their mothers on the maternity unit, there are very few indications for supplements. To assess whether a facility is inappropriately using fluids or artificial feeds, any infants receiving supplements must have been diagnosed as:

- Infants whose mothers are severely ill (e.g., with psychosis, sepsis, eclampsia, or shock) or infected with HIV or herpes simplex virus type 1 if lesions are on the breast
- Infants with inborn errors of metabolism (e.g., galactosemia, phenylketonuria, maple syrup urine disease)
- Infants with acute water loss (e.g., during phototherapy for jaundice), if increased breastfeeding cannot provide adequate hydration
- Infants whose mothers are taking medication that is contraindicated when breastfeeding (e.g., cytotoxic drugs, certain radioactive drugs such as iodine-131, and antithyroid drugs other than propylthiouracil) or whose mothers are engaged in substance abuse
- Newborn infants at risk of hypoglycemia due to impaired metabolic adaptation or increased glucose demand (small for gestational age, late preterm, experienced hypoxic/ischemic stress, those who are ill, and those whose mothers are diabetic) if their blood sugar fails to respond to breastfeeding or breastmilk feeding

When breastfeeding has to be temporarily delayed or interrupted, mothers should be helped to establish or maintain lactation—for example, through manual or hand-pumped expression of milk in preparation for the moment when breastfeeding may be begun or resumed.

Modified from World Health Organization/United Nations Children's Fund. (1992). *Baby-Friendly Hospital Initiative. Part II: Hospital-level implementation.* Geneva, Switzerland: World Health Organization; World Health Organization/United Nations Children's Fund. (2009). *Acceptable medical reasons for use of breast-milk substitutes.* Geneva, Switzerland: World Health Organization.

Box 4-7 Possible Maternal Indications for Supplementing the Breastfed Infant

- Maternal illness or condition (psychosis, eclampsia, herpes simplex lesion on the breast until healed, postpartum hemorrhage/Sheehan syndrome, varicella-zoster [chickenpox] until the mother is non-infectious, active tuberculosis until 2 or more weeks of treatment have occurred, Lyme disease until mother has initiated treatment, retained placenta)
- Geographic separation (mother and baby at different hospitals, mother or baby remaining in the hospital, custody or visitation issues)
- Maternal medications or recreational drugs (certain diagnostic radiopharmaceuticals until cleared from maternal plasma, most street or recreational drugs except cigarettes and small amounts of alcohol, and a very small number of medications)
- Delayed lactogenesis II (after day 5 with signs of inadequate infant intake)
- Intolerable pain and/or extensive damage to the nipples
- Breast anomalies, surgery, insufficient glandular tissue

Modified from Lawrence, R. A. (1997). *A review of the medical benefits and contraindications to breastfeeding in the United States.* (Maternal and Child Health Technical Information Bulletin). Arlington, VA: National Center for Education in Maternal and Child Health; Powers, N. G., & Slusser, W. (1997). Breastfeeding update 2: Clinical lactation management. *Pediatrics in Review, 18,* 147–161; Wight, N. E. (2001). *Supplements and the breastfed infant: When are they needed and how should they be supplied?* Independent Study Module. Schaumburg, IL: La Leche League International.

Box 4-8 Possible Infant Indications for Supplementing the Breastfed Infant

- Hypoglycemia validated with laboratory measurements, after the infant has been shown to unsuccessfully transfer colostrum during suckling opportunities
- Impending or significant dehydration (usually picked up after hospital discharge)
- Weight loss of 7–10% after days 3–5 with evidence of delayed lactogenesis II
- Meconium stools at day 5
- Inability of infant to transfer sufficient milk in the presence of an adequate milk supply
- Hyperbilirubinemia when the infant cannot sustain feedings at the breast
- Preterm, low-birth-weight, late preterm, congenital anomalies, illness, or other conditions that preclude the infant from either feeding directly at breast or feeding at breast but being unable to transfer sufficient quantities of milk

Modified from Powers, N. G., & Slusser, W. (1997). Breastfeeding update 2: Clinical lactation management. *Pediatrics in Review, 18,* 147–161; Wight, N. E. (2001). *Supplements and the breastfed infant: When are they needed and how should they be supplied?* Independent Study Module. Schaumburg, IL: La Leche League International.

If supplementation is being considered, a thorough breastfeeding assessment and evaluation of the mother and infant should take place and should include a direct observation of a feeding at breast; an evaluation of the maternal milk supply; a labor, delivery, and feeding history; evaluation of the infant's positioning, latch, suck, and swallow; and assessment of the infant's overall condition (Walker, 1989). A number of indications or conditions present in the mother (**Box 4-7**) or the infant (**Box 4-8**) would alert the clinician to the possible need for either temporary or ongoing supplementation. The infant must always be fed.

Box 4-9 Hierarchy of Supplements

- Fresh mother's own milk/colostrum
- Refrigerated mother's own milk
- Frozen and thawed mother's own milk
- Fortified (if necessary) mother's own milk for preterm infants
- Pasteurized donor-banked human milk
- Hypoallergenic infant formula
- Elemental infant formula
- Cow's milk-based infant formula
- Soy infant formula
- Water or glucose water

What to Supplement

If it is determined that supplementation is necessary, what should be used? A hierarchy of supplemental feedings (**Box 4-9**) in descending order of preference can be used as a guide. Fresh expressed mother's own milk is always preferable (AAP, Section on Breastfeeding, 2012) unless very rare conditions or situations temporarily or permanently preclude its use. The practice of antenatal breast expression has been advanced as a mechanism to avoid the use of infant formula if supplementation should be required for babies of diabetic mothers. Large, credible randomized controlled trials of this practice have not been conducted (Chapman, Pincombe, & Harris, 2013). Two small studies of antenatal colostrum expression reported outcomes of a reduced reliance on infant formula following delivery and a faster arrival at full breastfeeding when compared to a control group (Gurneesh & Ellora, 2009; Singh, Chonan, & Sidhu, 2009). These small studies contained several methodological inconsistencies, however, making it difficult to determine the validity of their outcomes.

Some concern has been advanced regarding the possibility of inducing contractions or premature labor by the nipple stimulation experienced when expressing colostrum prenatally. Breastfeeding during pregnancy has not been proven to be unsafe, nor has antenatal colostrum expression, given the multitude of other factors, other than oxytocin release, that predispose or induce premature labor. Forster and colleagues (2011) reported that cardiotocographs performed after antenatal colostrum expression showed no signs of any fetal compromise. Due to the clear benefits of early colostrum feedings and the potential hazardous effects of early formula supplementation, antenatal colostrum expression should outweigh the unsupported risks of prenatal colostrum expression (Cox, 2010). Diabetic mothers may wish to express colostrum prenatally, freeze it, and bring it to the hospital in case their infant requires supplementation (Cox, 2006). Mothers can begin expressing colostrum daily by drawing it into a 1-mL or 3-mL syringe at 34–37 weeks for 3–5 minutes on each breast as long as they experience no uterine cramping and are not at risk for preterm labor. Prebirth hand expression of colostrum can also be performed by mothers who are scheduled for a cesarean section or during the early phase of labor induction or present in spontaneous labor, as long as contractions are irregular and labor progression is slow (Tozier, 2013). Provision of this prebirth colostrum to infants at risk for hypoglycemia has been shown to improve exclusive breastfeeding rates and decrease formula supplementation (Tozier, 2013). Many healthcare providers teach prenatal

Table 4-4 Comparison of Supplements on Selected Parameters

Supplement	Calories/ oz/28 cc	Allergic Potential	Effect on Milk Production	Effect on Bilirubin Levels	Effect on Blood Sugar
Expressed mother's milk	18 colostrum 20 or more mature	None	Increases	Normal	Stabilizes and increases
Cow's milk–based formula	20	High	Decreases	Lowers	Increases
Soy formula	20	Medium to high	Decreases	Lowers	Increases
Hydrolyzed formula	20	Low	Decreases	Lowers	Increases
Sterile water	0	None	Decreases	Increases	None
D_5W	6	None	Decreases	Increases	Bounces

hand expression of colostrum to assure that a ready supply of colostrum is available if the need arises for supplementation and as a mechanism to avoid the use of infant formula (Chapman, Pincombe, Harris, & Fereday, 2013). Many mothers find prenatal colostrum expression to be both positive and valuable. Brisbane and Giglia (2015) reported that mothers who engaged in prenatal colostrum expression felt competent and familiar with breast expression, enjoyed the security of having a supply of stored colostrum, and described the practice as helping to alleviate stress over milk supply in the immediate postpartum period. A few mothers experienced difficulty in performing hand expression prenatally; clinicians could monitor for this problem and intervene to assure that the technique does not become stressful.

The potential risks and benefits of supplementation must be considered within the overall goal of preserving breastfeeding (Academy of Breastfeeding Medicine, 2009). Each type of supplement (**Table 4-4**) should be considered in terms of its potential to provide appropriate nutrition, protect the maternal milk supply, and avoid feeding-related morbidities (Wight, 2001).

The amount of supplement to be provided also depends on the situation. Wight (2006) recommended 3–5 mL/kg of expressed breastmilk or breastmilk substitute during the early days. This volume is based on normal volumes of colostrum, the average size of the infant's stomach, and average volumes of milk typically ingested by newborns. If an infant needed an entire feeding supplemented, this amount may vary based on the infant's health status, weight, and feeding goals. For late preterm infants, Stellwagen, Hubbard, and Wolf (2007) recommended feeding volumes of 5–10 mL every 2–3 hours on day 1, 10–20 mL on day 2, and 20–30 mL on day 3.

How to Supplement

There are a number of different ways to supplement a breastfed infant. Healthcare providers often recommend that the supplement be delivered by bottle, because it presents a rapid and easy way to feed an infant. However, sucking on an artificial nipple is not the same as suckling from the breast. Perioral muscle function differs between bottle-feeding and breastfeeding (Inoue, Sakashita, & Kamegai, 1995). Artificial nipples that require mostly suction rather than mostly compression can contribute to reduced masseter muscle activity as the muscle adjusts to bottle-feeding (Sakashita, Kamegai, & Inoue, 1996).

Geddes and colleagues (2012) conducted a study on a new nipple (Calma) that requires only suction (vacuum) to remove milk from the bottle. Compression will not remove milk. A minimum vacuum of −29 mm Hg was required to initiate milk flow. The mean peak vacuum applied during feeding with this nipple was significantly weaker than the peak vacuum of a baby who is feeding at breast (−67 mm Hg compared with −122 mm Hg). The baseline vacuum applied to this nipple was also weaker than that which an infant applies at breast (−12 mm Hg compared with −31 mm Hg). Baseline vacuum elongates and positions the human nipple in the mouth and keeps it there, making sure vacuum is not lost following each suck. In another study of the same nipple, it was found that intraoral vacuum was significantly lower than with breastfeeding, the mean hold pressure (the vacuum that keeps the nipple in the mouth) was lower, and the peak vacuum was lower than with breastfeeding (Segami, Mizuno, Taki, & Itabashi, 2013). Conventional artificial nipples do not require any hold pressure at all.

Infants often release the vacuum completely on some artificial nipples so as to relieve the gradual buildup of negative pressure in the bottle, which slows or stops milk flow (Ross & Fuhrman, 2015). Infants who acquire the learned habit of releasing vacuum on an artificial nipple to vent the system and reestablish milk flow may inadvertently transfer this habit to the breast. Completely releasing the vacuum disengages the infant from the breast, forcing the infant to relatch multiple times during a breastfeeding. This practice may be difficult to effect for a preterm or late preterm infant, or any infant with weak sucking pressures. It could also lead to sore or damaged maternal nipples. These reduced vacuums are of concern if an infant fed with this nipple were to apply the same vacuums to the breast and be unable to sufficiently draw in, elongate, and hold the nipple in place, as well as generate sufficient vacuum for milk removal.

Buccinator muscles are recruited to compensate for altered tongue function during bottle-feeding. Changes in tongue function alter and weaken other muscles, such as the styloglossus and palatoglossus, used during sucking and swallowing. This change in oral muscle function may contribute to an infant experiencing difficulty in transitioning to the breast after being bottle-fed (Ferrante, Silvestri, & Montinaro, 2006). The mechanics of sucking differ between breastfeeding and bottle-feeding, with significantly fewer sucking movements seen during bottle-feeding compared with breastfeeding (Moral et al., 2010). There can be significant differences between bottle-feeding and breastfeeding in terms of swallowing and the stability of the suck–swallow–breathe cycle (Goldfield, Richardson, Lee, & Margetts, 2006). Mizuno and Ueda (2006) reported that sucking pressures for nutritive and non-nutritive sucking are exactly the opposite when comparing breastfeeding and sucking on an artificial nipple. Random, frequent, and uncoordinated swallowing seen with some bottle-feeding systems can contribute to desaturation, poor intake, and a delay in breastfeeding skill acquisition.

If supplementation is done by bottle, choice of an artificial nipple can be problematic. Nipple flow rates are not standardized, many nipples are too stiff for an infant with a weak suck, some have rapid flow rates that compromise ventilation, and none fit the anatomic shape of an infant's oral structures. Artificial nipple flow rates vary widely, from 6 mL/min to 60 mL/min (Jackman, 2013). High flow rates (especially in medically fragile infants) can increase bradycardia and desaturation episodes, contribute to poor use of oral musculature, inhibit the infant's ability to self-regulate milk flow, and reduce feeding efficiency. A flow rate that is too slow can cause fatigue and frustration in both the infant and the caregiver. Jackman (2013) tested 25 nipples for flow performance and found that nipples designated as "slow flow" demonstrated double or triple the flow rate of other artificial nipples. The chart of nipple flow rates in this study may aid clinicians in choosing an artificial nipple that is more appropriate when supplementing by bottle is unavoidable. In a study of 29 nipple types, wide variability was seen between nipples, with flow rates ranging from 2.10 mL/min to 85.34 mL/min, with flow rates for some nipples significantly differing from the rates claimed by their manufacturers (Pados, Park, Thoyre, Estrem, & Nix, 2015). Clinicians may also wish to consult this study for a listing of the tested nipples when making recommendations.

The mechanics of sucking on specific artificial nipples have been sparsely studied (Fadavi, Punwani, Jain, & Vidyasagar, 1997; Goldfield et al., 2006), and care must be taken in interpreting the results because nipple parameters (material, deflection, flow rates, types of openings, and extension capabilities) are changed frequently by manufacturers. Aizawa, Mizuno, and Tamura (2010) demonstrated that the angle of mouth opening on the breast was double that of infants feeding from a standard size artificial nipple. A partially closed mouth configuration (as often seen with artificial nipples) on the breast may result in nipple pain and damage, and reduced milk intake.

When choosing an artificial nipple for a breastfed infant, several considerations must be taken into account. Commercial nipples currently on the market are frequently made of silicone, a material that is more durable and often firmer than the latex-free plastic used for most single-use nipples. Infants who receive formula supplements in the hospital will experience a single-use nipple, but if supplementation continues postdischarge, the infant will be exposed to other nipples with different hole sizes, pliability, shape and size, and air exchange features.

The human nipple is not stationary during breastfeeding and has a mean movement of 4.0 ± 1.3 mm during infant sucking (Jacobs, Dickinson, Hart, Doherty, & Faulkner, 2007). If the strength required to alter the artificial nipple shape is beyond the infant's capacity, the tongue may be forced down, reinforcing an incorrect swallow pattern (Ferrante et al., 2006).

The length of the artificial nipple is also important. Jacobs and colleagues (2007) found on ultrasound scans that the nipple tip of the human nipple was usually not drawn into the mouth to a point where it rested directly under the junction of the hard and soft palates but was positioned approximately 5 mm in front of this spot. The artificial nipple should not be so long that it causes the infant to gag. Shorter, softer, more mobile nipples may result in a supplementation experience that does not compromise the transition to feeding at the breast. Nipples that are too short sit in the anterior portion of the mouth, while the majority of the force used for compression originates in the posterior portion of the tongue.

Artificial nipples are typically less elastic than the human nipple, may elongate only minimally (Nowak, Smith, & Erenberg, 1994), may have varying flow rates even among the same nipples from the same manufacturer (Mathew, 1988a, 1990) (which may or may not be appropriate for an individual infant), and may deliver milk using only vacuum or only compression rather than both. The "orthodontic" type of nipple may eliminate the central grooving of the tongue (Wolf & Glass, 1992). The tongue motion on an artificial nipple, especially a firm one, is more squeezing or piston-like (Weber, Woolridge, & Baum, 1986). Artificial nipples also increase the amount of air that an infant swallows (Ardran, Kemp, & Lind, 1958). Random, frequent, and uncoordinated swallowing seen with some bottle systems can provoke oxygen desaturation, poor intake, and a delay in breastfeeding skill acquisition, especially in a compromised infant. If a bottle is used, paced feedings may avoid fatigue and desaturation in less mature infants.

The shape of the artificial nipple influences the infant's mouth conformation. Peterson and Harmer (2010) recommend using an artificial nipple that has a gradual transition from the tip to the base in order to cause the mouth to open wider. The infant will need to encompass a portion of the nipple base and should be able to maintain the mouth in a wide-open position throughout the feeding. A wider nipple base (as compared to a narrow nipple base) may engage the masseter muscles more appropriately, as seen during feeding at the breast.

Because of these differences in the characteristics of artificial nipples, which can sometimes be quite subtle, questions may arise about an infant's ability to correctly suckle at breast if he or she has been exposed to an artificial nipple that requires different sucking dynamics. This phenomenon has been referred to as nipple confusion or nipple preference. Neifert, Lawrence, and Seacat (1995) defined nipple confusion as "an infant's difficulty in achieving the correct oral configuration, latching technique, and suckling pattern necessary for successful breastfeeding after bottle feeding or other exposure to an artificial nipple." The fact that nipple confusion occurs is probably best illustrated by infants who have difficulty changing between bottle nipples of varying designs. Although the term "confusion" may be inaccurate, it may be that it is the tactile and proprioceptive qualities of an object that influence or alter the infant's oral movements and acceptance (Wolf & Glass, 1992). These qualities may act as a "superstimulus" and simply overwhelm an infant's sensitive mouth.

Some infants have no difficulty alternating between the breast and an artificial nipple. Others may experience difficulty in rapidly adapting to a change or may take time to learn a different behavior. A subset of infants may be unable to differentiate between the sucking movements required to extract milk relative to the differing types of nipples presented to them. According to Sakashita and colleagues (1996), "Bottle feeding is a non-physiological condition and the physiological behavior is replaced by an adaptive change, the sucking action." There are a number of other variables whose interaction with one another and effect on any given infant require the clinician's attention (**Box 4-10**).

Box 4-10 Other Possible Effects of Feeding Bottles and Artificial Nipples on Selected Infant Parameters

- Muscles of mastication along with jaw development may be affected temporarily with short-term supplementation or permanently with long-term bottle use.
- Respiratory patterns and ventilation in both term and preterm (Shivpuri, Martin, Carlo, & Fanaroff, 1983) infants are affected during bottle-feeding (Mathew, 1988b, 1991a).
- As swallowing frequency increases, the time between swallows available for breathing decreases, and obstructed breathing can occur (Koenig, Davies, & Thach, 1990).
- Apnea and bradycardia can occur in both preterm (Mathew, 1991b) and term infants (Mathew, Clark, & Pronske, 1985).
- Transcutaneous oxygen pressure declines in preterm infants, resulting in desaturation with the use of fast-flow nipples (Meier, 1988; Meier & Anderson, 1987).
- Cardiac parameters can be adversely affected by bottle-feeding (Butte, Smith, & Garza, 1991; Zeskind, Marshall, & Goff, 1992).
- Bottle-fed neonates exhibit differences in physiological organization compared with breastfed infants; higher heart rates, lesser heart period variability, and lowered vagal tone are seen in bottle-fed infants (DiPietro, Larson, & Porges, 1987). Higher vagal tone as seen in breastfed infants is a reflection of better physiological status and enhanced nervous system organization, and it results in a subsequent improved behavioral repertoire (Porges, 1983).

There is currently no way to predict which infants will have difficulty and which ones will transition between breast and bottle effortlessly. In an effort to prevent or reduce latch, suck, and numerous other problems attributed to artificial nipples, alternatives to bottles may be recommended. These devices can be used temporarily to deliver nutrition, may be selected to assist with latch-on, or may be necessary for longer periods of time to deliver nutrients while an infant learns to feed at breast. Common devices include tube feeding setups, cups, spoons, droppers, syringes, and paladai. (For more information on devices, please refer to the additional reading and resources list at the end of this chapter.)

Tube feeding devices include commercial versions such as the Supplemental Nursing System and the Starter Supplemental Nursing System by Medela, Inc., and the Lact-Aid Nursing Trainer System by Lactaid International, both of which can be used for supplementation at the breast or with finger feeding. The Hazelbaker FingerFeeder can be used with one hand to finger feed an infant. Similarly configured devices can be created from gavage tubing, from a length of butterfly tubing (with the needle removed) attached to a 20-cc or 30-cc syringe (Edgehouse & Radzyminski, 1990), or from a 36-inch length of 5 French tubing threaded through an artificial nipple on a feeding bottle (Newman, 1990). Finger feeding with any of these tubing devices utilizes the tubing attached to a caregiver's finger in the infant's mouth (Bull & Barger, 1987). Finger feeding (as opposed to bottle-feeding) allows the caregiver to better pace a feeding, provides the feel of real skin rather than silicone or latex, helps establish proper oral conformation, and does not allow intake of milk from compression only.

Use of these devices is usually temporary because the mother uses them to establish the infant at breast and/or supplement the infant at breast (**Figure 4-4**). However, some mothers use tube feeding devices for longer-term breastfeeding, such as for adoptive nursing, if the mother has had a breast reduction or other surgery on the breasts, if she is experiencing insufficient breastmilk, or if the infant is not capable of feeding directly at the breast without assistance because of oral anomalies, genetic or anatomic problems, or neurological compromise. When using these devices, small boluses can be effective if needed to help the infant initiate and sustain sucking, as flow regulates suck. Flow rate can be adjusted

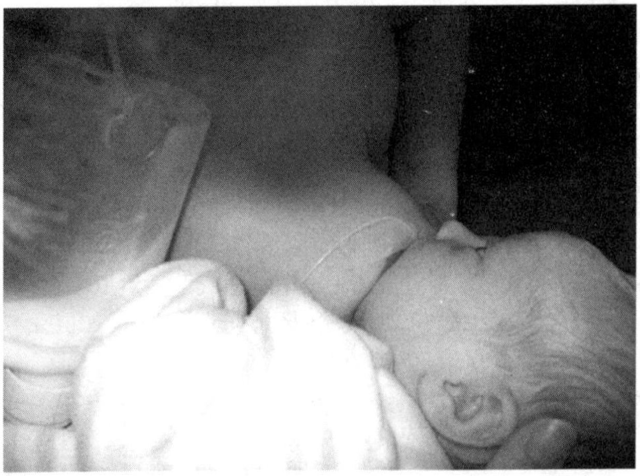

Figure 4-4 Infant feeding with assistance from a supplemental nutrition system.
Courtesy of Marsha Walker, RN, IBCLC.

to either augment or reduce the flow. If the infant is looking distressed, sputtering, coughing, or choking, then the flow needs to be reduced such that a comfortable ratio of sucking to swallowing is seen and the infant inhibits breathing only when swallowing (Wolf & Glass, 2008). Although some mothers may find these devices awkward or inconvenient, they have been shown to be an effective tool in addressing selected breastfeeding problems in term and preterm infants, and in extending the duration of breastfeeding (Borucki, 2005; Guoth-Gumberger, 2006; Oddy & Glenn, 2003).

Commercial infant feeding cups are available in hard and soft plastic in varying shapes and sizes. Some clinicians use a 28-mL medicine cup or a small party-favor-size Dixie cup with a rounded rim. Cup feeding allows the participation of the masseter and temporalis muscles, similar to the functioning of these muscles during breastfeeding (Gomes, Trezza, Murade, & Padovani, 2006). An electromyographic analysis of breast, cup, and bottle-feeding demonstrated that masseter muscle activity was significantly higher in breastfed infants compared to bottle-fed infants, while masseter muscle activity during cup feeding was between that of breastfeeding and bottle-feeding. These findings led the authors to conclude that cup feeding in healthy full-term neonates is an acceptable temporary substitute for feeding at the breast (Franca, Sousa, Aragao, & Costa, 2014). Cup feeding of supplements to breastfed infants has been shown to be safe, resulting in a lower incidence of desaturation episodes (especially in preterm infants) and helping to prolong breastfeeding, particularly if multiple supplements are required (Howard et al., 1999, 2003; Rocha, Martinez, & Jorge, 2002). Huang, Gau, Huang, and Lee (2009) demonstrated that full-term infants supplemented with bottles displayed more negative sucking behavior during attempts to latch to the breast and that mothers who used bottles to supplement breastfeeding had a lower perception of milk supply up to 4 weeks postpartum. Abouelfettoh, Dowling, Dabash, Elguindy, and Seoud (2008) showed that preterm infants who were supplemented by cup demonstrated more mature breastfeeding behaviors when compared to bottle-fed infants over 6 weeks and had a significantly higher proportion of breastfeedings 1 week after discharge. Cup feeding, however, can be slow and involve spillage, which must be accounted for when feeding fragile preterm infants. Some studies did not find nipple confusion lessened by cup feeding (Collins, Makrides, Gillis, & McPhee, 2008; Flint, New, & Davies, 2007). Cup feeding has the potential to delay discharge from the hospital for some preterm infants (Collins et al., 2008).

Small plastic spoons can be used to hand express colostrum into and spoon-feed a newborn unable to latch onto the breast (Hoover, 1998). Glass or plastic medicine droppers or soft plastic clinical droppers are useful to provide milk incentives at the breast for teaching latch-on (**Figure 4-5**). TB (tuberculin) syringes can be used for this purpose, or periodontal syringes may be selected to deliver larger quantities of milk on a temporary basis. A curved tip or periodontal syringe allows for a very precise control of milk flow. A paladai resembles a small gravy boat with a spout that is similar to cup feeding but reduces the spillage common with cup feeding (Malhotra, Vishwambaran, Sundaram, & Narayanan, 1999). Use of a paladai has more spillage than the use of a bottle and increases feeding time in preterm infants (Aloysius & Hickson, 2007).

All alternative feeding methods have strengths and weaknesses. Therefore they must be selected with the goals of establishing or returning the infant to feedings at the breast while preserving the milk supply.

Strengths and Limitations of Selected Alternative Feeding Methods

Supplementation should be undertaken with specific therapeutic goals in mind. Documentation when supplementing should include the indication, route of delivery, type of supplement, and amount ingested

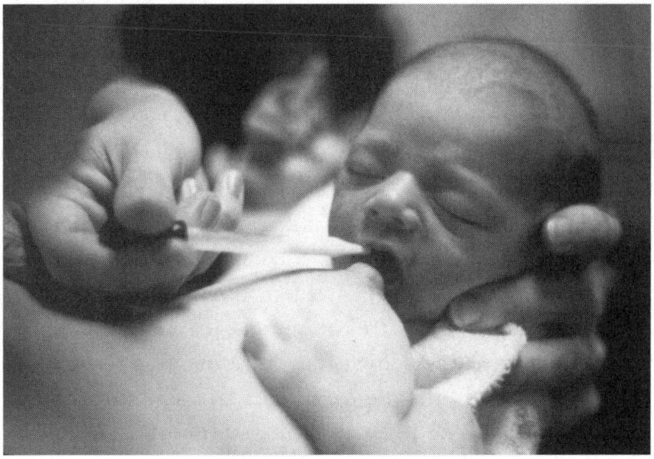

Figure 4-5 Assisting latch-on with a small clinic dropper.
Courtesy of Marsha Walker, RN, IBCLC.

by the infant. When a mother requests that her infant be supplemented, the clinician will need to ask why the mother is requesting this action, dispel any misconceptions, advise of potential risks and consequences, and educate other family members if they are the cause of the request. Mothers or staff may feel the need to supplement infants in the evening or at night because many infants are unsettled at these times. Mothers may state they are "feeding all the time," that the infant does not appear to be getting enough, and that the infant does not fall asleep after feeding. Rather than giving the infant a bottle of formula, clinicians should first directly assess a feeding at breast, recommend techniques to improve milk transfer, and recognize that they may be observing a normal diurnal feeding pattern that is common during the hospital stay and beyond. Benson (2001) demonstrated that the frequency of feeding in infants during the first 60 hours after birth was lowest between 3:00 am and 9:00 am and then gradually increased throughout the day to the highest frequency between 9:00 pm and 3:00 am. This is the precise time that staffing levels are at their lowest, lactation consultants are unavailable, and family members have either gone home or are as tired as the mother. Evening and night staffing that includes lactation consultants, staff nurses with additional breastfeeding management expertise, and staffing ratios that allow for more time per patient might alleviate unnecessary supplementation and its resulting side effects.

SUMMARY: THE DESIGN IN NATURE

Although circumstances and the environment surrounding the birth of an infant vary considerably, the process of lactation and the needs of an infant remain constant. Even after the umbilical cord is cut, the mother and newborn demonstrate a physiological attachment to each other. The mutual release of hormones when they touch each other, the explorations of each other's face, and the need to be with each other should be honored within the birthing environment. Minimizing birth interventions and constructing caretaking behaviors that facilitate and enhance close contact, promote early and frequent breastfeeding, and provide correct and consistent support, chart the course for a successful breastfeeding experience. See **Appendix 4-1**.

REFERENCES

Abouelfettoh, A. M., Dowling, D. A., Dabash, S. A., Elguindy, S. R., & Seoud, I. A. (2008). Cup versus bottle feeding for hospitalized late preterm infants in Egypt: A quasi-experimental study. *International Breastfeeding Journal, 3,* 27.

Academy of Breastfeeding Medicine. (2009). Hospital guidelines for the use of supplementary feedings in the healthy term breastfed neonate. Clinical Protocol #3. Revised 2009. *Breastfeeding Medicine, 4,* 175–182.

Academy of Breastfeeding Medicine. (2014). Guidelines for blood glucose monitoring and treatment of hypoglycemia in term and late-preterm neonates. Clinical Protocol #1. Revised 2014. *Breastfeeding Medicine, 9,* 173–179.

Adamkin, D. H., Committee on Fetus and Newborn, American Academy of Pediatrics. (2011). Clinical report: Postnatal glucose homeostasis in late-preterm and term infants. *Pediatrics, 127,* 575–579.

Agakidis, C., Agakidou, E., Philip Thomas, S., Murthy, P., & John Loyd, D. (2011). Labor epidural analgesia is independent risk factor for neonatal pyrexia. *Journal of Maternal and Fetal Neonatal Medicine, 24,* 1128–1132.

Aizawa, M., Mizuno, K., & Tamura, M. (2010). Neonatal sucking behavior: Comparison of perioral movement during breastfeeding and bottle-feeding. *Pediatrics International, 52,* 104–108.

Alkalay, A. L., Sarnat, H. B., Flores-Sarnat, L., Elashoff, J. D., Farber, S. J., Simmons, C. F. (2006). Population meta-analysis of low plasma glucose thresholds in full-term normal newborns. *American Journal of Perinatology, 23*(2), 115–119.

Allen, J. A., Perrine, C. G., & Scanlon, K. S. (2015). Breastfeeding supportive hospital practices in the US differ by county urbanization level. *Journal of Human Lactation,* [Epub ahead of print]. doi: 10.1177/0890334415578440

Aloysius, A., & Hickson, M. (2007). Evaluation of paladai cup feeding in breast-fed preterm infants compared with bottle feeding. *Early Human Development, 83,* 619–621.

Amar, A. P., Aryan, H. E., Meltzer, H. S., & Levy, M. L. (2003). Neonatal subgaleal hematoma causing brain compression: Report of two cases and review of the literature. *Neurosurgery, 52,* 1470–1474.

American Academy of Pediatrics, Section on Breastfeeding. (2012). Breastfeeding and the use of human milk. *Pediatrics, 129,* e827–e841.

American Academy of Pediatrics, Work Group on Cow's Milk Protein and Diabetes Mellitus. (1994). Infant feeding practices and their possible relationship to the etiology of diabetes mellitus. *Pediatrics, 94,* 752–754.

Amiel-Tison, C., Barrier, G., & Shnider, S. (1982). A new neurologic adaptive capacity scoring system for evaluating obstetric medication in full term infants. *Anesthesiology, 56,* 340–347.

Anderson, D. (2011). A review of systemic opioids commonly used for labor pain relief. *Journal of Midwifery & Women's Health, 56,* 222–239.

Anderson, G. C. (1976). *The transitional newborn* [videotape]. Chicago, IL: Aldine.

Anderson, G. C. (1989). Risk in mother–infant separation postbirth. *IMAGE: Journal of Nursing Scholarship, 21,* 196–199.

Anderson, G. C., Moore, E., Hepworth, J., & Bergman, N. (2003). Early skin-to-skin contact for mothers and their healthy newborn infants. *Cochrane Database of Systematic Reviews, 2,* CD003519.

Ardran, G. M., Kemp, F. H., & Lind, J. (1958). A cineradiographic study of bottle feeding. *British Journal of Radiology, 31,* 11–22.

Ball, H. L. (2008). Evolutionary paediatrics: A case study in applying Darwinian medicine. In S. Elton & P. O'Higgins (Eds.). *Medicine and evolution: Current applications, future prospects* (pp. 127–152). New York, NY: Taylor & Francis.

Ball, H. L., Ward-Platt, M. P., Heslop, E., Leech, S. J., & Brown, K. A. (2006). Randomised trial of infant sleep location on the postnatal ward. *Archives of Disease in Childhood, 91,* 1005–1010.

Baumgarder, D., Muehl, P., Fischer, M., & Pribbenow, B. (2003). Effect of labor epidural anesthesia on breastfeeding of healthy full-term newborns delivered vaginally. *Journal of American Board of Family Practice, 16,* 7–13.

Beilin, Y., Bodian, C. A., Weiser, J., Hossain, S., Arnold, I., Feierman, D. E., . . . Holzman, I. (2005). Effect of labor epidural analgesia with and without fentanyl on infant breastfeeding. *Anesthesiology, 103,* 1211–1217.

Benson, S. (2001). What is normal? A study of normal breastfeeding dyads during the first sixty hours of life. *Breastfeeding Review, 9,* 27–32.

Bergman, N. J. (2014). The neuroscience of birth—and the case for zero separation. *Curations, 37,* article 1440.

Bernis, C., & Varea, C. (2012). Hour of birth and birth assistance: From a primate to a medicalized pattern? *American Journal of Human Biology, 24,* 14–21.

Bertini, G., Dani, C., Tronchin, M., & Rubaltelli, F. F. (2001). Is breastfeeding really favoring early neonatal jaundice? *Pediatrics, 107*(3). Retrieved from http://www.pediatrics.org/cgi/content/full/107/3/e41

Bhutani, V. K., & Johnson, L. (2009). A proposal to prevent severe neonatal hyperbilirubinemia and kernicterus. *Journal of Perinatology, 29,* S61–S67.

Biro, M. A., Sutherland, G. A., Yelland, J. S., Hardy, P., & Brown, S. J. (2011). In-hospital formula supplementation of breastfed babies: A population-based survey. *Birth, 38,* 302–310.

Black, L. S. (2001). Incorporating breastfeeding care into daily newborn rounds and pediatric office practice. *Pediatric Clinics of North America, 48,* 299–319.

Blomquist, H. K., Jonsbo, F., Serenius, F., & Persson, L. A. (1994). Supplementary feeding in the maternity ward shortens the duration of breastfeeding. *Acta Paediatrica Scandinavica, 83,* 1122–1126.

Blyton, D. M., Sullivan, C. E., & Edwards, N. (2002). Lactation is associated with an increase in slow-wave sleep in women. *Journal of Sleep Research, 11,* 297–303.

Bolton, T. A., Chow, T., Benton, P. A., & Olson, B. H. (2009). Characteristics associated with longer breastfeeding duration: An analysis of a peer counseling support program. *Journal of Human Lactation, 25,* 18–27.

Borcherding, K. E., & Ruchala, P. L. (2002). Maternal hyponatremia. *AWHONN Lifelines,* 514–519.

Borucki, L. C. (2005). Breastfeeding mothers' experience using a supplemental feeding tube device: Finding an alternative. *Journal of Human Lactation, 21,* 429–438.

Brady, K., Bulpitt, D., & Chiarelli, C. (2014). An interprofessional quality improvement project to implement maternal/infant skin-to-skin contact during cesarean delivery. *Journal of Obstetric, Gynecologic, and Neonatal Nursing, 43,* 488–496.

Brazelton, T. B. (1961). Psychophysiologic reactions in the neonate. II. Effect of maternal medication on the neonate and his behavior. *Journal of Pediatrics, 58,* 513–518.

Brazy, J. E. (1988). Effects of crying on cerebral blood volume and cytochrome aa3. *Journal of Pediatrics, 112,* 457–461.

Brice, J. E., Moreland, T. A., & Walker, C. H. (1979). Effects of pethidine and its antagonists on the newborn. *Archives of Disease in Childhood, 54,* 356–361.

Bricker, L., & Lavender, T. (2002). Parenteral opioids for labor pain relief: A systematic review. *American Journal of Obstetrics and Gynecology, 186,* S94–S109.

Brimdyr, K., Cadwell, K., Widstrom, A-M., Svensson, K., Neumann, M., Hart, E. A., . . . Phillips, R. (2015). The association between common labor drugs and sucking when skin-to-skin during the first hour after birth. *Birth, 42,* 319–328.

Brisbane, J. M., & Giglia, R. C. (2015). Experiences of expressing and storing colostrum antenatally: A qualitative study of mothers in regional Western Australia. *Journal of Child Health Care, 19,* 206–215.

Brown, E. W., & Bosworth, A. W. (1922). Studies of infant feeding. VI. A bacteriological study of the feces and the food of normal babies receiving breast milk. *American Journal of Diseases in Childhood, 23,* 243.

Bull, P., & Barger, J. (1987). Fingerfeeding with the SNS [Newsletter article]. *Rental Roundup,* 25–34.

Bullen, C. L., Tearle, P. V., & Stewart, M. G. (1977). The effect of humanized milks and supplemented breast feeding on the faecal flora of infants. *Journal of Medical Microbiology, 10,* 403–413.

Businco, L., Bruno, G., & Giampietro, P. G. (1999). Prevention and management of food allergy. *Acta Paediatrica, 88* (suppl 430), 104–109.

Butte, N. F., Smith, E., & Garza, C. (1991). Heart rates of breast-fed and formula-fed infants. *Journal of Pediatric Gastroenterology and Nutrition, 13,* 391–396.

Bystrova, K., Widstrom, A. M., Matthiesen, A. S., Ransjo-Arvidson, A. B., Welles-Nystrom, B., Vorontsov, I., & Uvnas-Moberg, K. (2007). Early lactation performance in primiparous and multiparous women in relation to different maternity home practices: A randomized trial in St. Petersburg. *International Breastfeeding Journal, 8,* 2–9.

Cadwell, K., & Turner-Maffei, C. (2009). *Continuity of care in breastfeeding.* Sudbury, MA: Jones and Bartlett.

Caglar, M. K., Ozer, I., & Altugan, F. S. (2006). Risk factors for excess weight loss and hypernatremia in exclusively breastfed infants. *Brazilian Journal of Medical and Biological Research, 39,* 539–544.

Cakmak, H., & Kuguoglu, S. (2007). Comparison of the breastfeeding patterns of mothers who delivered their babies per vagina and via cesarean section: An observational study using the LATCH breastfeeding charting system. *International Journal of Nursing Studies, 44,* 1128–1137.

Camann, W. (2003). Spinal anesthesia in obstetrics: New concepts and developments. *Medscape Ob/Gyn Women's Health, 8*(2). Retrieved from http://www.medscape.com/viewarticle/464413

Camann, W. (2007). Labor analgesia and breastfeeding: Avoid parenteral narcotics and provide lactation support. *International Journal of Obstetric Anesthesia, 16,* 199–201.

Camann, W., & Trainor, K. (2012). Clear surgical drapes: A technique to facilitate the "natural cesarean delivery." *Anesthesia Analgesia, 115,* 981–982.

Cantani, A., & Micera, M. (2005). Neonatal cow milk sensitization in 143 case-reports: Role of early exposure to cow's milk formula. *European Review for Medical and Pharmacological Sciences, 9,* 227–230.

Casper, R. C., Gilles, A. A., Fleisher, B. E., Baran, J., Enns, G., & Lazzeroni, L. C. (2011). Length of prenatal exposure to selective serotonin reuptake inhibitor (SSRI) antidepressants: Effects on neonatal adaptation and psychomotor development. *Psychopharmacology (Berlin), 217,* 211–219.

Catassi, C., Bonucci, A., Coppa, G. V., Carlucci, A, & Giorgi, P. L. (1995). Intestinal permeability during the first month: Effect of natural versus artificial feeding. *Journal of Pediatric Gastroenterology and Nutrition, 21,* 383–386.

Cavlovich, F. E. (1994). Subgaleal hemorrhage in the neonate. *Journal of Obstetric, Gynecologic, and Neonatal Nursing, 24,* 397–404.

Centers for Disease Control and Prevention. (2008). Breastfeeding-related maternity practices at hospitals and birth centers—United States, 2007. *Morbidity and Mortality Weekly Report, 57,* 621–625.

Centers for Disease Control and Prevention. (2011). Vital signs: Hospital practices to support breastfeeding—United States, 2007 and 2009. *Morbidity and Mortality Weekly Report, 60,* 1020–1025.

Centers for Disease Control and Prevention. (2012). mPINC results. Retrieved from http://www.cdc.gov/breastfeeding/data/mpinc/index.htm

Centers for Disease Control and Prevention. (2014). mPINC results. Retrieved from http://www.cdc.gov/breastfeeding/data/mpinc/results-tables.htm

Chantry, C. J., Dewey, K. G., Peerson, J. M., Wagner, E. A., & Nommsen-Rivers, L. A. (2014). In-hospital formula use increases early breastfeeding cessation among first-time mothers intending to exclusively breastfeed. *Journal of Pediatrics, 164,* 1339–1345.

Chantry, C. J., Nommsen-Rivers, L. A., Peerson, J. M., Cohen, R. J., & Dewey, K. G. (2011). Excess weight loss in first-born breastfed newborns relates to maternal intrapartum fluid balance. *Pediatrics, 127,* e171–e179.

Chapman, T., Pincombe, J., & Harris, M. (2013). Antenatal breast expression: A critical review of the literature. *Midwifery, 29(3),* 203–210.

Chapman, T., Pincombe, J., Harris, M., & Fereday, J. (2013). Antenatal breast expression: Exploration and extent of teaching practices amongst International Board Certified Lactation Consultant midwives across Australia. *Women and Birth, 26,* 41–48.

Chen, Y. J., Yeh, T. F., & Chen, C. M. (2015). Effect of breastfeeding frequency on hyperbilirubinemia in breastfed term neonate. *Pediatrics International, 57,* 1121–1125.

Cheng, Y. W., Shaffer, B. L., & Caughey, A. B. (2006). Associated factors and outcomes of persistent occiput posterior position: A retrospective cohort study from 1976 to 2001. *Journal of Maternal–Fetal and Neonatal Medicine, 19,* 563–568.

Chezem, J. C., Friesen, C., & Boettcher, J. (2003). Breastfeeding knowledge, breastfeeding confidence, and infant feeding plans: Effects on actual feeding practices. *Journal of Obstetric, Gynecologic, and Neonatal Nursing, 32,* 40–47.

Chezem, J. C., Friesen, C., Montgomery, P., Fortman, T., & Clark, H. (1998). Lactation duration: Influences of human milk replacements and formula samples on women planning postpartum employment. *Journal of Obstetric, Gynecologic, and Neonatal Nursing, 27,* 646–651.

Chien, L. Y., Tai, C. J., Chu, K. H., Ko, Y. L., & Chiu, Y. C. (2007). The number of baby friendly hospital practices experienced by mothers is positively associated with breastfeeding: A questionnaire survey. *International Journal of Nursing Studies, 44,* 1138–1146.

Christensson, K., Siles, C., Moreno, L., Belaustequi, A., De La Fuente, P., Lagercrantz, . . . Winberg, J. (1992). Temperature, metabolic adaptation and crying in healthy full-term newborns cared for skin-to-skin or in a cot. *Acta Paediatrica, 81,* 488–493.

Christidis, I., Zotter, H., Rosegger, H., Engele, H., Kurz, R., & Kerbel, R. (2003). Infrared thermography in newborns: The first hour after birth. *Gynakologisch-Geburtshilfiche Rundschau, 43,* 31–35.

Cleary-Goldman, J., Negron, M., Scott, J., Downing, R. A., Camann, W., Simpson, L., & Flood, P. (2005). Prophylactic ephedrine and combined spinal epidural: Maternal blood pressure and fetal heart rate patterns. *Obstetrics and Gynecology, 106,* 466–472.

Coalson, D. W., & Glosten, B. (1991). Alternatives to epidural analgesia. *Seminars in Perinatology, 15,* 375–385.

Collins, C. T., Makrides, M., Gillis, J., & McPhee, A. J. (2008). Avoidance of bottles during the establishment of breast feeds in preterm infants. *Cochrane Database of Systematic Reviews, 8*(4), CD005252.

Connelly, K. P., Shropshire, L. C, & Salzberg, A. (1992). Gastric rupture associated with prolonged crying in a newborn undergoing circumcision. *Clinical Pediatrics, 31,* 560–561.

Cornblath, M., Hawdon, J. M., Williams, A. F., Aynsley-Green, A., Ward-Platt, M. P., Schwartz, R., & Kalhan, S. C. (2000). Controversies regarding definition of neonatal hypoglycemia: Suggested operational thresholds. *Pediatrics, 105,* 1141–1145.

Cornblath, M., Schwartz, R., Aynsley-Green, A., & Lloyd, J. K. (1990). Hypoglycemia in infancy: The need for a rational definition. *Pediatrics, 85,* 834–837.

Cotterman, K. J. (2004). Reverse pressure softening: A simple tool to prepare areola for easier latching during engorgement. *Journal of Human Lactation, 20,* 227–237.

Cox, S. G. (2006). Expressing and storing colostrum antenatally for use in the newborn period. *Breastfeeding Review, 14,* 11–16.

Cox, S. (2010). An ethical dilemma: Should recommending antenatal expressing and storing of colostrum continue? *Breastfeeding Review, 18,* 5–7.

Crivelli-Kovach, A., & Chung, E. K. (2011). An evaluation of hospital breastfeeding policies in the Philadelphia metropolitan area 1994–2009: A comparison with the baby-friendly hospital initiative 10 Steps. *Breastfeeding Medicine, 6,* 77–84.

Crossland, D. S., Richmond, S., Hudson, M., Smith, K., & Abu-Harb, M. (2008). Weight change in the term baby in the first 2 weeks of life. *Acta Paediatrica, 97,* 425–429.

Crowell, M. K., Hill, P. D., & Humenick, S. S. (1994). Relationship between obstetric analgesia and time of effective breastfeeding. *Journal of Nurse-Midwifery, 39,* 150–155.

Dahlenburg, G. W., Burnell, R. H., & Braybrook, R. (1980). The relation between cord serum sodium levels in newborn infants and maternal intravenous therapy during labor. *British Journal of Obstetrics and Gynecology, 87,* 519–522.

Daly, S. E. J., Owens, R. A., & Hartmann, P. E. (1993). The short-term synthesis and infant-regulated removal of milk in lactating women. *Experimental Physiology, 78,* 209–220.

DaMota, K., Banuelos, J., Goldbronn, J., Vera-Becerra, L. E., & Heinig, M. J. (2012). Maternal request for in-hospital supplementation of healthy breastfed infants among low-income women. *Journal of Human Lactation, 28,* 476–482.

Davanzo, R., Cannioto, Z., Ronfani, L., Monasta, L., & Demarini, S. (2012). Breastfeeding and neonatal weight loss in healthy term infants. *Journal of Human Lactation, 29,* 45–53.

De Carvalho, M., Hall, M., & Harvey, D. (1981). Effects of water supplementation on physiological jaundice in breastfed babies. *Archives of Disease in Childhood, 56,* 568–569.

De Carvalho, M., Klaus, M. H., & Merkatz, R. B. (1982). Frequency of breastfeeding and serum bilirubin concentration. *American Journal of Diseases in Childhood, 136,* 737–738.

De Carvalho, M., Robertson, S., & Klaus, M. (1985). Fecal bilirubin excretion and serum bilirubin concentrations in breastfed and bottle-fed infants. *Journal of Pediatrics, 107,* 786–790.

de Moura, E. G., Lisboa, P. C., & Passos, M. C. (2008). Neonatal programming of neuroimmunomodulation: Role of adipocytokines and neuropeptides. *Neuroimmunomodulation, 15,* 176–188.

De Rooy, L., & Hawdon, J. (2002). Nutritional factors that affect the postnatal adaptation of full-term small- and large-for-gestational-age infants. *Pediatrics, 109,* e42.

Declercq, E. R., Sakala, C., Corry, M. P., & Applebaum, S. (2002*). Listening to mothers: Report of the First National US Survey of Women's Childbearing Experiences.* New York: Maternity Center Association. Retrieved from http://www.childbirthconnection.org/pdfs/LtMreport.pdf

Declercq, E. R., Sakala, C., Corry, M. P., & Applebaum, S. (2006). *Listening to mothers survey II: Report of the Second National US Survey of Women's Childbearing Experiences.* New York, NY: Childbirth Connection. Retrieved from http://www.childbirthconnection.org/article.asp?ck=10396

Declercq, E. R., Sakala, C., Corry, M. P., Applebaum, S., & Herrlich, A. (2013). *Listening to mothers III pregnancy and birth: Report of the third national U.S. survey of women's childbearing experiences.* New York, NY: Childbirth Connection. Retrieved from http://transform.childbirthconnection.org/wp-content/uploads/2013/06/LTM-III_Pregnancy-and-Birth.pdf

Dewey, K. G., Nommsen-Rivers, L. A., Heinig, M. J., & Cohen, R. J. (2003). Risk factors for suboptimal infant breastfeeding behavior, delayed onset of lactation, and excess neonatal weight loss. *Pediatrics, 112,* 607–619.

DiFrisco, E., Goodman, K. E., Budin, W. C., Lilienthal, M. W., Kleinman, A., & Holmes, B. (2011). Factors associated with exclusive breastfeeding 2 to 4 weeks following discharge from a large, urban, academic medical center striving for Baby-Friendly designation. *Journal of Perinatal Education, 20,* 28–35.

DiGirolamo, A. M., Grummer-Strawn, L. M., & Fein, S. (2001). Maternity care practices: Implications for breastfeeding. *Birth, 28,* 94–100.

DiGirolamo, A. M., Grummer-Strawn, L. M., & Fein, S. B. (2008). Effect of maternity-care practices on breastfeeding. *Pediatrics, 122,* S43–S49.

Dinwiddie, R., Patel, B. D., Kumar, S. P., & Fox, W. W. (1979). The effects of crying on arterial oxygen tension in infants recovering from respiratory distress. *Critical Care Medicine, 7,* 50–53.

Dinwiddie, R., Pitcher-Wilmott, R., Schwartz, J. G., Shaffer, T. H., & Fox, W. W. (1979). Cardiopulmonary changes in the crying neonate. *Pediatric Research, 13,* 900–903.

DiPietro, J. A., Larson, S. K., & Porges, S. W. (1987). Behavioral and heart rate pattern differences between breast-fed and bottle-fed neonates. *Developmental Psychology, 23,* 467–474.

Doan, T., Gay, C. L., Kennedy, H. P., Newman, J., & Lee, K. A. (2014). Nighttime breastfeeding behavior is associated with more nocturnal sleep among first-time mothers at one month postpartum. *Journal of Clinical Sleep Medicine, 10,* 313–319.

Douma, M. R., Stienstra, R., Middeldorp, J. M., Arbous, M. S., & Dahan, A. (2015). Differences in maternal temperature during labour with remifentanil patient-controlled analgesia or epidural analgesia: A randomized controlled trial. *International Journal of Obstetric Anesthesia, 24,* 313–322.

Dowling, D. A., Meier, P. P., DiFiore, J. M., Blatz, M., & Martin, R. J. (2002). Cup-feeding for preterm infants: Mechanics and safety. *Journal of Human Lactation, 18,* 13–20.

Dozier, A. M., Howard, C. R., Brownell, E. A., Wissler, R. N., Glantz, J. C., Ternullo, S. R., . . . Lawrence, R. A. (2013). Labor epidural anesthesia, obstetric factors and breastfeeding cessation. *Maternal and Child Health Journal, 17,* 689–698.

Drewett, R. F., Woolridge, M. W., Jackson, D. A., Imong, S. M., Mangklabruks, A., Wongsawasdii, L., . . . Baum, J. D. (1989). Relationships between nursing patterns, supplementary food intake and breast milk intake in a rural Thai population. *Early Human Development, 20,* 13–23.

Dumas, L., Lepage, M., Bystrova, K., Matthiesen, A.-S., Welles-Nystrom, B., & Widstrom, A.-M. (2013). Influence of skin-to-skin contact and rooming-in on early mother–infant interaction: A randomized controlled trial. *Clinical Nursing Research, 22,* 310–336.

Edgehouse, L., & Radzyminski, S. G. (1990). A device for supplementing breastfeeding. *American Journal of Maternal/Child Nursing, 15,* 34–35.

Eidelman, A. I. (2001). Hypoglycemia and the breastfed neonate. *Pediatric Clinics of North America, 48,* 377–387.

Ekstrom, A., Widstrom, A.-M., & Nissen, E. (2003). Duration of breastfeeding in Swedish primiparous and multiparous women. *Journal of Human Lactation, 19,* 172–178.

Erlandsson, K., Dsilna, A., Fagerberg, I., & Christensson, K. (2007). Skin-to-skin care with the father after cesarean birth and its effect on newborn crying and prefeeding behavior. *Birth, 34,* 105–114.

Evron, S., Glezerman M., Sadan, O., Boaz, M., & Ezri, T. (2005). Remifentanil: A novel systemic analgesic for labor pain. *Anesthesia and Analgesia, 100,* 233–238.

Fadavi, S., Punwani, I. C., Jain, L., & Vidyasagar, D. (1997). Mechanics and energetics of nutritive sucking: A functional comparison of commercially available nipples. *Journal of Pediatrics, 130,* 740–745.

Fairbank, L., O'Meara, S., Renfrew, M. J., Woolridge, M., Sowden, A. J., & Lister-Sharp, D. A. (2000). Systematic review to evaluate the effectiveness of interventions to promote the initiation of breastfeeding. *Health Technology Assessment, 4,* 1–171.

Feldman-Winter, L., Procaccini, D., & Merewood, A. (2012). A model infant feeding policy for Baby-Friendly designation in the USA. *Journal of Human Lactation, 28,*304–311.

Ferrante, A., Silvestri, R., & Montinaro, C. (2006). The importance of choosing the right feeding aids to maintain breastfeeding after interruption. *International Journal of Orofacial Myology, 32,* 58–67.

Fildes, V. A. (1986). *Breasts, bottles and babies: A history of infant feeding.* Edinburgh, UK: Edinburgh University Press.

Flaherman, V. J., Bokser, S., & Newman, T. B. (2010). First-day newborn weight loss predicts in-hospital weight nadir for breastfeeding infants. *Breastfeeding Medicine, 5,* 165–168.

Fleschler, R., & Peskin, M. F. (2008). Selective serotonin reuptake inhibitors (SSRIs) in pregnancy: A review. *American Journal of Maternal/Child Nursing, 33,* 355–361.

Flint, A., New, K., & Davies, M. W. (2007). Cup feeding versus other forms of supplemental enteral feeding for newborn infants unable to fully breastfeed. *Cochrane Database of Systematic Reviews, 2,* CD005092.

Forster, D. A., McEgan, K., Ford, R., Moorhead, A., Opie, G., Walker, S., & McNamara, C. (2011). Diabetes and antenatal milk expressing: A pilot project to inform the development of a randomised controlled trial. *Midwifery, 27,* 209–214.

Forster, D. A., & McLachlan, H. L. (2007). Breastfeeding initiation and birth setting practices: A review of the literature. *Journal of Midwifery and Women's Health, 52,* 273–280.

Franca, E. C., Sousa, C. B., Aragao, L. C., & Costa, L. R. (2014). Electromyographic analysis of masseter muscle in newborns during suction in breast, bottle or cup feeding. *BMC Pregnancy Childbirth, 14,* 154.

Gagnon, A. J., Leduc, G., Waghorn, K., Yang, H., & Platt, R. W. (2005). In-hospital formula supplementation of health breastfeeding newborns. *Journal of Human Lactation, 21,* 397–405.

Gardella, C., Taylor, M., Benedetti, T., Hitti, J., & Critchlow, C. (2001). The effect of sequential use of vacuum and forceps for assisted vaginal delivery on neonatal and maternal outcomes. *American Journal of Obstetrics and Gynecology, 185,* 896–902.

Gartner, L. M. (1994). On the question of the relationship between breastfeeding and jaundice in the first 5 days of life. *Seminars in Perinatology, 18,* 502, 508–509.

Gartner, L. M., & Herschel, M. (2001). Jaundice and breastfeeding. *Pediatric Clinics of North America. 48,* 389–399.

Geddes, D. T., Sakalidis, V. S., Hepworth, A. R., McClellan, H. L., Kent, J. C., Lai, C. T., & Hartmann, P. E. (2012). Tongue movement and intra-oral vacuum of term infants during breastfeeding and feeding from an experimental teat that released milk under vacuum only. *Early Human Development, 88,* 443–449.

Gentile, S. (2007). Serotonin reuptake inhibitor–induced perinatal complications. *Paediatric Drugs, 9,* 97–106.

Gill, N. E., White, M. A., & Anderson, G. C. (1984). Transitional newborn infants in a hospital nursery: From first oral cue to first sustained cry. *Nursing Research, 33,* 213–217.

Gimeno, S. G., & deSouza, J. M. (1997). IDDM and milk consumption: A case-control study in Sao Paulo, Brazil. *Diabetes Care, 20,* 1256–1260.

Glover, J. (1990). Supplementation of breastfeeding infants and weight loss in hospital. *Journal of Human Lactation, 6,* 163–166.

Goer, H. (1995). *Obstetric myths versus research realities: A guide to the medical literature.* Westport, CT: Bergin & Garvey.

Goetzl, L., Cohen, A., Frigoletto, F., Ringer, S. A., Lang, J. M., & Lieberman, E. (2001). Maternal epidural use and neonatal sepsis evaluation in afebrile mothers. *Pediatrics, 108,* 1099–1102.

Goldfield, E. C., Richardson, M. J., Lee, K. G., & Margetts, S. (2006). Coordination of sucking, swallowing, and breathing and oxygen saturation during early infant breastfeeding and bottle-feeding. *Pediatric Research, 60,* 450–455.

Golub, M. S. (1996). Labor analgesia and infant brain development. *Pharmacology Biochemistry and Behavior, 55,* 619–628.

Gomes, C. F., Trezza, E. M. C., Murade, E. C. M., & Padovani, C. R. (2006). Surface electromyography of facial muscles during natural and artificial feeding of infants. *Journal of Pediatrics, (Rio J), 82,* 103–109.

Goodfellow, C. F., Hull, M. G. R., Swaab, D. F., Dogterom, J., & Buijs, R. M. (1983). Oxytocin deficiency at delivery with epidural analgesia. *British Journal of Obstetrics and Gynecology, 90,* 214–219.

Gorman, J. R., Kao, K., & Chambers, C. D. (2012). Breastfeeding among women exposed to antidepressants during pregnancy. *Journal of Human Lactation, 28,* 181–188.

Greenwell, E. A., Wyshak, G., Ringer, S. A., Johnson, L. C., Rivkin, M. J., & Lieberman, E. (2012). Intrapartum temperature elevation, epidural use, and adverse outcome in term infants. *Pediatrics, 129,* e447–e454.

Gross, J. B., Cohen, A. P., Lang, J. M., Frigoletto, F. D., & Lieberman, E. S. (2002). Differences in systemic opioid use do not explain fever incidence in parturients receiving epidural analgesia. *Anesthesiology, 97,* 157–161.

Gubler, T., Krahenmann, F., Roos, M., Zimmerman, R., & Ochsenbein-Kolble, N. (2013). Determinants of successful breastfeeding initiation in healthy term singletons: A Swiss university hospital observational study. *Journal of Perinatal Medicine, 41,* 331–339.

Guoth-Gumberger, M. (2006). Breastfeeding with the supplementary nursing system. Retrieved from http://www.breastfeeding-support.de/eng/sns-more.htm

Gurneesh, S., & Ellora, D. (2009). Effect of antenatal expression of breast milk at term to improve lactational performance: A prospective study. *Journal of Obstetrics and Gynecology India, 59,* 308–311.

Halamek, L. P., & Stevenson, D. K. (1996). Neonatal jaundice and liver disease. In A. Fanarof & R. Martin (Eds.), *Neonatal-perinatal medicine: Diseases of the fetus and infant* (6th ed., Vol. 2, pp. 1345–1389). St. Louis, MO: Mosby-Year Book.

Hale, T. (2008). *Medications and mother's milk* (13th ed.). Amarillo, TX: Hale Publishing.

Hall, R. T., Mercer, A. M., Teasley, S. L., McPherson, D. M., Simon, S. D., Santos, S. R., . . . Hipsh, N. E. (2002). A breastfeeding assessment score to evaluate the risk for cessation of breastfeeding by 7 to 10 days of age. *Journal of Pediatrics, 141,* 659–664.

Halpern, S. H., Levine, T., Wilson, D. B., MacDonell, J., Katsiris, S. E., & Leighton, B. L. (1999). Effect of labor analgesia on breastfeeding success. *Birth, 26,* 83–88.

Hamilton, B. E., Martin, J. A., & Ventura, S. J. (2011). *Births: Preliminary data for 2010. National vital statistics reports* (Vol. 60, no. 2). Hyattsville, MD: National Center for Health Statistics.

Hamza, J., Benlabed, M., Orhant, G., Escourrou, P., Curzi-Dascalova, L., & Gaultier, C. (1992). Neonatal pattern of breathing during active and quiet sleep after maternal administration of meperidine. *Pediatric Research, 4,* 412–416.

Handlin, L., Jonas, W., Petersson, M., Ejdeback, M., Ransjo-Arvidson, A-B., Nissen, E., & Uvnas-Moberg, K. (2009). Effects of sucking and skin-to-skin contact on maternal ACTH and cortisol levels during the second day postpartum-influence of epidural analgesia and oxytocin in the perinatal period. *Breastfeeding Medicine, 4,* 207–220.

Harris, D. L., Weston, P. J., & Harding, J. E. (2015). Lactate, rather than ketones, may provide alternative cerebral fuel in hypoglycaemic newborns. *Archives of Disease in Childhood—Fetal and Neonatal Edition, 100,* F161–F164.

Hawdon, J. M., Ward-Platt, M. P., & Aynsley-Green, A. (1992). Patterns of metabolic adaptation for term and preterm infants in the first neonatal week. *Archives of Disease in Childhood, 67,* 357–365.

Hayden, C. K., Shattuck, K. E., Richardson, C. V., Ahrendt, D. K., House, R., & Swischuk, L. E. (1985). Subependymal germinal matrix hemorrhage in full-term neonates. *Pediatrics, 75,* 714–718.

Heck, L. J., & Erenberg, A. (1987). Serum glucose levels in term neonates during the first 48 hours of life. *Journal of Pediatrics, 110,* 119–122.

Heinig, M. J., Follett, J. R., Ishii, K. D., Kavanagh-Prochaska, K., Cohen, R., & Panchula, J. (2006). Barriers to compliance with infant-feeding recommendations among low-income women. *Journal of Human Lactation, 22,* 27–38.

Henderson, J. J., Dickinson, J. E., Evans, S. F., McDonald, S. J., & Paech, M. J. (2003). Impact of intrapartum epidural analgesia on breastfeeding duration. *Australian and New Zealand Journal of Obstetrics and Gynaecology, 43,* 372–377.

Herrera, A. J. (1984). Supplemented versus unsupplemented breastfeeding. *Perinatology/Neonatology, 8,* 70–71.

Herrera-Gomez, A., Garcia-Martinez, O., Ramos-Torrecillas, J., de Luna-Bertos, E., Ruiz, C., & Ocana-Peinado, F. M. (2015). Retrospective study of the association between epidural analgesia during labour and complications for the newborn. *Midwifery, 31,* 613–616.

Higgins, J., Gleeson, R., Holohan, M., Cooney, C., & Darling, M. (1996). Maternal and neonatal hyponatremia: A comparison of Hartmann's solution with 5% dextrose for the delivery of oxytocin in labour. *European Journal of Obstetrics and Gynecology and Reproductive Biology, 68,* 47–48.

Hill, P. D., Humenick, S. S., Brennan, M. L., & Woolley, D. (1997). Does early supplementation affect longterm breastfeeding? *Clinical Pediatrics, 36,* 345–350.

Hiraishi, S., Agata, Y., Saito, K., Oguchi, K., Misawa, H., Fujino, N., Horiguchi, Y., & Yashiro, K. (1991). Inter-atrial shunt flow profiles in newborn infants: A colour flow and pulsed Doppler echocardiographic study. *British Heart Journal, 65,* 41–45.

Hirth, R., Weitkamp, T., & Dwivedi, A. (2012). Maternal intravenous fluids and infant weight. *Clinical Lactation, 3,* 59–63.

Holtrop, P. C., Madison, K. A., Kiechle, F. L., Karcher, R. E., & Batton, D. G. (1990). A comparison of chromogen test strip (Chemstrip bG) and serum glucose values in newborns. *American Journal of Diseases in Childhood, 144,* 183–185.

Hoover, K. (1998). Supplementation of the newborn by spoon in the first 24 hours. *Journal of Human Lactation, 14,* 245.

Hornell, A., Hofvander, Y., & Kylberg, E. (2001). Solids and formula: Association with pattern and duration of breastfeeding. *Pediatrics, 107*(3), e38.

Host, A. (1991). Importance of the first meal on the development of cow's milk allergy and intolerance. *Allergy Proceedings, 10,* 227–232.

Howard, C. R., de Blieck, E. A., ten Hoopen, C. B., Howard, F. M., Lanphear, B. P., & Lawrence, R. A. (1999). Physiologic stability of newborns during cup- and bottle-feeding. *Pediatrics, 104,* 1204–1207.

Howard, C. R., Howard, F. M., Lanphear, B., Eberly, S., deBlieck, E. A., Oakes, D., & Lawrence, R. A. (2003). Randomized clinical trial of pacifier use and bottle-feeding or cupfeeding and their effect on breastfeeding. *Pediatrics, 111,* 511–518.

Huang, Y.-Y., Gau, M.-L., Huang, C.-M., & Lee, J.-T. (2009). Supplementation with cup-feeding as a substitute for bottle-feeding to promote breastfeeding. *Chang Gung Medical Journal, 32,* 423–431.

Hudak, M. L., Tan, R. C., Committee on Drugs, Committee on Fetus and Newborn, & American Academy of Pediatrics. (2012). Neonatal drug withdrawal. *Pediatrics, 129,* e540–e560.

Hung, K. J., & Berg, O. (2011). Early skin-to-skin after cesarean to improve breastfeeding. *MCN American Journal of Maternal Child Nursing, 36,* 318–324.

Ingelfinger, J. R. (1991). Renal conditions in the newborn period. In J. P. Cloherty & A. R. Stark (Eds.), *Manual of neonatal care* (3rd ed., pp. 477–495). Boston, MA: Little, Brown and Company.

Inoue, I., Sakashita, R., & Kamegai, T. (1995). Reduction of masseter muscle activity in bottle-fed babies. *Early Human Development, 42,* 185–193.

Iqbal, M. M., Gundlapalli, S. P., Ryan, W. G., Ryals, T., & Passman, T. E. (2001). Effects of mood-stabilizing drugs on fetuses, neonates, and nursing infants. *Southern Medical Journal, 94,* 305–322.

Iyer, N. P., Srinivasan, R., Evans, K., Ward, L., Cheung, W. Y., & Matthes, J. W. (2008). Impact of early weighing policy on neonatal hypernatraemic dehydration and breastfeeding. *Archives of Disease in Childhood, 93,* 297–299.

Jackman, K. T. (2013). Go with the flow: Choosing a feeding system for infants in the neonatal intensive care unit and beyond based on flow performance. *Newborn & Infant Nursing Reviews, 13,* 31–34.

Jacobs, L. A., Dickinson, J. E., Hart, P. D., Doherty, D. A., & Faulkner, S. J. (2007). Normal nipple position in term infants measured on breastfeeding ultrasound. *Journal of Human Lactation, 23,* 52–59.

Jacobson, B., Eklund, G., Hamberger, L., Linnarsson, D., Sedvall, G., & Valverius, M. (1987). Perinatal origin of adult self-destructive behavior. *Acta Psychiatrica Scandinavica, 76,* 364–371.

Jacobson, B., Nyberg, K., Eklund, G., Bygdeman, M., & Rydberg, U. (1988). Obstetric pain medication and eventual adult amphetamine addiction in offspring. *Acta Obstetricia et Gynecologica Scandinavica, 67,* 677–682.

Jacobson, B., Nyberg, K., Gronbladh, L., Eklund, G., Bygdeman, M., & Rydberg, U. (1990). Opiate addiction in adult offspring through possible imprinting after obstetric treatment. *British Medical Journal, 301,* 1067–1070.

Jarvinen, K. M., Laine, S. T., Jarvenpaa, A. L., & Suomaiainen, H. K. (2000). Does low IgA in human milk predispose the infant to development of cow's milk allergy? *Pediatric Research, 48,* 457–462.

The Joint Commission. (2011). Perinatal care. Retrieved from http://www.jointcommission.org/perinatal_care

The Joint Commission. (2012). The Joint Commission expands performance measurement requirements. Retrieved from http://www.amnhealthcare.com/latest-healthcare-news/the-joint-commission-expands-performance-measurement-requirements/

Jonas, W., Johansson, L. M., Nissen, E., Ejdeback, M., Ransjo-Arvidson, A. B., & Uvnas-Moberg, K. (2009). Effects of intrapartum oxytocin administration and epidural analgesia on the concentration of plasma oxytocin and prolactin, in response to suckling during the second day postpartum. *Breastfeeding Medicine, 4,* 71–82.

Jordan, S. (2006). Infant feeding and analgesia in labour: The evidence is accumulating. *International Breastfeeding Journal, 1*, 25. Retrieved from http://www.internationalbreastfeedingjournal.com/content/1/1/25

Jordan, S., Emery, S., Bradshaw, C., Watkins, A., & Friswell, W. (2005). The impact of intrapartum analgesia on infant feeding. *BJOG: International Journal of Obstetrics and Gynaecology, 112*, 927–934.

Jordan, S., Emery, S., Watkins, A., Evans, J. D., Storey, M., & Morgan, G. (2009). Associations of drugs routinely given in labour with breastfeeding at 48 hours: Analysis of the Cardiff Births Survey. *BJOG: International Journal of Obstetrics and Gynaecology, 116*, 1622–1632.

Juvonen, P., Mansson, M., Kjellman, N. I., Bjorkstén, B., & Jakobsson, I. (1999). Development of immunoglobulin G and immunoglobulin E antibodies to cow's milk proteins and ovalbumin after a temporary neonatal exposure to hydrolyzed and whole cow's milk proteins. *Pediatric Allergy and Immunology, 10*, 191–198.

Karjalainen, J., Martin, J. M., Knip, M., Ilonen, J., Robinson, B. H., Savilahti, E., . . . Dosch, H. M. (1992). A bovine albumin peptide as a possible trigger of insulin-dependent diabetes mellitus. *New England Journal of Medicine, 327*, 302–307.

Karlberg, P. (1960). The adaptive changes in the immediate postnatal period with particular reference to respiration. *Journal of Pediatrics, 56*, 585–604.

Keefe, M. R. (1987). Comparison of neonatal nighttime sleep–wake patterns in nursery versus rooming-in environments. *Nursing Research, 36*, 140–144.

Keefe, M. R. (1988). The impact of infant rooming-in on maternal sleep at night. *Journal of Obstetric, Gynecologic, and Neonatal Nursing, 17*, 122–126.

Kent, J. C., Hepworth, A. R., Langton, D. B., & Hartmann, P. E. (2015). Impact of measuring milk production by test weighing on breastfeeding confidence in mothers of term infants. *Breastfeeding Medicine, 10*, 318–325.

Keppler, A. B. (1988). The use of intravenous fluids during labor. *Birth, 15*, 75–79.

Kieviet, N., Dolman, K. M., & Honig, A. (2013). The use of psychotropic medication during pregnancy: How about the newborn? *Neuropsychiatric Disease and Treatment, 9*, 1257–1266.

Kinsella, S. M., Pirlet, M., Mills, M. S., Tuckey, J. P., & Thomas, T. A. (2000). Randomized study of intravenous fluid preload before epidural analgesia during labour. *British Journal of Anaesthesiology, 85*, 311–313.

Klaus, M. H., Tooley, W. H., Weaver, K. H., & Clements, J. A. (1963). Lung volume in the newborn infant. *Pediatrics, 30*, 111–116.

Knip, M., Veijola, R., Virtanen, S. M., Hyoty, H., Vaarala, O., & Akerblom, H. K. (2005). Environmental triggers and determinants of beta cell autoimmunity and type I diabetes. *Diabetes, 54*, S125–S136.

Knip, M., Virtanen, S. M., & Akerblom, H. K. (2010). Infant feeding and the risk of type I diabetes. *American Journal of Clinical Nutrition, 91*(suppl), 1506S–1513S.

Koenig, J. S., Davies, A. M., & Thach, B. T. (1990). Coordination of breathing, sucking, and swallowing during bottle feedings in human infants. *Journal of Applied Physiology, 69*, 1623–1629.

Komara, C., Simpson, D., Teasdale, C., Whalen, G., Bell, S., & Giovanetto, L. (2007). Intervening to promote early initiation of breastfeeding in the LDR. *American Journal of Maternal/Child Nursing, 32*, 117–121.

Konetzny, G., Bucher, H. U., & Arlettaz, R. (2009). Prevention of hypernatraemic dehydration in breastfed newborn infants by daily weighing. *European Journal of Pediatrics, 168*, 815–818.

Kovach, A. C. (1997). Hospital breastfeeding policies in the Philadelphia area: A comparison with the Ten Steps to Successful Breastfeeding. *Birth, 24*, 41–48.

Krehbiel, D., Pomdron, P., Levy, F., & Prud'Homme, M. J. (1987). Peridural anesthesia disturbs maternal behavior in primiparous and multiparous parturient ewes. *Physiology and Behavior, 40*, 463–467.

Kroeger, M., & Smith, L. J. (2004). *Impact of birthing practices on breastfeeding: Protecting the mother and baby continuum*. Sudbury, MA: Jones and Bartlett.

Kruse, L., Denk, C. E., Feldman-Winter, L., & Rotondo, F. M. (2005). Comparing sociodemographic and hospital influences on breastfeeding initiation. *Birth, 32,* 81–85.

Kuhnert, B. R., Kuhnert, P. M., & Gross, T. L. (1982). The disposition of bupivacaine following epidural anesthesia for cesarean section. *Anesthesiology, 57,* 249–250.

Kumar, M., & Paes, B. (2003). Epidural opioid analgesia and neonatal respiratory depression. *Journal of Perinatology, 23,* 425–427.

Kurinij, N., & Shiono, P. H. (1991). Early formula supplementation of breastfeeding. *Pediatrics, 88,* 745–750.

Laine, K., Heikkinen, T., Ekbald, U., & Kero, P. (2003). Effects of exposure to selective serotonin reuptake inhibitors during pregnancy on serotonergic symptoms in newborns and cord blood monoamine and prolactin concentrations. *Archives of General Psychiatry, 60,* 720–726.

Lamp, J. M., & Macke, J. K. (2010). Relationships among intrapartum maternal fluid intake, birth type, neonatal output, and neonatal weight loss during the first 48 hours after birth. *Journal of Obstetric, Gynecologic, and Neonatal Nursing, 39,* 169–177.

Lang, S. (1994). Cup-feeding: An alternative method. *Midwives Chronicle and Nursing Notes, 107,* 171–176.

Lang, S., Lawrence, C. J., & L'E Orme, R. (1994). Cup feeding: An alternative method of infant feeding. *Archives of Disease in Childhood, 71,* 365–369.

Lawrence, R. A. (1997). *A review of the medical benefits and contraindications to breastfeeding in the United States.* (Maternal and Child Health Technical Information Bulletin). Arlington, VA: National Center for Education in Maternal and Child Health.

Leibovitch, L., Rymer-Haskel, N., Schushan-Eisen, I., Kuint, J., Strauss, T., & Maayan-Metzger, A. (2013). Short-term neonatal outcome among term infants after in utero exposure to serotonin reuptake inhibitors. *Neonatology, 104,* 65–70.

Leighton, B. L., & Halpern, S. H. (2002a). Epidural analgesia: Effects on labor progress and maternal and neonatal outcome. *Seminars in Perinatology, 26,* 122–135.

Leighton, B. L., & Halpern, S. H. (2002b). The effects of epidural analgesia on labor, maternal, and neonatal outcomes: A systematic review. *American Journal of Obstetrics and Gynecology, 186,* S69–S77.

Leng, G., Caquineau, C., & Sabatier, N. (2005). Regulation of oxytocin secretion. *Vitamins and Hormones, 71,* 27–58.

Lieberman, E., Cohen, A. P., Lang, J. M., Frigoletto, F., & Goetzl, L. (1999). Maternal intrapartum temperature elevation as a risk factor for cesarean section and assisted vaginal delivery. *American Journal of Public Health, 89,* 506–510.

Lieberman, E., Davidson, K., Lee-Parritz, A., & Shearer, E. (2005). Changes in fetal position during labor and their association with epidural analgesia. *Obstetrics and Gynecology, 105,* 974–982.

Lieberman, E., Eichenwald, E., Mathur, G., Richardson, D., Heffner, L., & Cohen, A. (2000). Intrapartum fever and unexplained seizures in term infants. *Pediatrics, 106,* 983–988.

Lieberman, E., Lang, J. M., Frigoletto, F., Richardson, D. K., Ringer, S. A., & Cohen, A. (1997). Epidural analgesia, intrapartum fever, and neonatal sepsis evaluation. *Pediatrics, 99,* 415–419.

Lieberman, E., Lang, J., Richardson, D. K., Frigoletto, F. D., Heffner, L. J., & Cohen, A. (2000). Intrapartum maternal fever and neonatal outcome. *Pediatrics, 105,* 8–13.

Lieberman, E., & O'Donoghue, C. (2002). Unintended effects of epidural analgesia during labor: A systematic review. *American Journal of Obstetrics and Gynecology, 186,* S31–S68.

Lind, J. N., Perrine, C. G., & Li, R. (2014). Relationship between use of labor pain medications and delayed onset of lactation. *Journal of Human Lactation, 30,* 167–173.

Lind, J. N., Petersen, E. E., Lederer, P. A., Phillips-Bell, G. S., Perrine, C. G., Li, R., . . . Anjohrin, S. (2015). Infant and maternal characteristics in neonatal abstinence syndrome—selected hospitals in Florida, 2010–2011. *Morbidity and Mortality Weekly Report, 64,* 213–216.

Lind, T. (1983). Fluid balance during labour: A review. *Journal of the Royal Society of Medicine, 76,* 870–875.

Livingstone, V. H., Willis, C. E., Abdel-Wareth, L., Thiessen, P., & Lockitch, G. (2000). Neonatal hyper natremic dehydration associated with breastfeeding malnutrition: Retrospective survey. *Canadian Medical Association Journal, 162,* 647–652.

Loftus, J. R., Hill, H., & Cohen, S. E. (1995). Placental transfer and neonatal effects of epidural sufentanil and fentanyl administered with bupivacaine during labor. *Anesthesiology, 83,* 300–308.

Lozoff, B., Brittenham, G. M., Trause, M. A., Kennell, J. H., & Klaus, M. H. (1977). The mother–newborn relationship: Limits of adaptability. *Journal of Pediatrics, 91,* 1–12.

Lucas, A. (1998). Programming by early nutrition: An experimental approach. *Journal of Nutrition, 128*(2 suppl), 401S–406S.

Ludington, S. M. (1990). Energy conservation during skin-to-skin contact between premature infants and their mothers. *Heart and Lung, 19,* 445–451.

Ludington-Hoe, S. M., Cong, X., & Hashemi, F. (2002). Infant crying: Nature, physiologic consequences, and select interventions. *Neonatal Network, 21,* 29–36.

Lundqvist-Persson, C. (2001). Correlation between level of self-regulation in the newborn infant and developmental status at two years of age. *Acta Paediatrica, 90,* 345–350.

Luopajarvi, K., Savilahti, E., Virtanen, S. M., Ilonen, J., Knip, M., Akerblom, H. K., & Vaarala, O. (2008). Enhanced levels of cow's milk antibodies in infancy in children who develop type I diabetes later in childhood. *Pediatric Diabetes, 9,* 434–441.

Macdonald, P. D., Ross, S. R., Grant, L., & Young, D. (2003). Neonatal weight loss in breast and formula fed infants. *Archives of Disease in Childhood—Fetal and Neonatal Edition, 88,* F472–F476.

Madan, J. C., Hoen, A. G., Lundgren, S. N., Farzan, S. F., Cottingham, K. L., Morrison, H. G., . . . Karagas, M. R. (2016). Association of cesarean delivery and formula supplementation with the intestinal microbiome of 6-week-old infants. *JAMA Pediatrics.* doi:10.1001/jamapediatrics.2015.3732.

Malhotra, N., Vishwambaran, L., Sundaram, K. R., & Narayanan, I. (1999). A controlled trial of alternative methods of oral feeding in neonates. *Early Human Development, 54,* 29–38.

Manganaro, R., Mami, C., Marrone, T., Marseglia, L., & Gemelli, M. (2001). Incidence of dehydration and hypernatremia in exclusively breastfed infants. *Pediatrics, 139,* 673–675.

Marshall, A. M., Nommsen-Rivers, L. A., Hernandez, L. L., Dewey, K. G., Chantry, C. J., Gregerson, K. A., & Horseman, N. D. (2010). Serotonin transport and metabolism in the mammary gland modulates secretory activation and involution. *Journal of Clinical Endocrinology and Metabolism, 95,* 837–846.

Martens, P. J., & Romphf, L. (2007). Factors associated with newborn in-hospital weight loss: Comparisons by feeding method, demographics, and birthing procedures. *Journal of Human Lactation, 23,* 233–241.

Martin, J. A., Hamilton, B. E., Osterman, M. J. K., Curtin, S. C., & Mathews, M. S. (2015). Births: Final data for 2013. *National Vital Statistics Reports, 64*(1). Hyattsville, MD: National Center for Health Statistics.

Martin, J. A., Hamilton, B. E., Ventura, S. J., Osterman, J. A., Kirmeyer, S. Mathews, T. J., & Wilson, E. (2011). Births: Final data for 2009. *National Vital Statistics Reports, 60*(1). Hyattsville, MD: National Center for Health Statistics.

Martin, J. A., Hamilton, B. E., Ventura, S. J., Osterman, M. H. S., Wilson, E. C., & Mathews, T. J. (2012). *Births: Final data for 2010. National Vital Statistics Reports,* 61(1). Hyattsville, MD: National Center for Health Statistics.

Mathew, O. P. (1988a). Nipple units for newborn infants: A functional comparison. *Pediatrics, 81,* 688–691.

Mathew, O. P. (1988b). Respiratory control during nipple feeding in preterm infants. *Pediatric Pulmonology, 5,* 220–224.

Mathew, O. P. (1990). Determinants of milk flow through nipple units: Role of hole size and nipple thickness. *American Journal of Diseases in Childhood, 144,* 222–224.

Mathew, O. P. (1991a). Breathing patterns of preterm infants during bottle feeding: Role of milk flow. *Journal of Pediatrics, 119,* 960–965.

Mathew, O. P. (1991b). Science of bottle feeding. *Journal of Pediatrics, 119,* 511–519.

Mathew, O. P., Clark, M. L., & Pronske, M. H. (1985). Apnea, bradycardia, and cyanosis during oral feeding in term neonates [Letter]. *Pediatrics, 106,* 857.

Matthews, M. K. (1989). The relationship between maternal labour analgesia and delay in the initiation of breastfeeding in healthy neonates in the early neonatal period. *Midwifery, 5,* 3–10.

Mayberry, L. J., Clemmens, D., & De, A. (2002). Epidural analgesia side effects, co-interventions, and care of women during childbirth: A systematic review. *American Journal of Obstetrics and Gynecology, 186,* S81–S93.

Meier, P. (1988). Bottle- and breast-feeding: Effects on transcutaneous oxygen pressure and temperature in preterm infants. *Nursing Research, 37,* 36–41.

Meier, P., & Anderson, G. C. (1987). Responses of small preterm infants to bottle- and breast-feeding. *American Journal of Maternal/Child Nursing, 12,* 97–105.

Merewood, A., Mehta, S. D., Chamberlain, L. B., Phillip, B. L., & Bauchner, H. (2005). Breastfeeding rates in US Baby-Friendly hospitals: Results of a national survey. *Pediatrics, 116,* 628–634.

Merry, H., & Montgomery, A. (2000). Do breastfed babies whose mothers have had labor epidurals lose more weight in the first 24 hours of life? Annual Meeting Abstracts. Academy of Breastfeeding Medicine, *News and Views, 6,* 21.

Mizuno, K., & Ueda, A. (2006). Changes in sucking performance from nonnutritive sucking to nutritive sucking during breast and bottle-feeding. *Pediatric Research, 59,* 728–731.

Moehler, E., Poustka, L., & Resch, F. (2007). Vacuum extraction and autonomic balance in human infants. *Journal of Perinatal Medicine, 35,* 347–349.

Moral, A., Bolibar, I., Seguranyes, G., Ustrell, J. M., Sebastia, G., Martinez-Barba, C., & Rios, J. (2010). Mechanics of sucking: Comparison between bottle feeding and breastfeeding. *BMC Pediatrics, 10,* 6.

Morgan, B. E., Horn, A. R., & Bergman, N. J. (2011). Should neonates sleep alone? *Biological Psychiatry, 70,* 817–825.

Moritz, M. L., Manole, M., Bogen, D. L., & Ayus, J. C. (2005). Breastfeeding-associated hypernatremia: Are we missing the diagnosis? *Pediatrics, 116,* e343–e347

Moses-Kolko, E. L., Bogen, D., Perel, J., Bregar, A., Uhl, K., Levin, B., & Wisner, K. L. (2005). Neonatal signs after late in utero exposure to serotonin reuptake inhibitors. *Journal of the American Medical Association, 293,* 2372–2383.

Mukhopadhyay, S., Lieberman, E. S., Puopolo, K. M., Riley, L. E., & Johnson, L. C. (2015). Effect of early-onset sepsis evaluations on in-hospital breastfeeding practices among asymptomatic term neonates. *Hospital Pediatrics, 5,* 203–210.

Mulder, P. J., Johnson, T. S., & Baker, L. C. (2010). Excessive weight loss in breastfed infants during the postpartum hospitalization. *Journal of Obstetric, Gynecologic, and Neonatal Nursing, 39,* 15–26.

Murray, E. K., Ricketts, S., & Dellaport, J. (2007). Hospital practices that increase breastfeeding duration: Results from a population-based study. *Birth, 34,* 202–211.

Neifert, M. R. (1998). The optimization of breastfeeding in the perinatal period. *Clinical Perinatology, 25,* 303–326.

Neifert, M. R. (1999). Clinical aspects of lactation: Promoting breastfeeding success. *Clinical Perinatology, 26,* 281–306.

Neifert, M. R. (2001). Prevention of breastfeeding tragedies. *Pediatric Clinics of North America, 48,* 273–297.

Neifert, M. R., Lawrence, R., & Seacat, J. (1995). Nipple confusion: Toward a formal definition. *Journal of Pediatrics, 126,* S125–S129.

Nelsom, J. M., Li, R., & Perrine, C. G. (2015). Trends of US hospitals distributing infant formula packs to breastfeeding mothers, 2007 to 2013. *Pediatrics, 135,* 1051–1056.

Newman, J. (1990). Breastfeeding problems associated with the early introduction of bottles and pacifiers. *Journal of Human Lactation, 6,* 59–63.

Nickel, N. C. (2011). *Breastfeeding friendly healthcare: A mixed methods evaluation of the implementation and outcomes of maternity practices to support breastfeeding.* Doctoral dissertation, University of North Carolina at Chapel Hill.

Nickel, N. C., Labbok, M. H., Hudgens, M. G., & Daniels, J. L. (2013). The extent that noncompliance with the Ten Steps to Successful Breastfeeding influences breastfeeding duration. *Journal of Human Lactation, 29,* 59–70.

Nicoll, A., Ginsburg, R., & Tripp, J. H. (1982). Supplementary feeding and jaundice in newborns. *Acta Paediatrica Scandinavica, 71,* 759–761.

Nissen, E., Lilja, G., Matthiesen, A.-S., Ransjo-Arvidsson, A. B., Uvnas-Moberg, K., & Widstrom, A. M. (1995). Effects of maternal pethidine on infants' developing breastfeeding behavior. *Acta Paediatrica, 84,* 140–145.

Nissen, E., Lilja, G., Winstrom, A.-M., & Uvnas-Moberg, K. (1995). Elevation of oxytocin levels early postpartum in women. *Acta Obstetricia et Gynecologica Scandinavica, 74,* 530–533.

Nissen, E., Widstrom, A. M., Lilja, G., Matthiesen, A. S., Uvnas-Moberg, K., Jacobsson, G., & Boréus, L. O. (1997). Effects of routinely given pethidine during labour on infants' developing breastfeeding behavior. Effects of dose-delivery time interval and various concentrations of pethidine/ norpethidine in cord plasma. *Acta Paediatrica, 86,* 201–208.

Noel-Weiss, J., Courant, G., & Woodend, A. K. (2008). Physiological weight loss in the breastfed neonate: A systematic review. *Open Medicine, 2,* 11–22.

Noel-Weiss, J., Woodend, A. K., Peterson, W. E., Gibb, W., & Groll, D. L. (2011). An observational study of associations among maternal fluids during parturition, neonatal output, and breastfed newborn weight loss. *International Breastfeeding Journal, 6,* 9.

Nordeng, H., Lindemann, R., Perminov, K. V., & Reikvam, A. (2001). Neonatal withdrawal syndrome after in utero exposure to selective serotonin reuptake inhibitors. *Acta Paediatrica, 90,* 288–291.

Nowak, A. J., Smith, W. L., & Erenberg, A. (1994). Imaging evaluation of artificial nipples during bottle feeding. *Archives of Pediatrics and Adolescent Medicine, 148,* 40–42.

Nyberg, K., Buka, S. L., & Lipsitt, L. P. (2000). Perinatal medication as a potential risk factor for adult drug abuse in a North American cohort. *Epidemiology, 11,* 715–716.

Oberlander, T. F., Misri, S., Fitzgerald, C. E., Kostaras, X., Rurak, D., & Riggs, W. (2004). Pharmacologic factors associated with transient neonatal symptoms following prenatal psychotropic medication exposure. *Journal of Clinical Psychiatry, 65,* 230–237.

Oddy, W. H., & Glenn, K. (2003). Implementing the Baby Friendly Hospital Initiative: The role of finger feeding. *Breastfeeding Review, 11,* 5–10.

O'Hana, H. P., Levy, A., Rozen, A., Greemberg, L., Shapira, Y., & Sheiner, E. (2008). The effect of epidural analgesia on labor progress and outcome in nulliparous women. *Journal of Maternal–Fetal and Neonatal Medicine, 21,* 517–521.

Okumus, N., Atalay, Y., Onal, E. E., Turkyilmaz, C., Senel, S., Gunaydin, B., . . . Unal, S. (2011). The effects of delivery route and anesthesia type on early postnatal weight loss in newborns: The role of vasoactive hormones. *Journal of Pediatric Endocrinology and Metabolism, 24,* 45–50.

Olza-Fernandez, I., Gabriel, M. A. M., Gil-Sanchez, A., Garcia-Segura, L. M., & Arevalo, M. A. (2014). Neuroendocrinology of childbirth and mother–child attachment: The basis of an etiopathogenic model of perinatal neurobiological disorders. *Frontiers in Neuroendocrinology, 35,* 459–472.

Omigbodun, A. O., Akindele, J. A., Osotimehin, B. O., Fatinikun, T., Fajimi, J. L., & Adeleye, J. A. (1993). Effect of saline and glucose infusions of oxytocin on neonatal bilirubin levels. *International Journal of Gynaecology and Obstetrics, 40,* 235–239.

Omigbodun, A. O., Fajimi, J. L., & Adeleye, J. A. (1991). Effects of using either saline or glucose as a vehicle for infusion in labour. *East African Medical Journal, 68,* 88–92.

Osterman, M. J. K., & Martin, J. A. (2011). Epidural and spinal anesthesia use during labor: 27-state reporting area, 2008. *National Vital Statistics Reports, 59*(5). Hyattsville, MD: National Center for Health Statistics.

Pados, B. F., Park, J., Thoyre, S. M., Estrem, H., & Nix, W. B. (2015). Milk flow rates from bottle nipples used for feeding hospitalized infants. *American Journal of Speech Language Pathology, 24,* 671–679.

Patrick, S. W., Dudley, J., Martin, P. R., Harrell, F. E., Warren, M. D., Hartmann, K. E., . . . Cooper, W. O. (2015). Prescription opioid epidemic and infant outcomes. *Pediatrics, 135,* 842–850.

Perrine, C. G., Scanlon, K. S., Li, R., Odom, E., & Grummer-Strawn, L. M. (2012). Baby-Friendly hospital practices and meeting exclusive breastfeeding intention. *Pediatrics, 130,* 54–60.

Peterson, A., & Harmer, M. (2010). *Balancing breast & bottle: Reaching your breastfeeding goals.* Amarillo, TX: Hale Publishing.

Petrova, A., Hegyi, T., & Mehta, R. (2007). Maternal race/ethnicity and one-month exclusive breastfeeding in association with the in-hospital feeding modality. *Breastfeeding Medicine, 2,* 92–98.

Philipp, B. L., Merewood, A., Miller, L. W., Chawla, N., Murphy-Smith, M. M., Gomes, J. S., . . . Cook, J. T. (2001). Baby-Friendly Hospital Initiative improves breastfeeding initiation rates in a US hospital setting. *Pediatrics, 108,* 677–681.

Piper, S., & Parks, P. L. (1996). Predicting the duration of lactation: Evidence from a national survey. *Birth, 23,* 7–12.

Piper, S., & Parks, P. L. (2001). Use of an intensity ratio to describe breastfeeding exclusivity in a national sample. *Journal of Human Lactation, 17,* 227–232.

Ponkey, S. E., Cohen, A. P., Heffner, L. J., & Lieberman, E. (2003). Persistent fetal occiput posterior position: Obstetric outcomes. *Obstetrics and Gynecology, 101,* 915–920.

Poole, J. H. (2003). Analgesia and anesthesia during labor and birth: Implications for mother and fetus. *Journal of Obstetric, Gynecologic, and Neonatal Nursing, 32,* 780–793.

Porges, S. W. (1983). Heart rate patterns in neonates: A potential diagnostic window to the brain. In T. Field & A. Sostek (Eds.), *Infants born at risk: Physiological, perceptual, and cognitive processes* (pp. 3–22). New York, NY: Grune and Stratton.

Porges, S. W. (1992). Vagal tone: A physiologic marker of stress vulnerability. *Pediatrics, 90,* 498–504.

Powers, N. G., & Slusser, W. (1997). Breastfeeding update 2: Clinical lactation management. *Pediatrics in Review, 18,* 147–161.

Preer, G. L., Newby, P. K., & Philipp, B. L. (2012). Weight loss in exclusively breastfed infants delivered by cesarean birth. *Journal of Human Lactation, 28,* 153–158.

Radzyminski, S. (2003). The effect of ultra low dose epidural analgesia on newborn breastfeeding behaviors. *Journal of Obstetric, Gynecologic, and Neonatal Nursing, 32,* 322–331.

Rahm, V.-A., Hallgren, A., Hogberg, H., Hurtig, I., & Odlind, V. (2002). Plasma oxytocin levels in women during labor with or without epidural analgesia: A prospective study. *Acta Obstetricia et Gynecologica Scandinavica, 81,* 1033–1039.

Ransjo-Arvidson, A.-B., Matthiesen, A.-S., Lilja, G., Nissen, E., Widstrom, A. M., & Uvnas-Moberg, K. (2001). Maternal analgesia during labor disturbs newborn behavior: Effects on breastfeeding, temperature, and crying. *Birth, 28,* 5–12.

Reynolds, G. J., & Davies, S. (1993). A clinical audit of cot-side blood glucose measurement in the detection of neonatal hypoglycemia. *Journal of Pediatrics and Child Health, 29,* 289–291.

Righard, L., & Alade, M. (1990). Effect of delivery room routines on success of first breastfeed. *Lancet, 336,* 1105–1107.

Righard, L., & Alade, M. O. (1992). Sucking technique and its effects on success of breastfeeding. *Birth, 19,* 185–189.

Riley, L. E., Celi, A. C., Onderdonk, A. B., Roberts, D. J., Johnson, L. C., Tsen, L. C., . . . Lieberman, E. S. (2011). Association of epidural-related fever and noninfectious inflammation in term labor. *Obstetrics and Gynecology, 117,* 588–595.

Riordan, J., Gross, A., Angeron, J., Krumwiede, B., & Melin, J. (2000). The effect of labor pain relief medication on neonatal suckling and breastfeeding duration. *Journal of Human Lactation, 16,* 7–12.

Riordan, J., & Riordan, S. (2000). *The effect of labor epidurals on breastfeeding.* Unit 4/Lactation Consultant Series Two. Schaumburg, IL: La Leche League International.

Roca, A., Garcia-Esteve, L., Imaz, M. L., Torres, A., Hernandez, S., Botet, F., . . . Martin-Santos, R. (2011). Obstetrical and neonatal outcomes after prenatal exposure to selective serotonin reuptake inhibitors: The relevance of dose. *Journal of Affective Disorders, 135,* 208–215.

Rocha, N. M. N., Martinez, F. E., & Jorge, S. M. (2002). Cup or bottle for preterm infants: Effects on oxygen saturation, weight gain, and breastfeeding. *Journal of Human Lactation, 18,* 132–138.

Rodriguez, G., Ventura, P., Samper, M. P., Moreno, L., Sarria, A., & Pérez-González, J. M. (2000). Changes in body composition during the initial hours of life in breastfed healthy term newborns. *Biology of the Neonate, 77,* 12–16.

Rooth, G., Lysikiewicz, A., Huch, R., & Huch, A. (1983). Some effects of maternal pethidine administration on the newborn. *British Journal of Obstetrics and Gynecology, 90,* 28–33.

Rosenberg, K. D., Eastham, C. A., & Kasehagen, L. J., (2008). Sandoval AP. Marketing infant formula through hospitals: The impact of commercial hospital discharge packs on breastfeeding. *American Journal of Public Health, 98,* 290–295.

Rosenberg, K. D., Stull, J. D., Adler, M. R., Kasehagen, L. J., & Crivelli-Kovach, A. (2008). Impact of hospital policies on breastfeeding outcomes. *Breastfeeding Medicine, 3,* 110–116.

Rosenblatt, D. B., Belsy, E. M., Lieberman, B. A., Redshaw, M., Caldwell, J., Notarianni, L., . . . Beard, R. W. (1981). The influence of maternal analgesia on neonatal behavior: II. Epidural bupivacaine. *British Journal of Obstetrics and Gynecology, 88,* 407–413.

Ross, E., & Fuhrman, L. (2015). Supporting oral feeding skills through bottle selection. *Perspectives on Swallowing and Swallowing Disorders (Dysphagia), 24,* 50–57.

Rowe-Murray, H., & Fisher, J. R. W. (2002). Baby Friendly hospital practices: Cesarean section is a persistent barrier to early initiation of breastfeeding. *Birth, 29,* 124–131.

Rubaltelli, F. F. (1968). The frequency of neonatal hyperbilirubinemia in newborns with vacuum extractor. *Attualità di Ostetricia e Ginecología, 14,* 1–4.

Ruchala, P. L., Metheny, N., Essenpreis, H., & Borcherding, K. (2002). Current practice in oxytocin dilution and fluid administration for induction of labor. *Journal of Obstetric, Gynecologic, and Neonatal Nursing, 31,* 545–550.

Ruth-Sanchez, V., & Greene, C. V. (1997). Water intoxication in a three day old: A case presentation. *Mother and Baby Journal, 2,* 5–11.

Ryan, A. S., Wenjun, Z., & Acosta, A. (2002). Breastfeeding continues to increase into the new millennium. *Pediatrics, 110,* 1103–1109.

Saarinen, K. M., Juntunen-Backman, K., Jarvenpaa, A. L., Kuitunen, P., Lope, L., Renlund, M., . . . Savilahti, E. (1999). Supplementary feeding in maternity hospitals and the risk of cow's milk allergy: A prospective study of 6209 infants. *Journal of Allergy and Clinical Immunology, 104,* 457–461.

Saarinen, K. M., & Savilahti, E. (2000). Infant feeding patterns affect the subsequent immunological features in cow's milk allergy. *Clinical and Experimental Allergy, 30,* 400–406.

Sakashita, R., Kamegai, T., & Inoue, N. (1996). Masseter muscle activity in bottle feeding with the chewing type bottle teat: Evidence from electromyographs. *Early Human Development, 45,* 83–92.

Saland, J., McNamara, H., & Cohen, M. I. (1974). Navajo jaundice: A variant of neonatal hyperbilirubinemia associated with breastfeeding. *Journal of Pediatrics, 85,* 271–275.

Salas, A. A., Salazar, J., Burgoa, C. V., De-Villegas, C. A., Quevedo, V., & Soliz, A. (2009). Significant weight loss in breastfed term infants readmitted for hyperbilirubinemia. *BMC Pediatrics, 9,* 82.

Salisbury, A. L., Wisner, K. L., Pearlstein, T., Battle, C. L., Stroud, L., & Lester, B. M. (2011). Newborn neurobehavioral patterns are differentially related to prenatal maternal major depressive disorder and serotonin reuptake inhibitor treatment. *Depression and Anxiety, 28,* 1008–1019.

Scariati, P. D., Grummer-Strawn, L. M., & Fein, S. B. (1997). Water supplementation of infants in the first month of life. *Archives of Pediatrics and Adolescent Medicine, 151,* 830–832.

Segami, Y., Mizuno, K., Taki, M., & Itabashi, K. (2013). Perioral movements and sucking pattern during bottle feeding with a novel, experimental teat are similar to breastfeeding. *Journal of Perinatology, 33,* 319–323.

Semenic, S., Loiselle, C., & Gottlieb, L. (2008). Predictors of the duration of exclusive breastfeeding among first-time mothers. *Research in Nursing Health, 31,* 428–441.

Sepkoski, C. M., Lester, B. M., Ostheimer, G. W., & Brazelton, T. B. (1992). The effects of maternal epidural anesthesia on neonatal behavior during the first month. *Developmental Medicine and Child Neurology, 34,* 1072–1080.

Shaker, I. J., Schaefer, J. A., James, A. E., Jr, & White, J. J. (1973). Aerophagia, a mechanism for spontaneous rupture of the stomach in the newborn. *Annals of Surgery, 39,* 619–623.

Sharkey, J. T., Puttaramu, R., Word, R. A., & Olcese, J. (2009). Melatonin synergizes with oxytocin to enhance contractility of human myometrial smooth muscle cells. *Journal of Clinical Endocrinology and Metabolism, 2,* 421–442.

Shivpuri, C. R., Martin, R. J., Carlo, W. A., & Fanaroff, A. A. (1983). Decreased ventilation in preterm infants during oral feeding. *Journal of Pediatrics, 103,* 285–289.

Shrago, L. (1987). Glucose water supplementation of the breastfed infant during the first three days of life. *Journal of Human Lactation, 3,* 82–86.

Shrago, L. C., Reifsnider, E., & Insel, K. (2006). The neonatal bowel output study: Indicators of adequate breast milk intake in neonates. *Pediatric Nursing, 32,* 195–201.

Sievers, E., Haase, S., Oldigs, H.-D., & Schaub, J. (2003). The impact of peripartum factors on the onset and duration of lactation. *Biology of the Neonate, 83,* 246–252.

Simpson, K. R. (2011). Clinicians' guide to the use of oxytocin for labor induction and augmentation. *Journal of Midwifery and Women's Health, 56,* 214–221.

Simpson, K. R., & James, D. C. (2008). Effects of oxytocin-induced uterine hyperstimulation during labor on fetal oxygen status and fetal heart rate patterns. *American Journal of Obstetrics and Gynecology, 199,* 34.e1–34.e5.

Singh, G., Chonan, R., & Sidhu, K. (2009). Effect of antenatal expression of breast milk at term in reducing breast-feeding failures. *Medical Journal of Armed Forces India, 65,* 131–133.

Smith, J., Plaat, F., & Fisk, N. M. (2008). The natural cesarean: A woman-centered technique. *British Journal of Obstetrics and Gynecology, 115,* 1037–1042.

Sondergaard, C., Henriksen, T. B., Obel, C., & Wisborg, K. (2001). Smoking during pregnancy and infantile colic. *Pediatrics, 108,* 342–346.

Srinivasan, G., Pildes, R. S., Cattamanchi, G., Voora, S., & Lilien, D. (1986). Plasma glucose values in normal neonates: A new look. *Journal of Pediatrics, 109,* 114–117.

Stage, E., Mathiesen, E. R., Emmersen, P. B., Greisen, G., & Damm, P. (2010). Diabetic mothers and their newborn infants: Rooming-in and neonatal morbidity. *Acta Paediatrica, 99,* 997–999.

Steinbach, M. T. (1999). Traumatic birth injury: Intracranial hemorrhage. *Mother and Baby Journal, 4,* 5–14.

Stellwagen, L. M., Hubbard, E. T., & Wolf, A. (2007). The late preterm infant: A little baby with big needs. *Contemporary Pediatrics, 4*(11), 51–59. Retrieved from http://contemporarypediatrics.modernmedicine.com/news/late-preterm-infant-little-baby-big-needs

Stettler, N., Stallings, V. A., Troxel, A. B., Zhao, J., Schinnar, R., Nelson, S. E., . . . Strom, B. L. (2005). Weight gain in the first week of life and overweight in adulthood: A cohort study of European American subjects fed infant formula. *Circulation, 111,* 1897–1903.

Stratton, J. F., Stronge, J., & Boylan, P. C. (1995). Hyponatremia and non-electrolyte solutions in labouring primigravida. *European Journal of Obstetrics and Gynecology and Reproductive Biology, 59,* 149–151.

Svensson, K., Matthiesen, A. S., & Widstrom, A. M. (2005). Night rooming-in: Who decides? An example of staff influence on mother's attitude. *Birth, 32,* 99–106.

Swenne, I., Sandberg, E., & Ostenson, C. G. (1994). Inter-relationship between serum concentrations of glucose, glucagon, and insulin during the first two days of life in healthy newborns. *Acta Pediatrica, 83,* 915–919.

Tender, J. A. F., Janakiram, J., Arce, E., Mason, R., Jordan, T., Marsh, M., . . . Moon, R. Y. (2009). Reasons for in-hospital formula supplementation of breastfed infants from low-income families. *Journal of Human Lactation, 25,* 11–17.

Thompson, A. L. (2012). Developmental origins of obesity: early feeding environments, infant growth, and the intestinal microbiome. *American Journal of Human Biology, 24,* 350–360.

Thorley, V. (1997). Cup feeding: Problems created by incorrect use. *Journal of Human Lactation, 13,* 54–55.

Thorp, J. A., Hu, D. H., Albin, R. M., McNitt, J., Meyer, B. A., Cohen, G. R., & Yeast, J. D. (1993). The effect of intrapartum epidural analgesia on nulliparous labor: A randomized, controlled, prospective trial. *American Journal of Obstetrics and Gynecology, 169,* 851–858.

Torvaldsen, S., Roberts, C. L., Simpson, J. M., Thompson, J. F., & Ellwood, D. A. (2006). Intrapartum epidural analgesia and breastfeeding: A prospective cohort study. *International Breastfeeding Journal, 1,* 24.

Towner, D., Castro, M. A., Eby-Wilkens, E., & Hilbert, W. M. (1999). Effect of mode of delivery in nulliparous women on neonatal intracranial injury. *New England Journal of Medicine, 341,* 1709–1714.

Tozier, P. K. (2013). Colostrum versus formula supplementation for glucose stabilization in newborns of diabetic mothers. *Journal of Obstetric, Gynecologic, and Neonatal Nursing, 42,* 619–628.

Uchil, D., & Arulkumaran, S. (2003). Neonatal subgaleal hemorrhage and its relationship to delivery by vacuum extraction. *Obstetrical and Gynecological Survey, 58,* 687–693.

Unal, S., Arhan, E., Kara, N., Uncu, N., & Alliefendioglu, D. (2008). Breastfeeding-associated hypernatremia: Retrospective analysis of 169 term newborns. *Pediatrics International, 50,* 29–34.

Uras, N., Karadag, A., Dogan, G., Tonbul, A., & Tatli, M. M. (2007). Moderate hypernatremic dehydration in newborn infants: Retrospective evaluation of 64 cases. *Journal of Maternal–Fetal and Neonatal Medicine, 20,* 449–452.

U.S. Food and Drug Administration. (1998). FDA public health advisory: Need for CAUTION when using vacuum assisted delivery devices. Retrieved from http://www.fda.gov/MedicalDevices/Safety/AlertsandNotices/PublicHealthNotifications/ucm062295.htm

Vaarala, O., Knip, M., Paronen, J., Hamalainen, A. M., Muona, P., Vaatainen, M., . . . , Akerblom, H. K. (1999). Cow milk formula feeding induces primary immunization to insulin in infants at genetic risk for type I diabetes. *Diabetes, 48,* 1389–1394.

Van de Velde, M. (2015). Patient-controlled intravenous analgesia remifentanil for labor analgesia: Time to stop, think and reconsider. *Current Opinions in Anesthesiology, 28,* 237–239.

Van Dommelen, P., Boer, S., Unal, S., & van Wouwe, J. P. (2014). Charts for weight loss to detect hypernatremic dehydration and prevent formula supplementing. *Birth, 41,* 153–159.

Vandenplas, Y., Delree, M., Bougatef, A., & Sacre, L. (1989). Cervical esophageal perforation diagnosed by endoscopy in a premature infant: Review of recent literature. *Journal of Pediatric Gastroenterology and Nutrition, 8,* 390–393.

Vestermark, V., Hogdall, C. K., Birch, M., Plenov, G., & Toftager-Larsen, K. (1991). Influence of the mode of delivery on initiation of breastfeeding. *European Journal of Obstetrics and Gynecology and Reproductive Biology, 38,* 33–38.

Volmanen, P., Valanne, J., & Alahuhta, S. (2004). Breastfeeding problems after epidural analgesia for labour: A retrospective cohort study of pain, obstetrical procedures and breastfeeding practices. *International Journal of Obstetric Anesthesia, 13,* 25–29.

Vricella, L. K., Louis, J. M., Mercer, B. M., & Bolden, N. (2011). Impact of morbid obesity on epidural anesthesia complications in labor. *American Journal of Obstetrics and Gynecology, 205,* 370, e1–e6.

Waldenstrom, U., & Swenson, A. (1991). Rooming-in at night in the postpartum ward. *Midwifery, 7,* 82–89.

Walker, M. (1989). Functional assessment of infant breastfeeding patterns. *Birth, 16,* 140–147.

Walker, M. (1997). Do labor medications affect breastfeeding? *Journal of Human Lactation, 13,* 131–137.

Walker, M. (2007). *Still selling out mothers and babies: Marketing of breastmilk substitutes in the USA.* Weston, MA: National Alliance for Breastfeeding Advocacy.

Walker, N. C., & O'Brien, B. (1999). The relationship between method of pain management during labor and birth outcomes. *Clinical Nursing Research, 8,* 119–134.

Walters, M. W., Boggs, K. M., Ludington-Hoe, S., Price, K. M., & Morrison, B. (2007). Kangaroo care at birth for full term infants. *American Journal of Maternal/Child Nursing. 32,* 375–381.

Watson, J., Hodnett, E., Armson, A., Davies, B., & Watt-Watson, J. (2012). A randomized controlled trial of the effect of intrapartum intravenous fluid management on breastfed newborn weight loss. *Journal of Obstetric, Gynecologic, and Neonatal Nursing, 41,* 24–32.

Weber, F., Woolridge, M. W., & Baum, J. D. (1986). An ultrasonographic study of the organization of sucking and swallowing by newborn infants. *Developmental Medicine and Child Neurology, 28,* 19–24.

Weiner, P. C., Hogg, M. I. J., & Rosen, M. (1977). Effects of naloxone on pethidine-induced neonatal depression. *British Medical Journal, 2,* 228–231.

Welle-Strand, G. K., Skurtveit, S., Jansson, L. M., Bakstad, B., Bjarko, L., & Ravndal, E. (2013). Breastfeeding reduces the need for withdrawal treatment in opioid-exposed infants. *Acta Paediatrica, 102,* 1060–1066.

Wen, S. W., Liu, S., Kramer, M. S., Marcoux, S., Ohlsson, A., Sauve, R., & Liston, R. (2001). Comparison of maternal and infant outcomes between vacuum extraction and forceps deliveries. *American Journal of Epidemiology, 153,* 103–107.

Widstrom, A-M., Lilja, G., Aaltomaa-Michalias, P., Dahllof, A., Lintula, M., & Nissen, E. (2011). Newborn behavior to locate the breast when skin-to-skin: A possible method for enabling early self-regulation. *Acta Paediatrica, 100,* 79–85.

Widstrom, A. M., Ransjo-Arvidsson, A.-B., Christensson, K., Matthiesen, A. S., Winberg, J., & Uvnas-Moberg, K. (1987). Gastric suction in healthy newborn infants. *Acta Paediatrica Scandinavica, 76,* 566–572.

Wieczorek, P. M., Guest, S., Balki, M., Shah, V., & Carvalho, J. C. A. (2010). Breastfeeding success rate after vaginal delivery can be high despite the use of epidural fentanyl: An observational cohort study. *International Journal of Obstetric Anesthesia, 19,* 273–277.

Wight, N. E. (2001). *Supplements and the breastfed infant: When are they needed and how should they be supplied?* [Independent study module]. Schaumburg, IL: La Leche League International.

Wight, N. E. (2006). Hypoglycemia in breastfed neonates. *Breastfeeding Medicine, 1,* 253–262.

Wiklund, I., Norman, M., Uvnas-Moberg, K., Ranjo-Arvidson, A. B., & Andolf, E. (2009). Epidural analgesia: Breastfeeding success and related factors. *Midwifery, 25,* e31–e38.

Williams, A. F. (1997). *Hypoglycemia of the newborn: Review of the literature.* Geneva, Switzerland: World Health Organization.

Wojcicki, J. M., Holbrook, K., Lustig, R. H., Caughey, A. B., Munoz, R. F., & Heyman, M. B. (2011). Infant formula, tea, and water supplementation of Latino infants at 4–6 weeks postpartum. *Journal of Human Lactation, 27,* 122–130.

Wolf, L. S., & Glass, R. P. (1992). *Feeding and swallowing disorders in infancy.* Tucson, AZ: Therapy Skill Builders.

Wolf, L. S., & Glass, R. P. (2008). The Goldilocks problem: Milk flow that is not too fast, not too slow, but just right. In C. W. Genna (Ed.), *Supporting sucking skills in breastfeeding infants* (pp. 131–152). Sudbury, MA: Jones and Bartlett.

Woods, A. B., Crist, B., Kowalewski, S., Carroll, J., Warren, J., & Robertson, J. (2012). A cross-sectional analysis of the effect of patient-controlled epidural analgesia versus patient controlled analgesia on postcesarean pain and breastfeeding. *Journal of Obstetric, Gynecologic, and Neonatal Nursing, 41,* 339–346.

World Health Organization. (1998). *Evidence for the ten steps to successful breastfeeding.* Geneva, Switzerland: Author.

World Health Organization/United Nations Children's Fund. (1989). *Protecting, promoting and supporting breastfeeding: The special role of maternity services.* Geneva, Switzerland: World Health Organization.

World Health Organization/United Nations Children's Fund. (1992). *Baby-friendly hospital initiative. Part II: Hospital-level implementation*. Geneva, Switzerland: World Health Organization.

World Health Organization/United Nations Children's Fund. (2009). *Acceptable medical reasons for use of breast-milk substitutes*. Geneva, Switzerland: World Health Organization.

Wright, A., Rice, S., & Wells, S. (1996). Changing hospital practices to increase the duration of breastfeeding. *Pediatrics, 97,* 669–675.

Yamauchi, Y., & Yamanouchi, I. (1990a). Breastfeeding frequency during the first 24 hours after birth in full-term neonates. *Pediatrics, 86,* 171–175.

Yamauchi, Y., & Yamanouchi, I. (1990b). The relationship between rooming-in/not rooming-in and breastfeeding variables. *Acta Paediatrica (Oslo), 79,* 1017–1022.

Yang, W-C., Zhao, L-L., Li, Y-C., Chen, C-H., Chang, Y-J., Fu, Y-C., & Wu, H-P. (2013). Bodyweight loss in predicting neonatal hyperbilirubinemia 72 hours after birth in term newborn infants. *BMC Pediatrics, 13,* 145.

Zeiger, R. S. (2003). Food allergen avoidance in the prevention of food allergy in infants and children. *Pediatrics, 111*(suppl), 1662–1671.

Zeskind, P. S. (1980). Adult responses to the cries of low-risk and high-risk infants. *Infant Behavior and Development, 3,* 167–177.

Zeskind, P. S., Marshall, T. R., & Goff, D. M. (1992). Rhythmic organization of heart rate in breast-fed and bottle-fed newborn infants. *Early Development and Parenting, 1,* 79–87.

Zeskind, P. S., & Stephens, L. E. (2004). Maternal selective reuptake inhibitor use during pregnancy and newborn neurobehavior. *Pediatrics, 113,* 368–375.

ADDITIONAL READING AND RESOURCES

Sources for Improving Hospital Care of the Breastfeeding Mother and Infant

Arizona Model Hospital Policy Resource Guide, http://www.azdhs.gov/phs/bnp/gobreastmilk/documents/AzBSBS-Model-Hospital-Policy-Guide.pdf

Baby-Friendly USA, Inc. (administers the Baby-Friendly certifying process for hospitals in the United States)
125 Wolf Road, Suite 103
Albany, NY 12205
Phone: (508) 888-8092
Email: Info@babyfriendlyusa.org
Website: http://www.babyfriendlyusa.org

"Breastfeeding Best Practice Guidelines for Nurses" includes evidence-based nursing practice guidelines for providing lactation care and services and is available from the Registered Nurses of Ontario. http://rnao.ca/bpg/guidelines/breastfeeding-best-practice-guidelines-nurses

Centers for Disease Control and Prevention. (2011). Vital signs: Hospital practices to support breastfeeding—United States 2007 and 2009. *Morbidity and Mortality Weekly Report, 60*(30), 1020–1025.

Centers for Disease Control and Prevention. (2013). *Strategies to prevent obesity and other chronic diseases: The CDC guide to strategies to support breastfeeding mothers and babies.* Atlanta, GA: U.S. Department of Health and Human Services. http://www.cdc.gov/breastfeeding/pdf/BF-Guide-508.PDF

Hospital Breastfeeding Toolkit—Illinois, http://www.scribd.com/doc/118247333/Hospital-Breastfeeding-Toolkit-Illinois

Maryland Hospital Breastfeeding Policy Recommendations, http://phpa.dhmh.maryland.gov/mch/Documents/MarylandHospitalBreastfeedingPolicyRecommendations.pdf

Model Hospital Policy Recommendations On-Line Toolkit, http://www.cdph.ca.gov/healthinfo/healthyliving/childfamily/Pages/MainPageofBreastfeedingToolkit.aspx

New York State Model Hospital Breastfeeding Policy, https://www.health.ny.gov/community/pregnancy/breastfeeding/docs/model_hospital_breastfeeding_policy_implementation_guide.pdf

Sample Hospital Breastfeeding Policy for Newborns from the American Academy of Pediatrics Section on Breastfeeding Academy of Breastfeeding Medicine. Protocol #7: Model Breastfeeding Policy, http://www.bfmed.org/Media/Files/Protocols/English%20Protocol%207%20Model%20Hospital%20Policy.pdf

Smith, L. J., & Kroger, M. (2010). *Impact of birthing practices on breastfeeding* (2nd ed.). Sudbury, MA: Jones & Bartlett Learning.

U.S. Department of Health and Human Services. (2011). *The Surgeon General's call to action to support breastfeeding.* Washington, DC: Author. Retrieved from http://www.surgeongeneral.gov/library/calls/breastfeeding/index.html

Alternative Devices for Supplementing the Breastfed Infant

Books

Genna, C. W. (2009). *Selecting and using breastfeeding tools.* Amarillo, TX: Hale Publishing.

Peterson, A., & Harmer, M. (2010). *Balancing breast and bottle: Reaching your breastfeeding goals.* Amarillo, TX: Hale Publishing.

Wolf, L. S., & Glass, R. P. (1992). *Feeding and swallowing disorders in infancy.* Tucson, AZ: Therapy Skill Builders.

Cups

Ameda Baby Cup, Ameda
475 Half Day Rd.
Lincolnshire, IL 60069
Phone: (877) 992-6332
Website: http://www.ameda.com

Flexi-Cut Cup (uses a cutout design to prevent neck extension), New Visions
1124 Roberts Mountain Rd.
Faber, VA 22938
Phone: (800) 606-7112
Website: http://www.new-vis.com

Foley Cup, Foley Development, Inc.
PO Box 50
Conway, MI 49722
Phone: (888) 463-2688
Website: http://www.foleycup.com

Soft Feeder, Medela, Inc.
1101 Corporate Dr.
McHenry, IL 60050
Phone: (800) 435-8316 or (815) 363-1166
Website: http://www.medela.com

Suckle Cup, Maternal Concepts
130 North Public St.
Elmwood, WI 54740
Phone: (800) 310-5817
Website: http://www.maternalconcepts.com

Tube-Feeding Devices

Hazelbaker FingerFeeder, Aidan and Eva
5115 Olentangy River Rd.
Columbus, OH 43235
Phone: (614) 451-1154
Website: http://www.fingerfeeder.com/index.html

Human Lactation Center, Resources on Crying, Secrets of Baby Behavior
http://lactation.ucdavis.edu/products/index.html

Lact-Aid International, Inc. (Lact-Aid nursing training device)
PO Box 1066
Athens, TN 37371
Phone: (866) 866-1239
Website: http://www.lact-aid.com

Supplemental Nursing System, Medela, Inc.
1101 Corporate Dr.
McHenry, IL 60050
Phone: (800) 435-8316 or (815) 363-1166
Website: http://www.medela.com

Appendix 4-1

Summary Interventions Based on Peripartum Factors, Birthing Practices, and Early Caretaking Behaviors

1. Encourage mothers to attend prenatal childbirth preparation and breastfeeding classes.
2. Discuss potential effects on breastfeeding of common birth interventions and what actions parents may take to reduce adverse effects on breastfeeding.
3. After delivery, facilitate the breast-seeking behaviors of the infant; encourage the first breastfeeding within 60–80 minutes of birth. Avoid forcing the infant to the breast during this time by not pushing the infant's head into the breast or placing pressure on the occipital region of the head.
4. Keep mothers and babies together after delivery and around the clock unless the mother's or infant's condition does not permit or special circumstances arise.
5. Supplementation should occur for medical reasons, using the method least likely to cause disruption of feeding at the breast and with the lowest potential to provoke allergy or diabetes in a susceptible family. Mothers should be asked if there is a family history of allergy or diabetes.
6. If breastfeeding is delayed or interrupted, mothers should be helped to initiate and maintain their milk supply. Hand expression of colostrum may be more effective than the use of a breast pump.
7. Alternative feeding methods, equipment, techniques, and instructions should be selected with the goals of establishing or returning the infant to feeding at the breast while preserving the maternal milk supply.
8. When a mother requests that her baby be supplemented, clinicians should ascertain why the mother wishes this, learn what infant behaviors she interprets as indicating insufficient milk production or inadequate intake, and perform an assessment of a feeding at breast before supplementing the infant.
9. Clinicians should be aware of the possible side effects that many birth interventions can produce in the breastfeeding dyad. See **Boxes 4-11 through 4-13**.
10. Mothers can be given the checklist in **Box 4-14** to use as a tool to assure that they acquire the skills and competence they need to breastfeed their infant postdischarge. Areas that remain unchecked indicate where clinicians need to focus their assessment and teaching efforts. Mothers can be instructed to check off each item as they master the skill or are informed of the information.

Box 4-11 Possible Labor Medication Side Effects

- Infant behavioral disorganization
- Difficulty modulating state control
- Sleepy baby
- Respiratory depression
- Decreased alertness
- Inhibition of sucking
- Less efficient sucking
- Lower neurobehavioral scores
- Increased incidence of sepsis workups
- Delay in effective breastfeeding
- Shorter duration of wakefulness
- Depressed visual and auditory attention
- Longer time to habituate to noise
- Decreased social responsiveness
- Decreased tone and reflexes
- Delayed rooting reflex
- Higher rates of instrument delivery
- Maternal and infant edema/water overload
- Increased use of oxytocin
- Increased incidence of intrapartum fever
- Unexplained neonatal seizures
- Increased incidence of jaundice
- Decreased spontaneous breast-seeking behaviors
- Disturbance of prefeeding sequence of behavior
- Altered sucking patterns
- Less time spent with baby during hospital stay
- Increased incidence of intracranial hemorrhage

Box 4-12 Possible Side Effects of Separation

- Reduced interaction between mother and baby
- Reduced opportunity to learn infant feeding cues
- Decreased access to the breast/fewer breastfeeds
- Increased use of supplementary feedings
- Can delay lactogenesis II
- Babies cry more
- Infants experience less quiet sleep
- Infants startle more
- Infants may have lower body and skin temperatures

- Infants can have lower blood glucose levels
- Is associated with reduced length of breastfeeding
- Care in nursery exposes infants to bright lights and loud noise
- Babies receive less contact with caregiver

Box 4-13 Possible Side Effects of Supplementation

- Decreases incidence of exclusive breastfeeding (in the hospital and long term)
- Can delay lactogenesis II
- Contributes to insufficient milk supply
- Water supplements can:
  - Contribute to weight loss
  - Increase hyperbilirubinemia
  - Exacerbate hypoglycemia
  - Result in caloric deprivation
- Infant formula supplements can:
  - Alter gut flora
  - Provoke sensitivity and allergy to cow's milk protein in susceptible families
  - Act as the environmental triggering event in the development of diabetes in susceptible families

Box 4-14 Checklist of What Mothers Need to Know Prior to Discharge

- ☐ I can position my baby correctly at both breasts.
- ☐ It does not hurt once the baby starts sucking.
- ☐ The baby can latch to each breast.
- ☐ I can tell when the baby is swallowing milk.
- ☐ I know how many times in 24 hours to feed the baby.
- ☐ I know how long to feed the baby on each side.
- ☐ I know when it is time to feed my baby.
- ☐ I know the five feeding cues to use if my baby is sleepy.
- ☐ I know how many diapers baby should have each day.
- ☐ I know how to tell if my baby is jaundiced.
- ☐ I know how to tell if a disposable diaper is wet.
- ☐ I know how much weight baby should gain weekly.
- ☐ I know that artificial nipples and pacifiers can confuse my baby and have been shown other ways to feed him if necessary.
- ☐ Someone will visit me a day or two after I get home, or . . .
- ☐ I will see my pediatrician or family doctor in two days.
- ☐ I know when and who to call for help with nursing.

II

Infant-Related Challenges to Breastfeeding

Chapter 5

First 24–48 Hours: Common Challenges

INTRODUCTION

Proper positioning of the mother and infant and a correct latch of the infant to the breast form the foundation of each breastfeeding encounter. Many problems stem from improper positioning, incorrect latch, and subsequent failure to transfer milk. Some problems innate to the infant or the mother require modification of positioning and latching techniques. This chapter explores positioning, latch, plus selected infant-related problems encountered during the first few days after birth. These days set the stage for successful breastfeeding and the mother's capacity to meet her breastfeeding goals.

CLINICIAN INFLUENCE

Advice given to mothers by healthcare professionals, family, and the media regarding infant care practices such as breastfeeding is a modifiable factor that can influence adherence to evidence-based guidelines. A recent study of more than 1,000 mothers found that approximately 20% of mothers reported receiving no advice from physicians regarding breastfeeding and 10–15% received advice that was not consistent with breastfeeding guidelines such as those promulgated by the American Academy of Pediatrics (Eisenberg, Bair-Merritt, Colson, Heeren, Geller, & Corwin, 2015). Approximately 14.9% of advice from birth hospital nurses was inconsistent with recommended guidelines, and 13.3% of mothers reported receiving no advice from such nurses. The prevalence of advice consistent with recommended guidelines can be improved with evidence-based hospital breastfeeding policies and incentives for physicians to discuss breastfeeding recommendations consistent with accepted national guidelines.

A breastfeeding mother benefits most when a nurse or lactation consultant remains with her for early feedings, ensuring that the infant is latched correctly and transferring milk. Nurses need to demonstrate appropriate positioning and latch, while allowing the mother to perform the task (Gill, 2001). Mothers find it helpful when clinicians offer prenatal information of the realities of breastfeeding, deliver practical help with positioning and latch-on, perform effective interventions for early problems, and offer enlightenment on questions such as how long and how often to breastfeed, when to switch breasts, and whether nipple shields and supplementing with bottles of formula will undermine breastfeeding (Graffy & Taylor, 2005). Inadequate, insensitive, or apathetic approaches to breastfeeding often culminate in a downward spiral of fatigue, frustration, and weaning by 2 weeks postpartum. Neutrality of clinicians regarding infant feeding negatively affects breastfeeding initiation and duration. Mothers who reported that hospital staff expressed no preference regarding infant feeding were more likely to be bottle-feeding at 6 weeks, especially if the mothers had intended to breastfeed for less than 2 months (DiGirolamo, Grummer-Strawn, & Fein, 2003).

Mothers are especially frustrated by inconsistent advice about breastfeeding techniques and the tendency of some clinicians to quickly support the use of a bottle when feeding difficulties are present—sometimes even offering a bottle before the infant goes to breast (Mozingo, Davis, Droppleman, & Merideth, 2000). Inconsistent advice, rushed encounters with mothers, lack of skilled nurses, unavailability of lactation consultants, and the promotion of unhelpful practices sabotage breastfeeding right from the start (McInnes & Chambers, 2008). A meta-synthesis of research examined mothers' perceptions and experiences of breastfeeding support. The study found that mothers actively seek realistic, accurate, and detailed information, especially practical help. The findings emphasized person-centered relationships and continuity of care as being especially effective in establishing supportive care and a trusting relationship with healthcare professionals (Schmied, Beake, Sheehan, McCourt, & Dykes, 2011). Failure to offer assistance with latch-on, failure to follow up after a feeding, inadequate assessment of breastfeeding technique, anecdotal descriptions of personal experience that differs from other professional information, and failure to provide information regarding community resources have been identified by mothers as behaviors by clinicians that are nonsupportive of learning to breastfeed (Hong, Callister, & Schwartz, 2003).

Clinicians must be mindful of interventions perceived by the mother as being unhelpful, discouraging, or ineffective (Ebersold, Murphy, Paterno, Sauvager, & Wright, 2007). Staff shortages and increasing demands on nurses can contribute to the inability of staff to provide the type of assistance and care that new mothers require. When mothers deem nurses to be too busy or rushed, they may feel disinclined to ask for the help they need (Hong et al., 2003). Mothers with low confidence levels are particularly vulnerable to insufficient and inadequate lactation care and services (Mantha, Davies, Moyer, & Crowe, 2008). Short postpartum hospital stays, inadequate staffing, and busy maternity units decrease contact between nurses and mothers, limiting teaching time and resulting in many mothers being discharged with unmet learning needs.

A study looking at the perceptions of 191 mothers who had initiated breastfeeding asked them to identify both the helpful advice they received and the information that they did not receive but wished they had (Leurer & Misskey, 2015). The results suggested that a number of the information gaps closely aligned with commonly cited reasons for abandoning breastfeeding—namely, perceived insufficient milk production, latching difficulties, and nipple discomfort. Information deficits mentioned by some mothers included:

- Lack of clarity regarding feeding length and frequency (how often and how long to feed infants in the early days, reading the infant's feeding cues, and reassurance that infants were receiving sufficient milk)
- Milk production issues (assessing adequacy of milk supply, ways to increase or decrease milk production, timing of lactogenesis II, managing engorgement)
- Ways to latch the infant effectively and different positions for feedings

- Milk expression (hand expression and pump use)
- Nipple discomfort (prevention and treatment of nipple pain)
- Prenatal discussion of the realities of breastfeeding (common challenges)

In the appendix to Chapter 4, Box 4-14 contains a checklist of what mothers need to know prior to hospital discharge and may help fill some of the gaps identified in maternal knowledge acquisition mentioned by these authors. Mothers value reassurance during their breastfeeding experience, but specifically state that what they really want is advice specific to their own infant and their own particular situation rather than general breastfeeding information (Miller et al., 2015). Individual analysis of a dyad's problem with adequate clinician's time for its resolution and written guidelines are most helpful for new mothers.

On busy maternity units, nurses can teach content that mothers and families are most in need of knowing (Ruchala, 2000), which may be different from or in addition to unit checklists. Some nurses find it helpful to teach mothers basic breastfeeding information and observe infant feeding with small groups of two or three mother–baby pairs to ensure that each mother has a core knowledge of breastfeeding and each infant has been assessed for successful milk transfer. Clinicians must also refrain from telling mothers what to do, and instead acknowledge the mothers' feelings and help them develop their own solutions. Karl, Beal, O'Hare, and Rissmiller (2006) described a compelling role for the nurse during the newborn period as an "attacher." Facilitating physical closeness and regular contact between mother and baby strengthens the attachment system between them, providing an oxytocin-rich environment that has a physiological and psychological positive effect on both of them.

Weddig, Baker, and Auld (2011) conducted a study to assess the variations in breastfeeding knowledge and practices of nurses on hospital maternity units. Substantial differences were noted between hospitals with the Baby-Friendly designation (bestowed by the Baby-Friendly Hospital Initiative, a program of the World Health Organization and UNICEF), as well as those working toward it, and those hospitals without such a designation or that were not working toward it. A glaring difference and barrier to evidence-based lactation care was the lack of breastfeeding policies seen in many of the hospitals. Descriptions of such practices as less than 5 minutes of skin-to-skin contact following delivery, random formula supplementation, frequent pacifier use, lack of support for rooming-in, little to no actual observation and assessment of latch and milk transfer, and measured times at the breast were reported. Nurses in non–Baby-Friendly hospitals stated that they did not have time to observe a feeding and relied on mothers' reports about the adequacy of feedings. Poor documentation resulted in relying on personal communication between nurses to track problems. Inconsistency and lack of continuity of care resulted when transitioning responsibility from one nurse to another. This study illustrated a significant disparity between nurses' intentions to support breastfeeding and their knowledge of how to do so. Lack of Baby-Friendly standards and education hampers a proper start to breastfeeding. These types of institutional barriers result in a precarious start to breastfeeding. In contrast, if staff nurses are provided with research-based knowledge regarding breastfeeding and the use of human milk, they can and will integrate breastfeeding care practices into their daily clinical routines (Spatz, Froh, Flynn-Roth, & Barton, 2015). Such knowledge translates into nurses who are empowered to help mothers successfully breastfeed, who advocate for the breastfeeding family, who are motivated to go beyond what is needed, and who share this knowledge with others in their community (Froh, Flynn-Roth, Barton, & Spatz, 2015).

It is especially important that mothers who anticipate or who are having difficulty with breastfeeding have access to a lactation consultant with the International Board Certified Lactation Consultant (IBCLC) credential. Castrucci, Hoover, Lim, and Maus (2006) showed a positive association between delivering an infant at a hospital using IBCLC-certified lactation consultants and breastfeeding at hospital discharge. The U.S. Lactation Consultant Association has determined that optimal IBCLC lactation consultant staffing is 1.3 full-time equivalent (FTE) per 1,000 deliveries each year in a Level I hospital, 1.6 FTE per 1,000 deliveries in a Level II hospital, and 1.9 FTE per 1,000 deliveries in a Level III hospital (U.S. Lactation Consultant Association, 2010; Mannel & Mannel, 2006).

POSITIONING OF THE MOTHER

When the mother is first learning to breastfeed, she needs to be positioned comfortably herself before putting the infant to breast. Typically, she may be in a sitting position on a bed, chair, or couch. She also may be reclining in a bed or lying on her side. Her back and arms can be supported with pillows when necessary so that her posture is relaxed. Some mothers appreciate a footstool when sitting in a chair, which tilts the mother's pelvis back, prevents her from feeling the need to lean forward, and elevates the infant so that the mother is not compelled to lean down or over her infant. Some mothers use commercial pillows designed to provide an inclined and/or firmer support surface than bed pillows, finding that they reduce back strain and facilitate an easier latch (Humenick, Hill, & Hart, 1998; see **Figure 5-1**). For other mothers, pillows simply get in the way.

A mother who experiences a cesarean birth may wish to breastfeed in a side-lying position, sitting upright with a pillow in her lap, or placing the infant to her side in a clutch or football hold (Frantz & Kalmen, 1979). A pillow under her knees or elevation of the knee gatch in a hospital bed may also be helpful. If an intrathecal or epidural catheter remains in place for continued pain relief after birth, care must

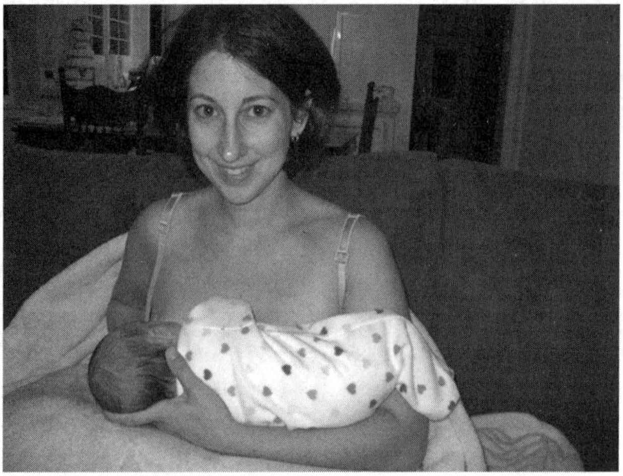

Figure 5-1 Commercial pillow for firm surface support.
Courtesy of Marsha Walker, RN, IBCLC.

be taken in positioning the mother and placing pillows behind her back such that the catheter is not dislodged. Mothers may have a number of areas of postpartum pain, including the perineum, back, cesarean incision site, intravenous (IV) line site, muscle aches and strains, or headache. Positioning options should also take these considerations into account so that pain is not exacerbated in these areas, the mother can be medicated if needed, and she is able to remain comfortable during the time it takes to feed the infant.

Assistance with positioning and latch is usually necessary during the early days of learning for both primiparous and multiparous mothers because each infant and each situation are different. Under normal circumstances, once the mother and baby have mastered the art of positioning and latch, positioning techniques and latch approaches become integrated into daily life, mothers and babies work out a mutually comfortable arrangement, and special or intricate positioning and latch techniques are no longer needed.

Hand Positions

Most mothers and many babies find it helpful if the breast is supported during the early learning period. There are two common ways to hold the breast, scissors and C-hold, with a number of variations also available for special situations. The way in which a mother is positioned and how she holds her breast can affect the angle at which the infant approaches the breast and can distort and firm the shape of both the breast and the areola (Minchin, 1998).

1. Scissors or V-hold. The breast is held by the index and middle fingers separated over the top and bottom of the areola. Some mothers and babies thrive with this hand position. Others find that although this is not "wrong," it has some potential drawbacks:
   - The fingers may exert enough pressure over milk ducts to partially obstruct the milk flow.
   - If the areola is large and/or the mother's hands are small, the fingers may cover parts of the areola that should be in the infant's mouth, causing an incorrect latch-on to only the nipple.
   - Too much pressure from one or the other finger could distort the nipple shape in the infant's mouth by tipping it up or down.
   - Pressure toward the chest wall from either or both fingers could exert enough traction on the nipple/areola to keep the infant from drawing sufficient tissue far enough into the mouth or pull the nipple out of the infant's mouth such that the infant applies vacuum to just the tip of the nipple.
2. C-hold. The breast is supported by four fingers underneath the breast and the thumb rests on top (**Figure 5-2**). This position helps keep the infant's jaw from having to support the weight of the breast. Women with large breasts may find that they cannot comfortably hold the breast in this manner and may benefit from folded towels or a rolled receiving blanket tucked under the

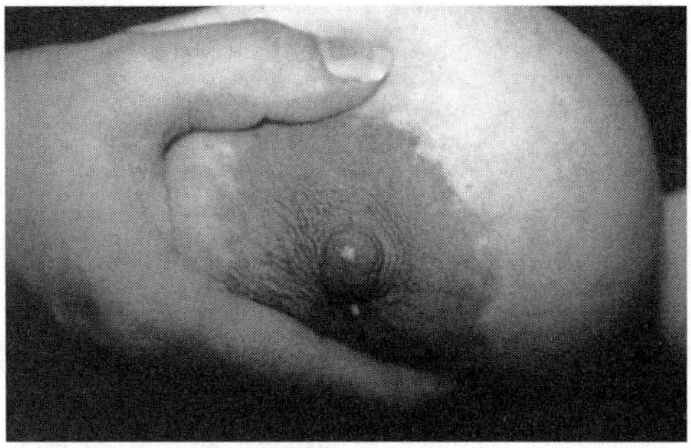

Figure 5-2 The C-hold.
Courtesy of Marsha Walker, RN, IBCLC.

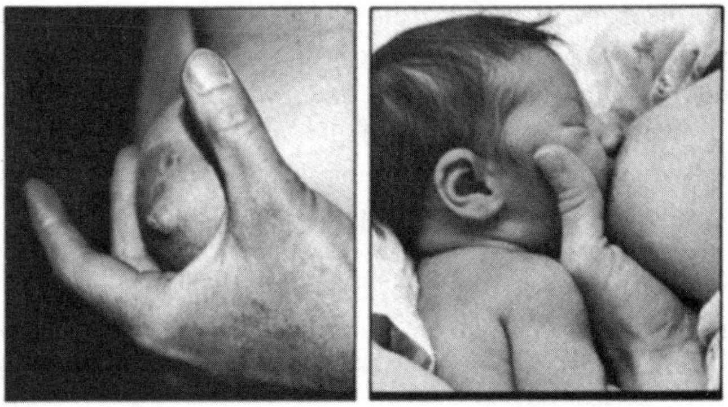

Figure 5-3 The Dancer hand position. This position supports the baby's mouth while gently compressing the cheeks.
Photo courtesy of Childbirth Graphics, copyright 1984 Sarah Coulter Danner.

breast for support. The support from the C-hold often helps to firm a very soft breast, stabilizing it during the latch and controlling the angle of the nipple/areola as it is presented to the infant (Chute, 1992).

- U-hold or Dancer hand position. This is a C-hold rotated 90 degrees such that the thumb is placed on the lateral margin of the breast and the four fingers rest on the medial aspect of the breast or vice versa (**Figure 5-3**). This hand position is often recommended for preterm infants, infants with a weak suck, or infants with muscular or neurological problems that prevent them from executing normal jaw movements (Danner & Cerutti, 1984). The entire jaw is supported simultaneously with the breast. The thumb and index finger are in a position to be placed on both cheeks of the infant and can be gently pressed inward to cause contact between the buccal surfaces of the mouth and the nipple. This action fills the gap in a preterm infant's mouth between the buccal surface inside the mouth and the nipple, causing all parts of the infant's mouth to come in contact with the breast.
- A modified C-hold with an index finger slipped under the infant's chin provides support for jaw instability when an infant's mandible exhibits excessive jaw excursion to the point where contact is lost with the nipple. In this situation, smacking sounds may be heard, indicating that the infant's jaw movement is excessive. A finger that is moved slightly back from the chin can also be gently placed under where the base of the tongue attaches to provide external support for the tongue.
- There is a great variety of shapes, sizes, and tissue elasticity of breasts, as well as numerous variations in the anatomic structure and function of infants' mouths. Although most of these combinations eventually accommodate to each other, some mismatches require more attention to positioning and alterations of standard positioning and latch techniques (Escott, 1989). In particular, the breast can be shaped (**Figure 5-4**) and adjusted to present a better match to the long axis of the infant's mouth depending on how the infant is positioned (Wiessinger, 1998).

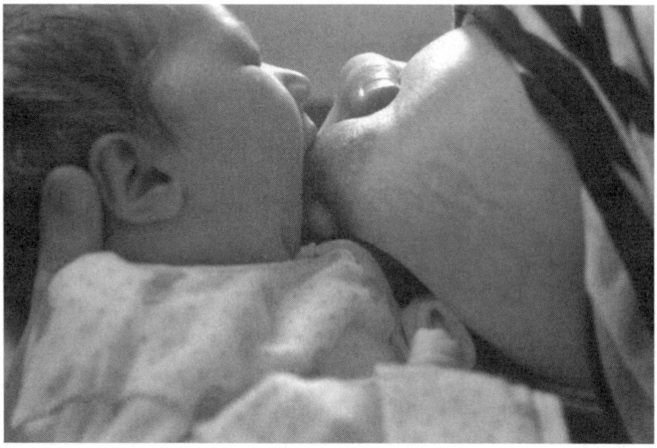

Figure 5-4 Shaping the breast.

- The breast can be shaped into a horizontal or vertical oval by the use of a U-hold or scissors hold modified to a more vertical position.
- Sometimes presenting "less" breast tissue (as with large or very soft breasts) for the latch results in more tissue being drawn into the infant's mouth.
- In very small infants, an elastic areola can be shaped with the index finger and thumb to present tissue in a manner more easily grasped by a tiny mouth.

POSITIONING OF THE INFANT

Poor positioning can compromise an infant's ability to feed effectively. Proper head, neck, and trunk alignment are important to smooth feeding performance (Shrago & Bocar, 1990). The head and neck are typically in neutral alignment, with the overall body position being one of slight flexion, including the hips (Wolf & Glass, 1992). There is a strong interaction between head and neck position and feeding function. Proper positioning during feeding affects respiratory mechanisms, oral motor control, swallowing, and the development of head and neck postural responses (Bosma, 1988). Blair, Cadwell, Turner-Maffei, and Brimdyr (2003) found that no one attribute of positioning (head flexion, body alignment, etc.) was more important than others in relation to the degree of nipple pain experienced by the mother. It appears that all attributes work together to achieve a position that is compatible for good milk transfer in each individual mother–baby pair.

Coca, Gamba, de Sousa e Silva, and Abrao (2009) found an increased proportion of mothers experienced nipple trauma when newborns were positioned with heads bent, chins placed away from the breast, and lips turned inward. Women whose infants were incorrectly positioned in this study were 1.94 times more at risk for developing nipple trauma compared with mothers whose infants were positioned correctly. Goyal, Banginwar, Ziyo, and Toweir (2011) described an increased association between poor positioning and cracked nipples, mastitis, and sore nipples. Kronborg and Vaeth (2009) found that ineffective positioning and latch contributed to early breastfeeding problems. Early problems were positively associated with later breastfeeding problems. Proper positioning is an important skill to be taught to new mothers but requires ongoing monitoring and assessment to prevent or remedy early problems with breastfeeding.

Four common positions for breastfeeding exist, with many variations available to suit special circumstances. A mother does not need to know all these positions but can be assisted to find which position or positions work best for her and her infant. Before her discharge from the hospital, the mother should be able to demonstrate at least one position in which she is comfortable and in which she can position the baby by herself on both sides or with minimal help.

1. Cradle hold. The infant is held completely facing the mother, typically on a slight angle with the head and shoulders a little higher than the hips (**Figure 5-5**). The infant lays on his or her side in direct contact with the mother's midriff. The infant's head rests on the upper forearm. The breast should not be pushed sideways to the infant. The infant is well supported by the mother's arm

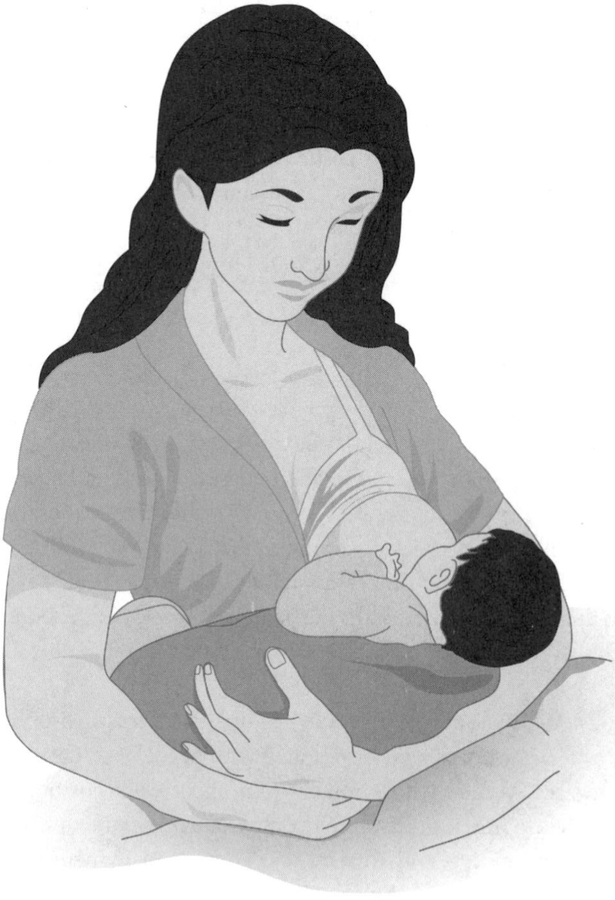

Figure 5-5 The cradle position.

across his or her back, tucking the hips into flexion and molding or wrapping the infant's body around her waist. This positioning should place the infant's nose at about the level of the nipple and the lower lip and chin below the nipple. The infant's head and neck should be straightly aligned with the shoulders and hips. Some mothers find this position awkward at first, with the infant's head difficult to control and position and the breast difficult to embrace in a C-hold without disrupting the contact between the infant's mouth and the breast.

2. Cross-cradle hold. The infant is in the same position as in the cradle hold but is held with the mother's opposite arm (**Figure 5-6**). The neck and shoulders of the infant are supported with the mother's hand, her fingers rest back behind the ears, there is no pressure on the occipital region of the head, and the mother's forearm supports the infant's back. This gives the mother more control over positioning the infant's head and may be easier to learn at first. The breast is accessed by the mother's hand without having to be inserted between the infant and the breast

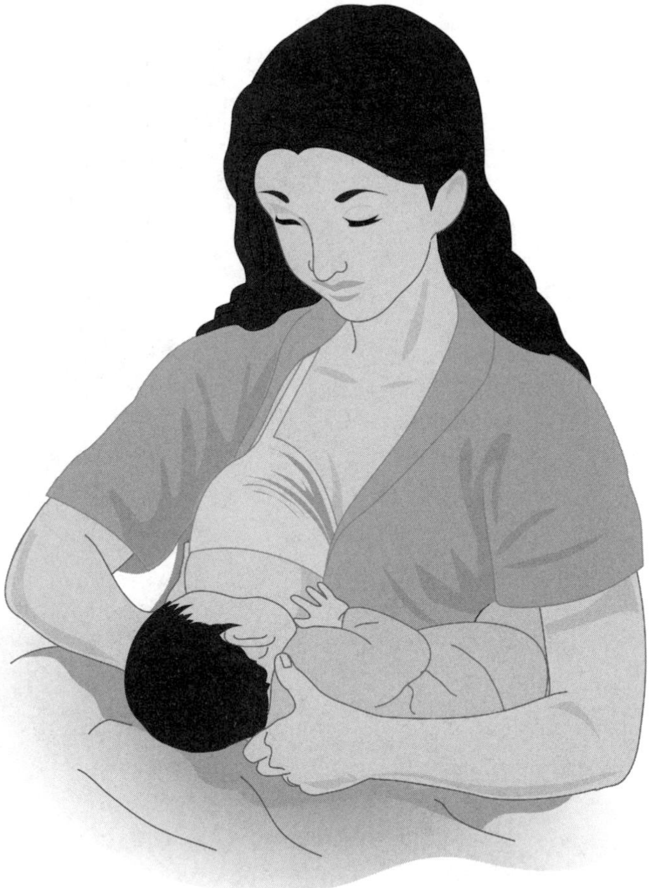

Figure 5-6 The cross-cradle hold.

tissue, and the nipple/areola is more visible to the mother. Some mothers start the feeding with the cross-cradle hold and, once the infant is positioned, change to the cradle hold. This position is frequently used as a learning position for a full-term infant or to position a small or preterm infant who tends to "roll" up when placed in a cradle hold.

3. Clutch or football hold. The infant is positioned on a pillow to the side of the mother turned slightly sideways or sitting partially upright (**Figure 5-7**). The mother's hand and wrist support the infant's back and shoulders, and her fingers rest behind the infant's ears. This position may be much easier for some mothers, giving them the most control over the infant's head and allowing the best visualization of the nipple/areola. Care should be taken that the weight of the breast is not placed on the infant's chest, that the infant is not placed so low that he or she pulls down on the nipple, or that the mother leans down over the infant. This position is also good for both the mother and the infant as they learn their respective breastfeeding skills. This position is also used for small or preterm infants.

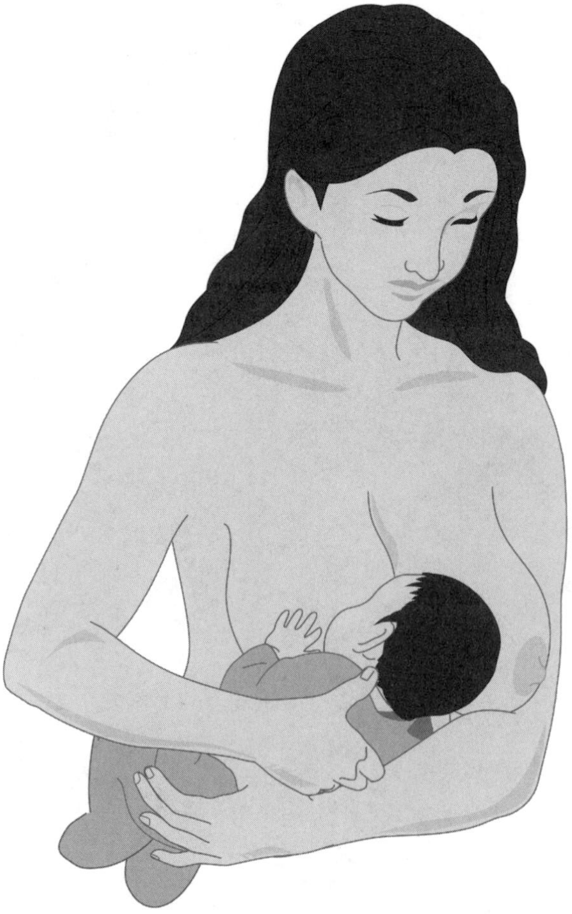

Figure 5-7 The football or clutch hold.

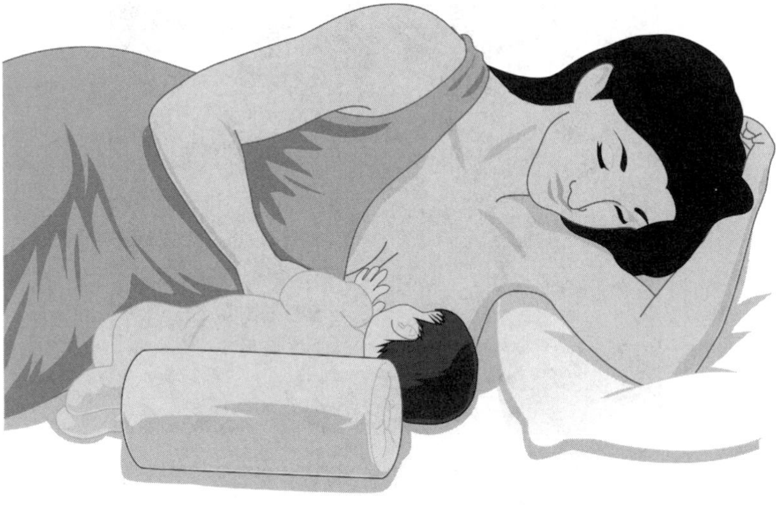

Figure 5-8 The side-lying position.

4. Lying down. Many mothers find this position an especially restful way to feed their infants, although some mothers may find it difficult to learn at first. The mother lies on her side with the infant's body on his or her side and completely facing and in contact with her (**Figure 5-8**). The infant's head may be resting on the bed or on the mother's forearm that supports the infant's back and hips. Some mothers place a rolled towel or blanket behind the infant to keep the infant on his or her side and place a pillow behind their own backs for support. Mothers can offer the top breast by adjusting their position such that they are turned further prone, thus avoiding having to move the infant and themselves to the other side.

Marmet and Shell (2008) described a number of therapeutic positions that function to compensate for sucking problems or for use in infants with anatomic variations, neurological deficits, respiratory issues, state control problems, young gestational age, or sensory integration variations:

- Infant and mother sitting. Useful in infants older than 6 weeks to help bring down an elevated tongue, for infants with a cleft palate, to help improve alertness in a sleepy infant, for velopharyngeal inadequacy, or repeated ear infections. The infant sits facing the mother's breast with legs straddled over the mother's leg.
- Mother supine and infant prone. The prone position is frequently used for positioning sick or preterm infants because it improves oxygenation and has been shown to increase sucking pressures when bottle-feeding (Mizuno, Inoue, & Takeuchi, 2000). With the mother supine and the infant prone, infants who need to bring their tongue forward, such as with tongue-tie or infants who have difficulty handling a fast flow of milk, may feed better.
- Mother semireclining and infant semiprone. This position may be helpful for infants with upper respiratory problems such as tracheomalacia or laryngomalacia (**Figure 5-9**). It is also helpful for infants with a receding chin or for a mother who has had a cesarean delivery. This position is also referred to within the biological nurturing concept.

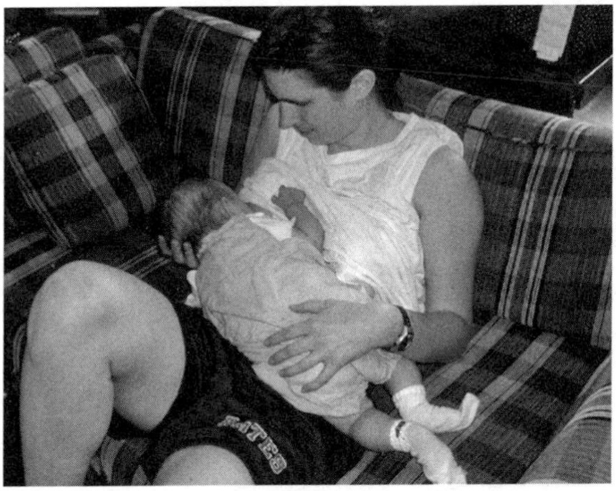

Figure 5-9 Semireclining position of mother and semiprone position of infant.

Biological Nurturing

Biological nurturing is a concept that involves how certain feeding positions and behaviors are associated with the release of primitive neonatal reflexes necessary to establish successful breastfeeding (Colson, de Pooy, & Hawdon, 2003; Colson, Meek, & Hawdon, 2008). It is any mother–baby behavior at the breast where the infant is in close chest contact with the mother's body contours.

- For the infant, biological nurturing means:
  - Mouthing, licking, smelling, nuzzling, and nestling at the breast
  - Sleeping at the breast
  - Groping and rooting at the breast
  - Latching onto the breast
  - Sucking and swallowing breastmilk through active feeding
- For the mother, biological nurturing means:
  - Holding the infant in close contact with a maternal body contour
  - Offering unrestricted access to the breast with as much skin-to-skin contact as the mother desires

Extended holding in postures where the mother leans back and the infant lies prone in close frontal apposition with maternal body contours (ventral positioning) is thought to aid in the release of primitive neonatal reflex-like movements necessary for successful breastfeeding.

Primitive neonatal reflexes is a collective name given to more than 50 unconditioned reflex responses and spontaneous behaviors to environmental stimuli such as rooting, sucking, swallowing; head, cheek, tongue, and lip reflexes; hand-to-mouth; stepping; and crawling. A greater number of primitive neonatal reflexes and a reduction in feeding problems at the breast were observed when mothers were in full biological nurturing postures (Colson et al., 2008). Biological nurturing positions also work well for the late preterm infant. Colson and colleagues (2003) noticed that although infants appeared to be asleep in the biological nurturing position, they were often actively feeding with strong sucking and swallowing. Thus an infant may not need to be fully awake to engage in nutritive sucking and swallowing.

The maternal semireclined position with the infant in a prone position adhering to her body contours may also be an effective intervention for the infant who "fights" at the breast. Clinicians have seen infants who arch away from the breast, bob their heads, and engage in erratic and jerky movements at the breast, preventing latch-on. To counteract the effects of gravity on positioning, mothers are taught to hold their infants close, often using pressure or holds that suppress or limit the expression of the neonatal reflexes used in breastfeeding (Colson, 2010). Placing the mother and infant into a biological nurturing position may use gravity to assist in moving the infant's chin and tongue forward and stop the movements that are preventing the infant from latching on. This type of ventral positioning may allow the full expression of the complete array of newborn reflexes by reducing the negative effect of gravity. Biological nurturing during the first 72 hours may also trigger higher peak concentrations of oxytocin at an earlier time, helping to offset oxytocin aberrations caused by oxytocin infusion during labor epidurals.

In a study of 86 mother–infant dyads, the release of all the rhythmic reflexes, the gravity reflex, and the total number of primitive neonatal reflexes in the group of infants exposed to synthetic oxytocin during labor was significantly lower than that in the non-exposed group of infants (Gabriel et al., 2015). These effects may occur due to large doses of synthetic oxytocin adversely affecting the central nervous system of the infant, reducing the expression of the oxytocin receptor or causing its desensitization. A study of 47 full-term healthy infants showed that the group of infants exposed to synthetic oxytocin during labor was 11.5 times more likely to demonstrate low/medium prefeeding cues compared to the group of unexposed infants (Bell, White-Traut, & Rankin, 2013). Prefeeding cues are oral–motor neurobehaviors that communicate feeding readiness, and the ability to self-comfort and regulate behavioral state. The higher the dose of oxytocin infusion during labor epidurals, the lower the oxytocin levels in mothers during breastfeeding on day 2 (Jonas et al., 2009).

Assisted by their mothers, babies in biological nurturing positions utilize antigravity reflexes to locate the breast and latch without complicated trunk and head support. Biological nurturing research seemed to show that breastfeeding continues to be mediated by newborn reflexive behavior well after birth, that numerous types of positions may either support or hinder these reflexes, and that by inhibiting or overriding instinctive maternal behaviors, common breastfeeding instruction may be counterproductive (Romano & Goer, 2008).

Clinicians may find that this type of prone positioning of the infant with a semireclining mother is a good option when other positions are found to be problematic for individual mother–baby pairs. If the dyad is struggling with finding a comfortable pain-free position, changing to this type of positioning may remedy the problem.

Sudden unexpected postnatal collapse has been described in breastfed newborns both in the delivery suite and in the postpartum hospital room (Friedman, Adrouche-Amrani, & Holzman, 2015). While rare, this event has been linked to positions where the infant's nose is occluded by pendulous breast tissue, the infant is face down or prone on the mother's chest or breast, the mother is on a cell phone or not paying attention to the location of the infant's nose, the mother has fallen asleep, or the infant's neck is in deep flexion. It is important that clinicians and mothers are aware of the head positioning of the infant both while breastfeeding and during maternal holding. During skin-to-skin holding, the infant's head should be turned to the side with the nares clearly visible and the head slightly extended.

LATCH

Latch has been described as possibly the single most important moment and movement in breastfeeding (Brandt, Andrews, & Kvale 1998). McAllister, Bradshaw, and Ross-Adjie (2009) demonstrated that 2 variables of hospital care were significantly associated with the duration of breastfeeding in their sample of 266 mothers—formula supplementation (negative) and the ability of the mother to be able to independently latch the baby to the breast upon discharge (positive). Teaching in the hospital should assure that the mother can successfully latch the infant to the breast, a skill that should be monitored and documented during the hospital stay. Once the infant is positioned correctly, the infant's lips can be brushed gently against the areola if his or her mouth is not already opening in anticipation. When it is opened like a yawn, the infant's mouth is moved to the breast, with the chin and lower lip making contact first, followed by the upper lip and tip of the nose. The infant's mouth must open wide, ranging up to approximately 160 degrees. Only the lower jaw can move to achieve this type of opening, so the infant's head must tilt back far enough to accommodate the dropping of the jaw (Cadwell, 2007). Some mothers and infants find an easier latch when the mother shapes the breast to offer the areola under the nipple as the first contact point, making that area more accessible. The lower lip and chin can be planted well down on the areola with the infant's mouth rolled the rest of the way on as the upper lip makes contact just above the nipple. An infant who is crying or who has an elevated tongue tip will need to be calmed, and the tongue can be stroked down and forward before latching.

In an effort to aid or hasten latch-on, some mothers, helpers, or healthcare providers push on the back of the infant's head as the infant is brought to the breast. Pushing on the occiput may cause the infant to compensate by extending the head, biting the nipple, or detaching from the breast. Increasing neck flexion causes the airway to become more prone to collapse, interfering with breathing. Anatomic structures change their relative positions when pressure is exerted on the occiput. The hyoid bone should move up and forward, which happens with slight extension of the head to facilitate swallowing. Excessive flexion with distortion of the cervical vertebrae can impinge on the proper movement of the hyoid bone, which has six other connections involved in sucking, swallowing, and breathing. Forcing the infant's head onto the breast may disturb placement of the tongue, encouraging it to elevate rather than cupping and moving down and forward (Widström & Thringstrom-Paulsson, 1993). Too much flexion of the neck, nose-first attachment to the breast, and continued pressure on the occiput create a scenario for nipple pain and poor milk transfer.

Blair and colleagues (2003) looked at positioning and latching behaviors of infants whose mothers reported varying degrees of nipple pain. Several factors of the latch and positioning of the infant combined to contribute to the soreness experienced by the mothers in the study, including the observations that only 18% of 92 infants had the optimal angle of mouth opening of 160 degrees (**Figure 5-10**), just 36.6% had both their nose and chin on or in close proximity to the breast, and merely 34.4% had their nose opposite the mother's nipple at latch. Poor attachment to the breast that leaves the nipple in the anterior portion of the mouth can contribute to sore nipples as well as obstructed milk flow (Morton, 1992), resulting in weight loss, hyperbilirubinemia, and low milk supply.

A deep latch or attachment to the breast is important to ensure uniform drainage of all the mammary lobes. Mizuno and colleagues (2008) found on examination of milk from three milk ducts in each breast that each duct contained milk with differing compositions. They measured the degree of emptying in three milk ducts from each breast of 37 breastfeeding mothers. Findings confirmed that the changes

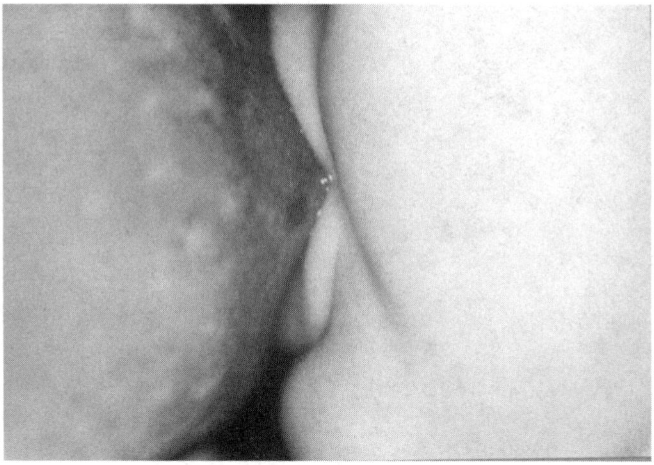

Figure 5-10 Optimal angle of mouth opening.

in the degree of emptying of each mammary lobe differed by the depth of attachment of the infant at the breast as measured by the creamatocrit of milk obtained before and after breastfeeding. A deep attachment was defined as the nipple and approximately 0.7–1.3 cm of the areola in the infant's mouth and the angle of the open mouth greater than 130 degrees. If the depth of attachment was shallow, milk was excreted unevenly from different mammary lobes.

Milk retention in a lobe can predispose a breast to plugged ducts and mastitis. If the depth of attachment is deep, the lobes drain uniformly, leaving a reduced risk of plugged ducts and mastitis. If a lobe is poorly drained over an extended period of time, less milk will be made in that lobe, reducing the amount of milk that the breast produces. Thus, achieving a deep latch is important in preventing breast problems and milk supply issues.

Problems with Latch

A number of indicators of poor positioning or latch should be checked before hospital discharge, if the mother reports nipple pain or damage, if there is a low milk supply, or if weight gain problems arise. A mother and infant who are experiencing difficulties with latch should be checked for the following:

- Body position of the infant
  - Misalignment of the head, trunk, and hips
  - Infant not tucked close and facing the mother, hips extended or back arched, neck flexed, or nose buried in the breast tissue
  - Head too high over the breast
  - Nose or chin not touching the breast
- Mouth and tongue
  - Angle of the infant's mouth opening less than 160 degrees (**Figure 5-11**)
  - Upper (tight labial frenulum) or lower lip not flanged

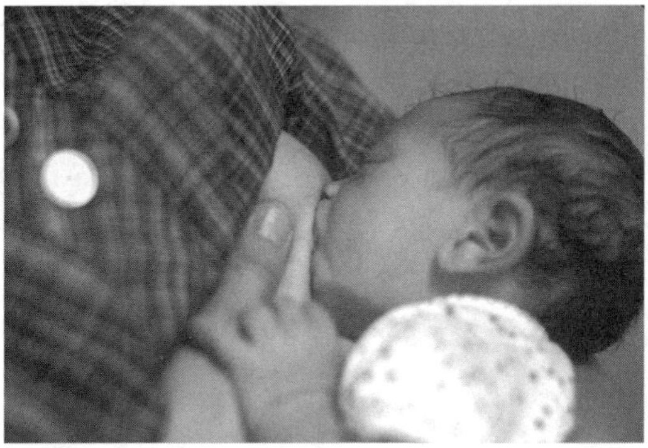

Figure 5-11 Mouth angle less than 160 degrees.

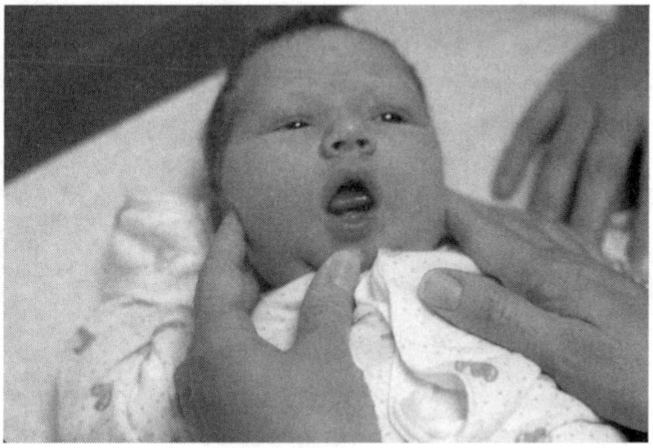

Figure 5-12 Flat tongue.

- Tongue not down, cupped, and forward
  - Humped (anterior to posterior direction)
  - Bunched (compressed in a lateral direction)
  - Retracted (tip behind alveolar ridges)
  - Elevated
  - Flat (**Figure 5-12**)
  - Short or tight lingual or labial frenulum
  - Large tongue, protruding tongue, short tongue
- Palate
  - High or arched
  - Bubble
  - Cleft (hard, soft)
- Cheeks
  - Drawn in, dimpled, or hollowed with each suck
  - Cheek line not a smooth arc (**Figure 5-13**)
- Jaw
  - Retrognathia or receding jaw (**Figure 5-14**; can position the tongue posteriorly where it leads to obstruction of the airway; can contribute to sore nipples unless chin is brought very close to the breast)
  - Large jaw excursions (cannot close over the areola)
  - Small jaw excursions (cannot open over the areola)
  - Lack of graded jaw excursions heard as clicking or smacking sounds
  - Jaw asymmetry or tilted jaws (may include torticollis; Wall & Glass, 2006)
- Lips
  - Poor occlusion of lips around the areola (milk leaking from the sides of the mouth)
  - Lips do not form a seal, preventing the creation of a pressure gradient between breast and mouth

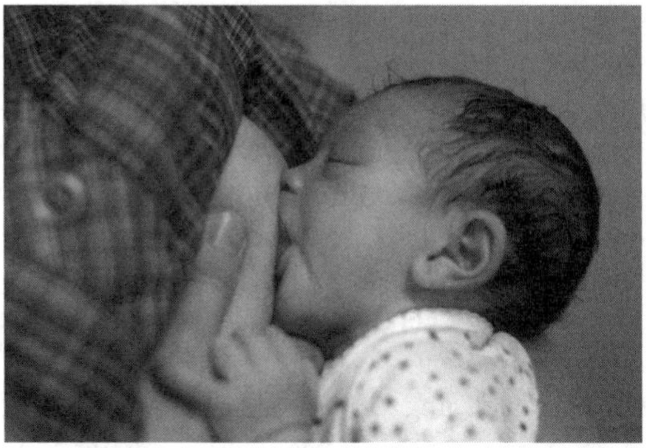

Figure 5-13 Cheek line not in a smooth arc.

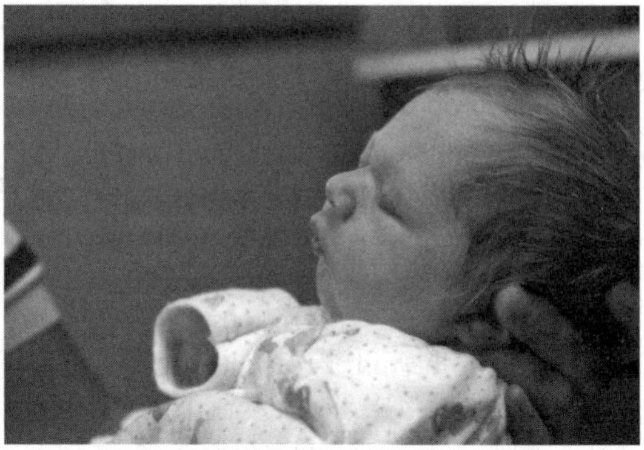

Figure 5-14 Receding jaw.

- Nipple
  - Slides back and forth within the infant's mouth during the feeding
  - Pops in and out of mouth (may indicate tongue-tie)
  - Creased in a horizontal, vertical, or oblique plane
  - Distorted shape or flattened
  - Blanched or in spasm after the infant releases the nipple
  - Pain, blisters, maceration, fissures, cracks, bleeding, craters
  - Flat, dimpled, retracted
  - Edematous areola that envelops the nipple
  - Engorged breast that flattens the nipple
- Rhythmicity or coordination of suck–swallow–breathe
  - Diminished suck-to-swallow ratio less than 1–3:1
  - High respiratory rate, stridor
  - Coughing or choking

Other situations may occur that cause problems with latch. These are described in the sections that follow.

State and Feeding Readiness

Many breastfeeding recommendations from the past and, to some extent, those used currently tend to lead to insufficient breastmilk and a hungry infant. Feeding schedules that are determined by the clock rather than infant feeding readiness cues can result in an over-hungry crying infant (Millard, 1990), or one who remains underfed because scheduled feeds coincide with deep sleep states. An infant in a deep sleep state cannot feed, nor can a vigorously crying infant organize his or her behavior to latch and feed effectively. Infants can breastfeed in the other four states: light sleep, drowsy, quiet alert, and active alert. Infants feed best in a quiet alert state but should be put to breast whenever feeding cues are demonstrated. The quiet alert state may be difficult for some newborns to achieve and may require organizational maturation before they develop competency in alerting themselves to feed from a sleeping state. Other infants may experience state control problems as a result of maternal labor medications, becoming more competent at state control as the drugs clear their body and the effects of the medications diminish.

Some newborns require help in achieving a state that is optimal for latch, whereas other infants demonstrate state organization and sucking competency with a minimum of effort on the part of the mother. The ability of infants to suck appropriately, demonstrate alertness and stamina, and possess the ability to self-regulate and respond to maternal soothing behaviors are major influences on the initial pattern and the ultimate duration of breastfeeding (Lothian, 1995). Sucking behavior in the early neonatal period affects the breastfeeding duration at 3 and 6 months. Vigorously feeding infants are much more likely to be fully breastfed and to breastfeed longer than infants described by their mothers as "procrastinators," who are at a higher risk for short-term breastfeeding (Mizuno, Fujimaki, & Sawada, 2004). Karl (2004) used an arousal model (Als, 1995) to describe behavioral breastfeeding difficulties on a continuum, with the quiet alert state as a neutral arousal reference and newborns unable to manage their state well enough to latch being viewed as either under-aroused (the sleepy infant) or over-aroused (the fussy or reluctant nurser).

Infants experiencing state overload appear to be sleeping but may be shut down or closed down in an attempt to block out negative stimuli that have raised their arousal levels beyond that which they can manage. A shut-down infant may appear to be asleep, and parents may have difficulty differentiating between these two states (**Table 5-1**). Increasing stimulation to an infant who is shut down further exacerbates the problem. Parents need to become knowledgeable regarding infant states and how best to assist their infant in achieving a latchable state. One of the most effective interventions for modulating infant arousal levels in over-aroused, under-aroused, and shut-down infants is the use of a combination of vestibular (upright rocking) and skin-to-skin tactile stimulation that affect state organization itself (Anderson, 1991). In an effort to encourage infant self-regulation and to positively modulate infant state, skin-to-skin care can be initiated directly after birth, which is the normal mammalian postnatal condition (Ferber & Makhoul, 2004).

Previous or Concurrent Use of Artificial Nipples and Pacifiers

Milk transfer from the breast to the infant is contingent upon the smooth functioning of a group of interrelated behaviors, intact anatomic structures, and coordinated physiological actions. Some infants have been observed to have difficulty in latching and sucking from the breast if artificial nipples and/or

Table 5-1 Differentiation Between Sleeping Infants and Over-Aroused, Shut-Down Infants

Sleeping Infant Descriptors	Shut-Down Infant Descriptors
Relaxed muscle tone	Tense muscle tone (not relaxed)
Peaceful facial expression	May reflect internal tension with furrowed eyebrows
Normal skin color	Color flushed or pale
Eyelids fluttering in light sleep	Eyes held tightly closed

Data from Karl, D. J. (2004). Using principles of newborn behavioral state organization to facilitate breastfeeding. *MCN: The American Journal of Maternal/Child Nursing, 29*, 292–298.

pacifiers have been introduced before breastfeeding is well established (Neifert, Lawrence, & Seacat, 1995). Popularly known as "nipple confusion," this phenomenon has several definitions:

- Type A: A neonate's difficulty in establishing the necessary oral configuration, latching technique, and sucking pattern to extract milk from the breast after exposure to an artificial teat. Type B: Older infants who have already established breastfeeding but begin to refuse the breast or prefer the bottle (Neifert, Lawrence, & Seacat, 1995).
- The infant's response to the various mechanical and flow characteristics of an artificial nipple compared with the breast, which causes the infant to prefer one feeding mechanism over the other (Dowling & Thanattherakul, 2001).
- The infant's difficulty with or preference for one feeding mechanism over another after exposure to artificial nipples (Zimmerman & Thompson, 2015).

Zimmerman and Thompson (2015) reviewed 14 articles supporting and refuting the concept of nipple confusion. This review of the literature found evidence that supported the concept of nipple confusion when breastfed infants were offered the artificial nipples on feeding bottles, but did not support the contention that pacifier use caused nipple confusion.

Nipple confusion may result from a combination of infant factors and equipment factors (Ross & Fuhrman, 2015). The shape and size of artificial nipples vary, with shorter nipples sitting farther forward in the oral cavity and longer nipples positioned farther back in the oral cavity, Because compressive forces of the tongue originate in the back or posterior portion of the tongue (Eishima, 1991), shorter artificial nipples may alter tongue movements such that when breastfeeding is attempted following the use of a short nipple, tongue mechanics may place compression incorrectly on the maternal nipple–areolar complex. The width of the artificial nipple at its base near the collar changes the angle of the infant's chin during feeding, which may alter the amount of vacuum the infant generates (Segami, Mizuno, Taki, & Itabashi, 2013). If replicated at the breast, this altered vacuum application may affect the infant's ability to generate enough vacuum to transfer milk. The shape of the artificial nipple has a direct effect on how the infant's oral structures engage in the sucking process, with a wider nipple base engaging the masseter muscles more, as in feeding at the breast (Gomes, Da Costa Gois, Oliveira, Thomson, & Cardoso, 2013). Healthy full-term infants may or may not be able to alter their sucking rate, pressure, and mouth configuration to regulate milk flow from an artificial nipple. Preterm infants, late preterm infants, infants challenged during the birth process, and medically fragile infants may not be resilient feeders and may demonstrate a limited ability to self-regulate milk flow from an artificial nipple or configure and adapt their oral structures to multiple feeding modalities.

Pacifier use is associated with a reduced length of breastfeeding (DiGirolamo, Grummer-Strawn, & Fein, 2008). This may be due to interference with proper sucking or may be an indicator of breastfeeding problems where a pacifier is used to soothe an infant who is not adequately transferring milk. In a study involving 670 mothers, 79% of the infants were given a pacifier, most commonly to soothe the infant or help put the baby to sleep. However, some mothers used a pacifier to stretch the length of time between breastfeedings, to help take the infant off the breast following a feeding, and to reduce non-nutritive sucking at the breast. The study reported that infants given a pacifier prior to 4 weeks of age and those using pacifiers on most days had a 3-fold risk of shorter breastfeeding duration (Mauch, Scott, Magarey, & Daniels, 2012).

Pacifier shape, length, and material, just as with other artificial nipples, can have an impact on the mechanics of sucking (Nowak, Smith, & Erenberg, 1995). Characteristics of the nipple can impact tongue and lip position as well as their movements during sucking. Orthodontic-shaped nipples may interfere with the central grooving of the tongue, whereas pacifiers with a ball-shaped tip may result in reduced functional sucking activity (Wolf & Glass, 1992). Levrini, Merlo, and Paracchini (2007) evaluated the distribution of stress on the palate using three different types of pacifiers, showing that pacifiers with different geometrical shapes caused a different stress distribution on the palate. Orthodontic-shaped pacifiers distributed the stress on the palate during sucking over a wider area than pacifiers that were narrow or that had a bulblike tip. The latter two types of pacifiers concentrate stress on the central part of the palate that could lead to a narrowing of the palatal arch. Not only could sucking be affected, but the eventual position of the child's dentition and speech may also be involved.

The concept of human imprinting has been advanced to help explain the observation of nipple preference. Mobbs (1989) discusses imprinting as an aspect of learning that takes place early in life. It is known that nonhuman mammals imprint or demonstrate a one-nipple preference; for example, the piglet and kitten establish their preferred teat and drive away others who would use it. Displacing sucking from the breast to an artificial nipple could change the imprint and memory within the oral cavity, causing oral tactile recognition to be decoyed to an artificial nipple (Mobbs, Mobbs, & Mobbs, 2015).

The human infant is thought to be programmed to seek and attach to a suitable object on which to imprint using its most powerful sense organs at birth—the nose and mouth. Olfaction is one of the guides to the nipple directly after birth (Varendi & Porter, 2001). Within minutes of birth, maternal breast odors elicit preferential head orientation of the infant, contributing to successful nipple localization. The chemical profile of breast secretions overlaps somewhat with that of amniotic fluid. Lactating women emit odor cues that release activity in newborns. Such cues may be carried in various substrates, including milk or areolar secretions.

A study by Doucet, Soussignan, Sagot, and Schaal (2007) examined the responses of infants facing their mothers' breasts with the goal of sorting out the source(s) of active volatile compounds emitted by the lactating breast. Infants (aged 3–4 days) were presented their mother's breast in 2 consecutive trials of 90 seconds each: a scentless condition (breast entirely covered with a transparent film) paired with 1 of 4 odorous conditions (fully exposed breast, $n = 15$; nipple only exposed, $n = 15$; areola only exposed, $n = 13$; and milk exposed, $n = 12$). The infants were more orally activated when facing any of the odorous breast conditions than when facing the scentless breast. They cried earlier and longer and opened their eyes less when facing the scentless breast. Nipple, areola, and milk odors appeared to be equivalent to the whole breast odor in stimulating oral activity and in delaying crying onset. This study showed that volatile compounds originating in areolar secretions or milk release mouthing, stimulate eye opening, and delay and reduce crying in newborns.

The early attraction to the breast may also be a reflection of prenatal exposure and the recognition of a familiar scent (Mizuno & Ueda, 2004; Porter & Winberg, 1999). Infants are able to discriminate between their mother's scent on a breast pad and that of an unfamiliar woman (Macfarlane, 1975). Olfactory breast-associated cues are so important that both 3- to 4-day-old breastfeeding and bottle-feeding infants orient toward a pad worn on a breast rather than an unused or clean pad (Makin & Porter, 1989). Preferences to mother's milk odor lasts as long as 2 weeks, with 14-day-old bottle-fed infants responding preferentially to a breast pad from an unfamiliar lactating woman rather than a pad treated with their own familiar formula (Porter, Makin, Davis, & Christensen, 1991). Washing the breast or separating the infant from the mother before the infant becomes oriented to the biologically relevant chemical signal from the breast could be one precursor that inhibits correct latch (Varendi, Porter, & Winberg, 1994). For this reason the use of scented pacifiers should be avoided in breastfed infants. One of the first ways an infant recognizes his or her mother is through the distinctive features of her nipple. As with birds, who are known to be preferentially selective to supernormal size stimuli, a human infant may experience a mishap in attaching to the mother's nipple by fixating on an artificial nipple whose large, rigid features predominate when there is a choice between sizes (Mobbs, 1989).

Zanardo and Straface (2015) reported that in 70 mothers, the mean temperature of the areolar skin was significantly higher than the temperature of the adjacent breast tissue. This warmth was thought to act as a thermal signal to help guide the newborn directly to the nipple. The elevated temperature of the areola is also thought to favor or act as an odor fixative on the surface of the areola to enhance the olfactory stimulatory effect on the infant. This thermal feature of the areola can be triggered by infant crying, with optimal odor release occurring in anticipation of the infant arriving at the nipple.

Tongue placement and the sequential movements of the tongue are crucial to the infant latching to the breast, drawing the nipple/areola into the mouth by forming a teat, and covering the lower gum to prevent nipple damage. The extrusion reflex has been defined as the forward movement of the cupped tongue over the lower gum so as to grasp the breast at the start of the formation of a teat (Stephens & Kotowski, 1994). With an artificial nipple, the teat is already formed and is inserted into a fully or partially closed mouth. This can lead to the extrusion reflex being diminished or extinguished from lack of use. If the extrusion reflex does not occur in the latch sequence of events at the breast, a teat cannot be formed. Consequently, the infant will apply the gums to the breast first rather than the tongue, resulting in nipple pain and poor milk transfer. One of the prime motoric differences between sucking on an artificial nipple and sucking at the breast may be in the initiation of sucking (Wolf & Glass, 1992).

The muscles involved with breastfeeding are also affected by the use of artificial nipples. Masseter muscle activity is significantly weakened by the use of artificial nipples (Gomes, Thomson, & Cardoso, 2009). Weakening the muscles involved with breastfeeding by the use of artificial nipples may make effective milk transfer at the breast more difficult. Muscles involved with breastfeeding are either immobilized (masseter, orbicularis oris), overactive (chin muscle), or malpositioned (tongue is pushed backward) during artificial nipple use (Inoue, Sakashita, & Kamegai, 1995).

Gestational Age

Developmental maturity and feeding behaviors may vary depending on the gestational age of the infant, postnatal age of the infant (days since birth), and any growth rate abnormalities. Sucking patterns vary, change, and mature along a continuum of gestational age, postnatal age, and health status.

In measurements taken on an artificial nipple, preterm infants compared with full-term infants generally demonstrated lower sucking pressures, less fluid consumption per suck, fewer sucks per feeding, and an inability to maintain the suction for long periods of time (Medoff-Cooper, Weininger, & Zukowsky, 1989). As gestational age increases, feeding behavioral organization improves, with more reliable maximum sucking pressures starting an upward trend at 34 weeks (Medoff-Cooper, 1991). Preterm breastfed infants who are encouraged to feed at breast can catch up and exhibit similar milk consumption to those born after a longer gestation (Nyqvist, 2001). Infants of lower gestational ages often lack the strength and endurance to engage in a correct latch and sustain it. Gestational age and birth weight classifications (Hankins, Clark, & Munn, 2006) and their effects on breastfeeding typically include the following categories:

- Preterm: less than 34 weeks. Latch may be complicated by poor initiation of sucking with excessive rooting, inability to close the mouth/wide jaw excursions, lapping at the nipple, oral defensiveness, elevated tongue tip, oral/facial hypotonia, a closed mouth, weak suck (suboptimal or immature sucking pressure), and jaw instability. If the infant cannot form a teat and draw it into his or her mouth, the infant's gums may contact the breast at the base of the nipple rather than farther back on the areola, interfering with efficient milk removal (Meier et al., 2000).
- Late preterm: 34 0/7 to 36 6/7 weeks. Latch may be complicated by respiratory instability in some breastfeeding positions, little energy reserve or stamina, immature state regulation, sleepiness, low tone, depressed sucking vacuum, or uncoordinated sucking (Wight, 2003).
- Early term: 37 0/7 to 38 6/7 weeks. Latch may be compromised by the increased risk from severe respiratory distress syndrome.
- Term: 39 0/7 to 41 6/7 weeks. Latch may be compromised by maternal labor medications, an overstimulating environment, high ambient temperature (Elder, 1970), or artificial nipple use.
- Postterm: 42 weeks or more. The infant may be lethargic; may have trouble sustaining sucking; may have experienced hypoxia (with depressed suck), birth injury, or trauma; and is prone to hypoglycemia.
- Macrosomia or large for gestational age (LGA): 4,000 g or more (8 lb, 14 oz). The infant may have experienced birth trauma and may be susceptible to hypoglycemia.
- Normal birth weight: 2,500–3,999 g (5 lb, 9 oz to 8 lb, 13 oz).
- Low-birth-weight: less than 2,500 g (< 5 lb, 9 oz).
- Very low-birth-weight: less than 1,500 g (< 3 lb, 5 oz).
- Small for gestational age (SGA): can occur in term, near-term, and preterm infants; mostly defined as two standard deviations below the mean for gestational age or as below the 10th percentile; sometimes referred to as intrauterine growth retardation. One may see poorer reflex performance with rooting and sucking, poor tone, difficulty coming to an alert state, stress when handled, and an easily fatigued infant (Als, Tronick, Adamson, & Brazelton, 1976).

Birth Trauma, Medications, Conditions, and Events

Events or conditions experienced during birth, such as hypoxia, brachial plexus injuries, fractured clavicle, vacuum extraction, facial muscle trauma, or deep or aggressive suctioning, can impinge on achieving a correct latch. Congenital conditions not discovered prenatally may first become apparent when an infant experiences feeding difficulties. Epidural analgesia (0.25% bupivacaine) is associated with insufficient milk and early formula supplementation, because infants may have difficulty in executing correct and effective suckling that results in diminishing maternal milk production (Volmanen, Valanne, & Alahuhta, 2004).

Fernandez and colleagues (2012) demonstrated a negative relationship between the amount of intrapartum oxytocin received by laboring mothers and difficulties seen with latch and sucking.

Newborns whose mothers received higher doses of oxytocin experienced the blunting of several primitive neonatal reflexes related to breastfeeding (sucking, jaw jerk, swallowing, and gazing). The inhibitory effect on sucking was observed 24 to 48 hours after birth and oxytocin has a known effect on the regulation of ingestive behaviors. Mothers who received higher doses of intrapartum oxytocin were also unlikely to be exclusively breastfeeding at 3 months. Bai, Wu, and Tarrant (2013) found an association between intrapartum interventions and breastfeeding duration. Mothers who experienced at least three intrapartum interventions (such as induction of labor, opioid medication, and emergency cesarean) demonstrated a median duration of 1 month less than mothers with no intrapartum interventions.

Widström and colleagues (1987) observed that organized breastfeeding behaviors in full-term infants develop in a predictable way during the first hours of life. These behaviors are initially expressed as spontaneous sucking (low at 15 minutes after birth, maximal at 45 minutes postdelivery, and absent by 2–2½ hours after birth when asleep) and rooting movements (low at 15 minutes and maximal at 60 minutes after birth) when placed on the mother's chest immediately at birth. They progress to hand-to-mouth movements (observed at a mean time of 34 ± 2 minutes), more intense rooting and sucking activity, and breast-seeking behaviors, and they culminate in attachment to the breast. Unmedicated infants found the breast unassisted and started vigorous suckling at 55 ± 4 minutes after delivery.

In order to provide a more detailed analysis of the behavioral sequence a newborn infant engages in to locate and latch to the nipple, Widström, Lilja, Aaltomaa-Michalias, Dahllòf, Lintula, and Nissen (2011) delineated 9 distinct stages of infant behavior during uninterrupted skin-to-skin care in the first hour following birth. These stages include:

1. Birth cry: follows birth and facilitates lung expansion and aeration
2. Relaxation phase: no movements of the infant for a few minutes, possibly from high oxytocin levels, which may contribute to slight sedation
3. Awakening: small movements of the head and shoulders
4. Activity: mouthing and sucking movements are seen and the rooting reflex becomes more apparent
5. Rest: rest phases may be seen between periods of activity
6. Crawling: crawling movements began in search of the nipple/areola
7. Familiarization: touching and licking the areola with massaging-like motions of the hand begins an acquaintance with the food source
8. Suckling: the infant attaches to the breast and begins to suckle; infants whose mothers have received labor medications may take longer for this to happen
9. Sleep: about 1H to 2 hours following birth, infants generally fall into a restful sleep

Facilitating skin-to-skin contact, not only immediately after delivery but for up to 3 hours following birth, increases the likelihood that infants will leave the hospital exclusively breastfed (Bramson et al., 2010; Crenshaw et al., 2012).

Although newborn human infants and other mammals both crawl to the breast soon after birth to feed, this "instinctive" behavior is easily disturbed. Separation of the infant from the mother before the first attachment to the breast has occurred can disrupt subsequent correct latch to the breast (Righard & Alade, 1990). Infants separated from their mothers before they have suckled from the breast may have more difficulty in latching and exhibit an incorrect latch and suck at the subsequent feeding.

Combinations of these factors may cause difficulties in latching and staying attached to the breast. Babies whose mothers have been heavily medicated during labor may need more time to travel through the 9 stages of skin-to-skin contact, with bathing and wrapping being delayed.

A young infant who is reluctant to feed at breast may be unable to do so because of residual conditions still present from the delivery. The normal overlap or overriding of the cranial bone plates generally self-corrects within a couple of days after birth. Traction on the head during either a vaginal or a cesarean delivery, and the possible resulting hyperextension of the neck, may displace the occipital bone forward, potentially compromising the jugular foramen and/or the foramen magnum (Smith, 2004). The jugular foramina provide passage out of the skull for three nerves:

1. The glossopharyngeal (IX) cranial nerve works with the vagus nerve to help control swallowing and airway function along with function of the tongue. It also works with the hypoglossal (XII) nerve to control the tongue. The hypoglossal nerve exits the skull through the hypoglossal canals located beside and beneath the joint surfaces of the occiput.
2. The vagus (X) nerve also helps maintain a normal heart rate.
3. The spinal accessory (XI) nerve innervates major neck muscles such as the sternocleidomastoid and a portion of the trapezius.

Pressure on these nerves is thought to contribute to some feeding problems. Abnormal presentations such as face, mentum (chin), arm, footling breech, or breech may also set the stage for compressive forces on nerves that are responsible for normal feeding activities.

An infant whose head is misshapen (one side of the head higher than the other) or whose bones are out of alignment may signal the need for closer inspection of the infant's feeding capacity. Fascia or connective tissue surrounds, supports, and connects one type of tissue to another and affects the normal range of motion for structures. Observations of infants and their limiting movements have led to a number of forms of bodywork for infants to correct these limitations. Craniosacral therapy (CST) is a gentle form of massage that focuses on the bones, connective tissues, and fluid that surround the brain and spinal cord to relieve constrictions that may be impinging on the functioning of these structures (Upledger, 2003a, 2003b). About 5 g of pressure is used to evaluate and correct mobility restrictions or misalignments along the cranial sutures (Brussel, 2001). Practitioners of CST may be chiropractors, massage therapists, physical therapists, physicians, dentists, or allied healthcare providers who have taken courses in CST.

Chiropractic treatment has also been described as an intervention to remediate cervical spine dysfunction due to birth or birth trauma. Such dysfunction may impede normal motion and function of the infant anatomy necessary for proper latch and sucking. Chiropractic treatment is designed to correct restrictions of motion in joints and stimulate optimal nervous system function. Coordination between the perioral muscles and the temporomandibular joint (TMJ) is important for optimal sucking. Restriction of motion in the TMJ or hypertonicity of the muscles that control this joint can interfere with the infant's ability to latch or create a vacuum. Chiropractic care has been used to improve restrictions in TMJ mobility and facilitate optimal latch and sucking (Holleman, Chiro, Nee, & Knaap, 2011).

Myofascial release is another therapy intended to produce and improve changes in tissue mobility. Most evidence on the usefulness or outcomes of CST is anecdotal or consists of case studies (Hewitt, 1999; Turney, 2002). Holtrop (2000) described resolution by cranial adjusting of sucking dysfunction in a

6-month-old infant with an inward dishing at the occipitoparietal junction and upper cervical (C1–C2) asymmetry and fixation. Although the available health outcome research consists mainly of low-grade evidence (Green, Martin, Bassett, & Kazanjian, 1999), Vallone (2004) suggested that biomechanical dysfunction based on articular or muscular integrity may influence the ability of an infant to suckle successfully and that intervention via soft tissue work, cranial therapy, and spinal adjustments may have a direct result in improving the infant's ability to suckle efficiently. Wescott (2004) believed that cranial osteopathy is a useful treatment when dealing with instances of breastfeeding problems resulting from birth trauma. If parents are interested in these forms of therapy, the practitioners of these treatment modalities should be qualified to provide them safely.

Some infants experience troublesome breastfeeding due to a nervous system that does not respond appropriately to sensory stimuli. Sensory-processing difficulties were first described in the 1960s by A. Jean Ayers, who was working with neurologically involved children (Ayers, 1977). Sensory integration has evolved over time and is now defined as the ability of the nervous system to accept sensory information, process it, and respond with motor and behavioral responses that are appropriate to the context (Weiss-Salinas & Williams, 2001). The nervous system is designed to modulate environmental stimuli and provide graded responses. However, with sensory-processing difficulties, there may be poor coordination, sensory defensiveness (extreme reactions to ordinary sensations), or sensory-modulation difficulties (extremes in activity, emotional levels, and arousal levels) (Reisman, 2002). An infant can be hypersensitive to some stimuli and hyposensitive to others (Genna, 2001). Indications of sensory-integration disturbance may first be manifested in the newborn as feeding difficulties and should be followed and remedied (**Box 5-1**). Infants with poor tactile processing who fail to root, attach to the breast, or ignore the breast may benefit from use of a nipple shield. The shield may present a stronger tactile signal to such an infant, helping to trigger rooting and mouth opening (Genna, 2013).

Some infants may simply become overwhelmed by multiple people handling them, loud noise, bright lights, radio, television, and ringing telephones. As a result, they may basically shut down until the environment becomes quieter.

Box 5-1 Possible Indicators of Sensory-Integration Difficulties

Hyperactive gag reflex
Shallow latch (breast not drawn deeply into mouth)
Low oral muscle tone
Poor sucking rhythmicity
Excessive jaw compression
Malpositioning of the tongue
Unusual posturing
Avoidance of certain positions (arching of the back)
Increased tone, withdrawal responses from the breast
Latch refusal, tonic bite
Passive at breast
Mother's belief that the infant does not like to breastfeed or does not like her

Oral aversion or oral–tactile hypersensitivity may be another manifestation of sensory integration difficulties but can often have iatrogenic origins. These conditions and the ensuing aversive responses can be caused by prematurity, immaturity, illness, delayed oral feeding, and unpleasant oral–tactile experiences (Wolf & Glass, 1992). The possibility of oral aversion resulting in maladaptive imprinting, faulty sucking techniques, and dysphagia (difficulty in swallowing) should be taken into account when an infant is reluctant to breastfeed (Healow & Hugh, 2000). Suctioning, intubation, and gavage feeding are all invasive to the oral cavity. Petechiae and bruises on the posterior palates of infants who were suctioned with a standard bulb syringe after a vaginal delivery have been reported (Black, 1993). Conditioned dysphagia from aggressive suctioning and procedures can be acquired and learned when a negative stimulus is associated with swallowing (Di Scipio, Kaslon, & Ruben, 1978). Other intrusions into a newborn's mouth that may contribute to oral-aversive behaviors include gastric lavage, use of artificial nipples or pacifiers, digital assessment of the mouth, finger feeding, use of latex gloves or finger cots, unpleasant-tasting fluids, and repeated suctioning with a bulb syringe.

Latch difficulties may be an early marker of a congenital condition previously called benign congenital hypotonia. Although not identifying a disease, this general descriptive term refers to an infant with low muscle tone at birth and a generalized floppiness. Diagnostic advances have been able to identify specific neurological disorders and myopathies such as central core disease, congenital muscular dystrophy, and spinal muscle atrophy, resulting in this term being phased out in favor of the more accurate diagnoses (Prasad & Prasad, 2003). An accurate diagnosis is important, because some neuromuscular disorders carry the risk of malignant hyperthermia (Thompson, 2002). The "floppy baby" referred to here represents a neuromuscular disorder of unknown origin that is nonprogressive and tends to improve over time. The infant feels like a rag doll with general weakness and flaccidity of the muscles. The infant may be unable to lift his or her head, has a weak cry, displays poor reflexes, shows poor suckling, has hypermobile joints, demonstrates an underactive gag reflex, has a high arched palate, demonstrates fasciculations of the tongue, and has an open mouth. Mothers may describe decreased fetal movements during the pregnancy. Some infants are born with joint contractures (arthrogryposis) of the ankles, knees, elbows, or wrists. An affected infant may also have congenitally dislocated hips and weakness in the anterior neck muscles, causing the head to lag when lifted. Sucking difficulties may be found with inactive lip, cheek, and tongue muscles as well as lack of sensory input from hand-to-mouth movements (Cohen, 1998). Such hypotonia may originate from an insult to the central nervous system that was not severe enough to cause permanent damage. It can also result from perinatal asphyxia, intraventricular hemorrhage, and prematurity. Clinicians may wish to look at the labor and delivery records to check for hypoxia, difficult delivery, or vacuum extraction in such cases.

Age-appropriate hypotonia may be expected to be seen in preterm and late preterm infants. Hypotonia commonly occurs in infants with Down syndrome. All infants with low tone should be well supported in positions that do not require extra effort to maintain their latch on the breast. Their efforts need to be directed to sucking, not supporting their body position. Mothers may need both hands to support the infant and the breast and may find that well-placed pillows or the use of a sling may help provide extra body support for the infant (Thomas, Marinelli, Hennessy, & Academy of Breastfeeding Medicine Protocol Committee, 2007). There are many additional ways to help infants with low tone to breastfeed.

Infant hypotonia is one of a number of symptoms of vitamin B_{12} deficiency. Infants of mothers who have undergone gastric bypass surgery should be checked for congenital B_{12} deficiency and monitored during their early months of breastfeeding (Celiker & Chawla, 2009). Vitamin B_{12} deficiency can also occur in breastfeeding infants whose mothers are vegetarians. Problems may not show up until the infant is several months old, with not only hypotonia being present but other symptoms, such as failure to thrive, lethargy, microcephaly, or developmental delay (Chalouhi et al., 2008; Honzik et al., 2010). Clinicians may find it prudent to determine the vitamin B_{12} status of mothers who have undergone gastric bypass surgery, gastric banding, or any other of these types of procedures and to monitor vegetarian mothers and their infants for B_{12} deficiencies. While most of the symptoms are reversible with treatment, permanent neurological damage can result in infants who are not promptly treated. Problems latching to the breast in these situations may determine the need to assess for hypotonia as well as the B_{12} status of both the mother and the infant.

Drug-exposed infants experiencing neonatal abstinence syndrome (NAS) present an almost completely opposite picture; that is, they may be hypertonic, be irritable, demonstrate abnormal movements, be hypersensitive, thrash at the breast, clamp down on the nipple, be unable to modulate their state to feed well, be difficult to position at breast, and pull back from the breast if experiencing nasal stuffiness (Jansson, Velez, & Harrow, 2004). Intrauterine drug exposure may temporarily impact the development of brainstem respiratory and swallow centers, transiently altering the suck–swallow–breathe cycle. During the early days after birth, some of these infants may ingest a lower volume of milk per sucking burst and/or demonstrate less rhythmical swallowing, especially if they have been opiate exposed in utero (Gewolb, Fishman, Qureshi, & Voce, 2004).

According to the Substance Abuse and Mental Health Services Administration (2014), among pregnant women aged 15 to 44, 5.4% were current illicit drug users based on data averaged across 2012 and 2013. This was lower than the rate among women in this age group who were not pregnant (11.4%). Among pregnant women aged 15 to 44, the average rate of current illicit drug use in 2012–2013 (5.4%) was not significantly different from the rate averaged across 2010–2011 (5.0%). Current illicit drug use in 2012–2013 was lower among pregnant women aged 15 to 44 during the third trimester than during the first and second trimesters (2.4% vs. 9.0% and 4.8%, respectively). The rate of current illicit drug use in the combined 2012–2013 data was 14.6% among pregnant women aged 15 to 17, 8.6% among women aged 18 to 25, and 3.2% among women aged 26 to 44. These rates were not significantly different from those in the combined 2010–2011 data (20.9% among pregnant women aged 15 to 17, 8.2% among pregnant women aged 18 to 25, and 2.2% among pregnant women aged 26 to 44). Clearly, substance abuse remains a significant problem, especially among younger mothers. In a worrisome trend, the abuse of prescription pain medications has seen a rampant increase among pregnant women (Epstein et al., 2013).

Mothers on methadone maintenance or other treatments for opioid dependence who are receiving proper care and counseling through substance abuse treatment programs should be encouraged to breastfeed with close follow-up (American Academy of Pediatrics, 2012). Early and consistent education for mothers and clinicians on the benefits of breastfeeding and how breastfeeding can compensate for some of the adverse effects of in utero exposure to opioids and other substances of abuse such as tobacco is most important (Pritham, 2013):

- Breastfeeding reduces the incidence of sudden infant death syndrome (SIDS), possibly because of its positive effects on breathing and arousal mechanisms.
- Breastfeeding may compensate for the psychomotor and cognitive performance delays seen in drug-exposed infants.

- The act of breastfeeding may positively affect the infant's central nervous system by reducing pain, stress, and anxiety.
- The act of breastfeeding may improve cardiac vagal tone and heart rate variability, thereby improving the infant's autonomic regulation.
- Infants who are breastfed are discharged from the hospital sooner than those who are formula-fed and are less apt to require treatment for NAS.
- Breastfeeding that is initiated at birth and continued for at least 72 hours has been shown to reduce the severity of NAS and the need for pharmacological treatment (Dryden, Young, Hepburn, & Mactier, 2009).

Boston Medical Center in Boston, Massachusetts, relies on an illicit drug use and breastfeeding policy that requires certain criteria be met in order for mothers to be encouraged to breastfeed. These criteria include that 10 weeks before birth a urine toxicology screen be done. If it is negative and the mother is compliant for a minimum of 12 weeks with an addiction recovery program, attends standard prenatal visits, and has a negative urine screen upon arrival to the labor and delivery service, then the mother is encouraged to breastfeed (Wachman, Byun, & Philipp, 2010).

Allegaert and van den Anker (2014) recommend that breastfeeding be added to any clinical pathway regarding the treatment of NAS. Infants experiencing in utero exposure to opioids may need to be medicated as the infants withdraw from opioids, because 60–90% of opiate-exposed infants develop NAS (Kandall, 1995) even with the low amounts of the medication received through breastmilk (Begg, Malpas, Hackett, & Ilett, 2001; Jansson, Choo, Velez, Lowe, & Huestis, 2008). NAS is a result of the abrupt discontinuation of fetal exposure to licit or illicit substances used or abused during pregnancy. Neonates with NAS demonstrate a range of symptoms, including central nervous system irritability, gastrointestinal dysfunction, respiratory distress, and vague autonomic symptoms such as mottling, yawning, sneezing, and fever (Kocherlakota, 2014). Dryden, Young, Hepburn, and Mactier (2009) demonstrated that breastfeeding was associated with reduced odds of the infant requiring treatment for NAS. Abdel-Latif and colleagues (2006) documented that breastfeeding has a significant positive impact on the neonate that included reduced NAS severity, delayed onset of NAS, and decreased need for pharmacological treatment regardless of gestational age and the type of drug exposure. McQueen, Murphy-Oikonen, Gerlach, and Montelpare (2011) found that predominantly breastfed infants had lower mean NAS scores, suggesting a decreased severity and duration of NAS symptoms when compared to infants who were combination fed or predominantly formula fed. Thus, breastfeeding is to be encouraged and supported because these infants are extremely vulnerable and can benefit greatly not only from the receipt of breastmilk but by the act of breastfeeding itself (Bagley, Wachman, Holland, & Brogly, 2014).

Jansson and colleagues (2004) identified eight potential challenges to breastfeeding presented by methadone-exposed infants and suggestions for handling them (**Table 5-2**). Wachman and colleagues (2010) reported that breastfeeding rates remained low among opioid-dependent women, even when receiving exemplary lactation care and services. This may be due to the significant challenges that these women face during their recovery from drug dependency as well as the difficulty of breastfeeding a drug-exposed infant who may be irritable and demonstrate feeding problems.

Table 5-2 Challenges to Breastfeeding in Methadone-Exposed Infants

Challenge	Intervention
1. Irritability/crying	Feed when in a drowsy state or before full crying appears Swaddle Vertical rocking Hold baby's hand Gentle cupping of head if tolerated "Tame" the environment by dimming lights and minimizing noise
2. State lability • Rapid fluctuation between states • Not achieving quiet alert state	Minimize stimulation Bring infant from sleep to quiet alert state slowly Watch for signs of stress
3. Hypertonicity • Generalized, often with asymmetries • Clenched jaw and poor gape (mouth opening) • Easily overstimulated ▪ Neck arching ▪ Side-to-side head thrashing • Arched posture	Gradual oral stimulation Respond to overstimulation cues (irritability, hiccups, tremors, excessive gas, gaze aversion, tachypnea [rapid breathing], mottling) Head support Wrap baby in a soft blanket to restrain thrashing movements Avoid the clutch hold and have baby facing the mother Use ventral positioning
4. Suck-and-swallow incoordination • Poor or disorganized suck patterns	Feeding therapy referral to occupational therapist, physical therapist, or speech-language pathologist Mothers may need to pump their milk Alternative feeding devices may be required until baby can feed at breast
5. Hypersensitivity	Feed in a dim, quiet room with comfortable, constant temperature Gentle and minimal handling Swaddling Have mother breastfeed in a side-lying position Artificial nipples may not be well tolerated and should be avoided Shape the breast to fit the long axis of the baby's mouth if he or she does not open wide enough to latch Wrap a soft blanket around baby's arms, upper body, and back of head to minimize thrashing
6. Nasal stuffiness (may cause detaching from the nipple, pulling back of baby's head, arching, and stiffening)	May require gentle nasal suctioning with saline drops
7. Vomiting	Small, frequent feeds and frequent burping
8. Pull-down (may appear to be sedated or asleep in an effort to avoid stimuli and create a tolerable environment)	Baby may actually be in an awake or hypersensitive state; vigorous stimulation in an attempt to wake baby should be avoided Soft handling, gentle talking, and skin-to-skin contact

Data from Jansson, L. M., Velez, M., & Harrow, C. (2004). Methadone maintenance and lactation: A review of the literature and current management guidelines. *Journal of Human Lactation, 20,* 62–71.

Rooming-in should be encouraged as it may promote more effective mothering behaviors and reduce the severity of the infant's withdrawal symptoms (Hilton, 2012). Oxytocin, which is released each time the infant is put to breast, may help the mother relax, increase feelings of love for the infant, reduce stress and pain, and generally help her cope with an infant who may be irritable and difficult to feed and calm.

Recently, buprenorphine (Buprenex, Subutex) has been used to treat opioid-abusing mothers during pregnancy. Infants seem to experience a less severe course of NAS when their mothers were treated with buprenorphine (Kakko, Heilig, & Sarman, 2008). Due to its poor oral bioavailability, buprenorphine is considered compatible with breastfeeding as the infant dose would be subclinical (Hale, 2012). Ilett and colleagues (2012) concluded that the dose of buprenorphine and norbuprenorphine that a breastfeeding infant receives via milk is generally less than 1% of the weight-adjusted maternal dose and unlikely to cause any acute adverse effects in the infant. The Center for Substance Abuse Treatment (2004) panel recommends breastfeeding for mothers undergoing buprenorphine treatment unless other contraindications exist. While these mothers often stop breastfeeding within a week, recent studies have shown that mothers treated with buprenorphine (O'Connor et al., 2011) and provided with excellent lactation support services (Wachman et al., 2010) breastfeed far longer.

Women receiving methadone treatment face opposition, stigma, misinformation from peers and healthcare professionals, and logistical challenges in their efforts to breastfeed (Demirci, Bogen, & Klionsky, 2015). In their study, Demirci and colleagues (2015) found that mothers feared the passage of methadone into their milk and lacked support and correct information from the healthcare community. Correction of misinformation, positive support from clinicians, and educating family and friends regarding the importance of breastfeeding are modifiable barriers to breastfeeding success. The Academy of Breastfeeding Medicine has published a protocol on breastfeeding and substance abuse that may be a helpful resource for educating clinicians on the importance of breastfeeding for this vulnerable and fragile population of infants and mothers (Reece-Stremtan, Marinelli, & Academy of Breastfeeding Medicine, 2015). The use of laser acupuncture combined with pharmacological therapy has been shown to significantly shorten the length of morphine therapy as well as significantly reduce the length of hospital stay in infants who were drug exposed in utero (Raith et al., 2015).

Infants who are exposed to other drugs during pregnancy may also exhibit stress or abstinence behaviors. Prenatal use of less potent opiates, some nonopiate central nervous system depressants, alcohol, marijuana, or tobacco can generate side effects in the newborn (Lester et al., 2002).

The overall smoking rate during the last 3 months of pregnancy in 2012 and 2013 in the United States was 15.4% (Substance Abuse and Mental Health Services Administration, 2014). Women who smoke are less likely to breastfeed than those who do not smoke and are more likely to wean earlier than nonsmoking mothers (Liu, Rosenberg, & Sandoval, 2006). There may be a number of explanations for this:

- Smoking > 10 cigarettes daily was reported to decrease milk production and alter milk composition (Hopkinson, Schanler, Fraley, & Garza, 1992).
- Mothers who smoke may perceive that their milk supply is inadequate (Hill & Aldag, 1996).
- The milk of smoking breastfeeding mothers has a lower fat content than the milk of mothers who do not smoke (Powers, 1999). Cigarette smoking during pregnancy is associated with lower milk-fat content and lower polyunsaturated fatty acids in the first 6 months of lactation

(Agostoni et al., 2003). Docosahexaenoic acid (DHA) levels were found to be lower in the milk of mothers who smoked. Bachour, Yafawi, Jaber, Choueiri, and Abdel-Razzak (2012) found that smoking resulted in a 26% decrease in the lipid concentration of the milk of mothers who smoked. These authors also report a 12% decrease in the milk-protein content of mothers who smoke. Alterations of this magnitude in the milk of mothers who smoke agree with previous studies that show a slower growth rate in breastfeeding infants of mothers who smoke (Vio, Salazar, & Infante, 1991). Clinicians may need to be more vigilant with infants of mothers who smoke, making sure that growth parameters remain in the normal range. Mothers who smoke may need to feed their infants more frequently to assure that growth does not falter. They can also employ the use of alternate massage during feedings to boost calorie and fat intake.

- Mothers who experience chronic exposure to nicotine may boost dopamine activity in the tuberoinfundibular tract, which functions to inhibit prolactin release (Bahadori, Riegiger, Farrell, Uitz, & Moghadasian, 2013). Such a side effect of smoking may serve to limit milk production.
- Mothers who smoked five or more cigarettes daily had infants who exhibited behaviors such as colic and crying that may contribute to early weaning (Matheson & Rivrud, 1989).
- Smoking mothers perceived a strong risk of harming the infant by smoking and weaned earlier due to concerns regarding the toxic effects of nicotine on the composition and quantity of their milk. Mothers did not receive a strong message from healthcare providers that the benefits of breastfeeding superseded the harm of smoking, as many smoking mothers remain unaware that the benefits of breastfeeding outweigh the potential harm posed to their infants by nicotine in their breastmilk (Goldade et al., 2008).
- In 102 samples of breastmilk purchased over the Internet, 58% had detectable levels of nicotine or cotinine, 4% had levels indicating active smoking, and 97% had detectable levels of caffeine. Sellers of breastmilk may misrepresent or be unaware of health behaviors that affect the content of their milk (Geraghty et al., 2015). Mothers and clinicians should be aware of potential contamination of breastmilk purchased over the Internet.

Tobacco-exposed infants have been shown to demonstrate neurotoxic effects such as greater excitability, greater hypertonia, the need for more handling, and signs of withdrawal or abstinence (Law et al., 2003). Smoking-exposed infants may demonstrate poor self-regulation with all side effects persisting up to a month after birth (Stroud et al., 2009). Yolton and colleagues (2009) examined the relationship between prenatal tobacco smoke exposure and infant neurobehavior. While finding significant differences out to 5 weeks in infant neurobehavior due to tobacco exposure, these authors found that infant neurobehavioral outcomes differed by race. Among white infants, as prenatal tobacco smoke exposure increased, infants were more excitable, more aroused, and less able to calm themselves. They also showed a reduced capacity to focus their attention during the neurobehavioral assessment with increased agitation. As tobacco exposure increased with black infants, they became less responsive during the neurobehavioral exam, were less able to interact socially, and were less affected by the manipulation of the examiner. These alterations in behavior may cause early breastfeeding to be more difficult due to over- or under-aroused infants. Clinicians may need to take these alterations in neurobehavioral profiles into account when working with infants of mothers who smoke.

Postnatal exposure to the nicotine in breastmilk can alter autonomic cardiovascular control in infants. Heart rate variability has been shown to decrease as the amount of nicotine in breastmilk increases (Dahlstrom, Ebersjo, & Lundell, 2008). Shorter times between the mother smoking a cigarette and the onset of breastfeeding increase the concentration of nicotine in breastmilk (Dahlstrom, Ebersjo, & Lundell, 2004). Mothers who smoke can be advised to smoke immediately after a breastfeeding to prolong the interval between nicotine intake and breastfeeding. Nicotine is not stored in breastmilk, and levels peak in breastmilk 30 to 60 minutes after cessation of smoking (Mennella & Beauchamp, 1998). Even passive smoke in the household increases the nicotine levels in breastmilk. Although mothers who smoke should be encouraged to breastfeed, they should also be helped to eliminate smoking from their homes. The following may provide potential motivations to stop smoking:

- Infants spend significantly less time sleeping during the hours immediately after breastfeeding when their mothers have recently smoked (Mennella, Yourshaw, & Morgan, 2007).
- Smoking is a leading risk factor for SIDS (Anderson, Johnson, & Batal, 2005).
- Nicotine-induced disruptions in sleep may contribute to long-term behavioral and learning deficits (DiFranza, Aligne, & Weitzman, 2004) because sleep promotes learning in infants (Gomez, Bootzin, & Nadel, 2006) and deprivation of active sleep impairs learning and the formation of new memories in animal models (McDermott et al., 2003).

Breastfeeding has been shown to be a protective factor against increases in smoking after childbirth. Supporting mothers who stop smoking during pregnancy so that they can breastfeed for at least 3 months can have lasting benefits for smoking reduction (Shisler et al., 2015). Breastfeeding also reduces children's susceptibility to the respiratory side effects of tobacco smoke exposure, as it appears to protect against asthma-related symptoms in early childhood (Liu et al., 2015).

Approximately 6% of pregnant women experience exposure to selective serotonin reuptake inhibitors (SSRIs), a commonly prescribed family of antidepressant medications (Andrade et al., 2008; Cooper, Willy, Pont, & Ray, 2007). Mothers taking antidepressant medications during pregnancy are less likely to breastfeed than mothers not taking such medications (Gorman, Kao, & Chambers, 2012). Infants born to mothers who were treated prenatally for depression with SSRIs, such as the commonly prescribed paroxetine (Paxil), fluoxetine (Prozac), citalopram (Celexa), and sertraline (Zoloft), can demonstrate a wide range of neurobehavioral alterations (Lattimore et al., 2005), including increased tremulousness and difficulty achieving more alert states (Zeskind & Stephens, 2004). As many as 35% of women use some type of psychotropic medication during pregnancy (Goldberg & Nissim, 1994). A neonatal behavioral syndrome, termed poor neonatal adaptation, has been described in infants whose mothers have been treated with SSRIs; it includes tremors, shaking, agitation, spasms, hyper- or hypotonia, irritability, hypoglycemia, temperature instability, and sleep disturbances. Respiratory system involvement includes indrawing, apnea/bradycardia, and tachypnea (Jordan et al., 2008). These signs appear during the 1st day of life and resolve within 3 to 5 days (Ferreira et al., 2007). Other differences observed in the exposed group were higher rates of vomiting, tachycardia, and jaundice. Some studies report an increase in persistent pulmonary hypertension (Yonkers et al., 2009). Salisbury and colleagues (2011) compared the neurobehavioral profile of infants born to mothers who had a major depressive disorder without SSRI exposure and those infants whose mothers had both a major depressive disorder and were treated with

SSRIs. The authors found different neurobehavioral profiles between the two groups of infants. Full-term infants of mothers with a major depressive disorder and SSRI treatment had a lower gestational age, lower quality of movements, and more central nervous system signs of stress. Infants of mothers with a major depressive disorder but no treatment with SSRIs had higher quality of movement scores but lower attention scores. Any or all of these signs may disturb early breastfeeding behaviors, necessitating close observation and a potential need for intense breastfeeding support. While short-term adverse outcomes for term infants are generally mild and time limited, preterm or unstable infants should be more closely monitored for adverse effects (Kendall-Tackett & Hale, 2010). Some of the signs and symptoms of withdrawal are seen in healthy non–drug-exposed infants or are indicative of other types of underlying problems. A withdrawal scoring sheet may be helpful to identify the drug-withdrawing infant from a collection of symptoms that persist over time (http://newborns.stanford.edu/ScoringSheet.html). The Neonatal Intensive Care Unit Network Neurobehavioral Scale was developed to provide a comprehensive assessment of neurological integrity and behavioral function in drug-exposed infants and to identify the types and ranges of withdrawal and stress behaviors likely to be seen in these infants (Lester, Tronick, & Brazelton, 2004). Use of this scale is intended to ensure a home environment sensitive to infant tolerance for stimulation and handling and to provide the clinician with insight regarding positioning, handling, and environmental conditions that are most beneficial in caring for these infants during hospitalization (Boukydis, Bigsby, & Lester, 2004). Depressive symptoms early in pregnancy have been associated with reduced concentrations of DHA in breastmilk (Keim et al., 2012). This study recommends early screening for major depression during pregnancy and looking at ways to improve the DHA status of these mothers to reduce both the burden of perinatal depression and the alteration of the breastmilk of these mothers.

Hale, Kendall-Tackett, Cong, Votta, and McCurdy (2010) found that discontinuation syndrome (poor adaptation, jitteriness, irritability, and poor gaze control) was seen in a small number of infants whose mothers took antidepressants during pregnancy. Six symptoms (jitteriness, vomiting, irritability, low body temperature, shivering, and problems with eating and sleeping) were 2 to 8 times more likely to be reported in infants whose mothers took antidepressants while pregnant compared to taking these medications during lactation. Infants were shown to have much lower odds of experiencing these symptoms if their mothers took antidepressants during pregnancy with mid-range or long half-lives (sertraline or fluoxetine) instead of ones with a short half-life. Clinicians should be watchful for these manifestations and be ready to manage them in mothers who have a history of antidepressive medication use. Some mothers who can switch to a longer acting agent may be able to reduce the odds of their infant experiencing symptoms associated with the discontinuation syndrome. Sertraline (Zoloft) and paroxetine (Paxil) have shown a better neonatal safety profile during breastfeeding compared to other antidepressive drugs (Orsolini & Bellantuono, 2015). Formula feeding has been shown to increase the risk of an infant experiencing poor neonatal adaptation when exposed to maternal antidepressants compared to breastfeeding or mixed feeding (Kieviet et al., 2015).

Marshall and colleagues (2010) reported that mothers taking SSRIs were at a two-fold greater risk of delayed lactogenesis II (onset of copious milk secretion). This delay in the milk coming in was related to the disruption that the SSRIs caused in serotonin within the breast. Serotonin is a regulator of lactation homeostasis. Increased vigilance is warranted to ensure adequate infant milk intake in the early days following delivery. Mothers with a history of SSRI treatment should be informed that a delay in lactogenesis II might occur and a feeding plan to anticipate this should be in place prior to discharge from the hospital.

Early feeding resistance in some infants may have an organic basis. Abadie and colleagues (2001) described a set of feeding behaviors in bottle-fed infants that they attributed to poor organic perinatal control of oroesophageal motility: early onset of poor sucking and swallowing skills, refusal to feed, excessive regurgitation, and occasional cough or pallor attacks during bottle-feeding. Some infants also displayed minor facial dysmorphism (retrognathia and arched palate) and mild hypotonia of the tongue base or larynx. The congenital nature of these behaviors combined with manometric findings in the esophagus led to the suspicion that these feeding behaviors were the result of prenatal factors, because central control of the coordinated peristalsis of esophageal motility, sucking, and swallowing originates in a central pattern generator in the brainstem (Jean, 2001). Also, retrognathia and arched palate are anatomic variations that have been observed in children with poor fetal sucking movements (Sherer, Metlay, & Woods, 1995).

Persistent and unresolved difficulties with latching may result in an infant who never achieves latch, early weaning from the breast, or a mother who pumps her milk and provides it to her baby in a bottle. Clinicians have the option of using a nipple shield to achieve latch. Although early shield design and use often yielded unwanted and detrimental outcomes to breastfeeding (Desmarais & Browne, 1990), more recent data have described beneficial outcomes. Central to such outcomes are the use of ultrathin silicone shields, critical assessment by a skilled lactation consultant, and continuous follow-up, both in the hospital and postdischarge. Many infants who otherwise may have been unable to breastfeed can and have benefited from the judicious use of this tool.

NIPPLE SHIELDS

Nipple shields can be quite helpful as an intervention in certain breastfeeding situations (Brigham, 1996; Wilson-Clay, 2003) and may help prolong the duration of breastfeeding when mothers encounter certain types of breastfeeding problems (Ekstrom, Abrahamsson, Eriksson, & Martensson, 2014). An understanding of what shields can and cannot accomplish is essential to the clinical decision-making process. Shields can:

- Therapeutically supply oral stimulation that an infant cannot obtain from the mother's nipples due to inability to latch or transfer milk
- Create a nipple shape in the infant's mouth
- Allow extraction of milk by expression with minimal suction, with negative pressure inside the shield tip keeping milk available
- Compensate for weak infant suction
- Present a stable nipple shape that remains during pauses in sucking bursts
- Maintain the nipple in a protruded position
- Affect the rate of milk flow
- Shields cannot:
    - Correct milk transfer problems or weight gain if the mother has inadequate milk volume
    - Fix damaged nipples if the cause is not discovered and remedied
    - Replace skilled intervention and close follow-up

While high-level research on shield use is lacking (McKechnie & Eglash, 2010), shield use can aid learning to feed at breast, allows supplementation to occur at breast (i.e., thread tubing under or alongside of the shield), encourages nipple protractility, does not overwhelm the mother with gadgets, and avoids the infant fighting the breast. Shield use may prevent premature termination of breastfeeding. Use of shields does not affect maternal prolactin levels, and infants are able to gain weight appropriately while using a nipple shield (Chertok, Schneider, & Blackburn, 2006).

The clinician must also consider some of the disadvantages of nipple shield use. It is sometimes used as a substitute for skilled care or as a quick fix but may not correct the underlying problem; may exacerbate or mask the original problem; may lead to insufficient milk volume, inadequate weight gain, or weaning; can be problematic without follow-up; may prevent proper extension of the nipple back into the infant's mouth (Minchin, 1998); could pinch the nipple and areola, causing abrasion, pain, skin breakdown, and internal trauma to the breast if not applied properly; could create nipple shield addiction (DeNicola, 1986), after which the infant will not feed at breast without the shield in place; might predispose the nipple to damage when the infant is put to breast without the shield, because the infant may chew rather than suckle; and could be discarded as a useful intervention in select situations. One case report noted nipple damage with the use of a 24-mm nipple shield due to excessively high intraoral vacuum generated by the infant when using the shield (Perrella, Lai, & Geddes, 2015). Blisters were noted on the nipple tip that corresponded to the openings on the nipple shield. When sucking pressures were measured, the intraoral vacuum was as much as 307% higher than reference values. While the distinct pattern of nipple blisters suggested high intraoral vacuum, outside of a research setting there is no clinical screening tool available to assess for excessive vacuum generation. This condition might be suspected when the mother continues to complain of nipple pain when using the shield. Clinicians might recommend changing to a larger nipple shield (28 mm), alternating breastfeeding positions to vary pressure at the nipple base, offering shorter but more frequent feedings, and breastfeeding when the infant is in a drowsy state.

The teat portion of a nipple shield is much stiffer than the maternal nipple, may be larger than the mother's nipple, presents a different texture to the infant, and does not deflect and elongate like a human nipple. The texture of an oral object in the infant's mouth can modulate the sucking instructions from the suck central pattern generator. When presented with either a smooth or a textured pacifier, healthy term infants were seen to reorganize and change their non-nutritive sucking pattern depending on the texture presented to them (Oder, Stalling, & Barlow, 2013). The act of sucking on a nipple shield produces sensory cues from Merkel cells that line the lip vermillion and buccal mucosa. These oral mechanoreceptors encode specific information regarding such features as the shape, texture, curvature, and edges to create a neural image of the object in the infant's mouth. The brain then modulates the timing and output from the suck central pattern generator according to the cues it has received from the Merkel cells. Central pattern generators are located in the brain stem reticular formation and are composed of networks of interneurons that produce rhythmic motor patterns such as breathing, walking, and sucking (Marder & Bucher, 2001). The oral tactile input from the Merkel cells is a learned form of perceptual recognition that governs the imprinting process. If the Merkel cells have encoded a nipple shield rather than the maternal nipple during a critical window of learning, would it then alter how the infant sucks in the absence of a shield? Should a shield be avoided during the early hours and days so that the Merkel cells encode the maternal nipple as the imprinted object to avoid altering suck instructions from the suck central pattern generator? Little is known regarding their effect on infant feeding behaviors relative to the imprinting that may be affected by presenting a superstimulus to an infant during a sensitive or critical period of time. Because most nipple shields cover the part of the areola that contains the glands of Montgomery, might nipple shields either mask or eliminate the infant's use of olfaction to locate and identify the mother's specific odor? How important are the pheromones of the mother? Would a nipple shield with a cut-out section present better olfaction guidance to the breast?

Eglash, Ziemer, and McKechnie (2010) surveyed 490 healthcare professionals regarding nipple shield use in their practices. The most common reason for shield use was to aid infants younger than 35 weeks gestational age to latch and feed. Many other reasons were given for shield use including as a way to transition an infant from bottle to breast. Most of the respondents were concerned regarding the lack of follow-up once shield use was started. Most mothers reported positive experiences with nipple shield use (Chertok, 2009). Follow-up is crucial during shield use to assure ongoing monitoring of appropriate infant growth, abundant maternal milk supply, and ongoing efforts to correct the original problem that resulted in shield use to begin with.

Hanna, Wilson, and Norwood (2013) described the experience of 81 mothers with breastfeeding difficulties who were given nipple shields to aid in the initiation of breastfeeding. Most were given nipple shields for problems with infant latch, but other reasons included nipple pain and damage, flat nipples, disorganized suck, or a combination of reasons. Most mothers found the shield to be helpful and its use allowed them to avoid premature weaning. Some problems with shields were mentioned such as difficulty with the adherence of the shield, shield too big for the infant's mouth, and longer feeding times. With the added use of a nipple shield, 31% of the mothers in this study reached the Healthy People-recommended goal of breastfeeding for 6 months. There was a significant positive relationship between use of the nipple shield at week 5 and total weeks of breastfeeding. Powers and Tapia (2004) found in a telephone survey of 202 breastfeeding women that most used a shield due to flat nipples and an infant with disorganized sucking.

Use of a nipple shield could be considered in situations involving latch difficulty, oral cavity problems, upper airway problems, prematurity (Clum & Primomo, 1996), and damaged nipples when other avenues to achieve latch have been attempted and failed to produce the desired outcome and when discharge or weaning is imminent. (A complete list of such situational examples is provided in **Appendix 5-1**.)

Shield Composition and Dimensions

Shields exclusively composed of rubber are no longer seen today, and standard bottle nipples placed over the mother's nipple or attached to a glass or plastic base are not appropriate interventions (**Figure 5-15A**). Silicone shields are extremely thin and flexible, with a firmer nipple portion. Because the silicone is so thin, more stimulation reaches the areola and milk volume is not as seriously depleted as with the other designs (Auerbach, 1990). Due to the increasing incidence of latex allergy in the general population, latex-containing shields should be avoided. Silicone shields (**Figure 5-15B**) are available in a number of shapes and sizes, ranging from 16 mm to 28 mm (**Table 5-3**).

Few data exist in the literature regarding shield selection and instructions for their use. (A summary of shield-use instructions is presented in Appendix 5-1.) The height of the nipple portion of the shield should not exceed the length of the infant's mouth from the juncture of the hard and soft palates to lip

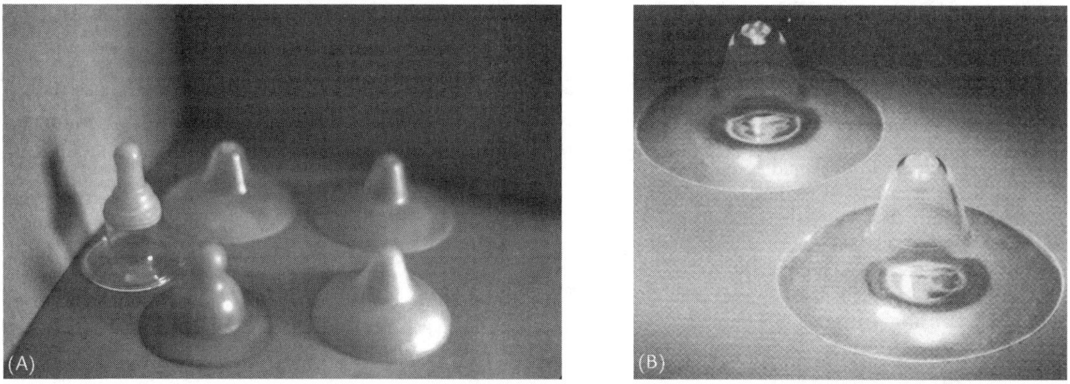

Figure 5-15 (A) Old-style nipple shields; (B) modern silicone nipple shields.

Table 5-3 Dimensions of Silicone Nipple Shields

Product	Size	Number of Holes
Avent	21 mm	3
Medela		
Standard	16 mm	4
	20 mm	
	24 mm	
Contact	16 mm	
	20 mm	
	24 mm	
Ameda	24 mm	5
Ardo	20 mm	4
	24 mm	
Mamivac		4
Conical	18 mm	
	20 mm	
	28 mm	
Cherry shaped	18 mm	
	22 mm	
Nuk	20 mm	4
	24 mm	
Lansinoh	24 mm	4

closure (Wilson-Clay & Hoover, 2002). If the height of the teat of a shield is greater than this length, the infant's jaw closure and tongue compression will fall on the shaft of the teat, and not over the breast. The teat must be large enough to allow for the expansion of the nipple during sucking. If the height of the teat is too short for the nipple, it may abrade against the inside of the teat or extrude through the teat holes.

The base diameter should fit the mother's nipple and better results occur with the shortest teat height and smallest base diameter.

Most nipple shields are conical shaped, but Mamivac makes a shield that has a cherry-shaped or more bulb-like tip. The cherry-shaped teat may be more appropriate for some infants and can be tried if a conical-shaped nipple shield does not provide the desired results.

Weaning From the Shield

There is no set time to wean an infant (or mother) from shield use. Extended use of the ultrathin silicone shield has not been shown to be detrimental (Bodley & Powers, 1996). Mothers start the shield-weaning process simply by encouraging skin-to-skin contact next to the nipple, starting the feed with the shield and then removing it, and gradually trying feeds without the shield. The tip of the shield should not be cut off in an attempt to present less and less of the device to the infant. Rough edges may scrape the infant's mouth, and the altered shape and consistency of the shield may not be appropriate to the desired outcome.

Follow-Up on Shield Use

Clinicians should provide proper written instructions for the mother and referrals if a shield is recommended as an interim measure to assist with breastfeeding. If a mother is discharged from the hospital using a shield, a community referral must be made to a lactation consultant or the nurse practitioner at the pediatrician's office for daily follow-up. Weight checks may need to be obtained twice a week. The pediatrician should be alerted to the problem that required use of the shield in the first place and should be aware of suggestions for discontinuing its use.

RELUCTANT NURSER

The mother is likely to experience frustration and anxiety over an infant who cannot feed at her breast. If breastfeeding attempts are internalized as failure, the mother may experience disappointment and disconnection from her infant rather than the beginnings of connection and competence (Driscoll, 1992). The mother's perception of the neonate's competence at breast serves as a primary reinforcer in her persistence with breastfeeding. An infant who does not latch to the breast generally presents a reality clash with a mother's expectation of breastfeeding as automatic and pleasing (Mozingo et al., 2000). It acts as a stressor that can lead directly to weaning if sensitive, consistent, and evidence-based interventions are not received. Mothers whose infants experience difficulty latching or sucking are significantly less likely to be breastfeeding at all at 12 weeks (Taveras et al., 2004). Positive feedback in the form of an infant who breastfeeds well reinforces the mother's decision to breastfeed and increases maternal self-esteem (Matthews, 1991). Problems related to latch include the infant who is reluctant to or unable to latch to the breast, with interventions for the reluctant nurser varying depending on what is contributing to the problem (**Box 5-2**).

Sleepy Infant

An infant who is "unavailable" to feed can be especially worrisome to both the mother and the clinician. With hospital stays of 48 hours or less being the norm for full-term healthy infants, many infants can be discharged without ever having actually fed at the breast. Infants "cycle" through active sleep, quiet sleep, and waking. Infant sleep cycles are 60 minutes long (adult cycles are 90 minutes long). Initially, newborns may wake with each cycle (every 1–2 hours), sometimes giving the impression that they are not receiving enough milk, when they are simply moving from one state to another. Babies do not sleep like adults. During the neonatal period, babies fall asleep in "rapid eye movement" (REM) sleep and then move more slowly to "deeper" forms of sleep. They spend about equal amounts of time in active and quiet sleep, alternating with

Box 5-2 Problem of the Reluctant Nurser

Problem Description

- Baby may latch to the breast only after many attempts
- Baby may be unable to latch
- Baby may completely refuse to latch to breast, either falling asleep or aggressively pushing away with an arched body
- Baby may exhibit rapid side-to-side head movements and may or may not latch to breast
- Baby may have a one-sided preference

Contributing Factors

- Poor positioning at breast
- Hypertonia (jaw clenching, pursed lips, neck and back hyperextension, tongue retraction or elevation)
- Interruption in the organized sequence of prefeeding behaviors immediately after birth
- Infrequent feeds leading to an over-hungry baby and excessive or prolonged crying, resulting in behavioral disorganization
- Drug-induced interference that prolongs the period of state disorganization in the newborn (epidural, butorphanol [Stadol], nalbuphine hydrochloride [Nubain], meperidine [Demerol])
- Interference with imprinting on the breast from separation, artificial nipples, or pacifiers
- Fetal history of breech presentation, extension in utero, protracted labor, cervical spine pain or damage, precipitous delivery, dislocated hip, fractured clavicle, or asymmetrical positioning in utero with right-sided preference
- Excessive pressure on the occipital region of baby's head from pushing the head forward into the breast
- Vigorous or deep suctioning or intubation that causes swelling or discomfort in the mouth or throat with resulting clenched mouth, tongue thrusting, neck extension, or pushing away from the breast
- Oral aversion or other sensory-integration problems
- Vacuum extraction, forceps, shoulder dystocia with misalignment of head, neck, and shoulders
- Cephalohematoma
- Short or tight lingual frenulum
- Flat or inverted nipples
- Upper airway disorders

(*continues*)

Management	Rationale
Check the positioning of baby at breast: • Baby completely facing mother with head, neck, and spine aligned • Mouth in front of and slightly below where nipple points • Baby brought to breast and held close • Mother does not lean forward or maneuver the breast sideways	Poor positioning increases the number of latch attempts needed before obtaining milk, which can frustrate both mother and baby. Improper positioning increases the chances that the baby will not attach to the breast, leading to sore nipples, engorgement, insufficient milk production, and slow weight gain.
Positioning may vary depending on the symmetry of the baby. Babies with a rightsided preference may need to be held in a football hold for the right breast and in a cradle or prone position for the left breast.	Positioning in utero and delivery events influence breastfeeding patterns.
Some babies do better when the mother is in a sidelying position. Breech babies may feed better sitting upright in a clutch hold (**Figure 5-16**). Babies with delivery trauma such as a cephalohematoma may be more comfortable and feed better when held with the affected side up. Babies with a fractured clavicle may feed better in a clutch hold if the weight of the breast is kept off the chest or in a cradle hold with the affected side up.	Several different positions may need to be explored to find one that is satisfactory.
Allow the baby time on the mother's breast immediately after delivery. Let baby seek and find the nipple before removal from the mother's chest.	This provides the opportunity for the prefeeding sequence of behaviors to occur, which increases the likelihood of proper attachment to the breast.
Keep the mother and baby together. Place the baby skin to skin on the mother's chest (Meyer & Anderson, 1999). Instruct the mother to feed her baby on cue: when he stirs at breast, when she sees rapid eye movements under the eyelids, when she sees movements of the tongue and mouth, when baby exhibits hand-to-mouth movements, or when baby makes small sounds.	This reestablishes and/or repatterns the initial sucking sequence that may not have occurred immediately post-delivery. With the baby in close, the mother can feel the infant's feeding cues and place him to breast before he becomes over hungry and when he is most likely to latch on.
An alternative technique is to place mother and baby in a bath, allowing baby to repattern in the warm water. To keep baby warm and soothed, a helper can gently pour warm water over the baby's back as he creeps to the breast and attaches (Harris, 1994).	
Place a warm towel over baby's neck; massage the shoulders and arms. This is helpful after a precipitous delivery, forceps, or vacuum extraction. It is also soothing to a high-tone baby.	Baby may be in pain from overriding cervical vertebrae. This helps relax the cervical structures and decrease tone in a high-tone baby.
For rapid side-to-side head movements, touch the midline of baby's upper lip with a dropper of colostrum or D5 (**Figure 5-17**). Move baby onto the breast as he follows the dropper to the nipple. When his mouth is wide open, place a few drops of water or colostrum on his tongue to elicit sucking and swallowing.	The dropper acts to provide external control and food incentives for attachment and sucking at breast.

Box 5-2 Problem of the Reluctant Nurser (*Continued*)

Management	Rationale
An arching baby can be placed either in the football hold or with the mother lying on her side. The mother can also use a sling to help position the baby in flexion.	These techniques help to flex the back and hips to avoid arching and jaw clenching.
If this does not calm the baby, place him on a receiving blanket, have two adults pick up the corners of the blanket, and rock the baby from side to side like a hammock. Then put the baby to breast.	
Provide latch and sucking incentives to the baby, which can include: • A periodontal syringe placed in the side of the baby's mouth that delivers a small amount of colostrum or sugar water with each suck until the baby demonstrates rhythmic suck and swallow at breast. • A syringe or soft clinic dropper can be used to elicit sucking (**Figure 5-18**). • Butterfly tubing attached to a 10-cc syringe and taped to the breast can provide these incentives as well as a supplement if needed.	This helps prevent the baby from pulling away from the breast before he latches on or swallows.
A baby who is crying hard or has been crying for a period of time may not be able to organize himself to feed. Allow this baby to suck on a finger or place the tubing on a finger and allow baby to suck (**Figure 5-19**) a little colostrum or sugar water by finger feeding him before putting him to breast.	
Avoid pacifiers and bottles. If the baby will not suck on a finger, place some colostrum in a 28-cc medicine cup and have the baby sip from the cup until he calms down and has a little food in his stomach.	
If the baby will not open his mouth wide enough for painless latch-on or clenches his jaw, hold the baby's jaw between your thumb and index finger and move the jaw a small amount from side to side. If the lower lip is rolled under, keeping the mouth from achieving a large enough gape, or the mouth is not open to > 130 degrees, gently pull down on the chin to evert the lower lip and encourage a more open mouth (**Figure 5-20**).	This helps inhibit jaw clenching. Pulling down on the chin too hard may dislodge the baby from the breast or cause him to bite down to stay attached.
Hand express milk into a spoon and spoon feed the baby.	Skipped feedings can lead to insufficient fluid and inadequate caloric intake.
If nothing else works, try the judicious use of a nipple shield.	Shield use may allow a baby who is experiencing difficulty latching or who may never latch without assistance to learn breastfeeding skills.

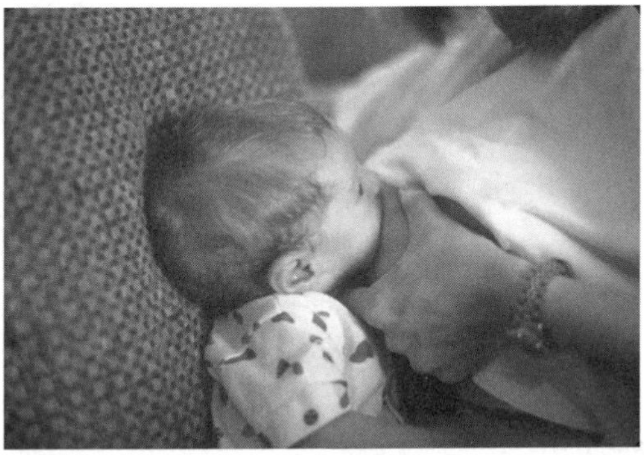

Figure 5-16 Upright hold.

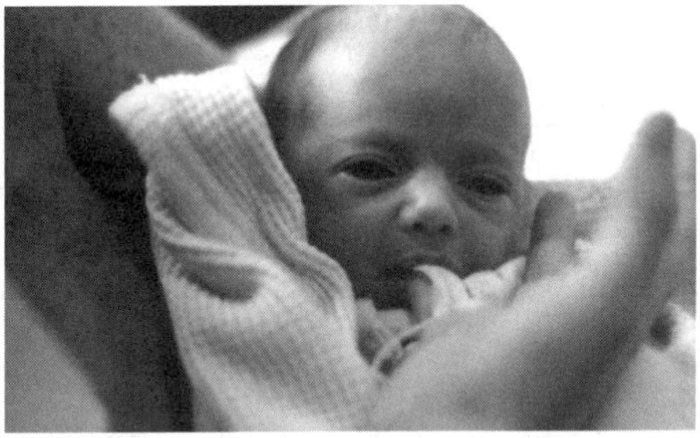

Figure 5-19 Tubing taped to the finger to elicit sucking.

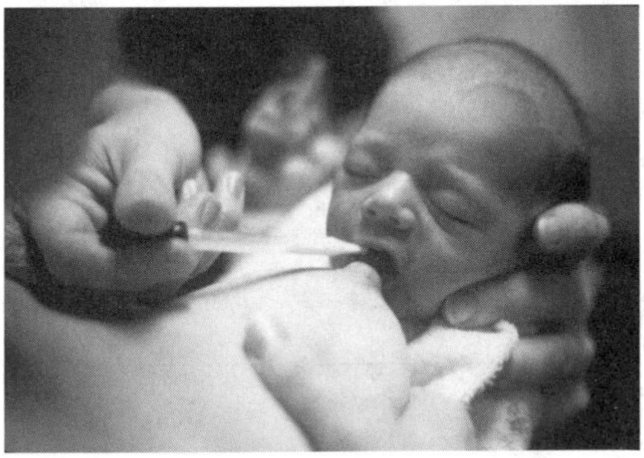

Figure 5-17 Use of dropper to orient infant to breast.

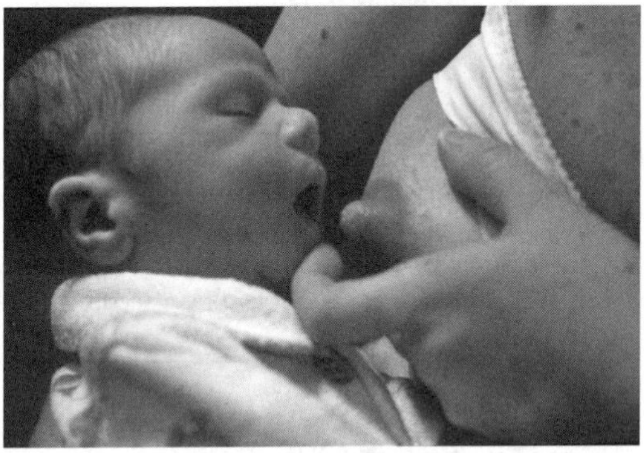

Figure 5-20 Gentle traction on the chin to encourage an open mouth.

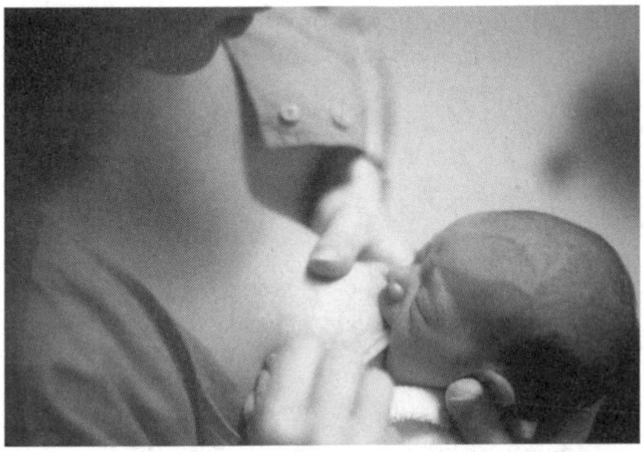

Figure 5-18 Use of soft clinic dropper to elicit sucking.

a period of 50 to 60 minutes (Peirano, Algarin, & Uauy, 2003). Babies, like adults, are more likely to wake up when they are in lighter forms of sleep than if they are in deeper forms of sleep. If something happens to disturb them in this lighter sleep such as a ringing phone or being put down into a bassinet or crib, babies are more likely to wake. During active sleep, infants' eyelids will flutter and their faces and bodies will twitch. Mothers can be instructed to wait to put newborns down until they are in a deeper sleep state (20 minutes or so after a feeding). This helps break a cycle of repeated awakenings each time the baby is put down. As long as the infant has actually transferred sufficient milk, these types of awakenings may be reduced by either extended skin-to-skin holding or waiting to transfer the infant to a bassinet or crib until he has entered a deeper sleep state.

Sleep architecture in newborns during the first days after birth shows both ultradian (biological rhythms that occur less frequently than every 24 hours) and circadian (biological rhythms that occur every 24 hours) cyclicity (Freudigman & Thoman, 1994) that is responsive to a number of variables, including mode of delivery (Freudigman & Thoman, 1998), maternal labor medications, gestational age, and the surrounding environment. The earliest postnatal sleep patterns differ between vaginally and cesarean-born infants. The diurnal sleep pattern of infants is disrupted by a cesarean delivery such that infants born by cesarean section have shown significantly less active sleep. During the first 2 days, vaginally born infants show significant day/night differences with more wakefulness, shorter mean sleep periods, and shorter longest sleep periods during the daytime on both days (Freudigman & Thoman, 1998). This presents as a vaginally born infant having more opportunities to breastfeed, whereas a cesarean-born infant may not demonstrate breastfeeding cues as frequently. Heavier infants of diabetic mothers have been shown to have higher amounts of quiet and motionless sleep (Sadeh, Dark, & Vohr, 1996), which may limit optimal breastfeeding opportunities. An increase in quiet sleep on the day of birth compared to 24 hours later can be seen as a temporary adaptive response to the stress of the birth process (Carroll, Denenberg, & Thoman, 1999). Jaundiced newborns tend to sleep more than nonjaundiced infants, which may have origins in increased carbon monoxide production. Carbon monoxide is formed from the breakdown of heme to bilirubin and is produced at a rate equal to the rate of bilirubin synthesis. Increased carbon monoxide production in jaundiced infants may likely play a role in increased sleep states due to the regulatory effects on sleep circadian rhythm and REM sleep via the cholinergic system activation (Ozkan, Tuzan, Kumral, Yesilirmak, & Duman, 2008). The first 2 hours after delivery offer the earliest opportunity for imprinting and latch to take place. However, most newborn infants do not fall into a deep sleep state for the next 24 hours after that point. Infants experience sleep cycles during this time, which makes it important that infants be kept with their mothers to take advantage of feeding opportunities during sleep–wake transition times.

Many mothers may be under the impression that crying indicates when it is time to feed an infant. In reality, crying is a late sign of hunger, and a sleepy infant may not come to a full arousal state and cry. Feeding cues in some infants can be very subtle and easily overlooked. Maternal labor medications can interfere with state control in infants, making it difficult to feed a sleepy infant. When such an infant arouses, he or she may go from sound sleep to hard crying, bypassing the graded levels of arousal in between. Sleeping is not an indication that an infant is receiving sufficient amounts of milk. Some parents have been told never to wake a sleeping infant, believe that sleeping is an indication that the infant is content, work toward causing the infant to sleep as much as possible, and have unrealistic expectations regarding the nature of newborn sleep.

The sleep organization of breastfed and formula-fed infants is different (Butte, Jensen, Moon, Glaze, & Frost, 1992), changes over time, and is influenced by maturation, development, nutrition, and caretaking patterns. Over the first 4 months of life, non-rapid-eye-movement (NREM) sleep (light sleep) increases to about 60% and REM sleep (deep sleep) decreases to approximately 40% of total sleep (Roffwarg, Muzio, & Dement, 1966). Breastfed infants typically show more spontaneous arousals from sleep (McKenna, Mosko, Dungy, & McAninch, 1990), especially in the early morning, spend more time in NREM sleep, and demonstrate accelerated maturation of the central nervous system compared with formula-fed infants.

Many infant training programs (Pinilla & Birch, 1993) exist to cause young infants to lengthen their nighttime sleep bouts, especially during the early months of life, when they are also at higher risk for SIDS (Schechtman, Harper, Wilson, & Southall, 1992). Parents should be aware that sleep training books and programs may not be in the best interest of a young infant. Arousal from sleep is a survival mechanism that can be impaired by the major risk factors for SIDS such as prone sleeping and maternal smoking. Horne, Parslow, Ferens, Watts, and Adamson (2004) found that 2- to 3-month-old formula-fed infants are less arousable in active sleep than breastfed 2- to 3-month-old infants. They also state that breastfeeding during the critical risk period for SIDS (2–4 months) remains very important, because reduced arousability in active sleep could impair the ability of an infant to respond to a life-threatening situation.

The establishment of organized sleep states and a normal sleep pattern during the neonatal period contribute to brain development and plasticity. The consolidation of the circadian sleep–wake cycle typically occurs between 1 and 4 months in term infants and somewhat later in preterm infants. Human milk contains a number of bioactive sleep-promoting components that include melatonin, tryptophan, nucleosides/nucleotides, and vitamin B_{12}. Some of these show circadian rhythms. Human milk has the capability to function in a manner that may synchronize the infant to consolidate a circadian sleep–wake cycle (Arslanoglu, Bertino, Nicocia, & Moro, 2012).

Some infants whose breastfeeding needs are not met at night, when it is "not all right" to breastfeed, may be unable to differentiate when it is permissible or not permissible to breastfeed and refuse to breastfeed during the day. Young breastfed infants during the early weeks of life need to feed at night. This ensures adequate weight gain and an abundant milk supply. Feeding very young infants cereal at night to make them sleep longer is a misconception, does not cause longer sleep (Macknin, Medendorp, & Maier, 1989), and displaces breastmilk from the diet. An infant who is very sleepy in the early days of life is a challenge to the breastfeeding mother (Walker, 1997). She needs to know when the infant is actually swallowing milk (**Box 5-3**) and how to know that the infant is getting enough milk (**Table 5-4**).

These data assume that infants have not experienced breastfeeding difficulties or any interventions that might disrupt the normal acquisition of early breastfeeding skills. The length of time for meconium to transition to the typical breastfed stool varies with gestational age, pattern of feedings, amount of intake, and supplementation with other fluids. Transitioning stool color serves as one of a number of indicators of sufficient breastmilk intake and infant wellbeing (Salariya & Robertson, 1993). Parents and clinicians often find it easier and more accurate to use a handout that illustrates stool color and

Box 5-3 Signs of Swallowing

- Hearing a puff of air from the nose
- Hearing a "ca" sound
- Hearing a swallow in the throat
- Feeling the areola drawn farther into the infant's mouth
- Seeing the areola move toward the infant's lips
- Observing the infant's jaw drop lower than during non-nutritive sucking
- Feeling the swallow by placing fingers on the infant's throat
- Hearing swallowing by listening with a stethoscope on the infant's throat

Table 5-4 Signs of Sufficient Breastmilk Intake

Age	Wet Diapers	Color	Urates	Stools	Color	Volume	Consistency	Weight Gain
Day 1	1	Pale	Possible	1	Black	≥ 15 g	Tarry/sticky	< 5% loss
Day 2	2–3	Pale	Possible	1–2	Greenish/ black	≥ 15 g	Changing	< 5% loss
Day 3	3–4	Pale	Possible	3–4	Greenish/ yellow	≥ 15 g	Soft	≤ 8–10% loss
Day 4	≥ 4–6 disposable ≥ 6–8 cloth	Pale	None	4 large 10 small	Yellow/ seedy		Soft/liquid	15–30 g/day

Modified from Powers, N. G., & Slusser, W. (1997). Breastfeeding update 2: Clinical lactation management. *Pediatrics in Review, 18,* 147–161; Black, L. S. (2001). Incorporating breastfeeding care into daily newborn rounds and pediatric office practice. *Pediatric Clinics of North America, 48,* 299–319; Neifert, M. R. (2001). Prevention of breastfeeding tragedies. *Pediatric Clinics of North America, 48,* 273–297.

consistency changes (**Figure 5-21**), as well as a diaper log, which ensures adequate intake or signals a need for clinical intervention.

Drowsiness at breast may also be related to the normal release of metabolic hormones that occurs when an infant breastfeeds. One such hormone, cholecystokinin (CCK), is a gastrointestinal hormone that enhances gut maturation, promotes glucose-induced insulin release, is released mainly in response to fat in the diet, enhances sedation, and is thought to play a role in regulating food intake by signaling satiety (Marchini & Linden, 1992). Breastfed infants have higher plasma concentrations of CCK during the first 5 days than do formula-fed infants (Marchini, Simoni, Bartolini, & Linden, 1993). During the breastfeeding episode, CCK has the effect of inducing sleepiness in both the mother and the infant (Uvnas-Moberg, Widström, Marchini, & Winberg, 1987). CCK levels in infants demonstrate two peaks related to breastfeeding. The first increase is seen immediately after breastfeeding, most likely due to activation of the vagal nerve; it is followed by a decline at 10 minutes and then a secondary rise at 30–60 minutes after feeding due to the stimulation effect of food on the CCK-producing cells (Uvnas-Moberg, Marchini, & Winberg, 1993). The interval between these two peaks, especially at about 10 minutes after the feed on the first side, may subsequently determine the optimal timing for placing the infant on the second breast because he or she may more easily arouse at that point in the CCK cycle. Interventions to help sleepy infants to breastfeed depend on the contributing factors and may change over time (**Box 5-4**).

FUSSY INFANT

An infant who is fussy at the breast or who fusses and is fretful after a feeding is a cause of significant anxiety in a new mother. Many mothers interpret a fussing infant or one who is not satisfied after a feeding to mean an insufficient milk supply (Hillervik-Lindquist, Hofvander, & Sjolin, 1991; Sjolin, Hofvander, & Hillervik, 1977, 1979; Verronen, 1982). In fact, the major cause of supplementation and premature weaning is perceived (or real) insufficient milk (Bevan, Mosley, Lobach, & Salimano, 1984; Bloom, Goldbloom, Robinson, & Stevens, 1982; Hill, 1991). Newborns may temporarily lack the refined skills for abundant milk transfer and indeed remain hungry after a feeding. Normal fluctuations in milk

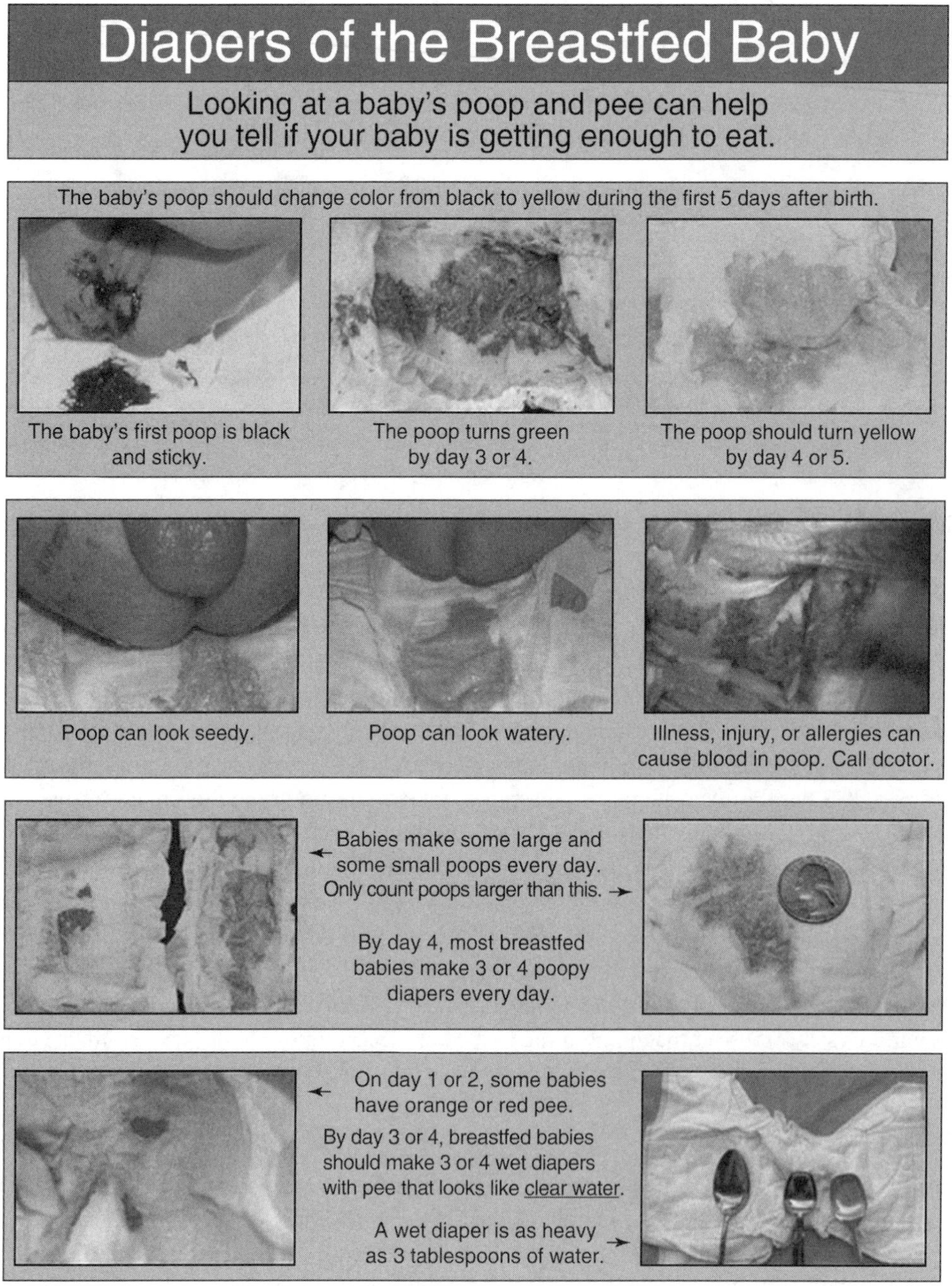

Figure 5-21 Diapers of the breastfed baby.

Box 5-4 Problem of the Sleepy Baby

Problem Description

- Baby does not wake or fuss on a regular enough basis to indicate hunger
- Baby falls asleep at breast after a few sucks
- Baby sucks sporadically at breast, falls asleep, wakes when put down, but continues to feed poorly
- Baby falls asleep before taking second breast

Contributing Factors

- Maternal illness or certain prenatal medications
- Birth complications with increased levels of endorphins
- Prematurity
- Neonatal illness
- Congenital anomalies
- Operative delivery
- Birth trauma
- Maternal labor medications with resulting state disorganization
- Overstimulating environment
- Invasive procedures
- Prolonged crying
- Increased levels of cholecystokinin (CCK)
- Hyperbilirubinemia
- Phototherapy

Management	Rationale
Keep mother and baby together.	This decreases crying, which is a behavioral sign of stress. Separated infants cry 10 times more often than when kept with their mother (Michelsson, Christensson, Rothganger, & Winberg, 1996).
Suggest skin-to-skin contact as much as possible: Baby can be carried in a sling once home so that breastfeeding cues are immediately recognized.	Mothers can respond immediately to these subtle cues. This helps to repattern the baby to suck at breast if artificial nipples have been used or if the mother was medicated during labor and delivery.
Teach alerting techniques to use when feeding cues are observed: • Talk to the baby with variable pitch. • Tickle or stroke the palms or soles. • Rub the baby's face. • Put his hand to his mouth. • Allow him to smell a nursing pad with colostrum on it.	These activities stimulate the trigeminal nerve (5th cranial nerve), which is the sensory arm for rooting and sucking. The trigeminal has input into the reticular activating system—the alarm clock of the brain. Sucking action decreases above 27°C (80°F) room temperature. Allows baby's movements to awaken him.

(continues)

Box 5-4 Problem of the Sleepy Baby *(continued)*

Management	Rationale
• Sit the baby upright. • Unwrap the baby; change the diaper. • Move in any direction with uneven rhythms.	
Provide incentives at breast to entice the baby to wake and feed: • Place a dropper of colostrum or D5 into the side of the baby's mouth while latching. • Use a feeding-tube device, butterfly tubing taped to breast and connected to a 10-cc syringe, gavage tubing taped to breast, or periodontal syringe (**Figure 5-22**) to deliver boluses at breast.	Establishing flow of fluid will often initiate and help sustain sucking.
If the baby is overstimulated and is shutting out the noise and light by sleeping, modify the environment and attempts at stimulation: • Provide a quiet, dim room. • Do some gentle walking. • Pat baby's back at the rate of his heartbeat, gradually slowing the patting to 72 beats per minute. • Feed the baby for short periods of time with timeouts. • Avoid talking to the baby or rubbing his head while at breast. • Avoid jiggling the baby. • Tug back gently on the nipple to induce a suck as long as the nipples are not sore. • Use alternate massage if baby dozes at breast between sucking bursts. • Avoid caretaking behaviors that promote sleep such as tight wrapping, solitary sleeping in a bassinet, use of a pacifier, rocking the bassinet, high ambient temperature, ignoring cries or feeding cues.	These modifications help supply behavioral organization to a disorganized or dysmature baby.
If baby refuses the second breast at a feeding, suggest that the mother offer it after 10 minutes or after about an hour or when she sees feeding cues again.	CCK levels usually fall at these times and baby may start to cycle into a lighter sleep state.
To help parents and clinicians keep track of feedings and diaper counts, a log can be given to parents to fill out for a week or so until the problem is resolved (**Figure 5-23**).	Recording feedings and diaper counts helps parents recognize when to seek help and avoid more serious problems such as dehydration and jaundice.

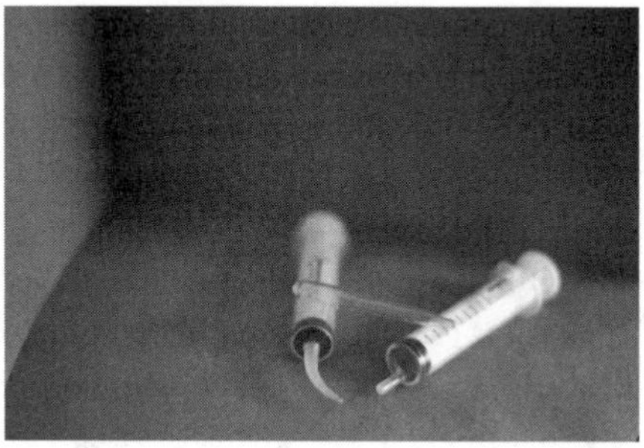

Figure 5-22 Periodontal syringes.

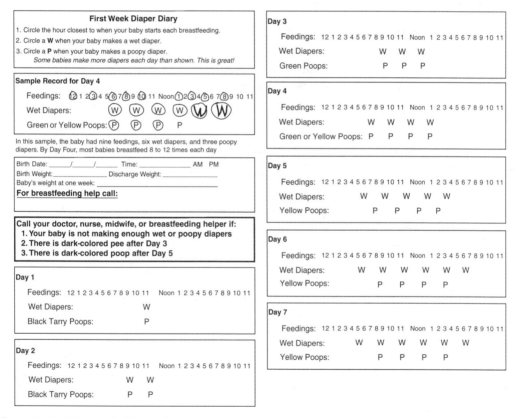

First Week Diaper Diary

1. Circle the hour closest to when your baby starts each breastfeeding.
2. Circle a **W** when your baby makes a wet diaper.
3. Circle a **P** when your baby makes a poopy diaper.

Some babies make more diapers each day than shown. This is great!

Sample Record for Day 4

Feedings: (12) 1 2 (3) 4 5 (6) 7 (8) 9 (10) 11 Noon (1) 2 (3) 4 (5) 6 7 (8) 9 10 11

Wet Diapers: (W) (W) (W) (W) (W) (W)

Green or Yellow Poops: (P) (P) (P) P

In this sample, the baby had nine feedings, six wet diapers, and three poopy diapers. By Day Four, most babies breastfeed 8 to 12 times each day

Birth Date: _____/_____/_____ Time: __________ AM PM

Birth Weight: __________ Discharge Weight: __________

Baby's weight at one week: __________

For breastfeeding help call:

Call your doctor, nurse, midwife, or breastfeeding helper if:
1. **Your baby is not making enough wet or poopy diapers**
2. **There is dark-colored pee after Day 3**
3. **There is dark-colored poop after Day 5**

Day 1

Feedings: 12 1 2 3 4 5 6 7 8 9 10 11 Noon 1 2 3 4 5 6 7 8 9 10 11

Wet Diapers: W

Black Tarry Poops: P

Day 2

Feedings: 12 1 2 3 4 5 6 7 8 9 10 11 Noon 1 2 3 4 5 6 7 8 9 10 11

Wet Diapers: W W

Black Tarry Poops: P P

Day 3

Feedings: 12 1 2 3 4 5 6 7 8 9 10 11 Noon 1 2 3 4 5 6 7 8 9 10 11

Wet Diapers: W W W

Green Poops: P P P

Day 4

Feedings: 12 1 2 3 4 5 6 7 8 9 10 11 Noon 1 2 3 4 5 6 7 8 9 10 11

Wet Diapers: W W W W

Green or Yellow Poops: P P P P

Day 5

Feedings: 12 1 2 3 4 5 6 7 8 9 10 11 Noon 1 2 3 4 5 6 7 8 9 10 11

Wet Diapers: W W W W W

Yellow Poops: P P P P

Day 6

Feedings: 12 1 2 3 4 5 6 7 8 9 10 11 Noon 1 2 3 4 5 6 7 8 9 10 11

Wet Diapers: W W W W W W

Yellow Poops: P P P P

Day 7

Feedings: 12 1 2 3 4 5 6 7 8 9 10 11 Noon 1 2 3 4 5 6 7 8 9 10 11

Wet Diapers: W W W W W W

Yellow Poops: P P P P

Figure 5-23 First-week diaper diary.

supply, growth or appetite spurts, or infant temperament can also influence an infant's behavior surrounding the feeding process. Maternal analgesia during labor has been described to have an effect on infant behavior, including increased crying (Ransjo-Arvidson et al., 2001). Maternal smoking during pregnancy has also been reported as contributing to infants who have more fussy periods and more intense reactions to events surrounding them (Kelmanson, Erman, & Litvina, 2002). Exposure to tobacco smoke and its metabolites has been linked to increased levels of plasma and intestinal motilin (a peptide that stimulates contractions in the gastrointestinal tract) in infants whose mothers smoked during pregnancy or who are exposed to second-hand smoke. Elevated levels of motilin have been linked with an increased risk of gastrointestinal dysregulation, including colic and acid reflux (Shenassa & Brown, 2004). There is a common perception that breastfed infants cry more, which may be related to the faster emptying of the stomach when it contains breastmilk, leading to the signal of fussing or crying as a hunger cue. However, changing an infant over to formula feeding may not reduce crying but may merely redistribute it away from evening and nighttime hours, giving the impression that the breastfed infant was not fed enough (Barr, Kramer, Pless, Boisjoly, & Leduc, 1989). Failure to address the cause of an unhappy breastfed infant can quickly lead to a downward spiral of formula supplementation, true insufficient milk, and weaning (**Box 5-5**).

On the other end of the spectrum, infant fussiness may be related to a cluster of symptoms variously described as hyperlactation (oversupply) and/or overactive letdown reflex, which often occur together, usually well after the mother has established an abundant milk supply. Sometimes an infant is fussy at breast and between feeds because of gastroesophageal reflux.

Box 5-5 Problem of the Fussy Baby

Problem Description

- Baby may fuss during a feeding
- Baby may fuss following a feeding or fall asleep at the breast and fuss when put down
- Baby may fuss between feedings, startle easily, or appear irritable
- Baby may resist being put to the breast, arch away from the breast, push back with the arms, extend the head, or turn away from the breast
- Once latched, baby may choke, gag, or repeatedly come on and off the breast
- Baby may stiffen when approaching the breast or flail his or her arms and legs

Contributing Factors

- Birth trauma or pain (fractured clavicle/humerus), vacuum extraction, forceps, cephalohematoma
- Intracranial hemorrhage
- Oral aversion (suctioning, intubation, gloved finger)
- Prenatal or perinatal medications
- Illicit drug use by mother or chemically dependent mother
- Sensory sensitivity
- Sensory overload
- Faulty imprinting on an artificial nipple
- Baby may be hungry due to poor feeding skills or limited milk transfer
- Insufficient milk supply
- Gastroesophageal reflux

Management	Rationale
Fussing or arching during feeding may indicate air in the baby's stomach, signaling that the baby needs to burp.	Babies swallow air when they cry; burping the baby may relieve his stomach discomfort.
If baby is overhungry, mother can express a small amount of colostrum or milk and feed the baby prior to latching attempts.	This helps to calm the baby by taking the edge off of hunger.
Offer more nighttime breastfeedings.	Many babies feed better at night because they prefer the darker, quieter environment.
Babies with birth injuries may be fussy; mothers should be instructed to: • Position baby to avoid further trauma or pain to injury. • Provide appropriate pain medication to a baby who is in pain.	Pain relief contributes to better organized feeding skills.

The sleepy infant, the reluctant nurser, and the fussy infant may all describe the same infant at different times. The fussy infant may respond to any of the interventions described for the sleepy infant or an infant who is reluctant to breastfeed. An infant who is fussy and reluctant to latch can be the infant with birth trauma who falls asleep at the breast. Too often, one intervention is attempted one time for one problem but does not work immediately, so another approach is tried, confusing the infant and the parents, leaving the problem unresolved, and allowing the situation to continue to deteriorate. Inconsistent information combined with recommendations to keep trying a variety of interventions with no systematic evaluation and follow-up is a recipe for early weaning.

A written care plan for infants and mothers experiencing problems, which is modified as needed until the problem resolves, is a more logical approach to early problematic breastfeeding situations (**Box 5-6**). Some hospitals have a whiteboard in patient rooms and use this to write the breastfeeding plan for each day of the hospital stay. This keeps the plan in prominent sight for both the mother and staff. During the time a mother and infant are in the hospital, charting systems should record breastfeeding progress and expected outcomes (Bassett, 2001; **Figure 5-24**). Variances from the expected behaviors are recorded, and a feeding plan should be devised to address outstanding issues. Some hospitals use care plans or care maps to organize teaching within short hospital maternity stays (Zander, 1991, 1992). A pathway is a collaborative plan of care that:

- Identifies critical components of intervention and care that must occur to achieve a predetermined length of stay
- Sequences major interventions to achieve the anticipated length of stay
- States the desired patient outcomes
- Ensures consistency of patient care
- Eliminates duplication or omission of information
- Provides objectives that are to be met each day to avoid information overload on the day of discharge
- Becomes a systematic plan of care so that each nurse has responsibility for a part of the total patient education plan

Box 5-6 Care Plan for the Infant Who Won't Latch On

Occasionally, there are times when an infant has difficulty latching on to the breast. Having a step-by-step plan to guide you will help you through those feeds. The goals are to stimulate milk production and make sure your infant has adequate nourishment.

Suggestions

1. Work with your infant in short increments of time.
2. Undress the infant to the diaper; take off your top and bra to maximize skin-to-skin contact. This will help keep infant awake and more alert during feeds.
3. Spend time snuggled with your infant skin-to-skin, with no attempt to latch on.
4. Make sure you are comfortable, with supporting pillows all around.
5. Watch closely for feeding cues. When your infant demonstrates interest in feeding, attempt to put him or her to breast. Wait until infant's mouth opens wide (you can gently tickle the lower lip with your nipple) and the tongue is down. Express a bit of breastmilk onto the nipple to entice infant. Quickly pull your infant to the breast, leading with the chin so that he or she gets a big mouthful of breast tissue.
6. Use your dominant hand to pull your infant to the breast quickly:
   - *Right handed:* Football (clutch) hold on the right side
   - *Left handed:* Cross-cradle (transverse) hold on the left side
7. If your infant cries, arches away, or pulls back, stop immediately; calm him or her by allowing infant to suck on your finger (nail side against the tongue). When infant's suck becomes rhythmical and infant is calm, try again. Try ventral positioning by leaning back at a 35-degree angle and placing the baby on his tummy to feed. If he or she is crying and arching away, try only three times at that feeding.
8. Work with your infant as long as he or she is calm and willing to work to go to breast. Do not push infant's tolerance level or try to get him or her to attach to the breast while screaming. You can try each breast and each position—you never know which one will work.
9. Use verbal positive reinforcement when your infant latches on.
10. If your infant does not latch on at that time, feed expressed breastmilk with a small cup or hollow-handled medicine spoon. Pump your breasts and save the milk for the next feed (breastmilk is safe at room temperature for 8–10 hours).
11. When your infant shows interest in the breast, try again. As long as you continue to pump your breasts, attempt to put your infant to breast, and feed him or her without a bottle nipple, you will maintain your milk supply.
12. Attempt to put your infant to breast at every feeding—at least 8 times in 24 hours.
13. Attempt feeding your infant before your infant is fully awake or crying to feed.
14. A successful latch-on during the night is common.

Mother's signature Date

Lactation consultant's signature Date

Data from parental care plan for infants who won't latch handout developed for Breastfeeding Support Consultants, 1996.

Nutrition and Elimination

Criteria for assessment of newborn infant at the breast

position:

- Mother states that she is comfortable: back, feet, and arms supported (head supported in side-lying)
- Infant's head and body supported at the level of the breast (pillows usually helpful with cradle and football to support mother's arm that is holding infant's head and body)
- Infant turned completely on side with nose, chin, chest, abdomen, and knees touching mother (cradle and side lying)
- Infant's head in neutral position (hip, shoulder, and ear aligned)
- Infant kept close by support from mother's arm and hand along the infant's back and buttock
- Mother's breast supported with cupped hand; thumb and fingers will be back from areola

Latch:

- Mouth wide open (like a yawn)
- Lips visible and flanged outward
- ¾–1" of areola covered by the infant's lips (usually most or all of the areola)
- Tongue over lower gum line
- No clicking or smacking sounds
- No indrawing or dimpling of cheek
- Mother states she is comfortable (no persistent nipple pain)

Suck and Swallow:

- Chin moves in rhythmic motion
- Bursts of sucking, swallowing, and rests

First Side X Second Side		Date																
		Time																
	Breast																	
RIGHT SIDE	POSITION	Reverse arm hold																
		Cradle																
		Football																
		Sidelying																
	BABY RESPONSE	Latch achieved																
		Minimal sucking																
		Sustained sucking																
		Sucking & swallowing																
		No latch achieved																
		Too sleepy																
		Reluctant																
LEFT SIDE	POSITION	Reverse arm hold																
		Cradle																
		Football																
		Sidelying																
	BABY RESPONSE	Latch achieved																
		Minimal sucking																
		Sustained sucking																
		Sucking & swallowing																
		No latch achieved																
		Too sleepy																
		Reluctant																
ASSISTANCE	Independent																	
	Minimum																	
	Moderate																	
	Maximum																	
	Feeding observed by nurse																	
	Feeding reported by patient																	
	Formula																	
		RN initials																
STOOLS	Meconium																	
	Transitional																	
	Curdy																	
	Yellow																	
	Green																	
	for each stool																	
URINE	Normal																	
	Uric acid crystals																	
	for each void																	

Figure 5-24 Assessment of newborn at breast.

Data from original developed by the Ottawa Hospital, ON, Canada.

Accompanying a pathway would be a list of criteria for referral to a lactation consultant (Backas, 1998) for more specialized and intensive work with the mother and baby to create the in-hospital and discharge feeding plan (**Box 5-7** and **5-8**).

Mothers of infants who do not respond to a standard feeding plan need individualized plans with interventions based on what the infant responds to best during feedings. Because the mother is a partner in the development of feeding plans, any plans that are formulated should be done so with her input and assurances that the plan can be carried out (Cadwell & Turner-Maffei, 2004). Critical thinking

Box 5-7 Criteria for Referral to In-Hospital Lactation Consultant

On Admission to Postpartum

- Multiple birth
- Maternal history of breast surgery/biopsy
- Maternal–infant separation due to maternal illness
- Maternal breast or nipple pathology/anomaly
- Adolescent 19 years of age or younger
- Maternal insulin-dependent diabetes mellitus
- History of previous unsuccessful breastfeeding experience
- Newborn admitted to special care nursery
- Newborn low-birth-weight (less than 2,500 g at birth)
- Newborn with birth weight 9 pounds or greater
- Newborn repetitive low blood sugar
- Newborn repetitive low body temperature
- Newborn less than 38 0/7 weeks' gestation
- Sibling required phototherapy as a newborn
- Newborn with cleft lip/palate
- Newborn anomaly with potential feeding impact

After Admission to Postpartum—Mother/Newborn Experiencing Any of the Following Problems

- Failure to latch on
- Repeated difficult latch-on
- No/poor suckling
- Newborn weight loss of 7% or more of birth weight
- Anytime use of breast pump is initiated
- Sore nipples
- Newborn having significant jaundice with or without receiving phototherapy (TSB plotting greater than 75th percentile on risk assessment)
- Newborn receiving phototherapy
- At any time upon the mother's request after the postpartum nurse has provided education and intervention

Beth Allen, RNC, IBCLC, Manager, Lactation Center, Northside Hospital, Atlanta, GA, 2012.

Box 5-8 Situations in Which Consultation With an Expert in Lactation Management May Be Helpful

- Maternal request/anxiety
- Previous negative breastfeeding experience
- Mother has flat/inverted nipples
- Mother has history of breast surgery
- Multiple births (twins, triplets)
- Infant is premature (< 37 weeks' gestation)
- Infant has congenital anomaly, neurological impairment, or other medical condition that affects the infant's ability to breastfeed
- Maternal or infant medical condition for which breastfeeding must be temporarily postponed or for which milk expression is required
- Documentation, after the first few feedings, that there is difficulty in establishing breastfeeding (e.g., poor latch-on, sleepy infant)
- Hyperbilirubinemia

Reproduced from Academy of Breastfeeding Medicine. (2013). *Clinical protocol number 5: Peripartum breastfeeding management for the healthy mother and infant at term, revision 2013.* Retrieved from www.bfmed.org/Media/Files/Protocols/Protocol_5_revised2013.pdf

(Bandman & Bandman, 1988) is necessary to start the problem-solving process (Burns & Grove, 1993) for the creation of a feeding plan tailored to each mother–baby unit's unique needs. The problem-solving process involves the following steps:

- Gathering and evaluating data
- Defining the problem
- Determining and evaluating potential options
- Choosing an approach and taking action
- Evaluating the outcomes of the action (Nichols & Zwelling, 1997)

A feeding plan also includes short- and long-term goals, outcome criteria, evaluation of the plan, and revisions as needed. For example, a common occurrence during a 48-hour hospital stay for many newborns and their mothers is an infant with ineffective latch and feeding, with the resulting question: "How long should the infant go before we supplement?" There is no one right answer to this question or situation; it depends on the status of the infant and the availability of skilled intervention. A feeding plan could resemble the sample in Box 5-4 depending on the factors contributing to the problem.

Decision Trees/Clinical Algorithms

Many hospital maternity units and outpatient settings use clinical algorithms (Babic, Kokol, & Stiglic, 1999; Babic, Sprogar, Zorman, Kokol, & Turk, 1999) or decision trees as guidelines, tools for decision support, and strategies to strengthen the intervention choice process. Algorithms can be used by staff nurses as a quick reference for needed interventions and as a tool for determining when to refer to the lactation consultant (Cobb, 2002). The decision trees featured in **Figures 5-25, 5-26, 5-27,** and **5-28** are examples of comprehensive and effective breastfeeding and postpartum checklists and flowcharts. Additional algorithms are available in **Appendix 5-2**.

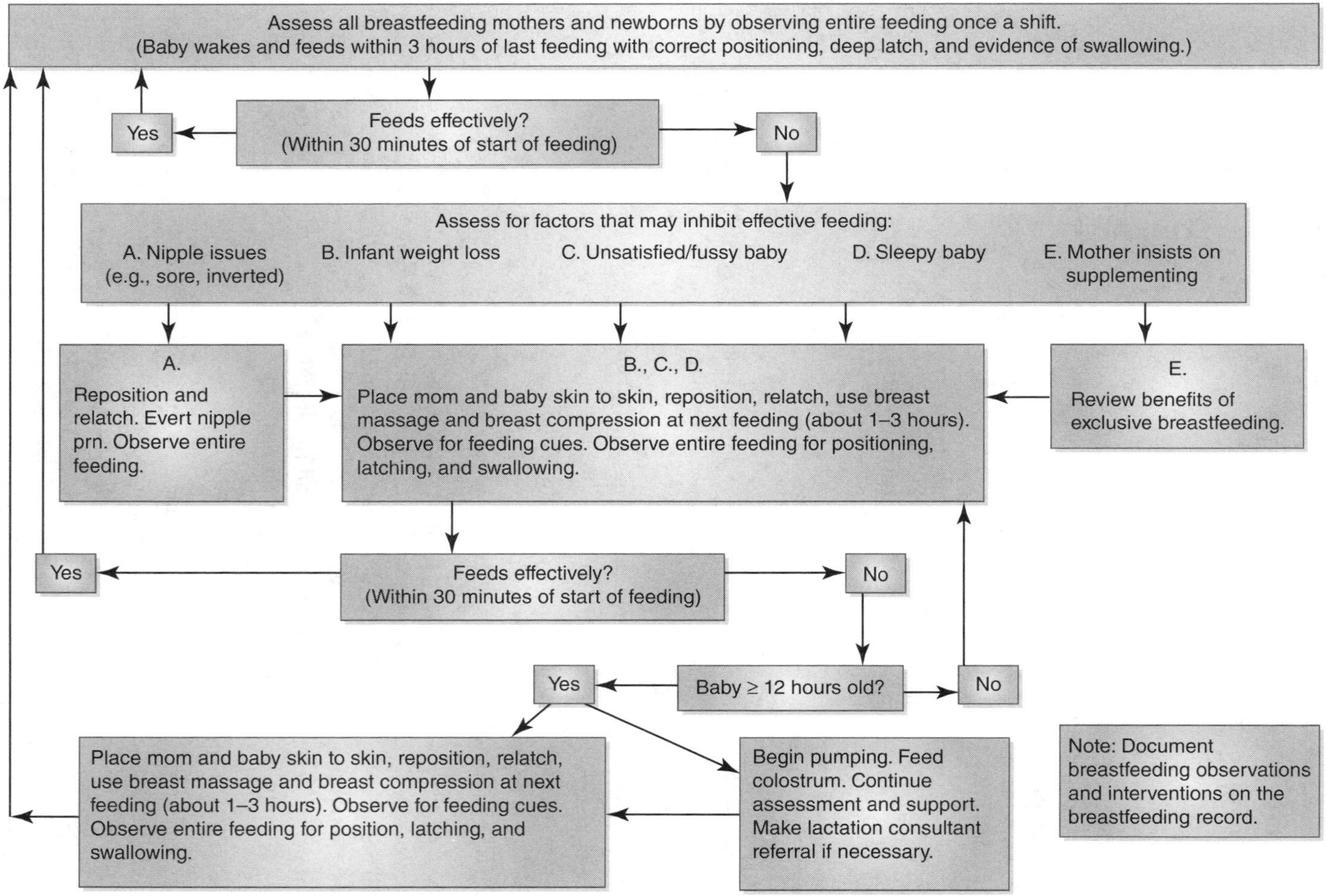

Figure 5-25 Breastfeeding decision tree and checklist. For use with normal newborns of more than 37 weeks' gestational age.

Checklist

Normal breastfeeding:

- ☐ Baby wakes and breastfeeds about every 1½ to 3 hours.
- ☐ Baby nurses 8–12 times in 24 hours.
- ☐ Baby may have frequent nursing sessions over a 4- to 5-hour period followed by a 4- to 5-hour sleep.
- ☐ Baby wakes more frequently to nurse at night compared to daytime, during the early days.
- ☐ Baby nurses better during quiet alert state.
- ☐ Baby learns to nurse more effectively when kept skin to skin with mom.
- ☐ When feeding cues are observed, place baby skin to skin with mom and offer breast.
- ☐ Avoid pacifier unless requested by mom. Pacifiers are associated with masked feeding cues, fewer breastfeeding sessions per day, lower breastmilk intake, and shorter breastfeeding duration.
- ☐ Rooming-in associated with shorter time to effective latch, increased milk supply, and longer breastfeeding duration.

Signs of milk transfer:

- ☐ Mom has contractions.
- ☐ Mom is thirsty.
- ☐ Mom gets drowsy.
- ☐ Baby switches from non-nutritive suck to long "suck/swallows."
- ☐ Baby has one or more wet diapers and one or more stools during the first 24 hours.
- ☐ Baby has two or more wet diapers and two or more stools during the second 24 hours.
- ☐ Baby has three or more wet diapers and two or more stools during the third 24 hours.
- ☐ Baby has four or more wet diapers and two or more stools during the fourth 24 hours.

Exclusive breastfeeding in the early postpartum period is associated with:

- ☐ Shorter time to effective latch.
- ☐ Greater milk supply and longer breastfeeding duration.
- ☐ Decreased exposure to foreign proteins.

The American Academy of Pediatrics (AAP) recommends exclusive breastfeeding for about 6 months, with the gradual introduction of iron-rich solid foods combined with breastmilk during the second half of the first year. The AAP recommends that breastfeeding continue for at least 12 months and, thereafter, for as long as mutually desired.

If there is a compelling clinical indication for supplementation, quantity should mimic the average intake of a breastfed baby:

Age in Hours	Amount/Feed	24-Hour Total*
<24	4–5 cc	1 oz
<48	15–20 cc	3–4 oz
<72	30 cc	8 oz
<96	60 cc	16 oz

*Based on 8 feedings/day

Figure 5-25 *(continued)*

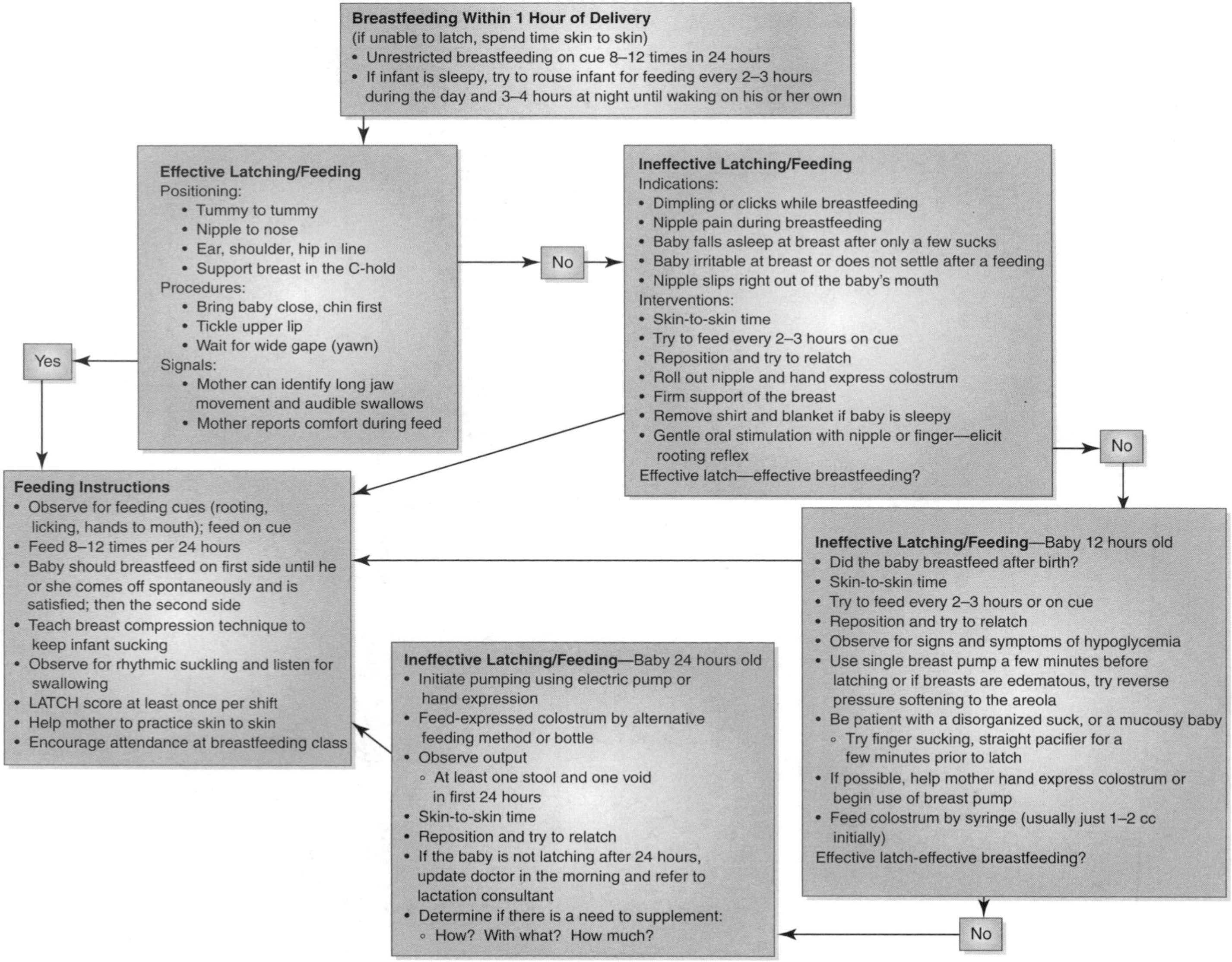

Figure 5-26 Breastfeeding guidelines for the first 24 hours through discharge for a healthy 37+ week infant.
Reproduced with permission from Winchester Hospital, Winchester, Massachusetts.

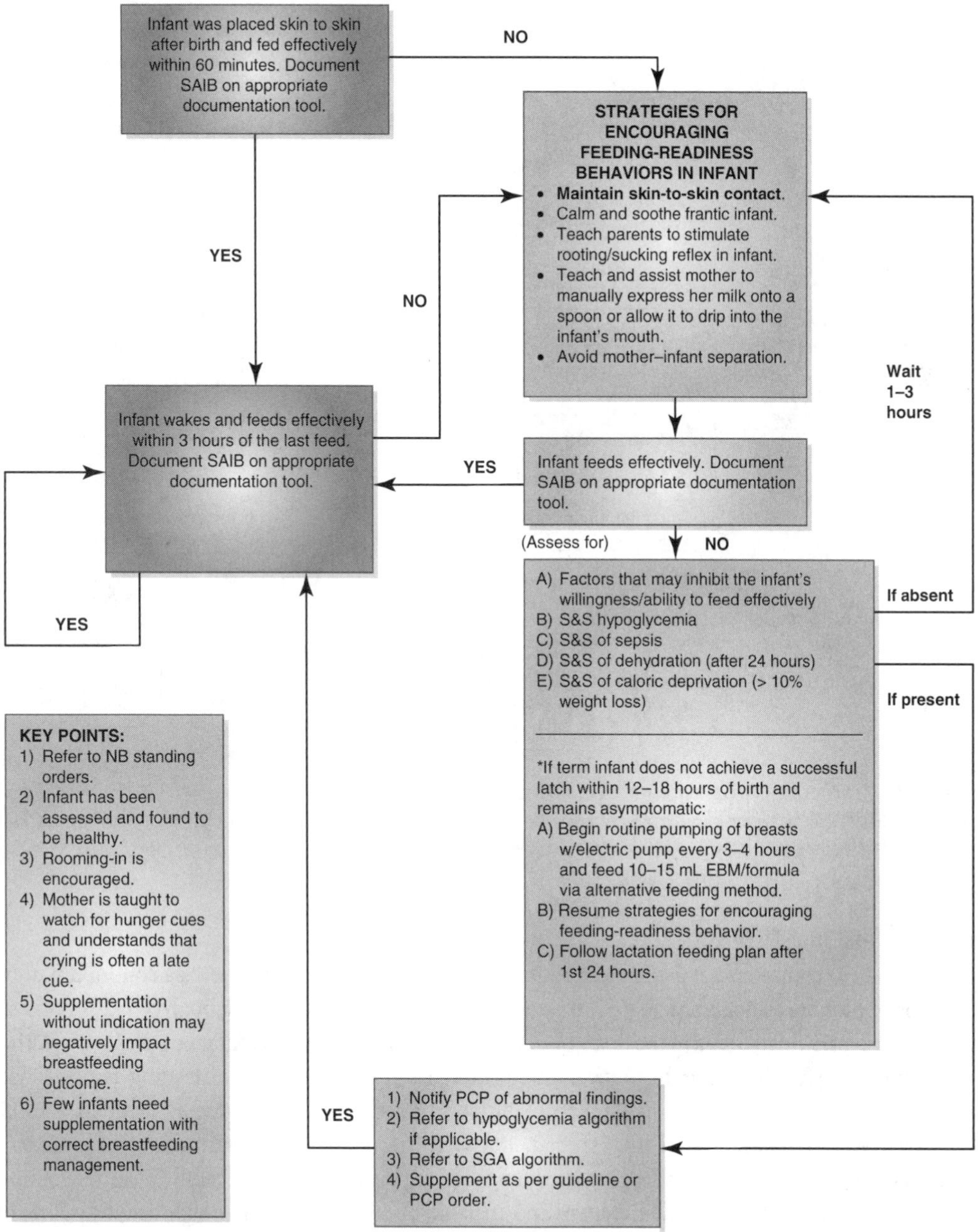

Figure 5-27 Breastfeeding flowchart for the term infant.
Elliot Hospital, Manchester, New Hampshire. Used with permission.

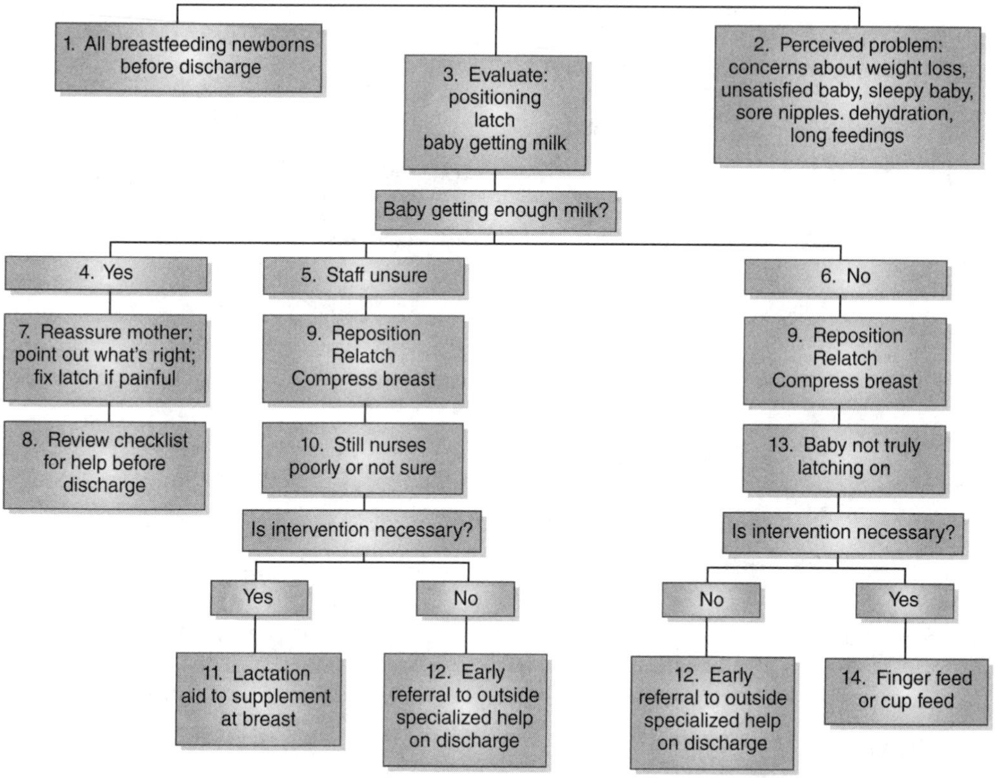

Figure 5-28 Immediate-postpartum decision tree.

Data by Jeannette Crenshaw for the Lamaze International Breastfeeding Support Specialist Training Program from: Newman, J. (1996). Decision tree and postpartum management for preventing dehydration in the breastfed baby. *Journal of Human Lactation, 12,* 129–135. Used with permission.

Problem of Hypoglycemia

Hypoglycemia is a common metabolic concern in the newborn infant and represents a continuum of blood glucose concentration, falling immediately after delivery and rising thereafter. Hypoglycemia is not a single number. Transient hypoglycemia in the first 3 hours after birth is normal with spontaneous recovery. Although breastfeeding in the first hour after birth is very important to the course of lactation, feeding a normal healthy newborn in the first hour after birth does not cause the blood glucose levels to rise (Sweet, Hadden, & Halliday, 1999). However, Chertok, Raz, Shoham, Haddad, and Wiznitzer (2009) found that infants of mothers with gestational diabetes who were breastfed immediately following birth had a significantly lower rate of borderline hypoglycemia than those not fed in the early postpartum period. They also had significantly higher mean blood glucose levels compared with those not breastfed immediately after delivery, and also had a mean blood glucose level that was higher than those infants who were formula fed for their first feed. An infant who misses this opportunity at breast does not require supplementation, nor does a healthy full-term breastfeeding infant require routine blood glucose monitoring (Adamkin & Committee on Fetus and Newborn, American Academy of Pediatrics, 2011). Adaptation in normal circumstances progresses in a pattern.

Physiological Adaptation After Birth

- The brain derives almost all of its energy from glucose.
- During gestation, glucose is stored in the fetus as glycogen, mostly in the liver but also in cardiac and skeletal muscle.
- Delivery terminates the glucose supply obtained from the mother in utero.
- Hepatic breakdown of the stored glycogen is triggered within minutes of the umbilical cord being cut by a surge in glucoregulatory hormones:
    - Increased epinephrine.
    - Increased insulin.
    - Increased norepinephrine.
    - Increased catecholamines.
    - Increased glucagon.
    - Increased corticosteroids.
    - Net effect is mobilization of glycogen and fatty acids.
- Liver glycogen stores are 90% depleted by 3 hours and gone by 12 hours (Hagedorn & Gardner, 1999).
- Activities that maintain glucose homeostasis are collectively called counter-regulation and consist of:
    - Glycogenolysis: the mobilization and release of glycogen from body stores to form glucose.
    - Gluconeogenesis: the production of glucose by the liver and kidneys from noncarbohydrate substrates such as fatty acids and amino acids.
    - Rate of glucose production is 4–6 mg/kg/min.
    - 3.7 mg/kg/min are needed to meet the energy requirements of the brain.
    - Approximately 70% of energy requirement is provided by glucose oxidation; the rest is provided by alternative fuels.
- Production of alternative brain fuels such as ketone bodies and lactate:
    - The lowest blood glucose values typically occur between 1 and 2 hours after birth (World Health Organization, 1997).
    - After 12 hours, the infant depends on glucose made from milk components (20–50%) and gluconeogenesis to maintain blood glucose (galactose, amino acids, glycerol, lactate) as well as free fatty acids from fat stores and milk.
    - Sixteen percent of infant's body weight is fat.
    - Breastmilk is more ketogenic (promotes production of ketones as an alternate brain fuel) than formula. Newborns convert energy stored in ketone bodies to high-energy phosphates. Ketone bodies provide fuel particularly to brain, heart, and skeletal muscle during the immediate newborn period of lower blood glucose levels.
    - Breastfed infants produce ketones as an adaptive mechanism. This may explain the healthy breastfed newborn with relatively low blood sugar who remains asymptomatic.
    - Lactate provides a useful source of cerebral fuel in most hypoglycemic infants, and those hypoglycemic babies with low plasma lactate concentrations may be at an increased risk for neurological side effects (Harris, Weston, & Harding, 2015).

A number of conditions or situations that put an infant at risk for hypoglycemia are as follows and are generally associated with clinical signs in the newborn. In these situations, it is generally assumed that infants are already being monitored and glucose measurements are being performed:

Preterm (AGA)	Discordant twin	Postmaturity
Preterm (SGA)	LGA	Hyperinsulinemia
Full term (SGA)	Asphyxia	Cold stress
Congestive heart failure	Sepsis	Rh disease
Erythroblastosis fetalis	Polycythemia	Microphallus or midline defect
Respiratory distress	Maternal glucose IV	Maternal epidural
Endocrine disorders	Inborn errors of metabolism	Diabetic mother
Maternal toxemia	Intrapartum fever	

(Depuy, Coassolo, Som, & Smulian, 2009)

Adamkin and the Committee on Fetus and Newborn, American Academy of Pediatrics (2011) therefore recommend that as a practical approach to hypoglycemia in the newborn, "at-risk" infants include those who are SGA, LGA, born to diabetic mothers, or are late preterm and should be managed according to the approach outlined in **Figure 5-29**. Blood glucose concentration should only be measured in term infants who have clinical manifestations or who are known to be at risk.

Schaefer-Graf and colleagues (2002) studied risk factors for hypoglycemia in LGA newborns of nondiabetic mothers. The antenatal 1-hour glucose test given during pregnancy was shown to be predictive of hypoglycemia in the newborn. An incremental risk of newborn hypoglycemia was seen with increasing 1-hour oral glucose tolerance test values with hypoglycemia rates of 2.5%, 9.3%, 22.0%, and 50% that were associated

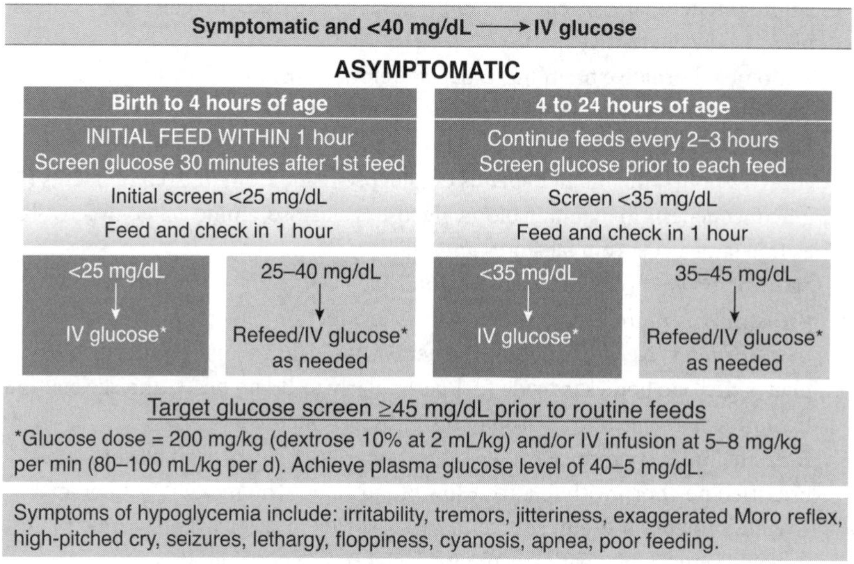

Figure 5-29 Screening and management algorithm for newborns with hypoglycemia.

Box 5-9 Signs and Symptoms of Hypoglycemia

- Abnormal cry
- Abnormal eye movements
- Apathy
- Apnea
- Cardiac arrest
- Congestive heart failure
- Cyanosis
- Diaphoresis
- Exaggerated reflexes
- Hypothermia
- Hypotonia
- Irregular breathing
- Irritability
- Jitteriness
- Lethargy
- Poor suck
- Refusal to feed
- Seizures
- Tachypnea
- Temperature instability
- Tremors
- Vasomotor instability (pallor)
- Vomiting

with maternal 1-hour glucose values of < 120, 120–179, 180–239, and > 240 mg/dL, respectively. Infants of mothers with high values may benefit from increased vigilance and placement in an at-risk category.

Signs and symptoms of hypoglycemia are subtle, nonspecific, and variable (**Box 5-9**). Jitteriness is a very common and usually benign finding in otherwise healthy full-term infants (D'Harlingue & Durand, 1991). In a study of 102 infants described as jittery, sucking on the clinician's finger stopped the jitteriness in 80% of infants. Of the other infants whose jitteriness did not stop, five were hypoglycemic and the rest were hypocalcemic (Linder et al., 1989). Nicholl (2003) recommended that if an infant appears jittery, first allow the infant to suck on a finger. The infant could also be put to breast to see if sucking would reduce the jitteriness. If the jitteriness remains, blood glucose and calcium should be measured, with blood glucose concentrations less than 1.5 mmol/L (< 27 mg/dL) being addressed immediately.

Problems With Glucose-Level Measurements

Whole blood glucose-level measurements are generally 10–15% lower than the corresponding plasma values. The normal blood glucose range for newborns during the first week is 27–108 mg/dL (1.5–6 mmol/L). The optimal method for measuring plasma glucose is the hexokinase, glucose oxidase, or dehydrogenase (enzymatic) method performed in a laboratory, but this method is often too slow for timely treatment. Therefore "point-of-care" devices are often used for measuring whole blood glucose concentration in the newborn nursery or neonatal intensive care units. Point-of-care glucose monitoring systems need to be accurate, precise, and versatile (Sirkin, Jalloh, & Lee 2002). Reagent strips and bedside machines will, on average, wrongly identify hypoglycemia in one of four infants who are, in fact, normoglycemic (World Health Organization, 1997). Low-birth-weight, low hematocrit, and parenteral feeding decrease the accuracy of point-of-care devices (Bellini, Serra, Risso, Mazzella, & Bonioli, 2007). Anemia falsely raises and polycythemia falsely depresses glucometer readings. Most current point-of-care glucometers are sufficient only for initial screening, and their values need to be confirmed with laboratory measurements and clinical assessment of the infant (Ho, Yeung, & Young, 2004; **Box 5-10**). Future improvements on glucose monitoring include subcutaneous microdialysis for long-term monitoring in the neonatal intensive care unit (Baumeister, Rolinski, Busch, & Emmrich, 2001) and near infrared spectroscopy (Gabriely et al., 1999) as a noninvasive method of glucose screening for all infants. It is important that devices used to measure neonatal glucose levels be specifically evaluated for use in this population.

There are a number of considerations when interpreting glucose measurements and choosing a course of action:

- Chemical reagent strips (e.g., Dextrostix) were not designed for use with a neonate but for use with adult diabetics.
- These methods usually underestimate blood glucose by ± 5–15 mg/dL, especially in the lower ranges.
- Laboratory follow-up and confirmation of glucose levels are necessary before treatment.
- Hematocrit should be considered because decreased glucose readings occur with a high hematocrit. Other conditions and substances can also affect glucose readings, such as altitude, hypoxia, and partial pressure of arterial oxygen.
- Use of maternal glucose intravenously (seen in older studies) contributed to the risk of hypoglycemia in the infant.
- Repeated heelsticks/venipunctures increase stress hormone response from pain and decrease blood glucose levels.
- Squeezing the heel causes hemolysis, which interferes with the assay, producing falsely low values (blood samples must be free flowing).
- Blood should be transported in a tube that contains a glycolytic inhibitor such as fluoride. This is because a long delay in laboratory processing of the blood sample can result in a falsely low concentration as red blood cells metabolize the glucose in the plasma.
- There is currently no point-of-care device or instrument that is reliable enough and accurate enough in the low range of blood glucose levels to qualify it as the sole method for newborn hypoglycemia screening.

Diwakar and Sasidhar (2002) demonstrated that term breastfed infants have their own distinct plasma glucose levels, which tend to show little significant variation between 3 and 72 hours of age.

Box 5-10 Glucose Screening Techniques and Equipment

Sampling techniques and their effect on glucose values when using bedside screening tools:

- Once in the sample tube, red blood cells continue to metabolize glucose.
- Bedside tools measure whole blood glucose concentrations, which can be 15% lower than plasma concentrations (which is where blood glucose is measured in a laboratory).
- Blood samples that are allowed to sit at room temperature for long periods of time may result in a glucose concentration drop of 18 mg/dL per hour.
- To avoid sampling errors, blood samples should be transported quickly to the laboratory, put on ice, or placed in a tube containing a glycolytic inhibitor.
- The infant's heel should be warmed to prevent venous stasis in heelstick samples that can lead to falsely low glucose values.

Screening Equipment

- Bedside or "point-of-care" glucose screening devices are commonly used as a rapid screening tool for neonatal hypoglycemia.
- One class of these devices is photometers that rely on reflectance-based technology to read reagent strips.
- The Dextrostix reagent strips were commonly used for many years to screen for neonatal hypoglycemia, despite the fact that this product was never intended to be used on neonates, as stated on the package insert, and that the results were inaccurate below 50 mg/dL. They were removed from the market in 1997.
- Meloy, Miller, Chandrasekaran, Summitt, and Gutcher (1999), in a study on the Accu-Check III reflectance meter, documented that the machine could correctly identify neonatal hypoglycemia only 76% of the time.
- More accurate and reliable equipment is available that utilizes electrochemical techniques or quantitative analysis, such as glucose oxidase meters.
- Even with reliable bedside screening devices, operational threshold values should be validated by laboratory analysis.

Modified from Cornblath, M., & Ichord, R. (2000). Hypoglycemia in the neonate. *Seminars in Perinatology, 24,* 136–149; Cowett, R. (1999). Neonatal hypoglycemia: A little goes a long way [Editorial]. *Journal of Pediatrics, 134,* 389–391; Meloy, L., Miller, G., Chandrasekaran, M., Summitt, C., & Gutcher, G. (1999). Accuracy of glucose reflectance testing for detecting hypoglycemia in term newborns. *Clinical Pediatrics, 38,* 717–724; National Association of Neonatal Nurses. (1994). *Neonatal hypoglycemia guidelines for practice.* Petaluma, CA: Author; Noerr, B. (2001). State of the science: Neonatal hypoglycemia. *Advances in Neonatal Care, 1,* 4–21; Thomas, C., Critchley, L., & Davies, M. (2000). Determining the best method for first-line assessment of neonatal blood glucose levels. *Journal of Paediatrics and Child Health, 36,* 343–348.

Prelacteal feeds were unnecessary, and satisfactory glucose levels were maintained even when infants remained unfed for up to 6 hours of age. Blood glucose concentrations tend to be lower during the first 24 hours. However, Hoseth, Joergensen, Ebbesen, and Moeller (2000) reported that with frequent effective breastfeeding, normal, healthy, full-term infants with no risk factors, who showed the lowest blood sugar levels at 1 hour of age, 1.4 mmol/L (25.2 mg/dL) to 1.9 mmol/L (28.7 mg/dL), developed no clinical signs of hypoglycemia. Defining hypoglycemia as a specific number does not take into account the multiple variables affecting blood glucose levels in the newborn. If a number such as 40 mg/dL were chosen as the cutoff point for treatment, this value could produce as much as a 20% incidence of diagnosis of hypoglycemia in full-term infants (Sexon, 1984).

Rather than a specific number, the concept of operational thresholds has been suggested to refine diagnosis and better handle glycemic changes in the newborn. Operational thresholds (i.e., blood glucose levels at which clinical interventions should be considered) have been delineated by Cornblath and colleagues (2000). These threshold values described for surveillance and intervention are different and should be separated from the targeted therapeutic values, which should be in the range of 72–90 mg/dL (4–5 mmol/L) (Kalhan & Peter-Wohl, 2000). They delineate a range of blood glucose values based on parameters that account for the status and age of the infant (**Table 5-5**).

Term Infant

- Healthy full-term infants from normal pregnancy and delivery who have no clinical signs do not require routine monitoring of glucose concentrations (Adamkin & Committee on Fetus and Newborn, American Academy of Pediatrics, 2011; Eidelman, 2001).

Breastfed Term Infant

- These infants tend to have lower concentrations of blood glucose than formula-fed infants but higher concentrations of ketone bodies.
- Breastfed infants who lose the most weight have the highest ketone bodies concentration.
- Provision of alternative fuels is a normal adaptive response to low nutrient intake during the establishment of breastfeeding.
- Breastfed infants may well tolerate lower plasma glucose levels without any significant clinical manifestation or sequelae.

Infant With Abnormal Clinical Signs

Symptomatic infant

- Plasma glucose should be measured.
- If the value is less than 45 mg/dL (2.5 mmol/L), clinical intervention should be started.

At-risk infants

- At-risk infants should be screened before any symptoms manifest (Wight, 2006).
- At-risk infants should be fed by 1 hour of age and screened 30 minutes after the feeding.
- Routine measurements should occur as soon as possible after birth, either on admission to the unit or within 30–60 minutes after birth.
- Screening should occur every 30 minutes for infants being treated for hypoglycemia and before feeding or any time there are abnormal signs.
- Plasma glucose of less than 36 mg/dL (2.0 mmol/L) requires close surveillance.

Table 5-5 Neonatal Hypoglycemia and Operational Thresholds for Clinical Intervention

Age	Threshold Glucose Infant Parameters	Postbirth Values for Intervention
Asymptomatic		
Full or near-term (34–37 weeks)	1st 24 hours	< 30–35 mg/dL
Healthy	After 24 hours	< 40–50 mg/dL
Full enteral feedings		
No risk factors		
Ill Infant		
Low-birth-weight	1st 24 hours	< 45–50 mg/dL
Preterm	After 24 hours	< 40–50 mg/dL
Sepsis		
Asphyxia		
Respiratory distress syndrome		
Symptomatic Infant		
Signs of hypoglycemia	Any age	< 45 mg/dL
Any gestational age		
At-Risk Infant		
Infant of diabetic mother	Any age	< 36 mg/dL
Sepsis		
Asphyxia		
Small for gestational age (SGA)		
Hyperinsulin		
Endocrine disorders		
Metabolic disorders		
Infants with glucose levels	Any age close monitoring	IV glucose therapy and < 20–25 mg/dL

Modified from Noerr, B. (2001). State of the science: Neonatal hypoglycemia. *Advances in Neonatal Care, 1,* 4–21; Cornblath, M., & Ichord, R. (2000). Hypoglycemia in the neonate. *Seminars in Perinatology, 24,* 136–149.

- Intervention is required if plasma glucose remains below this level, if the level does not increase after a feed, or if abnormal clinical signs develop.
- At very low glucose concentrations, less than 20–25 mg/dL (1.1–1.4 mmol/L), IV glucose infusion should aim to raise levels above 45 mg/dL (2.5 mmol/L).
- The therapeutic objective of 45 mg/dL is different from the threshold for intervention—36 mg/dL (2.0 mmol/L).

Breastfeeding Management

Breastfeeding protocols and caretaking activities during the hours after delivery should be designed to proactively reduce the likelihood of inducing hypoglycemia. Chertok and colleagues (2009) studied the effects of breastfeeding immediately after delivery compared with later initiation of breastfeeding on neonatal glucose levels of term infants born to mothers with gestational diabetes. The study also compared the glycemic levels of infants who breastfed with those who received formula for their first feed. The results showed that infants who were breastfed right after delivery had a significantly lower rate of borderline hypoglycemia than those not breastfed in the early minutes after birth. Infants breastfed immediately after birth had significantly higher mean blood glucose levels compared to infants who were not breastfed early. Breastfed infants additionally had a significantly higher mean blood glucose level compared to those who were fed formula for their first feed. Early breastfeeding when the infant is swallowing colostrum helps facilitate glycemic stability in infants, especially in those born to diabetic mothers. The clinician is well advised to see that effective breastfeeding takes places as soon as possible after delivery and ensure that the infant is swallowing colostrum at this time. Prevention activities also include the following:

- Breastfeed frequently, on cue, before sustained crying occurs, and avoid long intervals between feedings.
- Infants separated from their mothers have lower body temperatures, cry more, and have decreased blood glucose levels (Christensson et al., 1992; Durand et al., 1997). Christensson and colleagues (1992) reported that newborn infants separated from their mothers had blood sugar levels that were 10 mg/dL lower than infants kept in skin-to-skin contact at 90 minutes after birth. Environmental stress, such as hypothermia, can increase the energy demands of a newborn, which could exceed the infant's capacity to generate energy substrate (Kaplan & Eidelman, 1985). Walters, Boggs, Ludington-Hoe, Price, and Morrison (2007) demonstrated that healthy term infants placed skin to skin within 1 minute of birth had temperatures that rose and blood glucose levels in a satisfactory range (43–85 mg/dL), even in infants who had not fed before the study's glucose measurement at 60 minutes after birth (43–118 mg/dL).
    - Keep the infant in skin-to-skin contact with the mother during the early hours after birth. Skin-to-skin care heats the infant's entire body (peripheral and trunk) rather than just the trunk, which occurs under a radiant warmer (Christidis et al., 2003). This avoids the possibility of chilling during the early hours as does delaying the infant bath.
    - Keep the mother and infant together (even at night).
    - Do not allow the infant to cry.
    - Immediately respond to any cries.
- There is a normal dip in blood glucose in the first 1 to 4 hours after birth.
    - Avoid giving sugar water by mouth because it is metabolized rapidly, often before the infant can mount effective counter-regulatory activities. This may cause rebound hypoglycemia.
    - Avoid testing blood sugar during this time with reagent strips (in asymptomatic, low-risk infants).
    - Provide unlimited access to the breast and ensure colostrum/milk transfer.

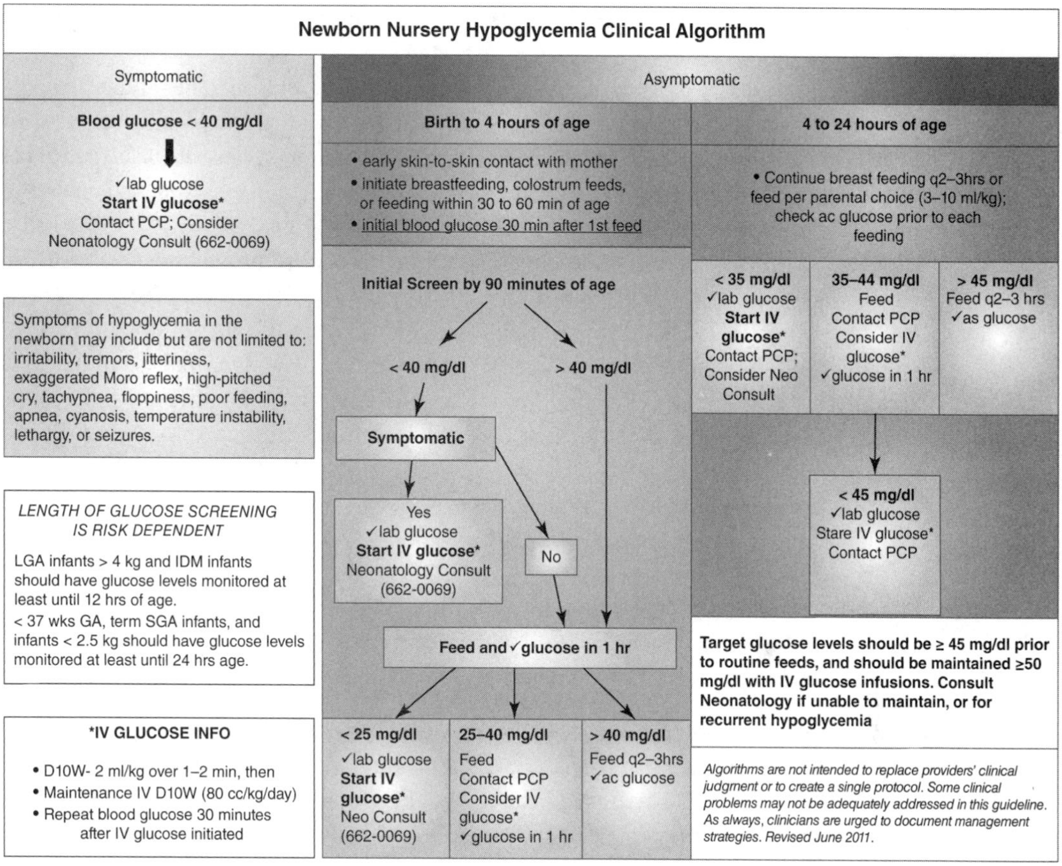

Figure 5-30 Newborn nursery hypoglycemia clinical algorithm.
Maine Medical Center.

- Feed expressed colostrum if the infant is unable to latch or feeds poorly. There do not appear to be any significant differences between glucose values for infants fed expressed colostrum versus formula supplementation (Tozier, 2013). Colostrum supplementation when necessary preserves exclusive breastfeeding, maintains acceptable levels of blood glucose, and reduces the risk for sensitizing infants to cow's milk protein and diabetes. **Figure 5-30** is a hypoglycemia algorithm that supports exclusive breastfeeding and the use of colostrum as a supplement.
- Infants with risk factors for hypoglycemia should be fed frequently.
  - The protein and fat in colostrum provide substrates for gluconeogenesis.
  - Colostrum and breastmilk enhance ketogenesis.

- Colostrum increases gut motility and gastric emptying time, causing rapid absorption of nutrients.
- If the infant is unable to latch or effectively transfer colostrum, have the mother hand express colostrum into a spoon and spoon-feed it to the infant (using a pump often results in little to no colostrum being retrievable to feed to the infant, because it sticks to the sides of the bottle). If the mother is unable to express colostrum and has expressed colostrum prenatally, use this to spoon feed the infant.
- Consider using an evidence-based hypoglycemia protocol to protect breastfeeding and appropriately manage hypoglycemia in the breastfed infant. The Academy of Breastfeeding Medicine developed a clinical protocol to use as a guideline for obtaining blood glucose levels in neonates who are at risk for developing hypoglycemia and to delineate appropriate interventions (Wight, Marinelli, & Academy of Breastfeeding Medicine, 2014). The Academy of Breastfeeding Medicine's clinical management is based on four basic principles:
    1. Monitoring those infants at highest risk
    2. Confirming that plasma glucose concentration is low and indeed responsible for the clinical manifestations present
    3. Demonstrating that the symptoms have responded after glucose therapy with restoration of the blood glucose to normoglycemic levels
    4. Observing and carefully documenting all of the above

Adamkin and the Committee on Fetus and Newborn, American Academy of Pediatrics (2011) have provided an algorithm and practical guidelines for managing hypoglycemia in the newborn. Lacking a specific concentration of glucose that can discriminate normal from abnormal glucose levels, this guideline recommends early identification of the at-risk infant and interventions to prevent unwanted problems. Nowhere in this guideline is infant formula recommended as a supplement to breastfeeding or as a means to treat low blood glucose concentrations in breastfed infants. A simplified and streamlined hypoglycemia algorithm (**Figure 5-31**) uses breastfeeding as the first-line treatment for newborn hypoglycemia and may be readily accepted by hospital staff, unlike more complicated algorithms (Csont, Groth, Hopkins, & Guillet, 2014).

Antenatal colostrum expression and/or colostrum expression during the early stage of labor is sometimes done by diabetic mothers in anticipation of the possible need to supplement the newborn for hypoglycemia (Tozier, 2013). The colostrum is stored in feeding syringes in the patient's refrigerator or placed on ice to be used during the early hours post birth if necessary. Some concerns about this practice have been raised by Forster and colleagues (2011) regarding increased admissions of newborns with hypoglycemia to the special care or neonatal intensive care nursery, decreased duration of pregnancy, and increased requirement for IV glucose. However, these same authors reported that the amount of colostrum obtained ranged between 5 mL and 310 mL depending on the number of expressions and the length of time between the start of expressing milk and the birth of the infant. Most women had a positive experience and would express antenatally again if the practice was proven beneficial. In a thorough review of the literature on antenatal colostrum expression, it was concluded that in the absence

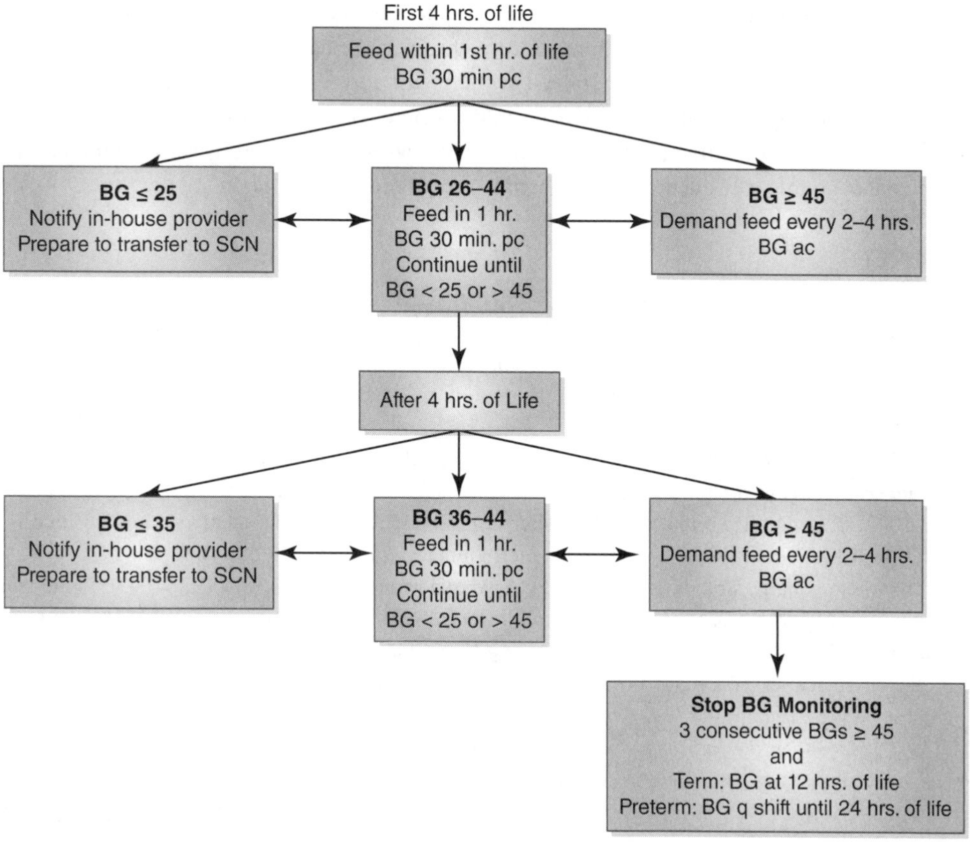

Figure 5-31 Simplified algorithm for blood gas protocol.
Csont, G. L., Groth, S., Hopkins, P., & Guillet, R. (2014). An evidence-based approach to breastfeeding neonates at risk for hypoglycemia. *Journal of Obstetric, Gynecologic, and Neonatal Nursing, 43,* 71–81.

of clear evidence to the contrary, prenatal expression of colostrum and the benefits of early colostrum feeding should outweigh the unsupported risks of teaching antenatal colostrum expression (Chapman, Pincombe, & Harris, 2013).

SUMMARY: THE DESIGN IN NATURE

Individual infants and their unique circumstances can present a challenge to breastfeeding that many mothers may not have anticipated. Birth trauma is not limited to the infant. Up to 34% of mothers have reported experiencing a traumatic delivery. The impact of this trauma can lead mothers down two very different breastfeeding paths. Some mothers are determined to persevere with breastfeeding to make up for a devastating childbirth, whereas others meet impediments to breastfeeding that cause sufficient distress for them to abandon breastfeeding attempts (Beck & Watson, 2008).

Clinicians may need to use their years of experience and tap into their knowledge base to initiate and preserve breastfeeding in difficult situations. Nature has programmed infants to be anatomically, physiologically, and metabolically competent to feed at the breast and consume mother's milk, but anatomy, perinatal events, and unforeseen circumstances may interfere with this process. Infants were born to be breastfed, but sometimes nature presents a different path that requires carefully selected interventions to reach the goal of an infant at the breast or breastmilk being provided to the infant.

REFERENCES

Abadie, V., Andre, A., Zaouche, A., Thouvenin, B., Baujat, G., & Schmitz, J. (2001). Early feeding resistance: A possible consequence of neonatal oro-oesophageal dyskinesia. *Acta Paediatrica, 90,* 738–745.

Abdel-Latif, M. E., Pinner, J., Clews, S., Cooke, F., Lui, K., & Oei, J. (2006). Effects of breast milk on the severity and outcome of neonatal abstinence syndrome among infants of drug-dependent mothers. *Pediatrics, 117,* e1163–e1169.

Academy of Breastfeeding Medicine. (2008). *Clinical protocol number 5: Peripartum breastfeeding management for the healthy mother and infant at term.* Retrieved from www.bfmed.org/Media/Files/Protocols/Protocol_5.pdf

Adamkin, D. H., & Committee on Fetus and Newborn, American Academy of Pediatrics. (2011). Clinical report: Postnatal glucose homeostasis in late-preterm and term infants. *Pediatrics, 127,* 575–579.

Agostoni, C., Marangoni, F., Grandi, F., Lammardo, A. M., Giovannini, M., . . . Galli, C. (2003). Earlier smoking habits are associated with higher serum lipids and lower milk fat and polyunsaturated fatty acid content in the first 6 months of lactation. *European Journal of Clinical Nutrition, 57,* 1466–1472.

Allegaert, K., & van den Anker, J. N. (2014). Neonatal abstinence syndrome: On the evidence to add breastfeeding to any clinical pathway. *Pediatric Critical Care Medicine, 15,* 579–580.

Als, H. (1995). *Manual for the naturalistic observation of newborn behavior, Newborn Individualized Developmental Care and Assessment Program (NIDCAP).* Boston. MA: Harvard Medical School.

Als, H., Tronick, E., Adamson, L., & Brazelton, T. B. (1976). The behavior of the full-term but underweight newborn infant. *Developmental Medicine & Child Neurology, 18,* 590–602.

American Academy of Pediatrics. (2012). Policy statement: Breastfeeding and the use of human milk. *Pediatrics, 129,* e827–e841.

Anderson, G. C. (1991). Current knowledge about skin-to-skin (kangaroo) care for preterm infants. *Journal of Perinatology, 11,* 216–226.

Anderson, M. E., Johnson, D. C., & Batal, H. A. (2005). Sudden infant death syndrome and prenatal maternal smoking: Rising attributed risk in the Back to Sleep era. *MBC Medicine, 3,* 4.

Andrade, S. E., Raebel, M. A., Brown, J., Lane, K., Livingston, J., Boudreau, D., . . . Platt, R. (2008). Use of antidepressant medications during pregnancy: A multisite study. *American Journal of Obstetrics and Gynecology, 198,* 194.e1–5.

Arslanoglu, S., Bertino, E., Nicocia, M., & Moro, G. E. (2012). WAPM working group on nutrition: Potential chronobiotic role of human milk in sleep regulation. *Journal of Perinatal Medicine, 40,* 1–8.

Auerbach, K. G. (1990). The effect of nipple shields on maternal milk volume. *Journal of Obstetric, Gynecologic, and Neonatal Nursing, 19,* 419–427.

Ayers, A. J. (1977). *Sensory integration and learning disorders.* Los Angeles, CA: Western Psychological Services.

Babic, S. H., Kokol, P., & Stiglic, M. M. (1999, June 18–20). *Fuzzy decision trees in the support of breastfeeding.* Presented at the 12th IEEE Symposium on Computer Based Medical Systems, Stamford, CT.

Babic, S. H., Sprogar, M., Zorman, M., Kokol, P., & Turk, D. M. (1999, June 18–20). *Evaluating breastfeeding advantages using decision trees.* Presented at the 12th IEEE Symposium on Computer Based Medical Systems, Stamford, CT.

Bachour, P., Yafawi, R., Jaber, F., Choueiri, E., & Abdel-Razzak, Z. (2012). Effects of smoking, mother's age, body mass index, and parity number on lipid, protein, and secretory immunoglobulin A concentrations of human milk. *Breastfeeding Medicine, 7*(3), 179–188.

Backas, N. (1998). *Working your way through the reimbursement maze. Medela rental roundup: The Medela messenger.* McHenry, IL: Medela.

Bagley, S. M., Wachman, E., Holland, E., & Brogly, S. B. (2014). Review of the assessment and management of neonatal abstinence syndrome. *Addiction Science & Clinical Practice, 9,* 19.

Bahadori, B., Riegiger, N. D., Farrell, S. M., Uitz, E., & Moghadasian, M. F. (2013). Hypothesis: smoking decreases breastfeeding duration by suppressing prolactin secretion. *Medical Hypotheses, 81,* 582–586.

Bai, D. L., Wu, K. M., & Tarrant, M. (2013). Association between intrapartum interventions and breastfeeding duration. *Journal of Midwifery and Women's Health, 58,* 25–32.

Bandman, E. L., & Bandman, B. (1988). *Critical thinking in nursing.* Norwalk, CT: Appleton & Lange.

Barr, R. G., Kramer, M. S., Pless, I. B., Boisjoly, C., & Leduc, D. (1989). Feeding and temperament as determinants of early infant crying/fussing behavior. *Pediatrics, 84,* 514–521.

Bassett, V. (2001). How one Canadian hospital developed a newborn critical path and documentation tool that supports moms and babies. *AWHONN Lifelines, 5,* 48–54.

Baumeister, F. A. M., Rolinski, B., Busch, R., & Emmrich, P. (2001). Glucose monitoring with long-term subcutaneous microdialysis in neonates. *Pediatrics, 108,* 1187–1192.

Beck, C. T., & Watson, S. (2008). Impact of birth trauma on breastfeeding: A tale of two pathways. *Nursing Research, 57,* 228–236.

Begg, E. J., Malpas, T. J., Hackett, L. P., & Ilett, K. F. (2001). Distribution of *R*- and *S*-methadone into human milk during multiple, medium to high oral dosing. *British Journal of Clinical Pharmacology, 52,* 681–685.

Bell, A. F., White-Traut, R., & Rankin, K. (2013). Fetal exposure to synthetic oxytocin and the relationship with prefeeding cues within one hour postbirth, *Early Human Development, 89,* 137–143.

Bellini, C., Serra, G., Risso, D., Mazzella, M., & Bonioli, E. (2007). Reliability assessment of glucose measurement by HemoCue analyzer in a neonatal intensive care unit. *Clinical Chemistry and Laboratory Medicine, 45,* 1549–1554.

Bevan, M., Mosley, D., Lobach, K., & Salimano, G. (1984). Factors influencing breastfeeding in an urban WIC program. *Journal of the American Dietetic Association, 84,* 563–567.

Black, L. S. (1993). *Baby-friendly newborn care.* Workshop for Lactation Specialists, Series VIII. Chicago, IL: La Leche League International.

Black, L. S. (2001). Incorporating breastfeeding care into daily newborn rounds and pediatric office practice. *Pediatric Clinics of North America, 48,* 299–319.

Blair, A., Cadwell, K., Turner-Maffei, C., & Brimdyr, K. (2003). The relationship between positioning, the breastfeeding dynamic, the latching process and pain in breastfeeding mothers with sore nipples. *Breastfeeding Review, 11,* 5–10.

Bloom, K., Goldbloom, R., Robinson, S., & Stevens, F., II. (1982). Factors affecting breastfeeding. *Acta Paediatrica Scandinavica, 300*(suppl), 9–14.

Bodley, V., & Powers, D. (1996). Long-term nipple shield use: A positive perspective. *Journal of Human Lactation, 12,* 301–304.

Bosma, J. F. (1988). Functional anatomy of the upper airway during development. In O. Mathew & G. Sant'Ambrogio (Eds.), *Respiratory function of the upper airway* (pp. 44, 47–86). New York, NY: Marcel Dekker.

Boukydis, C. F. Z., Bigsby, R., & Lester, B. M. (2004). Clinical use of the neonatal intensive care unit network neurobehavioral scale. *Pediatrics, 113,* 679–689.

Bramson, L., Lee, J. W., Moore, E., Montgomery, S., Neish, C., Bahjri, K., & Melcher, C. L. (2010). Effect of early skin-to-skin mother–infants contact during the first 3 hours following birth on exclusive breastfeeding during the maternity hospital stay. *Journal of Human Lactation, 26,* 130–137.

Brandt, K. A., Andrews, C. M., & Kvale, J. (1998). Mother–infant interaction and breastfeeding outcome 6 weeks after birth. *Journal of Obstetric, Gynecologic, and Neonatal Nursing, 27,* 169–174.

Brigham, M. (1996). Mothers' reports of the outcome of nipple shield use. *Journal of Human Lactation, 12,* 291–297.

Brussel, C. (2001). Considering craniosacral therapy in difficult situations. *Leaven, 37,* 82–83.

Burns, N., & Grove, S. K. (1993). *The practice of nursing research: Conduct, critique and utilization.* Philadelphia, PA: WB Saunders.

Butte, N. F., Jensen, C. L., Moon, J. K., Glaze, D. G., & Frost, J. D., Jr. (1992). Sleep organization and energy expenditure of breast-fed and formula-fed infants. *Pediatric Research, 32,* 514–519.

Cadwell, K. (2007). Latching-on and suckling of the healthy term neonate: Breastfeeding assessment. *Journal of Midwifery and Women's Health, 52,* 638–642.

Cadwell, K., & Turner-Maffei, C. (2004). *Case studies in breastfeeding: Problem-solving skills and strategies.* Sudbury, MA: Jones and Bartlett.

Carroll, D. A., Denenberg, V. H., & Thoman, E. B. (1999). A comparative study of quiet sleep, active sleep, and waking on the first 2 days of life. *Developmental Psychobiology, 35,* 43–48.

Castrucci, B. C., Hoover, K. L., Lim, S., & Maus, K. C. (2006). A comparison of breastfeeding rates in an urban birth cohort among women delivering infants at hospitals that employ and do not employ lactation consultants. *Journal of Public Health Management and Practice, 12,* 578–585.

Celiker, M. Y., & Chawla, A. (2009). Congenital B_{12} deficiency following maternal gastric bypass. *Journal of Perinatology, 29,* 640–642.

Center for Substance Abuse Treatment. (2004). *Clinical guidelines for the use of buprenorphine in the treatment of opioid addiction.* Treatment Improvement Protocol (TIP) series 40 (DHHS Publication No. [SMA] 04-3939). Rockville, MD: Substance Abuse and Mental Health Services Administration.

Chalouhi, C., Faesch, S., Anthoine-Milhomme, M. C., Fulla, Y., Dulac, O., & Cheron, G. (2008). Neurological consequences of vitamin B_{12} deficiency and its treatment. *Pediatric Emergency Care, 24,* 538–541.

Chapman, T., Pincombe, J., & Harris, M. (2013). Antenatal breast expression: A critical review of the literature. *Midwifery, 29,* 203–210.

Chertok, I. R. (2009). Reexamination of ultra-thin nipple shield use, infant growth and maternal satisfaction. *Journal of Clinical Nursing, 18,* 2949–2955.

Chertok, I. R., Raz, I., Shoham, I., Haddad, H., & Wiznitzer, A. (2009). Effects of early breastfeeding on neonatal glucose levels of term infants born to women with gestational diabetes. *Journal of Human Nutrition and Dietetics, 22,* 166–169.

Chertok, I. R., Schneider, J., & Blackburn, S. (2006). A pilot study of maternal and term infant outcomes associated with ultrathin nipple shield use. *Journal of Obstetrics, Gynecology & Neonatal Nursing, 35,* 265–272.

Christensson, K., Siles, C., Moreno, L., Belaustequi, A., De La Fuente, P., Lagercrantz, H., . . . Winberg, J. (1992). Temperature, metabolic adaption and crying in healthy full-term newborns cared for skin-to-skin or in a cot. *Acta Paediatrica, 81,* 488–493.

Christidis, I., Zotter, H., Rosegger, H., Engele, H., Kurz, R., & Kerbel, R. (2003). Infrared thermography in newborns: The first hour after birth. *Bynakol Geburtshilfliche Rundsch, 43,* 31–35.

Chute, G. E. (1992). Promoting breastfeeding success: An overview of basic management. *NAACOG's Clinical Issues in Perinatal & Women's Health Nursing: Breastfeeding, 3,* 570–582.

Clum, D., & Primomo, J. (1996). Use of a silicone nipple shield with premature infants. *Journal of Human Lactation, 12,* 287–290.

Cobb, M. A. B. (2002). A useful algorithm for nurses on a mother/baby unit: Promoting breastfeeding. *AWHONN Lifelines, 6,* 418–423.

Coca, K. P., Gamba, M. A., de Sousa e Silva, R., & Abrao, A. C. (2009). [Does breastfeeding position influence the onset of nipple trauma?]. *Revista de Escola de Enferm USP, 43,* 446–452.

Cohen, S. M. (1998). Congenital hypotonia is not benign: Early recognition and intervention is the key to recovery. *MCN: The American Journal of Maternal/Child Nursing, 23,* 93–98.

Colson, S. (2010). What happens to breastfeeding when mothers lie back? *Clinical Lactation, 1,* 11–14.

Colson, S. D., de Pooy, L., & Hawdon, J. M. (2003). Biological nurturing increases duration of breastfeeding for a vulnerable cohort. *MIDIRS Midwifery Digest, 13,* 92–97.

Colson, S. D., Meek, J. H., & Hawdon, J. M. (2008). Optimal positions for the release of primitive neonatal reflexes stimulating breastfeeding. *Early Human Development, 84,* 441–449.

Cooper, W. O., Willy, M. E., Pont, S. J., & Ray, W. A. (2007). Increasing use of antidepressants in pregnancy. *American Journal of Obstetrics and Gynecology, 196,* 544.e1–5.

Cornblath, M., Hawdon, J. M., Williams, A. F., Aynsley-Green, A., Ward-Platt, M. P., . . . Kalhan, S. C. (2000). Controversies regarding definition of neonatal hypoglycemia: Suggested operational thresholds. *Pediatrics, 105,* 1141–1145.

Cornblath, M., & Ichord, R. (2000). Hypoglycemia in the neonate. *Seminars in Perinatology, 24,* 136–149.

Cowett, R. (1999). Neonatal hypoglycemia: A little goes a long way [Editorial]. *Journal of Pediatrics, 134,* 389–391.

Crenshaw, J. T., Cadwell, K., Brimdyr, K., Widström, A-M., Svensson, K., Champion, J. D., . . . Winslow, E. H. (2012). Use of a video-ethnographic Intervention (PRECESS Immersion Method) to improve skin-to-skin care and breastfeeding rates. *Breastfeeding Medicine, 7,* 69–78.

Csont, G. L., Groth, S., Hopkins, P., & Guillet, R. (2014). An evidence-based approach to breastfeeding neonates at risk for hypoglycemia. *Journal of Obstetric, Gynecologic, and Neonatal Nursing, 43,* 71–81.

Dahlstrom, A., Ebersjo, C., & Lundell, B. (2004). Nicotine exposure in breastfed infants. *Acta Paediatrica, 93,* 810–816.

Dahlstrom, A., Ebersjo, C., & Lundell, B. (2008). Nicotine in breast milk influences heart rate variability. *Acta Paediatrica, 97,* 1075–1079.

Danner, S. C., & Cerutti, E. R. (1984). *Nursing your neurologically impaired baby.* Waco, TX: Childbirth Graphics.

Demirci, J. R., Bogen, D. L., & Klionsky, Y. (2015). Breastfeeding and methadone therapy: The maternal experience. *Substance Abuse, 36,* 203–208.

DeNicola, M. (1986). One case of nipple shield addiction. *Journal of Human Lactation, 2,* 28–29.

Depuy, A. M., Coassolo, K. M., Som, D. A., & Smulian, J. C. (2009). Neonatal hypoglycemia in term, nondiabetic pregnancies. *American Journal of Obstetrics and Gynecology, 200,* e45–e51.

Desmarais, L., & Browne, S. (1990). Inadequate weight gain in breastfeeding infants: Assessments and resolutions. *Lactation Consultant Series Unit 8.* Garden City Park, NY: Avery.

D'Harlingue, A. E., & Durand, D. J. (1993). Recognition, stabilization and transport of the high-risk newborn. In M. H. Klaus & A. A. Fanaroff (Eds.), *Care of the high risk neonate* (pp. 62–85). Philadelphia, PA: Saunders.

Di Scipio, W., Kaslon, J. K., & Ruben, R. J. (1978). Traumatically acquired conditioned dysphagia in children. *Annals of Otology, Rhinology, & Laryngology, 87,* 509–514.

DiFranza, J. R., Aligne, C. A., & Weitzman, M. (2004). Prenatal and postnatal environmental tobacco smoke exposure and children's health. *Pediatrics, 113,* 1007–1015.

DiGirolamo, A. M., Grummer-Strawn, L. M., & Fein, S. B. (2003). Do perceived attitudes of physicians and hospital staff affect breastfeeding decisions? *Birth, 30,* 94–100.

DiGirolamo, A. M., Grummer-Strawn, L. M., & Fein, S. B. (2008). Effect of maternity-care practices on breastfeeding. *Pediatrics, 122*(suppl 2), S43–S49.

Diwakar, K. K., & Sasidhar, M. V. (2002). Plasma glucose levels in term infants who are appropriate size for gestation and exclusively breastfed. *Archives of Disease in Childhood—Fetal and Neonatal Edition, 87,* F46–F48.

Doucet, S., Soussignan, R., Sagot, P., & Schaal, B. (2007). The "smellscape" of mother's breast: Effects of odor masking and selective unmasking on neonatal arousal, oral, and visual responses. *Developmental Psychobiology, 49,* 129–138.

Dowling, D., & Thanattherakul, W. (2001). Nipple confusion, alternative feeding methods, and breastfeeding supplementation: State of the science. *Newborn Infant Nursing Reviews, 1,* 217–223.

Driscoll, J. W. (1992). Breastfeeding success and failure: Implications for nurses. *NAACOG's Clinical Issues in Perinatal & Women's Health Nursing: Breastfeeding, 3,* 565–569.

Dryden, C., Young, D., Hepburn, M., & Mactier, H. (2009). Maternal methadone use in pregnancy: Factors associated with the development of neonatal abstinence syndrome and implications for healthcare resources. *British Journal of Obstetrics and Gynecology, 116,* 665–671.

Durand, R., Hodges, S., LaRock, S., Lund, L., Schmid, S., Swick, D., . . . Perez, A. (1997, March/April). The effect of skin-to-skin breastfeeding in the immediate recovery period on newborn thermoregulation and blood glucose values. *Neonatal Intensive Care,* 23–29.

Ebersold, S. L., Murphy, S. D., Paterno, M. T., Sauvager, M. D., & Wright, E. M. (2007). Nurses and breastfeeding: Are you being supportive? *Nursing for Women's Health, 11,* 482–487.

Eglash, A., Ziemer, A. L., & McKechnie, A. C. (2010). Health professionals' attitudes and use of nipple shields for breastfeeding women. *Breastfeeding Medicine, 5,* 147–151.

Eidelman, A. I. (2001). Hypoglycemia and the breastfed neonate. *Pediatric Clinics of North America, 48,* 377–387.

Eisenberg, S. R., Bair-Merritt, M. H., Colson, E. R., Heeren, T. C., Geller, N. L., & Corwin, M. J. (2015). Maternal report of advice received for infant care. *Pediatrics, 136,* e315–e322.

Eishima, K. (1991). The analysis of sucking behavior in newborn infants. *Early Human Development, 27,* 163–173.

Ekstrom, A., Abrahamsson, H., Eriksson, R-M., & Martensson, B. L. (2014). Women's use of nipple shields: Their influence on breastfeeding duration after a process-oriented education for health professionals. *Breastfeeding Medicine, 9,* 458–466.

Elder, M. S. (1970). The effects of temperature and position on the sucking pressure of newborn infants. *Child Development, 41,* 95–102.

Epstein, R. A., Bobo, W. V., Martin, P. R., Morrow, J. A., Wang, W., Chandrasekhar, R., & Cooper, W. O. (2013). Increasing pregnancy-related use of prescribed opioid analgesics. *Annals of Epidemiology. 23,* 498–503.

Escott, R. (1989, May). Positioning, attachment and milk transfer. *Breastfeeding Review, 1,* 31–36.

Ferber, S. G., & Makhoul, I. R. (2004). The effect of skin-to-skin contact (kangaroo care) shortly after birth on neurobehavioral responses of the term newborn: A randomized controlled trial. *Pediatrics, 113,* 858–865.

Fernandez, I. O., Gabriel, M. M., Martinez, A. M., Fernandez-Canadas Morillo, A., Lopez Sanchez, F., & Costarelli, V. (2012). Newborn feeding behaviour depressed by intrapartum oxytocin: A pilot study. *Acta Paediatrica, 101,* 749–754.

Ferreira, E., Carceller, A. M., Agogue, C., Martin, B. Z., St-Andre, M., Francoeur, D., & Berard, A. (2007). Effects of selective serotonin reuptake inhibitors and venlafaxine during pregnancy in term and preterm neonates. *Pediatrics, 119,* 52–59.

Forster, D. A., McEgan, K., Ford, R., Moorhead, A., Opie, G., Walker, S., & McNamara, C. (2011). Diabetes and antenatal milk expressing: A pilot project to inform the development of a randomized controlled trial. *Midwifery, 27,* 209–214.

Frantz, K. B., & Kalmen, B. A. (1979, December). Breastfeeding works for cesareans too. *RN, 42*(12), 39–47.

Freudigman, K., & Thoman, E. B. (1994). Ultradian and diurnal cyclicity in the sleep states of newborn infants during the first two postnatal days. *Early Human Development, 38,* 67–80.

Freudigman, K. A., & Thoman, E. B. (1998). Infants' earliest sleep/wake organization differs as a function of delivery mode. *Early Human Development, 32,* 293–303.

Friedman, F., Adrouche-Amrani, L., & Holzman, I. R. (2015). Breastfeeding and delivery room neonatal collapse. *Journal of Human Lactation, 31,* 230–232.

Froh, E. B., Flynn-Roth, R., Barton, S., & Spatz, D. L. (2015). The voices of breastfeeding resource nurses. *Journal of Obstetric, Gynecologic and Neonatal Nursing, 44,* 419–425.

Gabriel, M. A. M., Fernandez, I. O., Martinez, A. M. M., Armengod, C. G., Costarelli, V., Santos, I. M., . . . Murillo, L. G. (2015). Intrapartum synthetic oxytocin reduces the expression of primitive reflexes associated with breastfeeding. *Breastfeeding Medicine, 10,* 209–213.

Gabriely, I., Wozniak, R., Mevorach, M., Kaplan, J., Aharon, Y., & Shamoon, H. (1999). Transcutaneous glucose measurement using near-infrared spectroscopy during hypoglycemia. *Diabetes Care, 22,* 2026–2032.

Genna, C. W. (2001). Tactile defensiveness and other sensory modulation difficulties. *Leaven, 37,* 51–53.

Genna, C. W. (2013). *Supporting sucking skills in breastfeeding infants.* Burlington, MA: Jones & Bartlett Learning.

Geraghty, S. R., McNamara, K., Kwiek, J. J., Rogers, L., Klebanoff, M. A., Augustine, M., & Keim, S. A. (2015). Tobacco metabolites and caffeine in human milk purchased via the Internet. *Breastfeeding Medicine, 10,* 419–424.

Gewolb, I. H., Fishman, D., Qureshi, M. A., & Voce, F. L. (2004). Coordination of suck–swallow–respiration in infants born to mothers with drug-abuse problems. *Developmental Medicine and Child Neurology, 46,* 700–705.

Gill, S. L. (2001). The little things: Perceptions of breastfeeding support. *Journal of Obstetric, Gynecologic, and Neonatal Nursing, 30,* 401–409.

Goldade, K., Nichter, M., Nichter, M., Adrian, S., Tesler, L., & Muramoto, M. (2008). Breastfeeding and smoking among low-income women: Results of a longitudinal qualitative study. *Birth, 35,* 230–240.

Goldberg, H., & Nissim, R. (1994). Psychotropic drugs in pregnancy and lactation. *International Journal of Psychiatry in Medicine, 2,* 129–149.

Gomes, C. F., Da Costa Gois, M. L., Oliveira, B. C., Thomson, Z., & Cardoso, J. R. (2013). Surface electromyography in premature infants: A series of case reports and their methodological aspects. *Indian Journal of Pediatrics, 81,* 755–759.

Gomes, C. F., Thomson, Z., & Cardoso, J. R. (2009). Utilization of surface electromyography during the feeding of term and preterm infants: A literature review. *Developmental Medicine & Child Neurology, 51,* 936–942.

Gomez, R. L., Bootzin, R. R., & Nadel, L. (2006). Naps promote abstraction in language-learning infants. *Psychological Science, 17,* 670–674.

Gorman, J. R., Kao, K., & Chambers, C. D. (2012). Breastfeeding among women exposed to antidepressants during pregnancy. *Journal of Human Lactation, 28,* 181–188.

Goyal, R. C., Banginwar, A. S., Ziyo, F., & Toweir, A. A. (2011). Breastfeeding practices: Positioning, attachment (latch-on) and effective suckling: A hospital-based study in Libya. *Journal of Family and Community Medicine, 18,* 74–79.

Graffy, J., & Taylor, J. (2005). What information, advice, and support do women want with breastfeeding? *Birth, 32,* 179–186.

Green, C., Martin, C. W., Bassett, K., & Kazanjian, A. (1999). *A systematic review and critical appraisal of the scientific evidence on craniosacral therapy.* Vancouver, BC: British Columbia Office of Health Technology Assessment.

Hagedorn, M. I. E., & Gardner, S. L. (1999). Hypoglycemia in the newborn, part 1: Pathophysiology and nursing management. *Mother and Baby Journal, 4,* 15–21.

Hale, T. W. (2012). *Medications and mothers' milk* (15th ed.). Amarillo, TX: Hale Publishing.

Hale, T. W., Kendall-Tackett, K., Cong, Z., Votta, R., & McCurdy, F. (2010). Discontinuation syndrome in newborns whose mothers took antidepressants while pregnant or breastfeeding. *Breastfeeding Medicine, 5,* 283–288.

Hankins, G. D. V., Clark, S., & Munn, M. B. (2006). Cesarean section on request at 39 weeks: Impact on shoulder dystocia, fetal trauma, neonatal encephalopathy, and intrauterine fetal demise. *Seminars in Perinatology, 30,* 276–287.

Hanna, S., Wilson, M., & Norwood, S. (2013). A description of breastfeeding outcomes among U.S. mothers using nipple shields. *Midwifery, 29,* 616–621.

Harris, D. L., Weston, P. J., & Harding, J. E. (2015). Lactate, rather than ketones, may provide alternative cerebral fuel in hypoglycaemic newborns. *Archives of Disease in Childhood Fetal Neonatal Edition, 100,* F161–F164.

Harris, H. (1994). Remedial co-bathing for breastfeeding difficulties. *Breastfeeding Review, 2(10),* 465–468.

Healow, L. K., & Hugh, R. S. (2000). Oral aversion in the breastfed neonate. *Breastfeeding Abstracts, 20,* 3–4.

Hewitt, E. G. (1999). Chiropractic care for infants with dysfunctional nursing: A case series. *Journal of Clinical Chiropractic Pediatrics, 4,* 241–244.

Hill, P. (1991). The enigma of insufficient milk supply. *MCN: The American Journal of Maternal/Child Nursing, 16,* 312–316.

Hill, P. D., & Aldag, J. C. (1996). Smoking and breastfeeding status. *Research in Nursing & Health, 19,* 125–132.

Hillervik-Lindquist, C., Hofvander, Y., & Sjolin, S. (1991). Studies on perceived breast milk insufficiency. III. Consequences for breast milk consumption and growth. *Acta Paediatrica Scandinavica, 80,* 297–303.

Hilton, T. C. (2012). Breastfeeding considerations of opioid dependent mothers and infants. *MCN: The American Journal of Maternal/Child Nursing, 37,* 236–240.

Ho, H. T., Yeung, W. K. Y., & Young, B. W. Y. (2004). Evaluation of "point of care" devices in the measurement of low blood glucose in neonatal practice. *Archives of Disease in Childhood—Fetal and Neonatal Edition, 89*(4), F356–F359.

Holleman, A. C., Chiro, M., Nee, J., & Knaap, S. F. C. (2011). Chiropractic management of breastfeeding difficulties: A case report. *Journal of Chiropractic Medicine, 10,* 199–203.

Holtrop, D. P. (2000). Resolution of suckling intolerance in a 6-month-old chiropractic patient. *Journal of Manipulative Physiological and Therapeutics, 23,* 615–618.

Hong, T. M., Callister, L. C., & Schwartz, R. (2003). First-time mothers' views of breastfeeding support from nurses. *MCN: The American Journal of Maternal/Child Nursing, 28,* 10–15.

Honzik, T., Adamovicova, M., Smolka, V., Magner, M., Hruba, E., & Zeman, J. (2010). Clinical presentation and metabolic consequences in 40 breastfed infants with nutritional vitamin B_{12} deficiency: What have we learned? *European Journal of Paediatric Neurology, 14,* 488–495.

Hopkinson, J. M., Schanler, R. J., Fraley, J. K., & Garza, C. (1992). Milk production by mothers of premature infants: Influence of cigarette smoking. *Pediatrics, 90,* 934–938.

Horne, R. S. C., Parslow, P. M., Ferens, D., Watts, A., & Adamson, T. (2004). Comparison of evoked arousability in breast and formula fed infants. *Archives of Disease in Childhood, 89*(1), 22–25.

Hoseth, E., Joergensen, A., Ebbesen, F., & Moeller, M. (2000). Blood glucose levels in a population of healthy, breastfed, term infants of appropriate size for gestational age. *Archives of Disease in Childhood—Fetal and Neonatal Edition, 83,* F117–F119.

Humenick, S. S., Hill, P. D., & Hart, A. M. (1998). Evaluation of a pillow designed to promote breastfeeding. *Journal of Perinatal Education, 7,* 25–31.

Ilett, K. F., Hackett, L. P., Gower, S., Doherty, D. A., Hamilton, D., & Bartu, A. E. (2012). Estimated dose exposure of the neonate to buprenorphine and its metabolite norbuprenorphine via breastmilk during maternal buprenorphine substitution treatment. *Breastfeeding Medicine, 7,* 269–274.

Inoue, N., Sakashita, R., & Kamegai, T. (1995). Reduction of masseter muscle activity in bottle-fed infants. *Early Human Development, 42,* 185–193.

Jansson, L., Velez, M., & Harrow, C. (2004). Methadone maintenance and lactation: A review of the literature and current management guidelines. *Journal of Human Lactation, 20*(1), 62–71.

Jansson, L. M., Choo, R., Velez, M. L., Lowe, R., & Huestis, M. A. (2008). Methadone maintenance and long-term lactation. *Breastfeeding Medicine, 3,* 34–37.

Jean, A. (2001). Brain stem control of swallowing: Neuronal network and cellular mechanisms. *Physiological Review, 81,* 929–969.

Jonas, W., Johansson, L. M., Nissen, E., Ejdeback, M., Ransjo-Arvidson, A. B., & Uvnas-Moberg, K. (2009). Effects of intrapartum oxytocin administration and epidural analgesia on the concentration of plasma oxytocin and prolactin in response to suckling during the second day postpartum. *Breastfeeding Medicine, 4*(2), 71–82.

Jordan, A. E., Jackson, G. L., Deardorff, D., Shivakumar, G., McIntire, D. D., & Dashe, J. S. (2008). Serotonin reuptake inhibitor use in pregnancy and the neonatal behavioral syndrome. *Journal of Maternal–Fetal and Neonatal Medicine, 21,* 745–751.

Kakko, J., Heilig, M., & Sarman, I. (2008). Buprenorphine and methadone treatment of opiate dependence during pregnancy: Comparison of fetal growth and neonatal outcomes in two consecutive case series. *Drug and Alcohol Dependence, 96,* 69–78.

Kalhan, S., & Peter-Wohl, S. (2000). Hypoglycemia: What is it for the neonate? *American Journal of Perinatology, 17,* 11–18.

Kandall, S. (1995). Treatment options for drug-exposed infants. *NIDA Research Monographs, 149,* 78–99.

Kaplan, M., & Eidelman, A. I. (1985). Improved prognosis in severely hypothermic newborns treated by rapid rewarming. *Journal of Pediatrics, 105,* 515–518.

Karl, D. J. (2004). Using principles of newborn behavioral state organization to facilitate breastfeeding. *MCN: The American Journal of Maternal/Child Nursing, 29,* 292–298.

Karl, D. J., Beal, J. A., O'Hare, C. M., & Rissmiller, P. N. (2006). Reconceptualizing the nurse's role in the newborn period as an "attacher." *MCN: The American Journal of Maternal/Child Nursing, 31,* 257–262.

Keim, S. A., Daniels, J. L., Siega-Riz, A. M., Dole, N., Herring, A. H., & Scheidt, P. C. (2012). Depressive symptoms during pregnancy and the concentration of fatty acids in breast milk. *Journal of Human Lactation, 28,* 189–195.

Kelmanson, I. A., Erman, L. V., & Litvina, S. V. (2002). Maternal smoking during pregnancy and behavioural characteristics in 2–4 month-old infants. *Klinische Padiatrie, 214,* 359–364.

Kendall-Tackett, K., & Hale, T. W. (2010). The use of antidepressants in pregnant and breastfeeding women: A review of recent studies. *Journal of Human Lactation, 26,* 187–195.

Kieviet, N., Hoppenbrouwers, C., Dolman, K. M., Berkof, J., Wennink, H., & Honig, A. (2015). Risk factors for poor neonatal adaptation after exposure to antidepressants in utero. *Acta Paediatrica, 104,* 384–391.

Kocherlakota, P. (2014). Neonatal abstinence syndrome. *Pediatrics, 134,* e547–e556.

Kronborg, H., & Vaeth, M. (2009). How are effective breastfeeding technique and pacifier use related to breastfeeding problems and breastfeeding duration? *Birth, 36,* 34–42.

Kutner, L. (1986). Nipple shield consent form: A teaching aid. *Journal of Human Lactation, 2,* 25–27.

Lattimore, K. A., Donn, S. M., Kaciroti, N., Kemper, A. R., Neal, C. R., Jr., & Vazquez, D. M. (2005). Selective serotonin reuptake inhibitor (SSRI) use during pregnancy and effects on the fetus and newborn: A meta-analysis. *Journal of Perinatology, 25,* 595–604.

Law, K. L., Stroud, L. R., LaGasse, L. L., Niaura, R., Liu. J., & Lester, B. M. (2003). Smoking during pregnancy and newborn neurobehavior. *Pediatrics, 111,* 1318–1323.

Lester, B. M., Tronick, E. Z., & Brazelton, T. B. (2004). The neonatal intensive care unit network neurobehavioral scale procedures. *Pediatrics, 113,* 641–667.

Lester, B. M., Tronick, E. Z., LaGasse, L. L., Seifer, R., Bauer, C. R., Shankaran, S., . . . Maza, P. L. (2002). The Maternal Lifestyle Study (MLS): Effects of substance exposure during pregnancy on neurodevelopmental outcome in 1-month-old infants. *Pediatrics, 110,* 1182–1192.

Leurer, M. D., & Misskey, E. (2015). "Be positive as well as realistic": A qualitative description analysis of information gaps experienced by breastfeeding mothers. *International Breastfeeding Journal, 10,* 10.

Levrini, L., Merlo, P., & Paracchini, L. (2007). Different geometric patterns of pacifiers compared on the basis of finite element analysis. *European Journal of Paediatric Dentistry, 8,* 173–178.

Linder, N., Maser, A. M., Asli, I., Gale, R., Livoff, A., & Tamir, I. (1989). Suckling stimulation test for neonatal tremor. *Archives of Disease in Childhood, 64,* 44–46.

Liu, J., Rosenberg, K. D., & Sandoval, A. P. (2006). Breastfeeding duration and perinatal cigarette smoking in a population-based cohort. *American Journal of Public Health, 96,* 309–314.

Liu, Y. Q., Qian, Z., Wang, J., Lu, T., Lin, S., Zeng, X. W., . . . Dong, G. H. (2015). Breastfeeding modifies the effects of environment tobacco smoke (ETS) exposure on respiratory diseases and symptoms in Chinese children: The Seven Northeast Cities (SNEC) Study. *Indoor Air.* [Epub ahead of print]. doi: 10.1111/ina.12240

Lothian, J. A. (1995). It takes two to breastfeed: The baby's role in successful breastfeeding. *Journal of Nurse Midwifery, 40,* 328–334.

Macfarlane, A. (1975). Olfaction in the development of social preferences in the human neonate. In R. Porter & M. O'Connor (Eds.), *Parent–infant interaction* (pp. 103–113). Ciba Foundation Symposium 33. New York, NY: Elsevier.

Macknin, M. L., Medendorp, S. V., & Maier, M. C. (1989). Infant sleep and bedtime cereal. *American Journal of Diseases of Children, 143,* 1066–1068.

Makin, J. W., & Porter, R. H. (1989). Attractiveness of lactating females' breast odors to neonates. *Child Development, 60,* 803–810.

Mannel, R., & Mannel, R. S. (2006). Staffing for hospital lactation programs: Recommendations from a tertiary care teaching hospital. *Journal of Human Lactation, 22,* 409–417.

Mantha, S., Davies, B., Moyer, A., & Crowe, K. (2008). Providing responsive nursing care to new mothers with high and low confidence. *MCN: The American Journal of Maternal/Child Nursing, 33,* 307–314.

Marchini, G., & Linden, A. (1992). Cholecystokinin, a satiety signal in newborn infants? *Journal of Developmental Physiology, 17,* 215–219.

Marchini, G., Simoni, M. R., Bartolini, F., & Linden, A. (1993). The relationship of plasma cholecystokinin levels to different feeding routines in newborn infants. *Early Human Development, 35,* 31–35.

Marder, E., & Bucher, D. (2001). Central pattern generators and the control of rhythmic movements. *Current Biology, 11,* 986–996.

Marmet, C., & Shell, E. (2008). Therapeutic positioning for breastfeeding. In C. W. Genna (Ed.), *Supporting sucking skills in breastfeeding infants* (pp. 359–377). Sudbury, MA: Jones and Bartlett.

Marshall, A. M., Nommsen-Rivers, L. A., Hernandez, L. L., Dewey, K. G., Chantry, C. J., Gregerson, K. A., & Horseman, N. D. (2010). Serotonin transport and metabolism in the mammary gland modulates secretory activity and involution. *Journal of Clinical Endocrinology and Metabolism, 95,* 837–846.

Matheson, I., & Rivrud, G. N. (1989). The effect of smoking on lactation and infantile colic. *Journal of the American Medical Association, 261,* 42–43.

Matthews, M. K. (1991). Mothers' satisfaction with their neonates' breastfeeding behaviors. *Journal of Obstetric, Gynecologic, and Neonatal Nursing, 20,* 49–55.

Mauch, C. E., Scott, J. A., Magarey, A. M., & Daniels, L. A. (2012). Predictors of and reasons for pacifier use in first-time mothers: An observational study. *BMC Pediatrics, 12,* 7.

McAllister, H., Bradshaw, S., & Ross-Adjie, G. (2009). A study of in-hospital midwifery practices that affect breast-feeding outcomes. *Breastfeeding Review, 17,* 11–15.

McDermott, C. M., Lahoste, G. J., Chen, C., Musto, A., Bazan, N. G., & Magee, J. C. (2003). Sleep deprivation causes behavioral, synaptic, and membrane excitability alterations in hippocampal neurons. *Journal of Neuroscience, 23,* 9687–9695.

McInnes, R. J., & Chambers, J. A. (2008). Supporting breastfeeding mothers: Qualitative synthesis. *Journal of Advanced Nursing, 62,* 407–427.

McKechnie, A. C., & Eglash, A. (2010). Nipple shields: A review of the literature. *Breastfeeding Medicine, 5,* 309–314.

McKenna, J. J., Mosko, S., Dungy, C., & McAninch, J. (1990). Sleep and arousal patterns of co-sleeping human mother/infant pairs: A preliminary physiological study with implications for the study of sudden infant death syndrome (SIDS). *American Journal of Physical Anthropology, 83,* 331–347.

McQueen, K. A., Murphy-Oikonen, J., Gerlach, K., Montelpare, W. (2011). The impact of infant feeding method on neonatal abstinence scores of methadone-exposed infants. *Advances in Neonatal Care, 11,* 282–290.

Medoff-Cooper, B. (1991). Changes in nutritive sucking patterns with increasing gestational age. *Nursing Research, 40,* 245–247.

Medoff-Cooper, B., Weininger, S., & Zukowsky, K. (1989). Neonatal sucking as a clinical assessment tool: Preliminary findings. *Nursing Research, 38,* 162–165.

Meier, P. P., Brown, L. P., Hurst, N. M., Spatz, D. L., Engstrom, J. L., Borucki, L. C., & Krouse, A. M. (2000). Nipple shields for preterm infants: Effect on milk transfer and duration of breastfeeding. *Journal of Human Lactation, 16,* 106–113.

Meloy, L., Miller, G., Chandrasekaran, M., Summitt, C., & Gutcher, G. (1999). Accuracy of glucose reflectance testing for detecting hypoglycemia in term newborns. *Clinical Pediatrics, 38,* 717–724.

Mennella, J. A., & Beauchamp, G. K. (1998). Smoking and the flavor of breast milk. *New England Journal of Medicine, 339,* 1559–1560.

Mennella, J. A., Yourshaw, L. M., & Morgan, L. K. (2007). Breastfeeding and smoking: Short-term effects on infant feeding and sleep. *Pediatrics, 120,* 497–502.

Meyer, K., & Anderson, G. C. (1999). Using kangaroo care in a clinical setting with full term infants having breastfeeding difficulties. *MCN: The American Journal of Maternal/Child Nursing, 24,* 190–192.

Michelsson, K., Christensson, K., Rothganger, H., & Winberg, J. (1996). Crying in separated and nonseparated newborns: Sound spectrographic analysis. *Acta Paediatrica, 85,* 471–475.

Millard, A. V. (1990). The place of the clock in pediatric advice: Rationales, cultural themes, and impediments to breastfeeding. *Social Science & Medicine, 31,* 211–221.

Miller, A. S., Telford, A. C. J., Huizinga, B., Pinkster, M., ten Heggeler, J., & Miller, J. E. (2015). What breastfeeding mothers want: Specific contextual help. *Clinical Lactation, 6,* 117–123.

Minchin, M. (1998). *Breastfeeding matters* (4th ed., pp. 84–89, 142–147). St. Kilda, BC: Alma.

Mizuno, K., Fujimaki, K., & Sawada, M. (2004). Sucking behavior at breast during the early newborn period affects later breastfeeding rate and duration of breastfeeding. *Pediatrics International, 46,* 15–20.

Mizuno, K., Inoue, M., & Takeuchi, T. (2000). The effects of body positioning on sucking behaviour in sick neonates. *European Journal of Pediatrics, 159,* 827–831.

Mizuno, K., Nishida, Y., Mizuno, N., Taki, M., Murase, M., & Itabashi, K. (2008). The important role of deep attachment in the uniform drainage of breast milk from mammary lobe. *Acta Paediatrica, 97,* 1200–1204.

Mizuno, K., & Ueda, A. (2004). Antenatal olfactory learning influences infant feeding. *Early Human Development, 76,* 83–90.

Mobbs, E. G. (1989, May). Human imprinting and breastfeeding: Are the textbooks deficient? *Breastfeeding Review, 1*(14), 39–41.

Mobbs, E. J., Mobbs, G. A., & Mobbs, A. E. D. (2015). Imprinting, latchment and displacement: A mini review of early instinctual behavior in newborn infants influencing breastfeeding success. *Acta Paediatrica.* [Epub ahead of print]. doi: 10.1111/apa.13034

Morton, J. A. (1992). Ineffective suckling: A possible consequence of obstructive positioning. *Journal of Human Lactation, 8,* 83–85.

Mozingo, J. N., Davis, M. W., Droppleman, P. G., & Merideth, A. (2000). "It wasn't working": Women's experiences with short-term breastfeeding. *MCN: The American Journal of Maternal/Child Nursing, 25,* 120–126.

National Association of Neonatal Nurses. (1994). *Neonatal hypoglycemia guidelines for practice.* Petaluma, CA: Author.

Neifert, M. R. (2001). Prevention of breastfeeding tragedies. *Pediatric Clinics of North America, 48,* 273–297.

Neifert, M. R., Lawrence, R., & Seacat, J. (1995). Nipple confusion: Toward a formal definition. *Journal of Pediatrics, 126,* S125–S129.

Nicholl, R. (2003). What is the normal range of blood glucose concentrations for healthy term newborns? *Archives of Disease in Childhood, 88,* 238–239.

Nichols, F. H., & Zwelling, E. (1997). *Maternal–newborn nursing: Theory and practice.* Philadelphia, PA: Saunders.

Noerr, B. (2001). State of the science: Neonatal hypoglycemia. *Advances in Neonatal Care, 1,* 4–21.

Nowak, A. J., Smith, W. L., & Erenberg, A. (1995). Imaging evaluation of breast-feeding and bottle-feeding systems. *Journal of Pediatrics, 126,* S130–S134.

Nyqvist, K. H. (2001). The development of preterm infants' milk intake during breastfeeding: Influence of gestational age. *Journal of Neonatal Nursing, 7,* 48–52.

O'Connor, A., Alto, W., Musgrave, K., Gibbons, D., Llanto, L., Holden, S., & Karnes, J. (2011). Observational study of buprenorphine treatment of opioid-dependent pregnant women in a family medicine residency: Reports on maternal and infant outcomes. *Journal of the American Board of Family Medicine, 24,* 194–201.

Oder, A. L., Stalling, D. L., & Barlow, S. M. (2013). Short-term effects of pacifier texture on NNS in neurotypical infants. *International Journal of Pediatrics, 2013,* Article ID 168459. doi: 10.1155/2013/168459.

Orsolini, L., & Bellantuono, C. (2015). Serotonin reuptake inhibitors and breastfeeding: A systematic review. *Human Psychopharmacology, 30,* 4–20.

Ozkan, H., Tuzan, F., Kumral, A., Yesilirmak, D., & Duman, N. (2008). Increased sleep tendency in jaundiced infants: Role of endogenous CO. *Medical Hypotheses, 71,* 879–880.

Peirano, P., Algarin, C., & Uauy, R. (2003). Sleep–wake states and their regulatory mechanisms throughout early human development. *Journal of Pediatrics, 143,* S70–S79.

Perrella, S. L., Lai, C. T., & Geddes, D. T. (2015). Case report of nipple shield trauma associated with breastfeeding an infant with high intra-oral vacuum. *BMC Pregnancy and Childbirth, 15,* 155.

Pinilla, T., & Birch, L. L. (1993). Help me make it through the night: Behavioral entrainment of breast-fed infants' sleep patterns. *Pediatrics, 91,* 436–444.

Porter, R. H., Makin, J. W., Davis, L. B., & Christensen, K. M. (1991). An assessment of the salient olfactory environment of formula-fed infants. *Physiology & Behavior, 50,* 907–911.

Porter, R. H., & Winberg, J. (1999). Unique salience of maternal breast odors for newborn infants. *Neuroscience & Biobehavioral Reviews, 23,* 439–449.

Powers, D., & Tapia, V. B. (2004). Women's experiences using a nipple shield. *Journal of Human Lactation, 20,* 327–334.

Powers, N. G. (1999). Slow weight gain and low milk supply in the breastfeeding dyad. *Clinics in Perinatology, 26,* 399–430.

Powers, N. G., & Slusser, W. (1997). Breastfeeding update 2: Clinical lactation management. *Pediatrics in Review, 18,* 147–161.

Prasad, A. N., & Prasad, C. (2003). The floppy infant: Contribution of genetic and metabolic disorders. *Brain and Development, 25,* 457–476.

Pritham, U. A. (2013). Breastfeeding promotion for management of neonatal abstinence syndrome. *Journal of Obstetric, Gynecologic, and Neonatal Nursing, 42,* 517–526.

Raith, W., Schmolzer, G. M., Resch, B., Reiterer, F., Avian, A., Koestenberger, M., & Uriesberger, B. (2015). Laser acupuncture for neonatal abstinence syndrome: A randomized controlled trial. *Pediatrics, 136,* 876–884.

Ransjo-Arvidson, A. B., Matthiesen, A. S., Lilja, G., Nissen, E., Widström, A. M., & Uvnas-Moberg, K. (2001). Maternal analgesia during labor disturbs newborn behavior: Effects on breastfeeding, temperature, and crying. *Birth, 28,* 5–12.

Reece-Stremtan, S., Marinelli, K. A., & American Academy of Breastfeeding Medicine. (2015). ABM clinical protocol #21: Guidelines for breastfeeding and substance use or substance use disorder, revised 2015. *Breastfeeding Medicine, 10,* 135–141.

Reisman, J. (2002). Sensory processing disorders. *Minnesota Medicine, 85*(11), 48–51.

Righard, L., & Alade, M. O. (1990). Effect of delivery room routines on success of first breast-feed. *Lancet, 336,* 1105–1107.

Roffwarg, H. P., Muzio, J. N., & Dement, W. C. (1966). Ontogenetic development of the human sleep–dream cycle. *Science, 152,* 604–619.

Romano, A. M., & Goer, H. (2008). Research summaries for normal birth. *Journal of Perinatal Education, 17,* 55–60.

Ross, E., & Fuhrman, L. (2015). Supporting oral feeding skills through bottle selection. *Perspectives on Swallowing and Swallowing Disorders (Dysphagia), 24,* 50–57.

Ruchala, P. L. (2000). Teaching new mothers: Priorities of nurses and postpartum women. *Journal of Obstetric, Gynecologic, and Neonatal Nursing, 29,* 265–273.

Sadeh, A., Dark, I., & Vohr, B. R. (1996). Newborns' sleep–wake patterns: The role of maternal, delivery and infant factors. *Early Human Development, 44,* 113–126.

Salariya, E. M., & Robertson, C. M. (1993). The development of a neonatal stool colour comparator. *Midwifery, 9,* 35–40.

Salisbury, A. L., Wisner, K. L., Pearlstein, T., Battle, C. L., Stroud, L., & Lester, B. M. (2011). Newborn neurobehavioral patterns are differentially related to prenatal maternal major depressive disorder and serotonin reuptake inhibitor treatment. *Depression and Anxiety, 28,* 1008–1019.

Schaefer-Graf, U. M., Rossi, R., Buhrer, C., Siebert, G., Kjos, S. L., Dudenhausen, J. W., & Vetter, K. (2002). Rate and risk factors of hypoglycemia in large-for-gestational-age newborn infants of nondiabetic mothers. *American Journal of Obstetrics & Gynecology, 187,* 913–917.

Schechtman, V. L., Harper, R. M., Wilson, A. J., & Southall, D. P. (1992). Sleep state organization in normal infants and victims of the sudden infant death syndrome. *Pediatrics, 89,* 865–870.

Schmied, V., Beake, S., Sheehan, A., McCourt, C., & Dykes, F. (2011). Women's perceptions and experiences of breastfeeding support: A metasynthesis. *Birth, 38,* 49–60.

Segami, Y., Mizuno, K., Taki, M., & Itabashi, K. (2013). Perioral movements and sucking pattern during bottle feeding with a novel, experimental teat are similar to breastfeeding. *Journal of Perinatology, 33,* 319–323.

Sexon, W. R. (1984). Incidence of neonatal hypoglycemia: A matter of definition. *Journal of Pediatrics, 105,* 149–150.

Shenassa, E. D., & Brown M.-J. (2004). Maternal smoking and infantile gastrointestinal dysregulation. *Pediatrics, 114,* e497–e505.

Sherer, D. M., Metlay, L. A., & Woods, J. R. (1995). Lack of mandibular movement manifested by absent fetal swallowing: A possible factor in the pathogenesis of micrognathia. *American Journal of Perinatology, 12,* 30–33.

Shisler, S., Homish, G. G., Molnar, D. S., Schuetze, P., Colder, C. R., & Eiden, R. D. (2015). Predictors of changes in smoking from 3rd trimester to 9 months postpartum. *Nicotine Tobacco Research.* [Epub ahead of print]. doi: 10.1093/ntr/ntv057

Shrago, L., & Bocar, D. (1990). The infant's contribution to breastfeeding. *Journal of Obstetric, Gynecologic, and Neonatal Nursing, 19,* 209–215.

Sirkin, A., Jalloh, T., & Lee, L. (2002). Selecting an accurate point-of-care testing system: Clinical and technical issues and implications in neonatal blood glucose monitoring. *Journal for Specialists in Pediatric Nursing, 7,* 104–112.

Sjolin, S., Hofvander, Y., & Hillervik, C. (1977). Factors related to early termination of breastfeeding: A retrospective study in Sweden. *Acta Paediatrica Scandinavica, 66,* 505–511.

Sjolin, S., Hofvander, Y., & Hillervik, C. (1979). A prospective study of individual courses of breastfeeding. *Acta Paediatrica Scandinavica, 68,* 521–529.

Smith, L. (2004). Physics, forces, and mechanical effects of birth on breastfeeding. In M. Kroeger (Ed.), *Impact of birthing practices on breastfeeding: Protecting the mother and baby continuum.* Sudbury, MA: Jones and Bartlett.

Spatz, D. L., Froh, E. B., Flynn-Roth, R., & Barton, S. (2015). Improving practice at the point of care through the optimization of the breastfeeding resource nurse model. *Journal of Obstetric, Gynecologic, and Neonatal Nursing, 44,* 412–418.

Stephens, J., & Kotowski, J. (1994). The extrusion reflex: Its relevance to early breastfeeding. *Breastfeeding Review, 2,* 418–421.

Stroud, L. R., Paster, R. L., Papandonatos, G. D., Niaura, R., Salisbury, A. L., Battle, C., . . . Lester, B. (2009). Maternal smoking during pregnancy and newborn behavior: Effects at 10 to 27 days. *Journal of Pediatrics, 154,* 10–16.

Substance Abuse and Mental Health Services Administration. (2014). *Results from the 2013 National Survey on Drug Use and Health: Summary of National Findings.* NSDUH Series H-48, HHS Publication No. (SMA) 14-4863. Rockville, MD: Author.

Sweet, D. G., Hadden, D., & Halliday, H. L. (1999). The effect of early feeding on the neonatal blood glucose level at 1 hour of age. *Early Hum Development, 55,* 63–66.

Taveras, E. M., Li, R., Grummer-Strawn, L., Richardson, M., Marshall, R., Rêgo, V. H., . . . Lieu, T. A. (2004). Opinions and practices of clinicians associated with continuation of exclusive breastfeeding. *Pediatrics, 113,* e283–e290.

Thomas, C., Critchley, L., & Davies, M. (2000). Determining the best method for first-line assessment of neonatal blood glucose levels. *Journal of Paediatrics and Child Health, 36,* 343–348.

Thomas, J., Marinelli, K. A., Hennessy, M., & Academy of Breastfeeding Medicine Protocol Committee. (2007). ABM clinical protocol #16: Breastfeeding the hypotonic infant. *Breastfeed Medicine, 2,* 112–118.

Thompson, C. E. (2002). Benign congenital hypotonia is not a diagnosis. *Letters in Developmental Medicine and Child Neurology, 44,* 283–284.

Tozier, P. K. (2013). Colostrum versus formula supplementation for glucose stabilization in newborns of diabetic mothers. *Journal of Obstetric, Gynecologic, and Neonatal Nursing, 42,* 619–628.

Turney, J. (2002). Tackling birth trauma with cranio-sacral therapy. *Practicing Midwife, 5,* 17–19.

Upledger, J. E. (2003a). Applications of craniosacral therapy in newborns and infants, Part I. Retrieved from http://www.massagetoday.com/archives/2003/05/08.html

Upledger, J. E. (2003b). Applications of craniosacral therapy in newborns and infants, Part II. Retrieved from http://www.massagetoday.com/archives/2003/06/13.html

U.S. Lactation Consultant Association. (2010). International Board Certified Lactation Consultant Staffing Recommendations for the inpatient setting. Retrieved from http://uslca.org/wp-content/uploads/2013/02/IBCLC_Staffing_Recommendations_July_2010.pdf

Uvnas-Moberg, K., Marchini, G., & Winberg, J. (1993). Plasma cholecystokinin concentrations after breastfeeding in healthy 4 day old infants. *Archives of Diseases in Childhood, 68,* 46–48.

Uvnas-Moberg, K., Widström, A. M., Marchini, G., & Winberg, J. (1987). Release of GI hormones in mother and infant by sensory stimulation. *Acta Paediatrica Scandinavica, 76,* 851–860.

Vallone, S. (2004). Chiropractic evaluation and treatment of musculoskeletal dysfunction in infants demonstrating difficulty breastfeeding. *Journal of Clinical Chiropractic Pediatrics, 6(1),* 349–361.

Varendi, H., & Porter, R. H. (2001). Breast odour as the only maternal stimulus elicits crawling towards the odour source. *Acta Paediatrica, 90,* 372–375.

Varendi, H., Porter, R. H., & Winberg, J. (1994). Does the newborn baby find the nipple by smell? *Lancet, 344,* 989–990.

Verronen, P. (1982). Reasons for giving up and transient lactational crises. *Acta Paediatrica Scandinavica, 71,* 447–450.

Vio, F., Salazar, G., & Infante, C. (1991). Smoking during pregnancy and lactation and its effects on breastmilk volume. *American Journal of Clinical Nutrition, 54,* 1011–1016.

Volmanen, P., Valanne, F., & Alahuhta, S. (2004). Breastfeeding problems after epidural analgesia for labour: A retrospective cohort study of pain, obstetrical procedures and breastfeeding practices. *International Journal of Obstetric Anesthesia, 13,* 25–29.

Wachman, E. M., Byun, J., & Philipp, B. L. (2010). Breastfeeding rates among mothers of infants with neonatal abstinence syndrome. *Breastfeeding Medicine, 5,* 159–164.

Walker, M. (1997). Breastfeeding the sleepy baby. *Journal of Human Lactation, 13,* 151–153.

Wall, V., & Glass, R. (2006). Mandibular asymmetry and breastfeeding problems: Experience from 11 cases. *Journal of Human Lactation, 22,* 328–334.

Walters, M. W., Boggs, K. M., Ludington-Hoe, S., Price, K. M., & Morrison, B. (2007). Kangaroo care at birth for full term infants: A pilot study. *MCN: The American Journal of Maternal/Child Nursing, 32,* 375–381.

Weddig, J., Baker, S. S., & Auld, G. (2011). Perspectives of hospital-based nurses on breastfeeding initiation best practices. *Journal of Obstetric, Gynecologic, and Neonatal Nursing, 40,* 166–178.

Weiss-Salinas, D., & Williams, N. (2001). Sensory defensiveness: A theory of its effect on breastfeeding. *Journal of Human Lactation, 17,* 145–151.

Wescott, N. (2004). The use of cranial osteopathy in the treatment of infants with breastfeeding problems or sucking dysfunction. *Australian Journal of Holistic Nursing, 11,* 25–32.

Widström, A.-M., Lilja, G., Aaltomaa-Michalias, P., Dahllòf, A., Lintula, M., & Nissen, E. (2011). Newborn behaviour to locate the breast when skin-to-skin: A possible method for enabling early self-regulation. *Acta Paediatrica, 100,* 79–85.

Widström, A.-M., Ransjo-Arvidson, A. B., Christensson, K., Matthiesen, A. S., Winberg, J., & Uvnas-Moberg K. (1987). Gastric suction in healthy newborn infants. *Acta Paediatrica Scandinavica, 76,* 566–572.

Widström, A.-M., & Thringstrom-Paulsson, J. (1993). The position of the tongue during rooting reflexes elicited in newborn infants before the first suckle. *Acta Paediatrica, 82,* 281–283.

Wiessinger, D. (1998). A breastfeeding teaching tool using a sandwich analogy for latch-on. *Journal of Human Lactation, 14,* 51–56.

Wight, N. E. (2003). Breastfeeding the borderline (near-term) preterm infant. *Pediatric Annals, 32,* 329–336.

Wight, N. E. (2006). Hypoglycemia in breastfed neonates. *Breastfeeding Medicine, 1,* 253–262.

Wight, N., Marinelli, K. A., & Academy of Breastfeeding Medicine. (2014). ABM clinical protocol #1: Guidelines for blood glucose monitoring and treatment of hypoglycemia in term and late-preterm neonates. *Breastfeeding Medicine, 9,* 173–179.

Wilson-Clay, B. (1996). Clinical use of silicone nipple shields. *Journal of Human Lactation, 12,* 279–285.

Wilson-Clay, B. (2003). Nipple shields in clinical practice: A review. *Breastfeeding Abstracts, 22,* 11–12.

Wilson-Clay, B., & Hoover, K. (2002). *The breastfeeding atlas* (2nd ed.). Austin, TX: LactNews Press.

Wolf, L. S., & Glass, R. P. (1992). *Feeding and swallowing disorders of infancy: Assessment and management.* Tucson, AZ: Therapy Skill Builders.

World Health Organization. (1997). *Hypoglycemia of the newborn: Review of the literature* (pp. 30–31). Geneva, Switzerland: Author.

Yolton, K., Khoury, J., Xu, Y., Succop, P., Lanphear, B., Bernert, J. T., & Lester, B. (2009). Low-level exposure to nicotine and infant neurobehavior. *Neurotoxicology and Teratology, 31,* 356–363.

Yonkers, K. A., Wisner, K. L., Stewart, D. E., Oberlander, T. F., Dell, D. L., Stotland, N., . . . Lockwood, C. (2009). The management of depression during pregnancy: A report from the American Psychiatric Association and the American College of Obstetricians and Gynecologists. *General Hospital Psychiatry, 31,* 403–413.

Zanardo, V., & Straface, G. (2015). The higher temperature in the areola supports the natural progression of the birth to breastfeeding continuum. *PLoS One, 10*(3), e0118774.

Zander, K. (1991). Care maps: The core of cost/quality care. *New Definition, 6,* 9–11.

Zander, K. (1992). Quantifying, managing, and improving quality: How CareMaps link CQI to the patient. *New Definition, 7,* 1–3.

Zeskind, P. S., & Stephens, L. E. (2004). Maternal selective serotonin reuptake inhibitor use during pregnancy and newborn neurobehavior. *Pediatrics, 113,* 368–375.

Zimmerman, E., & Thompson, K. (2015). Clarifying nipple confusion. *Journal of Perinatology, 35,* 895–899.

ADDITIONAL READING AND RESOURCES

The Academy of Breastfeeding Medicine has developed protocols on common clinical issues, including the one on hypoglycemia referenced in this chapter, as guidelines for the care of breastfeeding infants and their mothers. Full-text versions of all the Academy of Breastfeeding Medicine's protocols are available at http://www.bfmed.org/Resources/Protocols.aspx.

Infant Sleep Resources

Heinig, M. J., Banuelos, J., Goldbronn, J., & Kampp, J. (2009). FitWIC baby behavior study. UC Davis Human Lactation Center, Department of Nutrition. Retrieved from http://www.nal.usda.gov/wicworks/Sharing_Center/gallery/FitWICBaby.htm

Clinical Algorithms

University of North Carolina Lactation Program, http://www.mombaby.org/index.php?c=2&s=30&p=623

Lee, K. G. (2008). Breastfeeding and the premature infant. In D. Brodsky & M. A. Ouellette (Eds.), *Primary care of the premature infant* (pp. 61–69). Philadelphia, PA: Saunders. https://www.preemietoolkit.com/pdfs/Nutrition_and_Feeding/Algorithm_For_Breastfeeding_The_Late_Preterm_Infant.pdf

Massachusetts Breastfeeding Coalition Lactation management for mobile platforms, http://massbreastfeeding.org/index.php/2009/breastfeeding-management/

BreastFeeding Inc.
Nipple and breast pain algorithm, http://www.breastfeedinginc.ca/product.php?prodID=42

Nursery at Lucile Packard Children's Hospital, Stanford School of Medicine, http://newborns.stanford.edu/Breastfeeding/

In Utero Drug Exposure

Neonatal Drug Withdrawal guidelines from the American Academy of Pediatrics, Sample Withdrawal Scoring Sheet—from Lucile Packard Children's Hospital, and a video clip of neonatal abstinence syndrome, http://newborns.stanford.edu/InUteroDrugs.html

Appendix 5-1

Summary Interventions on Nipple Shield Use

SITUATIONS FOR WHICH SHIELD USE IS COMMONLY ADVISED

Latch Difficulty

- Nipple anomalies (flat, retracted, fibrous, inelastic)
- Mismatch between small infant mouth and large nipple
- Infant from heavily medicated mother
- Birth trauma (vacuum extraction, forceps)
- Oral aversion (vigorous suctioning)
- Artificial nipple preference (pacifiers, bottles)
- To transition an infant from bottle to breast
- Infant with weak or disorganized suck (slips off nipple, preterm, neurological problems)
- Infant with high or low tone
- Delay in putting infant to breast

Oral Cavity Problems

- Cleft palate
- Channel palate (Turner syndrome, formerly intubated)
- Bubble palate
- Lack of fat pads (preterm, SGA)
- Low-threshold mouth
- Poor central grooving of the tongue
- Micrognathia (recessed jaw)

Upper Airway Problems

- Tracheomalacia
- Laryngomalacia

Damaged Nipples

- When all else fails and the mother states she is going to quit breastfeeding

INSTRUCTIONS FOR SHIELD USE

- Choose an appropriately sized shield.
- Drip expressed milk onto the outside of the teat to encourage the infant to latch.
- Warm the shield to help it stick.
- Apply the shield (may moisten the edges to help it adhere better) by turning it almost inside out.
- Hand express a little milk into the teat if necessary.
- Use a periodontal syringe to pre-fill the teat if the mother is unable to express colostrum or milk into the teat.
- Use alternate massage to help drain the breast.
- Tubing can be placed inside or outside of the shield for supplementation.
- Check the infant's latch with the shield: The mouth must not close on the shaft of the teat.
- Check that the infant is not just sucking on the tip of the teat.
- Some mothers may need more than one shield.
- Some mothers may need to pump after each feeding.
- Mothers should carefully check their breasts for plugged ducts and areas that are not draining well.
- If yeast is present on the areola, the shield should be boiled; otherwise, the shield should be washed in hot soapy water after each use, rinsed thoroughly, and air dried.
- Perform an infant weight check about every 3 days until the mother's milk supply is stable and the infant is gaining well.

CONSERVATIVE NIPPLE SHIELD GUIDELINES

Action	Rationale
Recommend a nipple shield if the clinical situation warrants it.	Not all special situations require a shield. Shield use may preserve breastfeeding in selected situations.
If a nipple shield is required during the initial hospital stay, wait at least 24-36 hours before introducing a shield, feeding the infant by spoon with expressed colostrum. For preterm and other special situations, shields could be introduced for persistent special issues.	Allow the infant to imprint on the maternal nipple first.
For healthy term infants, delay shield use if possible until after the mother and infant have been discharged home.	Some infants may latch and feed better following discharge, removing the need for a shield.
Recommend that the mother make an appointment with an IBCLC for continued follow-up.	Professional follow-up is required for assessing and monitoring any ongoing problems or issues that necessitated shield use.

Recommend an appropriately sized and shaped shield as the situation warrants. Start with a medium size shield. Use a larger one if the shield pinches, the maternal nipple is large, or there is pain. Use the smallest shield that gives the best results. A cut-out shield may be prudent for early use to allow olfaction to guide the infant to the breast. A cherry shaped shield may be helpful if the infant has difficulty latching to the conical shield.	Clinicians may need to try a number of different shields in order to secure the best fit and outcome.
Advise the mother to warm the shield under hot water prior to application, turn it almost inside out to apply, hand express colostrum or milk into the teat, or use a periodontal syringe to preload the teat with milk.	Warming helps the shield adhere better and promotes milk ejection. Proper application allows the maternal nipple to be drawn into the shield's teat. Milk in the teat provides immediate availability so that infants with a weak suck do not become fatigued while initiating milk flow.
Have the mother massage and compress the breast periodically during the feeding.	This may prevent milk stasis, plugged ducts, and mastitis.
Pump following feedings if milk production is low or the risk for a compromised milk supply is high.	Milk production must be monitored to assure an abundant supply and that the shield is not contributing to milk supply reduction.
Check to make sure that the shield is properly applied, that the infant is latched appropriately and is transferring milk, and that the mother knows how to clean the shield. Recommend frequent weight checks.	Shield use should not reinforce improper latching. Milk transfer monitoring is important to assure proper infant weight gain and an abundant milk supply.

Appendix 5-2

Additional Clinical Algorithms

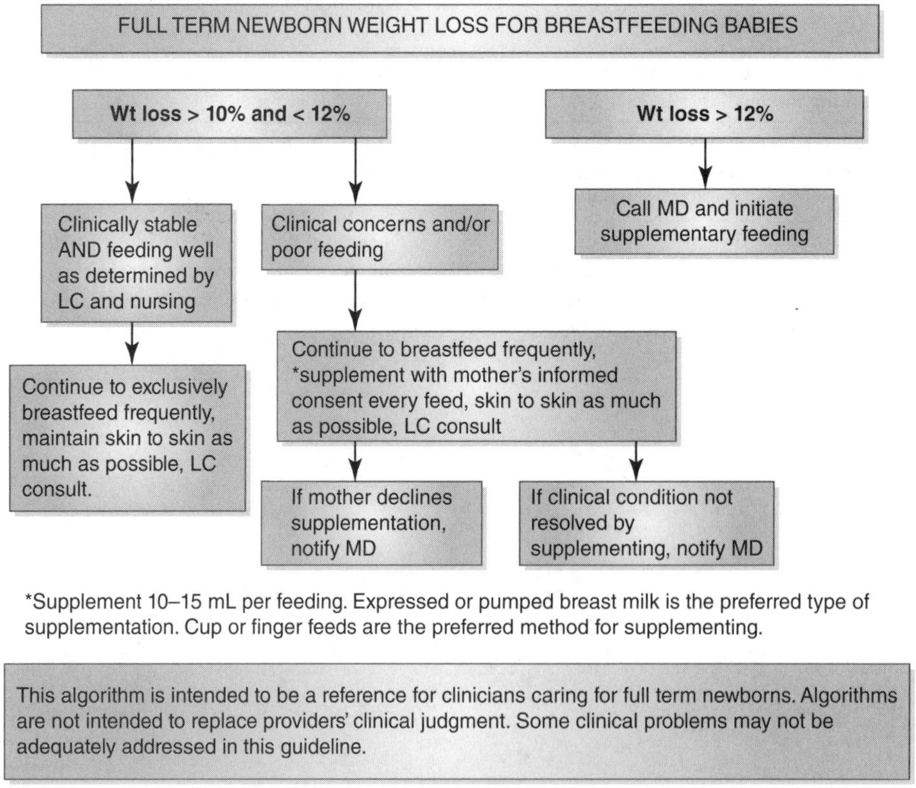

FULL TERM NEWBORN WEIGHT LOSS FOR BREASTFEEDING BABIES
Wt loss > 10% and < 12%
Wt loss > 12%
Clinically stable AND feeding well as determined by LC and nursing
Clinical concerns and/or poor feeding
Call MD and initiate supplementary feeding
Continue to exclusively breastfeed frequently, maintain skin to skin as much as possible, LC consult.
Continue to breastfeed frequently, *supplement with mother's informed consent every feed, skin to skin as much as possible, LC consult
If mother declines supplementation, notify MD
If clinical condition not resolved by supplementing, notify MD
*Supplement 10–15 mL per feeding. Expressed or pumped breast milk is the preferred type of supplementation. Cup or finger feeds are the preferred method for supplementing.
This algorithm is intended to be a reference for clinicians caring for full term newborns. Algorithms are not intended to replace providers' clinical judgment. Some clinical problems may not be adequately addressed in this guideline.

Figure 5-32 Full-term newborn weight loss for breastfeeding babies.
Used with permission of Massachusetts General Hospital.

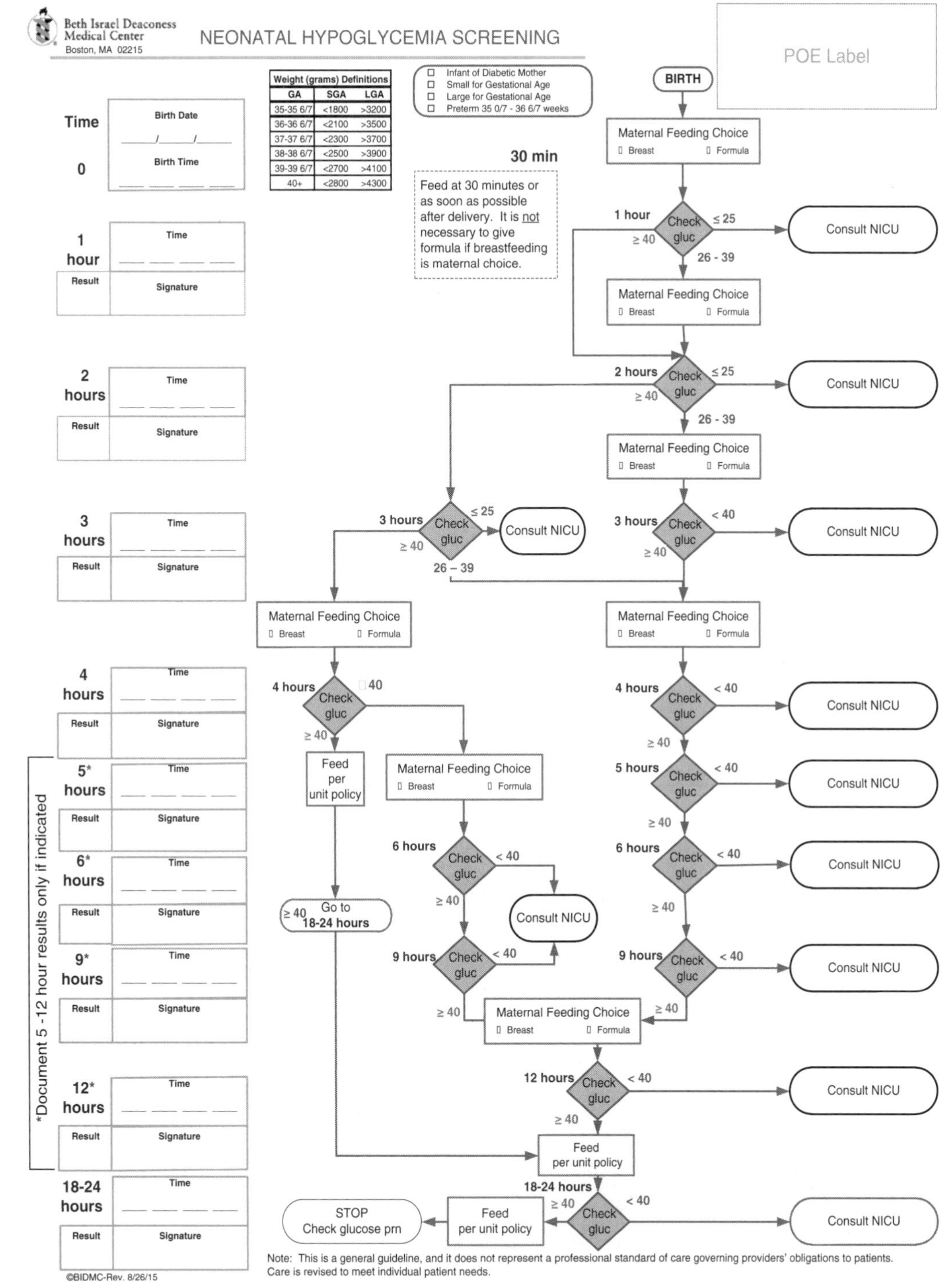

Figure 5-33 Neonatal hypoglycemia screening.

Used with permission: Courtesy of Beth Israel Deaconess Medical Center, Boston, Massachusetts, and Anna Jaques Hospital, Newburyport, Massachusetts.

Chapter 6

Beyond the Initial 48–72 Hours: Infant Challenges

INTRODUCTION

A number of breastfeeding problems and issues must be addressed immediately and throughout the initial hospital stay, whereas other issues may have their origins in the early days but become apparent after discharge. Some are conditions that require an ongoing need for specialized lactation support postdischarge. This chapter discusses situations that require close follow-up and intense support, including hyperbilirubinemia (jaundice), dehydration, weight gain/loss issues, and breastfeeding late preterm and preterm infants.

NEONATAL JAUNDICE

Neonatal jaundice is a common condition and generally self-limiting in the newborn. It is estimated that 60–70% of term infants will become visibly jaundiced—that is, they will have serum bilirubin levels exceeding 5–7 mg/dL (85–119 mmol/L)—in the first week of life (MacMahon, Stevenson, & Oski, 1998; Maisels & McDonagh, 2008). Neonatal hyperbilirubinemia increases during the hours after birth and usually peaks at 96–120 hours after discharge from the hospital. Approximately 5% reach levels > 17 mg/dL (290.7 mmol/L; Harris, Bernbaum, Polin, Zimmerman, & Polin. 2001), and around 2% of these newborns reach a total serum bilirubin level of > 20 mg/dL (342 mmol/L; Newman et al., 1999). Estimated rates of high-risk bilirubin levels (> 25 mg/dL [427 mmol/L]) vary from 1:700 (Newman et al., 1999) to 1:1,000 (Bhutani, Johnson, & Sivieri, 1999a). Jaundice is a frequent reason for readmission to the hospital during the first 2 weeks of life (Hall, Simon, & Smith, 2000; Maisels & Kring, 1998). Most jaundice in healthy full-term newborns is a benign condition that resolves over the first week or 2. However, extremely high levels of bilirubin (> 25–30 mg/dL [427.5–513 mmol/L]) can be toxic to the brain, producing a condition known as kernicterus. Kernicterus involves bilirubin toxicity to the basal ganglia and various brainstem nuclei when extreme amounts of bilirubin cross the blood–brain barrier, then infiltrate and destroy nerve cells.

Bilirubin Metabolism

Bilirubin is an orange or yellow pigment, 80–90% of which is derived from the breakdown of hemoglobin from aged or hemolyzed red blood cells. Heme is a constituent of hemoglobin that is released in association with the breakdown of aging red blood cells. Most heme in the newborn originates from fetal erythrocytes, is initially converted to biliverdin through the action of the enzyme heme oxygenase, and then is reduced further to bilirubin that is transported in the circulation tightly bound to albumin. In the liver, bilirubin is conjugated by another enzyme, uridine diphosphoglucuronosyl transferase (UDPGT); released into the bile duct; and delivered to the intestinal tract for elimination through the stool (also termed direct bilirubin). However, some unconjugated (indirect) bilirubin remains unbound to albumin and circulates as free bilirubin. Unbound, unconjugated bilirubin passes easily through lipid-containing membranes, like the blood–brain barrier, where in high amounts it is neurotoxic and can transiently or permanently affect neurons (Volpe, 2001).

The production, conjugation, and excretion of bilirubin are affected by conditions unique to the newborn that cause an imbalance in this metabolic process, predisposing the newborn to hyperbilirubinemia. As the newborn moves from the low oxygen environment of the uterus to the relatively high oxygen environment of room air, excess fetal red blood cells are no longer needed. Infants produce more bilirubin than they can eliminate, a situation exacerbated by prematurity, bruising or hematoma formation, infection, maternal glucose intolerance, weight loss, oxytocin exposure during labor, genetic modifiers of bilirubin metabolism, and all types of hemolysis. Alterations in and to this process include the following:

- Production: High bilirubin production (twice that of an adult) occurs because fetal erythrocytes are overabundant, have a short lifespan, and their breakdown rapidly creates an excess of heme for the newborn liver to process.
- Conjugation: Conjugation undergoes delays because the activity of UDPGT is limited and hepatic uptake of bilirubin is decreased.
- Excretion: The small intestine of the newborn delays bilirubin excretion through the activity of the enzyme beta-glucuronidase, which converts conjugated bilirubin back to its unconjugated state, allowing bilirubin to be reabsorbed back into circulation (enterohepatic circulation) (Steffensrud, 2004). The newborn bowel slowly becomes colonized with the bacteria needed to degrade bilirubin into urobilinogen that cannot be reabsorbed. The longer direct (conjugated) bilirubin remains in the intestine, the greater the likelihood of its conversion back to indirect bilirubin (unconjugated), which is sent back to the liver for reprocessing (Blackburn, 1995). At birth, the intestines can contain as much as 200 g of meconium, including up to 175 mg of bilirubin, half of which is in the indirect form, an amount that is 4 to 7 times the daily rate of bilirubin production at term (Bartoletti, Stevenson, Ostrander, & Johnson, 1979).
- Genetic predisposition: There are racial variations in bilirubin metabolism among the normal population (Beutler, Gelbart, & Demina, 1998). Mutation of a gene for the enzyme required for bilirubin conjugation contributes to the increased predisposition of some Asian infants (~20%) for severe neonatal hyperbilirubinemia (Akaba et al., 1998). UDPGT 1A1 was shown to be associated with hyperbilirubinemia in Asian infants but not Caucasian infants (Long, Zhang, Fang, Luo, & Liu, 2011). In a population of Asian infants, Chang, Lin, Liu, Yeh, and Ni (2009) found that male breastfed infants with a variant nucleotide 211 of the UGT 1A1 gene had a high risk for developing prolonged hyperbilirubinemia. Sato and colleagues (2013) studied 401 exclusively breastfed Japanese infants and classified them into 2 groups based on maximal weight

loss following birth and presence of polymorphic mutations of UGT 1A1 (genotypes G71R and TA 7). They demonstrated that the effect of G71R mutation on neonatal hyperbilirubinemia was significant in infants, with 5% or greater maximal weight loss, and its influence increases in parallel with the degree of maximal weight loss. This study indicates that optimal breastfeeding, breastfeeding management, and milk intake may overcome the genetic predisposition factor G71R for the development of hyperbilirubinemia in exclusively breastfed Asian infants. Prolonged jaundice, often termed breastmilk jaundice, has also been shown to occur in a significant number of infants of Asian descent with a particular genotype (UGT 1A1*6) (Maruo et al., 2014).

Other polymorphisms become risk factors in Asian infants who experience 10% or greater body weight loss during the neonatal period. Inadequate breastmilk intake may increase the bilirubin burden in infants with polymorphisms in the genes that are involved in the transport or metabolism of bilirubin (Sato et al., 2015). Multiple genetic modifiers of bilirubin metabolism may interact in the presence of breastfeeding in an infant of Asian descent (Yang et al., 2015), making it important to monitor breastfeeding not only in the hospital but also following discharge to assure adequate milk intake.

- Microbiological content of breastmilk: The microbiological content of breastmilk has been associated with the development of jaundice in breastfed infants. Breastmilk with high levels of *Bifidobacterium* species may be protective against neonatal jaundice, whereas low concentrations of these microorganisms may facilitate the development of jaundice (Tuzun, Kumral, Duman, & Ozkan, 2013).
- Weight loss: Birth weight loss during the first 3 days following birth may be a clinical indicator of a predisposition to significant jaundice at 72 hours. One study found that weight loss of 4.48% on day 1, 7.6% weight loss on day 2, and 8.15% weight loss on day 3 were useful cutoff values in predicting significant jaundice at 72 hours (Yang et al., 2013). These values may aid clinicians in determining the need for more intensive breastfeeding support during the hospital stay.

Classifications of Newborn Jaundice

Clinicians see jaundice in an infant when bilirubin pigment is deposited in subcutaneous tissue, producing the characteristic yellowing of the skin and sclera. The type of jaundice typically seen in full-term neonates is termed physiological jaundice, where bilirubin levels rise steadily during the first 3–4 days of life, peak around the 5th day, and decline thereafter. In preterm infants bilirubin levels may peak on day 6 or 7 and resolve over a more extended period of time. Total serum bilirubin levels are influenced by a number of factors such as race, gestational age, type of feeding, and drugs or medications given to the mother or infant. The newborn's age in hours is commonly used as the criteria to decide if a particular bilirubin level is acceptable or if further monitoring is necessary (Bhutani et al., 1999a). Other contributing factors to physiological jaundice include a previous sibling with jaundice, lack of effective breastfeeding, excessive weight or water loss after birth, infection, mother with diabetes, and bruising/hematoma (Dixit & Gartner, 2000). The incidence of hyperbilirubinemia can be higher in populations living at high altitudes (Leibson et al., 1989).

Jaundice that is not physiological or that is not related to breastfeeding or breastmilk is classified as pathological. Infants with risk factors should be monitored closely during the first days to weeks of life (Porter & Dennis, 2002). Characteristics of pathological jaundice include the following (Dennery, Seidman, & Stevenson, 2001; Melton & Akinbi, 1999):

- Appearance of jaundice within the first 24 hours after birth.
- Fast rising bilirubin levels (> 5 mg/dL/day [85 μmol/L]).
- Total serum bilirubin level higher than 17 mg/dL (290.7 μmol/L) in a full-term newborn.
- Bilirubin levels greater than 8 mg/dL (136 μmol/L) in the first 24 hours may be hemolytic in origin (Maisels, 2001).

Pathological causes may include:

- Sepsis.
- Rubella.
- Toxoplasmosis.
- Hemolytic disease (Rh isoimmunization, ABO blood group incompatibility).
- Erythrocyte disorders (glucose-6-phosphate-dehydrogenase deficiency). Glucose-6-phosphate-dehydrogenase deficiency occurs in 11–13% of African Americans (Kaplan & Hammerman, 2000) and is more common among mothers from Mediterranean countries and Southeast Asia. Screening for this disorder is not routinely performed and is associated with an increased incidence of hyperbilirubinemia and the need for phototherapy (Kaplan, Herschel, Hammerman, Hoyer, & Stevenson, 2004). It has also been associated with cases of kernicterus in the United States (Johnson & Brown, 1999; Penn, Enzmann, Hahn, & Stevenson, 1994; Washington, Ector, & Abboud, 1995).
- Extravasation of blood (cephalohematoma or subgaleal hemorrhage, such as from vacuum extraction, bruising).
- Inborn errors of metabolism.
- Hypothyroidism.
- Polycythemia (such as from delayed cord clamping, twin–twin transfusion).
- Intestinal defect or obstruction.
- Macrosomic infant of a diabetic mother.

Whereas total serum bilirubin levels of 15–20 mg/dL (255–340 |μmol/L) are not that unusual in some healthy, full-term normal infants, extreme hyperbilirubinemia, although rare, is of concern. Strong predictors of total serum bilirubin levels of at least 25 mg/dL are gestational age, bruising, family history, and a rapid rise in total serum bilirubin levels (Kuzniewicz, Escobar, Wi, Liljestrand, McCulloch, & Ne 2008). There is a set of common clinical risk factors for severe hyperbilirubinemia—the more risk factors present, the greater the risk for severe hyperbilirubinemia (**Box 6-1**).

Newman and colleagues (1999) studied the incidence of extremes in bilirubin levels in a sample of 50,000 term and near-term infants and found the following:

- Levels greater than 20 mg/dL (340 μmol/L) in 2% of the sample (1 in 50 infants)
- Levels of 25 mg/dL (425 μmol/L) or greater in 0.15% (1 in 650 infants)
- Levels of 30 mg/dL (510 μmol/L) or greater in 0.01% (1 in 10,000 infants)

Box 6-1 Clinical Risk Factors for Severe Hyperbilirubinemia

- Jaundice in the first 24 hours of life.
- Visible jaundice before discharge (48 hours). Dermal icterus is not visibly noticed as yellowing of the skin when total serum bilirubin levels are less than 4 mg/dL (68 μmol/L; Kramer, 1969). It progresses in a cephalocaudal pattern (Knudsen & Ebbesen, 1997) and is noticed in the face when the serum bilirubin reaches 5 mg/dL, progresses to the upper chest at 10 mg/dL, becomes visible on the abdomen at 12 mg/dL, and finally appears on the palms and soles when bilirubin levels are greater than 15 mg/dL. Although these observations do not replace transcutaneous measurements or laboratory blood analysis, they give the clinician an idea of how closely an infant should be monitored.
- Previous jaundiced sibling.
- Gestational age of 35–38 weeks. Late preterm infants are between 2.4 and 5.7 times more likely to develop significant hyperbilirubinemia (Newman, Xiong, Gonzales, & Escobar, 2000; Sarici et al., 2004), with their serum bilirubin levels peaking later, at 5–7 days, necessitating a longer period of follow-up. Readmission for hyperbilirubinemia is much more likely in these infants when they are discharged less than 48 hours after birth (Hall et al., 2000).
- Exclusive breastfeeding. Clinically, such cases usually involve infants who are not efficiently transferring milk.
- East Asian ethnicity.
- Bruising or cephalohematoma.
- Maternal age greater than 25 years.
- Male infant.

Data from American Academy of Pediatrics, Subcommittee on Neonatal Hyperbilirubinemia. (2001). Neonatal jaundice and kernicterus. *Pediatrics, 108,* 763–765.

Bilirubin levels in some infants can infrequently rise high enough to cause neurological consequences if not monitored closely or if interventions are not implemented to lower bilirubin levels. The term bilirubin encephalopathy is often used to describe the clinical manifestations of bilirubin toxicity, and the American Academy of Pediatrics (AAP, 2004) recommends that the term acute bilirubin encephalopathy be used to describe the acute manifestations of toxicity seen in the first weeks after birth and the term kernicterus be used as a pathological description of the yellow staining of the brainstem nuclei and basal ganglia (Cashore, 1998). The AAP (2004) recommends that the term kernicterus be reserved for the chronic and permanent clinical sequelae of bilirubin toxicity.

No exact bilirubin level or duration of hyperbilirubinemia exposure has been defined to locate the exact point at which neurotoxicity could occur. Furthermore, evidence to date cannot explicitly account for why some infants with extremes of bilirubin levels develop kernicterus and others do not, or why early signs of bilirubin encephalopathy appear reversible in some infants and are permanent in others (Hanko, Lindemann, & Hansen, 2001). Bilirubin entry into the brain is facilitated by numerous conditions, including displacement of bilirubin from its albumin binding, reduced albumin-binding capacity, and increased permeability of the blood–brain barrier. Bilirubin is oxidized in the brain by an enzyme whose activity increases with greater postnatal age (Hansen, 2000). The brain may be able to protect itself to an extent through bilirubin oxidation (Hansen, Allen, & Tommarello, 1999) that may be subject to genetic variability (Hansen, 2001). This protective effect may vary among infants, possibly accounting for the differing outcomes in infants with high bilirubin levels. Bilirubin encephalopathy proceeds along a continuum (**Table 6-1**), where early signs and symptoms may be subtle, nonspecific, transient, and potentially reversible to an advanced and chronic stage of permanent neurological injury (Volpe, 2001).

In a controlled study of 140 5-year-old children with a neonatal total serum bilirubin level of > 25 mg/dL, Newman and colleagues (Newman, Liljestrand, & Escobar, 2003; Newman et al., 2006) found no associations between bilirubin exposure and neurological abnormalities, IQ, behavioral problems, or frequency of parental concerns. These outcomes were repeated in a study by Vandborg, Hansen, Greisen, Jepsen, and Ebbesen (2012), who found no evidence of developmental delay in children between 1 and 5 years of age who had a gestational age > 35 weeks and had experienced at least one measure of total serum bilirubin level > 25 mg/dL during the first 3 weeks of life.

Although extreme levels of bilirubin have the potential to be neurotoxic, bilirubin actually has a physiological role in the body as an antioxidant (McDonagh, 1990). Bilirubin "protection" may be seen in infants with illnesses associated with free-radical production such as circulatory failure, neonatal asphyxia, aspiration, and sepsis, where the rate of bilirubin rise appears less in these infants, because bilirubin is consumed to cope with oxidative stress (Sedlak & Snyder, 2004). Neonatal blood plasma is better

Table 6-1 Continuum of Bilirubin Encephalopathy

Early (First 3–4 Days After Birth)	After First Week	Chronic (Kernicterus)
Lethargy	Increasing lethargy	Athetoid cerebral palsy
Decreased alertness	Increased irritability	High-frequency hearing loss
Poor feeding	Minimal feeding	Developmental delays
Weak suck	Fever	Motor delays
Excessive sleepiness	Shrill cry	Paralysis of upward gaze
High-pitched cry	Opisthotonus*	Dental dysplasia
Hypertonia	Seizures Apnea Retrocollis† Oculogyric crisis‡ Hypotonia Stupor, coma Rigidity	Mild mental retardation

*Opisthotonus is a spasm in which the heels and head are bent backward and the body is bowed forward.
†Retrocollis is torticollis with spasms affecting the posterior neck muscles.
‡Oculogyric crisis is a spasm causing upward fixation of the eyeballs lasting several minutes or hours.

Modified from Connelly, A. M., & Volpe, J. J. (1990). Clinical features of bilirubin encephalopathy. *Clinical Perinatology, 17,* 371–379; Dennery, P. A., Seidman, D. S., & Stevenson, D. K. (2001). Neonatal hyperbilirubinemia. *New England Journal of Medicine, 344,* 581–590; Maisels, M. J., & Newman, T. B. (1995). Kernicterus in otherwise healthy, breastfed term newborns. *Pediatrics, 96*(4pt1), 730–733; Volpe, J. J. (2001). Bilirubin and brain injury. In J. J. Volpe (Ed.), *Neonatal neurology.* Philadelphia, PA: Saunders.

protected against oxidative stress due in part to the elevated levels of bilirubin (Wiedemann, Kontush, Finckh, Hellwege, & Kohlschutter, 2003). Shekeeb, Kumar, Sharma, Narang, and Prasad (2008) showed that bilirubin acts as a physiological antioxidant until it reaches a concentration of 20 mg/dL in full-term normal neonates. Beyond that concentration, it is conjectured that bilirubin no longer acts as an antioxidant and cannot be considered physiological. For bilirubin to disrupt brain function, it must gain entry into the brain. Normally, the blood–brain barrier functions to block the passage of bilirubin into the brain, but this action is less mature in newborn infants. Bilirubin, once it has entered the brain, has a short half-life and is cleared from the brain by the action of an enzyme. However, this enzyme's activity is lower in the neonate and is subject to inter-individual differences and genetic variability, suggesting that vulnerability to bilirubin toxicity may in part have a genetic basis (Hansen, 2002). A number of factors can disrupt the blood–brain barrier, which is normally closed to albumin and bilirubin as long as it is bound to albumin (Hansen, 1994). These include hyperosmolality, hypercarbia, hypoxia, hyperoxemia, asphyxia, acidosis, prematurity, hypoalbuminemia, and bilirubin-displacing drugs.

Breastfeeding and Jaundice

Stevenson, Dennery, and Hintz (2001) consider breastfeeding as the "normal driving influence on the transitional pattern of hyperbilirubinemia with formula feeding representing an iatrogenic perturbation of the normal influences of human milk on the enterohepatic circulation of bilirubin." Neonatal jaundice is connected to breastfeeding in three groups seen in clinical practice:

1. The exclusively breastfed, healthy term infant during the 1st week after birth
2. Newborns who do not receive adequate amounts of breastmilk and have high concentrations of indirect bilirubin during the first postnatal week (referred to as nonfeeding jaundice, starvation jaundice, lack of breastfeeding jaundice)
3. Breastfed infants who experience a situation of prolonged unconjugated hyperbilirubinemia (called breastmilk jaundice)

Breastfeeding has long been associated with higher bilirubin levels and a more prolonged duration of jaundice compared with formula feeding (Dahms et al., 1973; Osborn, Reiff, & Bolus, 1984; Schneider, 1986). Breastfeeding practices at the time of these studies, however, may have contributed to this impression. Infants in the early studies may have experienced restricted milk intake due to:

- Hospital policies that ordered nothing by mouth for the first 24 hours
- Limited access to breastfeeding from restrictive schedules that allowed feedings only every 4 hours and usually not at night
- Short access times to the breast from advice that limited feedings to only a couple of minutes per side
- Supplementation with sterile water or sugar water that provided few to no calories

Fasting (lack of calories) can enhance the enterohepatic circulation of bilirubin as can the continued presence of a reservoir of bilirubin contained in unpassed meconium. Bertini, Dani, Tronchin, and Rubaltelli (2001) demonstrated that the development of early jaundice was not associated with breastfeeding per se, but rather with increased weight loss after birth subsequent to fasting or insufficient milk intake. A subpopulation of breastfed infants in their study experienced a high bilirubin level peak that was associated with mixed feeding (supplemented infants) and a higher weight loss. They also found a strong association between significant hyperbilirubinemia and vacuum extraction. Thus, what is sometimes termed early-onset breastfeeding jaundice is most likely a manifestation of inadequate breastfeeding that causes the exaggerated pattern of hyperbilirubinemia in the first 5 days of life (Gartner, 2001; Neifert, 1998).

Infrequent, inefficient breastfeeding reduces caloric intake, increases weight loss, delays meconium passage, and can drive bilirubin to levels where clinical intervention becomes necessary.

Hyperbilirubinemia that peaks between 6 and 14 days has been termed late-onset or breastmilk jaundice and can develop in up to one-third of healthy breastfed infants (AAP, 1994). Total serum bilirubin levels may range from 12 to 20 mg/dL (205.2–342 mmol/L) and are considered nonpathological. Hyperbilirubinemia can persist for up to 3 months (Gartner, 2001). It appears that it is normal for 20–30% of predominantly breastfed infants to be jaundiced at 3–4 weeks and for 30–40% of these infants to have bilirubin levels greater than 5 mg/dL (Maisels et al., 2014). The underlying cause of breastmilk jaundice is not clearly understood and may be multifactorial. It has been suggested that substances in breastmilk such as beta-glucuronidases and nonesterified fatty acids might inhibit normal bilirubin metabolism (Brodersen & Herman, 1963; Gartner & Herschel, 2001; Melton & Akinbi, 1999; Poland, 1981). Maruo, Nishizawa, Sato, Sawa, and Shimada (2000) suggested that a defect or mutation in the bilirubin UDPGT gene may cause an infant with such a mutation to be susceptible to jaundice that components in the mother's milk may trigger. Ota and colleagues (2011) describe pregnanediol as a contributor to breastmilk jaundice in carriers of the G71R polymorphic mutation. The milk of mothers whose infants experienced prolonged jaundice was found to have a decreased antioxidant capacity (Uras et al., 2010).

Managing Hyperbilirubinemia

Numerous methods are used to prevent or manage hyperbilirubinemia:

- One of the most successful methods for preventing hyperbilirubinemia has been the administration of high-titer anti-D immunoglobulin G, or RhoGAM, to reduce the incidence and severity of Rh isoimmunization disease (Rh incompatibility).
- Phototherapy is the most common therapy for high bilirubin levels. Its use is designed to prevent bilirubin toxicity, but it does not treat the underlying cause of the hyperbilirubinemia. Phototherapy uses light energy to change the shape and structure of bilirubin, which converts it to molecules that the body can excrete. Phototherapy works on bilirubin that is present in the skin and superficial subcutaneous tissue. Phototherapy has a number of side effects (Blackburn & Loper, 1992), some of which can affect breastfeeding (separation, lethargy, poor feeding, increased fluid requirement, poor state control). Conventional phototherapy lights can produce a change in the infant's thermal environment with increased heat contributing to insensible water loss. The new generation of light-emitting diode (LED) phototherapy devices should reduce this problem because they produce less heat (Dijk & Hulzebos, 2012). Phototherapy has been shown to induce DNA damage in lymphocytes, with the DNA damage increasing significantly with longer durations of phototherapy (Tatli, Minnet, Kocyigit, & Karadag, 2008). A fiberoptic blanket or band may be used—in lower urgency situations—allowing parents to hold, care for,

and breastfeed the infant. This also allows treatment to occur in the home rather than the infant being readmitted into the hospital. A rebound of 1 to 2 mg/dL (17 to 34 |µmol/L) can occur after phototherapy is discontinued and usually a follow-up bilirubin level is recommended 24 hours after discharge.

- Exchange transfusion is used in more extreme situations, usually for infants with hemolytic disease.
- Pharmacological agents have been tried over the years, with most being discarded as ineffective. A number of chemoprevention and treatment therapies have included heme oxygenase inhibitors such as metal meso- and protoporphyrins. Tin-mesoporphyrin (SnMP), blocks the action of heme oxygenase in converting hemoglobin to bilirubin. Its action is designed to shut off production of bilirubin at its source rather than remove it after it has been formed. It reduces blood bilirubin levels for 7–10 days after administration (Kappas, 2004). Its safety, indications for use, efficacy, and side effects of whole-scale inhibition of bilirubin production remain to be determined (Blackmon, Fanaroff, & Raju, 2004; Hansen, 2003). L-aspartic acid, a beta-glucuronidase inhibitor (and component in hydrolyzed infant formula), has been given experimentally to breastfed newborns. Gourley, Zhanhai, Kreamer, and Kosorok (2005) reported on a small number of infants whose fecal bilirubin excretion increased and jaundice decreased when given 5-mL doses of L-aspartic acid 6 times a day for 7 days after birth.

Changes in the Approach to and Prevalence of Hyperbilirubinemia and Kernicterus

The root cause for the development of kernicterus has been identified as a systems failure in neonatal care, especially during the 1st week after birth. A convergence of a number of changes and factors began contributing to an increasing number of infants being readmitted to the hospital for hyperbilirubinemia and an increase in reports of the development of acute bilirubin encephalopathy and kernicterus (Ross, 2003), including the following:

- A more relaxed approach to jaundice because studies did not reveal adverse developmental outcomes in infants who had experienced mild to moderate jaundice (Newman & Maisels, 1992; Watchko & Oski, 1983).
- More liberal treatment guidelines that postponed phototherapy in infants older than 72 hours of age until the total serum bilirubin level reached 20 mg/dL and for infants between 49 and 72 hours old until it reached 18 mg/dL (AAP, 1994).
- The practice of discharging healthy term newborns within 48 hours of birth, before many infants appear clinically jaundiced and after which bilirubin levels are most likely to rise (Braveman, Egerter, Pearl, Marchi, & Miller, 1995; Braveman, Kessel, Egerter, & Richmond, 1997; Britton, Britton, & Beebe, 1994; Liu, Clemens, Shay, Davis, & Novack, 1997):
  - Early hospital discharge is associated with increased hospital readmissions for jaundice (Brown et al., 1999; Grupp-Phelan, Taylor, Liu, & Davis, 1999).
  - Short hospital stays, minimal staffing, and lack of provider expertise in breastfeeding management provide limited time and often little guidance for mothers and infants to become proficient at breastfeeding.

    - Minimum criteria for discharge within 48 hours of birth includes an infant who has completed at least two successful feedings, with documentation that the infant is capable of coordinating sucking, swallowing, and breathing. The breastfeeding mother and infant should be assessed by trained staff regarding positioning, latch-on, and adequacy of swallowing (AAP, 2004), criteria that are not routinely performed in many hospital settings.
    - The shift in locus of care surrounding hyperbilirubinemia from the hospital to the community has created a need for early postdischarge observation (Palmer et al., 2003).
- A pattern of newborn follow-up care that consists of a 1- to 2-week postdischarge visit, occurring long after the period of high risk and the time for effective intervention has passed (Eaton, 2001); lack of adherence to an evidence-based follow-up schedule that recommends healthcare provider examinations and observations at age 72 hours if discharged before age 24 hours, a visit at 96 hours of age if discharged between 24 and 47.9 hours of age, and a visit at 120 hours of age if discharged between 48 and 72 hours of age (AAP, Subcommittee on Hyperbilirubinemia, 2004).
- An increase in reports of kernicterus (Johnson & Bhutani, 2003; Johnson & Brown, 1999):
    - Severe hyperbilirubinemia and kernicterus were the subjects of a report (Carter & Dixon, 2001).
    - Kernicterus was the subject of a sentinel event alert by the Joint Commission (2001) and a second alert of revised guidelines (2004).
    - Hyperbilirubinemia and kernicterus were discussed in a commentary by the AAP's subcommittee on hyperbilirubinemia (Eaton, 2001), emphasizing that many of the infants experiencing these conditions did not have obvious hemolytic disease and were healthy breastfeeding newborns (frequently not receiving adequate nutrition and hydration, most likely due to inefficient feeding skills), a significant portion of whom were less than 38 weeks' gestational age (near term).
    - In July 2003 the National Institute of Child Health and Human Development convened a group of experts to review the existing knowledge base regarding neonatal hyperbilirubinemia and the barriers to preventing kernicterus (Palmer, Keren, Maisels, & Yeargin-Allsopp, 2004).
    - A 5-year consortium funded by the Agency for Healthcare Research and Quality explored the barriers to implementing the 1994 AAP jaundice guideline in healthcare systems. Some of the major problems included discharge before breastfeeding was established, cumbersome reimbursement policies for blood tests, clinicians who would not see infants until 2 weeks postdischarge, and insurance carriers rejecting claims for the early visit (Ip, Glicken, Kulig, & O'Brien, 2003).

More recent reports show that the diagnosis of kernicterus has decreased to an estimated incidence of approximately 1.5 per 100,000 term newborn births and 4 per 100,000 births of preterm infants (Burke et al., 2009). Preterm infants with jaundice require close monitoring and a consistent breastfeeding plan of care with access to lactation consultant services.

Clinical Approaches to Breastfeeding Support: Practice Suggestions

Because all infants have an initial rise in bilirubin levels as they transition to extrauterine life, the goal of breastfeeding management strategies revolves around optimizing the skill sets mothers and newborns need to prevent bilirubin levels from becoming serious and to preserve breastfeeding if they do. Short postpartum stays provide increasingly less time for clinicians to teach and assess and for mothers and infants to practice their newly learned skills. The following measures optimize breastfeeding from the start and reduce the likelihood of severe hyperbilirubinemia from inadequate intake:

- Facilitate contact between mother and infant and avoid separation.
    - Encourage 24-hour rooming-in and breastfeeding at night to hasten excretion of bilirubin-laden meconium.
    - Minimize visitors who may cause a mother to delay or eliminate breastfeedings during their presence (Kovach, 2002).
- Recommend and ensure a minimum of 8 and a goal of 10–12 feedings each 24 hours (AAP, Subcommittee on Hyperbilirubinemia, 2004) (especially important for near-term infants and infants of mothers with diabetes or who are overweight or obese).
    - This takes advantage of the laxative effect of colostrum that stimulates gut motility and prevents the reabsorption of bilirubin.
    - Frequent feedings reduce the likelihood of large weight losses and dehydration that drive up bilirubin levels. The greater the frequency of feedings in the first days, the lower the peak bilirubin level (De Carvalho, Klaus, & Merkatz, 1982; Varimo, Simila, Wendt, & Kolvisto, 1986; Yamauchi & Yamanouchi, 1990). Infants who are breastfed fewer than 8 times per 24 hours *following discharge* are at an increased risk for hyperbilirubinemia (Chen, Yeh, & Chen, 2015). Discharge instructions should emphasize the importance of frequent feedings during the first 2 weeks of life.
    - Jaundice can contribute to or exacerbate early breastfeeding problems. Increased serum bilirubin levels can cause lethargy, excessive sleepiness, and poor feeding (Gartner & Herschel, 2001).
    - Sleepy infants or infants who are closed down should be placed skin to skin with their mother and moved to the breast when demonstrating behavioral feeding-readiness cues.
- Assess for infant swallowing at breast. Frequent attempts at feedings by themselves will not ensure adequate intake unless the infant is actually swallowing colostrum/milk. Document if and when swallowing takes place, making sure that the mother can state when the infant is swallowing.
    - If the infant is latched but not swallowing, recommend alternate massage to initiate and sustain a suck–swallow feeding pattern. If the infant pauses for an excessive amount of time between sucking bursts, the mother can use a nipple tug (i.e., simulate that she is going to remove the nipple from the infant's mouth by either pushing down on the areola enough to cause the infant to pull the nipple/areola back into his or her mouth or pull the infant slightly away from the breast without breaking suction). This is similar to the technique used to stimulate the suck of a bottle-fed infant by pulling back on the bottle but not breaking suction. As long as the mother's nipples are not sore or the tug does not create pain or damage, this may be a simple method of sustaining a sucking rhythm for an infant unable to do so. A tube-feeding device can also be taped or held at the breast to deliver colostrum/milk and prevent caloric deprivation from contributing to increased bilirubin levels (Auerbach & Gartner, 1987).

  - If the infant cannot latch or is unable to transfer milk, have the mother hand express colostrum into a spoon and spoon-feed this to the infant.
  - Avoid supplementation with formula, if possible, because this reduces feeding frequency, decreases milk intake, and diminishes milk production (unless the mother is concurrently expressing milk). Nondehydrated breastfed infants should not receive water or dextrose water because this practice does not reduce total serum bilirubin levels or prevent hyperbilirubinemia (AAP, Subcommittee on Hyperbilirubinemia, 2004; De Carvalho, Hall, & Harvey, 1981; Nicholl, Ginsburg, & Tripp, 1982).
- Occasionally, a breastfed infant may require supplementation due to the effects of phototherapy, the inability to effect breastmilk transfer, or the unavailability of the mother. The mother's colostrum/milk or banked human milk is the first option of choice (Herschel, 2003). If human milk is not on hand, a hydrolyzed casein formula may be a logical choice for use until the mother's colostrum/milk is accessible. A casein hydrolysate formula has been shown to better contribute to reduced bilirubin levels than standard infant formulas (Gourley, Kreamer, Cohnen, & Kosorok, 1999), perhaps because it contains a beta-glucuronidase inhibitor (Gourley, Kreamer, & Cohnen, 1997). It also reduces the risk of provoking allergies and diabetes in susceptible infants. Mothers should be instructed to pump milk to preserve lactation and provide milk for future supplementation if needed.
- Chen, Sadakata, Ishida, Sekizuka, and Sayama (2011) studied the effects of gentle baby massage on neonatal jaundice in full-term breastfed infants through a controlled clinical trial. Stool frequency was measured on days 1 and 2 and transcutaneous bilirubin levels were measured on the 2nd to 5th days. Results showed that stool frequency in the massaged infants on days 1 and 2 (4.6 and 4.3 respectively) was significantly higher than that in the control group (3.3 and 2.6 respectively). Transcutaneous bilirubin levels were lower in the massaged group on each day measured compared with the control group. Total bilirubin levels on day 4 were 11.7 ± 2.8 mg/dL in the massaged group compared with 13.7 ± 1.7 in the control infants. The higher stool output was thought to lower the bilirubin levels more quickly, as the reservoir of bilirubin present in meconium was more rapidly eliminated and enterohepatic circulation was maintained in a more physiological manner. Massage might further enhance the amount of milk ingested and improve the digestive process, which would provide more calories to the infant through activation of metabolic hormones. Infant massage as a potential preventive intervention is an enjoyable, no-cost possibility to help prevent high bilirubin levels in newborns.
- A bilirubin nomogram is currently in use to predict an infant's risk of developing clinically significant hyperbilirubinemia by plotting the total serum bilirubin level against the infant's age in hours predischarge (Bhutani, Johnson, & Sivieri, 1999b; Bhutani et al., 2000). Hyperbilirubinemia is defined as a bilirubin level greater than the 95th percentile at any age. Infants above the 75th percentile generally require an immediate total serum bilirubin measurement, whereas infants below the 40th percentile are at very low risk for developing subsequent hyperbilirubinemia. Although used to determine the timing and strategies of early interventions for lowering bilirubin levels (Bhutani, Johnson, & Keren, 2004), the nomogram, along with clinical risk factors, should be used to identify the need for increasingly intensive breastfeeding assistance.

A significant number of infants in the low and intermediate risk zones on a bilirubin nomogram remain at risk for readmission for high bilirubin levels, signaling the need for early postdischarge follow-up (Slaughter, Annibale, & Suresh, 2009).

- Maisels and colleagues (2009) recommend universal predischarge bilirubin screening using either total serum bilirubin or transcutaneous bilirubin measurements, combined with clinical risk factors and plotting of the infant on the hour-specific nomogram. The total serum bilirubin can be measured from the same blood sample that is drawn for metabolic screening purposes so the infant does not need to experience another heelstick. While the gold standard for measuring bilirubin levels is total serum bilirubin concentration obtained from a blood sample, an alternative for preliminary screening is the use of transcutaneous bilirubin measurements with a noninvasive device that relates the amount of light absorption by bilirubin (the yellow color of the skin) to the concentration of bilirubin in the skin (Bosschaart et al., 2012). Even though transcutaneous measurements are not equivalent to that which is obtained from a blood sample, they do provide immediate information about an infant's bilirubin level that is better than a visual estimate, which reduces the likelihood that clinically significant jaundice will be missed (Maisels, 2012). They also allow an observation of values that are crossing percentiles on the bilirubin nomogram that would alert the clinician to provide more intense monitoring of the infant. Maisels and colleagues (2009) provide an algorithm with recommendations for management and follow-up according to predischarge measurements, gestational age, and risk factors for subsequent hyperbilirubinemia. The Academy of Breastfeeding Medicine has a clinical protocol for jaundice in breastfeeding infants equal to or greater than 35 weeks' gestation (Academy of Breastfeeding Protocol Committee, 2010).
- The basic minimum criteria for discharge before 48 hours is the completion of two successful breastfeedings with documented swallowing and the ability of the mother to demonstrate competency regarding positioning, latch, and recognizing swallowing (AAP, 2004). Breastfeeding technique, maternal competency, and documentation of swallowing, with corrective strategies implemented if needed, should be initiated before weight loss and jaundice become excessive.

The 3rd and 4th days after birth are critical times for assessment of breastfeeding adequacy and for initiating interventions to correct problems. Interestingly, hospital stays of at least 3 days (including cesarean-born infants) were associated with a reduced risk of readmission for hyperbilirubinemia (Hall et al., 2000). Presumably, the extra time spent in the hospital improves the chances of skilled lactation services being made available and timely intervention for continued breastfeeding problems. As many as 22% of infants can still be experiencing suboptimal breastfeeding (< 10 on the Infant Breastfeeding Assessment Tool) on day 3 and up to 22% of mothers may encounter delayed lactogenesis II after discharge (i.e., greater than 72 hours with no evidence of the onset of copious milk production or engorgement; Dewey, Nommsen-Rivers, Heinig, & Cohen, 2003). With early discharge, follow-up must take place in the primary care provider's office, in a hospital outpatient setting, in a clinic, or in the home (Egerter, Braverman, & Marchi, 1998). The responsibility for detecting and monitoring jaundice has shifted to the parents, with some failing to keep follow-up appointments and many lacking a basic understanding of jaundice and how to recognize it. Although telephone follow-ups may answer early questions, they may fail to capture information from parents who are unable to assess if breastfeeding is adequate. A parent describing an infant as sleepy, lethargic, irritable, or not feeding well presents a dilemma to a clinician who cannot visually assess the infant and the breastfeeding parameters. These descriptors should not be summarily dismissed as typical newborn behaviors (Stokowski, 2002a). When mothers are taught to do so, they are capable of recognizing the progression of jaundice as well as the presence of significant jaundice (Madlon-Kay, 1997, 2002), but visual assessment is still unreliable in judging the intensity of worsening jaundice. Even nurses cannot rely on visual assessment of cephalocaudal progression of jaundice to estimate bilirubin levels, especially in late preterm infants.

Nevertheless, there is a strong relationship between the cephalocaudal progression of jaundice and rising bilirubin levels, which can persist up to 28 days (Maisels et al., 2014). Although actual bilirubin values should be determined by laboratory analysis, in a study of 76 infants, conjunctival icterus was always accompanied by cutaneous jaundice to at least the chest and more often than not a total serum bilirubin greater than 14.9 mg/dL (255 μmol/L), consistently in the 76–95% to more than 95% range on the Bhutani nomogram. Only a few infants with total serum bilirubin in the range of 10–14.9 mg/dL (171–255 μmol/L) had conjunctival icterus (Azzuqa & Watchko, 2015).

Jaundice extent also has poor overall accuracy for predicting the risk of development of significant hyperbilirubinemia (Keren, Luan, Tremont, & Cnaan, 2009). Transcutaneous bilirubin measurement is a noninvasive screening tool that eliminates a large number of unnecessary skin punctures and is more reliable than visual assessment. However, it cannot replace laboratory measurement of serum bilirubin (Carceller-Blanchard, Cousineau, & Delvin, 2009). Placing the infant in sunlight will not treat high bilirubin levels and may bleach the skin to the point where visual assessment of the skin is impeded. A better approach is to objectively teach parents about jaundice, providing them with a printed resource to refer to at home (Stokowski, 2002b).

With the proliferation of smartphones and their apps has come the ability to monitor a number of health-related parameters (e.g., heart rate, lung function, fitness). A new device called the BiliCam uses the smartphone's camera, an app, and a paper color calibration card to help parents monitor jaundice in their infant following discharge (de Greef et al., 2014). Although refinements are still being made to this app, it represents a low-cost, easy-to-use screening tool for clinicians and parents that is designed to be comparable to the transcutaneous bilirubin screening currently in clinical use.

Effect of Jaundice on Continued Breastfeeding and Maternal Behaviors

Earlier studies of the effect of neonatal jaundice on maternal behaviors suggested that the experience of neonatal jaundice and its treatments were associated with a set of behaviors described as the vulnerable child syndrome, in which mothers perceived their infant's current and subsequent medical conditions as more serious, resulting in a pattern of high healthcare use and diminished reliance on their own ability to remedy minor problems themselves. The blood tests, phototherapy, separation, supplementation or replacement of breastmilk with formula, and prolonged hospitalization also had an adverse effect on breastfeeding, resulting in the increased likelihood of early termination of breastfeeding (Elander & Lindberg, 1984; Kemper, Forsyth, & McCarthy, 1989, 1990). Mothers who lack an understanding of jaundice, who have language barriers, or whose healthcare provider does not provide clear explanations to eliminate maternal misconceptions may feel guilty, believing that they caused the jaundice (Hannon,

Willis, & Scrimshaw, 2001). Interactions with healthcare professionals are a crucial factor in mediating the impact of jaundice on the mother and the breastfeeding relationship. Conflicting orders, offhand comments about the mother's milk (or lack of milk), and recommendations to supplement or stop breastfeeding engender confusion, discontent, anger, and guilt, creating the impression that the mother is responsible for making her baby sick (Willis, Hannon, & Scrimshaw, 2002). Brethauer and Carey (2010) described the lived experience of mothers with a jaundiced infant. Mothers related a number of negative feelings and experiences that included physical and emotional exhaustion, being distressed by the infant's appearance, feeling out of control, having to exert heightened vigilance, and feeling discounted. Mothers also complained that healthcare providers all had different opinions, that mothers felt defensive and at fault, and that guidelines differed among multiple healthcare providers. Inconsistent information is highly distressful. Clinicians' actions that are consistent, current, and evidence-based favor continued breastfeeding, demonstrating that a high value is placed on the mother continuing to breastfeed her infant.

Use of a clinical pathway may work toward preserving breastfeeding and maternal confidence when an infant is readmitted. Spatz and Goldschmidt (2006) created a clinical pathway when it was noted that many breastfeeding infants admitted for jaundice, dehydration, or weight loss were admitted when no specialized lactation services were available (nights, weekends, holidays). The pathway provides the bedside nurse with an evidence-based, current, and consistent framework for clinical decision making and achieving the goals of effective milk transfer and preservation of the maternal milk supply. Clinicians will need to determine the infant's ability to effectively feed at breast; observe for milk transfer; select technology needed to assist latch and milk transfer, such as a tube-feeding device or nipple shield; and initiate maternal pumping 8–10 times each 24 hours with a goal of 500–1,000 mL/day. If the infant is being treated with phototherapy, breastfeeding should continue on a frequent basis.

HYPERNATREMIC DEHYDRATION

A breastfed infant with effective feeding skills receives adequate amounts of fluid when nursing frequently, transferring milk, gaining weight appropriately, and producing urine and stools within normal age-expected parameters. Young infants are especially susceptible to volume depletion because the immature kidney does not yet maximally concentrate urine or reserve water. This is commonly seen in conditions that involve acute excessive fluid loss such as gastroenteritis. However, case reports of hypernatremic dehydration in otherwise healthy breastfed infants continue to appear in the medical literature (Neifert, 2001) and usually present around 7–10 days of age, with a range of 3–21 days (Oddie, Richmond, & Coultard, 2001). Dehydration may coexist with high bilirubin levels (Tarcan, Tiker, Vatandas, Haberal, & Gurakan, 2005), because the common thread between the two may have an iatrogenic etiology with parents unaware of their infant's deteriorating condition. Weight loss in an infant of greater than 7% should alert the clinician to an increased risk for hypernatremia and signal the need for more intensive breastfeeding evaluation and interventions (Unal, Arhan, Kara, Uncu, & Aliefendioglu, 2008; Uras, Karadag, Dogan, Tonbul, & Tatli, 2007). In a systematic review of the literature, 1,485 cases of breastfeeding-associated neonatal hypernatremia were recognized, with 96% linked with a greater than 10% infant weight loss (Lavagno et al., 2016). Percentage of weight loss from birth weight can be quite high, ranging from 14% to 32% (Cooper, Atherton, Kahana, & Kotagal, 1995). Although jaundice is usually the most frequent diagnosis in early neonatal presentations to the emergency department, dehydration in infants younger than

8 days old is also not uncommon (Manganaro, Mami, Marrone, Marseglia, & Gemelli, 2001), especially because there seems to be a correlation between early discharge and an increase in emergency department visits by neonates (Liu et al., 2000; Millar, Gloor, Wellington, & Joubert, 2000). The incidence of rehospitalization for dehydration in the immediate neonatal period ranges from 1.2 to 3.4 per 1,000 live births, with about 5% of these dehydrated infants presenting with a cause for dehydration as something other than feeding problems—sepsis or meningitis, for example (Escobar et al., 2002). Escobar and colleagues (2002) noted that the following were the most important risk factors for dehydration:

- First-time mother
- Exclusive breastfeeding (no validation of effectiveness of feeding)
- A mother older than 35 years
- Infant's gestational age less than 39 weeks
- Cesarean-born infants whose initial hospital stay was less than 48 hours

They also noted that serious sequelae were avoided in their institution due to an integrated health-care system that provided early and easy access to follow-up and that the most effective preventive measure is to ensure successful initiation and continuation of breastfeeding, particularly among first-time mothers. Other risk factors include a delay in the first feeding after birth and a lack of attention to poor latch, delayed lactogenesis II, and nipple problems (Caglar, Ozer, & Altugan, 2006).

In one study, charts with standard deviation score (SDS) lines for weight loss in the first month were constructed for 2,359 healthy breastfed newborns and 271 infants with breastfeeding-associated hypernatremic dehydration. Many of the children with hypernatremic dehydration or those who eventually developed the condition fell below the –1 SDS line on day 3, the –2 SDS line on day 4, and the –2.5 SDS line on day 5. Even at an early age, the charts demonstrated that weight loss differed between healthy term breastfed newborns and those with hypernatremic dehydration (van Dommelen, Boer, Unal, & van Wouwe, 2014). Use of such a weight loss graph (**Figure 6-1**) may alert clinicians to the need for more intense breastfeeding support to improve breastmilk intake and help prevent unnecessary formula supplementation.

Dehydration usually has its origins in the initial hospital stay, with fewer than 8 breastfeedings each 24 hours, ineffective feedings with poor latch and little to no swallowing, maternal complaints of sore nipples, use of pacifiers, separation, and an infant at discharge who has experienced reduced colostrum intake and whose mother is unable to determine when swallowing occurs. A number of maternal and infant factors serve as red flags that can provide the setting for dehydration to occur and can alert the clinician of the need for close follow-up:

- **Maternal**
  - Issues with the breasts (previous insufficient milk; flat or retracted nipples; asymmetrical, hypoplastic, or tubular breasts; previous breast surgery; cracked or bleeding nipples).
  - Perinatal and delivery issues (urgent cesarean section, significant postpartum hemorrhage, hypertension, infection, diabetes, overweight/obesity, cystic fibrosis, heart disease, separation from the infant). Konetzny, Bucher, and Arlettaz (2009) reported that infants born by cesarean section had a 3.4 times higher risk for hypernatremia than those born vaginally.
  - Delay of lactogenesis II (copious milk production not evident by day 4, unrelieved severe engorgement).

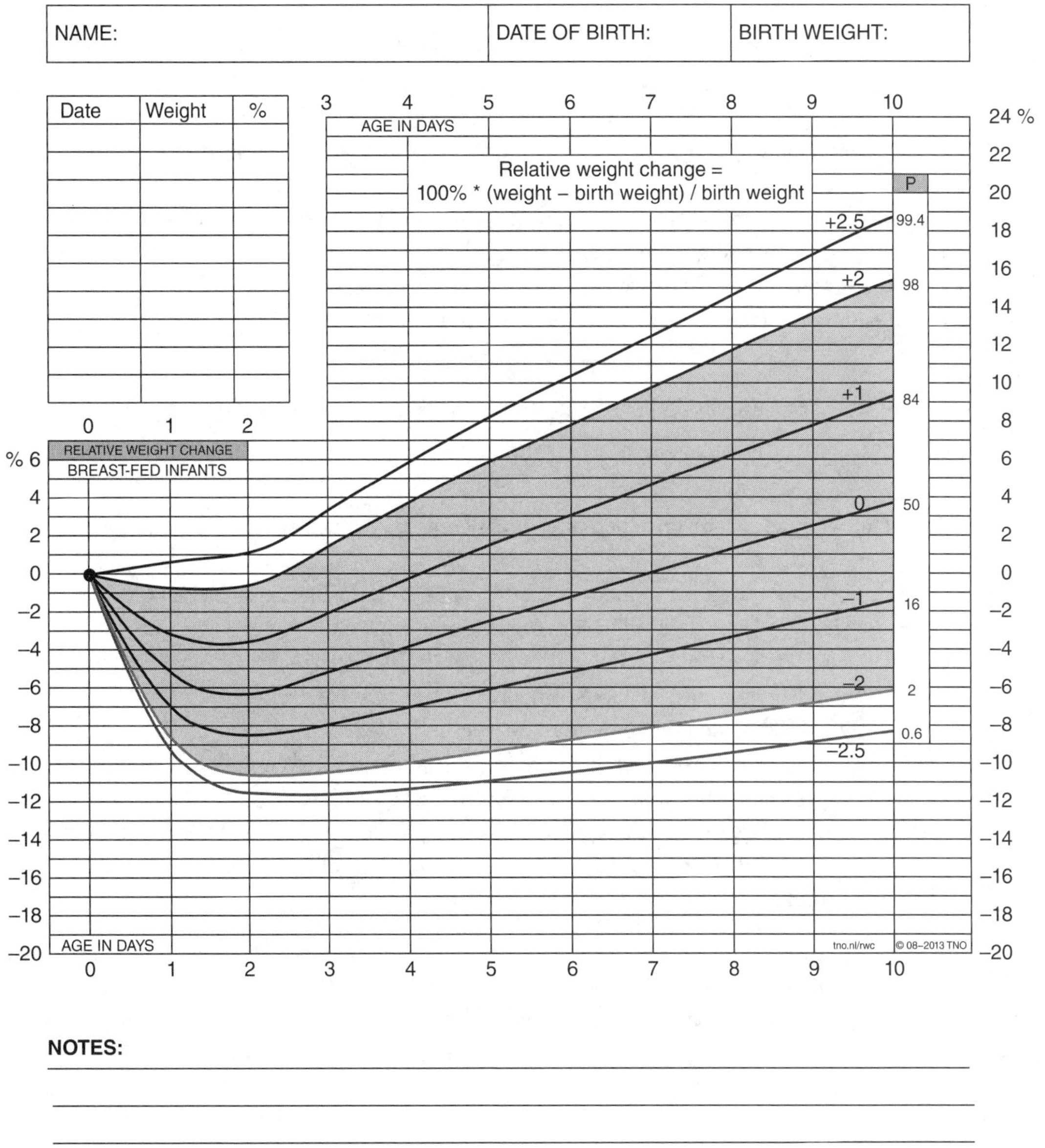

Figure 6-1 Weight loss graph.

Based on https://www.tno.nl/media/2889/graphbreastfedinfants.pdf

- **Infant**
  - Gestational age issues (preterm infants—especially the late preterm, 35- to 37-week-old infant who is discharged in 48 hours or less; small-for-gestational-age infants; post-term infants)
  - Oral anomalies (cleft lip, cleft of the hard or soft palate, bubble palate, micrognathia, ankyloglossia)
  - Infant state control problems (near term, maternal labor medications, closed down)
  - Birth issues (vacuum extraction, birth injuries)
  - Neuromotor issues (hypotonic, hypertonic, dysfunctional sucking)
  - Health issues (cardiac defect, infection, respiratory instability)
  - Newborn care issues (separation, pacifier use, crying)

Additional criteria can be used after discharge to evaluate the potential for or existence of dehydration:

- Sleepy, nondemanding infant who sleeps for long periods of time and is described by the parents as quiet or rarely crying.
- An infant who is fussy or unsettled after breastfeedings or who takes an excessive amount of time at each feeding.
- Diminished urine and stool outputs; persistence of meconium-like stools on day 4, urate crystals in the diaper after day 3, dark yellow or concentrated urine.
- Greater than a 7% weight loss along with other indicators, such as fewer than three stools per day, dry mucous membranes, feeding difficulties, and excessive sleeping.
- Birth weight not regained by 10–14 days of age; mild dehydration may coexist with a 3–5% weight loss, moderate dehydration may become apparent at 6–10% weight loss, and weight loss greater than 10% could be an indication of severe dehydration (Manganaro et al., 2001). However, some infants appear to lose a great deal of weight before discharge because they diurese excess fluid (especially if the mother has had a large amount of intravenous fluids) and/or pass a large meconium stool.

Clinical signs of dehydration can be subtle at first and may go unnoticed by parents who might only be aware of a sleepy infant who may be difficult to feed. Dehydration may not be noted until laboratory evaluation. Infants with hypernatremic dehydration have better preserved extracellular volume with less pronounced clinical signs of dehydration. Weight loss and inadequate stooling are sensitive indicators of dehydration among breastfed infants (Moritz, Manole, Bogen, & Ayus, 2005). As dehydration progresses, the clinician may observe the following signs:

- Clammy skin
- Skin turgor that goes from elastic to tenting
- Skin color that may be pale, with pallor progressing to gray or mottled skin
- Delayed capillary refill
- Decreased tears in eyes, progressing to sunken looking
- Dry lips and buccal mucosa
- Sunken anterior fontanel

- Fever (Maayan-Metzger, Mazkereth, & Kuint, 2003; Ng et al., 1999)
- Lethargy
- Increased pulse rate progressing to tachycardia
- High serum bilirubin concentrations (Liu et al., 2000)

The popular media have reported tragic consequences in a small number of infants who suffered severe hypernatremic dehydration, painting breastfeeding as the dangerous cause of this unfortunate outcome (Helliker, 1994). These preventable situations are caused by the lack of adequate breastfeeding, clinical mismanagement, a delay in seeking help, and failure of proper follow-up on the part of the healthcare system (Laing & Wong, 2002). Clinicians may mistakenly ascribe high sodium levels in breastmilk as the causative factor, reasoning that excessive intake of high-sodium breastmilk resulted in hypernatremic dehydration (Rand & Kolberg, 2001). Usually, poor breastfeeding management, lack of milk transfer, and inadequate follow-up contribute to poor intake in the infant and lack of milk drainage from the breast, with the resulting milk exhibiting high sodium levels indicative of involution. Breastfeeding is unlikely to be the direct cause of neonatal hypernatremia (Sofer, Ben-Ezer, & Dagan, 1993). Retrospective studies of dehydration usually identify problems with milk synthesis, difficulty with breastmilk removal, and low daily breastmilk intake as the overarching factors associated with the development of hypernatremia (Livingstone, Willis, Abdel-Wareth, Thiessen, & Lockitch, 2000). There appears to be an association between the degree of weight loss and the degree of hypernatremia (Macdonald, Ross, Grant, & Young, 2003). The triad of hypernatremia, a history of breastfeeding problems, and weight loss contribute to the "diagnosis" of breastfeeding difficulty–associated hypernatremia (BDAH) (Oddie, Craven, Deakin, Westman, & Scally, 2013). Mild hypernatremia (146–150 mmol/L) is commonly seen and has been documented in almost one-third of breastfed infants with all degrees of recorded weight loss (Marchini & Stock, 1997). Yaseen, Salem, & Darwich (2004) described decreased diaper output in the clinical presentation of exclusively breastfed infants admitted for dehydration. These infants were significantly more likely to have less than six voids and less than three stools in the 24 hours before admission. Failure to screen for the problems prenatally and immediately postdelivery and a lack of adequate follow-up combine to set the stage for poor outcomes (Moritz et al., 2005; Yidzdas et al., 2005). Weighing infants at 72–96 hours along with appropriate and timely lactation support facilitates early recognition of problems and helps decrease the incidence of hypernatremia as well as the severity while preserving breastfeeding (Iyer et al., 2008).

Treatment

Because hypernatremia in breastfed infants typically develops over a longer period of time as compared with acute dehydration from gastroenteritis, it is usually corrected over a longer period of time. If the dehydration is severe, the infant may be admitted into the hospital and receive intravenous fluids to improve cardiovascular function, making sure that the brain and kidneys are perfused while avoiding a too rapid infusion that could lead to seizures or cerebral edema (Molteni, 1994). An infant who is only mildly dehydrated may not be hospitalized. Both types of situations still require that the infant be fed, preferably pumped breastmilk from the mother. If human milk is not available and the mother is not producing sufficient amounts, formula supplementation is needed until her milk production can meet the needs of the infant.

Clinical Approaches to Breastfeeding Support: Practice Suggestions

- Lactation usually can and should be preserved, even if the underlying cause precludes full milk production.
- To improve milk production, the mother should be instructed to pump both breasts simultaneously with a high-quality electric breast pump at least 8–10 times per day (in the absence of an infant at breast or after breastfeedings). This pumped milk (or other supplement) should be offered to the infant during or after each breastfeeding. If the infant is hospitalized, the mother should be able to room-in with the infant and offer the breast frequently.
- If the infant is able to latch, supplemental milk can be provided to the infant through a tube-feeding device placed on the breast to improve sucking and increase milk production during the breastfeeding. The amount of supplement needed can initially be calculated by weighing the infant before and after a breastfeeding and offering the amount of supplement after each breastfeed that would provide a daily intake of 150–200 mL/kg/day. As the infant's sucking improves and the milk supply builds, more milk will be left in the supplementer device or less supplement will be taken by other means. Although use of a bottle to deliver supplements is not precluded, sucking on an artificial nipple weakens the suck or may further weaken a poor suck. A tube-feeding device can be placed on the breast in such a way as to make the delivery of milk easy enough to avoid stress in the mother and infant while not causing a too rapid delivery of milk that overwhelms the infant. Supplementing at breast and pumping also demonstrate the value clinicians place on breastfeeding, human milk, and the mother's efforts to preserve lactation and the breastfeeding experience.
- Weight gain of 56 g per day (double the normal daily weight increment) or more is not unusual during the period of catch-up growth and indicates sufficient intake. Infant formula can be replaced with breastmilk as the mother's supply improves. Pumping should continue until the infant no longer needs supplements and is gaining weight adequately on exclusive breastfeeding.
- Pacifiers should be avoided, because sucking efforts need to be channeled toward improving milk transfer from the breasts.
- Signs of infant swallowing should be taught to the mother. Efforts can be made to increase the volume of milk ingested by the infant at each feeding by using alternate massage.

SLOW WEIGHT GAIN

The definition of normative weight loss in the healthy, full-term, breastfeeding infant has generated conflicting opinions regarding what is normal and when interventions such as supplemental feedings are required. Methodological inconsistencies among numerous studies make it difficult to differentiate between physiological weight loss and a red flag (Tawia & McGuire, 2014; Thulier, 2016). MacDonald and colleagues (2003) demonstrated that a weight loss of up to 12% is experienced by about 95% of neonates. Noel-Weiss, Courant, and Woodend (2008) conducted a systematic review of the literature and within the 11 studies meeting the inclusion criteria, mean weight loss ranged from 5.7–6.6%, with a standard deviation of about 2%. Most infants in these studies regained their birth weight within the first 2 weeks postpartum, with the 2nd and 3rd days after birth being the days of maximum weight loss. Martens and

Romphf (2007) showed that the mean in-hospital weight loss of 812 healthy full-term newborns was 5.09% ± 2.89%, varying by feeding category. Exclusively breastfed infants' in-hospital weight loss was 5.49% ± 2.6%, partially breastfed infants' 5.52% ± 3.02%, and formula-fed infants' 2.43% ± 2.12%. Factors that significantly increased the percentage of weight loss included higher birth weight, female gender, epidural use, and longer hospital stay. Weight loss charts and early weight loss nomograms have been created to identify infants who may be on a trajectory for increased weight loss beyond what is physiologically expected (Bertini, Breschi, & Dani, 2015; Flaherman et al., 2015). Maternal obesity has also been associated with excess infant weight loss when compared with infants whose mothers are not obese (Mok et al., 2008).

Other factors can contribute to early newborn weight loss in the breastfed infant that are not indicators of insufficient feeding (normal diuresis, loss of meconium, hospital and birthing practices, large amounts of maternal intravenous fluid). Although weight loss per se is important to monitor, bowel output has been suggested as another indicator of sufficient breastmilk intake. Shrago, Reifsnider, & Insel (2006) found that more bowel movements per day during the first 5 days after birth were significantly associated with less initial weight loss, earlier transition to yellow bowel movements, earlier return to birth weight, and heavier weight at 14 days of age. Optimal bowel output in this study was a mean of four to five bowel movements per day with transition to yellow bowel movements at a mean of 6.8 days. However, relying on stool output alone may yield many false positives. Nommsen-Rivers, Heinig, Cohen, and Dewey (2008) demonstrated that diaper outputs when measured in the home setting showed too much overlap between infants with adequate versus inadequate breastmilk intake. This made it problematic to rely on diaper output as the only indicator of sufficient milk intake. Nommsen-Rivers and colleagues recommended that the parameters of fewer than four bowel movements on day 4 or delay of lactogenesis II beyond 72 hours after birth is suggestive of breastfeeding insufficiency. Monitoring of diaper output may provide an advance warning of pending weight loss or dehydration even though newborn diaper counts show wide variation.

After the initial weight loss during the first few days after birth, most breastfed infants regain their birth weight by 2 weeks. Up to 12% of infants may experience excess weight loss (greater than 10%) during this period, which has been closely linked with delayed lactogenesis II and suboptimal infant breastfeeding skills (Dewey et al., 2003). For the mother of an infant who does not demonstrate appropriate weight gain or who continues to lose weight, the expectation of a thriving infant and a successful breastfeeding experience is abruptly challenged. Between 2 and 6 weeks of age, the average breastfed female infant is expected to gain approximately 34 g/day and the male breastfed infant should gain about 40 g/day, with the minimum expected gain for both boys and girls being about 20 g/day (Nelson, Rogers, Ziegler, & Fomon, 1989). After this, the weight, length, and head circumference of infants are followed on growth charts.

In the United States between 1977 and 2000, the 1977 National Center for Health Statistics growth charts were used. These charts had a number of limitations, including the very few breastfed infants who were included in the reference data upon which the charts were constructed. Discrepancies were revealed when data became available on the normal growth of exclusively breastfed infants. In comparison with these charts, breastfed infants have a relatively rapid weight gain in the first 2–3 months followed by a drop in percentile ranking thereafter (Dewey, Heinig, Nommsen, Peerson, & Lonnerdal, 1992; Dewey et al., 1995), leading some healthcare providers to recommend supplementation for perceived growth faltering. The Centers for Disease Control and Prevention (CDC) produced new growth charts in 2000 to address some of the major concerns with the National Center for Health Statistics charts (Ogden et al., 2002). These charts, however, still fail to address the normal growth of the reference infant—one fed exclusively on breastmilk until about age 6 months and thereafter breastfed while receiving appropriate complementary foods (Dewey, 2001). With this in mind the World Health Organization (WHO) released new standards in April 2006 for assessing the growth and development of children from birth to age 5 years (de Onis, Garza, Onyango, & Martorell, 2006; WHO Multicentre Growth Reference Study Group, 2006). These new standards are designed to describe how all children should grow rather than providing a more limited snapshot of how children grew at a specified time and place (Garza & de Onis, 2004).

There are differences between the WHO and CDC charts, with the main differences occurring in infancy. The mean weight of infants included in the WHO standards is above the CDC median during the first 6 months of infancy, crosses it at approximately 6 months, and remains below the CDC median until about 32 months (de Onis, Garza, Onyango, & Borghi, 2007). These weight-for-age differences are especially important during infancy. The CDC charts cannot account for the rapidly changing weights of early infancy because the study design lacked empirical weight data between birth and 2 months of age. The infancy section of the WHO standard is based on a greater sample size and shorter measurement intervals, allowing it to account for the rapidly changing growth in early infancy and the physiological weight loss during the first few days. The WHO standards are based on exclusively breastfed infants, whereas the CDC charts included relatively few infants who were breastfed for more than a couple of months. Underweight will be higher when based on the WHO standard compared with the CDC reference during the first 6 months of infancy (de Onis, Onyango, Borghi, Garza, & Yang, 2006). When using the CDC charts, breastfed infants will show an apparent decline in weight for age after 6 months (van Dijk & Innis, 2009).

Danner, Joeckel, Michalak, Phillips, and Goday (2009) developed weight gain velocity charts to help align the differences between the CDC and WHO charting systems. In general, children on the WHO growth charts gain at a faster rate during the first 6 months of life, after which time the children on the CDC growth charts gain weight faster. The charts from the Danner study provide a reference for grams/day and grams/month weight gain in 5 different percentiles. These weight velocity charts are helpful in assessing adequacy of weight gain in short time intervals. Clinicians may find these growth velocity charts to be a helpful tool for assessing weight gain adequacy, especially if it appears that a breastfed infant is faltering anywhere on either of the charting systems. The WHO system may result in false positives for underweight in some breastfed infants during the first 6 months, with the potential of unnecessary supplementation or early use of complementary foods (Binns, James, & Lee, 2008; Cattaneo & Guoth-Gumberger, 2008).

Adequate growth and the need for supplementing breastfeeding should be based on more than a single measurement from either of the growth charting systems. Clinical, developmental, and behavioral assessments are also paramount in assessing growth adequacy. Changes in growth velocity as determined by three measurements over a suitable period of time may be a more reliable indicator of growth faltering (Cattaneo & Guoth-Gumberger, 2008).

The CDC recommends that clinicians in the United States use the 2006 WHO international growth charts to screen for normal growth in children who are less than 24 months old and use the CDC growth charts for children aged 2–19 years (Grummer-Strawn, Reinold, & Krebs, 2010). When using the WHO growth charts to screen for possible abnormal or unhealthy growth, use of the 2.3rd and 97.7th percentiles (or ± 2 standard deviations) are recommended, rather than the 5th and 95th percentiles.

A number of authors have conceptualized the problem from various starting points, with some offering schema or flow charts to provide a more encompassing framework.

- Desmarais and Browne (1990) coined the term impending failure to thrive to differentiate between infants who are normal but slow growing, those who are failing to thrive, and those who are at risk for inadequate weight gain without appropriate intervention. Overlapping maternal and infant conditions may result in a complex cause-and-effect scenario that clinicians must unravel to identify the root cause or causes of the problem.
- Lawrence and Lawrence (2010) use a schema to classify causes associated with infant behavior from those related to maternal problems. Infant causes were broadly classified as poor intake, low net intake, and high energy requirements. Maternal classifications included poor milk production and poor release of milk.
- Ramsay, Gisel, and Boutry (1993) related weight-gain problems to a history of alterations in normal feeding skills and behaviors. In their study, infants with growth faltering had a history of abnormally long durations of feeding times, poor appetite (did not provide clear hunger signals), delayed texture tolerance (in older infants), and difficult feedings (infants had difficulty latching to the breast, pushed out the nipple, and had frequent feedings that lasted an hour or more). They discussed the possibility that growth faltering correlated to a subgroup of infants with what was termed a feeding skills disorder and that mothers of these infants did not display faulty interactions with their infants. The term nonorganic failure to thrive is still sometimes used to refer to infants whose lack of expected weight gain is unrelated to underlying pathology. Failure to thrive has traditionally conjured a negative connotation of poor maternal–infant interaction, but these authors found that maternal–infant interaction was not related to poor intake.

Common in many studies of postnatal factors associated with slow infant weight gain are several elements: a history of feeding problems; a description of being a slow feeder; and reports of weak sucking, poor appetite, and taking in only small quantities of milk at a time (Hollen, Din, Jones, Emond, & Emmett, 2014; McDougall, Drewett, Hungin, & Wright, 2008). Emond, Drewett, Blair, and Emmett (2007) found that weak sucking was equally important in breastfed and bottle-fed infants. One in six infants in a cohort of 11,900 infants was reported by their parents to have weak sucking. Growth faltering was almost twice as likely in this group. Exhaustion while feeding may be another marker for potentially slow weight gain with infants demonstrating the above feeding behaviors being more likely to be biologically vulnerable (Hollen et al., 2014). Emond and colleagues caution that early onset and persistence of slow or difficult feeding may be a signal of inadequate intake, leading to possible growth faltering. Growth faltering may be transient or temporary. Subtle oromotor dysfunction has also been mentioned to be associated with some weight faltering as parents have described retrospectively that their infants with weight faltering were more likely to have had sucking difficulty and problems chewing and swallowing (Wright, Parkinson, & Drewett, 2006). Some early feeding difficulties may possibly be a marker of subtle neurological impairments and serve as a precursor to eventual poor weight gain. There is also some evidence that slow weight gain over the first

2 months is associated with developmental delay (Drewett, Emond, Blair, & Emmett, 2005; Emond, Blair, Emmett, and Drewett, 2007). Emond, et al. (2007) showed a 3-point IQ deficit in the slowest gaining 5% of term infants in the first 8 weeks, demonstrating that IQ deficit is associated with early rather than later growth faltering. With weak sucking associated with growth faltering, early weight gain issues in some infants may be a feeding-skills problem of neurophysiological origin. On the other hand, if the early weeks of life are a critical period for nutritional adequacy, then insufficient nutrition could impact brain growth and later cognitive functioning. Although this effect does not appear to be large, it is comparable in size with the effects of other variables that impinge on IQ such as bottle-feeding, prenatal cocaine use, and low-birth-weight (Anderson, Johnstone, & Remley, 1999; Corbett & Drewett, 2004).

Clearly, early growth faltering is an issue that requires close monitoring. Failure to thrive not only has a negative undertone (neglect or abuse) but also has differing definitions:

- A fall of 2 standard deviations on the weight chart in the first 8 weeks or a fall below the 3rd percentile for weight (Kien, 1985)
- The rate of weight gain is less than –2 standard deviation value during an interval of 2 months or longer for infants less than 6 months of age or for 3 months for an infant over 6 months and the weight for length is less than the 5th percentile (Foman & Nelson, 1993).
- The infant continues to lose weight after 10 days of life, does not regain birth weight by 3 weeks of age, or gains at a rate below the 10th percentile for weight gain beyond 1 month of age (Lawrence & Lawrence, 2010).

Because slow weight gain or growth faltering in a breastfed infant may be interpreted differently depending on which growth charts and parameters are used (Olsen, 2006), Powers (2001) suggested using a set of criteria to differentiate when a breastfed infant is gaining appropriately and when a feeding problem requires intervention:

- Newborn infant less than 2 weeks of age who is more than 10% below birth weight
- An infant whose weight is less than birth weight at 2 weeks of age
- After an initial void, an infant who has no urine output in any given 24-hour period
- An infant who does not have yellow milk stools by the end of the 1st week
- An infant who has clinical signs of dehydration
- Infants 2 weeks to 3 months of age whose weight gain is less than 20 g/day
- Unexplained weight loss at any age
- Completely flat growth curves at any age

Sometimes infants older than 3 or 4 months of age will be identified as suddenly experiencing growth faltering. It is important to differentiate whether this is the normal downward crossing of percentile rankings (i.e., the change in growth velocity and weight gain patterns typical for a healthy, well-nourished, breastfed infant when using standard growth charts) or a true problem. Lukefahr (1990) reported that when infants over 1 month of age presented with growth faltering, organic causes were actually present in about 50% of the cases. Growth faltering in length velocity or length for age may also indicate an organic cause or a nutrient deficiency such as a low vitamin B_6 status (Heiskanen, Siimes, & Salmenpera Perheentupa, 1995). Sucking becomes voluntary rather than reflexive around 3 or 4 months of age, and older infants can be highly distractible at breast. The clinician should check a number of issues, including organic or disease-based causes, as well as more common issues (Frantz, 1992) such as follows:

- Displacing sucking to fingers or other objects
- Changes in feeding patterns:
  - Limitations on the length and frequency of feedings if an infant is teething
  - Parents are using an infant training program or a sleep-through-the night regimen that limits or reduces the number of feeds per 24 hours
- Infant becomes so distractible that he or she shortens the feedings to the point of inadequate intake
- Busy maternal schedule or return to employment that reduces milk intake
  - Early introduction of less calorie-dense solid foods that displace breastmilk from the diet
- Mother experiences illness or severe dieting
- Mother begins taking oral contraceptives

Sometimes when an older infant who has been thriving at the breast slows or stops gaining weight, the etiology emerges as a combination of a mother with an abundant milk supply and rapid milk ejection reflex that allows an infant who is either a poor feeder, or who develops into a poor feeder, to easily obtain milk with minimal effort. When the milk production diminishes and the infant must execute correct and strong suckling, this oral motor skill emerges as less than optimal, reducing milk transfer and contributing to a flattening growth curve (Newman, 2004). Use of alternate massage may prove helpful. Breast compression can improve the pressure gradient between the breast and the infant's mouth, assisting in milk transfer.

In the presence of a slow-gaining breastfed infant, both infant (**Table 6-2**) and maternal (**Table 6-3**) assessments must be conducted to formulate a differential diagnosis, construct a problem-oriented management strategy, preserve the lactation and breastfeeding experience, and support the mother through an anxiety-provoking period of time (Powers, 1999). Slow weight gain per se is usually not "the problem" but is most often the result or manifestation of a problem. Simple faulty management, such as poor positioning, incorrect latch, insufficient number of feedings per 24 hours, or use of a pacifier to stretch out feeding times, should be assessed and corrected first. Late recognition of problems results in high rates of mothers abandoning breastfeeding (Harding, Cairns, Gupta, & Cowan, 2001; Oddie et al., 2001).

Once a history, physical exam, and breastfeeding assessment have been completed, the clinician may have formed an opinion of what factors may be contributing to the problem. A number of interacting maternal and infant factors may need to be accounted for or corrected as the feeding plan is developed. Mothers may have a sufficient milk supply but the infant is unable to transfer this milk effectively. Mothers may have low milk production with or without an infant who demonstrates effective feeding skills. The clinician will also need to determine if supplementation is necessary and how this would be accomplished while preserving lactation and breastfeeding. Powers (2010) suggested that supplementation may be considered or indicated by the clinical condition of the infant, by the amount of weight loss (greater than 10% in a newborn or young infant), failure to return to birth weight later than 2–3 weeks of age, average daily weight gain of less than 20 g, any amount of unexplained weight loss, weight and length curves that are completely flat at any age, and deceleration of head circumference that consecutively crosses percentiles.

Table 6-2 Infant Factors That May Contribute to Slow Weight Gain

Factor	Effect
Gestational age and growth	Preterm, late preterm, post-term, SGA, IUGR, and LGA infants may lack mature feeding skills. Provision of breastmilk is especially important for SGA infants because it promotes better catch-up growth in head circumference (brain growth) than supplementing with standard formula (Lucas et al., 1997). Many of these infants are known to exhibit weak sucking, a major contributor to slow weight gain.
Alterations in oral anatomy	Alterations such as ankyloglossia, cleft lip, cleft of hard or soft palate, bubble palate, facial growth anomalies such as micrognathia, and congenital syndromes that affect the oral structure may contribute to poor milk intake.
Alterations in oral functioning	Hypotonia, hypertonia, neurological pathology, and physiology may interfere with the performance, strength, or stamina of the structures involved in the suck-swallow-breathe cycle.
High energy requirements	Cardiac disease, respiratory involvement (bronchopulmonary dysplasia [BPD]), metabolic disorders that create a need for increased caloric intake, and volume restriction that places limits on intake may contribute to slow weight gain.
Known illness	Infection, trisomy 21, cystic fibrosis, and cardiac defects often put the infant at risk for poor growth because of the combination of a low endurance for feeding and high metabolic demands. Growth faltering may be apparent in the early months due to atopic dermatitis (Agostoni et al., 2000).
Maternal medications	Certain prenatal prescription medications or recreational drugs may interfere with normal sucking physiology.
Intrapartum factors	Cesarean delivery, hypoxia, anoxia, labor medications, state control difficulties, epidural analgesia, forceps, and vacuum extraction that affect brain function, anatomic structures, and nerves contribute to ineffective milk transfer.
Iatrogenic factors	Hospital routines that separate mothers and infants, provide inappropriate supplementation, offer pacifiers, or provide conflicting or poor breastfeeding instruction leave both mothers and infants lacking needed feeding skills.
Gastrointestinal or metabolic/malabsorption problems	Gastroesophageal reflux or other conditions that limit nutrient intake or metabolism may contribute to slow weight gain.

IUGR = intrauterine growth restriction; LGA = large for gestational age; SGA = small for gestational age.

In complicated situations, if an infant is being monitored for intake and output or if amounts of supplements are being calculated, intake at a feeding can be determined, if necessary, by taking a pre- and postfeed weight of the infant on an electronic scale sensitive to within 2 g (Meier et al., 1994). This can be useful in determining the intake at that particular feeding. Sometimes a mother can pump

Table 6-3 Maternal Factors That May Contribute to Slow Infant Weight Gain

Factor	Effect
Breast abnormalities	Previous breast surgery, insufficient glandular development, augmentation, reduction, and trauma may influence the ultimate volume of milk that the breasts will produce but do not preclude breastfeeding.
Nipple anomalies	Flat, retracted, inverted, oddly shaped, or dimpled nipples may make latching more difficult and reduce milk intake. Improper suckling on nipples may also damage them, further reducing infant milk intake.
Ineffective or insufficient milk removal	Improperly positioned/latched infant, ineffective suckling, and unresolved engorgement leave residual milk and reduce supply, making less milk available to the infant.
Delayed lactogenesis II	A mother who is overweight, is obese, or has diabetes may experience an initial delay in lactogenesis II. When copious milk production is delayed, frequency of feedings must increase to offset the volume deficit.
Poor breastfeeding management	Delayed or disrupted early feeding opportunities, separation, too few feedings, and illness may reduce feeding opportunities at breast. Failure to pump milk in the absence of an infant suckling at breast may interfere with proliferation and sensitivity of prolactin receptors.
Medications/drugs	Use of prescription or recreational drugs, labor medications, and IV fluids may delay lactogenesis II or interfere with infant suckling. Oral contraceptives can reduce lactose content and overall milk volume (Hale, 2003). Smoking may also decrease volume (Vio, Salazar, & Infante, 1991) and fat content of milk (Hopkinson, Schanler, Fraley, & Garza, 1992).
Hormonal alterations	Hypothyroidism, retained placenta, superimposed pregnancy, pituitary disorders, polycystic ovarian syndrome, theta lutein cysts (Hoover, Barbalinardo, & Platia, 2002), oral contraceptives, diabetes insipidus, assisted reproduction/difficulty conceiving, and other endocrine-related problems may interfere with the normal progression of milk production.
Milk ejection problems	Drugs, alcohol, smoking, stress, pain, and other factors that inhibit the letdown reflex reduce the amount of milk available to the infant.
Miscellaneous factors	Lack of vitamin B_{12} in a vegetarian diet, parenting programs that limit feedings, ineffective breast pump or pumping schedule, inadequate weight gain during pregnancy, postpartum hemorrhage, anemia, and cesarean delivery may contribute to slow infant weight gain (Evans, Evans, Royal, Esterman, & James, 2003).

her breasts after a feeding and take a postfeed weight to determine the approximate total amount of milk that was available at that particular feeding and determine if a supplement is required at that time (Meier, Lysakowski, Engstrom, Kavanaugh, & Mangurten, 1990). These procedures are not indicative of 24-hour intakes and milk production, but may help the clinician to gather data regarding whether the milk production is appropriate and the infant is unable to effect milk transfer or to help estimate recommended amounts of supplements based on approximate intake at a feeding. Because infants demonstrate a large feed-to-feed intake variability, a closer picture of intake and milk production would involve the mother performing a prefeed weight, breastfeeding her infant, performing a postfeed weight, pumping both breasts, and totaling the amounts over a 24-hour period of time. In a more urgent situation this may not be practical, and the clinician would work to correct mismanagement or feeding techniques while supplementing the infant during or after each breastfeeding with as much pumped milk or formula as the infant will take. In a less urgent situation, Powers (2010) recommended starting amounts of supplement that represent approximately 25% of normal intake and adjust up or down as weight gain improves. For example, a 6-lb, 9-oz (3.0 kg) infant would require 15–20 oz (450–600 mL) as a total daily intake. Supplementing with 4 oz divided into 6 to 8 feedings over a 24-hour period represents a conservative starting point.

Determining what and how to supplement can be considered on a basis of the most to least physiological. Supplements in order of preference are the mother's own expressed milk, mother's hindmilk if the supply permits, pasteurized donor milk (if indicated for an ill, preterm, or severely immunocompromised infant), and infant formula (type based on the family history of the presence of allergies or diabetes). Hindmilk, which is obtained farther into a breastfeeding, is also the fat-rich cream layer seen in stored breastmilk. This cream layer can be especially calorie-dense with up to 28–30 calories or more per ounce (Lucas, Gibbs, Lyster, & Baum, 1978). Although milk volume is most often the major factor affecting weight gain of exclusively breastfed infants (Aksit, Ozkayin, & Caglayan, 2002), the use of the hindmilk cream layer can boost caloric intake significantly while delivering a physiological volume of milk (Valentine, Hurst, & Schanler, 1994). Infants over 6 months of age can be supplemented with calorie-dense semisolid foods. The method of supplementation would preferably be directly at the breast using a tube-feeding device or tubing run through a nipple shield if the infant was unable to latch to the breast. If short-term or occasional supplements were indicated, other devices could be selected such as a cup, syringe, dropper, spoon, or bottle. During the creation of the feeding plan, the clinician has a number of techniques and equipment (see **Appendix 6-1**) from which to choose and, in conjunction with the mother, determine which combinations best suit the situation.

Clinical Approaches to Breastfeeding Support: Practice Suggestions

A common theme in the history of a breastfeeding infant with slow weight gain is the description of prolonged feedings (30–60 minutes), as in the study by Ramsay and colleagues (1993) and the case study in **Box 6-2**. Walshaw, Owens, Scally, and Walshaw (2008) reported that infants who fed for approximately 10 minutes on both breasts at each feeding gained more weight and breastfed exclusively for a longer duration than infants who spent more extended times at the breast. Little is known regarding the physiology of prolonged feedings. The highest amounts of breastmilk are available during the first 2 letdowns, usually occurring within 10 minutes of the start of a feeding. It may be that prolonged feedings reduce the pulsatile nature of oxytocin release, making reduced amounts of milk available as the feeding is prolonged (Walshaw, 2010). In the situation of low

Box 6-2 Case Study of Baby Briana

Briana had begun sleeping through the night at 4 weeks of age, fed about 6 times every 24 hours, took 1 hour to feed at breast, and took 1 hour to consume 2 oz of formula from a bottle. She had been seen by her family practice physician with no reports of organic or pathological conditions. Briana had been seen by a feeding team at a children's hospital who recommended that she be switched to high-calorie formula and fed by a fast-flow bottle nipple. She was also noted to have a tongue thrust. She produced four to five wet diapers per day and a bowel movement every few days.

A breastfeeding was observed showing good positioning and latch, but Briana took between 17 and 34 sucks per swallow. She would swallow only after a letdown. Briana's mother stated that she wished to continue breastfeeding and providing as much of her milk as possible for Briana but that she could pump little to no milk at that point. A phone call to the infant's physician revealed that if the weight loss could not be rectified, Briana would be admitted into the hospital for further testing. If formula supplementation was indicated, a standard formula could be used.

The initial goal was to reverse the weight loss immediately and avoid admission into the hospital. The longer term goal was to maximize milk production and help Briana improve her suckling to the point that she could consume most of her feedings at the breast within a reasonable length of time.

Techniques chosen

Nipple tug, alternate massage

Equipment chosen

Supplemental Nutrition System (SNS) tube-feeding device, electric breast pump with double collection kit, feeding and weight log, infant formula if no breastmilk was available for supplementation

Plan

1. Briana was to be fed 8–10 times every 24 hours with a 2:00 am night feeding to be added temporarily. This would add more opportunities for increasing intake.
2. The SNS (with the medium-size tubing) was to be used during each feeding, with 3–4 oz of formula as the supplement until pumped milk was available. Supplements were reduced to 1–2 ounces as Briana consumed more milk from the breast and left more supplement in the SNS. Nipple tug and alternate massage were chosen as initial techniques to strengthen the suck, maximize fat intake, and increase breastmilk volume. Supplementing at the breast would serve to stimulate milk production and reduce the amount of time for each feeding. The choice of these techniques and equipment was also designed to improve sucking efficiency so that a more efficient suck-to-swallow ratio was demonstrated. Because flow regulates suck, the SNS was chosen to initiate and maintain flow.
3. Briana's mother was to pump her breasts after as many feedings as possible during the day to maximize milk production. She pumped between 2 and 6 times per day, with total 24-hour volume pumped between 2 and 8 ounces.

weight gain, a feeding pattern may be suggested for infants who latch and suck at the breast that recommends:

- Frequent feedings (10–12 per 24 hours).
- Feeding on the first side using alternate massage until the infant will no longer suck and swallow when alternate massage is applied during a pause, or no longer than 10–15 minutes before switching to the other side. Prolonged feedings can frustrate and tire both mother and infant and may result in diminishing returns relative to milk intake.
- Feeding on the second breast using alternate massage as above.
- It has been shown that the fat content of breastmilk peaks 30 minutes following a feeding or pumping (Hassiotou et al., 2013). Clinicians may wish to recommend that mothers of slow gaining infants put the infant back to breast 30 minutes following a feeding to increase the infant's caloric intake by making available this high-fat milk.
- Additional milk can be supplied if needed by a tube-feeding device at the breast. This can be breastmilk that was pumped or hand expressed 30 minutes after a feeding.

The creation of the feeding plan and choice of interventions reflect the etiology of the problem (Box 6-2). The overarching goals of the management guidelines are to protect the milk supply and provide adequate nourishment to the infant to restore and support normal growth. Written feeding guidelines with short- and long-term goals for the parents are important to reinforce teaching and provide a mechanism for parents to remember the multiple tasks that must be accomplished. Feeding plans can be as simple as increasing the number of feedings and adding alternate massage on each breast at each feeding until weight gain improves. Other situations may be more complex, as described in the following sections.

BREASTFEEDING PRETERM INFANTS

In 2014, the premature birth rate (before 37 weeks' gestation) in the United States was 11.32% of live births (Hamilton, Martin, Osterman, & Curtin, 2015). Preterm births vary by race, with the rate of preterm birth being 10.14% in non-Hispanic white, 16.29% in non-Hispanic black, and 11.23% in Hispanic infants. Rates of preterm birth vary by state, with a low of 8.5% in California to a high of 15.99% in Mississippi. The preferred feeding modality for the almost half-million preterm infants born each year is human milk and breastfeeding (AAP, Section on Breastfeeding, 2012). Breastfeeding rates for preterm or low-birth-weight infants are low. In a survey of 124 neonatal intensive care units (NICUs), 50.3% of the 42,891 premature infants were not receiving any breastmilk when they were discharged from the hospital (Powers, Clark, Bloom, Thomas, & Peabody, 2001).

Parents benefit from receiving factual information regarding the therapeutic effects that human milk and breastfeeding will have on their infant so that their feeding decision is evidence based (Meier, 2001; Meier & Brown, 1997). The healthcare professional has an ethical responsibility to avoid withholding information because of the unfounded concern that to inform mothers of research-based options may make them feel guilty if they choose not to breastfeed. A study of preterm mothers whose initial intent was to formula feed but subsequently initiated lactation after the encouragement of NICU care providers found the mothers denied feeling forced or pressured into breastfeeding by staff who presented an unequivocal message regarding the importance of breastfeeding (Miracle, Meier, & Bennett, 2004a). Women who are subsequently made aware of the nutritional and immunological properties of human milk in relation to improved infant health outcomes often express anger and frustration with the healthcare professionals who failed to share this knowledge with them (Miracle, Meier, & Bennett, 2004b). Scrutiny of a number of other non-evidence-based assumptions has shown that clinicians need not fear encouraging the mother of a preterm infant to breastfeed (Rodriguez, Miracle, & Meier, 2005). Sisk, Lovelady, Dillard, and Gruber (2006) showed that lactation counseling for 196 mothers of preterm infants who both planned and did not plan to breastfeed did not increase anxiety, regardless of initial feeding plans. Eighty-five percent of the mothers who initially did not plan to breastfeed initiated milk expression and stated that pumping was worth the effort. The mothers in the group that initially did not plan to breastfeed were able to provide at least 50% of their infants' intake for the first 3 weeks, 48.8% for the 4th week, and 32.8% of the infants' intake for the entire hospitalization period. Mothers in both groups stated that "infant health benefits" was the most common reason for expressing milk. All the mothers in both groups stated that they were glad that the staff helped them with milk expression. The study used individual counseling sessions with lactation consultants who informed all mothers regarding the benefits of their breastmilk for their premature infants. This was followed immediately by a pumping session. Mothers were told that there would be no pressure to continue pumping if after attempting to do so they did not wish to continue. This approach was especially effective in changing mothers' feeding decisions for the period of hospitalization, as 85% of the mothers who initially planned to formula feed were able to provide their milk for infants who otherwise would never have received the nutritive and protective factors in breastmilk.

Early positive messages regarding the importance of breastmilk for preterm infants are a powerful motivator in helping mothers to change their feeding goals to exclusive breastmilk feeding for their preterm infant. Unfortunately, the mother's breastmilk may be inadequate for the maintenance of lactation beyond the first several weeks. The initial messages regarding the protective effects of human milk may need to transition to messages about the longer-term health benefits of continued breastfeeding once the immediate risks of necrotizing enterocolitis (NEC), sepsis, and other early risks have passed. Such education should begin prior to the day 29–72 period when breastfeeding goals may become less ambitious (Hoban et al., 2015). Some mothers may feel that the danger period is over by this time, and that their milk has helped overcome the initial risks of prematurity (Rossman, Kratovil, Greene, Engstrom, & Meier, 2013). As they return to employment and other duties, they may therefore become more comfortable with bottle- or formula feeding.

Why Use Human Milk for Preterm Infants?

Feeding human milk to preterm infants has a number of important short- and long-term health outcomes that are vital to share with the mother (**Box 6-3**). Knowing the importance of breastmilk to their infants may help mothers to not only provide their milk for their infants but also act as a motivator to continue pumping milk during discouraging times of long hospitalizations.

Necrotizing enterocolitis is a devastating and potentially lethal disease that is seen predominantly in preterm infants. Breastmilk given for less than 7 days significantly increases the infant's risk of developing NEC (Kimak, de Castro Antunes, Braga, Brandt, & de Carvalho Lima, 2015). The preterm fetal gut has not completed its maturation process; human milk contains components that enhance this maturation,

Box 6-3 Health Outcomes of Preterm Infants When Not Fed Their Own Mother's Milk

- Achievement of full enteral feedings later (Sisk, Lovelady, Gruber, Dillard, & O'Shea, 2008)
- Experience a significant increase in nosocomial infections (Schanler, 2007)
- More likely to develop necrotizing enterocolitis (Meinzen-Derr et al., 2009)
- Lower scores on tests of visual acuity (Morales & Schanler, 2007)
- Decreased neurocognitive performance (Horwood, Darlow, & Mogridge, 2001)
- Altered immune system function (Tarcan, Gurakan, Tiker, & Ozbek, 2004)
- Increased intestinal permeability and slower intestinal maturation (Taylor, Basile, Ebeling, & Wagner, 2009)

whereas infant formula does not. The gastrointestinal system plays a major role in serving as a barrier to pathogens and allergens and as a vehicle for nutrient absorption. However, the preterm gut faces threats and risks to its microbial development, especially if the infant was born by cesarean, is separated from the mother, is given antibiotics, and is fed formula. Gut maturation is significantly delayed in preterm infants who are fed formula (Reisinger et al., 2014). Artificially fed infants do not receive human milk components that promote the closure of the tight junctions between cells, increasing the risk that certain volumes of infant formula will act as a toxic dose for the premature intestine (Taylor et al., 2009). Because preterm infants cannot fully digest carbohydrates and proteins, human milk provides components that aid this process. When fed infant formula, undigested casein can reach the gut, attract neutrophils that provoke inflammation and the opening of the tight junctions between cells, allow intact proteins to engage in systemic invasion, and further damage a fragile gut, leading to NEC (Claud & Walker, 2001). Maayan-Metzger, Avivi, Schushan-Eisen, and Kuint (2012) found lower rates of both NEC and retinopathy of prematurity in infants fed human milk compared to those fed infant formula. Breastmilk has a microbiome of its own that provides an inoculum of microorganisms unique to the mother/baby dyad and works to make sure that the succession of microbial colonization in the gut is not altered resulting in dysbiosis. Dysbiosis is an alteration in the microbial composition or diversity in gut that can lead to inflammation, opening of the epithelial tight junctions, enteric symptoms, and increased permeability of the gut such that toxins, live bacteria, undigested foods, bacterial metabolites, and viruses are enabled to enjoy easy access into the infant's bloodstream.

Colostrum is important as the first feeding rather than formula. Premature infants have a reduced time of exposure to swallowed amniotic fluid, with its array of growth factors, in utero. Colostrum feedings help compensate for this shortcoming by providing high concentrations of secretory immunoglobulin A (IgA), growth factors, antioxidants, anti-inflammatory cytokines, and a host of other protective components that no manufactured formula contains. The early days of colostrum production is a critical exposure period for fragile infants, with mothers of the least mature infants producing the most protective colostrum (Meier, Engstrom, Patel, Jegier, & Bruns, 2010). Colostrum secretion is often prolonged in preterm mothers, suggesting that an extended colostral phase may serve as another protective mechanism for the compromised infant.

Johnson and colleagues (2010) found that in infants born at < 26 weeks' gestation, autism spectrum symptoms and disorders were more prevalent at 11 years of age in those who had not received breastmilk as infants. Vohr and colleagues (2006) found that every 10mL/kg/day increase in breastmilk intake contributed 0.53 points to the Bayley Mental Development Index, conferring a 5.3 IQ point advantage for infants consuming 110 mL/kg/day. Isaacs and colleagues (2010) showed that the percentage of breastmilk received by preterm infants was positively correlated to later IQ in a dose–response manner, especially in boys. Receipt of human milk in these preterm infants was seen to enhance brain development, particularly in white matter growth. Quigley and colleagues (2012) reported that cognitive development is enhanced at 5 years of age with any breastfeeding, but more significantly with at least 4 months of breastfeeding. This was especially true in infants born preterm. Breastfed children in this study were 1 to 6 months ahead of nonbreastfed children. This long-term advantage may optimize cognitive potential and decrease the need for costly early intervention and special education services in childhood.

Maternal Stresses

The large body of published evidence on the effects of human milk feeding in preterm infants shows that mother's milk is the milk of choice for the premature infant (Schanler & Atkinson, 1999). Scientific and medical advances have created a population of extremely low-birth-weight infants who are often critically ill. The use of human milk for these infants fills the gaps in their undeveloped host defenses and metabolic and gastrointestinal immaturity and produces long-term advantages in vision and neurodevelopment. Human milk provides protection from the conditions that preterm infants are most prone to develop, such as infection and NEC (Schanler, 2001).

Some clinicians may be concerned that providing breastmilk is too stressful to the mother, but evidence shows that the provision of breastmilk provides a mechanism for the mother to regain an element of control over an overwhelming situation. Fear, grief, remorse, anger, and guilt can be refocused into activities that allow the mother to exercise her unique role in the intimate care of her newborn. Rather than being considered as a visitor, the mother is part of the team who cares for her infant. Her milk provides both medication and nutrition, a contribution that is uniquely hers (Kavanaugh, Meier, Zimmermann, & Mead, 1997; Lang, 2002; Spanier-Mingolelli, Meier, & Bradford, 1998; Whiteley, 1996). Breastfeeding (or pumping breastmilk) is an oxytocin-releasing condition that further contributes to decreased stress and improved maternal–infant attachment (Feldman, Weller, Leckman, Kuint, & Eidelman, 1999). Expressing breastmilk for her tiny infant acts as a connection between mother and baby, conferring maternal identity in a time of stress. Davim, Enders, and da Silva (2010) found that mothers of preterm infants who could not immediately breastfeed following delivery experienced feeling of sorrow, disappointment, frustration, guilt, and concern about harming the baby while holding the baby for breastfeeding. However, once able to breastfeed, mothers reported feelings of fulfillment, pride, and satisfaction at the first breastfeeding experience. These emotions and feelings are important to facilitate as a motivation to help mothers continue breastfeeding through a difficult period of time as well as to counter the initial negative emotions. A hospitalized preterm infant provides limited opportunities to engage in the mothering role, whereas expressing milk helps fill a void in the maternal experience (Sweet, 2008). Although milk expression is time consuming and does not give the pleasurable feedback of an infant suckling at the breast, mothers find hope through this act. Mothers may also feel pressured to produce sufficient quantities of milk and may feel guilty if unable to do so. Therefore, it is important that breastfeeding and the provision of breastmilk be treated as a priority by hospital staff in the early days after a preterm birth. Failure to acknowledge the importance of milk expression and monitor it increases the risk of low milk production and interpretation by the mother that her milk is not valued. When they are presented with a supportive environment for breastfeeding and pumping in the NICU, many mothers will not only choose to breastfeed because they feel it is better for their baby, but also state that they will breastfeed subsequent infants (Sharp, Campbell, Chiffings, Simmer, & French, 2015).

Contraindications to Breastfeeding

Occasionally, a concern arises that the mother's medical condition and/or requirement for medications are incompatible with breastfeeding or pumping milk. Up to 1 million breastfeeding mothers may need to use medications and most can continue to breastfeed (Nice, 2012). However, there are a few contraindications to breastfeeding (Lawrence, 1997; Lawrence & Lawrence, 2001) and a few medications and drugs that are not compatible with breastfeeding. Medications that are not compatible may frequently be replaced with those that are (Anderson, Pochop, & Manoguerra, 2003). Maternal drugs that preclude breastfeeding include such drugs as antimetabolite or cytotoxic medications—anticancer drugs, I^{131}, and drugs of abuse such as heroin, cocaine, amphetamines, and phencyclidine. The most current resource on drugs in human milk is the database available at LactMed (http://toxnet.nlm.nih.gov/newtoxnet/lactmed.htm).

Maternal illnesses that preclude breastfeeding in the United States include HIV/AIDS (although pasteurization of the expressed milk inactivates the virus), human T-cell lymphotropic virus types I and II, and active tuberculosis before treatment (AAP, 2003). The AAP and Committee on Pediatric AIDS (2013) recommends that HIV-infected women should not breastfeed their infant or provide their milk for the nutrition of their own or other infants. Mothers in labor with an undocumented HIV status can be tested with a rapid HIV test and assisted to pump their milk and supported to provide skin-to-skin care for their infant until a confirmatory test is available and HIV infection is ruled out. Chantry and colleagues (2012), however, showed that flash heating of expressed breastmilk is a feasible and successful mechanism to provide safe breastmilk to infants of mothers with HIV. Hoque et al. (2013) demonstrated HIV inactivation by heating expressed breastmilk in a pan over a stove to 65°C (140°F). Cytomegalovirus (CMV) is ubiquitous and the most common cause of intrauterine and perinatal infections in the world (Numazaki, 1997). CMV infections transmitted through breastmilk are usually asymptomatic in term infants but may pose a potential problem for immunocompromised or extremely preterm infants. CMV DNA can be detected in the breastmilk of seropositive mothers and can be transmitted to an infant through breastmilk, with most preterm infants not manifesting clinical symptoms (Yasuda et al., 2003). However, if a number of conditions are simultaneously present, symptomatic CMV infections are possible (i.e., a high viral load in the milk, high CMV immunoglobulin G in the mother, extreme prematurity with few transplacentally acquired maternal antibodies, and whether the breastmilk of a seropositive mother had been heat treated or frozen and for how long; Jim et al., 2004). Lactoferrin in breastmilk is often protective against CMV in the early weeks when levels are high in colostrum and milk, but once these levels fall and/or viral loads increase beyond a certain threshold, transmission may occur. Local inflammation in the breast may also decrease lactoferrin levels when large amounts of virus are present in breastmilk.

Concomitant viral replication in the breast itself may lead to a local inflammation and passage of the virus into the milk (Lonnerdal & Iyer, 1995; van der Strate et al., 2001). Most breastmilk of seropositive mothers becomes positive for CMV DNA 2 weeks after delivery (Yasuda et al., 2003). DNA copy numbers increase to a peak at 3–6 weeks postpartum (Vochem, Hamprecht, Jahn, & Speer, 1998; Yasuda et al., 2003), with CMV excretion into breastmilk declining to undetectable levels by 8–12 weeks postpartum (Hamprecht, Maschmann, Jahn, Poets, & Goelz, 2008; Yasuda et al., 2003). Freezing breastmilk at −20°C (4°F) for 3–7 days usually decreases viral titers below the transmission threshold (AAP, 2003); however, freezing does not totally eliminate the risk of CMV transfer into the milk. The viral titer at the time of freezing, not the length of time frozen, correlates with the risk of transmission. Heat treatment or pasteurization eliminates CMV but alters some of the anti-infective properties of the milk (Lawrence, 2006).

Very low gestational age and infants with preexisting chronic diseases are conditions associated with symptomatic infection (Capretti et al., 2009). There is an apparent absence of long-term adverse outcomes in the small number of preterm infants who acquire CMV from breastmilk (Neuberger et al., 2004). CMV infection acquired through breastmilk seems to be transient, mild, and self-limiting. Jim and colleagues (2015) reported that transmission of CMV from seropositive mothers via breastmilk to preterm infants did not appear to have major adverse effects on clinical outcomes, growth, neurodevelopmental status, and hearing function at 12 and 24 months corrected age. Given that the peak time of CMV transmission into milk is 3–4 weeks postpartum, colostrum (the first week of milk) may be used fresh or frozen. Kurath, Halwachs-Baumann, Müller, and Resch (2010) performed a systematic literature review, finding a 22.8% mean rate of cytomegalovirus transmission through breastmilk, a mean risk of symptomatic disease of 3.7%, and that of sepsis-like symptoms at 0.7%. One recommendation is that if the mother is CMV seropositive, all maternal breastmilk should be frozen for at least 24 hours before feeding until the infant is greater than 32 weeks corrected age or feeding directly at the breast (California Perinatal Quality Care Collaborative, 2008).

A positive correlation has been reported between the acquisition of postnatal CMV infection and the amount of freeze-thawed breastmilk ingested. A significantly higher (10%) incidence of postnatal CMV infection was observed when infants were fed more than 60% freeze-thawed breastmilk out of the total oral intake, compared with a 4% CMV incidence when infants were fed 60% or less breastmilk out of the total oral intake during the first 8 postnatal weeks. Additionally, more than 60% freeze-thawed breastmilk feeding out of the total oral intake during the first 8 weeks was the independent risk factor for postnatal acquisition of CMV infection (Yoo et al., 2015). These findings would suggest that an increased cumulative viral load in freeze-thawed breastmilk plays a critical role in the acquisition of postnatal CMV infection via breastmilk. These authors also state that pasteurization starting from the second week after birth for at least the first 8 postnatal weeks for extremely preterm infants at the limit of viability might be necessary to effectively prevent CMV transmission through breastmilk. Another approach is to test mothers for their viral load of CMV; the milk from mothers with a high viral load could then be pasteurized, and infants from mothers with a low viral load could be fed freeze-thawed breastmilk.

Sufficient and Appropriate Milk

Milk production for preterm mothers is always a concern, as lactogenesis II may be delayed in some preterm mothers, causing low milk production in the early days (Cregan, De Mello, Kershaw, McDougall, & Hartmann, 2002). The volume of milk was further reduced when antenatal corticosteroids were administered between 28 and 34 weeks' gestation and delivery occurred 3–9 days later (Henderson, Hartmann, Newnham, & Simmer, 2008). However, pumping protocols that consider the physiology of milk production may help compensate for this by initiating early and frequent pumping (Hill, Aldag, & Chatterton, 2001). Written pumping instructions should be provided for the mother (Walker, 1992).

Preterm mother's milk is generally adequate for growth in infants weighing 1,500–1,800 g (about 3.5–4 lbs), with increased concentrations of nutrients associated with the degree of prematurity (Atkinson, 2000). If growth of infants weighing less than 1,500 g is deemed inadequate on human milk alone, powdered or liquid fortifiers are added to the mother's milk (Guerrini, 1994; Schanler, 1998; Schanler, Shulman, & Lau, 1997) and have been shown to improve growth and decrease hospital stays (Bhat & Gupta, 2003). Some controversy exists regarding the use of fortifiers due to the neutralization of preterm milk's bactericidal activities when fortifiers high in iron are combined with human milk (Chan, 2003). Fortification has been reported to cause azotemia, hypercalcinuria, increased infections, and increased NEC (Lucas et al., 1996).

The addition of preterm cow's milk–based formula to human milk decreased lysozyme activity by 41–74% (Quan et al., 1994). Mixing excessive amounts of powdered fortifier into human milk (beyond one packet per 25 mL of milk) can result in hypercalcemia or further complications of cardiac arrhythmia. Adding human milk fortifier to breastmilk increases the osmolality after mixing, which creates a greater risk for NEC (Janjindamai & Chotsampancharoen, 2006). Protein is often the limiting factor in preterm nutrition and is important for developing healthy lean body mass. Although fortifiers may result in short-term growth advantages, powdered formula products, powdered fortifiers, and powdered specialty infant formulas are not sterile. Intrinsic contamination of powdered infant formula with *Enterobacter sakazakii* and the subsequent morbidity and mortality in some preterm infants consuming these products have been reported (CDC, 2002). Fortification of human milk has been shown to result in increased bacterial colony counts, especially when held at room temperature during continuous feeding (Jocson, Mason, & Schanler, 1997). Commercial fortifiers are concentrated forms of protein and essential minerals such as calcium and phosphorus, not a source of additional calories.

Prolonged storage of fortified human milk decreases the availability of epidermal growth factor and other beneficial molecules to the infant. Fortified milk should be used immediately after its preparation (Askin & Diehl-Jones, 2005).

Fortified human milk, however, is more beneficial than preterm infant formula. Infants may gain more slowly on fortified human milk but remain healthier (Schanler, Shulman, & Lau, 1999). Many nurseries fractionate human milk to use the high-fat hindmilk as a concentrated source of lipids and additional calories, while staying within any volume tolerance limitations of an individual infant. The lipid content in human milk correlates with the caloric density of the milk, making it relatively simple to determine the lipid and caloric content of a mother's milk by using a measure called the creamatocrit (Lucas et al., 1978). Small point-of-care machines rather than cumbersome laboratory procedures can accurately determine lipid and calorie content of milk (Meier et al., 2006), allowing more individualized nutrition for these tiny infants.

The fortification of human milk can be implemented in two different forms: standard and individualized. The current concept and recommendations for optimization of human milk fortification is the "individualized fortification." There are two methods of individualized fortification, "targeted/tailored fortification" and the "adjustable fortification." Adjustable fortification uses blood urea nitrogen levels to manipulate fortifier strength, whereas targeted fortification analyzes breastmilk and fortifies macronutrients individually to achieve targeted intake. The use of individualized, adjustable fortification is generally recommended (Di Natale, Coclite, Di Ventura, & Di Fabio, 2011). The use of fortified human milk produces adequate growth in premature infants and satisfies the specific nutritional requirements of these infants.

The use of donor human milk for preterm infants has many advantages, such as preventing NEC, reducing feeding intolerance, and improving long-term outcomes. Common concerns, such as slow growth and loss of important biological components of donor human milk due to storage and pasteurization, should not be a reason for denial of donor milk (Arslanoglu, Ziegler, Moro, & World Association of Perinatal Medicine Working Group on Nutrition, 2010). One study showed that in-hospital growth of preterm infants can be adequate with predominantly human milk diets, both mother's own milk and donor milk derived; that donor milk use did not decrease the provision of mother's own milk but replaced formula in the first 2 weeks of life; and that oxygen requirements were less in extremely low-birth-weight infants when fed human milk compared with a diet containing formula (Verd et al., 2015). In a NICU that had established a donor human milk policy, not only did the proportion of infants fed exclusively human milk increase, but these infants also experienced a significantly earlier initiation of enteral feeding (Marinelli, Lussier, Brownell, Herson, & Hagadorn, 2014). Some mothers may be concerned with the use of donor human milk and be uncomfortable with the use of another mother's milk. Sensitively provided information, acknowledging that mother's own milk is superior to donor milk, reminding mothers that use of donor human milk is usually temporary, and helping mothers understand the donor milk is safe and preferable to formula helps to reduce maternal anxiety regarding its use (Esquerra-Zwiers et al., 2016). While donor human milk is important to the preterm infant who requires it, pasteurization of donor milk removes all microbial life from the product, which means that the recipient infant does not receive an inoculum of maternal bacteria to properly program the gut's immune system. Therefore it would be important to have the mother express whatever colostrum and milk that she can during those early critical weeks of life when the bacterial colonization of the preterm gut is taking place (Groer, Gregory, Louis-Jacques, Thibeau, & Walker, 2015). The Mothers' Milk Bank of New England provides recommendations for making the use of pasteurized donor human milk a NICU standard of care (Butler & Bar-Yam, 2012).

Infant Stresses

Preterm infants are at a great feeding disadvantage due to their neurological immaturity, muscle hypotony, short awake times, and nascent feeding skills. Many healthcare providers have traditionally thought that feeding at breast was harder work than feeding from a fast-flow artificial nipple. Prerequisites for feeding at breast were (and still are in some nurseries) based on attaining a certain weight or gestational age or demonstrating the ability to consume an entire bottle-feeding before being permitted to feed at breast. These clinical practices should be reexamined (Callen, Pinelli, Atkinson, & Saigal, 2005) as closer scrutiny has shown that preterm infants demonstrate better oxygenation during feedings at breast as compared with feeding from a bottle. These infants exhibit fewer episodes of desaturation, bradycardia, temperature instability, and apnea, and are physiologically ready to breastfeed before they are ready to bottle-feed (Blaymore-Bier, 1997; Meier, 1988; Meier & Anderson, 1987; Meier & Pugh, 1985). Chen, Wang, Chang, and Chi (2000) found that apnea and desaturation occurred only during bottle-feeding in their study of 25 preterm infants who served as their own controls. This is primarily related to their ability to pace their own feeding by controlling the milk flow rate to allow time for breathing between sucking bursts. Berger, Weintraub, Dollberg, Kopolovitz, and Mandel (2009) demonstrated that preterm infants feeding at the breast do not expend more energy than when fed by a bottle. There was no significant difference in resting energy expenditure when infants at 32 weeks' gestation were fed by bottle or breast. Longer feeding times at the breast did not increase resting energy expenditure and thus were not more tiring than bottle-feeding. Thus, there appears no reason to delay feeding directly from the breast until a preterm infant can feed from a bottle.

Cardiorespiratory patterns of preterm infants during bottle-feeding can show decreases in minute ventilation, decreased breathing frequency, prolonged airway closure, decreased $tcpO_2$, increased apnea, increased bradycardia, and decreased sucking pressures (Koenig, Davies, & Thach, 1990; Matthew, 1988, 1991; Shivpuri, Martin, Carlo, & Fanaroff, 1983). The risk of bottle-feeding to the preterm infant's physiological regulation and stability extends right up to the days immediately before discharge from the NICU. Preterm infants continue to have desaturation events during bottle-feeding, spending as much as 20% of their feeding time with oxygen levels less than 90% (Thoyre & Carlson, 2003). Under optimal conditions, many preterm infants could have the capacity for intake of adequate volumes of breastmilk that are sufficient for appropriate growth at the time, irrespective of attaining fully mature sucking patterns (Nyqvist, 2008).

Hospital Lactation Care and Services

Care of the preterm infant can be quite complex. Many NICUs use care paths or clinical pathways (California Perinatal Quality Care Collaborative, 2008; Dougherty & Luther, 2008; Forsyth et al., 1998); specific breastfeeding protocols; records that support intentional, planned, and prevention-focused interventions (Baker & Rasmussen, 1997); or a combination of approaches to address the challenges of providing mother's milk for these infants while transitioning them to breast. Early transfer of care to the infant's parents eases the transition from NICU to home (Nyqvist & Kylberg, 2008). Multiple activities occur simultaneously that include provisions for maternal milk expression, feeding of mother's milk to the infant, transitioning the infant to feedings at the breast, and provision of discharge guidelines to extend the duration of breastfeeding or the use of mother's milk.

Coordinated and comprehensive services have been established by some nurseries to prevent fragmented attempts at breastfeeding an infant shortly before discharge and to avoid the common problem of insufficient milk production (Hurst, 2007). Concerted efforts by NICUs to improve breastfeeding outcomes often result in more infants being fed increased amounts of human milk, including banked human milk, and more infants discharged home breastfeeding (Montgomery et al., 2008). Structured and successful hospital models base their interventions on evidence so that all NICU staff comply with policies that are directed or coordinated by a nurse or physician (Hurst, Myatt, & Schanler, 1998; Meier et al., 1993). Castrucci, Hoover, Lim, and Maus (2007) reported that delivering at a hospital where an International Board Certified Lactation Consultant (IBCLC) was present increased the odds of breastfeeding among mothers of infants admitted to the NICU by 34%. Introduction of an IBCLC service in an NICU increased the proportion of infants given their own mother's milk from 31% to 47% (Gonzalez et al., 2003). Mannel and Mannel (2006) recommend

1 full-time equivalent IBCLC per 235 infant admissions to the NICU to provide the following level of services:

- Direct consult times that include direct patient interaction, documentation, and staff interaction
- First visit after delivery: 60 minutes (promote milk expression, review milk expression, facilitate acquisition of breast pump)
- Follow-up visit at 4–5 days postpartum: 60 minutes (assess milk production, pumping efficacy, infant status, kangaroo care)
- Follow-up visit at 10–14 days: 30 minutes (assess milk production, infant status, kangaroo care)
- Follow-up visit to initiate direct breastfeeding: 90 minutes
- Follow-up visit before discharge: 90 minutes (assess breastfeeding, discharge teaching)

NICUs with optimal breastfeeding support engage in a set of practices that are known to result in improved levels of mothers initiating breastfeeding and successfully expressing milk volumes adequate for infant needs both in hospital and after discharge (**Box 6-4**) (Nyqvist & Kylberg, 2008; Spatz, 2004). The first oral feeding at breast is significantly associated with the infant receiving any breastmilk at discharge (Casavant, McGrath, Burke, & Briere, 2015). Clinicians may wish to make every effort to support the preterm infant receiving the first oral feeding as one that is done at the mother's breast, even if little milk is transferred and the infant is not yet ready for discharge. Some units have instituted a care-by-parent program before discharge to improve readiness for independent parenting (Costello & Chapman, 1998). Domanico, Davis, Coleman, and Davis (2011) showed that the NICU design can have a significant effect on infant and family outcomes. A single-family room floor plan compared to a multi-patient, open-bay ward resulted in more mothers sustaining lactation during the hospital stay of their infants, their infants averaging significantly more of their hospital stay receiving their mother's milk, and more infants being discharged breastfeeding from the single-family room floor plan. The quiet, more hygienic environment resulted in fewer apneic episodes, reduced nosocomial sepsis, and earlier transition to enteral feedings. Using a multipronged approach to improving breastmilk feeding rates in an inner-city NICU, these rates increased from 22% to 88% over a 5-year period when IBCLC services were added to the NICU, electric breast pumps were made available for home use, mandatory staff training was instituted, and all mothers admitted to the hospital were contacted prenatally or within 24 hours of delivery by the IBCLC for lactation counseling and support (Dereddy, Talati, Smith, Kudumula, & Dhanireddy, 2015).

Many NICUs belong to the Vermont Oxford Network (VON), a voluntary collaboration of NICUs worldwide whose database holds information on more than 1.5 million infants and provides benchmarking data for NICUs to use for practice improvement. A systematic quality improvement effort by NICUs can result in significant improvements in the rate of the use of mother's own milk at the initiation of enteral feeds as well as the rate of infants being discharged on human milk feedings. One such comprehensive quality improvement effort resulted in 3.1-fold greater odds of the infants receiving mother's own milk at discharge; with this program, despite the increased use of human milk feedings, there was no increase in the percentage of infants discharged with severe growth restriction, nor did the use of donor human milk decrease the use of mother's own milk at discharge (Fugate, Hernandez, Ashmeade, Miladinovic, & Spatz, 2015).

Box 6-4 Hospital Practices Supportive of NICU Breastfeeding Care

- Provide evidence-based information about breastfeeding, breastmilk, and infant formula for informed decision making.
- Communicate the staff's valuing of breastfeeding.
- Have a written breastfeeding policy communicated to and followed by all staff (nurses and physicians).
- Provide current and consistent breastfeeding/pumping guidelines.
- Involve the mother in all feeding plans.
- Encourage mothers to assume responsibility for feeding tasks such as performing pre- and post-feed weights and fractionating their milk.
- Teach, assess, and monitor milk expression, storage, and transport.
- Initiate skin-to-skin care (kangaroo care).
- Introduce the breast early with frequent learning opportunities.
- Work to have the first oral feeding done at the mother's breast
- Use a demand or semi-demand breastfeeding strategy.
- Teach positioning; assess latch, sucking, and swallowing.
- Use assistive devices as needed.
- Measure milk transfer.
- Supplement without bottles if possible.
- Support the father's presence and provide guidelines for his help with breastfeeding.
- Create a feeding plan for the postdischarge period.
- Refer parents to community sources for breastfeeding support.

Modified from Nyqvist, K. H., & Kylberg, E. (2008). Application of the Baby Friendly Hospital Initiative to neonatal care: Suggestions by Swedish mothers of very preterm infants. *Journal of Human Lactation, 24,* 252–262; Spatz, D. L. (2004). Ten steps for promoting and protecting breastfeeding for vulnerable infants. *Journal of Perinatal & Neonatal Nursing, 18,* 385–396; Rodriguez, N. A., Miracle, D. J., & Meier, P. P. (2005). Sharing the science on human milk feedings with mothers of very-low-birth-weight infants. *Journal of Obstetric, Gynecologic, and Neonatal Nursing, 34,* 109–119; Meier, P. P., Engstrom, J. L., Mingolelli, S. S., Miracle, D. J., & Kiesling, S. (2004). The Rush Mothers' Milk Club: Breastfeeding interventions for mothers with very-low-birth-weight infants. *Journal of Obstetric, Gynecologic, and Neonatal Nursing, 33,* 164–174.

A large component of discharge readiness on the part of both parent and infant centers around feeding issues. Most mothers express some anxiety regarding caring for the infant and breastfeeding at home without the constant presence of a trained NICU staff. Follow-up phone calls are especially important during the first 24–72 hours postdischarge (Elliott & Reimer, 1998) because mothers of preterm infants are more likely to abandon breastfeeding efforts earlier than mothers of term infants (Furman, Minich, & Hack, 1998; Lefebvre & Ducharme, 1989). Two impediments to breastfeeding duration beyond a few weeks are compromised milk production and failure to transition the infant to the breast, both of which have their origins in hospital practices and policies (Bier et al., 1993; Hill, Hanson, & Mefford, 1994; Hill, Ledbetter, & Kavanaugh, 1997; Kavanaugh, Mead, Meier, & Mangurten, 1995). Mothers' reports of dwindling volumes of pumped milk, the infant's resistance or refusal to latch, uncertainty regarding whether the infant received enough milk at each feeding, and a weak suck that fails to transfer sufficient amounts of milk, with the further reduction of breast stimulation, provide continuing challenges postdischarge.

Mothers' concerns over an inadequate milk supply and whether the infant consumed an adequate volume of milk at a feeding are different problems requiring different approaches to resolve.

Barriers to continued breastfeeding change across time. Callen and colleagues (2005) reported that nipple and breast problems were most prevalent at NICU discharge, as was low milk volume, whereas poor breastfeeding technique of the infant was most prevalent at 1 month. From discharge to 3 months, many infants had difficulty breastfeeding because they were difficult to arouse, slept through feedings, or fell asleep at the breast before completing a feeding. Some infants would fight at the breast and have difficulty latching. Many of these problems are interrelated. A focus on assisting mothers and infants to fully establish breastfeeding before discharge would help reduce the problems of faulty breastfeeding technique. Pineda (2011) found that direct feedings at the breast were linked to the provision of breastmilk at discharge and more success with breastfeeding during the NICU stay. A prospective, nonrandomized trial in 71 infants ranging in age from 26 to 36 weeks' gestation assessed the development of breastfeeding skills as a mechanism to develop feeding recommendations. Efficient rooting and latching were observed as early as 28 weeks and nutritive sucking at 30.6 weeks, with 80% of these infants establishing full breastfeeding at a mean of 36 weeks and as early as 33.4 weeks. Although maturation is important for preterm infants to establish mature patterns of sucking, swallowing, and breathing, experience or practice feeding at the breast also seems important for these infants to acquire early breastfeeding skills (Hedberg Nyqvist, 2001). When possible, preterm infants should receive their first oral feeding at breast before using bottles. This practice is facilitated when mothers have clear breastfeeding goals. Mothers of infants who received their first oral feeding at breast rather than by bottle are more likely to provide more than one direct breastfeed per day throughout the entire feeding progression in the hospital and to provide direct breastfeeding at discharge (Briere, McGrath, Cong, Brownell, & Cusson, 2015).

The provision of peer counselors in the NICU has been shown to be an effective intervention in improving breastfeeding outcomes for preterm infants (Rossman et al., 2011). The shared experience of a peer counselor who had a preterm infant herself can provide a special type of support and empowerment for preterm mothers during an extremely stressful period of time.

Clinical Approaches to Breastfeeding Support: Practice Suggestions

Breastfeeding for the preterm infant and mother is different than for a healthy term infant. Length of the infant's stay in the hospital is significantly correlated to the probability of being breastfed at discharge—the shorter the stay, the higher the probability of being breastfed at the time of final discharge (Kirchner, Jeitler, Waldhor, Pollak, & Wald, 2009). A number of barriers and complex medical situations can present themselves on the route from birth to breastfeeding. This journey may take time, commitment, and adjustment to a very different reality from what was imagined. Strategies for the clinician are as follows:

1. Provide human milk oral care/oropharyngeally administered colostrum. Colostrum as oral immune therapy is an emerging intervention that is inexpensive, well tolerated by even the smallest and sickest infants, and has been shown to modulate the immature immune system.
   - Oropharyngeal administration of mother's own colostrum involves placing small amounts of colostrum directly onto the oral mucosa, with the expectation that the immune components

will be absorbed by the mucous membranes. This can be done even when the infant is on a ventilator. The risk of acquiring a nosocomial infection is highest for the lowest-birth-weight infants, but this risk can be modified by the use of the mother's own milk. Because extremely preterm infants are often clinically unstable and may have comorbidities that cause bowel hypoperfusion, enteral feedings are usually precluded during the early days following birth. As a consequence, the mother's colostrum, which contains the highest concentrations of protective factors, is unavailable to an infant who can take nothing by mouth. Administering small amounts of the mother's own colostrum to the mucosa of the oral cavity with a small syringe allows the potent immune factors in colostrum, such as cytokines, lactoferrin, secretory IgA, and human milk oligosaccharides, to be absorbed by the oropharyngeal-associated lymphoid tissue (OFALT), which includes the tonsils and adenoids, as well as by the gut-associated lymphoid tissues (GALT) and the bronchial-associated lymphoid tissues (Rodriguez, Meier, Groer, & Zeller, 2009). The safety of this procedure was shown in a study in which 0.1 mL (approximately 7 drops) of colostrum was placed along the left buccal mucosa (the mucous membranes that line the inside cheeks of the mouth) and 0.1 mL of colostrum was placed along the right buccal mucosa beginning within the first 48 hours of life (Rodriguez et al., 2010). Oxygen saturations were stable or increased during this procedure, with no episodes of apnea, bradycardia, hypotension, or any other adverse effects being reported. The infants were thought to taste the colostrum, as they were observed sucking on the breathing tube. Mothers were seen to react positively to this infant behavior, offering a psychological boost to the mothers. The human milk oligosaccharides in colostrum serve to inhibit bacterial adhesion to mucosal surfaces and may be important as a protective mechanism against pneumonia in ventilator-dependent infants. The administration of oropharyngeal colostrum has also been shown to reduce the occurrence of clinical sepsis (Lee et al., 2015), reduce the time to full enteral feeding (Rodriguez, Groer, & Zeller, 2011), and contribute to reaching goal birth weights sooner (Seigel et al., 2013).

- Human milk oral care is a process whereby fresh colostrum/human milk is applied to the oral mucosa of the infant with a swab. The nurse, parent, or family member dips a sterile cotton applicator or sponge swab into freshly expressed human milk and then applies the swab to the infant's lips and oral mucosa several times per day. This procedure has been shown to be enjoyable for the infant, contributes to improving the infant's immune function, and acts as a motivating factor for the mother to continue pumping her milk (Froh, Deatrick, Curley, & Spatz, 2015). Mothers who engage in this caregiving procedure feel that they are contributing to their infant's care and that their milk is being used for a special purpose and not just being frozen away for use some time in the future.

2. Initiate and sustain milk production. In the absence of an infant at the breast, mothers of preterm infants may need to pump milk (Auerbach & Walker, 1994) for weeks or even months until their infants are fully established at breast or to provide as much breastmilk as possible under very trying circumstances. Mothers will need to do the following:
   - Secure an efficient breast pump. The most efficient pumps have been shown to be fully automated, multiuser (hospital-grade) pumps that cycle about 48–50 times per minute, with vacuums that do not exceed 240 mm Hg and that use a double collection kit to pump both

breasts simultaneously (Hill, Aldag, & Chatterton, 1999; Mitoulas, Lai, Gurrin, Larsson, & Hartmann, 2002). Mothers should be instructed in how to use the pump and receive specific guidelines for cleaning the collection kit. Although these pumps can be rented, many low-income women cannot afford the expense and their health insurance (if they have it) may reject such a claim. As of August 1, 2012, many health plans will be covering breast pumps with no cost sharing as part of the Affordable Health Care for America Act. Mothers should first check with their health insurers to see if the cost of a pump will be covered. Local Special Supplemental Nutrition Program for Women, Infants, and Children (WIC) agencies may have electric pumps to loan. Some institutions may have a grant-funded program to ensure such pumps are available to all women who need them (Philipp, Brown, & Merewood, 2000). Some insurance carriers may provide a pump that is inadequate or ineffective for the needs of the mother of a hospitalized preterm or ill infant. Clinicians may need to help mothers secure the correct type of pump for their situation by advocating for use of these devices with insurers.

- Use a double collection kit. Mothers tend to pump a greater quantity of milk with simultaneous pumping in a shorter period of time. Simultaneous breast pumping with added breast massage while pumping yields more milk per expression session than sequential pumping with no breast massage (Jones, Dimmock, & Spencer, 2001).
- Select a properly fitted flange or breastshield. When the vacuum is exerted on the maternal nipple, it is drawn into the tunnel of the breastshield and must be able to move freely. The tunnel can vary in size from 21.0–40.0 mm depending on the manufacturer and the number of breastshield options available with each pump (Walker, 2010a). Nipple sizes can range from less than 12 mm at the base to more than 23 mm (Stark, 1994; Wilson-Clay & Hoover, 2002; Ziemer & Pidgeon, 1993). Nipples swell during pumping (Wilson-Clay & Hoover, 2002). If blanching at the nipple–areolar junction is observed or pain is experienced by the mother, reduced milk flow could occur. A standard size breastshield is 24–25 mm, but many women actually require a larger shield of 27–30 mm for pain-free and effective pumping, especially during the early weeks of frequent milk expression (Meier, Motykowski, & Zuleger, 2004). The clinician should observe a milk expression session to determine if the breastshield is properly fitted, especially in the presence of pain or reduced milk removal. Some mothers may require different sizes of shields for each breast or shield size adjustment as lactation progresses and the breasts change size. Some mothers who cannot obtain a good fit might benefit from the Pumpin Pal (http://www.pumpinpal.com)—an angled breastshield that may better accommodate some breasts.
- Start breastmilk expression soon after delivery. The timing of when breastmilk expression is begun relative to delivery can have an important influence on pumped milk volume. Early initiation of pumping within 6 hours of delivery is associated with lactation continuing after the infant reaches 40 weeks corrected age (Furman, Minich, & Hack, 2002; Meier & Brown, 1996; Neifert & Seacat, 1988). Initiation of milk expression within 6 hours of delivery may not be associated with an increased milk volume unless milk expression was initiated within the first hour of birth (Parker, Sullivan, Krueger, & Mueller, 2015).

Parker, Sullivan, Krueger, Kelechi, and Mueller (2012) studied the effects of early initiation of milk expression on the onset of lactogenesis stage II and milk volume in mothers of very low-birth-weight infants. Mothers were randomized to initiate milk expression within 60 minutes of birth in group one, and in group two, mothers initiated milk expression between 1 and 6 hours following delivery. Milk volume and timing of lactogenesis stage II were compared between the two groups. Group one produced significantly more milk than group two during the first 7 days postdelivery as well as when measured at week 3. Group one also demonstrated a significantly earlier lactogenesis stage II. Clinicians may wish to recommend that mothers of preterm infants start milk expression within an hour of birth if possible if the infant cannot be put to breast during that time.

Ohyama, Watabe, and Hayasaka (2010) found that manual expression yielded twice as much colostrum as did electric pumping during the first 48 hours following delivery in mothers who delivered between 29 and 39 weeks. Net milk yield was 2 mL (range, 0–12.6 mL) in the hand expression group and 0.6 mL (range, 0–7.2 mL) in the pumping group. Mothers in this study alternated between manual expression and using a double electric pump every 3 hours for 7 expression sessions, such that every other expression session was done by hand. The most effective way to remove colostrum in the early hours following delivery appears to be by manual expression.

3. Pump milk frequently. Frequent pumping during the 1st week after birth is important to optimize the eventual amount of milk that will be available to the infant. Good milk production has been associated with five or more expressions and at least 100 minutes of pumping per day (Hopkinson, Schanler, & Garza, 1988). Fewer pumping sessions per 24 hours may produce sufficient amounts of milk for mothers intending to provide milk for preterm infants of higher gestational ages, for mothers intending to provide milk for short periods of time, or for mothers who plan to combine breastfeeding with formula use. However, clinical experience has shown that mothers who intend to produce a full milk supply, exclusively breastfeed at discharge, breastfeed multiples, or have a sufficient volume to fractionate and use hindmilk need to pump about 8–12 times per 24 hours during the first 10–14 days after birth. Hill and colleagues (1999) showed that optimal milk output has been associated with the following:
    - An output of greater than 3,500 mL/week (500 mL/day [17–18 oz/day]) is achieved with more than 44 pumping sessions per week.
    - Adequate milk production is achieved in weeks 4 and 5 if milk volumes of 3,500 mL/week have been achieved by week 2.
    - High milk production by 10–14 days of 800–1,000 mL provides a 50% oversupply. This can help compensate for the typical milk volume decrease seen during the 2nd month of milk expression (Hill, Brown, & Harker, 1995; Hurst et al., 1998). The maternal prolactin response to a breast pump, although evident, may not be the same as how prolactin release responds to a vigorously nursing infant, necessitating more frequent pumping during the early phase of lactation where the breasts calibrate how much milk they will eventually be able to produce. Many mothers will not be able to produce the high volume of milk known to optimize the chances for full lactation during the entire course of the infant's hospitalization as well as

for the many months postdischarge (Bishara, Dunn, Merko, & Darling, 2009). Additional interventions may be necessary. Morton and colleagues (2007a) reported that pump-dependent mothers of preterm infants who hand expressed greater than 5 times per day as well as used an electric pump approximately 5 times per day during the first 3 days postpartum produced significantly larger volumes of milk than mothers who only used an electric pump. Breast massage while pumping has been shown to significantly increase the amount of milk pumped at each session, suggesting that milk volumes appear to be associated with the completeness of breast emptying rather than with increased frequency or duration of pumping (Morton et al., 2007b). Clinicians may wish to assure that preterm mothers are taught hand expression techniques and that these techniques are used in conjunction with a hospital-grade electric breast pump. While the combination of the electric breast pump and hand expression techniques results in higher milk yields, exclusive hand expression has been shown to produce significantly less cumulative daily milk production during the first 7 days postpartum and beyond (Lussier et al., 2015).

If a mother is producing 1,700 mL of milk per week by week 2, her likelihood of reaching the minimum volume of 3,500 mL/wk is only 50%. If she is producing less than 1,700 mL/week at week 2, the mother may need intensive help in salvaging the milk supply (Ehrenkranz & Ackerman, 1986).

- Monitor pumping frequency and milk volumes. A pumping log should be maintained that accounts for the number of times a mother pumps, what time of day she pumps, and the volume she pumps from each breast. This allows for quick intervention if milk production falters.

4. Address low milk volume immediately. Some suggestions follow:
    - Add another pumping session at night when prolactin levels are highest. Preterm mothers tend to have lower basal prolactin levels than full-term mothers (Hill et al., 2009). Additional pumping sessions expose the breasts to higher than basal levels of prolactin multiple times during the day, perhaps compensating for the uncompleted preparation of the breasts provoked by an early delivery. Frequent pumping is extremely important for its effect on prolactin exposure. Pumping no more than 5 times per day may not provide sufficient prolactin exposure for many mothers.
    - Massage each breast methodically while pumping to maximize the volume and fat content per expression. Thorough breast draining is important because the degree of emptiness influences the amount of milk that is replaced (Daly, Kent, Owens, & Hartmann, 1996). Milk remaining in the breast can lead to both a down-regulation in milk volume and an increased risk for milk stasis, engorgement, and mastitis. Mothers can continue pumping for 2 minutes after what appear to be the final drops of milk to ensure as complete drainage as possible. Most mothers have one breast that produces more milk than the other, and this breast dominance continues over time. Pumping instructions should specify to continue pumping for 2 minutes after both breasts have stopped flowing to ensure the nondominant breast is adequately drained (Hill, Aldag, Zinaman, & Chatterton, 2007).
    - Warm the pump flange and the breast. Kent, Geddes, Hepworth, and Hartmann (2011) found that warmed pump flanges resulted in a larger amount of available milk removal.

Yigit and colleagues (2012) studied whether warming the breast prior to pumping would increase the volume of milk expressed from a warmed breast compared with the other breast that was not warmed. Mothers placed a warm compress (40.5°C [104.9°F]) on one breast prior to pumping with an electric breast pump. The amount of milk obtained from warmed breasts was significantly higher than that obtained from the nonwarmed breasts. Warming probably has an enhancing effect on the milk ducts or milk flow, allowing more milk to be pumped, rather than increasing actual breastmilk production.

- Music therapy has been used to improve milk output in preterm mothers. In one study, mothers of preterm infants who listened to soothing music before and during pumping sessions showed greater milk output and demonstrated lower cortisol levels as a measure of reduced stress compared to mothers who did not listen to music (Ak, Lakshmanagowda, & Goturu, 2015). In another study looking at the effect of music therapy on milk production of mothers of preterm infants, not only did these mothers produce significantly more milk, but they also produced milk that was significantly higher in fat content during the first 6 days of the study (Keith, Weaver, & Vogel, 2012). A soothing music intervention may be very helpful to preterm mothers by both reducing stress levels and increasing oxytocin levels (Nilsson, 2009).
- Pump at the infant's bedside or while holding the infant skin to skin.
- Facilitate kangaroo care, which has been shown to contribute to higher milk volumes (Hurst, Valentine, Renfro, Burns, & Ferlic, 1997).
- Check that the breastshield/flange of the pump is not constricting or strangulating the nipple. If necessary, change to a larger breastshield, especially if the mother states that her nipples are sore.
- Check that the mother is using a fully automated hospital-grade electric breast pump and that it is working correctly and efficiently.
- Mothers should be instructed to use their own maximum comfortable vacuum setting as soon as the first letdown is detected because most of the milk is removed during the first two milk ejections (Kent et al., 2008).
- Assess for breaks in the pumping schedule or a worsening of the infant's condition.
- Ask if the mother is using oral or injected contraceptives because these have the capacity to diminish milk production.
- If there is an impaired letdown response, milk removal may become inefficient. An infant at breast takes about 56 ± 4 seconds to elicit the letdown response. A breast pump can take up to 147 ± 13 seconds (Kent, Ramsay, Doherty, Larsson, & Hartmann, 2003). Stress and fatigue may further delay milk letdown. Relaxation rituals (Fehrer, Berger, Johnson, & Wilde, 1989) or breast massage before pumping may contribute to milk release. Oxytocin nasal spray before pumping can provide a temporary boost to milk ejection. Fewtrell, Loh, Blake, Ridout, and Hawdon (2006) performed a study that looked at the use of nasal oxytocin prior to pumping by preterm mothers and the resulting milk output. Mothers were randomized to either use the oxytocin spray or a placebo while pumping with an Ameda Elite electric breast pump. Mothers used the spray 2 to 5 minutes before pumping. The

oxytocin group produced more milk over the first 2 days, with the placebo group matching and exceeding the volume of the oxytocin group by day 5. Many mothers reported a drop in milk output when they stopped using the spray, even though a few of the mothers were actually using the placebo. While oxytocin nasal spray might not result in higher milk volumes over the course of the time a mother is pumping, it may give mothers a boost during those early days when establishing high volumes of milk is so important. Oxytocin nasal spray is no longer available as a packaged nasal spray, but compounding pharmacies can mix oxytocin into a nasal spray form (Gross, 1995). The original preparation, Syntocinon, contained 40 units/mL. The current prescription is written for a 15-mL nasal spray using standard oxytocin. The dosage is 1 to 2 sprays in the nares, followed by breastfeeding in 1 to 2 minutes (Lawrence & Lawrence, 2010).

- Other medications and interventions (Gabay, 2002) include the use of metoclopramide (Reglan) (Ehrenkranz & Ackerman, 1986; Toppare et al., 1994), acupuncture (Clavey, 1996), domperidone (Motilium) where available (da Silva, Knoppert, Angelini, & Forret, 2001), and human growth hormone (Gunn et al., 1996).
- Metoclopramide stimulates prolactin release from the pituitary and is dose related. Metoclopramide is a dopamine antagonist and increases serum prolactin by blocking the inhibitory effect of dopamine on prolactin secretion. Doses of 30–45 mg/day are most effective, with many studies showing 66–100% increases in milk production. Other studies report conflicting results and varying methodologies (Anderson & Valdes, 2007), with some showing no improvement in milk production when mothers take sufficient doses of metoclopramide (Hansen, McAndrew, Harris, & Zimmerman, 2005). Mothers who do not respond to metoclopramide therapy may already have elevated levels of prolactin, may be overweight or obese with a blunted prolactin response to suckling, or have other factors that affect the response to prolactin-enhancing therapy. Parity may also influence the effect of metoclopramide on prolactin response (Brown, Fernandes, Grant, Hutsul, & McCoshen, 2000). Hale (2003) suggested ascertaining serum prolactin levels before commencing metoclopramide therapy to determine the advisability of instituting such an intervention. Maternal gastric cramping and diarrhea are infrequent side effects, and therapy for longer than 4 weeks may be accompanied by depression in some mothers. Domperidone is a peripheral dopamine antagonist but unlike metoclopramide, it does not enter the brain compartment and it has few central nervous system side effects such as depression. It is effective in raising serum prolactin levels and increasing milk production in many but not all women (da Silva et al., 2001; Wan et al., 2008). Knoppert and colleagues (2012) reported a significant increase in milk volume when taking domperidone. A dose of domperidone of 20 mg 3 times daily, instead of 10 mg 3 times daily was associated with a clinical, but not statistically significant increase in milk production. In a study comparing metoclopramide and domperidone, use of domperidone resulted in slightly higher milk volumes, and mothers taking metoclopramide reported slightly more side effects (Ingram, Taylor, Churchill, Pike, & Greenwood, 2012).
- Electroacupuncture at Shaoze (SI 1) has been shown to increase milk production and prevent a postpartum drop in prolactin levels (Wei, Wang, Han, & Li, 2008). Acupressure

applied at GB20 (in a depression between the upper portion of the sternocleidomastoid muscle and the trapezius on the same level with GV16), acupoint LI4 (on the dorsum of the hand), between the first t20 and second d20 (in a depression between the upper portion of the sternocleidomastoid muscle and the trapezius on the same level) has been shown to increase milk production. This intervention can be applied by the mother as a cost-effective, simple method of improving milk volume (Esfahani, Berenji-Sooghe, Valiani, & Ehsanpour, 2015).

Many herbal remedies such as fenugreek and milk thistle have been proposed as popular remedies for low milk production but lack the rigor of studies showing safety, proper dosing, and both intended and unintended effects in mothers of preterm infants. However, Di Pierro, Callegari, Carotenuto, and Tapia (2008) reported that standardized *Silybum marianum* (milk thistle) extract (micronized silymarin, 420 mg/day) improved the milk production in term mothers who were producing marginally adequate amounts of milk.

- Recombinant human prolactin (r-hPRL) has been shown to be an effective galactagogue (Page-Wilson, Smith, & Welt, 2007). In one study of mothers with prolactin deficiency and mothers of preterm infants with lactation insufficiency, peak prolactin increased in mothers treated with r-hPRL every 12 hours (Powe et al., 2010).
- Another study of mothers with documented prolactin deficiency and mothers with lactation insufficiency that developed while they were pumping breastmilk for their preterm infants, found that r-hPRL not only increased milk volume (by 73 to 146 mL/day; 2.4 to 5 oz/day), but also enhanced the anti-infective properties of the milk (Powe et al., 2011).
- The use of mothers' colostrum/milk from days 4 to 14 for early trophic feedings (to stimulate intestinal maturity) yielded an unexpected association with improved breastmilk production (Schanler, Shulman, Lau, Smith, & Heitkemper, 1999). This serves to point out the powerful influence of psychological effects on maternal milk production. Just knowing that her milk is being used for her own baby shows that there may be a two-part effect in beginning early feedings with breastmilk instead of formula (Morton, 2002). Trophic feeds with breastmilk not only improve infant feeding tolerance (Schanler et al., 1999) but also enhance the maternal milk supply.
- Primiparous mothers or mothers with no prior lactation experience may produce lower volumes of milk. Hill, Aldag, Chatterton, and Zinaman (2005) reported that preterm mothers with no prior nursing experience produced 25% less milk than did mothers with previous nursing experience during days 6 and 7 and that lower gestational ages resulted in lower milk output. Therefore, mothers with no prior lactations and whose infants are of lower gestational ages constitute a subgroup that requires more vigilant monitoring of their milk production.
- A technique called "power pumping" can be recommended for improving milk output or to rescue a faltering milk supply. The mother pumps for 10–12 minutes, rests for 10–12 minutes, and repeats this process for 1 hour once a day. Some mothers do this twice a day. Power pumping takes advantage of the fact that almost half of the available milk is presented during the first letdown, which removes the milk made available during the time

the milk ducts stay dilated. Pumping 5 or 6 times within an hour with breaks in between "tricks" the breast into making this large amount of milk available at each of these mini pumping sessions.

- Have the mother try a different brand of double electric breast pump. Sometimes a different suction curve may provide a boost to milk output.
- Mothers can listen to music while pumping. Keith, Weaver, and Vogel (2012) showed that preterm mothers who listened to music while pumping not only produced more milk than mothers who did not listen to music, but the fat content of their milk was higher.

Facilitating Early and Frequent Skin-to-Skin Contact Between Mother and Infant

"The relationship between skin-to-skin contact and breastfeeding is fundamental," say Kirsten, Bergman, and Hann (2001). The American Academy of Pediatrics recommends skin-to-skin care for preterm infants along with continuous cardiovascular monitoring and verification of correct head positioning for airway patency and stability of the endotracheal tube (Baley & Committee on Fetus and Newborn, 2015). In industrialized countries, structured interventions that focus on skin-to-skin care and support in the establishment of an abundant milk supply improve the rates of breastfeeding at discharge (Bell, Geyer, & Jones, 1995). Efforts in the NICU should assure that preterm infants have access to skin-to-skin care by parents.

Studies of the effects of skin-to-skin contact or kangaroo care on breastfeeding show that:

- Breastfeeding duration is extended (Charpak, Ruiz-Pelaez, de Figueroa, & Charpak, 2001; Flacking, Ewald, & Wallin, 2011; Ludington-Hoe, Thompson, Swinth, Hadeed, & Anderson, 1994; Whitelaw, Histerkamp, Sleath, Acolet, & Richards, 1988).
- Breastmilk production is enhanced (Blaymore-Bier et al., 1996; Hurst et al., 1997; Thompson, 1996).
- The number of breastfeeds per day is increased (Syfrett, Anderson, Behnke, Neu, & Hilliard, 1993).
- The breastfeeding competence of the infant is greatly improved (Hedberg Nyqvist, 2001; Koepke & Bigelow, 1997; Widstrom et al., 1988).
- More preterm infants are discharged on exclusive breastfeeding (Cattaneo et al., 1998; Hann, Malan, Kronson, Bergman, & Huskisson, 1999; Hurst et al., 1997).
- With a mean contact of 4.47 hours per day, exclusive breastfeeding is increased at discharge, as well as at 1.5, 3, and 6 months (Hake-Brooks & Anderson, 2008).
- The stability of the cardiorespiratory system is enhanced, hypoglycemia is decreased, and hypothermia is reduced (Bergman, Linley, & Fawcus, 2004).

Implementing Suckling at the Breast

To avoid delays in a preterm infant going to breast, many NICUs have abandoned the requirement of a certain age or weight attainment and simply place the infant at a recently pumped breast when the infant is stable and extubated (Meier, 2001; Narayanan, Mehta, Choudhury, & Jain, 1991). Guidelines from the international network on kangaroo mother care recommend that direct breastfeeding be started as soon as the infant shows a sucking ability (Cattaneo, Davanzo, Uxa, & Tamburlini, 1998). Infants engage in non-nutritive suckling, mouthing, and licking the nipple tip with no expectation of measurable intake but enjoy an introduction to the breast and a taste of their mother's milk. The infant also experiences the positive benefits of non-nutritive suckling (as with a pacifier) but without the side effects of an artificial nipple (Pinelli & Symington, 2000). Infants can next engage in non-nutritive suckling at the breast during gavage feedings. These experiences help shape the desired behavior and make progress toward sucking on a partially full breast with the expectation of a small intake. Even infants weighing less than 1,000 g who are on nasal continuous positive airway pressure can be placed in skin-to-skin contact at the breast and be encouraged to engage in non-nutritive suckling before and during gavage feedings.

The capacity for increasing intake at the breast develops over time (Hedberg Nyqvist, 2001). It is a function of a number of combined parameters that include gestational age, age in days since birth, the presence or absence of medical complications, maturation of sucking behavior, and especially unlimited access to the breast for repeated learning opportunities. Using the Preterm Infant Breastfeeding Behavior Scale to describe the maturational steps to full breastfeeding, Hedberg Nyqvist, Sjoden, and Ewald (1999) found that healthy preterm infants demonstrated rooting and sucking on the first contact with the breast. Effective rooting, areolar grasp, and latching were observed as early as 28 weeks, and repeated bursts of 10 or more sucks and maximum bursts of 30 or more sucks were seen as early as 32 weeks. Infants pace their feeds by controlling the length of sucking bursts and pauses between bursts to avoid oxygen desaturation and bradycardia from the repeated swallowing seen with artificial nipples. These researchers discussed this type of functional behavior in relation to the repeated opportunities for oral contact with the maternal nipple, exposure to the taste and smell of breastmilk, and the natural extension and modification of activities already performed in utero. The responses elicited by this type of stimulation can alter the trajectory for breastfeeding behaviors that is in line with the assumption that appropriate contingent stimuli and contextual support may reveal an infant's motor behavior that would not otherwise be apparent at a particular time. Given that neuronal mapping is taking place, whereby the brain's sensory and motor pathways are being established, it is important that feeding directly at the breast be used as a model template for this neuromotor development.

Interventions to improve sucking at the breast can also include osteopathy in the cranial field or osteopathic manipulation. Lund and colleagues (2011) reported that a number of osteopathic manipulations have the ability to improve poor sucking at the breast. They report on preterm twins whose poor sucking was corrected by a series of manipulations. These may have contributed to the stabilization of the muscles that support the hyoid bone and helped relieve possible entrapment of the hypoglossal nerve. In one study, infants who received sensory–motor–oral stimulation and non-nutritive suckling were able to begin oral feeding 8 days earlier, wean off the gavage tube 8 days earlier, and be discharged from the hospital 10 days earlier (Rocha, Moreira, Pimenta, Ramos, & Lucena, 2007).

Transitioning to Full Feedings at the Breast

Breastfeeding outcomes are optimal if infants transition to the breast before or shortly after discharge. Mothers should be advised of why feedings at the breast are more advantageous than continuing to provide pumped milk by bottle or to supplement with formula (Buckley & Charles, 2006). The sheer amount of time involved in slow feeding sessions at the breast, pumping milk, and monitoring adequate intake may overwhelm a mother as she attempts to transition her infant to exclusive feedings at the breast.

Proper positioning and support at the breast helps to compensate for a number of feeding skill deficits experienced by preterm infants.

1. Place the infant in a clutch (football) or cross-cradle position. These positions afford the best visualization for the mother; support the infant's head, neck, and trunk; allow the mother to adjust the angle of the infant's head to keep the airway from collapsing; and promote maximum chest expansion so the infant is not curled forward, restricting breathing movements.
2. The breast should be supported and "held" in the infant's mouth because preterm infants generate low levels of vacuum, frequently losing grasp on the nipple/areola. The Dancer hand position provides jaw and breast support, and the mother can slightly compress the infant's cheeks if necessary to keep the mouth in contact with the nipple.
3. Weak sucking pressures are not unusual and can result in difficulties staying attached to the nipple as well as initiating and sustaining milk flow and transfer. To compensate for low generation of vacuum, a small ultra-thin silicone nipple shield has been shown to reduce the frequent losing of the nipple and increase the amount of milk transferred per feeding (Clum & Primomo, 1996; Meier et al., 2000). Once the nipple has been drawn into the shield, a vacuum in the semirigid teat keeps the nipple elongated, reducing the workload on the infant of having to repeatedly draw the nipple/areola back into the mouth. A pool of milk remains available at the tip of the shield, rewarding the infant for any compression or vacuum exerted (Wilson-Clay & Hoover, 2002). Many NICUs use non-nutritive sucking opportunities and oral stimulation programs that have been shown to improve breastfeeding rates at discharge and through the first 6 months (Pimenta et al., 2008).
4. Music therapy has been shown to improve sucking in preterm infants, especially live music when a lullaby is sung by a parent or when the infant is exposed to entrained rhythms from a Gato box that simulates the heartbeat sound that the infant would hear in utero (Loewy, Stewart, Dassier, Telsey, & Homel, 2013). Live, organized, entrained, rhythmic sounds are able to improve sustained sucking patterns. This noninvasive therapy can help tame the chaotic acoustic environment of a NICU into a more organized and therapeutic environment. Akca and Aytekin (2014) studied the effect of soothing noise on the sucking outcomes of full-term infants as measured by the LATCH breastfeeding assessment tool. In the experimental group, 64 infants were exposed to the song "Don't Let Your Baby Cry 2" from the album *Colic* released by Othan Osman of the On Music Production Company; the 63 infants in the control group were not exposed to the music. The music was played during the first breastfeeding after birth and again 24 hours later. The LATCH scores in the experimental group (8.61 ± 1.37) were found to be significantly higher than those in the control group (6.52 ± 1.79). Music therapy interventions may be a low-cost, noninvasive method of improving sucking and overall feeding outcomes.

Ensuring Adequate Intake

- If the infant needs additional milk or a mother has a low milk supply, expressed milk or formula can be provided with a tube-feeding device run under a nipple shield or placed next to the breast.
- Supplementary or complementary feedings may be necessary until the infant is taking in all the requirements at breast. Test weighing (pre- and postfeed weights) has been used in some nurseries and research settings where accurate measurements of intake are necessary to determine how much supplement to provide (Meier et al., 1994; Meier, Engstrom, Fleming, Streeter, & Lawrence, 1996; Scanlon, Alexander, Serdula, Davis, & Bowman, 2002). Pre- and postfeed weighing is an accurate mechanism to ascertain the amount of breastmilk ingested at the breast, making the calculation for supplementation more precise (Haase, Barreira, Murphy, Mueller, & Rhodes, 2009).
- To avoid using a bottle to supplement, especially in the absence of the mother, some nurseries follow protocols for providing additional milk through a nasogastric tube (Kliethermes, Cross, Lanese, Johnson, & Simon, 1999; Stine, 1990) or by cup feeding (Lang, Lawrence, & Orme, 1994). When compared with bottle-feeding, cup feeding is less physiologically stressful (Howard et al., 1999; Marinelli, Burke, & Dodd, 2001), but spillage or drooling of milk can be a problem (Dowling, Meier, DiFiore, Blatz, & Martin, 2002) if not accounted for. Abouelfettoh, Dowling, Dabash, Elguindy, and Seoud (2008) demonstrated that infants cup fed in the hospital showed significantly more mature breastfeeding behaviors for 6 weeks after discharge compared with those who were supplemented with bottles. Cup-fed preterm infants had higher Preterm Infant Breastfeeding Behavior Scale scores than infants supplemented with bottles and had a significantly higher number of breastfeedings 1 week after discharge.
- Garpiel (2012) compared four supplemental feeding methods to determine the optimal method to facilitate the transition to effective breastfeeding in preterm infants—nasogastric tube with pacifier, bottle with preterm nipple, cup feeding with 30-mL medicine cup, and the Haberman Feeder (Medela). The infants in the nasogastric tube with pacifier group had significantly better breastfeeding ability at discharge compared with the other three groups, as well as a significantly higher breastfeeding frequency than infants in the bottle group. Infants in the bottle-supplemented group demonstrated a reduction in breastmilk intake per pre- and postbreastfeeding test weights after the supplemental bottle was introduced. Consequently, the mothers reduced their breastfeeding frequency, believing that it would expedite their infants' hospital discharge. Infants in the group that used the nasogastric with pacifier feeding method tolerated it better than infants in the bottle group. Bottle-supplemented infants had almost 4 times the number of apnea, bradycardia, and oxygen desaturation events during feedings. The variables of frequency of skin-to-skin and breastfeeding sessions were positively correlated with breastfeeding ability at discharge. Higher levels of breastfeeding ability at discharge were predictive of continued breastfeeding at 4 weeks postdischarge.

- Semi-demand breastfeeding can be used during the transition period. In this practice, mothers feed their infant directly at breast, and perform pre- and post-feed weights, after which the need for subsequent supplementation is determined. The remaining milk (and fortifier if needed) can be provided during night tube feedings (Davanzo, Strajn, Kennedy, Crocetta, & De Cunto, 2014).
- Nutrition after discharge is designed to avoid growth failure. Some recommendations include fortifying mother's pumped milk with powdered preterm discharge formula, which may be an off-label use of the product. Few data exist as to the safety and efficacy of this practice (Griffin & Cooke, 2007). Feeding plans for the discharged preterm infant should emphasize direct breastfeeding, use of expressed fortified human milk if needed, continued milk expression, and ongoing professional clinical lactation services (Groh-Wargo & Thompson, 2014).

Creating a Feeding Plan for Postdischarge Management

In preparation for discharge, infants are usually transitioned to cue-based feedings when they can consume about 50% or more of their feedings, either at the breast or through a combination of breastfeeding and supplementation (Meier, 2003). Cue-based oral feedings often result in an earlier transition to full oral feedings (Kirk, Alder, & King, 2007). As the time for discharge approaches, feeding plans can be modified to arrange for the mother to stay for a longer visit of perhaps 8 hours, during which time the infant is fed on cue, intake per feed is measured by pre- and postfeed weights, and any needed supplementation is provided as an extra feeding or divided over the following feedings in the absence of the mother (Spatz, 2004). Any equipment needed for discharge is secured at this point, including a rented scale. Some mothers find that the use of a tube-feeding device at the breast helps their infant to consume the required amount of milk while improving sucking skills, eliminating the need for bottles. Many mothers are given a 24-hour minimum intake that their infant should consume and use the scale to calculate when and if the infant should be supplemented. Once the infant demonstrates the ability to take all feedings from the breast, the scale may be used twice weekly until the infant consistently shows an average daily weight gain of 15–30 g. If the mother has rented a breast pump, she should be instructed to keep it until the infant is fully established at breast. This may actually be 2–4 weeks after discharge when the infant reaches approximately term-corrected age (Hill et al., 1994, 1997).

Although a major concern of mothers of term infants is whether they are producing sufficient amounts of milk, preterm mothers' anxiety centers around whether their infant is consuming adequate amounts of milk (Kavanaugh et al., 1995). Even though the infant may be home, immature feeding skills may still persist—slipping off the nipple, falling asleep at breast at the beginning of a feeding, undependable feeding-cue signals, and fussing after a feeding—that indicate to the mother her infant may not be getting enough. Mothers may find that they can use alternate massage at this point to increase the volume and fat content per feeding and use the nipple tug to strengthen the infant's suck. Mothers may also find that hand expressing or pumping just until the milk lets down facilitates improved milk intake by the infant. The infant's low sucking pressure could be inadequate for some mothers to trigger the letdown reflex, resulting in little to no milk transfer (Hurst, 2005).

BREASTFEEDING LATE PRETERM INFANTS

The late preterm birth (34–36 weeks) rate was 6.82% in 2014 (Hamilton, Martin, Osterman, & Curtin, 2015). These infants are not just smaller versions of a full-term infant. Research and clinical experience are finding that preterm birth, by even just 1 week, raises the risk for neonatal morbidity and mortality (Kramer et al., 2000; Raju, Higgins, Stark, & Leveno, 2006; Wang, Dorer, Fleming, & Catlin, 2004). In July 2005, a National Institutes of Health panel recommended that this group of infants be referred to as late preterm rather than near term to better convey their greater vulnerabilities and need for closer monitoring and follow-up. The designation near term was thought to mislead parents and clinicians into thinking that these infants are almost term and could thus be treated similarly to term infants (Raju et al., 2006). Defining this population of infants helps clarify expectations of parents and clinicians as to how these infants behave and how better to anticipate care based on their unique vulnerabilities. Late preterm infants are at an increased risk for airway instability, apnea, bradycardia, excessive sleepiness, large weight loss, dehydration, feeding difficulties, weak sucking, jaundice, hypoglycemia, hypothermia, immature self-regulation, respiratory distress, sepsis, prolonged artificial milk supplementation, hospital readmission, and breastfeeding failure during the neonatal period (Adamkin, 2006; Engle, Tomashek, Wallman, & Committee on Fetus and Newborn, American Academy of Pediatrics, 2007). Even though some late preterm infants may look like full-term infants, late preterm infants are physiologically, metabolically, and neurologically immature and have limited compensatory mechanisms to adjust to the extrauterine environment.

The last 6 weeks of gestation are a unique period of growth and development for the fetus. At birth, the brain mass of 34- to 35-week late preterm infants is approximately 60% that of term infants, myelination is markedly underdeveloped, and neuronal connections and synaptic junctions are not fully developed. At the end of 36 weeks of gestation, the brain weight of a premature infant is about 80% that of a term infant's brain weight (Kinney, 2006), affecting such functions as arousal, sleep–wake behavior, and the coordination of feeding with breathing. Late preterm infants are born precisely at the time when rapid brain development is occurring (Hallowell & Spatz, 2012). The immature brainstem adversely impacts upper airway and lung volume control, laryngeal reflexes, and the chemical control of breathing and sleep mechanisms. Ten percent of these infants experience significant apnea of prematurity (Darnall, Ariagno, & Kinney, 2006). With their diminished muscle tone, late preterm infants are more prone to positional apnea due to airway obstruction. Their immature autonomic system may demonstrate exaggerated responses to stressful stimuli with rapid or lower heart rates, abnormal breathing, skin mottling, frequent startling, regurgitation, or simply shutting down. Their ability to self-regulate may be limited. They may appear to be irritable, difficult to console, and/or not very responsive to their parents' overtures.

Mothers of late preterm infants may be at increased risk for delayed lactogenesis II. Preterm birth itself often compromises the initiation of lactation, delaying the onset of copious milk production (Cregan et al., 2002) and presenting a prolonged colostral phase to an infant with immature feeding skills. Late preterm infants with limited breastfeeding skills and reduced breastfeeding efficiency and whose mothers present colostrum for an extended period of time are at risk for slow or no weight gain, dehydration, and hyperbilirubinemia. Their mothers are at risk for insufficient milk production.

Late preterm infants are at a disadvantage in terms of feeding skills. They are born with low energy stores (both subcutaneous and brown fat). They have high energy demands, poor feeding abilities, and are sleepy, with fewer and shorter awake periods. They tire easily when feeding, have a weak suck and low tone, demonstrate an inability to sustain sucking, and may have a small mouth, with uncoordinated oral–motor movements. They are easily overstimulated and may shut down before consuming adequate amounts of colostrum or milk. They may take only small volumes of milk during the early days in the hospital, which are often sufficient for that period of time, but exhibit feeding difficulties and slow weight gain when higher volumes of milk intake become necessary for normal growth. Although some infants may demonstrate adequate muscle tone initially, this tone may be rapidly depleted during a feeding, indicating decreased endurance. Postural stability may be immature, creating a less efficient feeding pattern. Late preterm infants experience reduced tone in the muscles involved with feeding, which, coupled with neurological immaturity of the suck–swallow–breathe cycle, can result in uncoordinated and ineffective milk intake at the breast. If treated like a normal term newborn, they are at an increased risk for inadequate nourishment. They may go through the motions of feeding but may transfer little if any milk for their efforts.

The creation of a breastfeeding plan of care for late preterm infants is directed by their vulnerabilities (Walker, 2008). Breastfeeding management options for this population are often extrapolated from those used with either full-term infants or with infants less than 34 weeks of gestation, neither of which may be completely appropriate for the unique needs of the late preterm population. An in-hospital feeding plan appears in **Table 6-4**. Breastfeeding interventions are designed to accomplish three goals: prevent adverse outcomes, establish the mother's milk supply, and ensure adequate infant intake.

Careful positioning for breastfeeding is necessary to avoid apnea, bradycardia, or desaturation, especially for younger infants with decreased muscle tone. They are more prone to positional apnea due to airway obstruction and should not be fed in positions that cause excessive flexion of the neck or trunk. The traditional cradle hold is one of the positions to avoid early on because infants can become so flexed that full rib cage expansion is impeded and the risk of airway collapse is increased. Some infants may prefer slight extension in their neck to keep their airway open. Clutch holds are a better choice for the late preterm infant (Meier, Firman, & Degenhardt, 2007). If infants have poor muscle tone, mothers may find that using the Dancer hand position helps stabilize the jaw so the infant does not keep slipping off the nipple or does not bite or clench the jaws to keep from sliding off the breast (Danner & Cerutti, 1984). Some infants may need assistance in opening their mouths wide enough to draw in the entire nipple plus part of the areola because they do not exhibit spontaneous mouth opening or do not open their mouths wide enough. Eliciting the rooting reflex may help, as mouth opening is a central component of this reflex. For some infants, mothers can be instructed to gently exert downward pressure on the chin to open the mouth and turn out the lower lip (Wolf & Glass, 1992).

Colson, de Rooy, and Hawdon (2003) described a strategy called biological nurturing that involved holding late preterm newborn infants so that their chest, abdomen, and legs were closely flexed around a maternal body contour and unrestricted access to the breast was offered, with abundant skin-to-skin contact. Mothers were encouraged to hold the infant in a biological nurturing position between feedings. The authors suggested that during the 40 weeks of a full-term pregnancy, mothers

Table 6-4 Sample In-Hospital Breastfeeding Plan for Mothers

Plan	Details
Feed your infant frequently. This helps keep infant's blood sugar from falling and bilirubin from becoming too high.	Within 1 hour after birth. Once every hour for the next 3–4 hours. Every 2–3 hours until 12 hours of age. At least 8 times each 24 hours during the hospital stay.
Place infant skin to skin on your chest.	This keeps the infant warm and the blood sugar from falling. It lets you breastfeed at the first sign of feeding cues.
Watch for rapid eye movements under the eyelids.	This is a sign that the infant may be ready to feed.
Move infant to breast when infant shows feeding cues. This helps increase the amount of milk infant takes at a feeding.	Sucking movements of the mouth and tongue. Rapid eye movements under the eyelids. Hand-to-mouth movements. Body movements. Small sounds.
Make sure you know how to tell when infant is swallowing.	The infant's jaw drops and holds for a second. You hear a "ca" sound. You feel a drawing action on the areola and see it move toward infant's mouth. You hear the infant swallow. You feel the swallow when you place a finger on the infant's throat. Your nurse hears the swallow when a stethoscope is placed on the infant's throat.
Use alternate massage if the infant does not swallow after every 1–3 sucks.	Massage and squeeze the breast each time the infant stops between sucks. Do this on each breast at each feeding. This helps get more colostrum into the infant, avoids fatigue, and keeps the infant sucking longer.
If your infant does not swallow when at the breast, hand express colostrum into a teaspoon and spoon-feed 2 teaspoons to the infant using the above guidelines.	Using a breast pump sometimes makes it hard to collect the small amounts of expressed colostrum. Spoon-feeding the infant ensures that he or she is well nourished until able to efficiently feed at the breast.

Data from Walker, M. (2009). *Breastfeeding the late preterm infant: Improving care and outcomes*. Amarillo, TX: Hale Publishing.

cannot put their infants down, so physiologically the infant could continue to be incubated or gestated in the mothers' arms during the early days after a late preterm birth. When mothers picked up on feeding cues, infants who appeared to be asleep were observed to be actively sucking at the breast. After the infant was seen to complete a suck–swallow cycle, another cycle was more easily triggered, suggesting that flow regulates suck and that the more swallows achieved, the more sucking that followed. This study suggested that mothers assume an approximately 30-degree semireclining position with the entire frontal aspect of the infant's body draped prone around a natural contour of the mother's body. Breastfeeding in a ventral or abdominal position elicited a system of primitive neonatal reflexes that avoided arching away from the breast and aided latch and sucking as gravity pulled the chin and tongue forward (Colson, Meek, & Hawdon, 2008). Ventral positioning elicited more primitive neonatal feeding reflexes than traditional dorsal positions and triggered antigravity reflexes that inhibited erratic movements of arms and legs or flailing at the breast. Ventral positioning may be tried if the infant arches from the breast, flails, shows erratic movements of the arms and legs, cannot latch to the breast, or if it appears that gravity is overcoming the infant's ability to attach to the breast.

If the infant cannot obtain adequate colostrum or milk directly from the breast with the use of frequent cue-based feeds, with the addition of alternate massage, with help from milk incentives at the breast, or with a nipple shield in place, supplementation may be required. The best supplement is expressed colostrum/milk or banked human milk if available. Feeding volumes of 5–10 mL every 2–3 hours on the 1st day, 10–20 mL on day 2, and 20–30 mL on day 3 are suggested (Stellwagen, Hubbard, & Wolf, 2007). Mothers can hand express colostrum into a spoon and spoon-feed this to the infant (Hoover, 1998). One teaspoon equals 5 mL. If a pump is used to express colostrum, small amounts may cling to the sides of the collection container, leaving little for actual use. Pumping into a small container, such as an Ameda diaphragm or the Medela colostrum collection container that has been placed between the valve and the collection bottle of either an Ameda or Medela breast pump, may yield a greater quantity of usable colostrum. Cup feeding of late preterm infants has been shown to significantly increase the likelihood of their being exclusively breastfed at discharge and at 3 and 6 months after discharge, without increasing the length of the hospital stay or compromising weight gain (Yilmaz, Caylan, Karacan, Bodur, & Gokcay, 2014).

Mothers of late preterm infants will often need to express their milk, just as mothers of infants born before 34 weeks do. If the infant is unable to feed at the breast, is unable to transfer enough colostrum or milk at feedings, is in the earliest gestation range of late preterm infants (34 weeks), or is separated from the mother, written pumping instructions should be provided. These should include the following (Walker, 2010b):

- Begin expressing milk within 1 hour of birth and no later than 6 hours following delivery.
- Hand express colostrum as frequently as possible during the first 3 days. This can be expressed into a spoon and spoon-fed to the infant or pulled into a syringe and fed to the infant if he/she is in a special care nursery.
- Double pump with a hospital-grade electric pump 8 times per 24 hours for 10–15 minutes each time.
- Massage and compress the breasts while pumping.

Once lactogenesis II occurs:

- Mothers should use the maximum comfortable vacuum on the pump.
- While double pumping with the electric pump, mothers should massage and compress each breast, making sure that all four quadrants are massaged and any lumps or blockages are addressed.
- Once the spray of milk stops, the mother can turn off the pump and massage each breast for 1 to 2 minutes, then resume pumping with the pump or hand express out as much of the remaining milk as possible.

- To further boost milk production if needed, power pumping can be done.
- Mothers should keep a pumping log and clinicians should check to see that an adequate volume of milk continues to be produced.

Clinicians and mothers find it beneficial to mutually create an individualized breastfeeding plan for use after discharge. A number of policy statements and practice guidelines are available that pertain to breastfeeding the late preterm infant (Briere, Lucas, McGrath, Lussier, & Brownell, 2015). A sample plan appears in **Box 6-5**. It can and should be modified to provide mothers with the tools they need to successfully breastfeed their infants. A different type of discharge feeding plan suggests separating each day into periods of breastfeeding (during the day) and bottle-feeding and pumping (during the night) (Meier, Patel, Wright, & Engstrom, 2013). Initial postdischarge feeding plans may need to be modified over time. Clinicians will need to follow these families closely.

Box 6-5 Sample Discharge Breastfeeding Plan for a Late Preterm Infant

Your milk and feeding at the breast are very important to your late preterm infant.

Even though your infant may look full term, he or she is not fully developed and may need some extra help and time learning to breastfeed. Your milk contains ingredients that provide protection from disease and help promote your infant's brain development that was interrupted by an early birth. Your infant may tire easily before a feeding is finished and may seem to sleep a lot. These guidelines will help get breastfeeding off to a good start.

Feed your infant on cue 8–12 times over 24 hours. Preterm infants are not always reliable in telling you when they need to feed. Sleeping is not an indication that the infant is getting enough milk. Use these signs as a cue to feed if your infant is very sleepy:

- Sucking movements of the mouth and tongue
- Rapid eye movements under the eyelids
- Hand-to-mouth movements
- Body movements
- Small sounds

Place your infant in a clutch or cross-cradle position. If your infant has difficulty attaching to the breast, flails at the breast, or arches away from the breast, use a semireclining position. Recline to a 30-degree angle, and place your infant on his or her tummy with the mouth directly over the nipple. This allows gravity to bring the infant's chin and tongue forward and help the infant latch.

As your infant latches on, make sure his or her mouth is wide open.

You should hear or feel your infant swallowing every 1–3 sucks during most of the feeding.

Use alternate massage on each breast at each feeding to keep the infant sucking and increase the amount of milk he or she receives at each feeding. Thoroughly massage and compress each part of the breast so that milk does not back up and set the stage for plugged ducts or an infection.

If you are not sure how much milk your infant is getting at each feeding, you can weigh the infant before and after a feeding. This information will help you determine whether you need to offer a supplement.

Record each feeding, any use of a supplement, the amount of pumped milk, the number of wet diapers, and the number of bowel movements on your feeding log until the infant is reliably feeding and gaining weight.

If your infant does not latch to the breast, try the following:

- Gently roll your nipple between your fingers to make it easier for the infant to grasp.
- As you bring your infant to breast, have a helper place a tube-feeding device or dropper in the corner of the infant's mouth and deliver a small amount of milk as the infant attempts to latch. If the infant swallows and attempts to latch again, another small amount of milk can be given. Repeat the process until the infant no longer attempts to latch. These practice sessions should not last longer than 10 minutes to avoid tiring both you and your infant.
- Finish the feeding by finger or cup feeding.
- If the attempts at latching do not work, you may find that a silicone nipple shield allows the infant to latch and sustain sucking at the breast. Moisten the shield with warm water, turn it almost inside-out as you apply it to the breast, apply a little breastmilk to the outside of the shield, hand express milk into the shield tunnel, and bring the infant to breast. If the infant latches, continue using alternate massage throughout the feeding.

The infant should have at least 6 wet diapers and 3 or more bowel movements each day by the fifth day after birth. Bowel movements should start turning yellow by day 4. Meconium-stained diapers on day 5 may indicate that the infant is not getting enough milk. Uric acid crystals (red stains) on day 4 in wet diapers may also indicate that the infant is not transferring enough milk at the breast.

Take your infant to the physician's office 2 days after coming home from the hospital for a weight check and to make sure he or she is not jaundiced. A weight check should be performed every 3 days or so to ensure that your infant continues to gain about ½ to 1 ounce per day.

If the infant cannot feed long enough at each feeding or is not gaining well, supplements of expressed breastmilk can be given by tube feeding at the breast, finger feeding, cup feeding, or bottle-feeding. If you do not have enough milk to use as a supplement, a hydrolyzed formula can be used until your milk production has increased. Continue to pump your milk 2–3 times each day to use as a supplement and to improve your milk supply.

Try "power pumping" for an hour once or twice each day. Pump for 5–10 minutes until the milk stops spraying from the first letdown. Wait 10 minutes or so, and then pump again until the milk stops spraying.

Almost half of the milk that is available in the breast is pumped with the first letdown. Power pumping takes advantage of these "first" letdowns to mimic frequent feedings and helps increase your milk production. Depending on how your infant is doing at the breast, pumping should continue until he or she is 40–42 weeks corrected age, with weaning off the pump occurring over the first month at home.

Data from Walker, M. (2009). *Breastfeeding the late preterm infant: Improving care and outcomes.* Amarillo, TX: Hale Publishing.

SUMMARY: THE DESIGN IN NATURE

Whereas many breastfeeding problems remain iatrogenic, others are created by circumstances surrounding the birth of the infant. Mothers and clinicians require patience and persistence, because there is frequently no quick fix for some of these issues. Most of these problems and situations do not require avoiding or abandoning breastfeeding, just better breastfeeding management.

REFERENCES

Abouelfettoh, A. M., Dowling, D. A., Dabash, S. A., Elguindy, S. R., & Seoud, I. A. (2008). Cup versus bottle feeding for hospitalized late preterm infants in Egypt: A quasi-experimental study. *International Breastfeeding Journal, 3,* 27.

Academy of Breastfeeding Medicine Protocol Committee. (2010). ABM clinical protocol #22: Guidelines for management of jaundice in the breastfeeding infant equal to or greater than 35 weeks gestation. *Breastfeeding Medicine, 5,* 87–93.

Adamkin, D. H. (2006). Feeding problems in the late preterm infant. *Clinics in Perinatology, 33,* 831–837.

Agostoni, C., Grandi, F., Scaglioni, S., Gianni, M. L., Torcoletti, M., Radaelli, G., . . . Riva, E. (2000). Growth pattern of breastfed and nonbreastfed infants with atopic dermatitis in the first year of life. *Pediatrics, 106,* e73.

Ak, J., Lakshmanagowda, P. B., & Goturu, J. (2015). Impact of music therapy on breast milk secretion in mothers of premature newborns. *Journal of Clinical & Diagnostic Research, 9,* CC-04-CC06.

Akaba, K., Kimura, T., Sasaki, A., Tanabe, S., Ikegami, T., Hashimoto, M., . . . Hayasaka, K. (1998). Neonatal hyperbilirubinemia and mutation of the bilirubin uridine diphosphate-glucuronosyltransferase gene: A common missense mutation among Japanese, Koreans and Chinese. *Biochemistry & Molecular Biology International, 46,* 21–26.

Akca, K., & Aytekin, A. (2014). Effect of soothing noise on sucking success of newborns. *Breastfeeding Medicine, 9,* 538–542.

Aksit, S., Ozkayin, N., & Caglayan, S. (2002). Effect of sucking characteristics on breast milk creamatocrit. *Paediatric Perinatal Epidemiology, 16,* 355–360.

American Academy of Pediatrics (AAP). (1994). Practice parameter: Management of hyperbilirubinemia in the healthy term newborn. *Pediatrics, 94*(4 pt 1), 558–562.

American Academy of Pediatrics (AAP). (2003). *Red book.* Report of the Committee on Infectious Diseases (26th ed.). Elk Grove Village, IL: Author.

American Academy of Pediatrics (AAP). (2004). Policy statement: Hospital stay for healthy term newborns. *Pediatrics, 113,* 1434–1436.

American Academy of Pediatrics (AAP), Committee on Pediatric AIDS. (2013). Infant feeding and transmission of human immunodeficiency virus in the United States. *Pediatrics, 131,* 391–396.

American Academy of Pediatrics (AAP), Section on Breastfeeding. (2012). Breastfeeding and the use of human milk. *Pediatrics, 129,* e827–e841.

American Academy of Pediatrics (AAP), Subcommittee on Hyperbilirubinemia. (2004). Clinical practice guideline: Management of hyperbilirubinemia in the newborn infant 35 or more weeks of gestation. *Pediatrics, 114,* 297–316.

American Academy of Pediatrics (AAP), Subcommittee on Neonatal Hyperbilirubinemia. (2001). Neonatal jaundice and kernicterus. *Pediatrics, 108,* 763–765.

Anderson, J. W., Johnstone, B. M., & Remley, D. T. (1999). Breastfeeding and cognitive development: A meta-analysis. *American Journal of Clinical Nutrition, 70,* 525–535.

Anderson, P. O., Pochop, S. L., & Manoguerra, A. S. (2003). Adverse drug reactions in breastfed infants: Less than imagined. *Clinical Pediatrics, 42,* 325–340.

Anderson, P. O., & Valdes, V. (2007). A critical review of pharmaceutical galactagogues. *Breastfeeding Medicine, 2,* 229–242.

Arslanoglu, S., Ziegler, E. E., Moro, G. E., & World Association of Perinatal Medicine Working Group on Nutrition. (2010). Donor human milk in preterm infant feeding: Evidence and recommendations. *Journal of Perinatal Medicine, 38,* 347–351.

Askin, D. B., & Diehl-Jones, W. L. (2005). Improving on perfection: Breast milk and breast-milk additives for preterm neonates. *Newborn Infant Nursing Review, 5,* 10–18.

Atkinson, S. A. (2000). Human milk feeding of the micropremie. *Clinics in Perinatology, 27,* 235–247.

Auerbach, K. G., & Gartner, L. M. (1987). Breastfeeding and human milk: Their association with jaundice in the neonate. *Clinics in Perinatology, 14,* 89–107.

Auerbach, K. G., & Walker, M. (1994). When the mother of a premature infant uses a breast pump: What every NICU nurse needs to know. *Neonatal Network, 13,* 23–29.

Azzuqa, A., & Watchko, J. F. (2015). Bilirubin concentrations in jaundiced neonates with conjunctival icterus. *Journal of Pediatrics, 167,* 840–844.

Baker, B. J., & Rasmussen, T. W. (1997). Organizing and documenting lactation support of NICU families. *Journal of Obstetric, Gynecologic, and Neonatal Nursing, 26,* 515–521.

Baley, J., & Committee on Fetus and Newborn. (2015). Skin-to-skin care for term and preterm infants in the neonatal ICU. *Pediatrics, 136,* 596–599.

Bartoletti, A. L., Stevenson, D. K., Ostrander, C. R., & Johnson, J. D. (1979). Pulmonary excretion of carbon monoxide in the human infant as an index of bilirubin production. Part I: Effects of gestational age and postnatal age and some common neonatal abnormalities. *Journal of Pediatrics, 94,* 952–955.

Bell, E. H., Geyer, J., & Jones, L. (1995). A structured intervention improves breastfeeding success for ill or preterm infants. *MCN: The American Journal of Maternal/Child Nursing, 20,* 309–314.

Berger, I., Weintraub, V., Dollberg, S., Kopolovitz, R., & Mandel, D. (2009). Energy expenditure for breastfeeding and bottle-feeding preterm infants. *Pediatrics, 124,* e1149–e1152.

Bergman, N. J., Linley, L. L., & Fawcus, S. R. (2004). Randomized controlled trial of skin-to-skin contact from birth versus conventional incubator for physiological stabilization in 1200 g to 2199 g neonates. *Acta Paediatrica, 93,* 779–785.

Bertini, G., Breschi, R., & Dani, C. (2015). Physiological weight loss chart helps to identify high-risk infants who need breastfeeding support. *Acta Paediatrica, 104,* 1024–1027.

Bertini, G., Dani, C., Tronchin, M., & Rubaltelli, F. F. (2001). Is breastfeeding really favoring early neonatal jaundice? *Pediatrics, 107,* e41. Retrieved from http://www.pediatrics.org/cgi/content/full/107/3/e41

Beutler, E., Gelbart, T., & Demina, A. (1998). Racial variability in the UDP-glucuronosyltransferase 1 (UGT1A1) promoter: A balanced polymorphism for regulation of bilirubin metabolism? *Proceedings of the National Academy of Sciences of the United States of America, 95,* 8170–8174.

Bhat, B. A., & Gupta, B. (2003). Effects of human milk fortification on morbidity factors in very low birth weight infants. *Annals of Saudi Medicine, 23,* 28–31.

Bhutani, V. K., Gourley, G. R., Adler, S., Kreamer, B., Dalin, C., & Johnson, L. H. (2000). Noninvasive measurement of total serum bilirubin in a multiracial predischarge newborn population to assess the risk of severe hyperbilirubinemia. *Pediatrics, 106,* e17. Retrieved from http://www.pediatrics.org/cgi/content/full/106/2/e17

Bhutani, V. K., Johnson, L. H., & Sivieri, E. M. (1999a). Risk assessment of hyperbilirubinemia in nearterm newborns. *Pediatrics, 104*(suppl 3), 741.

Bhutani, V. K., Johnson, L., & Sivieri, E. M. (1999b). Predictive ability of a predischarge hour-specific serum bilirubin for subsequent significant hyperbilirubinemia in healthy term and near-term newborns. *Pediatrics, 103,* 6–14.

Bhutani, V. K., Johnson, L. H., & Keren, R. (2004). Diagnosis and management of hyperbilirubinemia in the term neonate: For a safer first week. *Pediatric Clinics of North America, 51,* 843–861.

Bier, J. B., Ferguson, A., Anderson, L., Solomon, E., Voltas, C., Oh, W., & Vohr, B. R. (1993). Breastfeeding of very low birth-weight infants. *Journal of Pediatrics, 23,* 773–778.

Binns, C., James, J., & Lee, M. K. (2008). Why the new WHO growth charts are dangerous to breastfeeding. *Breastfeeding Review, 16,* 5–7.

Bishara, R., Dunn, M. S., Merko, S. E., & Darling, P. (2009). Volume of foremilk, hindmilk, and total milk produced by mothers of very preterm infants born at less than 28 weeks of gestation. *Journal of Human Lactation, 25,* 272–279.

Blackburn, S. (1995). Hyperbilirubinemia and neonatal jaundice. *Neonatal Network, 14,* 15–25.

Blackburn, S. T., & Loper, D. L. (1992). *Maternal, fetal, and neonatal physiology: A clinical perspective.* Philadelphia, PA: W. B. Saunders.

Blackmon, L. R., Fanaroff, A. A., & Raju, T. N. K. (2004). Research on prevention of bilirubin-induced brain injury and kernicterus: National Institute of Child Health and Human Development conference executive summary. *Pediatrics, 114,* 229–233.

Blaymore-Bier, J. A. (1997). Breastfeeding infants who were extremely low birth weight. *Pediatrics, 100,* e3.

Blaymore-Bier, J. A., Ferguson, A. E., Morales, Y., Liebling, J. A., Archer, D., Oh, W., & Vohr, B. R. (1996). Comparison of skin-to-skin contact with standard contact in low-birth-weight infants who are breastfed. *Archives of Pediatric and Adolescent Medicine, 150,* 1265.

Bosschaart, N., Kok, J. H., Newsum, A. M., Ouweneel, D. M., Mentink, R., van Leeuwen, T. G., & Aalders, M. C. G. (2012). Limitations and opportunities of transcutaneous bilirubin measurements. *Pediatrics, 129,* 689–694.

Braveman, P., Egerter, S., Pearl, M., Marchi, K., & Miller, C. (1995). Early discharge of newborns and mothers: A critical review of the literature. *Pediatrics, 96,* 716–726.

Braveman, P., Kessel, W., Egerter, S., & Richmond, J. (1997). Early discharge and evidence-based practice: Good science and good judgment. *Journal of the American Medical Association, 278,* 334–336.

Brethauer, M., & Carey, L. (2010). Maternal experience with neonatal jaundice. *MCN: The American Journal of Maternal/Child Nursing, 35,* 8–14.

Briere, C-E., Lucas, R., McGrath, J. M., Lussier, M., & Brownell, E. (2015). Establishing breastfeeding with the late preterm infant in the NICU. *Journal of Obstetric, Gynecologic, and Neonatal Nursing, 44,* 102–113.

Briere, C-E., McGrath, J. M., Cong, X., Brownell, E., & Cusson, R. (2015). Direct-breastfeeding premature infants in the neonatal intensive care unit. *Journal of Human Lactation, 31,* 386–392.

Britton, J. R., Britton, H. L., & Beebe, S. A. (1994). Early discharge of the term newborn: A continued dilemma. *Pediatrics, 94,* 291–295.

Brodersen, R., & Herman, L. S. (1963). Intestinal reabsorption of unconjugated bilirubin. *Lancet, 1,* 1242.

Brown, A. K., Damus, K., Kim, M. H., King, K., Harper, R., Campbell, D., . . . Harin, A. (1999). Factors relating to readmission of term and near-term neonates the first two weeks of life. Early discharge survey group of the health professional advisory board of the greater New York chapter of the March of Dimes. *Journal of Perinatal Medicine, 27,* 263–275.

Brown, T. E., Fernandes, P. A., Grant, L. J., Hutsul, J. A., & McCoshen, J. A. (2000). Effect of parity on pituitary prolactin response to metoclopramide and domperidone: Implications for the enhancement of lactation. *Journal of the Society for Gynecologic Investigation, 7,* 65–69.

Buckley, K. M., & Charles, G. E. (2006). Benefits and challenges of transitioning preterm infants to at-breast feedings. *International Breastfeeding Journal, 1,* 13.

Burke, B. L., Robbins, J. M., MacBird, T., Hobbs, C. A., Nesmith, C., & Tilford, J. M. (2009). Trends in hospitalizations for neonatal jaundice and kernicterus in the United States, 1988–2005. *Pediatrics, 123,* 524–532.

Butler, N., & Bar-Yam, N. (2012). *Use of pasteurized donor human milk as NICU standard of care.* Newton, MA: Mothers' Milk Bank of New England. Retrieved from http://www.milkbankne.org/files/MBNE_NICU.pdf

Caglar, M. K., Ozer, I., & Altugan, F. S. (2006). Risk factors for excess weight loss and hypernatremia in exclusively breastfed infants. *Brazilian Journal of Medical and Biological Research, 39,* 539–544.

California Perinatal Quality Care Collaborative. (2008). *Nutritional support of the VLBW infant.* Retrieved from https://www.cpqcc.org/sites/default/files/NUTRITIONAL_SUPPORT_OF_THE_VLBW_INFANT_-_REVISED_2008EntireToolkit.pdf

Callen, J., Pinelli, J., Atkinson, S., & Saigal, S. (2005). Qualitative analysis of barriers to breastfeeding in very-low-birthweight infants in the hospital and postdischarge. *Advances in Neonatal Care, 5,* 93–103.

Capretti, M. G., Lanari, M., Lazzarotto, T., Gabrielli, L., Pignatelli, S., Corvaglia, L., . . . Faldella, G. (2009). Very low birth weight infants born to cytomegalovirus-seropositive mothers fed with their mother's milk: A prospective study. *Journal of Pediatrics, 154,* 842–848.

Carceller-Blanchard, A., Cousineau, J., & Delvin, E. E. (2009). Point of care testing: Transcutaneous bilirubinometry in neonates. *Clinical Biochemistry, 42,* 143–149.

Carter, K., & Dixon, K. (2001). Kernicterus in full-term infants—United States, 1994–1998. *Morbidity and Mortality Weekly Report, 50,* 491–494.

Casavant, S. G., McGrath, J. M., Burke, G., & Briere, C. E. (2015). Caregiving factors affecting breastfeeding duration within a neonatal intensive care unit. *Advances in Neonatal Care, 15,* 421–428.

Cashore, W. J. (1998). Bilirubin metabolism and toxicity in the newborn. In P. A. Polin & W. W. Fox (Eds.), *Fetal and neonatal physiology.* Philadelphia, PA: W. B. Saunders.

Castrucci, B. C., Hoover, K. L., Lim, S., & Maus, K. C. (2007). Availability of lactation counseling services influences breastfeeding among infants admitted to neonatal intensive care units. *American Journal of Health Promotion, 21,* 410–415.

Cattaneo, A., Davanzo, R., Uxa, F., & Tamburlini, G. (1998). Recommendations for the implementation of the kangaroo mother care for low birthweight infants. *Acta Paediatrica, 87,* 440–445.

Cattaneo, A., Davanzo, R., Worku, B., Surjono, A., Echeverria, M., Bedri, A., . . . Tamburlini, G. (1998). Kangaroo mother care for low birthweight infants: A randomized controlled trial in different settings. *Acta Paediatrica, 87*(9), i976–i985.

Cattaneo, A., & Guoth-Gumberger, M. (2008). The new WHO child growth standards: Possible effects on exclusive breastfeeding in the first six months. *Breastfeeding Review, 16,* 9–12.

Centers for Disease Control and Prevention (CDC). (2002). *Enterobacter sakazakii* infections associated with the use of powdered infant formula—Tennessee, 2001. *Morbidity and Mortality Weekly Report, 51,* 298–300.

Chan, G. (2003). Effects of powdered human milk fortifiers on the antimicrobial actions of human milk. *Journal of Perinatology, 23,* 620–623.

Chang, P. F., Lin, Y. C., Liu, K., Yeh, S. J., & Ni, Y. H. (2009). Prolonged unconjugated hyperbilirubinemia in breastfed male infants with a mutation of uridine diphosphate-glucuronosyl transferase. *Journal of Pediatrics, 155,* 860–863.

Chantry, C. J., Young, S. L., Rennie, W., Nqonyani, M., Mashio, C., Israel-Ballard, K., . . . Koniz-Booher, P. (2012). Feasibility of using flash-heated breastmilk as an infant feeding option for HIV-exposed, uninfected infants after 6 months of age in urban Tanzania. *Journal of Acquired Immune Deficiency Syndromes, 60,* 43–50.

Charpak, N., Ruiz-Pelaez, J. G., de Figueroa, C. Z., & Charpak, Y. (2001). A randomized, controlled trial of kangaroo mother care: Results of follow-up at 1 year of corrected age. *Pediatrics, 108,* 1072–1079.

Chen, C-H., Wang, T-M., Chang, H-H., & Chi, C-S. (2000). The effect of breast- and bottle-feeding on oxygen saturation and body temperature in preterm infants. *Journal of Human Lactation, 16,* 21–27.

Chen, J., Sadakata, M., Ishida, M., Sekizuka N., & Sayama, M. (2011). Baby massage ameliorates neonatal jaundice in full-term newborn infants. *Tohoku Journal of Experimental Medicine, 223,* 97–102.

Chen, Y. J., Yeh, T. F., & Chen, C. M. (2015). Effect of breastfeeding frequency on hyperbilirubinemia in breastfed term neonate. *Pediatrics International, 57,* 1121–1125.

Claud, E. C., & Walker, A. (2001). Hypothesis: Inappropriate colonization of the premature intestine can cause neonatal necrotizing enterocolitis. *FASEB Journal, 15,* 1398–1403.

Clavey, S. (1996). The use of acupuncture for the treatment of insufficient lactation (Que Ru). *American Journal of Acupuncture, 24,* 35–46.

Clum, D., & Primomo, J. (1996). Use of a silicone nipple shield with premature infants. *Journal of Human Lactation, 12,* 287–290.

Colson, S. D., de Rooy, L., & Hawdon, J. M. (2003). Biological nurturing increases duration of breastfeeding for a vulnerable cohort. *MIDIRS Midwifery Digest, 13,* 92–97.

Colson, S. D., Meek, J. H., & Hawdon, J. M. (2008). Optimal positions for the release of primitive neonatal reflexes stimulating breastfeeding. *Early Human Development, 84,* 441–449.

Connelly, A. M., & Volpe, J. J. (1990). Clinical features of bilirubin encephalopathy. *Clinical Perinatology, 17,* 371–379.

Cooper, W. O., Atherton, H. D., Kahana, M., & Kotagal, U. R. (1995). Increased incidence of severe breastfeeding malnutrition and hypernatremia in a metropolitan area. *Pediatrics, 96*(5, pt 1), 957–960.

Corbett, S. S., & Drewett, R. F. (2004). To what extent is failure to thrive in infancy associated with poorer cognitive development? A review and meta-analysis. *Journal of Child Psychology & Psychiatry, 45,* 641–654.

Costello, A., & Chapman, J. (1998). Mothers' perceptions of the care-by-parent program prior to hospital discharge of their preterm infants. *Neonatal Network, 17,* 37–42.

Cregan, M. D., De Mello, T. R., Kershaw, D., McDougall, K., & Hartmann, P. E. (2002). Initiation of lactation in women after preterm delivery. *Acta Obstetrica et Gynecologica Scandinavica, 81,* 870–877.

da Silva, O. P., Knoppert, D. C., Angelini, M. M., & Forret, P. A. (2001). Effect of domperidone on milk production in mothers of premature newborns: A randomized double blind, placebo-controlled trial. *Canadian Medical Association Journal, 164,* 17–21.

Dahms, B. B., Krauss, A. N., Gartner, L. M., Klain, D. B., Soodalter, J., & Auld, P. A. (1973). Breastfeeding and serum bilirubin values during the first 4 days of life. *Journal of Pediatrics, 83,* 1049–1054.

Daly, S. E., Kent, J. C., Owens, R. A., & Hartmann, P. E. (1996). Frequency and degree of milk removal and the short-term control of human milk synthesis. *Experimental Physiology, 81,* 861–875.

Danner, E., Joeckel, R., Michalak, S., Phillips, S., & Goday, P. S. (2009). Weight velocity in infants and children. *Nutrition in Clinical Practice, 24,* 76–79.

Danner, S. C., & Cerutti, E. R. (1984). *Nursing your neurologically impaired baby.* Rochester, NY: Childbirth Graphics.

Darnall, R. A., Ariagno, R. L., & Kinney, H. C. (2006). The late preterm infant and the control of breathing, sleep, and brainstem development: A review. *Clinics in Perinatology, 33,* 883–914.

Davanzo, R., Strajn, T., Kennedy, J., Crocetta, A., & De Cunto, A. (2014). From tube to breast: The bridging role of semi-demand breastfeeding. *Journal of Human Lactation, 30,* 405–409.

Davim, R. M., Enders, B. C., & da Silva, R. A. (2010). Mothers' feelings about breastfeeding their premature babies in a rooming-in facility. *Revista da Escola de Enfermagem USP, 44,* 713–718.

De Carvalho, M., Hall, M., & Harvey, D. (1981). Effects of water supplementation on physiological jaundice in breastfed infants. *Archives of Disease in Childhood, 56,* 568–569.

De Carvalho, M., Klaus, M. H., & Merkatz, R. B. (1982). Frequency of breastfeeding and serum bilirubin concentration. *American Journal of Diseases of Children, 136,* 737–738.

de Greef, L., Goel, M., Seo, M. J., Larson, E. C., Stout, J. W., Taylor, J. A., & Patel, S. N. (2014). BiliCam: Using mobile phones to monitor newborn jaundice. *2014 ACM International Joint Conference on Pervasive and Ubiquitous Computing (UbiComp 2014).*

de Onis, M., Garza, C., Onyango, A. W., & Borghi, E. (2007). Comparison of the WHO Child Growth Standards and the CDC 2000 growth charts. *Journal of Nutrition, 137,* 144–148.

de Onis, M., Garza, C., Onyango, A. W., & Martorell, R. (Eds.). (2006). WHO Child Growth Standards. *Acta Paediatrica Supplement, 450*, 1–101.

de Onis, M., Onyango, A. W., Borghi, E., Garza, C., & Yang, H. (2006). Comparison of the World Health Organization (WHO) Child Growth Standards and the National Center for Health Statistics/WHO International Growth Reference: Implications for child health programmes. *Public Health and Nutrition, 9*, 942–947.

Dennery, P. A., Seidman, D. S., & Stevenson, D. K. (2001). Neonatal hyperbilirubinemia. *New England Journal of Medicine, 344,* 581–590.

Dereddy, N. R., Talati, A. J., Smith, A., Kudumula, R., & Dhanireddy, R. (2015). A multipronged approach is associated with improved breast milk feeding rates in very low birth weight infants of an inner-city hospital. *Journal of Human Lactation, 31,* 43–46.

Desmarais, L., & Browne, S. (1990). Inadequate weight gain in breastfeeding infants: Assessments and resolutions. In K. G. Auerbach (Ed.), *Lactation consultant series.* Garden City Park, NY: Avery Publishing Group.

Dewey, K. G. (2001). Nutrition, growth and complementary feeding of the breastfed infant. *Pediatric Clinics of North America, 48,* 87–104.

Dewey, K. G., Heinig, M. J., Nommsen, L. A., Peerson, J. M., & Lonnerdal, B. (1992). Growth of breastfed and formula-fed infants from 0 to 18 months: The DARLING study. *Pediatrics, 89,* 1035–1041.

Dewey, K. G., Nommsen-Rivers, L. A., Heinig, M. J., & Cohen, R. J. (2003). Risk factors for suboptimal infant breastfeeding behavior, delayed onset of lactation, and excess neonatal weight loss. *Pediatrics, 112,* 607–619.

Dewey, K. G., Peerson, J. M., Brown, K. H., Krebs, N. F., Michaelsen, K. F., Persson, L. A., . . . Yeung, D. L. (1995). WHO working group on infant growth: Growth of breastfed infants deviates from current reference data: A pooled analysis of US, Canadian, and European data sets. *Pediatrics, 96,* 495–503.

Di Natale, C., Coclite, E., Di Ventura, L., & Di Fabio, S. (2011). Fortification of maternal milk for preterm infants. *Journal of Maternal–Fetal and Neonatal Medicine, 24*(suppl 1), 41–43.

Di Pierro, F., Callegari, A., Carotenuto, D., & Tapia, M. M. (2008). Clinical efficacy, safety and tolerability of BIO-C (micronized Silymarin) as a galactagogue. *Acta Biomedica, 79,* 205–210.

Dijk, P. H., & Helzebos, C. V. (2012). An evidence-based view on hyperbilirubinemia. *Acta Paediatrica, 101*(suppl 464), 3–10.

Dixit, R., & Gartner, L. (2000). The jaundiced newborn: Minimizing the risks. *Patient Care, 34,* 45–69.

Domanico, R., Davis, D. K., Coleman, F., & Davis, B. O. (2011). Documenting the NICU design dilemma: Comparative patient progress in open-ward and single family room units. *Journal of Perinatology, 31,* 281–288.

Dougherty, D., & Luther, M. (2008). Birth to breast—a feeding care map for the NICU: Helping the extremely low birth weight infant navigate the course. *Neonatal Network, 27,* 371–377.

Dowling, D. A., Meier, P. P., DiFiore, J. M., Blatz, M., & Martin, R. J. (2002). Cup feeding for preterm infants: Mechanics and safety. *Journal of Human Lactation, 18,* 13–20.

Drewett, R. F., Emond, A., Blair, P., & Emmett, P. (2005). The importance of slow weight gain in the first 2 months in identifying children who fail to thrive. *Journal of Reproductive and Infant Psychology, 23,* 309–317.

Eaton, A. P. (2001). Early postpartum discharge: Recommendations from a preliminary report to Congress [Commentary]. *Pediatrics, 107,* 400–404.

Egerter, S. A., Braverman, P. A., & Marchi, K. S. (1998). Follow-up of newborns and their mothers after early hospital discharge. *Clinics in Perinatology, 25,* 471–481.

Ehrenkranz, R., & Ackerman, B. (1986). Metoclopramide effect on faltering milk production by mothers of premature infants. *Pediatrics, 78,* 614–619.

Elander, G., & Lindberg, T. (1984). Hospital routines in infants with hyperbilirubinemia influence the duration of breastfeeding. *Acta Paediatrica Scandinavia, 73,* 708–712.

Elliott, S., & Reimer, C. (1998). Postdischarge telephone follow-up program for breastfeeding preterm infants discharged from a special care nursery. *Neonatal Network, 17,* 41–45.

Emond, A., Drewett, R., Blair, P., & Emmett, P. (2007). Postnatal factors associated with failure to thrive in term infants in the Avon Longitudinal Study of Parents and Children. *Archives of Disease in Childhood, 92,* 115–119.

Emond, A. M., Blair, P. S., Emmett, P. M., & Drewett, R. F. (2007). Weight faltering in infancy and IQ levels at 8 years in the Avon Longitudinal Study of Parents and Children. *Pediatrics, 120,* e1051–e1058.

Engle, W. A., Tomashek, K. M., Wallman, C., & Committee on Fetus and Newborn, American Academy of Pediatrics. (2007). "Late-preterm" infants: A population at risk. *Pediatrics, 120,* 1390–1401.

Escobar, G. J., Gonzales, V. M., Armstrong, M. A., Folck, B. F., Xiong, B., & Newman, T. B. (2002). Rehospitalization for neonatal dehydration. *Archives of Pediatrics and Adolescent Medicine, 156,* 155–161.

Esfahani, M. S., Berenji-Sooghe, S., Valiani, M., & Ehsanpour, S. (2015). Effect of acupressure on milk volume of breastfeeding mothers referring to selected health care centers in Tehran. *Iranian Journal of Nursing and Midwifery Research, 20,* 7–11.

Esquerra-Zwiers, A., Rossman, B., Meier, P., Engstrom, J., Janes, J., & Patel, A. (2016). "It's somebody else's milk": Unraveling the tension in mothers of preterm infants who provide consent for pasteurized donor human milk. *Journal of Human Lactation, 32,* 95–102.

Evans, K. C., Evans, R. G., Royal, R., Esterman, A., & James, S. (2003). Effect of caesarean section on breast milk transfer to the normal term newborn over the first week of life. *Archives of Disease in Childhood—Fetal and Neonatal Edition, 88,* F380–F382.

Fehrer, S., Berger, L., Johnson, J., & Wilde, J. (1989). Increasing breastmilk production for premature infants with a relaxation/imagery audiotape. *Pediatrics, 83,* 57–60.

Feldman, R., Weller, A., Leckman, J. F., Kuint, J., & Eidelman, A. I. (1999). The nature of the mother's tie to her infant: Maternal bonding under conditions of proximity, separation, and potential loss. *Journal of Child Psychology & Psychiatry, 40,* 929–939.

Fewtrell, M. S., Loh, K. L., Blake, A., Ridout, D. A., & Hawdon, J. (2006). Randomised, double blind trial of oxytocin nasal spray in mothers expressing breast milk for preterm infants. *Archives of Disease in Childhood—Fetal and Neonatal Edition, 91,* F169–F174.

Flacking, R., Ewald, U., & Wallin, L. (2011). Positive effect of kangaroo mother care on long-term breastfeeding in very preterm infants. *Journal of Obstetric, Gynecologic, and Neonatal Nursing, 40,* 190–197.

Flaherman, V. J., Schaefer, E. W., Kuzniewicz, M. W., Li, S. X., Walsh, E. M., & Paul, I. M. (2015). Early weight loss nomograms for exclusively breastfed newborns. *Pediatrics, 135,* e16–e23.

Foman, S. J., & Nelson, S. E. (1993). Size and growth. In S. J. Foman (Ed.), *Nutrition of normal infants.* St. Louis, MO: Mosby.

Forsyth, T. J., Maney, L. A., Ramirez, A., Raviotta, G., Burts, J. L., & Litzenberger, D. (1998). Nursing case management in the NICU: Enhanced coordination for discharge planning. *Neonatal Network, 17,* 23–34.

Frantz, K. B. (1992). The slow-gaining breastfeeding infant. *NAACOG's Clinical Issues in Perinatal and Women's Health Nursing: Breastfeeding, 3,* 647–655.

Froh, E. B., Deatrick, J. A., Curley, M. A. Q., & Spatz, D. L. (2015). Making meaning of pumping for mothers of infants with congenital diaphragmatic hernia. *Journal of Obstetric, Gynecologic, and Neonatal Nursing, 44,* 439–449.

Fugate, K., Hernandez, I., Ashmeade, T., Miladinovic, B., & Spatz, D. L. (2015). Improving human milk and breastfeeding practices in the NICU. *Journal of Obstetric, Gynecologic, and Neonatal Nursing, 44,* 426–438.

Furman, L., Minich, N., & Hack, M. (2002). Correlates of lactation in mothers of very low birth weight infants. *Pediatrics, 109,* 695–696.

Furman, L., Minich, N. M., & Hack, M. (1998). Breastfeeding of very low birth weight infants. *Journal of Human Lactation, 14,* 29–34.

Gabay, M. P. (2002). Galactagogues: Medications that induce lactation. *Journal of Human Lactation, 18,* 274–279.

Garpiel, S. J. (2012). Premature infant transition to effective breastfeeding: A comparison of four supplemental feeding methods. *Journal of Obstetric, Gynecologic, and Neonatal Nursing, 41*(s1), S143.

Gartner, L. M. (2001). Breastfeeding and jaundice. *Journal of Perinatology, 21,* S25–S29.

Gartner, L. M., & Herschel, M. (2001). Jaundice and breastfeeding. *Pediatric Clinics of North America, 48,* 389–399.

Garza, C., & de Onis, M. (2004). WHO Multicentre Growth Reference Study Group. Rationale for developing a new international growth reference. *Food and Nutrition Bulletin, 24*(suppl 1), S5–S14.

Gonzalez, K. A., Meinzen-Derr, J., Burke, B. L., Hibler, A. J., Kavinsky, B., Hess, S., . . . Morrow, A. L. (2003). Evaluation of a lactation support service in a children's hospital neonatal intensive care unit. *Journal of Human Lactation, 19,* 286–292.

Gourley, G. R., Kreamer, B. L., & Cohnen, M. (1997). Inhibition of beta-glucuronidase by casein hydrolysate formula. *Journal of Pediatric Gastroenterology, 25,* 267–272.

Gourley, G. R., Kreamer, B., Cohnen, M., & Kosorok, M. R. (1999). Neonatal jaundice and diet. *Archives of Pediatrics and Adolescent Medicine, 153,* 184–188.

Gourley, G. R., Zhanhai, L., Kreamer, B. L., & Kosorok, M. R. (2005). A controlled, randomized, doubleblind trial of prophylaxis against jaundice among breastfed newborns. *Pediatrics, 116,* 385–391.

Griffin, I. J., & Cooke, R. J. (2007). Nutrition of preterm infants after hospital discharge. *Journal of Pediatric Gastroenterology and Nutrition, 45*(suppl 3), S195–S203.

Groer, M. W., Gregory, K. E., Louis-Jacques, A., Thibeau, S., & Walker, W. A. (2015). The very low birth weight infant microbiome and childhood health. *Birth Defects Research (Part C), 105,* 252–264.

Groh-Wargo, S., & Thompson, M. (2014). Managing the human-milk–fed, preterm, VLBW infant at NICU discharge: The sprinkles dilemma. *Infant Child and Adolescent Nutrition, 6,* 262–269.

Gross, M. S. (1995). Letter. *ILCA Globe, 3,* 5.

Grummer-Strawn, L. M., Reinold, C., & Krebs, N. F. (2010). Use of World Health Organization and CDC growth charts for children 0–59 months in the United States. *Morbidity and Mortality Weekly Report, 59*(rr09), 1–15. Retrieved from http://www.cdc.gov/mmwr/preview/mmwrhtml/rr5909a1.htm

Grupp-Phelan, J., Taylor, J. A., Liu, L. L., & Davis, R. L. (1999). Early newborn hospital discharge and readmission for mild and severe jaundice. *Archives of Pediatrics and Adolescent Medicine, 153,* 1283–1288.

Guerrini, P. (1994). Human milk fortifiers. *Acta Paediatrica, 402*(suppl), 37–39.

Gunn, A. J., Gunn, T. R., Rabone, D. L., Breier, B. H., Blum, W. F., & Gluckman, P. D. (1996). Growth hormone increases breast milk volumes in mothers of preterm infants. *Pediatrics, 98,* 279–282.

Haase, B., Barreira, J., Murphy, P. K., Mueller, M., & Rhodes, J. (2009). The development of an accurate test weighing technique for preterm and high-risk hospitalized infants. *Breastfeeding and Medicine, 4,* 151–156.

Hake-Brooks, S. J., & Anderson, G. C. (2008). Kangaroo care and breastfeeding of mother–preterm infant dyads 0–18 months: A randomized, controlled trial. *Neonatal Network, 27,* 151–159.

Hale, T. W. (2003). Medications in breastfeeding mothers of preterm infants. *Pediatric Annals, 32,* 337–347.

Hall, R. T., Simon, S., & Smith, M. T. (2000). Readmission of breastfed infants in the first 2 weeks of life. *Journal of Perinatology, 20,* 432–437.

Hallowell, S. G., & Spatz, D. L. (2012). The relationship of brain development and breastfeeding in the late preterm Infant. *Journal of Pediatric Nursing, 27,* 154–162.

Hamilton, B. E., Martin, J. A., Osterman, M. J. K., & Curtin, S. C. (2015). Births: Preliminary data for 2014. *National Vital Statistics Reports, 64*(6). Hyattsville, MD: National Center for Health Statistics. Retrieved from http://www.cdc.gov/nchs/data/nvsr/nvsr64/nvsr64_06.pdf and http://www.cdc.gov/nchs/data/nvsr/nvsr64/nvsr64_06_supplemental_and_expanded_tables.pdf

Hamprecht, K., Maschmann, J., Jahn, G., Poets, C. F., & Goelz, R. (2008). Cytomegalovirus transmission to preterm infants during lactation. *Journal of Clinical Virology, 41,* 198–205.

Hanko, E., Lindemann, R., & Hansen, T. W. R. (2001). Spectrum of outcome in infants with extreme neonatal jaundice. *Acta Paediatrica, 90,* 782–785.

Hann, M., Malan, A., Kronson, M., Bergman, N., & Huskisson, R. (1999). Kangaroo mother care. *South African Medical Journal, 89,* 37.

Hannon, P. R., Willis, S. K., & Scrimshaw, S. C. (2001). Persistence of maternal concerns surrounding neonatal jaundice: An exploratory study. *Archives of Pediatrics and Adolescent Medicine, 155,* 1357–1363.

Hansen, T. W. (2000). Bilirubin oxidation in the brain. *Molecular and Genetic Metabolism, 71,* 411–417.

Hansen, T. W. (2001). Bilirubin brain toxicity. *Journal of Perinatology, 21,* S48–S51.

Hansen, T. W. (2003). Recent advances in the pharmacotherapy for hyperbilirubinemia in the neonate. *Expert Opinion in Pharmacotherapy, 4,* 1939–1948.

Hansen, T. W., Allen, J. W., & Tommarello, S. (1999). Oxidation of bilirubin in the brain: Further characterization of a potentially protective mechanism. *Molecular and Genetic Metabolism,* 68, 404–409.

Hansen, T. W. R. (1994). Bilirubin in the brain. *Clinical Pediatrics, 33,* 452–459.

Hansen, T. W. R. (2002). Mechanisms of bilirubin toxicity: Clinical implications. *Clinics in Perinatology, 29,* 765–778.

Hansen, W. F., McAndrew, S., Harris, K., & Zimmerman, M. B. (2005). Metoclopramide effect on breastfeeding the preterm infant: A randomized trial. *Obstetrics & Gynecology, 105,* 383–389.

Harding, D., Cairns, P., Gupta, S., & Cowan, F. (2001). Hypernatremia: Why bother weighing breastfed babies? *Archives of Disease in Childhood—Fetal and Neonatal Edition, 85,* F145.

Harris, M. C., Bernbaum, J. C., Polin, J. R., Zimmerman, R., & Polin, R. A. (2001). Developmental follow-up of breastfed term and near-term infants with marked hyperbilirubinemia. *Pediatrics, 107,* 1075–1080.

Hassiotou, F., Hepworth, A. R., Williams, T. M., Twigger, A-J., Perrella, S., Lai, C. T. . . . .Hartmann, P. E. (2013). Breastmilk cell and fat contents respond similarly to removal of breastmilk by the infant. *PLoS One, 8,* e78232.

Hedberg Nyqvist, K. (2001). The development of preterm infants' milk intake during breastfeeding. *Journal of Neonatal Nursing, 7,* 48–52.

Hedberg Nyqvist, K., Sjoden, P.-O., & Ewald, U. (1999). The development of preterm infants' breastfeeding behavior. *Early Human Development, 55,* 247–264.

Heiskanen, K., Siimes, M. A., & Salmenpera Perheentupa, J. (1995). Low vitamin B_6 status associated with slow growth in healthy breastfed infants. *Pediatric Research, 38,* 740–746.

Helliker, K. (1994, July 22). Dying for milk: Some mothers try in vain to breastfeed, starve their infants. *Wall Street Journal,* pp. 1, 4.

Henderson, J. J., Hartmann, P. E., Newnham, J. P., & Simmer, K. (2008). Effect of preterm birth and antenatal corticosteroid treatment on lactogenesis II in women. *Pediatrics, 121,* e92–e100.

Herschel, M. (2003). *Jaundice and breastfeeding.* Independent study module #12. Schaumburg, IL: La Leche League International.

Hill, P. D., Aldag, J. C., & Chatterton, R. T. (1999). Effects of pumping style on milk production in mothers of non-nursing preterm infants. *Journal of Human Lactation, 15,* 209–216.

Hill, P. D., Aldag, J. C., & Chatterton, R. T. (2001). Initiation and frequency of pumping and milk production in mothers of non-nursing preterm infants. *Journal of Human Lactation, 17,* 9–13.

Hill, P. D., Aldag, J. C., Chatterton, R. T., & Zinaman, M. (2005). Primary and secondary mediators' influence on milk output in lactating mothers of preterm and term infants. *Journal of Human Lactation, 21,* 138–150.

Hill, P. D., Aldag, J. C., Demirtas, H., Naeem, V., Parker, N. P., Zinaman, M. J., & Chatterton, R. T., Jr. (2009). Association of serum prolactin and oxytocin with milk production in mothers of preterm and term infants. *Biological Research for Nursing,* 10, 340–349.

Hill, P. D., Aldag, J. C., Zinaman, M. D., & Chatterton, R. T. (2007). Comparison of milk output between breasts in pump-dependent mothers. *Journal of Human Lactation, 23,* 333–337.

Hill, P. D., Brown, L. P., & Harker, T. L. (1995). Initiation and frequency of breast expression in breastfeeding mothers of LBW and VLBW infants. *Nursing Research, 44,* 352–355.

Hill, P. D., Hanson, K. S., & Mefford, A. L. (1994). Mothers of low birthweight infants: Breastfeeding patterns and problems. *Journal of Human Lactation, 10,* 169–176.

Hill, P. D., Ledbetter, R. J., & Kavanaugh, K. (1997). Breastfeeding patterns in low-birth-weight infants after hospital discharge. *Journal of Obstetric, Gynecologic, and Neonatal Nursing, 26,* 190–197.

Hoban, R., Bigger, H., Patel, A. L., Rossman, B., Fogg, L. F., & Meier, P. (2015). Goals for human milk feeding in mothers of very low birth weight infants: How do goals change and are they achieved during the NICU hospitalization? *Breastfeeding Medicine, 10,* 305–311.

Hollen, L. I., Din, Z. U., Jones, L. R., Emond, A. M., & Emmett, P. (2014). Are diet and feeding behaviors associated with the onset of and recovery from slow weight gain in early infancy? *British Journal of Nutrition, 111,* 1696–1704.

Hoover, K. (1998). Supplementation of the newborn by spoon in the first 24 hours. *Journal of Human Lactation, 14,* 245.

Hoover, K. L., Barbalinardo, L. H., & Platia, M. P. (2002). Delayed lactogenesis II secondary to gestational ovarian theca lutein cysts in two normal singleton pregnancies. *Journal of Human Lactation, 18,* 264–268.

Hopkinson, J. M., Schanler, R. J., Fraley, J. K., & Garza, C. (1992). Milk production by mothers of premature infants: Influence of cigarette smoking. *Pediatrics, 90,* 934–938.

Hopkinson, J. M., Schanler, R. J., & Garza, C. (1988). Milk production by mothers of premature infants. *Pediatrics, 81,* 815–820.

Hoque, S. A., Hoshino, H., Anwar, K. S., Tanaka, A., Shinagawa, M., Hayakawa, Y., . . . Ushijima, H. (2013). Transient heating of expressed breast milk up to 65°C inactivates HIV-1 in milk: A simple, rapid, and cost-effective method to prevent postnatal transmission. *Journal of Medical Virology, 85,* 187–193.

Horwood, L. J., Darlow, B. A., & Mogridge, N. (2001). Breast milk feeding and cognitive ability at 7–8 years. *Archives of Disease in Childhood—Fetal and Neonatal Edition, 84,* F23–F27.

Howard, C. R., de Blieck, E. A., ten Hoopen, C. B., Howard, F. M., Lanphear, B. P., & Lawrence, R. A. (1999). Physiologic stability of newborns during cup- and bottle-feeding. *Pediatrics, 104,* 1204–1207.

Hurst, N. (2005). Assessing and facilitating milk transfer during breastfeeding for the premature infant. *Newborn Infant Nursing Review, 5,* 19–26.

Hurst, N. M. (2007). The 3 M's of breastfeeding the preterm infant. *Journal of Perinatal & Neonatal Nursing, 21,* 234–239.

Hurst, N. M., Myatt, A., & Schanler, R. J. (1998). Growth and development of a hospital-based lactation program and mother's own milk bank. *Journal of Obstetric, Gynecologic, and Neonatal Nursing, 27,* 503–510.

Hurst, N. M., Valentine, C. J., Renfro, L., Burns, P., & Ferlic, L. (1997). Skin-to-skin holding in the neonatal intensive care unit influences maternal milk volume. *Journal of Perinatology, 17,* 213–217.

Ingram, J., Taylor, H., Churchill, C., Pike, A., & Greenwood, R. (2012). Metoclopramide or domperidone for increasing maternal breast milk output: A randomized controlled trial. *Archives of Disease in Childhood—Fetal and Neonatal Edition, 97,* F241–F245.

Ip, S., Glicken, S., Kulig, J., & O'Brien, R. (2003, January). *Management of neonatal hyperbilirubinemia.* Evidence Report/Technology Assessment (No. 65, prepared by Tufts–New England Medical Center Evidence-Based Practice Center under contract No. 290-97-0019). AHRQ Publication No. 03-E011. Rockville, MD: U.S. Department of Health and Human Services, Agency for Healthcare Research and Quality.

Isaacs, E. B., Fischi, B. R., Quinn, B. T., Chong, W. K., Gadian, D. G., & Lucas, A. (2010). Impact of breast milk on IQ, brain size and white matter development. *Pediatric Research, 67,* 357–362.

Iyer, N. P., Srinivasan, R., Evans, K., Ward, L., Cheung, W. Y., & Matthes, J. W. (2008). Impact of an early weighing policy on neonatal dehydration and breastfeeding. *Archives of Disease in Childhood, 93,* 297–299.

Janjindamai, W., & Chotsampancharoen, T. (2006). Effect of fortification on the osmolality of human milk. *Journal of the Medical Association of Thailand, 89,* 1400–1403.

Jim, W. T., Chiu, N. C., Ho, C. S., Shu, C. H., Chang, J. H., Hung, H. Y. . . . Chuu, C. P. (2015). Outcome of preterm infants with postnatal cytomegalovirus infection via breast milk: A two year prospective follow-up study. *Medicine (Baltimore), 94,* e1835.

Jim, W.-T., Shu, C.-H., Chiu, N.-C., Kao, H. A., Hung, H. Y., Chang, J. H., . . . Huang, F. Y. (2004). Transmission of cytomegalovirus from mothers to preterm infants by breast milk. *Pediatric Infectious Disease Journal, 23,* 9.

Jocson, M. A. L., Mason, E. O., & Schanler, R. J. (1997). The effects of nutrient fortification and varying storage conditions on host defense properties of human milk. *Pediatrics, 100,* 240–242.

Johnson, L., & Bhutani, V. K. (2003). Reply to the editor. *Journal of Pediatrics, 142,* 214–215.

Johnson, L., & Brown, A. K. (1999). A pilot registry for acute and chronic kernicterus in term and near term infants. *Pediatrics, 104,* 736.

Johnson, S., Hollis, C., Kochhar, P., Hennessy, E., Wolke, D., & Marlow, N. (2010) Autism spectrum disorders in extremely preterm children. *Journal of Pediatrics, 156,* 525–531.

Joint Commission. (2001, April). Kernicterus threatens healthy newborns. *Sentinel Event Alert,* 18.

Joint Commission. (2004, April). Revised guidance to help prevent kernicterus. *Sentinel Event Alert,* 31.

Jones, E., Dimmock, P. W., & Spencer, S. A. (2001). A randomized controlled trial to compare methods of milk expression after preterm delivery. *Archives of Disease in Childhood—Fetal and Neonatal Edition, 85,* F91–F95.

Kaplan, M., & Hammerman, C. (2000). Glucose-6-phosphate dehydrogenase–deficient neonates. A potential cause for concern in North America. *Pediatrics, 106,* 1478–1480.

Kaplan, M., Herschel, M., Hammerman, C., Hoyer, J. D., & Stevenson, D. K. (2004). Hyperbilirubinemia among African American, glucose-6-phosphate dehydrogenase–deficient neonates. *Pediatrics, 114,* e213–e219.

Kappas, A. (2004). A method for interdicting the development of severe jaundice in newborns by inhibiting the production of bilirubin. *Pediatrics, 113,* 119–123.

Kassing, D. (2002). Bottle-feeding as a tool to reinforce breastfeeding. *Journal of Human Lactation, 18,* 56–60.

Kavanaugh, K., Mead, L., Meier, P., & Mangurten, H. H. (1995). Getting enough: Mother's concerns about breastfeeding a preterm infant after discharge. *Journal of Obstetric, Gynecologic, and Neonatal Nursing, 24,* 23–32.

Kavanaugh, K., Meier, P., Zimmermann, B., & Mead, L. (1997). The rewards outweigh the efforts: Breastfeeding outcomes for mothers of preterm infants. *Journal of Human Lactation, 13,* 15–21.

Keith, D. R., Weaver, B. S., & Vogel, R. L. (2012). The effect of music-based listening interventions on the volume, fat content, and caloric content of breast milk produced by mothers of premature and critically ill infants. *Advances in Neonatal Care, 12,* 112–119.

Kemper, K., Forsyth, B., & McCarthy, P. (1989). Jaundice, terminating breastfeeding, and the vulnerable child. *Pediatrics, 84,* 773–778.

Kemper, K. J., Forsyth, B. W., & McCarthy, P. L. (1990). Persistent perceptions of vulnerability following neonatal jaundice. *American Journal of Diseases of Children, 144,* 238–241.

Kent, J. C., Geddes, D. T., Hepworth, A. R., & Hartmann, P. E. (2011). Effect of warm breastshields on breast milk pumping. *Journal of Human Lactation, 27,* 331–338.

Kent, J. C., Mitoulas, L. R., Cregan, M. D., Geddes, D. T., Larsson, M., Doherty, D. A., & Hartmann, P. E. (2008). Importance of vacuum for breastmilk expression. *Breastfeeding Medicine, 3,* 11–19.

Kent, J. C., Ramsay, D. T., Doherty, D., Larsson, M., & Hartmann, P. E. (2003). Response of breasts to different stimulation patterns of an electric breast pump. *Journal of Human Lactation, 19,* 179–186.

Keren, R., Luan, X., Tremont, K., & Cnaan, A. (2009). Visual assessment of jaundice in term and late preterm infants. *Archives of Disease in Childhood—Fetal and Neonatal Edition, 94,* F317–F322.

Kien, C. L. (1985). Failure to thrive. In W. A. Walher & J. B. Watkins (Eds.), *Nutrition in pediatrics.* Boston, MA: Little, Brown.

Kimak, K. S., de Castro Antunes, M. M., Braga, T. D., Brandt, K. G., & de Carvalho Lima, M. (2015). Influence of enteral nutrition on occurrences of necrotizing enterocolitis in very-low-birth-weight infants. *Journal of Pediatric Gastroenterology and Nutrition, 61,* 445–450.

Kinney, H. C. (2006). The near-term (late preterm) human brain and risk for periventricular leukomalacia: A review. *Seminars in Perinatology, 30,* 81–88.

Kirchner, L., Jeitler, V., Waldhor, T., Pollak, A., & Wald, M. (2009). Long hospitalization is the most important risk factor for early weaning from breast milk in premature babies. *Acta Paediatrica, 98,* 981–984.

Kirk, A. T., Alder, S. C., & King, J. D. (2007). Cue-based oral feeding clinical pathway results in earlier attainment of full oral feeding in premature infants. *Journal of Perinatology, 27,* 572–578.

Kirsten, G. F., Bergman, N. J., & Hann, F. M. (2001). Kangaroo mother care in the nursery. *Pediatric Clinics of North America, 48,* 443–452.

Kliethermes, P. A., Cross, M. L., Lanese, M. G., Johnson, K. M., & Simon, S. D. (1999). Transitioning preterm infants with nasogastric tube supplementation: Increased likelihood of breastfeeding. *Journal of Obstetric, Gynecologic, and Neonatal Nursing, 28,* 264–273.

Knoppert, D. C., Page, A., Warren, J., Seabrook, J. A., Carr, M., Angelini, M., . . . Dasilva, O. P. (2012). The effect of two different domperidone dosages on maternal milk production. *Journal of Human Lactation, 29*(1), 38–44.

Knudsen, A., & Ebbesen, F. (1997). Cephalocaudal progression of jaundice in newborns admitted to neonatal intensive care units. *Biology of the Neonate, 71,* 357–361.

Koenig, J. S., Davies, A. M., & Thach, B. T. (1990). Coordination of breathing, sucking, and swallowing during bottle-feedings in human infants. *Journal of Applied Physiology, 69,* 1623–1629.

Koepke, J. E., & Bigelow, A. E. (1997). Observations of newborn suckling behavior. *Infant Behavior and Development, 20,* 93.

Konetzny, G., Bucher, H. U., & Arlettaz, R. (2009). Prevention of hypernatraemic dehydration in breastfed newborn infants by daily weighing. *European Journal of Pediatrics, 168,* 815–818.

Kovach, A. C. (2002). A 5-year follow-up study of hospital breastfeeding policies in the Philadelphia area: A comparison with the ten steps. *Journal of Human Lactation, 18,* 144–154.

Kramer, L. I. (1969). Advancement of dermal icterus in the jaundiced newborn. *American Journal of Diseases of Children, 118,* 454–458.

Kramer, M. S., Demissie, K., Yang, H., Platt, R. W., Sauvé, R., & Liston, R. (2000). The contribution of mild and moderate preterm birth to infant mortality. Fetal and Infant Health Study Group of the Canadian Perinatal Surveillance System. *Journal of the American Medical Association, 284,* 843–849.

Kurath, S., Halwachs-Baumann, G., Müller, W., & Resch, B. (2010). Transmission of cytomegalovirus via breast milk to the prematurely born infant: A systematic review. *Clinical Microbiology and Infection, 16,* 1172–1178.

Kuzniewicz, M. W., Escobar, G. J., Wi, S., Liljestrand, P., McCulloch, C., & Newman, T. B. (2008). Risk factors for severe hyperbilirubinemia among infants with borderline bilirubin levels: A nested case-control study. *Journal of Pediatrics, 153,* 234–240.

Laing, I. A., & Wong, C. M. (2002). Hypernatremia in the first few days: Is the incidence rising? *Archives of Disease in Childhood—Fetal and Neonatal Edition, 87,* F158–F162.

Lang, S. (2002). *Breastfeeding special care babies* (2nd ed.). Edinburgh, UK: Bailliere Tindall.

Lang, S., Lawrence, C. J., & Orme, R. L. (1994). Cup feeding: An alternative method of infant feeding. *Archives of Disease in Childhood, 71,* 365–369.

Lavagno, C., Camozzi, P., Tenzi, S., Lava, S. A. G., Simonetti, G. D., Bianchetti, M. G., & Milani, G. P. (2016). Breastfeeding-associated hypernatremia: A systematic review of the literature. *Journal of Human Lactation, 32,* 67–74.

Lawrence, R. A. (1997). *A review of the medical benefits and contraindications to breastfeeding in the United States.* Maternal and Child Health Technical Information Bulletin. Arlington, VA: National Center for Education in Maternal and Child Health.

Lawrence, R. A., & Lawrence, R. M. (2010). *Breastfeeding: A guide for the medical profession* (7th ed.). St. Louis, MO: Mosby.

Lawrence, R. M. (2006). Cytomegalovirus in human breast milk: Risk to the premature infant. *Breastfeeding and Medicine, 1,* 99–107.

Lawrence, R. M., & Lawrence, R. A. (2001). Given the benefits of breastfeeding, what contraindications exist? *Pediatric Clinics of North America, 48,* 235–251.

Lee, J., Kim, H-S., Jung, Y. H., Choi, K. Y., Shinj, S. H., Kim, E-K., & Choi, J-H. (2015). Oropharyngeal colostrum administration in extremely premature infants: An RCT. *Pediatrics, 135,* e357–e366.

Lefebvre, F., & Ducharme, M. (1989). Incidence and duration of lactation and lactational performance among mothers of low-birth-weight and term infants. *Canadian Medical Association Journal, 140,* 1159–1164.

Leibson, C., Brown, M., Thibodeau, S., Stevenson, D., Vreman, H., Cohen, R., . . . Moore, L. G. (1989). Neonatal hyperbilirubinemia at high altitude. *American Journal of Diseases of Children, 143,* 983–987.

Liu, L. L., Clemens, C. J., Shay, D. K., Davis, R. L., & Novack, A. H. (1997). The safety of newborn early discharge: The Washington State experience. *Journal of the American Medical Association, 278,* 293–298.

Liu, S., Wen, S. W., McMillan, D., Trouton, K., Fowler, D., & McCourt, C. (2000). Increased neonatal admission rate associated with decreased length of hospital stay at birth in Canada. *Canadian Journal of Public Health, 91,* 46–50.

Livingstone, V. H., Willis, C. E., Abdel-Wareth, L. O., Thiessen, P., & Lockitch, G. (2000). Neonatal hypernatremic dehydration associated with breastfeeding malnutrition: A retrospective survey. *Canadian Medical Association Journal, 162,* 647–652.

Loewy, J., Stewart, K., Dassier, A-M., Telsey, A., & Homel, P. (2013). The effects of music therapy on vital signs, feeding, and sleep in premature infants. *Pediatrics, 131,* 902–918.

Long, J., Zhang, S., Fang, X., Luo, Y., & Liu, J. (2011). Neonatal hyperbilirubinemia and Gly71Arg mutation of UGT1A1 gene: A Chinese case control study followed by systematic review of existing evidence. *Acta Paediatrica, 100,* 966–971.

Lonnerdal, B., & Iyer, S. (1995). Lactoferrin: Molecular structure and biological function. *Annual Review of Nutrition, 15,* 93–110.

Lucas, A., Fewtrell, M. S., Davies, P. S. W., Bishop, N. J., Clough, H., & Cole, T. J. (1997). Breastfeeding and catch-up growth in infants born small for gestational age. *Acta Paediatrica, 86,* 564–569.

Lucas, A., Fewtrell, M. S., Morley, R., Lucas, P. J., Baker, B. A., Lister, G., & Bishop, N. J. (1996). Randomized outcome trial of human milk fortification and developmental outcome in preterm infants. *American Journal of Clinical Nutrition, 64,* 142–151.

Lucas, A., Gibbs, J. A., Lyster, R. L., & Baum, J. D. (1978). Creamatocrit: Simple clinical technique for estimating fat concentration and energy value of human milk. *British Medical Journal, 1,* 1018–1020.

Ludington-Hoe, S. M., Thompson, C., Swinth, J., Hadeed, A. J., & Anderson, G. C. (1994). Kangaroo care: Research results, and protocol implications and guidelines. *Neonatal Network, 13,* 19–27.

Lukefahr, J. L. (1990). Underlying illness associated with failure to thrive in breastfed infants. *Clinical Pediatrics, 29,* 468–470.

Lund, G. C., Edwards, G., Medlin, B., Keller, D., Beck, B., & Carreiro, J. E. (2011). Osteopathic manipulative treatment for the treatment of hospitalized premature infants with nipple feeding dysfunction. *Journal of the American Osteopathic Association, 111,* 44–48.

Lussier, M. M., Brownell, E. A., Proulx, T. A., Bielecki, D. M., Marinelli, K. A., Bellini, S. L., & Hagadorn, J. I. (2015). Daily breastmilk volume in mothers of very low birth weight neonates: A repeated-measures randomized trial of hand expression versus electric breast pump expression. *Breastfeeding Medicine, 10,* 312–317.

Maayan-Metzger, A., Avivi, S., Schushan-Eisen, I., & Kuint, J. (2012). Human milk versus formula feeding among preterm infants: Short-term outcomes. *American Journal of Perinatology, 29,* 121–126.

Maayan-Metzger, A., Mazkereth, R., & Kuint, J. (2003). Fever in healthy asymptomatic newborns during the first days of life. *Archives of Disease in Childhood—Fetal and Neonatal Edition, 88,* F312–F314.

Macdonald, P. D., Ross, S. R. M., Grant, L., & Young, D. (2003). Neonatal weight loss in breast and formula fed infants. *Archives of Disease in Childhood—Fetal and Neonatal Edition, 88,* F472–F476.

MacMahon, J. R., Stevenson, D. K., & Oski, F. A. (1998). Physiologic jaundice. In H. W. Taeusch & R. A. Ballard (Eds.), *Avery's diseases of the newborn* (7th ed.). Philadelphia, PA: W. B. Saunders.

Madlon-Kay, D. J. (1997). Recognition of the presence and severity of newborn jaundice by parents, nurses, physicians, and icterometer. *Pediatrics, 100,* e3.

Madlon-Kay, D. J. (2002). Maternal assessment of neonatal jaundice after discharge. *Journal of Family Practice, 51,* 445–448.

Maisels, M. J. (2001). Neonatal hyperbilirubinemia. In M. H. Klaus & A. A. Fanaroff (Eds.), *Care of the high-risk neonate.* Philadelphia, PA: W. B. Saunders.

Maisels, M. J. (2012). Noninvasive measurements of bilirubin. *Pediatrics, 129,* 779–781.

Maisels, M. J., Bhutani, V. K., Bogen, D., Newman, T. B., Stark, A. R., & Watchko, J. F. (2009). Hyperbilirubinemia in the newborn infant > 35 weeks' gestation: An update with clarifications. *Pediatrics, 124,* 1193–1198.

Maisels, M. J., Clune, S., Coleman, K., Gendelman, B., Kendall, A., McManus, S., & Smyth, M. (2014). The natural history of jaundice in predominantly breastfed infants. *Pediatrics, 134,* e340–e345.

Maisels, M. J., & Kring, E. (1998). Length of stay, jaundice, and hospital readmission. *Pediatrics, 101,* 995–998.

Maisels, M. J., & McDonagh, A. F. (2008). Phototherapy for neonatal jaundice. *New England Journal of Medicine, 358,* 920–928.

Maisels, M. J., & Newman, T. B. (1995). Kernicterus in otherwise healthy, breastfed term newborns. *Pediatrics, 96*(4pt1), 730–733.

Malhotra, N., Vishwambaran, L., Sundaram, K. R., & Narayanan, I. (1999). A controlled trial of alternative methods of oral feeding in neonates. *Early Human Development, 54,* 29–38.

Manganaro, R., Mami, C., Marrone, T., Marseglia, L., & Gemelli, M. (2001). Incidence of dehydration and hypernatremia in exclusively breastfed infants. *Journal of Pediatrics, 139,* 673–675.

Mannel, R., & Mannel, R. S. (2006). Staffing for hospital lactation programs: Recommendations from a tertiary care teaching hospital. *Journal of Human Lactation, 22,* 409–417.

Marchini, G., & Stock, S. (1997). Thirst and vasopressin secretion counteract dehydration in newborn infants. *Journal of Pediatrics, 130,* 736–739.

Marinelli, K. A., Burke, G. S., & Dodd, V. L. (2001). A comparison of the safety of cupfeedings and bottlefeedings in premature infants whose mothers intend to breastfeed. *Journal of Perinatology, 21,* 350–355.

Marinelli, K. A., Lussier, M. M., Brownell, E., Herson, V. C., & Hagadorn, J. I. (2014). The effect of a donor milk policy on the diet of very low birth weight infants. *Journal of Human Lactation, 30,* 310–316.

Martens, P. J., & Romphf, L. (2007). Factors associated with newborn in-hospital weight loss: Comparisons by feeding method, demographics, and birthing procedures. *Journal of Human Lactation, 23,* 233–241.

Maruo, Y., Morioka, Y., Jugito, H., Nakahara, S., Yanagi, T., Matsui, K., . . . Takeuchi, Y. (2014). Bilirubin uridine diphosphate-glucuronosyltransferase variation is a genetic basis of breastmilk jaundice. *Journal of Pediatrics, 165,* 36–41.

Maruo, Y., Nishizawa, K., Sato, H., Sawa, H., & Shimada, M. (2000). Prolonged unconjugated hyperbilirubinemia associated with breast milk and mutations of the bilirubin uridine diphosphate-glucuronosyltransferase gene. *Pediatrics, 106,* e59.

Matthew, O. (1988). Respiratory control during nipple feeding in preterm infants. *Pediatric Pulmonology, 5,* 220–224.

Matthew, O. (1991). Breathing patterns of preterm infants during bottle-feeding: Role of milk flow. *Journal of Pediatrics, 119,* 960–965.

McDonagh, A. F. (1990). Is bilirubin good for you? *Clinics in Perinatology, 17,* 359–369.

McDougall, P., Drewett, R. F., Hungin, P., & Wright, C. M. (2008). The detection of early weight faltering at the 6–8 week check and its association with family factors, feeding and behavioral development. *Archives of Disease in Childhood, 94,* 549–552.

Meier, P. P. (1988). Bottle- and breastfeeding: Effects on transcutaneous oxygen pressure and temperature in preterm infants. *Nursing Research, 37,* 36–41.

Meier, P. P. (2001). Breastfeeding in the special care nursery: Prematures and infants with medical problems. *Pediatric Clinics of North America, 48,* 425–442.

Meier, P. P. (2003). Supporting lactation in mothers with very low birth weight infants. *Pediatric Annals, 32,* 317–325.

Meier, P. P., & Anderson, G. C. (1987). Responses of small preterm infants to bottle- and breastfeeding. *MCN: The American Journal of Maternal/Child Nursing, 12,* 97–105.

Meier, P. P., & Brown, L. P. (1996). State of the science: Breastfeeding for mothers and low birth weight infants. *Nursing Clinics of North America, 31,* 351–365.

Meier, P. P., & Brown, L. P. (1997). Defining terminology for improved breastfeeding research. *Journal of Nurse Midwifery, 42,* 65–66.

Meier, P. P., Brown, L., Hurst N., Spatz, D. L., Engstrom, J. L., Borucki, L. C., & Krouse, A. M. (2000). Nipple shields for preterm infants: Effect on milk transfer and duration of breastfeeding. *Journal of Human Lactation, 16,* 106–114.

Meier, P. P., Engstrom, J. L., Crichton, C. L., Clark, D. R., Williams, M. M., & Mangurten, H. H. (1994). A new scale for in-home test-weighing for mothers of preterm and high risk infants. *Journal of Human Lactation, 10,* 163–168.

Meier, P. P., Engstrom, J. L., Fleming, B., Streeter, P. L., & Lawrence, P. B. (1996). Estimating milk intake of hospitalized preterm infants who breastfeed. *Journal of Human Lactation, 12,* 21–26.

Meier, P. P., Engstrom, J. L., Mangurten, H. H., Estrada, E., Zimmerman, B., & Kopparthi, R. (1993). Breastfeeding support services in the neonatal intensive care unit. *Journal of Obstetric, Gynecologic, and Neonatal Nursing, 22,* 338–347.

Meier, P. P., Engstrom, J. L., Mingolelli, S. S., Miracle, D. J., & Kiesling, S. (2004). The Rush Mothers' Milk Club: Breastfeeding interventions for mothers with very-low-birth-weight infants. *Journal of Obstetric, Gynecologic, and Neonatal Nursing, 33,* 164–174.

Meier, P. P., Engstrom, J. L., Patel, A. L., Jegier, B. J., & Bruns, N. E. (2010). Improving the use of human milk during and after the NICU stay. *Clinics in Perinatology, 37,* 217–245.

Meier, P. P., Engstrom, J. L., Zuleger, J. L., Motykowski, J. E., Vasan, U., Meier, W. A., . . . Williams, T. M. (2006). Accuracy of a user-friendly centrifuge for measuring creamatocrits on mothers' milk in the clinical setting. *Breastfeeding Medicine, 1,* 79–87.

Meier, P. P., Firman, L. M., & Degenhardt, M. (2007). Increased lactation risk for late preterm infants and mothers: Evidence and management strategies to protect breastfeeding. *Journal of Midwifery and Women's Health, 52,* 579–587.

Meier, P. P., Lysakowski, Y., Engstrom, J. L., Kavanaugh, K. L., & Mangurten, H. H. (1990). The accuracy of test weighing for preterm infants. *Journal of Pediatric Gastroenterology and Nutrition, 10,* 62–65.

Meier, P. P., Motykowski, J. E., & Zuleger, J. L. (2004). Choosing a correctly-fitted breastshield for milk expression. *Medela Messenger, 21,* 1, 8–9.

Meier, P., Patel, A. L., Wright, K., & Engstrom, J. L. (2013). Management of breastfeeding during and after the maternity hospitalization for late preterm infants. *Clinical in Perinatology, 40,* 689–705.

Meier, P. P., & Pugh, E. J. (1985). Breastfeeding behavior of small preterm infants. *MCN: The American Journal of Maternal/Child Nursing, 10,* 396–401.

Meinzen-Derr, J., Poindexter, B., Wrage, L., Morrow, A. L., Stoll, B., & Donovan, E. F. (2009). Role of human milk in extremely low birth weight infants' risk of necrotizing enterocolitis or death. *Journal of Perinatology, 29,* 57–62.

Melton, K., & Akinbi, H. T. (1999). Neonatal jaundice: Strategies to reduce bilirubin-induced complications. *Postgraduate Medicine, 106,* 167–168, 171–174, 177–178.

Millar, K. R., Gloor, J. E., Wellington, N., & Joubert, G. I. E. (2000). Early neonatal presentations to the pediatric emergency department. *Pediatric Emergency Care, 16,* 145–150.

Miracle, D. J., Meier, P. P., & Bennett, P. A. (2004a). Making my baby healthy: Changing the decision from formula to human milk feedings for very-low-birth-weight infants. *Advances in Experimental Medicine and Biology, 554,* 317–319.

Miracle, D. J., Meier, P. P., & Bennett, P. A. (2004b). Mothers' decisions to change from formula to mother's milk for very-low-birth-weight infants. *Journal of Obstetric, Gynecologic, and Neonatal Nursing, 33,* 692–703.

Mitoulas, L. R., Lai, C. T., Gurrin, L. C., Larsson M., & Hartmann, P. E. (2002). Efficacy of breast milk expression using an electric breast pump. *Journal of Human Lactation, 18,* 344–352.

Mok, E., Multon, C., Piguel, L., Barroso, E., Goua, V., Christin, P., . . . Hankard, R. (2008). Decreased full breastfeeding, altered practices, perceptions, and infant weight change of prepregnant obese women: A need for extra support. *Pediatrics, 121,* e1319–e1324.

Molteni, K. H. (1994). Initial management of hypernatremic dehydration in the breastfed infant. *Clinical Pediatrics, 33,* 731–740.

Montgomery, D., Schmutz, N., Baer, V. L., Rogerson, R., Wheeler, R., Rowley, A. M., . . . Christensen, R. D. (2008). Effects of instituting the "BEST Program" (Breast Milk Early Saves Trouble) in a level III NICU. *Journal of Human Lactation, 24,* 248–251.

Morales, Y., & Schanler, R. J. (2007). Human milk and clinical outcomes in VLBW infants: How compelling is the evidence of benefit? *Seminars in Perinatology, 31,* 83–88.

Moritz, M. L., Manole, M. D., Bogen, D. L., & Ayus, J. C. (2005). Breastfeeding-associated hypernatremia: Are we missing the diagnosis? *Pediatrics, 16,* e343–e347.

Morton, J., Hall, J. Y., Thairu, L., Nomanbhoy, S., Bhutani, R., Carlson, S., . . . Rhine, W. D. (2007a). Early hand expression affects breastmilk production in pump-dependent mothers of preterm infants. Retrieved from http://www.abstracts2view.com/pasall/view.php?nu=PAS07L1_37

Morton, J., Hall, J. Y., Thairu, L., Nomanbhoy, S., Bhutani, R., Carlson, S., . . . Stevenson, D. K. (2007b). Breast massage maximizes milk volumes of pump-dependent mothers. Retrieved from http://www.abstracts2view.com/pasall/view.php?nu=PAS07L1_32

Morton, J. A. (2002). Strategies to support extended breastfeeding of the premature infant. *Advances in Neonatal Care, 2,* 267–282.

Narayanan, I., Mehta, R., Choudhury, D. K., & Jain, B. K. (1991). Sucking on the "emptied" breast: Non-nutritive sucking with a difference. *Archives of Disease in Childhood, 66,* 241–244.

Neifert, M. (1998). The optimization of breastfeeding in the perinatal period. *Clinics in Perinatology, 25,* 303–326.

Neifert, M. A., & Seacat, J. (1988). Practical aspects of breastfeeding the premature infant. *Perinatology and Neonatology, 12,* 24–30.

Neifert, M. R. (2001). Prevention of breastfeeding tragedies. *Pediatric Clinics of North America, 48,* 273–297.

Nelson, S. E., Rogers, R. R., Ziegler, E. E., & Fomon, S. J. (1989). Gain in weight and length during early infancy. *Early Human Development, 19,* 223–239.

Neuberger, P., Hamprecht, K., Vochem, M., Maschmann, J., Speer, C. P., Jahn, G., . . . Goelz, R. (2006). Case-control study of symptoms and neonatal outcome of human milk–transmitted cytomegalovirus infection in premature infants. *Journal of Pediatrics, 148,* 326–331.

Newman, J. (2004). Case study: Slow weight gain after initial rapid gain. *ABM News and Views, 10,* 23–24.

Newman, T. B., Escobar, G. J., Gonzalez, V. M., Armstrong, M. A., Gardner, M. N., & Folck, B. F. (1999). Frequency of neonatal bilirubin testing and hyperbilirubinemia in a large health maintenance organization. *Pediatrics, 104,* 1198–1203.

Newman, T. B., Liljestrand, P., & Escobar, G. J. (2003). Infants with bilirubin levels of 30 mg/dl or more in a large managed care organization. *Pediatrics, 111,* 1303–1311.

Newman, T. B., Liljestrand, P., Jeremy, R. J., Ferriero, D. M., Wu, Y. W., Hudes, E. S., & Escobar, G. J. (2006). Jaundice and Infant Feeding Study Team. Outcomes among newborns with total serum bilirubin levels of 25 mg per deciliter or more. *New England Journal of Medicine, 354,* 1889–1900.

Newman, T. B., & Maisels, M. J. (1992). Evaluation and treatment of jaundice in the term newborn: A kinder, gentler approach. *Pediatrics, 89,* 809–818.

Newman, T. B., Xiong, B., Gonzales, V. M., & Escobar, G. J. (2000). Prediction and prevention of extreme neonatal hyperbilirubinemia in a mature health maintenance organization. *Archives of Pediatrics and Adolescent Medicine, 154,* 1140–1147.

Ng, P. C., Chan, H. B., Fok, T. F., Lee, C. H., Chan, K. M., Wong, W., & Cheung, K. L. (1999). Early onset hypernatraemic dehydration and fever in exclusively breastfed infants. *Journal of Pediatrics and Child Health, 35,* 585–587.

Nice, F. J. (2012). Medications and breastfeeding: current concepts. *Journal of the American Pharmacists Association, 52,* 86–94.

Nicholl, A., Ginsburg, R., & Tripp, J. H. (1982). Supplementary feeding and jaundice in newborns. *Acta Paediatrica Scandinavica, 71,* 759–761.

Nilsson, U. (2009). Soothing music can increase oxytocin levels during bed rest after open-heart surgery: A randomized control trial. *Journal of Clinical Nursing, 18,* 2153–2161.

Noel-Weiss, J., Courant, G., & Woodend, A. K. (2008). Physiological weight loss in the breastfed neonate: A systematic review. *Open Medicine, 2,* e11–e22.

Nommsen-Rivers, L. A., Heinig, M. J., Cohen, R. J., & Dewey, K. G. (2008). Newborn wet and soiled diaper counts and timing of onset of lactation as indicators of breastfeeding inadequacy. *Journal of Human Lactation, 24,* 27–33.

Numazaki, K. (1997). Human cytomegalovirus infection of breast milk. *FEMS Immunology and Medical Microbiology, 18,* 91–98.

Nyqvist, K. H. (2008). Early attainment of breastfeeding competence in very preterm infants. *Acta Paediatrica, 97,* 776–781.

Nyqvist, K. H., & Kylberg, E. (2008). Application of the Baby Friendly Hospital Initiative to neonatal care: Suggestions by Swedish mothers of very preterm infants. *Journal of Human Lactation, 24,* 252–262.

Oddie, S., Richmond, S., & Coultard, M. (2001). Hypernatremic dehydration and breastfeeding: A population study. *Archives of Disease in Childhood, 85,* 318–320.

Oddie, S. J., Craven, V., Deakin, K., Westman, J., & Scally, A. (2013). Severe neonatal hypernatremia: A population based study. *Archives of Disease in Children—Fetal Neonatal Edition, 98,* F384–F387.

Ogden, C. L., Kuczmarski, R. J., Flegal, K. M., Mei, Z., Guo, S., Wei, R., . . . Johnson, C. L. (2002). Centers for Disease Control and Prevention 2000 growth charts for the United States: Improvements to the 1977 National Center for Health Statistics version. *Pediatrics, 109,* 45–60.

Ohyama, M., Watabe, H., & Hayasaka, T. (2010). Manual expression and electric breast pumping in the first 48 h after delivery. *Pediatrics International, 52,* 39–43.

Olsen, E. M. (2006). Failure to thrive: Still a problem of definition. *Clinical Pediatrics, 45,* 1–6.

Osborn, L. M., Reiff, M. I., & Bolus, R. (1984). Jaundice in the full term neonate. *Pediatrics, 73,* 520–525.

Ota, Y., Maruo, Y., Matsui, K., Mimura, Y., Sato, H., & Takeuchi, Y. (2011). Inhibitory effect of 5 beta-pregnane-3 alpha, 20 beta-diol on transcriptional activity and enzyme activity of human bilirubin UDP-glucuronosylttransferase. *Pediatric Research, 70,* 453–457.

Page-Wilson, G., Smith, P. C., & Welt, C. K. (2007). Short-term prolactin administration causes expressible galactorrhea but does not affect bone turnover: Pilot data for a new lactation agent. *International Breastfeeding Journal, 2,* 10.

Palmer, R. H., Clanton, M., Ezhuthachan, S., Newman, C., Maisels, J., Plsek, P., & Salem-Schatz, S. (2003). Applying the "10 simple rules" of the Institute of Medicine to management of hyperbilirubinemia in newborns. *Pediatrics, 112,* 1388–1393.

Palmer, R. H., Keren, R., Maisels, M. J., & Yeargin-Allsopp, M. (2004). National Institute of Child Health and Human Development (NICHD) conference on kernicterus: A population perspective on prevention of kernicterus. *Journal of Perinatology, 24,* 723–725.

Parker, L. A., Sullivan, S., Krueger, C., Kelechi, T., & Mueller, M. (2012). Effect of early breast milk expression on milk volume and timing of lactogenesis stage II among mothers of very low birth weight infants: A pilot study. *Journal of Perinatology, 32,* 205–209.

Parker, L. A., Sullivan, S., Krueger, C., & Mueller, M. (2015). Association of timing of initiation of breastmilk expression on milk volume and timing of lactogenesis stage II among mothers of very low-birth-weight infants. *Breastfeeding Medicine, 10,* 84–91.

Penn, A. A., Enzmann, D. R., Hahn, J. S., & Stevenson, D. K. (1994). Kernicterus in a full term infant. *Pediatrics, 93,* 1003–1006.

Philipp, B. L., Brown, E., & Merewood, A. (2000). Pumps for peanuts: Leveling the playing field in the NICU. *Journal of Perinatology, 4,* 249–250.

Pimenta, H. P., Moreira, M. E., Rocha, A. D., Gomes, S. C., Jr., Pinto, L. W., & Lucena, S. L. (2008). Effects of non-nutritive sucking and oral stimulation on breastfeeding rates for preterm, low birth weight infants: A randomized clinical trial. *Journal of Pediatrics, 84,* 423–427.

Pineda, R. (2011). Direct breastfeeding in the neonatal intensive care unit: Is it important? *Journal of Perinatology, 31,* 540–545.

Pinelli, J., & Symington, A. (2000). Non-nutritive sucking for promoting physiologic stability and nutrition in preterm infants. *Cochrane Database System Review, 2.*

Poland, R. L. (1981). Breast-milk jaundice. *Journal of Pediatrics, 99,* 86–88.

Porter, M. L., & Dennis, B. L. (2002). Hyperbilirubinemia in the term newborn. *American Family Physician, 65,* 599–606, 613–614.

Powe, C. E., Allen, M., Puopolo, K. M., Merewood, A., Worden, S., Johnson, L. C., . . . Welt, C. K. (2010). Recombinant human prolactin for the treatment of lactation insufficiency. *Clinical Endocrinology (Oxford), 73,* 645–653.

Powe, C. E., Puopolo, K. M., Newburg, D. S., Lonnerdal, B., Chen, C., Allen, M., . . . Welt, C. K. (2011). Effects of recombinant human prolactin on breast milk composition. *Pediatrics, 127,* e359–366.

Powers, N., Clark, R. H., Bloom, B. T., Thomas, P., & Peabody, J. (2001). Site variation in rates of breast-milk feedings in neonates discharged from intensive care units [Abstract]. *Academy of Breastfeeding Medical News and Views, 7,* 37.

Powers, N. G. (1999). Slow weight gain and low milk supply in the breastfeeding dyad. *Clinics in Perinatology, 26,* 399–430.

Powers, N. G. (2001). How to assess slow growth in the breastfed infant: Birth to 3 months. *Pediatric Clinics of North America, 48,* 345–363.

Powers, N. G. (2010). Low intake in the breastfed infant: Maternal and infant considerations. In J. Riordan & K. Wambach (Eds.), *Breastfeeding and human lactation* (4th ed.). Sudbury, MA: Jones & Bartlett Learning.

Quan, R., Yang, C., Rubinstein, S., Norman J., Lewiston, N. J., Sunshine, P., Stevenson, D. K., & Kerner Jr., J. A. (1994, June). The effect of nutritional additives on anti-infective factors in human milk. *Clinical Pediatrics, 33,* 325–328.

Quigley, M. A., Hockley, C., Carson, C., Kelly, Y., Renfrew, M. J., & Sacker, A. (2012). Breastfeeding is associated with improved child cognitive development: A population-based cohort study. *Journal of Pediatrics, 160,* 25–32.

Raju, T. N., Higgins, R. D., Stark, A. R., & Leveno, K. J. (2006). Optimizing care and outcome for late-preterm (near-term) infants: A summary of the workshop sponsored by the National Institute of Child Health and Human Development. *Pediatrics, 118,* 1207–1214.

Ramsay, M., Gisel, E. G., & Boutry, M. (1993). Non-organic failure to thrive: Growth failure secondary to feeding-skills disorder. *Developmental Medicine & Child Neurology, 35,* 285–297.

Rand, S. E., & Kolberg, A. (2001). Neonatal hypernatremic dehydration secondary to lactation failure. *Journal of the American Board of Family Practice, 14,* 155–158.

Reisinger, K. W., de Vaan, L., Kramer, B. W., Wolfs, T. G., van Heurn, L. W., & Derikx, J. P. (2014). Breastfeeding improves gut maturation compared with formula feeding in preterm babies. *Journal of Pediatric Gastroenterology and Nutrition, 59,* 720–724.

Rocha, A. D., Moreira, M. E., Pimenta, H. P., Ramos, J. R., & Lucena, S. L. (2007). A randomized study of the efficacy of sensory–motor–oral stimulation and non-nutritive sucking in very low birthweight infant. *Early Human Development, 83,* 385–388.

Rodriguez, N. A., Groer, M. W., & Zeller, J. M. (2011). A randomized controlled trial of the oropharyngeal administration of mother's colostrum to extremely low birth weight infants in the first days of life. *Neonatal Intensive Care, 24,* 31–35.

Rodriguez, N. A., Meier, P. P., Groer, M. W., & Zeller, J. M. (2009). Oropharyngeal administration of colostrum to extremely low birth weight infants: Theoretical perspectives. *Journal of Perinatology, 29,* 1–7.

Rodriguez, N. A., Meier, P. P., Groer, M. W., Zeller, J. M., Engstrom, J. L., & Fogg, L. (2010). A pilot study to determine the safety and feasibility of oropharyngeal administration of own mother's colostrum to extremely low birth weight infants. *Advances in Neonatal Care, 10,* 206–212.

Rodriguez, N. A., Miracle, D. J., & Meier, P. P. (2005). Sharing the science on human milk feedings with mothers of very-low-birth-weight infants. *Journal of Obstetric, Gynecologic, and Neonatal Nursing, 34,* 109–119.

Ross, G. (2003). Hyperbilirubinemia in the 2000s: What should we do next? *American Journal of Perinatology, 20,* 415–424.

Rossman, B., Engstrom, J. L., Meier, P. P., Vonderheid, S. C., Norr, K. F., & Hill, P. D. (2011). "They've walked in my shoes": Mothers of very low birth weight infants and their experiences with breastfeeding peer counselors in the neonatal intensive care unit. *Journal of Human Lactation, 27,* 14–24.

Rossman, B., Kratovil, A. L., Greene, M. M., Engstrom, J. L., & Meier, P. P. (2013). "I have faith in my milk": The meaning of milk for mothers of very low birth weight infants hospitalized in the neonatal intensive care unit. *Journal of Human Lactation, 29,* 359–365.

Sachs, H. C., & Committee on Drugs. (2013). The transfer of drugs and therapeutics into human breastmilk: An update on selected topics. *Pediatrics, 132,* e796–e809.

Sarici, S. U., Serdar, M. A., Korkmaz, A., Erdem, G., Oran, O., Tekinalp, G., . . . Yigit, S. (2004). Incidence, course, and prediction of hyperbilirubinemia in near-term and term newborns. *Pediatrics, 113,* 775–780.

Sato, H., Uchida, T., Toyota, K., Kanno, M., Hashimoto, T., Watanabe, M., . . . Hayasaka K. (2013). Association of breastfed neonatal hyperbilirubinemia with UGT1A1 polymorphisms: 211G>A (G71R) mutation becomes a risk factor under inadequate feeding. *Journal of Human Genetics, 58,* 7–10.

Sato, H., Uchida, T., Toyota, K., Nakamura, T., Tamiya, G., Kanno, M., . . . Hayasaka, K. (2015). Association of neonatal hyperbilirubinemia in breastfed infants with UGT1A1 or SLCOs polymorphisms. *Journal of Human Genetics, 60,* 35–40.

Scanlon, K. S., Alexander, M. P., Serdula, M. K., Davis, M. K., & Bowman, B. A. (2002). Assessment of infant feeding: The validity of measuring milk intake. *Nutrition Review, 60,* 235–251.

Schanler, R. J. (1998). Fortified human milk: Nature's way to feed premature infants. *Journal of Human Lactation, 14,* 5–11.

Schanler, R. J. (2001). The use of human milk for premature infants. *Pediatric Clinics of North America, 48,* 207–219.

Schanler, R. J. (2007). Mother's own milk, donor human milk, and preterm formulas in the feeding of extremely premature infants. *Journal of Pediatric Gastroenterology and Nutrition, 45*(suppl 3), S175–S177.

Schanler, R. J., & Atkinson, S. A. (1999). Effects of nutrients in human milk on the recipient premature infant. *Journal of Mammary Gland Biology and Neoplasia, 4,* 297–307.

Schanler, R. J., Shulman, R. J., & Lau, C. (1997). Growth of premature infants fed fortified human milk. *Pediatric Research, 41,* 240A.

Schanler, R. J., Shulman, R. J., & Lau, C. (1999). Feeding strategies for premature infants: Beneficial outcomes of feeding fortified human milk versus preterm formula. *Pediatrics, 103,* 1150–1157.

Schanler, R. J., Shulman, R. J., Lau, C., Smith, E. O., & Heitkemper, M. M. (1999). Feeding strategies for premature infants: Randomized trial of gastrointestinal priming and tube-feeding methods. *Pediatrics, 103,* 434–439.

Schneider, A. P., II. (1986). Breast milk jaundice in the newborn: A reality. *Journal of the American Medical Association, 255,* 3270–3274.

Sedlak, T. W., & Snyder, S. H. (2004). Bilirubin benefits: Cellular protection by a biliverdin reductase antioxidant cycle. *Pediatrics, 113,* 1776–1782.

Seigel, J. K., Smith, P. B., Ashley, P. L., Cotton, C. M., Herbert, C. C., King, B. A., . . . Bidegain, M. (2013). Early administration of oropharyngeal colostrum to extremely low birth weight infants. *Breastfeeding Medicine, 8,* 491–495.

Sharp, M., Campbell, C., Chiffings, D., Simmer, K., & French, N. (2015). Improvement in long-term breastfeeding for very preterm infants. *Breastfeeding Medicine, 10,* 145–149.

Shekeeb, S. M., Kumar, P., Sharma, N., Narang, A., & Prasad, R. (2008). Evaluation of oxidant and antioxidant status in term neonates: A plausible protective role of bilirubin. *Molecular and Cellular Biochemistry, 317,* 51–59.

Shivpuri, C. R., Martin, R. J., Carlo, W. A., & Fanaroff, A. A. (1983). Decreased ventilation in preterm infants during oral feeding. *Journal of Pediatrics, 103,* 285–289.

Shrago, L. C., Reifsnider, E., & Insel, K. (2006). The neonatal bowel output study: Indicators of adequate breast milk intake in neonates. *Pediatric Nursing, 32,* 195–201.

Sisk, P. M., Lovelady, C. A., Dillard, R. G., & Gruber, K. J. (2006). Lactation counseling for mothers of very low birth weight infants: Effect on maternal anxiety and infant intake of human milk. *Pediatrics, 117,* e67–e75.

Sisk, P. M., Lovelady, C. A., Gruber, K. J., Dillard, R. G., & O'Shea, T. M. (2008). Human milk consumption and full enteral feeding among infants who weigh < 1250 grams. *Pediatrics, 121,* e1528–e1533.

Slaughter, J., Annibale, D., & Suresh, G. (2009). False-negative results of pre-discharge neonatal bilirubin screening to predict severe hyperbilirubinemia: A need for caution. *European Journal of Pediatrics, 168,* 1461–1466.

Sofer, S., Ben-Ezer, D., & Dagan, R. (1993). Early severe dehydration in young breastfed newborn infants. *Israeli Journal of Medical Science, 29,* 85–89.

Spanier-Mingolelli, S. R., Meier, P. P., & Bradford, L. (1998). "Making the difference for my baby": A powerful breastfeeding motivator for mothers of preterm and high risk infants [Abstract]. *Pediatric Research, 43,* 269.

Spatz, D. L. (2004). Ten steps for promoting and protecting breastfeeding for vulnerable infants. *Journal of Perinatal & Neonatal Nursing, 18,* 385–396.

Spatz, D. L., & Goldschmidt, K. A. (2006). Preserving breastfeeding for the rehospitalized infant: A clinical pathway. *MCN: The American Journal of Maternal/Child Nursing, 31,* 45–51.

Stark, Y. (1994). *Human nipples: Function and anatomical variations in relationship to breastfeeding.* Master's thesis. Pasadena, CA: Pacific Oaks College.

Steffensrud, S. (2004). Hyperbilirubinemia in term and near-term infants: Kernicterus on the rise? *Newborn and Infant Nursing Review, 4,* 191–200.

Stellwagen, L. M., Hubbard, E. T., & Wolf, A. (2007). The late preterm infant: A little baby with big needs. *Contemporary Pediatrics, 4*(11), 51–59.

Stevenson, D. K., Dennery, P. A., & Hintz, S. R. (2001). Understanding newborn jaundice. *Journal of Perinatology, 21,* S21–S24.

Stine, M. J. (1990). Breastfeeding the premature newborn: A protocol without bottles. *Journal of Human Lactation, 6,* 167–170.

Stokowski, L. A. (2002a). Early recognition of neonatal jaundice and kernicterus. *Advances in Neonatal Care, 2,* 101–114.

Stokowski, L. A. (2002b). Family teaching toolbox: Newborn jaundice. *Advances in Neonatal Care, 2,* 115–116.

Sweet, L. (2008). Expressed breast milk as "connection" and its influence on the construction of "motherhood" for mothers of preterm infants: A qualitative study. *International Breastfeeding Journal, 3,* 30.

Syfrett, E. B., Anderson, G. C., Behnke, M., Neu, J., & Hilliard, M. E. (1993, November). *Early and virtually continuous kangaroo care for lower risk preterm infants: Effect on temperature, breastfeeding, supplementation, and weight.* Presented at the Proceedings of the Biennial Conference of the Council of Nurse Researchers, American Nurses Association, Washington, DC.

Tarcan, A., Gurakan, B., Tiker, F., & Ozbek, N. (2004). Influence of feeding formula and breast milk fortifier on lymphocyte subsets in very low birth weight premature newborns. *Biology of the Neonate, 86,* 22–28.

Tarcan, A., Tiker, F., Vatandas, N. S., Haberal, A., & Gurakan, B. (2005). Weight loss and hypernatremia in breastfed babies: Frequency in neonates with non-hemolytic jaundice. *Journal of Pediatrics and Child Health, 41,* 484–487.

Tatli, M. M., Minnet, C., Kocyigit, A., & Karadag, A. (2008). Phototherapy increases DNA damage in lymphocytes of hyperbilirubinemic neonates. *Mutation Research, 654,* 93–95.

Tawia, S., & McGuire, L. (2014). Early weight loss and weight gain in healthy, full-term, exclusively breastfed infants. *Breastfeeding Review, 22,* 31–42.

Taylor, S. N., Basile, L. A., Ebeling, M., & Wagner, C. L. (2009). Intestinal permeability in preterm infants by feeding type: Mother's milk versus formula. *Breastfeeding Medicine, 4,* 11–15.

Thompson, N. M. (1996). Relactation in a newborn intensive care setting. *Journal of Human Lactation, 12,* 233–235.

Thoyre, S. M., & Carlson, J. (2003). Occurrence of oxygen desaturation events during preterm infant bottle feeding near discharge. *Early Human Development, 72,* 25–36.

Thulier, D. (2016). Weighing the facts: A systematic review of expected patterns of weight loss in full-term, breastfed infants. *Journal of Human Lactation, 32,* 28–34.

Toppare, M. F., Laleli, Y., Senses, D. A., Kitaper, F., Kaya, I. S., & Dilmen, U. (1994). Metoclopramide for breast milk production. *Nutrition Research, 14,* 1019–1029.

Tuzun, F., Kumral, A., Duman, N., & Ozkan, H. (2013). Breast milk jaundice: Effect of bacteria present in breast milk and infant feces. *Journal of Pediatric Gastroenterology and Nutrition, 56,* 328–332.

Unal, S., Arhan, E., Kara, N., Uncu, N., & Aliefendioglu, D. (2008). Breastfeeding-associated hypernatremia: Retrospective analysis of 169 term newborns. *Pediatrics International, 50,* 29–34.

Uras, N., Karadag, A., Dogan G., Tonbul, A., & Tatli, M. M. (2007). Moderate hypernatremic dehydration in newborn infants: Retrospective evaluation of 64 cases. *Journal of Maternal–Fetal and Neonatal Medicine, 20,* 449–452.

Uras, N., Tonbul, A., Karadag, A., Dogan, D. G., Erel, O., & Tatli, M. M. (2010). Prolonged jaundice in newborns is associated with low antioxidant capacity in breast milk. *Scandinavian Journal of Clinical and Laboratory Investigation, 70,* 433–437.

Valentine, C. J., Hurst, N. M., & Schanler, R. J. (1994). Hindmilk improves weight gain in low birth weight infants fed human milk. *Journal of Pediatric Gastroenterology and Nutrition, 18,* 474–477.

van der Strate, B. W. A., Harmsen, M. C., Schafer, P., Swart, P. J., The, T. H., Jahn, G., . . . Hamprecht, K. (2001). Viral load in breast milk correlates with transmission of human cytomegalovirus to preterm neonates, but lactoferrin concentrations do not. *Clinical and Diagnostic Laboratory Immunology, 8,* 818–821.

van Dijk, C. E., & Innis, S. M. (2009). Growth-curve standards and the assessment of early excess weight gain in infancy. *Pediatrics, 123,* 102–108.

Van Dommelen, P., Boer, S., Unal, S., & van Wouwe, J. P. (2014). Charts for weight loss to detect hypernatremic dehydration and prevent formula supplementing. *Birth, 41,* 153–159.

Vandborg, P. K., Hansen, B. M., Greisen, G., Jepsen, M., & Ebbesen, F. (2012). Follow-up of neonates with total serum bilirubin levels > 25 mg/dl: A Danish population-based study. *Pediatrics, 130,* 61–66.

Varimo, P., Simila, S., Wendt, L., & Kolvisto, M. (1986). Frequency of breastfeeding and hyperbilirubinemia [letter]. *Clinical Pediatrics, 25,* 112.

Verd, S., Porta, R., Botet, F., Gutierrez, A., Ginovart, G., Barbero, A. H., . . . Plata, I. I. (2015). Hospital outcomes of extremely low birth weight infants after introduction of donor milk to supplement mother's milk. *Breastfeeding Medicine, 10,* 150–155.

Vio, F., Salazar, G., & Infante, C. (1991). Smoking during pregnancy and lactation and its effects on breast milk volume. *American Journal of Clinical Nutrition, 54,* 1011–1016.

Vochem, M., Hamprecht, K., Jahn, G., & Speer, C. P. (1998). Transmission of cytomegalovirus to preterm infants through breast milk. *Pediatric Infectious Diseases Journal, 17,* 53–58.

Vohr, B. R., Poindexter, B. B., Dusick, A. M., McKinley, L. Y, Wright, L. L., Langer, J. C, & Poole, W. K., (2006). Beneficial effects of breast milk in the neonatal intensive care unit on the developmental outcome of extremely low birth weight infants at 18 months of age. *Pediatrics, 118,* e115–e123.

Volpe, J. J. (2001). Bilirubin and brain injury. In J. J. Volpe (Ed.), *Neonatal neurology.* Philadelphia, PA: W. B. Saunders.

Walker, M. (1992). Breastfeeding the premature infant. *NAACOG's Clinical Issues in Perinatal and Women's Health Nursing, 3,* 620–633.

Walker, M. (2008). Breastfeeding the late preterm infant. *Journal of Obstetric, Gynecologic, and Neonatal Nursing, 37,* 692–701.

Walker, M. (2009). Breastfeeding the late preterm infant: *Improving care and outcomes.* Amarillo, TX: Hale Publishing.

Walker, M. (2010a). Breast pumps and other technologies. In Riordan, J., Wambach, K. (Eds.), *Breastfeeding and human lactation.* (4th ed.) Sudbury, MA: Jones and Bartlett.

Walker, M. (2010b). Breastfeeding management for the late preterm infant: Practical interventions for "little imposters." *Clinical Lactation, 1,* 22–26.

Walshaw, C. A. (2010). Are we getting the best from breastfeeding? *Acta Paediatrica, 99,* 1292–1297.

Walshaw, C. A., Owens, J. M., Scally, A. J., & Walshaw, M. J. (2008). Does breastfeeding method influence infant weight gain? *Archives of Disease in Childhood, 93,* 292–296.

Wan, E. W., Davey, K., Page-Sharp, M., Hartmann, P. E., Simmer, K., & Ilett, K. F. (2008). Dose-effect study of domperidone as a galactagogue in preterm mothers with insufficient milk supply, and its transfer into milk. *British Journal of Clinical Pharmacology, 66,* 283–289.

Wang, M. L., Dorer, D. J., Fleming, M. P., & Catlin, E. (2004). Clinical outcomes of near-term infants. *Pediatrics, 114,* 372–376.

Washington, E. C., Ector, W., & Abboud, M. (1995). Hemolytic jaundice due to G6PD deficiency causing kernicterus in a female newborn. *Southern Medical Journal, 88,* 776–779.

Watchko, J. F., & Oski, F. A. (1983). Bilirubin 20 mg/dL: Vingintiphobia. *Pediatrics, 71,* 660–663.

Wei, L., Wang, H., Han, Y., & Li, C. (2008). Clinical observation on the effects of electroacupuncture at Shaoze (SI 1) in 46 cases of postpartum insufficient lactation. *Journal of Traditional Chinese Medicine, 28,* 168–172.

Whitelaw, A., Histerkamp, G., Sleath, K., Acolet, D., & Richards, M. (1988). Skin to skin contact for very low birthweight infants and their mothers. *Archives of Disease in Childhood, 63,* 1377.

Whiteley, W. (1996). A parent's experience of a special care baby unit. Emotional dimensions of prematurity. *Professional Care of Mother and Child, 6,* 141–142.

WHO Multicentre Growth Reference Study Group. (2006). *WHO child growth standards: Length/height-for-age, weight-for-age, weight-for-length, weight-for-height and body mass index-for-age: Methods and development.* Geneva, Switzerland: World Health Organization.

Widstrom, A. M., Marchini, G., Matthiesen, A. S., Werner, S., Winberg, J., & Uvnas-Moberg, K. (1988). Nonnutritive sucking in tube-fed preterm infants: Effects on gastric motility and gastric contents of somatostatin. *Journal of Pediatric Gastroenterology and Nutrition, 7,* 517.

Wiedemann, M., Kontush, A., Finckh, B., Hellwege, H. H., & Kohlschutter, A. (2003). Neonatal blood plasma is less susceptible to oxidation than adult plasma owing to its higher content of bilirubin and lower content of oxidizable fatty acids. *Pediatric Research, 53,* 843 –849.

Willis, S. K., Hannon, P. R., & Scrimshaw, S. C. (2002). The impact of the maternal experience with a jaundiced newborn on the breastfeeding relationship. *Journal of Family Practice, 51,* 465.

Wilson-Clay, B., & Hoover, K. (2002). *The breastfeeding atlas.* Austin, TX: LactNews Press.

Wolf, L. S., & Glass, R. P. (1992). *Feeding and swallowing disorders in infancy.* Tucson, AZ: Therapy Skill Builders.

Wright, C. M., Parkinson, K. N., & Drewett, R. F. (2006). How does maternal and child feeding behavior relate to weight gain and failure to thrive? Data from a prospective birth cohort. *Pediatrics, 117,* 1262–1269.

Yamauchi, Y., & Yamanouchi, I. (1990). Breastfeeding frequency during the first 24 hours after birth in full-term neonates. *Pediatrics, 86,* 171–175.

Yang, H., Wang, Q., Zheng, L., Lin, M., Zheng, X-B., Lin, F., & Yang, L-Y. (2015). Multiple genetic modifiers of bilirubin metabolism involvement in significant neonatal hyperbilirubinemia in patients of Chinese descent. *PLoS One, 10,* e0132034.

Yang, W-C., Zhao, L-L., Li, Y-C., Chen, C-H., Chang, Y-J., Fu, Y-C., & Wu, H-P. (2013). Bodyweight loss in predicting neonatal hyperbilirubinemia 72 hours after birth in term newborn infants. *BMC Pediatrics, 13,* 145.

Yaseen, H., Salem, M., & Darwich, L. (2004). Clinical presentation of hypernatremic dehydration in exclusively breastfed neonates. *Indian Journal of Pediatrics, 71,* 1059–1062.

Yasuda, A., Kimura, H., Hayakawa, M., Ohshiro, M., Kato, Y., Matsuura, O., . . . Morishima, T. (2003). Evaluation of cytomegalovirus infections transmitted via breast milk in preterm infants with a realtime polymerase chain reaction assay. *Pediatrics, 111,* 1333–1336.

Yidzdas, H. Y., Satar, M., Tutak, E., Narl, N., Büyükçelik, M., & Özlü, F. (2005). May the best friend be an enemy if not recognized early: Hypernatremic dehydration due to breastfeeding. *Pediatric Emergency Care, 21,* 445–448.

Yigit, F., Cigdem, Z., Temizsoy, E., Cingi, M. E., Korel, O., Yildirim, E., & Ovali, F. (2012). Does warming the breasts affect the amount of breastmilk production? *Breastfeeding Medicine, 7,* 487–488.

Yilmaz, G., Caylan, N., Karacan, C. D., Bodur, I., & Gokcay, G. (2014). Effect of cup feeding and bottle feeding on breastfeeding in late preterm infants: A randomized controlled study. *Journal of Human Lactation, 30,* 174–179.

Yoo, H. S., Sung, S. I., Jung, Y. J., Lee, M. S., Han, Y. M., Ahn, S. Y., . . . Park, W. S. (2015). Prevention of cytomegalovirus transmission via breastmilk in extremely low birth weight infants. *Yonsei Medical Journal, 56,* 998–1006.

Ziemer, M., & Pidgeon, J. (1993). Skin changes and pain in the nipple during the first week of lactation. *Journal of Obstetric, Gynecologic, and Neonatal Nursing, 22,* 247–256.

ADDITIONAL READING AND RESOURCES

Breastfeeding Preterm Infants

Arnold, L. D. W. (2002). The cost-effectiveness of using banked donor milk in the neonatal intensive care unit: Prevention of necrotizing enterocolitis. *Journal of Human Lactation, 18,* 172–177.

Arnold, L. D. W. (2008). US health policy and access to banked donor human milk. *Breastfeeding Medicine, 3,* 221–229.

Arnold, L. D. W. (2010). *Human milk in the NICU: Policy into practice.* Sudbury, MA: Jones and Bartlett.

California Perinatal Quality Care Collaborative. (2008). Nutritional support of the VLBW infant. Retrieved from https://www.cpqcc.org/sites/default/files/NUTRITIONAL_SUPPORT_OF_THE_VLBW_INFANT_-_REVISED_2008EntireToolkit.pdf

Callen, J., & Pinelli, J. (2005). A review of the literature examining the benefits and challenges, incidence and duration, and barriers to breastfeeding in preterm infants. *Advances in Neonatal Care, 5,* 72–88.

Callen, J., Pinelli, J., Atkinson, S., & Saigal, S. (2005). Qualitative analysis of barriers to breastfeeding in very-low-birthweight infants in the hospital and postdischarge. *Advances in Neonatal Care, 5,* 93–103.

Hoover, K., & Wilson-Clay, B. Pumping milk for your premature baby and pumping record. Patient teaching sheets. Retrieved from http://www.breastfeedingmaterials.com/products/pumpingforpreterm

Hurst, N. (2005). Assessing and facilitating milk transfer during breastfeeding for the premature infant. *Newborn and Infant Nursing Reviews, 5,* 19–26.

Meier, P. P., Engstrom, J. L., Mingolelli, S. S., Miracle, D. J., & Kiesling, S. (2004). The Rush Mothers' Milk Club: Breastfeeding interventions for mothers of very low birth weight infants. *Journal of Obstetric, Gynecologic, and Neonatal Nursing, 33,* 164–174.

Nyqvist, K. H. (2005). Breastfeeding support in neonatal care: An example of the integration of international evidence and experience. *Newborn and Infant Nursing Reviews, 5,* 34–48.

Wight, N. E., Morton, J. A., & Kim, J. H. (2008). *Best medicine: human milk in the NICU.* Amarillo, TX: Hale Publishing.

Resources on Jaundice

For Health Providers

American Academy of Pediatrics Predischarge Assessment of the Risk for Severe Hyperbilirubinemia in Newborns 35 or More Weeks of Gestation
http://www.aap.org/en-us/professional-resources/practice-support/Vaccine-Financing-Delivery/Documents/Hyperbilirubinemia_SAMPLE.pdf

BiliTool for Jaundice Risk Assessment
http://www.bilitool.org

California Perinatal Quality Control Collaborative
https://www.cpqcc.org/qi-tool-kits/severe-hyperbilirubinemia-prevention-shp

CDC Jaundice Materials for Clinicians and to Distribute to Patients
http://www.cdc.gov/ncbddd/jaundice/index.html

For Parents

Fast Facts for Families: What You Should Know About Jaundice Management
http://www.cdc.gov/ncbddd/jaundice/documents/JaundiceMgmtBrochure.pdf

Jaundice in Newborns Q&A
http://www.healthychildren.org/English/news/Pages/Jaundice-in-Newborns.aspx

Resources on Premature Infants

For Parents

PreemieCare
http://www.preemiehelp.com

University of California–San Diego Health
http://health.ucsd.edu/specialties/obgyn/maternity/newborn/nicu/spin/parents/Pages/default.aspx

For Providers

Videos

Breastmilk Solutions, Dr. Jane Morton
http://www.breastmilksolutions.com/index.html

Stanford School of Medicine Getting Started with Breastfeeding
http://newborns.stanford.edu/Breastfeeding/index.html

Human Milk Supplementation

Human Milk Banking Association of North America, for ordering banked human milk
http://www.hmbana.org

Mothers' Milk Bank of New England, use of pasteurized donor human milk as NICU standard of care
http://www.milkbankne.org/files/MBNE_NICU.pdf

University of California–San Diego Health System Supporting Premature Infant Nutrition (SPIN) Program
http://health.ucsd.edu/specialties/obgyn/maternity/newborn/nicu/spin/Pages/default.aspx

Resources on Late Preterm Infants

For Parents

The Diaper Diary (for keeping track of output) and Pumping Milk for Your Premature Baby
http://www.breastfeedingmaterials.com/

Directory to find the name and contact information of a lactation consultant with the IBCLC credential
http://uslca.org/resources/find-an-ibclc

Guoth-Gumberger, M. Breastfeeding with the supplementary nursing system (Rosenheim, Germany) http://www.breastfeeding-support.de

Late Preterm Infant: What Parents Need to Know AWHONN

https://www.acog.org/-/media/Districts/District-II/PDFs/PretermBirthAWHONNWhatParentsNeedToKnow.pdf?la=en

Massachusetts Breastfeeding Coalition Zip Milk: To locate International Board Certified Lactation Consultants and other sources of breastfeeding support in Massachusetts, Louisiana, North Carolina, Georgia, New Hampshire, Wisconsin, and New Jersey

http://zipmilk.org/index.php?state=clear

For Providers

Academy of Breastfeeding Medicine. (2011). ABM Clinical Protocol #10: Breastfeeding the late preterm infant (34 0/7 to 36 6/7 weeks gestation) (First revision June 2011). *Breastfeeding Medicine, 6*(3), 151–156. Retrieved from http://www.bfmed.org/Media/Files/Protocols/Protocol%2010%20Revised%20English%206.11.pdf

California Perinatal Quality Care Collaborative. (2007). Care and management of the late preterm infant toolkit. Retrieved from https://www.cpqcc.org/qi-tool-kits/care-and-management-late-preterm-infant

Parent Guide: Going Home With Your Late Preterm Infant Contemporary Pediatrics, available to healthcare providers as handout for parents

http://www.modernmedicine.com/modernmedicine/Parent+Guides/Parent-Guide-Going-home-with-your-late-preterm-inf/ArticleStandard/Article/detail/473739?contextCategoryId=6465

Walker, M. (2009). *Breastfeeding the late preterm infant: Improving care and outcomes.* Amarillo, TX: Hale Publishing

Appendix 6-1

Summary of Interventions for Slow Infant Weight Gain

Breastfeeding Techniques and Equipment Useful in Slow Weight-Gain Situations

Rationale	Technique
Cross-cradle or clutch position	This provides good visualization for the mother and may be easier for her to manipulate and support the infant's head and body.
Ventral or laid-back position	Ventral positioning is used for infants with upper airway or breathing problems such as laryngomalacia or tracheomalacia, and for infants who have difficulty latching in other positions.
Dancer hand position	This position offers additional jaw support for hypotonia and excessive jaw movement, and slightly decreases intraoral space. A variation is just a finger placed under the chin.
Sublingual pressure	The index finger is placed gently under the chin where the tongue attaches to the floor of the mouth to keep the tongue from losing contact with the nipple. It can be used when clicking or smacking sounds are heard, indicating that the tongue is losing contact with the nipple.
Nipple tug	The mother pulls back slightly on her areola when the infant pauses (or pulls infant slightly away from her) without breaking the suction and only if the nipples are not sore. This causes the infant to pull the nipple/areola back into the mouth, strengthening the suck and sustaining the suckling.
Alternate massage/ breast compressions	The mother massages and compresses the breast during the pause between sucking bursts to increase the volume and fat content of the feeding, to encourage the infant to begin another sucking burst, and to sustain and increase the number of sucks and swallows per burst.
Finger feeding	A length of tubing attached to a bottle, syringe, or feeding tube device is placed on the index finger. The infant draws the finger into the mouth and receives milk after each suck.

Equipment for Use in Slow Weight-Gain Situations

Device	Rationale
Tube-feeding device	Any commercial devices—such as the Medela Supplemental Nutrition System (SNS); the starter SNS; the Lact-Aid Nursing Trainer System from Lact-Aid International, or ones constructed from butterfly tubing (with the needle removed) attached to a syringe; a length of number 5 French tubing run from a bottle of expressed milk; or a gavage feeding setup—can be attached to the breast to deliver supplement as the infant breastfeeds. This encourages proper suckling, improves the maternal milk supply, and avoids artificial nipples. The flow of milk into the infant's mouth stimulates further sucking (flow regulates suck). If an infant is unable to latch to the breast, the tubing can be run underneath and through an opening in a nipple shield.
Nipple shield	A thin silicone nipple shield may help an infant latch to the breast, especially one with a weak suck. Sometimes milk transfer is enhanced when combined with alternate massage.
Periodontal syringe, dropper	These are usually used to provide an incentive at breast for encouraging the infant to latch-on or to sustain sucking. They are a slow mechanism to provide meaningful amounts of supplementary milk, and if used as such, generally prolong feedings and exhaust the infant and the parents.
Cup	A small 28-cc medicine cup, a paladai (Malhotra, Vishwambaran, Sundaram, & Narayanan, 1999), or other small cup with a smooth, rounded edge can be a quick and safe way to increase milk intake after practice sessions at the breast (Howard et al., 1999). The milk is not poured into the infant's mouth, but the infant is supported in an upright position and allowed to sip milk at his or her own pace.
Spoon or spoon-like device	The Medela Soft Feeder or a medicine-dispensing device with a spoon-like shape can be used for small amounts of supplement.
Standard bottle/ nipple	Standard bottle nipples may deliver a fast flow of milk and contribute to weakening the suck of an infant who may already be demonstrating sucking variations. A slow- to medium-flow round nipple made of soft silicone may be a reasonable choice (Kassing, 2002).
Specialty bottle/ nipple	A device such as the Haberman Feeder from Medela has a nipple with a valve that releases milk only with sucking effort and reduces the amount of negative pressure required to withdraw milk. Adjustments are graduated from an easy to a more difficult flow to strengthen the suck and avoid flooding the infant's mouth with milk.
Breast pump	A hospital-grade electric breast pump with a double collection kit can be used to increase milk production, especially helpful for use in longer term situations. Some mothers can use a personal use category of breast pump for pumping on a shorter term basis.
Electronic scale	An electronic scale that is accurate to within 2 g can be used for monitoring intake (for example, Olympic Smart Scale, Medela Baby Weigh Scale). These scales are often used during the initial assessment of the slow weight gain and can be rented by the mother to monitor intake at feedings and help determine the need for supplements after each feeding and over a 24-hour period.
Feeding logs	Depending on the complexity of the situation, mothers may need to keep track of a number of parameters such as the number of feeds per 24 hours, the amount of milk transferred from the breast to the infant by pre- and postfeed weights, the amount of milk pumped, the amount of supplement consumed, daily weights, and diaper counts of urine and stool output.

Chapter 7

Physical, Medical, and Environmental Problems and Issues

INTRODUCTION

Although it is the dream of all parents and the hope of all clinicians that infants are able to sail through breastfeeding with fair winds and few obstacles, this is not always the case. There are a number of conditions and situations that do not preclude breastfeeding but may complicate the process. Even if direct feeding at the breast is not possible for some infants, almost all infants benefit from receiving human milk.

TWINS AND HIGHER ORDER MULTIPLES

It is both possible and desirable to breastfeed twins and higher order multiples. In 2013, there were 132,324 births of twins in the United States. The triplet and higher order multiple birth rate declined 4% from 2012 to 2013, to 119.5 per 100,000 births. The 4,700 births that occurred in triplet and higher order multiple deliveries included 4,364 triplets, 270 quadruplets, and 66 quintuplets—the lowest numbers reported in a decade (Martin, Hamilton, Osterman, Curtin, & Mathews, 2015).

Multiple births are more common with increasing maternal age and with the use of infertility therapy. There is a high risk of adverse outcomes in multiple births. One of every eight twins and one of every three triplets are born very preterm (less than 32 weeks of gestation), compared with fewer than 2 of every 100 singletons. Accordingly, death during infancy is much more common among twins (29.8 per 1,000) and triplets (59.6 per 1,000) than among singletons (6.0 per 1,000). In response to the unparalleled rise in higher order multiple births during the 1980s and 1990s and their attendant risk of poor outcome, the American Society of Reproductive Medicine published guidelines intended to reduce the incidence of triplets and higher order multiples resulting from assisted reproductive therapy by limiting the number of embryos transferred (Practice Committee of the American Society for Reproductive Medicine, & Practice Committee of Society for Assisted Reproductive Technology, 2009).

In an analysis of a survey of more than 1,800 higher order multiples births conducted by the Mothers of Supertwins organization, 69.6% of the respondents stated that they initiated breastfeeding, with the average time that at least some breastmilk was provided ranging from 11 to 14 weeks (Ross, 2012). Increased breastfeeding rates for mothers of multiples may be achieved with highly motivated mothers who have access to lactation help and support groups (Damato, Dowling, Madigan, & Thanattherakul, 2005;

Gromada & Spangler, 1998). Mothers who wish to breastfeed their infants due to the improved health outcomes from the use of breastmilk may need extensive education on the importance of providing their milk to multiple infants (Friedman, Flidel-Rimon, Lavie, & Shinwell, 2004). Although mothers of multiples elect to breastfeed at similar rates to mothers with singleton pregnancies (Bowers & Gromada, 2003), they and their infants are at an increased risk for a number of complications—the higher the plurality, the greater the likelihood of poor perinatal outcomes. These infants tend to be born both preterm and small for gestational age (**Table 7-1**).

Geraghty, Pinney, Sethuraman, Roy-Chaudhury, and Kalkwarf (2004) evaluated the feeding practices of four groups of mothers: mothers of term singletons, mothers of preterm singletons, mothers of term multiples, and mothers of preterm multiples. By 3 days postpartum, mothers of preterm multiples provided breastmilk less often than all other groups. This trend continued for the first 6 months of life, showing that the duration of any breastmilk feeding was significantly shorter for preterm multiples than for all other groups (12 weeks for preterm multiples, 19 weeks for preterm singletons, 24 weeks for term singletons, and 24 weeks for term multiples). The combination of multiple gestation and preterm delivery resulted in lower breastmilk feeding rates and a shorter duration of breastfeeding by mothers of preterm multiples. This suggests the need for more intensive breastfeeding support and follow up for this especially vulnerable population.

The inability to synthesize sufficient amounts of milk for multiples does not appear to account for the less optimal breastfeeding outcomes in preterm multiples. Milk yields in mothers of twins measured between 2 and 6 months ranged from 1,680 to 3,000 mL/day. Mothers of multiples are capable of producing sufficient amounts of milk for two or more infants over long periods of time (Biancuzzo, 1994; Liang, Gunn, & Gunn, 1997). The milk yield of one mother of triplets was 3,080 mL/day at 2.5 months (Saint, Maggiore, & Hartmann, 1986). Mean daily weight gains of quadruplets during the 1st month after discharge varied from 30 to 54 g, indicative of adequate milk supply as a result of optimal breastfeeding management (Mead, Chuffo, Lawlor-Klean, & Meier, 1992). Berlin reported that a mother of quadruplets expressed 108 oz per 24 hours during the time the infants were in the neonatal intensive care unit (NICU), validating the capacity of the breasts to respond to the increased needs of multiple infants. In a case study

Table 7-1 Comparison of Gestational Age and Birth Weight in Multiple Births*

Plurality	Mean Gestational Age (weeks)	Mean Birth Weight (g)
Singleton	38.8 (± 2.5)	3,332 (± 573) [~7 lbs 4 oz]
Twins	35.3 (± 3.7)	2,347 (± 645) [~5 lbs 3 oz]
Triplets	32.2 (± 3.8)	1,687 (± 561) [~ 3 lbs 12 oz]
Quadruplets	29.4 (± 4.0)	1,309 (± 522) [~ 2 lbs 14 oz]
Quintuplets	28.5 (± 4.7)	1,105 (± 777) [~ 2 lbs 7 oz]

*Values in parentheses are standard deviations.

Data from Martin, J. A., Hamilton, B. E., Sutton, P. D., Ventura, S. J., Menacker, F., & Munson, M. L. (2003). *Births: Final data for 2002. National Vital Statistics Reports, 52*. Hyattsville, MD: National Center for Health Statistics.

of a mother of quintuplets, banked donor human milk was also used when the infants required more milk than the mother could provide. This allowed the infants to be fed human milk exclusively, which contributed to the relative lack of medical complications in these infants (Szucs, Axline, & Rosenman, 2009). Michaels and Wanner (2013) describe a mother with a right mastectomy who delivered twin boys at 37+ weeks' gestation, with both infants going to breast within 2 hours of delivery. The early course of breastfeeding was complicated by milk production that did not meet the needs of the infants and required formula supplementation. After 3.5 weeks she was prescribed a regimen of 30 mg domperidone 3 times per day. At 8 weeks the mother desired to further improve her milk production and the domperidone dosage was increased to 120–160 mg daily. By 3 months she was able to eliminate formula supplementation as she was producing all of the milk the infants required. Even with overwhelming challenges, mothers of multiples should be provided every opportunity to breastfeed and provide as much milk as possible for their infants.

Prenatal Preparation for Breastfeeding Multiples

Although most mothers are aware early in their pregnancy that they are carrying more than one infant, they may question their ability to breastfeed multiple infants. Clinicians should reassure parents that the provision of breastmilk and breastfeeding remains both possible and optimal (Sollid, Evans, McClowry, & Garrett, 1989). Breastmilk provides the same protective factors to multiples as to singletons (Flidel-Rimon & Shinwell, 2002) and can promote the development of a close maternal attachment to each infant (Gromada, 1981). Other prenatal considerations are as follows:

- Maternal nutritional management. Because preterm birth and growth-restricted infants are two common outcomes of a multiple pregnancy, maternal nutrition and weight gain are especially important factors in optimizing the duration of the pregnancy and reducing the incidence of low or very-low-birth-weight infants (Leonard, 1982). Mothers carrying multiple infants usually benefit from nutritional counseling to ensure adequate intake of energy and nutrients to achieve weight gain targets of 35–44 lbs for a twin pregnancy (Roem, 2003) and a 50-lb weight gain for a triplet pregnancy (Brown & Carlson, 2000). Optimal rates of fetal growth and birth weights in a twin pregnancy are achieved at rates of maternal weight gain that vary by gestational period and by maternal pregravid body mass index (Luke et al., 2003; **Table 7-2**).
- An identified source of breastfeeding support. A mother will need access to a lactation consultant and/or other resources for breastfeeding support with specific expertise in managing the breastfeeding of multiples (Leonard, 2000; Storr, 1989). She will also require information regarding prenatal classes specific to multiple births (Moxley & Haddon, 1999) and information on the extent of lactation care and services she can expect where she delivers her infants. Efforts should be made to designate a case manager or other healthcare provider who coordinates both breastfeeding management and the other support services needed by a multiple-birth family. This helps reduce confusion, miscommunication, and fragmented care that contribute to poor breastfeeding outcomes (Leonard, 2003).

Table 7-2 Weight Gain in Twin Pregnancies by Pregravid Weight and Gestational Period

Pregravid Weight Status	Gestational Period	Weight Gain
Underweight	0–20 weeks 20–28 weeks 28 weeks to delivery	1.25–1.75 lbs/week 1.5–1.75 lbs/week 1.25 lbs/week
Normal weight	0–20 weeks 20–28 weeks 28 weeks to delivery	1.0–1.5 lbs/week 1.25–1.75 lbs/week 1.0 lb/week
Overweight	0–20 weeks 20–28 weeks 28 weeks to delivery	1.0–1.25 lbs/week 1.0–1.5 lbs/week 1.0 lb/week
Obese	0–20 weeks 20–28 weeks 28 weeks to delivery	0.75–1.0 lb/week 0.75–1.25 lbs/week 0.75 lb/week

- Written and video resources. A mother should have a working knowledge of breastfeeding with specific written materials relevant to how multiple births affect breastfeeding (Gromada, 1999) and have viewed a video with her partner and family so that family members understand their role. She should also be provided with community and online support sources specific to parenting multiples.
- Equipment resources. Mothers need written information on where to secure an electric breast pump, digital scale, "V" or horseshoe-shaped pillow for simultaneous feeding of two infants, equipment for transporting twins or higher order multiples, and so forth. She should also check if her health insurance covers the cost of a pump rental and lactation care and services.
- Exploring and setting breastfeeding goals. Discuss the mother's plans for how much breastfeeding she would like to accomplish (Auer & Gromada, 1998). There are many different ways to breastfeed multiples:
  - Some mothers of twins and triplets are able to provide breastmilk for and/or breastfeed exclusively all of the infants (Leonard, 2000; Liang et al., 1997).
  - Mothers may combine feeding at the breast, bottle-feeding expressed breastmilk, and/or bottle-feeding (or other alternative feeding technique) infant formula depending on the number of infants, their health status, in-hospital experience, and the mother's milk production (Biancuzzo, 1994; Hattori & Hattori, 1999). This may change over time as the infants become more proficient at the breast, the milk supply increases, or one or more infants do not tolerate infant formula or experience other health problems.
  - Even small amounts of breastmilk are important to multiple infants, especially if born preterm or with other health concerns. Some mothers use a rotation plan of feeding two triplets at the breast simultaneously (one on each breast), followed by the third infant who is given both breasts. This rotation may help the smaller infant who feeds from both breasts, which may contain the higher fat-content milk.

    - Donor breastmilk from a milk bank in the Human Milk Banking Association of North America network can be secured if mothers cannot produce sufficient volumes of milk.
- Securing at-home help. Expectant parents of multiples need to secure regular and reliable sources of ongoing help at home. This is especially important for parents of higher order multiples and if the mother has experienced a cesarean delivery, extended bedrest, or other complications of a multiple pregnancy. These sources may be family, friends, postpartum doulas, postpartum support agencies, volunteers from church organizations, or grandparent organizations. Some parents may not be able to afford at-home help and need to explore other community services for which they may be eligible, such as homemaker and home health aid services. This type of help is often necessary for many months, especially with higher order multiples.

Managing the In-Hospital Experience

Once the infants are born, a breastfeeding plan should be created, taking into account the number of infants, the status of the infants, the mother's health and comfort needs, the mother's desires, and the agreed-upon short- and long-term goals. Overarching goals include the initiation and maintenance of optimal milk production and establishing feeding at the breast or breastmilk feeding (if one or more infants are unable to feed directly from the breast) of all infants.

Healthy Full-Term Multiples

Flexible rooming-in should be encouraged, with the timing and amount of rooming-in individualized to each family (Leonard, 2002). Healthy twins and triplets can be kept skin to skin and breastfed on cue, with feeding sessions assisted and documented by a nurse, lactation consultant, or other caregiver skilled in preterm multiple breastfeeding. Cue-based feeding takes into account the differing needs and feeding skills of each infant (Gromada, 1992). Mothers benefit from the presence of the father and other helpers such as student nurses, peer counselors, or even family members who can assist with holding and positioning the infants. Each infant should have his or her own color-coded documentation forms to track intake and output and to record breastfeeding assessments. Breastfeeding should be initiated at the earliest opportunity, with one infant at a time. This allows each infant to be properly positioned and latched and to ensure that each infant is swallowing milk. It also helps with maternal attachment to each infant. Simultaneous breastfeeding may be better postponed until the infants demonstrate effective breastfeeding skills that can be validated with an assessment tool. The mother thus becomes acquainted with each infant's breastfeeding style and needs, helping her acquire competence and confidence in her ability to breastfeed each baby. Simultaneous breastfeeding at this point could mask problems, especially the ability of each infant to sustain nutritive sucking and swallowing. If the infants are not in the mother's room, they should be brought to her on cue for all feedings. In the absence of maternal complications, healthy multiples should have early access to the breast and breastfeed between 8 and 12 times each 24 hours (Gromada & Spangler, 1998). Supplements, pacifiers, and bottles should be avoided except for medical reasons. Infants should not alternate between feeding at the breast and being bottle-fed. This practice has the potential to delay the acquisition of effective feeding skills at the breast and to interfere with the initiation and maintenance of an abundant milk supply.

In some situations the infants may be full term and healthy, but the mother's postpartum recovery may be affected by complications of the pregnancy or delivery. It is not unusual to encounter a mother of multiples who has pregnancy-induced hypertension or preeclampsia and is receiving magnesium sulfate ($MgSO_4$) to treat this, has experienced a cesarean delivery, is on a patient-controlled analgesia (PCA) pump for pain medication, and is experiencing weakness from extended bedrest or heavy blood loss. A mother on $MgSO_4$ (and pain medications) may be temporarily unable to orient herself and organize her time to attend to all the tasks she is expected to accomplish. She may be weak and need physical help in positioning and actually holding the infants at the breast. She may need someone else to watch for infant feeding readiness cues and initiate each breastfeeding session. If the mother is pumping for preterm or ill infants in the NICU, she may also need to be reminded about each pumping session and require someone to physically hold the breastshields to her breast and operate the pump. Many of these mothers are unable to absorb verbal teaching, keep records, or remember details about each infant's condition until the effects of the medications have worn off.

Clinicians and parents should anticipate that lactogenesis II and copious milk production may be delayed by factors common to multiple births and known to affect the timing of these events such as an urgent cesarean section (Dewey, Nommsen-Rivers, Heinig, & Cohen, 2003), extreme stress (Chen, Nommsen-Rivers, Dewey, & Lonnerdal, 1998; Dewey, 2001), presence of diabetes, severe postpartum hemorrhage (Willis & Livingstone, 1995), anemia (Henly et al., 1995), ineffective or infrequent breast drainage, and unrelieved severe engorgement. Use of $MgSO_4$ has been suggested as a contributor to poor milk production and a later onset of lactation (Haldeman, 1993; Hale & Ilett, 2002). Although the amount of magnesium transferred to breastmilk is almost clinically irrelevant (Hale, 2012), sedation, hypotonia, and poor sucking have been reported in infants whose mothers received $MgSO_4$ prenatally or during the intrapartum period (Finnegan, 1982; Fuentes & Goldkrand, 1987; Riaz, Porat, Brodsky, & Hurt, 1998), adding yet another dimension to ineffective breast drainage and a delay in lactogenesis II.

Preterm Multiples

If the infants have been born preterm, they may be separated from their mother in a special-care nursery or NICU, may or may not be capable of feeding at the breast, or may be too preterm or ill to be brought out to the mother. They may be placed in separate beds, separate nurseries, or transported to different hospitals depending on their acuity and availability of beds where they were born. If the infants are unable to transfer milk effectively at breast or cannot be fed at the breast, the mother should begin pumping her milk within about 6 hours of delivery, preferably within 1 hour if possible. Mothers who hand express or pump within an hour or 2 of giving birth may yield enough colostrum for each infant's first feeding. After that, mothers should pump milk with an electric pump, a double collection kit, and a breastshield large enough to accommodate the nipple comfortably within the nipple tunnel. Breastmilk production can be maximized by early pumping, expressing 8–12 times each 24 hours, and massaging and compressing the breast while pumping (Hill, Aldag, & Chatterton, 2001; Jones, Dimmock, & Spencer, 2001). Combining milk expression techniques may result in greater milk output (Morton, Hall, Wong, Thairu, Benitz, & Rhine, 2009). These researchers demonstrated that in pump-dependent preterm mothers, those that used hand expression greater than five times per day, as well as using an electric pump five times per day during the first 3 days postpartum produced significantly larger volumes of milk than mothers who only used an electric pump. Furthermore, massaging each breast while using an electric breast pump significantly increased the amount of milk pumped at each session. Over the course of the 8-week study, mothers that combined early hand expression of colostrum in the first 3 days following birth and who used breast massage and compression while pumping and hand expression if needed, produced more milk than term mothers (average 955 mL per day). This was independent of pumping frequency in mothers who frequently used hand expression.

Parents can be encouraged to practice skin-to-skin care with their newborns, either one or two at a time and shared between the mother and father, helping to facilitate milk production, earlier feedings at the breast, and parental self-confidence (Dombrowski et al., 2000). Cobedding twins or pairs of multiples involves keeping two infants snuggled together in the same bassinet. This practice enhances stabilization, reduces stress levels, often results in better breastfeeding, and tends to keep them awake at the same time (Nyqvist & Lutes, 1998). Breastfeeding is also improved as mothers synchronize breastfeeding with the twins' behavioral states (Nyqvist, 2002). If the mother is unable to walk to the special care nursery or NICU, she should be transported in her bed or wheelchair when ready to see and touch her infants. Parents will need to discuss how the expressed colostrum should be distributed among the infants if early volumes are limited. Options include small amounts evenly distributed among all infants, all colostrum given to the sickest infant, or rotating complete colostrum feedings among the infants.

Oropharyngeal administration of the mother's own immune-boosting colostrum should be practiced if the infant is unable to feed directly at breast or is unable to be enterally fed. Human milk oral care can be administered by the parents several times per day (see Chapter 6).

As the infants move toward direct feeding at the breast, a breastfeeding plan for each infant is necessary and adapted as needed to account for variations in their conditions, specific feeding problems, pumping schedule, equipment needs, the parents' needs, and the needs and care of older children. Within the plan would be strategies to address ineffective suckling, need for complemental or supplemental feedings, limited milk transfer, and the effect of any congenital anomalies on breastfeeding (LaFleur & Niesen, 1996). Milk transfer in healthy multiples should be carefully assessed before giving additional formula directly after or in between breastfeedings. Unnecessary formula feeding can depress the infant's appetite, prolong intervals between breastfeeds, reduce sucking efficiency, prolong feeding sessions, and extend the time it takes to establish exclusive breastfeeding (Biancuzzo, 1994). Every effort should be made to provide opportunities for each infant to feed directly from the breast prior to discharge while the mother still has access to specialized staff.

Direct breastfeeding—that is having the infants gain experience feeding directly from the breast prior to discharge—is an important intervention that can improve breastfeeding outcomes of infants in a NICU. In a study of 66 mothers of preterm infants, Pineda (2011) found that of those mothers who continued to provide breastmilk until discharge, 100% had put their infants directly to breast at least once during the hospital stay. All mothers who initiated breastmilk feedings but did not put the infants to breast during the NICU stay were no longer providing breastmilk for their infants at NICU discharge. There was a positive association between having the first oral feeding at breast and an increased frequency of later breastfeeds, an increased duration of breastmilk feedings, and trends toward increased success with breastmilk feedings at hospital discharge. This study emphasizes the importance of assuring that infants in the NICU are provided with abundant opportunities to feed directly from the breast, even if these attempts must be followed up with supplementation. Mothers of multiples need every advantage they can obtain to increase their breastfeeding success.

Hospital Discharge

Before discharging the mother or any of the infants, mothers need a clear plan of how to feed and care for themselves and their infants. All household helpers and nursing equipment should be in place and/or in the home before discharge, including an electric breast pump, collection containers if milk will be transported to the infants remaining in the hospital, digital scale for pre- and post-feed intake assessments and periodic weight checks, nipple shields if needed for infants with a weak suck, alternative feeding equipment if needed, special pillow for simultaneous infant feeding if needed, and a designated location for feedings.

Ideally, all infants would be discharged at the same time, but this is not always possible. Each infant may come home at a different time with some infants admitted into different hospitals, making visiting, breastfeeding, and milk transport a logistical nightmare. When one or more infants come home and one or more remain in the hospital, the mother can use the following plans:

- Bring the at-home infants along with a caregiver to the hospital while visiting those infants who remain hospitalized; this might be very likely when the mother lives a great distance from the hospital.
- For briefer visits, the infants at home can be left with a caregiver while the mother visits the hospital.
- In the event that the mother is unwell or unable to visit the hospital, her pumped milk can be brought to the infants by the father or other helper; in some instances, hospital employees who live near the mother have transported milk to the hospitalized infants.
- A mother can breastfeed the infant at home on one side while pumping the other breast, maintaining a connection to the infant(s) still hospitalized, as mother and infant work as a team to provide milk for the absent infant.
- Mothers may feel torn between the infants at home and those in the hospital. Some units have "video conferencing" capabilities where a camera can transmit images of the infants to the mother at home.

Feeding Rotations

Mothers usually adopt a breast rotation pattern that best fits everyone's needs. Mothers can alternate breasts for each feeding, rotate infants and breasts every 24 hours, or "assign" breasts to each infant.

It is important to ensure that each breast is producing its maximum capacity of milk by avoiding the assignment of one breast to a poorly feeding infant. Most mothers offer one breast per feeding (or the third triplet can be offered both sides after two have been fed). Mothers of odd-numbered sets of multiples may need to alternate breasts and infants more frequently than each 24 hours because infants' bilateral development is enhanced when fed in different positions. Pacifiers may be a temptation to use when all infants are crying at once or to calm an infant until it is his or her turn at breast. However, pacifiers have the potential to alter an infant's mouth conformation and introduce poor breastfeeding technique into the breastfeeding plan. Mothers of multiples do not need the increased chance of problems that pacifiers could produce.

Separate and Simultaneous Feedings

Whereas some mothers with healthy full-term infants are ready for simultaneous feedings early in the postpartum period, many mothers prefer to feed one infant at a time, allowing them to become acquainted with each one individually. It may be difficult for some mothers to sort out the different feeding sensations of each infant when they are being fed simultaneously, especially if one infant is not feeding efficiently. An infant with feeding difficulties, chronic health problems, or special needs may require being fed separately until feeding skills have been mastered. Infants who cannot meet their full nutritional needs at the breast may need to be fed individually if the mother must use a nipple shield or tube-feeding device, or must weigh the baby pre- and postfeed to determine supplementation quantities.

Simultaneous feeding saves time and works well when all infants are skilled at feeding, the mother enjoys it, and each infant copes well with his or her sibling at the other breast. Some mothers, however, feel awkward or do not enjoy the sensation of two infants who may be suckling with different rhythms and reserve simultaneous feedings for times when both are crying or when time constraints exist. Birth anomalies such as torticollis or plagiocephaly may also play a part in determining how some of the infants are best positioned for feedings. Plural births experience a higher incidence and risk of plagiocephaly. Breastfeeding may help prevent occipital plagiocephaly as breastfed infants are repositioned more frequently and sleep for shorter periods of time (Losee, Mason, Dudas, Hua, & Mooney, 2007). When feeding simultaneously, some mothers begin with the infant with greater latching difficulties while both hands are free, followed by a more-skilled infant. Occasionally, a skilled infant can be put to breast to elongate and shape the nipple/areola, elicit milk ejection, and be removed from that breast and placed on the other breast, while the less-skilled infant takes advantage of a nipple that has been elongated for him or her with milk readily available. Mothers of higher order multiples may breastfeed two infants at a time while bottle-feeding the third.

Mothers typically use a combination of single and simultaneous feedings and move from feeding on cue to more scheduled feedings, especially with three or more infants. Some mothers use a modified demand schedule where one infant is fed on cue and the other(s) simultaneously or sequentially immediately afterward. Some mothers wake the other infant or infants when the first one rouses, coordinating simultaneous feeds, or she may prefer sequential feeding of one infant right after the other.

Simultaneous feeding positions may be easier initially when using special pillows that are shaped to accommodate two infants. These are firmer than bed pillows and angled such that the infants are not flat but slightly elevated and semi-lying on their sides. Narrow rocking chairs or recliners may not have enough room to use such pillows. There are four basic simultaneous feeding positions and many variations that mothers devise to best suit their needs:

1. Double cradle (crisscross): Each infant is held in the cradle position with their bodies crisscrossed, either one over the other or parallel to the mother's thighs.
2. Double clutch or football: Often an easier position to learn initially, each infant lies tucked under an arm or lies on a pillow perpendicular to the mother's body.
3. Combination (one infant in the cradle position, one in the clutch position): This positioning may be a little more discrete, but care should be taken that the infant's head in the clutch position does not overly compress the other infant's abdomen.
4. Laid-back positioning of the mother with ventral (prone) positioning of the infants.

Partial Breastfeeding and Breastmilk Feeding Options

Mothers of multiples are more likely to supplement or complement with bottles, infant formula, or expressed breastmilk given by bottle or alternative feeding method. This is especially common with higher order multiples and if early effective breastfeeding or breastmilk expression was adversely impacted by maternal and/or infant complications. Complements and supplements are least likely to diminish milk production if each multiple is breastfeeding 7–10 times per day. Certain feeding patterns are more likely to result in diminished milk production and early weaning unless the feeding plan includes pumping breastmilk for the complements and supplements:

- Alternating breast and bottle such that all infants feed at breast for one feeding and all are bottle-fed the next feeding
- All infants receive a complement after each breastfeeding
- Breastfeeding one or more multiples and supplementing the others at each feeding
- One infant exclusively breastfeeds and the other exclusively bottle-feeds

Some infants with chronic health problems may never accomplish direct feeding at the breast but can still receive pumped human milk. Over time, most mothers are able to decrease the number of complements and supplements and may offer alternative feeds on a daily or weekly basis to sleep for a few uninterrupted hours or if milk production cannot keep pace with the increasing needs of the infants. Checklists that include feeding and pumping logs should be kept to ensure adequate intake and growth of all of the infants. Many parents will paint a fingernail or toenail a different color on each infant to easily and rapidly tell them apart if needed and to color code their individual records.

Each infant is an individual and may present a range of feeding behaviors that change over time. The infants may experience growth spurts at different times, may gain weight differently, may come to prefer one breast over the other, may start solids at different times, and may wean at different times.

Prolonging Breastfeeding and the Provision of Breastmilk

New breastfeeding issues continue to arise over the course of the breastfeeding experience. Mothers of twins list numerous explanations for the cessation of breastfeeding or expressing (Damato, Dowling, Standing, & Schuster, 2005): return to work, inadequate milk supply, breast or nipple problems, time burdens of either nursing or pumping or both, presence of older siblings, maternal illness, fatigue, poor infant feeding behaviors, infant sleepiness, and/or desire to have more time for other things. Infants from multiple births do not meet the national breastfeeding goals outlined in the Healthy People 2020 recommendations of 81.9% initiation rate and 60% continuation rate at 6 months. Geraghty, Khoury, and Kalkwarf (2004) reported a continuous decline in the amount of breastmilk received by multiples with 64% of twins receiving at least some breastmilk at 3 days of life and 25% of twin infants receiving some breastmilk at 6 months. Fifty-five percent of triplets received some breastmilk within the first month of life, with only 15% receiving any breastmilk at 6 months.

Some mothers find increasing time burdens if it becomes difficult to nurse infants simultaneously as they grow larger and must nurse one infant at a time. A major factor in continued breastfeeding is the length of time required to feed each infant (Flidel-Rimon & Shinwell, 2006). Some infants remain very slow feeders, and interventions to accelerate feedings may prove helpful (alternate massage, supplementing at breast, scheduled feedings). Mothers who have been on extended bedrest during the pregnancy may have difficulty meeting the physical demand of caring for infants, pumping, and breastfeeding due to the deconditioning that happens during prolonged periods of inactivity. Mothers may find that the large amounts of help they enjoyed during the early weeks have dwindled, making it more difficult to attend to multiple infants and other responsibilities.

Breast pumps should be checked periodically to make sure they are functioning properly. A vacuum gauge should be used to occasionally ensure that a pump is generating maximum amounts of vacuum because some pumps may lose vacuum-generating capacity, especially if a mother is not using a multi-user breast pump.

Damato, Dowling, Madigan, and Thanattherakul (2005) found that the percentage of breastmilk feedings at 1 month after expected delivery date was predictive of continued breastfeeding at 6 months after expected delivery date. Intensive breastfeeding interventions and support are frequently necessary to ensure breastfeeding continues. Often, the first 5–9 weeks of breastfeeding are the most difficult and require the most time investment. At 5 weeks the effort put into breastfeeding equals the same effort as bottle-feeding, but between 8 and 9 weeks the effort to breastfeed becomes less than that to bottle-feed. If mothers can sustain breastfeeding for 1–2 months, breastfeeding becomes less time consuming than bottle-feeding, not only with bottle preparation but also in better health and decreased trips to the pediatrician or hospital. Knowing this may help mothers set a goal and provide hope that things will improve. Mothers who feed their infants solely at the breast, especially during the first 2 months postpartum, are more likely to continue feeding human milk at later time points and to feed human milk for longer durations (Geraghty, Khoury, & Kalkwarf, 2005).

ANOMALIES, DISEASES, AND DISORDERS THAT CAN AFFECT BREASTFEEDING

Ankyloglossia

Ankyloglossia, or tongue-tie, is a congenital oral anomaly, whose prevalence or incidence is between 1.7% and 10.7%, or about 1 to 4 infants per 100 in consecutive births and as high as 25% in infants identified as having breastfeeding difficulties (Ballard, Auer, & Khoury, 2002; Hogan, Westcott, & Griffiths, 2005; Masaitis & Kaempf, 1996; Messner, Lalakea, Aby, Macmahon, & Bair, 2000). The wide range in prevalence can be attributed to different diagnostic criteria used in the studies.

There is no standard test or criteria for the definition or recognition of ankyloglossia, and it may be described in terms of physical characteristics of the infant's oral anatomy or include signs of functional impairment. It is generally described as a condition in which the normal range of motion of the tongue is restricted due to an abnormal attachment of the lingual frenulum (or frenum). The International Affiliation of Tongue-Tie Professionals defines tongue-tie as the embryological remnant of tissue in the midline between the undersurface of the tongue and the floor of the mouth that restricts normal tongue movement (International Affiliation of Tongue-Tie Professionals, 2014). When the cells of the lingual frenulum do not undergo complete apoptosis during the embryological period, the residual tissue may restrain the movements of the tongue (Knox, 2010). The lingual frenulum (or frenum) may be too short, thick, and taut after birth or may not have receded, remaining attached too far along the base of the tongue. The frenula are strong cords of tissue at the front and center of the mouth that guide the development of mouth structures during gestation. There are a number of frena, such as the lingual frenum (under the tongue), the maxillary frenum (under the upper lip), and the buccal frenum, which connects the buccal mucosa (inner check) to the alveolar mucosa.

Development of the tongue begins in the floor of the primitive oral cavity when the embryo is 4 weeks old and the external face is developing. Important during fetal development, the frenula continue after birth to help guide and position the baby teeth as they come in. Children with tongue-tie may be unable to protrude the tongue, touch the roof of the mouth, or move the tongue from side to side. If the lingual frenum extends to the tip of the tongue, a V-shaped notch or heart shape can be seen at the tip.

Ankyloglossia is often familial, not preventable, and usually seen as an isolated condition in an otherwise normal, healthy infant. However, some malformations of the tongue that happen during embryogenesis are seen in combination with a high arched palate, recessed chin, and/or other congenital defects and syndromes (Emmanouil-Nikoloussi & Kerameos-Foroglou, 1992a, 1992b). Maternal cocaine use has been described as a risk factor for tongue-tie (Harris, Friend, & Tolley, 1992). Because tongue-tie is a midline defect and can be associated with a number of genetic syndromes, failure to see improved breastfeeding after correction of ankyloglossia may signal the need to evaluate the infant further for a posterior tongue-tie or for other causes of poor neurological or mechanical control of the tongue.

Problems Associated with Tongue-Tie

A number of pathologies may be associated with tongue-tie, including the following:

- Breastfeeding difficulties. With the rising breastfeeding initiation rates and improved assessment techniques, case studies, small noncontrolled case series, and clinician concerns regarding breastfeeding difficulties associated with tongue-tie have proliferated (Berg, 1990a; Fleiss, Burger, Ramkumar, & Carrington, 1990; Huggins, 1990; Marmet, Shell, & Marmet, 1990; Notestine, 1990; Ward, 1990; Wilton, 1990). Ankyloglossia is associated with a 25–60% incidence of difficulties with breastfeeding. Among lactation experts, ankyloglossia has become a recognized cause of breastfeeding difficulties that include poor latching, inadequate milk transfer by the infant, slow weight gain, and distress while feeding and, in the mother, sore/macerated nipples (Palmer, 2003), diminished milk production, displeasure with continuous feedings, and premature weaning (Berg, 1990b; Griffiths, 2004; Jain, 1995; Walker, 1989). Infants with tongue-tie have been shown to achieve latch scores that are significantly lower than those of infants without this abnormality. In one study, latch scores of severely tongue-tied infants were never greater than 8 (Puapornpong, Raungrongmorakot, Mahasitthiwat, & Ketsuwan, 2014). Lalakea and Messner (2003a) found that latching difficulties of tongue-tied infants occurred significantly more frequently in the tongue-tied group (25%) than in controls (3%).

  For every day of maternal pain during the first 3 weeks of breastfeeding, there is a 10–26% risk of cessation of breastfeeding (Schwartz et al., 2002), making it a priority to immediately address conditions that cause maternal nipple pain such as ankyloglossia. The prevalence of persistent nipple pain in mothers whose infants have ankyloglossia is between 36% and 80%. Only 3% of mothers of normal infants have intractable pain or difficulty in achieving latch at 6 weeks, but 25% of mothers of infants with ankyloglossia have these problems (Messner et al., 2000). Some infants may also present with a high arched palate because the tongue's contact with the palate during gestation typically gives the palate its characteristic shape. A tongue that cannot assume its normal position may contribute to an alteration in the oral cavity's shape, acting as a further contributor to sore nipples in the mother and possible diminished milk transfer in the infant. Mothers themselves describe obvious differences between breastfeeding older children who are unaffected and breastfeeding a subsequent infant with tongue-tie. After tongue-tie release, most mothers note an improvement in breastfeeding and a reduction in nipple trauma (Lalakea & Messner, 2003a). Mothers having difficulty breastfeeding from nipple pain due to infant ankyloglossia show a significant long-term benefit from frenulotomy (or frenotomy). Khoo, Dabbas, Sudhakaran, Ade-Ajayi, and Patel (2009) showed that pre-frenulotomy nipple pain was associated with an increased likelihood of not breastfeeding at 3 months. A mother with short nipples and inelastic breast tissue may present a problem for latching by the infant whose tongue cannot execute the maneuvers necessary to draw the nipple and areola deeply into the mouth (Genna, 2013). Even a mother's erect nipples may not be able to compensate for the infant's tongue alteration (Henry & Hayman, 2014).

- Shorter sucking bursts. Sucking burst durations have been reported to be much shorter in infants with tongue-tie and in those prone to malpositioning of the nipple in the infant's mouth (Garbin et al., 2013). Following frenotomy, the sucking burst duration lengthened, more milk was transferred during feeding at the breast, and respiratory rates (which had been higher during pre-frenotomy sucking) normalized to a lower rate. Frenotomy has been shown to not only increase the number of sucks per burst but also decrease the pause length between sucking bursts and improve the suck–swallow–breathe coordination (Martinelli, Marchesan, Gusmao, Honorio, & Berretin-Felix, 2015).
- Respiratory compromise. Researchers reported that tongue-tie can also be associated with displacement of the epiglottis and larynx, resulting in decreased oxygen saturation during feeding (Mukai, Mukai, & Asaoka, 1991). Young infants with ankyloglossia are often observed to come off of the breast frequently, pause for long periods of time between sucking bursts, and choke, cry, or fall asleep at the breast. Some of the improvement seen after frenotomy may also be due to the resolution of respiratory and circulatory compromise that could have been contributing to the altered breastfeeding patterns.
- Frustration in mothers. Mothers have described frustration and disappointment with breastfeeding a tongue-tied infant, especially if the condition is not identified by knowledgeable healthcare providers. Resolution of tongue-tie can lead to relief in mothers and a more pleasurable breastfeeding experience (Edmunds, Fulbrook, & Miles, 2013).
- Speech problems. Many of the shapes that the tongue engages in during feeding are also seen in speech production. It has been suggested that the matrix of tongue movements during human speech is derived from the wide range and variety of tongue movements found in suckling and feeding (Hiimae & Palmer, 2003). Controversy exists (even among speech therapists) regarding whether or not the anomaly interferes with speech (Messner & Lalakea, 2000). Some children with ankyloglossia develop normal speech as they learn to compensate for limited tongue mobility, even without speech therapy (Wright, 1995). Up to 50% of children with ankyloglossia referred for otolaryngology evaluation have articulation difficulties, with the rate

and range of articulation errors causing their speech to be difficult to understand (Fletcher & Meldrum, 1968; Lalakea & Messner, 2003b; Messner & Lalakea, 2002). Tongue-tie impacts tongue-tip mobility, affecting the sounds made by l, r, t, s, d, n, th, sh, and z. Although problematic to predict which infants with tongue-tie are likely to experience articulation problems later, the following characteristics are common in children with speech problems:

- V-shaped notch at the tip of the tongue
- Inability to protrude the tongue past the upper gums
- Inability to touch the roof of the mouth
- Difficulty moving the tongue from side to side

The release of a tongue-tie has been shown to have a positive effect on articulation, with z-plasty surgery having a better impact on speech/articulation than simple tongue-tie release (Yousefi et al., 2015).

- Dental and orthodontic problems. Pressure from a tight lingual frenulum can cause a diastasis or gap between the two lower central incisors, just as a taut labial frenulum (under the upper lip) can result in a large gap between the two upper central incisors. Restriction of normal tongue movements may result in a tongue thrust, forcing the tongue forward during a swallow instead of moving it up and back against the roof of the mouth. This can establish a pattern of abnormal swallowing (Palmer, 2001), affecting not only breastfeeding but also the ultimate positioning of the teeth.
- Slow weight gain or failure to thrive. Forlenza, Black, McNamara, and Sullivan (2010) reported on an extreme case of failure to thrive in an infant with severe ankyloglossia who was below his birth weight at 6 months of age. Feeding problems, poor latch, sore nipples, weight loss, and the mother's description of a "short tongue" were repeatedly ignored by healthcare providers. Milk transfer measured by pre- and postfeeding weights increased from 5 mL prior to frenotomy to 56 mL immediately after the first procedure and to a maximum of 190 mL after the second procedure for extension of the frenotomy. This illustrates the importance of taking ankyloglossia seriously. Tongue mobility is crucial for normal breastfeeding and the avoidance of sustained feeding problems in breastfed infants.
- Aerophagia (excessive intake of air into the stomach), bloating, excessive gas, and signs of reflux. Kotlow (2011) reported that infants who presented with a history of excessive gas, unresolved reflux, and bloating found relief when maxillary and lingual ties were revised. Infants who present with colic or reflux symptoms, especially of long unresolved duration, may benefit from an oral assessment for lingual and maxillary ties.

Controversies in Diagnosis and Management

Disagreement exists among a number of healthcare disciplines regarding the definition of ankyloglossia and its management. In a survey of medical experts, significant differences of opinion existed regarding ankyloglossia's association with breastfeeding difficulties, altered speech patterns, dental problems, and whether correction was needed or helpful (Messner & Lalakea, 2000).

Buryk, Bloom, and Shope (2011) conducted a randomized trial with 30 infants in the frenotomy group and 28 infants in a sham procedure group. There was an immediate improvement following frenotomy in maternal nipple pain, and an increase in the infants' breastfeeding scores. These effects were not seen in the sham procedure group, where mothers continued to experience painful nipples and infants' breastfeeding scores showed no improvement.

Berry, Griffins, and Westcott (2012) conducted a similar randomized, double-blind trial with one group of infants receiving a frenotomy and the other group no frenotomy. Seventy-eight percent of mothers in the frenotomy group reported an immediate improvement in breastfeeding compared with 47% of the mothers whose infants received the sham procedure. The majority of blinded mothers were able to correctly identify when the tongue-tie had been divided through changes in the way their infants fed.

Even though all breastfeeding difficulties seen in infants with ankyloglossia cannot be attributed to this condition with certainty, the severity of the problems generally support that the overall benefits of the procedure outweigh the minimal risks (Argiris, Vasani, Wong, Stimpson, Gunning, & Caulfield, 2011). Most mothers report an improvement in breastfeeding within 2 weeks of the procedure, if not immediately.

Frenotomy has been shown to produce a significant decline in breastfeeding symptom severity. A Breastfeeding Symptom Survey was created to help mothers recognize breastfeeding symptoms related to tongue-tie as early as possible. Results of this survey are intended to bring relevant symptoms to the attention of the lactation consultant or healthcare provider, thereby prompting them to determine the underlying cause of the symptoms and implement immediate interventions (Ochi, 2014). However, lack of universal improvement in breastfeeding following frenulotomy suggests that further investigation may be in order to ascertain if another surgery is needed or if other problems should be investigated (Sethi, Smith, Kortequee, Ward, & Clark, 2013).

The location and tightness of the frenulum can vary significantly, and the degree of tightness can influence consequences and outcomes. A number of schemata have been advanced to confirm the presence of ankyloglossia and grade its severity as a mechanism to validate intervention:

- The Assessment Tool for Lingual Frenulum Function (Hazelbaker, 1993) evaluates the infant's tongue with scores of 0 to 2 on five appearance items and seven function items, with frenotomy recommended when the score totals 8 or less on appearance and 11 or less on function. However, not all items on this tool have good interrater reliability (Madlon-Kay, Ricke, Baker, & DeFor, 2008). Amir, James, and Donath (2006) found that the first three items on the function score that assess the mobility of the tongue (forward extension, lateral movement, and tongue elevation) were reliable indicators for frenotomy when the score was less than or equal to 4.
- The Frenotomy Decision Rule for Breastfeeding Infants (Srinivasan, Dobrich, Mitnick, & Feldman, 2006) evaluates the need for frenotomy based on:
  - Mother with nipple pain/trauma, AND/OR inability to maintain latch, AND/OR poor infant weight gain, AND a visible frenulum restricting tongue movement, leading to:
    - Tongue unable to touch roof of mouth, OR
    - Tongue unable to cup examining finger, OR
    - Tongue cannot protrude beyond gum line
  - This approach found no relationship between actual length of the frenulum and breastfeeding problems, but the extent of breastfeeding difficulties determined if surgical correction was necessary. Frenotomy based on these criteria improved the LATCH score, reduced nipple pain almost immediately, and extended breastfeeding.

- Ankyloglossia was described and graded in relation to abnormalities of the lingual frenulum and to variations in the origin of the free portion of the tongue (Mukai et al., 1991).
- Ankyloglossia has been categorized by the length of the free tongue (length of the tongue from insertion of the lingual frenulum into the base of the tongue to the tip of the tongue). The normal range of the free tongue was defined as greater than 16 mm (Kotlow, 1999):
  - Class I: Mild ankyloglossia, 12–16 mm
  - Class II: Moderate, 8–11 mm
  - Class III: Severe, 3–7 mm
  - Class IV: Complete, less than 3 mm
- Structural guidelines were also advanced that described criteria for the normal range of motion and behavior of the tongue:
  - The tip of the tongue should be capable of protruding outside the mouth without clefting.
  - The tip of the tongue should be able to sweep the upper and lower lips without straining.
  - When the tongue is moved backward, it should not blanch the tissue behind the teeth.
  - The tongue should not place excessive forces on the lower central incisors.
  - The lingual frenulum should allow a normal swallowing pattern.
  - The lingual frenulum should not create a gap between the lower central incisors.
  - The underside of the infant's tongue should not exhibit abrasion or erosion.
  - The frenulum should not prohibit the infant from achieving a proper latch to the nipple/areola.
  - Speech difficulties should not be created from limited tongue movements.
- Tongue-ties were divided into four types according to how close to the tip of the tongue the leading edge of the frenulum was attached (Coryllos, Genna, & Salloum, 2004):
  - Type 1—the frenulum is attached to the tip of the tongue, in front of the alveolar ridge.
  - Type 2—the frenulum is attached 2–4 mm behind the tongue tip and attaches on or just behind the alveolar ridge.
  - Type 3—the frenulum attaches to the mid-tongue and the middle floor of the mouth. This is a tighter and less elastic frenulum.
  - Type 4—the frenulum is very thick, shiny, and highly inelastic because it is essentially attached against the base of the tongue. This situation can result in difficulties with bolus formation and swallowing because the tongue is unable to assume a cupped shape and form a central groove to channel milk to the back of the throat for the swallow. This tongue would have difficulty engaging in an anterior-to-posterior peristaltic wave with a resulting presentation of limited milk intake and sore or macerated maternal nipples. Although less common in occurrence, this type of tongue-tie is not immediately visible when the infant opens his or her mouth and can go unnoticed until breastfeeding problems become symptomatic.
- A lingual frenulum protocol with scores for infants was devised as a two-part evaluation to assess and diagnose anatomic alterations in the lingual frenulum. The first part consists of a clinical history of breastfeeding and family history; the second part is a clinical evaluation of the anatomic and functional aspects of the tongue, including assessment at breast. When the sum

of the history and clinical examination is equal to or more than 9, then the lingual frenum is considered altered (Martinelli, Marchesan, & Berretin-Felix, 2012).

- The Bristol Tongue Assessment Tool (BTAT) assesses four aspects of the tongue; tongue tip appearance, attachment of the frenulum to the lower gum ridge, lift of the tongue with the mouth wide open (crying), and protrusion of the tongue. The scores of the items are summed and can range from 0 to 8. Scores of 0–3 indicate more severe reduction of tongue function (Ingram et al., 2015).

Anterior and Posterior Tongue-Ties

Differentiating between the various grades or types of tongue-tie can be challenging, especially being able to recognize a posterior or submucosal tongue-tie. Anterior ankyloglossia is much more common and more easily managed than posterior ankyloglossia (Hong et al., 2010). Clinical signs of an anterior tongue-tie include a frenum that (Knox, 2010):

- Is thin and transparent
- Appears as a thin membrane
- Is reminiscent of mucosal tissue
- Attaches toward the anterior portion of the tongue

A posterior tongue-tie can be described as follows (Knox, 2010):

- A thick posterior fibrous strand in the midline between the underside of the tongue and the floor of the mouth
- No abnormality may be visible, with the tongue appearing to be flat
- Thick, white, and fibrous-looking frenum
- On palpation, the tissue is taut and firm and may feel like a ridge or bump when the gloved finger is moved laterally over the frenum
- Thick posterior frenum tissue may remain after the anterior membrane has been clipped

A posterior tongue-tie does not necessarily present with a heart-shaped tongue, as the tongue tip may actually be capable of elevation and extension over the lower gum. The tip of the tongue may curl under. Coryllos, Genna, and Fram (2013) describe markers of a posterior tongue-tie that include:

- The presence of a faint white line from the base of the tongue to the floor of the mouth that resists when pressed
- A deep crease down the middle of the tongue's underside
- Tremors of the tongue or jaw toward the end of a feeding, indicating that the infant is working too hard at feeding
- Resistance being felt when a gloved finger is pressed against where the tongue base meets the floor of the mouth
- Tongue retraction when the infant opens the mouth widely

Other markers or side effects of ankyloglossia include (Genna, 2013):

- Sucking blisters on the infant's lips from the sweeping action of the tongue or from compensation behaviors in which the infant uses the lips to apply pressure for holding the breast in the mouth
- Nipple abrasions resulting from the posterior tongue retracting and rubbing against the nipple
- Excessive jaw excursions
- Popping on and off the breast during a feeding

Dr. James Murphy palpates the oral cavity to identify tongue-tie by using the "Murphy Maneuver." With this technique, the pinky finger is inserted pad-side down into the left side of the infant's mouth under the tongue, and is gently swept across the floor of the mouth to the right. Normal frenulum anatomy is indicated by free movement of the finger, whereas encountering a "speed bump" indicates a tethered frenulum. A small bump can cause a slight lateral movement of the tongue; it rarely needs surgical treatment. A significant bump, in contrast, will cause the tongue to be dragged to the right side of the mouth; it is associated with a high likelihood of the need for treatment (Murphy, 2009).

Surgical revision of posterior tongue-tie may be even more important for improving breastfeeding mechanics. One study showed that among those infants with anterior ankyloglossia, 78% demonstrated some degree of improvement in breastfeeding following surgery; by comparison, 91% of those with posterior ankyloglossia showed some degree of breastfeeding improvement. Maxillary lip-tie release provided 100% improvement in breastfeeding (Pransky, Lago, & Hong, 2015).

Some practitioners may resist intervention and instead recommend waiting for the infant to outgrow the condition and/or place the infant on a bottle if breastfeeding difficulties cannot be resolved. Delays in surgical correction, even with intensive lactation counseling and education, usually do not improve breastfeeding (Hogan et al., 2005; Marmet et al., 1990). An infant with ankyloglossia can obtain milk from a bottle by a chewing motion that would be problematic at breast; however, placing such an infant on a bottle will not resolve the possible tongue thrust, faulty swallowing, open bite, and articulation errors that may still manifest themselves if the condition remains uncorrected. This infant might also experience problems swallowing semisolid foods when they are introduced. Visual and digital assessment of the infant's tongue reveals the extent of the problem with the mother often presenting with sore or macerated nipples (Ricke, Baker, Madlon-Kay, & DeFor, 2005), poor drainage of the breasts with possible resulting milk stasis, and descriptions of feeding sessions that are frustrating and lengthy. The infant may pop on and off the breast, make a clicking or smacking sound while nursing as the tongue loses contact with the nipple–areolar complex, dribble milk from the corners of the mouth because the tongue cannot form a central groove to channel milk to the back of the throat, and fatigue quickly during feedings (Fernando, 1998). Knox (2010) and the United Kingdom's National Institute for Health and Clinical Excellence (2005) recommend that frenotomy be considered when a thin anterior frenum is present that is associated with clinical signs and symptoms. A posterior tongue-tie is more likely to be associated with breastfeeding difficulties than thin anterior ones.

When Should Treatment Occur?

Treatment should occur within 24 hours of diagnosis (Knox, 2010) because of the time-sensitive nature for establishing an abundant milk supply, assuring adequate infant milk intake, and the necessity to alleviate any nipple pain being experienced by the mother. Steehler, Steehler, and Harley (2012) found that in a sample of 91 mothers of infants who underwent frenotomy for ankyloglossia, 80.4% strongly believed that the procedure benefited their infant's ability to breastfeed. However, this belief differed depending on when the procedure was performed. If frenotomy was performed in the 1st week of life, 86% of mothers thought it significantly improved breastfeeding. But if frenotomy was performed after the 1st week of life, 74% of mothers reported that the procedure significantly improved their infant's ability to breastfeed.

The Infant Breastfeeding Assessment Tool score was significantly higher in infants after undergoing a frenotomy (3.33 ± 1.51 prior to frenotomy vs. 9.19 ± 2.44 after frenotomy) compared to a nonsurgical control group of tongue-tied infants (4.17 ± 0.75 pre-intervention vs. 6.00 ± 1.73 post-intervention). For those undergoing frenotomy, a 94% improvement was noted by mothers of infants younger than 30 days versus a 68% improvement in infants older than 30 days (Sharma & Jayaraj, 2015).

The time-sensitive nature of the frenotomy procedure has been noted in other studies, in that a delay beyond 4 weeks from referral to assessment of tongue-tie is more likely to result in abandonment of breastfeeding (Donati-Bourne, Batool, Hendrickse, & Bowley, 2015). Earlier tongue-tie division has been shown to result in quicker recovery of appropriate feeding patterns (Blenkinsop, 2003). In a study of 31 tongue-tied infants, researchers found that frenotomy performed prior to day 8 had a greater impact on improving weight gain compared to frenotomy performed after day 8 (Praborini, Purnamasari, Munandar, & Wulandari, 2015). Even though latch was improved in infants undergoing frenotomy after day 8, it resulted in only small increases in weight. This may signal the need for rapid assessment and intervention when ankyloglossia is suspected and confirmed.

Geddes and colleagues (2008) performed ultrasound scans on the oral cavities of 24 infants with ankyloglossia before and after frenotomy. Total milk production of their mothers increased significantly after frenotomy, which serves to alert the clinician to ensure milk production remains adequate before and after surgery but especially in mothers if frenotomy is not performed. Milk intake, milk transfer, and the LATCH assessment scores increased significantly and the mothers' pain decreased significantly after surgery. Ultrasound scans identified two types of tongue movements, with infants compressing either the base or the tip of the nipple. These movements resolved following frenotomy, as did maternal nipple pain. Some mothers, depending on their breast anatomy, milk production, and milk ejection characteristics, may not experience sore nipples and their infants may breastfeed and gain weight adequately in spite of the presence of ankyloglossia (Geddes et al., 2010).

Kumar and Kalke (2012) remind clinicians that infants with ankyloglossia are at an increased risk for breastfeeding difficulties and that when such difficulties are present, a prompt referral is necessary to an experienced lactation consultant. This also constitutes the necessity for a referral for frenotomy, as there is strong evidence that frenotomy often results in rapid improvement of those difficulties.

Surgical Intervention

Clipping the frenulum, or frenotomy (without repair), is a simple procedure typically used for infants under 4 months of age that has a feeding improvement rate of up to 95% (Hogan et al., 2005). It is an office procedure performed by a doctor or dentist, without anesthesia or at the most perhaps topical benzocaine applied to each side of the frenulum. The procedure is usually brief and bloodless, with hemostasis (if needed) achieved by simple pressure or breastfeeding, which lengthens the tongue and acts as an analgesic and antiseptic. Frenuloplasty is a procedure often performed on older children (or in cases of severe ankyloglossia in infants) involving a more complete release of the frenulum with a plastic closure (z-plasty flap closure or a horizontal to vertical plasty). Complex cases can be referred to an oral surgeon or an ear, nose, and throat specialist. Some frenotomies can also be performed using a dental laser in a dentist's office or with an electrocautery needle (Kotlow, 2004a, 2004b; Naimer, Biton, Vardy, & Zvulunov, 2003).

Complications of frenotomy and frenuloplasty were historically reported to include concerns about pain, infection, excessive bleeding, scarring at the surgical site and restricted mobility of the tongue, too much tongue mobility, or damage to the orifices of the submandibular and lingual salivary glands. Current practitioners, however, report few if any complications and less pain than a vaccine injection (Ballard et al., 2002; Coryllos et al., 2004; Griffiths, 2004; Lalakea & Messner, 2003a). Frenotomy is a safe and effective early intervention for problems attributed to ankyloglossia (Segal, Stephenson, Dawes, & Feldman, 2007), especially given the association between nipple pain and the cessation of breastfeeding. Approximately 80% or more of infants will respond positively to frenotomy, with a low risk of harm being reported (Bowley & Arul, 2014). Because the procedure is minor and has a high success rate in alleviating breastfeeding difficulties, it could be considered an effective tool to help prolong both exclusive and partial breastfeeding (Dollberg, Marom, & Botzer, 2014).

Instructions for the frenotomy procedure can be found in a number of sources, including from the Academy of Breastfeeding Medicine Protocol Committee, Ballard, Chantry, and Howard (2004); Coryllos et al. (2004); Lalakea & Messner (2002); and Marmet et al. (1990). A video with a demonstration of the complete procedure along with follow-up breastfeeding management is also available (Jain, 1996).

Maxillary Lip-Tie

Ankyloglossia or tongue-tie is not the only alteration in oral frenal attachments. An abnormal frenulum attachment may also occur as a maxillary lip-tie. The maxillary frenum is the cord attaching the upper lip to the gum tissue. It can interfere with latching if its range of motion restricts the upward and outward movement of the lip away from the gum. A restriction in the maxillary frenulum would impact the ability of the upper lip to flare out and upward during the latch, potentially curling under and leading to lack of a seal around the breast, excessive intake of air, poor milk transfer due to reduced vacuum, and sore nipples.

Kotlow (2011) has developed a clinical classification of maxillary lip-tie. Clinicians may wish to check for this condition if an infant cannot flare out the upper lip, if the mother describes an infant with excessive gas, colic-like symptoms, bloating, reflux, or excessive fussiness; or experiences poor milk transfer, or nipple pain. A maxillary lip-tie appears as an excessive amount of vertical upper lip tissue and in many forms, ranging from small and string-like in appearance to a wide fan-like band. If a small crease is observed between the nose and upper lip when placing a finger into the infant's mouth, this is a sign that the lip is being tethered to the upper gum line (Kotlow, 2013).

When maxillary lip-tie is present, the maxillary frenulum can be clipped or revised with a dental laser just as the lingual frenulum. This release becomes important not just for proper breastfeeding but also in older infants whose upper central incisors (two front teeth) have erupted. When these infants nurse at night, milk may pool in the pockets created by the lip-tie and result in the development of dental caries on the outer surfaces of these teeth (Kotlow, 2013).

Breastfeeding Management

Ankyloglossia can be initially identified in the hospital before discharge with a typical presentation of a difficult or poor latch and persistent maternal nipple pain (Ballard et al., 2002). Infants may also present with sucking blisters on the upper and/or lower lip. This combination of breastfeeding difficulties is an indication to check the infant's lingual frenulum. Parents should be advised of the condition, its possible ramifications if left uncorrected (Karabulut et al., 2008), and options for and possible side effects of correction. Clipping the frenulum at this point improves latch, strength and rhythmicity of suckling, and milk transfer, and eliminates the clicking sounds and popping on and off the breast. Maternal nipple pain is significantly diminished (Dollberg, Botzer, Grunis, & Mimouni, 2006), removing a major roadblock to maternal breastfeeding plans. Once discharged, undiagnosed or uncorrected ankyloglossia may result in significantly more and severe complications. Ricke and colleagues (2005) reported that breastfeeding infants who were tongue-tied were three times more likely to be exclusively bottle-fed at 1 week than matched control infants with no tongue-tie. If surgical intervention is delayed or not an option (for religious, cultural, or personal reasons) or if parents are unable to locate a healthcare professional willing to perform the procedure, a breastfeeding plan would include the following:

- Positioning of the infant that would encourage gravity assistance for the tongue to move down and forward (semiprone, completely vertical, or an upright clutch hold)
- Latch modifications that might include stroking the infant's tongue down and forward, chin or jaw support, and techniques to evert flat nipples before latch
- Using a nipple shield for relief from the pain and adequate milk transfer to the infant
- Pumping milk to follow each feeding to ensure an adequate supply and to provide as a supplement if the infant is unable to transfer sufficient amounts of milk or if the maternal nipples are too sore or damaged
- Checking the weight frequently to ensure adequate infant growth
- Paying close attention to articulation achievements as the infant begins to vocalize

If surgical intervention is an option, the mother should be informed of the following:

- Frenotomy usually provides immediate relief from nipple pain and markedly improved infant latch and milk transfer.
- Infants engage in compensatory tongue movements, resulting in varied patterns of tongue, mouth, head, neck, and body movements while breastfeeding.
- If ankyloglossia has remained uncorrected for a period of time (usually more than 5 days), the infant may need time to retrain the tongue and develop suckling strength. To help infants learn the use of a newly mobilized tongue, they may benefit from having the tongue stroked down and forward before each feeding. To encourage extension of the tongue, tongue "exercises" can be used such as dipping a cotton swab in breastmilk or a flavoring and touching the tip and sides of the tongue to encourage forward and lateral movement. To improve suckling strength,

a nipple tug can be used several times during each feeding if the maternal nipples are not sore (the mother pulls back slightly on the nipple or pulls the infant slightly away from the breast while latched, not enough to break suction but enough to cause the infant to draw the nipple/areola deeper into the mouth). If the nipples are sore, the tugging can be done with a clean finger in the infant's mouth, pulling back slightly without breaking suction to encourage the infant to exert more vacuum.

Follow up on all maternal and infant breastfeeding complications of ankyloglossia should take place immediately after the surgical procedure until resolved and should be ongoing if no interventions are used to correct the defect. Maternal complications include the following:

- Damage or infection to the nipples may require topical medication and hand expression rather than mechanical expression, unless pumping remains comfortable. A mother with flat nipples may wish to evert the nipple before placing the infant at breast to avoid further pain or damage.
- Milk stasis or mastitis may respond well to use of alternate massage during breastfeedings and/or pumping with breast massage between feeds. Inflammatory conditions may also respond well to systemic nonsteroidal anti-inflammatory medications.
- Diminished milk production is addressed by frequent feedings at breast with alternate massage and pumping milk until adequate production is established. The pump flange should be large enough to avoid causing pain to the nipples.

Infant issues may include the following:

- The infant should be assessed during a feeding to ensure milk transfer and adequate intake, with pre- and postfeed weights taken if needed. Weight checks should take place every 3 to 4 days until an acceptable weight gain pattern is established. Infants having difficulty with milk transfer may need to be temporarily supplemented with pumped breastmilk.
- After a frenotomy, a white patch under the tongue at the surgical site is normal for about 48 hours. Pain medication and antibiotics are rarely, if ever, required.
- Many practitioners recommend that for the best results following a frenotomy and especially after the division of a posterior tongue-tie, that stretching exercises be done to prevent adhesions from forming that would revert the tongue back to its restrictive condition. The International Affiliation of Tongue-Tie Professionals recommends elevating the tongue 5 to 8 times daily for a week after the procedure. The stretching can be done for 3 seconds at every feeding until complete healing, which can take close to 14 days (Edmunds, Hazelbaker, Murphy, & Philipp, 2012).

Cleft Lips and Palates

As the fourth most common congenital disability, oral clefting represents a significant feeding challenge to the infant, to his or her parents, and to the interdisciplinary healthcare team involved in caring for such an infant over an extended period of time (Edmondson & Reinhartsen, 1998). It may occur in isolation or as part of 150–300 syndromes (Cohen & Bankier, 1991). Up to 13% of infants with clefting have other birth defects. Some genetic influence may be present (Merritt, 2005a) as once one child is affected, parents have a 40% chance of having another affected child. In the United States the prevalence for cleft lip with or without cleft palate is 2.2–11.7 per 10,000 births. Cleft palate alone results in a prevalence rate of 5.5–6.6 per 10,000 births (Forrester & Merz, 2004). It is most prevalent among Native Americans (3.6/1,000 births) and less commonly seen in Asians (1.7–2.1/1,000 births), whites (1/1,000 births), and African Americans (0.3/1,000 births; Lewanda & Jabs, 1994). Each year in the United States, 2,651 infants are born with a cleft palate and 4,437 babies are born with a cleft lip, with or without a cleft palate (Parker et al., 2010). About 70% of all orofacial clefts are isolated clefts.

Although cleft lip and palate are frequently associated with each other, they develop separately at differing gestational ages, allowing a child to present with one or any combination of clefting. Approximately 50% have a combined cleft lip and palate, whereas 30% have an isolated cleft palate and 20% have an isolated cleft lip. Cleft lip results when the two sides of the lip fail to fuse during the 5th to 8th weeks of gestation. This may also include a split in the upper gum (alveolar ridge) and upper jaw. Cleft palate occurs when the palatine processes do not join during the 6th to 12th weeks of gestation.

The etiology of clefting is not well understood and most likely results from a combination of genetic and environmental factors. Gene variants have been identified that may contribute to oral clefts and triple the risk of recurrence in affected families (Zucchero et al., 2004). A few of the numerous recognized teratogens have been identified as being associated with cleft defects, including alcohol consumption during the embryonic period and ingestion of drugs, such as phenytoin and retinoids, and illicit drugs, such as cocaine. Ultrasound can detect clefts as early as 17 weeks of gestation. Some data have shown that mothers who take multivitamins containing folic acid or consume vitamin-enriched cereals from 2 months before conception through the 1st trimester can reduce the risk of clefting by 25–50% (Shaw, Lammer, Wasserman, O'Malley, & Tolarova, 1995; Tolarova & Harris, 1995).

A breakdown of cleft lip and/or palate shows three groups: sporadic occurrence (75–80%), familial (10–15%), and clefting associated with syndromes (1–5%). Additional anomalies present in 44–64% of all infants with oral clefting (Sprintzen, Siegel-Sadewitz, Amato, & Goldberg, 1985). Routine screening for associated malformations in infants with clefting may find cardiac, skeletal, and central nervous system anomalies along with possible effects seen in the eyes, ears, digestive system, and urogenital system (Rawashdeh & Jawdat Abu-Hawas, 2008).

Clefting may be diagnosed prenatally, is usually apparent at birth, and requires sensitive and supportive care from the healthcare team. Parents need immediate help with feeding techniques and plans before discharge. Mothers need to be shown how to feed the infant, how to determine sufficient intake, what problems to anticipate, and how to handle problems, as provision of breastmilk for these infants tends to be of a shorter duration (Smedegaard, Marxen, Moes, Glassou, & Scientsan, 2008). Feeding challenges are usually the first priority for parents. Many mothers discharged from the hospital lack adequate information, are in need of specific feeding instructions, and experience dissatisfaction with the type and amount of information and follow-up they received (Byrnes, Berk, Cooper, & Marazita, 2003; Oliver & Jones, 1997; Trenouth & Campbell, 1996; Young, O'Riordan, Goldstein, & Robin, 2001). Mothers of infants with clefting are eager for information and quite responsive to the needs of their infant (Coy, Speltz, & Jones, 2002).

Feeding directly from the breast may be an option for infants with an isolated cleft of the lip, a narrow or small posterior clefting of the palate, or a small submucous cleft (Curtin, 1990). Reid, Reilly, and Kilpatrick (2007) found that infants with cleft lip generate the greatest amount of suction followed by those with cleft palate and those with cleft lip and palate, whereas infants with cleft lip and palate generate reduced amounts of compression. However, with greater involvement of the palate, generation of intraoral suction is significantly compromised, and with a bilateral cleft palate, it may be difficult or impossible to compress the nipple between the tongue and any part of the roof of the mouth.

Poor feeding skills are common, especially if the cleft palate is associated with a syndrome or Pierre Robin sequence (Reid, Kilpatrick, & Reilly, 2006). Sucking parameters are altered in cleft-involved infants. Masarei and colleagues (2007) showed that sucking was less efficient in cleft-involved infants, with shorter sucks, a faster rate of sucking, more sucks per swallow, and a greater proportion of intraoral positive-pressure generation than infants without clefting. This may necessitate assisted milk delivery and a modification of feeding management, including short- or long-term breastmilk expression (Stockdale, 2000).

Human milk is very important to infants with clefting. Children with cleft lip and palate are at an increased risk for otitis media and hearing, speech, language, social, dental, and academic difficulties. The greater the degree of hearing loss at 12 months, the lower the language scores for expressive skills and comprehension (Jocelyn, Penko, & Rode, 1996). Children with clefts who are breastfed or receive breastmilk for less than a month have been shown to require special education services in significantly higher numbers, demonstrating that a short duration of breastmilk intake is associated with poorer school performance (Erkkila, Isotalo, Pulkkinen, & Haapanen, 2005). The provision of breastmilk, even if the infant cannot feed directly from the breast, has been shown to reduce middle ear infections and improve the amount of time infants are free from effusion, contributing to the reduction of conductive hearing loss. Protection against otitis media extends well beyond the period of breastmilk feeding (Paradise, Elster, & Tan, 1994). Aniansson, Svensson, Becker, and Ingvarsson (2002) demonstrated a significant correlation during the first 18 months of life between a longer duration of feeding with breastmilk and a lower incidence of acute and secretory otitis media, concluding that premature cessation of human milk feeding can contribute to an increased incidence of both acute and secretory otitis media. While infants with a cleft lip are more likely to receive breastmilk exclusively, unfortunately infants with a cleft palate or combined cleft lip and palate are less likely to receive any breastmilk at all (Kaye et al., 2016). Feeding infants with a cleft palate is difficult no matter how they are fed, but breastmilk is a very important aspect of nutritional support, immune function, and future health of the infant.

Feeding methods and feeding management guidelines can be selected based on the variety of sizes and positions of the clefts, the anatomic shape and size of the maternal nipple/areola, the breastmilk supply and rate of milk flow, the choice of specialized equipment and techniques, and when surgical interventions are planned. Breastfeeding is important to infants with clefts to aid in the development of muscles for feeding as well as those for speech (Merritt, 2005b).

A number of specialized feeding devices and common equipment can be selected and combined to best match the infant's needs and contribute to a tailored approach for each individual situation:

- Palatal obturator. An obturator is a Silastic or acrylic device that acts as an artificial palate that, when custom molded, fills or occludes the palatal cleft. They are fabricated by a pediatric dentist or prosthodontist for a hard palate cleft and are not used for submucous clefts or clefts of the soft palate (Osuji, 1995). Some infants are fitted for the obturator within the first few days after birth to act as the initial orthopedic treatment in facilitating or directing the desired development of the oral cavity. The device supports the palatal shelves as they grow and keeps the tongue out of the cleft, helping to normalize tongue activity and positioning and preventing the tongue from widening the cleft. It simultaneously acts as a feeding appliance to create a seal over the palatal cleft, providing a mechanism for generating negative intraoral pressure and a surface against which the tongue can compress the nipple (Crossman, 1998). Use of an obturator has been shown to reduce feeding times, enhance the volume of milk consumed (Turner et al., 2001), develop some weak intraoral negative pressure (Kogo et al., 1997), and allow an infant to feed directly at breast for at least some of his or her required intake. Turner and Moore (1995) and Humenczuk (1998) described highly motivated breastfeeding mothers whose infants could obtain 25–50% of their milk at the breast with early insertion of a palatal obturator, with the rest of the infants' nutritional requirements provided through the SpecialNeeds Feeder (formerly called the Haberman Feeder). The appliance should be checked for rough edges if the mother complains of sore nipples while breastfeeding when the obturator is in place. Studies of obturator use have yielded conflicting opinions and data (Goyal, Chopra, Bansal, & Marwaha, 2014), but if a higher volume of milk is ingested, it indicates improved sucking performance and an encouraging step toward more successful breastfeeding.

- The SpecialNeeds Feeder (Haberman Feeder). The SpecialNeeds Feeder nipple has a slit rather than cross-cut opening and is attached to a milk reservoir with a one-way valve, allowing milk but not air to enter the reservoir chamber. The chamber is pliable so that milk can be gently squeezed into the infant's mouth as needed. Around the base of the nipple are markings to indicate how to position the nipple to achieve variations in flow rate. The nipple shank is available in a standard length and a shorter preemie length. Milk can be extracted from this device by compression only so that an infant who cannot generate vacuum can obtain milk through the compressive force generated by the jaw and gums (Haberman, 1988).
- Mead-Johnson Cleft Lip/Palate Nurser. This feeder has a long, soft, thin-walled nipple with a crosscut design to direct the milk flow past the cleft. If the nipple is too long for the infant, a standard nipple with a single hole or an orthodontic nipple can be substituted. The bottle is soft and is easily squeezed in rhythm to the infant's sucking and swallowing movements. The bottle is gently pulsed, not continually squeezed, to overcome the lack of vacuum and to ensure that milk is not aspirated from a rapid or forceful injection of milk into the back of the throat. A flexible or squeezable bottle may be easier for parents to use and results in an increased volume of milk intake and good weight outcomes when assisted feeding is needed (Shaw, Bannister, & Roberts, 1999).
- Pigeon Cleft Palate Nipple. The Pigeon Nipple works by compression only. The nipple has a firm side that is oriented toward the roof of the mouth and a softer side that is placed on the tongue. A small notch at the base of the nipple serves as an air vent. This notch should be uppermost under the baby's nose when feeding. Tightening the nipple and collar slows the flow of milk. Loosening it makes the flow faster. If the nipple collapses, it should be loosened and retightened. A plastic one-way valve fits into the nipple to keep milk in the nipple. The valve should be placed with the flat side toward the tip of the nipple. When the baby begins to suck,

milk flows readily. The infant controls the flow of milk and no squeezing of the bottle is needed. The Pigeon Baby Bottle is specifically shaped to fit the air vents and one-way valve of the Pigeon Cleft Palate Nipple.

- Ross Cleft Palate Assembly (Abbott Nutrition). This nipple tapers to a small narrow tube and frequently is used after surgical repair of the palate or to hasten feedings when they routinely take longer than 40 minutes. It provides a continuous flow of milk and must be used carefully to avoid milk flow that the infant is unable to handle. A catheter-tipped plunger syringe, Brecht feeder, or Asepto syringe with a length of soft tubing is also sometimes used after surgery.
- Angled bottles. These usually make it easier to feed infants in an upright position.
- Supplemental nursing system (SNS) or the Lact-Aid Nursing Trainer System. Both tube-feeding devices deliver supplemental milk at the breast, can be squeezed to facilitate milk flow, and can be suspended around the mother's neck at varying heights for gravity-assisted flow. Some infants with a small cleft may have enough intact palate toward which the breast and tubing can be directed.
- Nipple shields. These have also been used in some situations because they provide a firm teat. Once milk is drawn into or expressed into the teat, weak suckling or compression will withdraw the milk.
- Spoons, cups, and syringes. These devices are sometimes used by parents for delivering extra milk. In one study, the use of a disposable syringe to feed 1- to 14-week-old infants with cleft lip and palate resulted in a faster feeding time, less spillage and regurgitation, and a weight gain similar to a control group of infants without cleft lip and palate (Ize-Iyamu & Saheeb, 2011).
- Hospital-grade electric breast pump with a double collection kit. Most mothers of infants with clefting, especially when the infant has a cleft palate, will need to express milk, sometimes for an extended period of time (Stockdale, 2000).
- Digital scale. A rented digital scale can be used for pre- and postfeed weights to monitor intake of the recommended amount of milk each 24 hours until feeding and weight gain are well established.

Pre- and Postoperative Considerations

Primary surgical closure of the cleft lip may take place as early as 2–3 days of age and usually within the first 3 months of life. Early lip closure has the potential to alter the palatal dimensions, which is why early lip closure may be accompanied by the use of a palatal obturator to prevent palatal collapse immediately after lip surgery (Kramer, Hoeksma, & Prahl-Andersen, 1994). Repair of the palate usually takes place in the second half of the first year. Some surgeons currently repair the palate before 6 months of age, with feeding directly from the breast a possibility as a result. A study of 21 infants undergoing palate repair within the 1st month of life and returning to breastfeeding or bottle-feeding after recovery from anesthesia showed no short-term adverse outcomes, although long-term effects on facial development and speech were not evaluated (Denk, 1998).

Although opinions vary (Redford-Badwal, Mabry, & Frassinelli, 2003), most infants can feed directly from the breast immediately after cleft lip repair surgery without disrupting the integrity of the suture line (Weatherly-White, Kuehn, Mirrett, Gilman, & Weatherley-White, 1987). Returning to direct breastfeeding rather than using spoon, dropper, bottle, or tube and syringe feedings post-surgery after both cleft lip and cleft palate repair has been shown to be advantageous to infants in that they require less sedation, fewer intravenous fluids and hospital days, and are capable of gaining weight while avoiding disruption of the surgical repair (Cohen, Marschall, & Schafer, 1992; Darzi, Chowdri, & Bhat, 1996).

With the possibility of direct breastfeeding after cleft repair, mothers need to ensure that they have an abundant milk supply that can be sustained over a protracted period of time. It is to the infant's advantage to be put to breast before surgical repairs, even if he or she is unable to secure all the milk needed for growth. At a minimum, this facilitates familiarity with the breast and a soft soothing breast for comfort sucking, with most milk provided through assisted delivery devices as necessary. Although infants with cleft palates may not be able to support normal growth through exclusive feeding at the breast, imprinting on the breast is desirable. This keeps open the option for some feedings at the breast after lip and/or palate repair.

Feeding and Breastfeeding Management

There is a paucity of information describing breastfeeding and breastfeeding outcomes in the cleft population (Reid, 2004). However, breastfeeding directly at the breast for the provision of breastmilk is possible and should be encouraged (Donovan, 2012). Evidence-based guidelines for breastfeeding infants with clefting help increase the likelihood that these infants will receive breastmilk and enjoy feeding at the breast (Reilly et al., 2013). A combination of feeding methods is generally used to provide an optimal feeding environment for infants with clefting. Clarren, Anderson, and Wolf (1987) described an approach that considered the parameters of the feeding deficit in terms of the anatomic defect and then matched the deficits to the specific feeding devices or techniques. They based their recommendations on assessment of how the deficit affects the normal feeding parameters of generation of negative pressure and the ability to engage in mechanical movements. Infants with a cleft lip, cleft palate, or a combination of both who do not have concomitant health problems or other syndromes that would affect feeding generally swallow normally but suck abnormally. Reflux of milk through the nose without sequelae is not diagnostic of a swallowing problem. Infants with cleft palate can ingest excessive amounts of air because there is no separation between the nasal and oral cavities. This leads to bloating, choking, gagging, fatigue with feeding, prolonged feeding times, and spitting up (Cooper-Brown et al., 2008). Generation of negative pressure is generally precluded when there is a cleft in the lip and alveolus, the bony palate, or a combination, unless the deficit can be plugged. Problems with the actual muscular movements used by the infant in the mechanics of feeding occur in the following three cleft-related defects:

1. Bilateral cleft lip when there is significant anterior projection of the premaxilla makes it difficult for the infant to stabilize the nipple.
2. Wide or extensive palatal clefts involve so much of the palate that there is little to no surface against which the tongue can press the nipple.
3. Retroplaced tongues may be actively inserted into the palatal cleft; they may not cup and move down and forward, contributing to an inability to perform coordinated movements.

Cleft Lip Only

Clefts of the lip can range from a small unilateral notch to bilateral clefts that extend into the nares with projection of the premaxilla. Presurgical orthopedic appliances or treatments may be placed to help mold the nose. In the absence of any coexisting problems, infants with an isolated cleft lip demonstrate appropriate mechanical movements of the tongue and jaw to compress the nipple, form a bolus, and swallow normally, but negative pressure or vacuum could be compromised by the lack of an intact upper lip to form a seal. Evidence has shown that infants with cleft lip can generate suction and breastfeed successfully (Choi, Kleinheinz, Joos, & Komposch, 1991; Garcez & Giugliani, 2005). The most frequently seen problems are the presence of weak suction, difficulty in latching to the breast, and breastmilk escaping through the nostrils.

Techniques. Positioning at the breast is most important for these infants. Typically, for a unilateral defect, the breast should enter the mouth from the side on which the defect is located so that the nipple/areola approximates the section of the palate that is most intact. A cleft in the lip may be sealed by breast tissue or by the mother's thumb pushing the tissue over the gap. An infant with a bilateral defect often feeds best when directly facing the breast in a straddle position with the breast tipped down or angled slightly to one side of the mouth (Danner, 1992a). Some infants feed more efficiently when their throat is level with or slightly higher than the breast such that the nape of the neck is level with or slightly higher than the areola. Other infants can obtain more milk by having the mother lean over them, allowing gravity to assist in keeping the breast in the infant's mouth (Danner, 1997).

Because the infant with a cleft palate is usually unable to generate sufficient intraoral negative pressure to hold the breast in his or her mouth, the mother needs to support the breast and the infant's head to keep the infant from falling off the breast. Substantial chin support is needed such as with the Dancer hand position.

Positioning for feeding by bottle is also a concern. Proper position of the head and neck is important, with the head usually at an angle between 40 and 60 degrees to minimize nasal regurgitation of milk. The infant's chin may need to be supported, especially if the jaw is small. Infants tend to swallow a lot of air and may need to be burped frequently. The bottle is squeezed rhythmically when the infant sucks or every 3–5 sucks if the infant experiences breathing difficulties while feeding. It is important that the artificial nipple is placed on top of the tongue as it is inserted, because there is a tendency for the tongue to be pushed or drawn backward into the mouth, obstructing the airway and preventing proper sucking movements.

The use of the Dancer hand position helps to stabilize the infant's mouth. If the mother presses her thumb and forefinger gently against the infant's cheeks, this causes the buccal surfaces of the cheek to maintain contact with the nipple, improving oral suction.

Some mothers with an abundant milk supply can hand express milk into the infant's mouth. This may partially meet the needs of the infant, but many infants require supplemental milk after feeding at the breast.

Listening plays a key role in breastfeeding the challenged infant. Swallowing at breast is a reassuring sign that milk intake has occurred. A nonreassuring sign is the soft hissing or "kissing" sound of air going through the cleft (Biancuzzo, 1998; Glass & Wolf, 1999).

Infants can be positioned in a clutch or very upright cradle or cross-cradle position. Some infants prefer to straddle the mother's thigh, facing the breast with the neck slightly extended and lower jaw pressing close into the breast. The mother's breast tissue may occlude the cleft with no further adjustment, or the mother may need to either cover the cleft with her thumb or press breast tissue over the cleft to prevent an air leak. If the lip curls under, the mother can lift and reposition it. The infant's head and the mother's breast need to be securely held during the entire feeding, allowing the breast tissue to conform to the defect and prevent the infant from losing his or her grip on the nipple/areola. Because the infant may be unable to generate the initial suction necessary to draw the nipple/areola far into the mouth and elongate these tissues to form a teat, some mothers report that they manually form or shape the nipple and place it into the infant's mouth as an assisted form of latching (Grady, 1977; Styer & Freeh, 1981). The mother can use alternate massage to initiate and sustain sucking and improve both volume and fat content of each feeding. If the infant tires easily, the mother can hand express milk directly into the infant's mouth.

Equipment. If feedings take longer than 30–45 minutes and/or the infant is not gaining weight adequately, a Lact-Aid Nursing Trainer or SNS device may be used to deliver more milk in a shorter period of time while still feeding at the breast. If weight gain is an ongoing issue, consider using pumped hindmilk in the supplementing device at breast or secured to a finger for finger feeding. Extra milk can also be delivered by periodontal syringe while sucking on the breast or on a finger, by cup, or by bottle using an artificial nipple with a large soft base that occludes the cleft and offers variable flow options. Feedings using a disposable syringe have been shown to result in adequate weight gain, faster feeding times, less spillage, and decreased nasal regurgitation (Ize-Iyamu & Saheeb, 2011).

Cleft of the Soft Palate, Submucous Cleft, or Bifid Uvula

Many infants with soft palate clefting may breastfeed normally. Others may breastfeed well until the head grows larger and the unseen gap in the underlying musculature widens. Some infants may regurgitate milk through their nose when the soft palate does not seal against the tongue. Paradise and colleagues (1994) rated the severity or degree of nasal regurgitation as an indicator of the degree of impairment of palatal function (none, mild, moderate, and severe) but provided no data on whether this aspect was predictive of breastfeeding outcomes. Miller (1998) anecdotally found that breastfeeding success before surgical repair of the palate seemed inversely proportional to the size of the cleft in the soft palate, not the total size of the entire cleft. When there is difficulty with palatal movement, oral suction may be interrupted prematurely, a click may be heard when the seal is broken, intermittent airway obstruction is possible with noisy breathing, the volume of fluid per suck may be reduced, and feeding can become inefficient (Wolf & Glass, 1992). Weight gain should be monitored closely, as with all types of cleft defects.

Techniques. Any feeding at the breast should be done in an upright position to reduce nasal regurgitation. Breastfeeding in a side-lying position may exacerbate this problem. Alternate massage may be helpful to improve volume and fat intake per suck and per feeding. The infant's head position may need to be adjusted and modified to reduce the possibility of airway obstruction or swallowing difficulties.

Equipment. Palatal obturators are not used for soft palate clefts. Weight gain may be monitored by pre- and postfeed weights on a digital scale. Hindmilk supplements may be needed for weight gain and can be delivered through tube-feeding devices; milk may need to be pumped if the infant is unable to obtain adequate amounts from direct feedings at the breast. If the mother chooses to use an artificial nipple, she may find that a standard nipple with a longer nipple shaft is efficient and effective. An angled bottle also allows the infant to be more easily fed in an upright position.

Isolated Cleft of the Bony (Hard) Palate

The generation of both vacuum and compression is affected depending on the location and size of the cleft. Effective vacuum and compression of the nipple/areola is not possible with a large midline cleft. With a narrow or posterior cleft, enough intact palate may exist for the generation of sufficient vacuum to position and stabilize the nipple in the anterior portion of the mouth or to the opposite side of the mouth, where the tongue would find an opposing surface against which to elongate and compress the breast. However, this may increase the likelihood of sore or damaged nipples. Feedings at breast may be sufficient enough for at least a partial intake of milk but may need to be supplemented.

Techniques. Upright positioning is recommended. The mother may need to manually shape and insert her nipple/areola into the infant's mouth if sufficient vacuum cannot be generated to draw in and hold the nipple/areola in place. Hand expression of milk directly into the infant's mouth improves intake at each feeding. If the cleft is unilateral (not midline), the infant may do better with the breast entering the mouth from the side on which the defect is located, thus directing the nipple to the area of the palate that is intact (Danner, 1992a). The breast must be held in the infant's mouth with chin support, and the infant must be held to the breast for the entire feeding.

Equipment. With a large cleft, extra milk can be provided at breast through a Lact-Aid Nursing Trainer, SNS, or tubing attached to a syringe. These devices normally require an infant to generate suction to cause the milk to flow. The SNS or Lact-Aid Nursing Trainer may need to be suspended in a higher position with the tubing straighter and of a larger size, and on the SNS, both tubes may need to be open for optimal milk flow. Pressure usually needs to be applied to the milk container suspended between the mother's breasts in rhythm with the infant's sucking. Pressure should be applied just after the gums compress the areola to sequence the milk bolus to enter the infant's mouth at the same time any milk flows from the breast (Danner, 1997). The tubing may need to be taped to the breast on the same axis that the breast enters the infant's mouth such that the tubing is placed to the side of the nipple where the intact palate is or where the nipple and tubing can be compressed along the alveolar ridge. The tubing can also be taped to the underside of the mother's areola, whichever gives the best results. A nipple shield may be used and tubing can be attached either under or on top of the shield for the delivery of additional milk. If the infant needs to be further supplemented, a SpecialNeeds Feeder (Haberman Feeder) or other flexible bottle arrangement can be used to ensure adequate intake per feeding in a reasonable amount of time.

Cleft Lip and Palate

When a cleft lip and palate are present, the cleft is usually quite large with little to no intact palate for compression, making the generation of vacuum impossible (Wolf & Glass, 1992). Some milk intake may be possible in a few infants, but the majority of milk needs to be delivered with assistive devices. Palatal obturators may be used, which occlude the cleft and allow compression and some suction. Nipple shields may also be tried. Infants may fatigue quickly when being fed or become fussy with hunger and small milk intakes. Weight checks should be frequent because weight gain can be rapidly compromised by the infant's limited ability to consume milk in a reasonable amount of time.

Techniques. The infant with a bilateral cleft can be positioned to directly face the breast by straddling the mother's lap. The breast, nipple, and areola need to be shaped and guided to the side with the most intact tissue and pointed slightly downward. The mother can elicit the milk-ejection reflex and hand express milk into the infant's mouth, at least for the beginning of the feeding. She then follows with pumped milk through either a tube-feeding device at the breast or her choice of an assistive feeding device. The amount of milk needed by the infant each day should be calculated and a plan designed to ensure adequate intake. Infants have an easier time accomplishing any feeding at breast if they are at least put to the breast intermittently, even if they receive the bulk of their milk from a feeding device. Many mothers reserve the breastfeeding time as cuddle time without the pressure and expectation of large milk intakes.

Equipment. Mothers may use a digital scale for determining the amount of milk taken from the breast to calculate how much to offer as a supplement. Daily weights are taken to ensure appropriate weight gain. Mothers need an electric pump with a double collection kit, and pumping times should be built into the daily feeding plan. If the mother uses a bottle for assisted milk delivery, she should choose one with a nipple that does not deliver milk so fast that it compromises swallowing and breathing and one that works to stimulate sucking patterns as close to those of breastfeeding as possible (Noble & Bovey, 1997). The flow rate of an artificial nipple should be similar to that from the breast, 0.1–0.5 cc per suck (Wolf & Glass, 1992). Usually, a squeezable bottle with a standard-size nipple hole is sufficient. Cutting larger holes or cross-cuts into the nipple may create a rapid and irregular flow of milk. Infants showing signs of being overwhelmed by a fast flow of milk may need to rest each three to five sucks by removing the bottle from the infant's mouth or using a nipple with a smaller hole (Richard, 1991). A SpecialNeeds Feeder (Haberman Feeder) is also a good choice because it delivers milk with compression and allows the feeder to gently squeeze the milk reservoir if needed. Milk does not flow back into the bottle and ingested air is minimized.

Parents of infants affected by any type of clefting need individual information and support from healthcare professionals with expertise in feeding these special infants. This expert help is needed immediately at the time of diagnosis and until feedings become manageable. Many mothers receive inaccurate and conflicting information and must rely on their own skills to manage the early feedings (Lindberg & Berglund, 2014). These mothers may be challenged by the burden of expressing their milk and need clear guidelines on how to balance feedings, pumping, and the other aspects of their day-to-day lives.

SYNDROMES AND CONGENITAL ANOMALIES

Pierre Robin Sequence

Pierre Robin sequence (PRS) is characterized by the presence of three congenital anomalies: micrognathia or retrognathia (a small or posteriorly positioned mandible located about 10–12 mm behind the superior arch), glossoptosis (a normal-sized tongue that is displaced into the pharynx, causing obstruction of the airway), and a wide U-shaped cleft palate. It occurs in approximately 1 in 8,850 live births (Sheffield, Reiss, Strohm, & Gilding, 1987) and is termed a sequence rather than a syndrome. In approximately 80% of newborns with PRS, the triad of anomalies occurs as part of an underlying genetic condition. About 40% of infants with PRS have Stickler syndrome (a tissue disorder that includes not only clefting but also cataracts or retinal detachment, a flat face, a small jaw, and skeletal abnormalities, hearing loss, and cardiac problems) with another 15% experiencing velocardiofacial syndrome (an autosomal dominant condition that includes not only clefting but abnormalities of the heart, learning disabilities, hearing loss, speech problems, leg pain, and behavior extremes). Hyoid bone abnormalities have been observed in some infants with PRS and are associated with swallowing dysfunction (El Amm & Denny, 2008). Infants with PRS should always be evaluated for other underlying or associated conditions (Prows & Bender, 1999).

The single defect that initiates the cascade of anomalies is micrognathia. The abnormally small mandible during fetal development displaces the tongue to such a posterior position that it prevents the palatal shelves from fusing, creating the cleft in the palate. The small mandible can be caused by mechanical factors in utero such as fibroids or a transverse position; by teratogens such as alcohol, isotretinoin (Accutane), or tobacco; and/or by genetic factors such as chromosome abnormalities or gene mutations. The primary problem upon birth is airway obstruction, with prone positioning used to bring the tongue forward to create a patent airway. If this simple positioning is not effective, other interventions may be used as needed such as a nasopharyngeal airway, continuous positive airway pressure, surgery, or tracheostomy (Marques et al., 2001).

The chronic airway resistance caused by PRS requires infants to exert increased breathing and cardiac efforts that consume additional calories. The method of feeding is determined by the degree and type of medical interventions needed and by the general management of airway obstruction. With or without the presence of a cleft palate, airway obstruction remains a prime cause of oral feeding problems (Marcellus, 2001). Some infants may require ongoing nasogastric feedings until oral feedings are fully established. Although most airway obstruction is obvious within several hours of birth, some infants with PRS may present with late airway obstruction as evidenced by failure to thrive and oxygen desaturation, necessitating close follow-up for weight gain upon hospital discharge (Wilson et al., 2000). Mothers may wish to provide supplementation at the breast to strengthen feeding and speech muscles and to familiarize the infant with the breast, making it easier to feed at the breast in the future.

Techniques

If the micrognathia is mild and there is no cleft, some direct feeding at the breast may be possible with alternate massage, concurrent with or followed by supplement delivered through a tube-feeding device. Infants should be placed in a prone or ventral position to bring the tongue forward when feeding at the breast. Feedings should be limited to 15–20 minutes to avoid excessive fatigue. Lingual massage may be helpful to relax and bring the tongue forward. Positioning of the infant with micrognathia and airway instability is usually prone but is complicated when a nasopharyngeal airway is in place. Osteopathic manipulative treatment and cranial manipulation therapy have been described as being helpful in mild cases; they manipulate the muscles that control the mandible. Altering the forces on the mandible can help bring it forward to improve its structure and function (Summers, Ludwig, & Kanze, 2014).

Equipment

Cleft palate feeders may be used to deliver all or part of the required milk. Some mothers use a nipple shield, which does not require suction to draw it into the infant's mouth. The mother expresses milk into the shield reservoir for the infant to remove by compression and follows with any supplement by bottle that is needed. Some infants require nasogastric feeding to accomplish adequate weight gain.

A palatal obturator can be used to (Radhakrishnan & Sharma, 2011):

- Prevent the tongue from entering the defect, which can interfere with the growth of the palatal shelves toward the midline
- Position the tongue correctly for proper jaw development
- Contribute to proper speech development
- Reduce the passage of milk into the nasopharynx
- Decrease the incidence of otitis media

Modified from Radhakrishnan & Sharma, 2011.

Choanal Atresia

Choanal atresia is a congenital anomaly of the anterior skull base characterized by narrowing or blockage of the nasal airway by membranous or bony tissue. The condition is thought to occur when the thin tissue separating the nose and mouth remains after the infant is born. It occurs in approximately 1 in 7,000–8,000 live births, with about 60% demonstrating unilateral blockage. Unilateral choanal atresia may be asymptomatic until a respiratory infection occurs or the mother notices that the infant exhibits periodic mouth breathing, chest retraction when breathing through the nose, difficulty coordinating breathing while suckling at the breast (sputtering, choking, coughing), or circumoral cyanosis (bluish lips). The infant may "pace" the feedings by using shorter sucking bursts and pausing longer between bursts to breathe. Mothers should be instructed to watch for circumoral cyanosis and remove the infant from the breast to allow breathing between sucking bursts if the infant does not do so. Bilateral choanal atresia is more serious because both sides of the nose are blocked and, if completely occluded, cause acute breathing problems and cyanosis. Infants may breathe through their mouths; however, the work of mouth breathing is costly to the infant and could only shortly delay, not remove, the need for surgery.

Bilateral choanal atresia is identified in the hospital shortly after birth and usually requires immediate placement of an airway. Surgery is generally performed early in the newborn period, and stents may be placed to maintain the integrity of the surgically created airway. The length of the stents may need to be adjusted to accommodate feedings at the breast, and the mother may need to experiment with positions until she and her infant find one that is comfortable and effective. Stents may not be placed in many cases, however, as their use is controversial. Postsurgical outcomes have been found to be comparable with or without stents (Kwong, 2015). This makes breastfeeding much easier.

Feeding at the breast with bilateral choanal atresia is usually not possible until a patent airway has been established. Until then, feedings are delivered through an oral-gastric tube. Mothers whose infants present with choanal atresia (especially bilateral) should begin pumping breastmilk as soon as possible and continue to do so until the infant is completely established at the breast.

Bilateral choanal atresia is also commonly associated as a component of other congenital anomalies, such as CHARGE syndrome. CHARGE syndrome is a nonrandom association of anomalies caused by a mutation in the CHD7 gene on chromosome 8 that includes:

C Coloboma, a cleft of the iris plus a number of other eye malformations
H Heart malformations
A Atresia choanae and possibly cleft lip and palate
R Retarded growth, although birth weights and lengths are usually normal
G Genitourinary problems
E Ear anomalies, along with dysfunction of cranial nerves that can result in facial palsy, swallowing problems, and reflux

Cranial nerve dysfunction is a primary clinical feature of CHARGE syndrome, which is seen as weak sucking, swallowing difficulty, gastroesophageal reflux, and aspiration (Dobbelsteyn, Peacocke, Blake, Crist, & Rashid, 2008; White, Giambra, Hopkin, Daines, & Rutter, 2005). Affected infants are at high risk for aspiration and may also demonstrate oral aversion or defensiveness either as a primary sensory disorder or as secondary to delayed or negative oral sensory and unpleasant feeding experiences (Dobbelsteyn, Marche, Blake, & Rashid, 2005). Depending on the number and severity of the problems, some infants may be able to partially breastfeed but may only be able to receive expressed milk through gastrostomy feeding tubes.

There are many other more rare craniofacial anomalies, most of which occur as components of syndromes that have greater or lesser effects on feeding management in the involved infants. Feeding problems are frequent with infants who require interventions for airway management, especially in infants with mandibular hypoplasia (Perkins, Sie, Milczuk, & Richardson, 1997).

UPPER AIRWAY PROBLEMS

Laryngomalacia

This generally benign congenital abnormality of the laryngeal cartilage is the most common cause of noninfective stridor in infancy (Solomons & Prescot, 1987; Wood, 1984). It accounts for 65–75% of cases of stridor in children under 1 year of age and is 8 times more common than tracheomalacia. It may be accompanied by tracheomalacia, although the two have different etiology and pathophysiology (Mair & Parsons, 1992; Solomons & Prescot, 1987). The malacia, or softening, is thought to be a delay in the maturation of the structures that support the larynx, causing the epiglottis to prolapse over the larynx during inspiration. This partial obstruction typically causes stridor upon inspiration that is usually more apparent when the infant is in the supine position, crying, feeding, excited, or has an upper respiratory infection. The flexible supraglottic soft tissue structures that are drawn in during inspiration blow out passively during expiration so that there is no resistance to air escaping and no expiratory stridor.

Stridor typically is heard during the first few weeks of life but may not become obvious in some infants until they are between 4 and 6 weeks of age, because until then the flow of air upon inspiration may not be strong enough to generate the typical sound of stridor. Stridor generally increases over the first 6 months with a gradual disappearance by about 2 years of age. The intensity of stridor may fluctuate during the day with periods of quiet respiration (Gibson, 2004). Infants with laryngomalacia generally breathe and sleep better prone. When sitting, they should be at least at a 30-degree angle with their heads positioned to relieve or reduce the obstruction. They should be held in an upright position for 30 minutes after feedings and not fed lying down. Chronic airway obstruction contributes to increased energy expenditure in the infant, which, in combination with feeding difficulties, may result in poor weight gain (Ayari, Aubertin, Girschig, Van den Abbeele, & Mondain, 2012).

Infants with laryngomalacia are at an increased risk of developing gastroesophageal reflux (GER; Belmont & Grundfast, 1984; Bibi et al., 2001), thought to occur as a result of the more negative intrathoracic pressures necessary to overcome the inspiratory obstruction. This may cause wide swings in intrathoracic and abdominal pressures that overcome the antireflux barrier. Depending on the severity of GER, failure to gain weight or weight loss can occur, heightening the anxiety of parents already concerned about their infant's noisy breathing (Milczuk & Johnson, 2000). Crying exacerbates the obstruction and increases the work of breathing. Occasionally, an infant will experience a more clinically severe lesion where there is sufficient interference with ventilation that feeding and growth are impaired. Crowing respirations may be heard, and chest retractions that are severe enough to cause chest wall deformities represent the extremes. Rarely, clinical hypoxemia may be seen with oxygen saturation below 90% and supplemental oxygen prescribed, or in severe cases nasotracheal intubation or even tracheostomy may be needed.

Breastfeeding Management

Laryngomalacia has the potential to disrupt the normal sequence of suck, swallow, and breathe as the infant attempts to coordinate breathing with sucking and swallowing. Noisy respiration may be identified before hospital discharge but may be ascribed to residual fluid in the airways that typically clears on its own. Once lactogenesis II occurs, both the increased amount of milk and the pressure from the milk-ejection reflex may result in an infant who chokes, coughs, sputters, and frequently comes off the breast during a feeding. Latching and feeding in certain positions may exacerbate the problem. Avelino, Liriano, Fujita, Pignatari, and Weckx (2005) reported that breastfeeding infants with laryngomalacia frequently have difficulties when feeding, especially problems with choking. Infants may have difficulty gaining weight, feedings may be prolonged and difficult, infants may engage in breath holding with brief periods of circumoral cyanosis, and stridor may become more apparent over the first 3–4 weeks. The increased work of breathing may cause an infant to become fatigued at breast before accomplishing sufficient milk intake. An infant may have more prominent airway obstruction on one side if the laryngomalacia is more pronounced on that side.

Glass and Wolf (1994) suggested feeding position modifications and pacing techniques to improve feeding efficiency and to reduce the stress and work of feeding. Pacing is done by removing the breast every four to five suck–swallows to allow regular times for breathing. Pacing may only be necessary during high-flow-rate periods of the feeding (i.e., with the initial milk-ejection reflex and several of the following ones) until there is less pressure and a decreased flow rate further into the feeding as the breast drains. Supine positions for feeding should be avoided because they allow the epiglottic soft tissues to fall backward into the laryngeal outlet. Infants may feed better when the head is allowed to extend slightly to open the airway. Mothers may wish to recline and place the infant in a prone or ventral position for feeding. Sucking bursts may be short and rest periods longer as the infant compensates. Some infants also feed better with the use of a nipple shield. The shield helps control the fast flow of milk, allowing the infant to better pace swallowing with pauses for breathing.

Tracheomalacia

Tracheomalacia is a congenital developmental defect in the tracheal wall cartilage where the softened tracheal rings cannot prevent the airway from collapsing during expiration. The most common congenital tracheal abnormality, it occurs in approximately 1 in 2,100 children. With type 1, tracheomalacia becomes apparent shortly after birth. Tracheomalacia can be acquired from events outside the trachea, such as an abnormality of the blood vessels surrounding the trachea (vascular ring) or a tumor in the neck or throat causing pressure on the airway and changes in the cartilage (type 2). Type 3 tracheomalacia is an actual breakdown of the tracheal cartilage from prolonged intubation or chronic or recurrent tracheal infections. Infants with tracheomalacia demonstrate stridor on expiration and coughing, and they have worsening breathing when crying and feeding and when an upper respiratory infection is present. They frequently have GER and begin wheezing around 4 weeks of age. Wheezing can be mistaken for asthma, cystic fibrosis, or bronchiolitis, but infants with tracheomalacia are generally healthy, happy wheezers.

Tracheomalacia, laryngomalacia, and bronchomalacia can occur in isolation or in combination with each other. Malacia lesions may occur in association with other disorders such as congenital heart disorders, tracheoesophageal fistula, and various syndromes (Masters et al., 2002). Most children outgrow type 1 tracheomalacia between the ages of 1 and 3 years but may need to be monitored more closely if they have respiratory infections—an important reason to ensure adequate breastmilk intake to reduce this risk.

Breastfeeding Management

Many of these infants breathe and sleep better when prone. Some breastfeed better in a prone or semiprone position, which both eases breathing and allows gravity to slow the flow of milk during milk ejection and when the breast is very full. Some infants also feed better with the use of a nipple shield.

The shield helps control the fast flow of milk, allowing the infant to better pace swallowing with pauses for breathing. Infants should remain upright after feedings because they have a tendency to swallow air and experience GER. Most of the same feeding recommendations suggested for laryngomalacia also apply to tracheomalacia. Weight gain must be followed closely because the work of breathing burns calories and places these infants at an increased risk for slow weight gain or weight loss.

Mothers who have infants with breathing difficulties must ensure that their breasts are adequately drained at each feeding to prevent milk stasis, engorgement, or mastitis. Whereas alternate massage is often used to assist in weight gain and to increase feeding efficiency, this technique may not be appropriate while an infant with tracheomalacia or laryngomalacia is attached to the breast. It may be more helpful to massage and compress the breast during pacing pauses as well as toward the end of a feeding when the breast has been partially drained. Mothers should check for areas of the breast that are not draining well and manually massage those areas to improve milk drainage. Some mothers may also need to express milk if the infant remains a poor feeder or needs supplements.

Tracheostomy

Tracheostomy involves a surgical procedure to place a tube into the trachea with an opening in the throat called a stoma. In severe cases of respiratory compromise or obstructed airway, this procedure may be performed so that the infant may breathe through the stoma. The stoma is kept clear and the air entering it is kept moist so that secretions do not dry and block the opening. As long as the infant is capable of breastfeeding, nursing at the breast is both possible and desirable. If the infant is unable to breastfeed directly at the breast, expressed milk should be provided. Mothers may need to express their milk during the time surrounding the surgery and recovery period until the infant can be reestablished at the breast. Care must be taken when positioning the infant at the breast such that the stoma is not obstructed by clothing, head positioning, or the mother's hand. The mother should be able to see the throat throughout the feeding, with some mothers preferring the cradle or cross-cradle hold to better visualize the stoma area (Merewood & Philipp, 2001). Some infants may prefer a more flexed head position. Many mothers will use a covering with a filter or a specially designed humidifier during feedings as insurance that dribbled milk or milk that is spit up does not inadvertently enter the stoma.

GASTROINTESTINAL DISORDERS, ANOMALIES, AND CONDITIONS

Tracheoesophageal Fistula and Esophageal Atresia

These are congenital anomalies of the gastrointestinal tract that occur early in fetal development. Their incidence is reported to be between 1 in 1,500 and 1 in 4,500 live births (Clark, 1999), with approximately 30–40% of these infants having other coexisting congenital defects. Esophageal atresia (EA) with or without tracheoesophageal fistula (TEF) is the most common congenital anomaly of the esophagus. TEF/EA may be part of a complex known as the VATER or VACTERL association, where vertebral, anal, cardiac, radial, renal, and/or limb anomalies are also present. An infant with TEF/EA should be examined for such additional anomalies (Spoon, 2003). While most of the cases are sporadic, the incidence is higher in twins. There is a strong association between maternal diabetes and multisystem anomalies, with the incidence of VACTERL association in infants of diabetic mothers five times greater than that of infants from nondiabetic mothers (Loffredo, Wilson, & Ferencz, 2001). In normal development, the trachea and esophagus completely separate from each other. When they do not, a fistula (abnormal opening or connection) may be present between the esophagus and trachea or an atresia may be present, which usually involves the esophagus ending in a blind pouch with no connection to the stomach. The following are five common classifications based on the esophageal configuration and the presence or absence of a fistula:

- Type A—esophageal atresia: The proximal and distal ends of the esophagus end in blind pouches, neither connected to each other nor with a fistula present.
- Type B—tracheoesophageal fistula: The proximal or upper segment of the esophagus is connected to the trachea.
- Type C—esophageal atresia: A fistula in the distal section of the esophagus and the upper portion of the esophagus end in a blind pouch. This is the most common form, occurring in about 85% of all TEF cases (Ryckman & Balistreri, 2002).
- Type D—The upper and lower portions of the esophagus are connected to the trachea but not to each other.

- Type E—This anomaly resembles the letter H in that there is a small fistula connecting the esophagus to the trachea at about the midpoint of the esophagus. The fistula varies in size, with some no more than pinpoint size. This is the only configuration that may not be apparent at birth if the fistula is small. The esophagus and trachea are essentially intact, feeding is possible, but the infant may demonstrate frequent coughing and respiratory infections.

Infants with TEF/EA may also have tracheomalacia, abnormal esophageal peristalsis, and GER. This defect may be picked up on prenatal ultrasound and can be suspected if the mother has polyhydramnios. If polyhydramnios is present or the infant is symptomatic, a feeding tube is usually passed to ensure patency of the esophagus before the infant breastfeeds. At birth, infants may have frothy saliva and mucus in the mouth and nose and exhibit choking and coughing with noticeable drooling, respiratory distress, cyanosis, and, if fed, choking and gagging with milk regurgitated through the mouth and nose. Strains of *Pseudomonas* and *Serratia* have been isolated in the section of the esophagus that is present in these infants, making it very important that breastmilk is used when enteral feedings are started.

Surgical repair is generally performed in the 1st few days after birth, with parenteral nutrition provided before and immediately after surgery and enteral feedings, including breastfeeding, started about 5–7 days postoperatively. If a transanastomotic feeding tube has been placed, feeding through the tube is started gradually, usually beginning 48 hours after the surgery (Pinheiro, Simoes e Silva, & Pereira, 2012). When the infant can swallow saliva, oral feedings can be started.

Long delays before normal feeding begins can result in oral aversion and lack of feeding skills. The presence of a nasogastric feeding tube reduces the infant's oral sense of pleasure and can lead to a reduction of sucking and swallowing reflexes (Conforti, Valfre, Falbo, Bagolan, & Cerchiari, 2015).The infant may be given sham feedings by mouth in conjunction with gastrostomy feeding to accustom the infant to associate oral feeding with satiety and decrease later feeding difficulties. Sham feedings before surgical repair can promote appropriate and early development of the sucking and swallowing mechanism. Such therapy can result in earlier development of oral feeding mechanisms and a shorter time to full oral feedings (Golonka & Hayashi, 2008).

Gastrostomy is usually placed for nutrition in more complex situations where repair can be delayed for many months, with the possibility of sham breastfeeding. Milk drains out of the stoma, but the infant experiences the process of feeding and the comfort and enjoyment of "feeding" at the breast. The mother will need to pump breastmilk for the gastrostomy feeds (Wolf & Glass, 1992).

GER is common among these infants, as is esophageal dysmotility. Deficient peristalsis in the esophagus is a contributor to GER and esophageal emptying is accomplished by gravity. This may mean that the best position to breastfeed an infant with this condition is completely upright. The infant can straddle the mother's thigh and can sit on a pillow if needed to avoid having the mother leaning down during feedings.

Colic

Infantile colic is a set of behaviors typically described in healthy infants as episodes of irritability and hard, unexplained, and inconsolable crying, often with clenched fists, a red face, and drawn-up legs (Lucassen et al., 1998). It begins in the early weeks of life, peaks between 5 and 8 weeks of age, and usually resolves spontaneously between 4 and 6 months of age. The prevalence of colic is estimated to be between 5% and 28% (Lucassen et al., 2001). Some clinicians use the "rule of threes" as the criterion for defining colic, which states that the behaviors persist for 3 or more hours each day, for 3 or more days each week, for 3 or more weeks (Wessel, Cogg, Jackson, Harris, & Detwiler, 1954).

Colic has been attributed to various independent causes such as infant temperament (Canifet, Jackobsson, & Hagander, 2002), type of feeding, cow's milk allergies, lactose intolerance, maternal smoking (Sondergaard, Henriksen, Obel, & Wisborg, 2001), and maternal anxiety or depression (Barr, 1996). The physiological relationship between maternal smoking (or tobacco exposure) and colic shows that smoking is linked to increased plasma and intestinal motilin (gastrointestinal hormone that stimulates gastric and intestinal motility) levels, and higher than average motilin levels are linked to elevated risks of colic (Shenassa & Brown, 2004). Daily maternal smoking during pregnancy increases the risk of infant colic, with exclusive breastfeeding being somewhat protective (Canivet, Ostergren, Jakobsson, Dejin-Karlsson, & Hagander, 2008). The prevalence of colic has been shown to be twofold higher in infants of smoking mothers but less among those infants who were breastfed (Reijneveld, Brugman, & Hirasing, 2000). An increased number of cigarettes smoked per day is associated with an increased risk for infant colic. Nicotine replacement therapy during pregnancy increases the risk for infantile colic to the same extent as infant exposure to tobacco smoke (Milidou, Henriksen, Jensen, Olsen, & Sondergaard, 2012).

Cohen Engler, Hadash, Shehadeh, and Pillar (2012) studied the relationship between breastmilk melatonin and infant colic. Melatonin has a relaxing effect on the smooth muscle of the gastrointestinal tract and is secreted during the night in adults but not in infants. Their study found that melatonin was present in breastmilk, showing a clear circadian rhythm. Exclusively breastfed infants had a lower incidence of colic attacks and a lower severity of irritability attacks than infants who were not exclusively breastfed.

Allergy to cow's milk protein in breastfed infants has been implicated in colic and GER. Bovine whey proteins are present in human milk (Axelsson, Jakobsson, Lindberg, & Benediktsson, 1986; Cant, Marsden, & Kilshaw, 1985; Stuart, Twiselton, Nicholas, & Hide, 1984), and ingestion by susceptible infants could provoke symptoms of colic (Jakobsson & Lindberg, 1983; Kilshaw & Cant, 1984; Lothe & Lindberg, 1989; Lothe, Lindberg, & Jakobsson, 1982). Eliminating cow's milk protein from the maternal diet may reduce or resolve the colic (Hill et al., 1995; Jakobsson, Borulf, Lindberg, & Benediktsson, 1983; Jakobsson & Lindberg, 1978). However, elimination of cow's milk from the diet of a breastfeeding mother may not always remedy this problem. In one study, infants with a negative skin prick test for cow's milk allergy were not helped by such a maternal elimination, but infants with a positive skin prick test for cow's milk allergy did benefit from this intervention (Moravej, Imanieh, Kashef, Handjani, & Eghterdari, 2010).

A low-allergen diet with maternal elimination of common allergenic foods (cow's milk, eggs, peanuts, tree nuts, wheat, soy, and fish) showed a reduction in infant distressed behavior among breastfed infants presenting with colic in the first 6 weeks (Hill et al., 2005). However, even with the reduction in crying, the infants still met the criteria for the definition of colic. Switching a fussy breastfed infant to a protein hydrolysate formula, lactose-reduced formula, or soy formula has not been shown to improve colic symptoms (Lucassen, 2010). The use of soy protein–based infant formula is also not recommended for the prevention of colic or allergy (Kleinman, 2013).

Although primary lactose intolerance is rare, occasionally excessive crying, gassiness, and green frothy stools may have their origin in a transient lactose intolerance as a result of disruption in lactase production. Lactase is a brush border, small intestinal enzyme that breaks down lactose. Its production could be disrupted from illness, antibiotic use, or encounters with cow's milk protein. A functional lactase deficiency could result from low-fat feedings that cause rapid gastric emptying (Anonymous, 1986) with large quantities of lactose being presented to the small intestinal brush border for digestion. The ability of lactase to handle the high load of lactose may simply be overwhelmed (Lawlor-Smith & Lawlor-Smith, 1998). A high lactose load in breastmilk feedings has been described as occurring due to limited or timed feedings on the first breast, leading to a reduced fat and increased lactose intake (Woolridge & Fisher, 1988). If some colic symptoms are an artifact of breastfeeding routines, then management should consist of ensuring that the infant finishes the first side before being offered the second breast, the use of alternate massage should be encouraged to optimize fat intake, and perhaps offering the drained breast again to further increase fat content of the feed. Rather than substitute a lactose-free formula into the infant's diet, it is possible to add a commercial preparation of lactase to expressed breastmilk that converts lactose to simple sugars before the feeding (Buckley, 2000).

Savino, Bailo et al. (2005) found a difference in the colonization patterns of lactobacilli in the intestines of breastfed colicky and noncolicky infants. *Lactobacillus brevis* and *Lactococcus lactis* were found only in colicky infants, whereas *L. acidophilus* was found only in noncolicky infants. Colicky infants are also more frequently colonized by anaerobic Gram-negative bacteria, but it is not known whether gut microflora differences are the cause of colic or its consequence (Savino et al., 2004). Oral administration of the probiotic *Lactobacillus reuteri* improved colicky symptoms in breastfed infants within 1 week of treatment compared with simethicone, which had little effect (Savino, Pelle, Palumeri, Oggero, & Miniero, 2007). A meta-analysis of 12 randomized controlled trials of the administration of *L. reuteri* to colicky exclusively breastfed infants showed that the probiotic may be effective in treating excessive crying (Sung et al., 2013). Crying time reduction was seen in breastfed colicky infants who received an extract based on *Matricaria recutita* (German chamomile), *Foeniculum vulgare* (fennel), and *Melissa officinalis* (lemon balm; Savino, Cresi, Castagno, Silvestro, & Oggero, 2005).

Although excessive crying usually resolves over the first 3 months of life, a subgroup of infants with persistent colic symptoms has been identified (Clifford, Campbell, Speechley, & Gorodzinsky, 2002). In some infants, feeding problems have been shown to occur simultaneously with crying problems (Asnes & Mones, 1982; Berkowitz, Naveh, & Berant, 1997; Dellert, Hyams, Treem, & Geertsma, 1993; Feranchak, Orenstein, & Cohn, 1994; Nelson, Chen, Syniar, & Christoffel, 1997). There are limited data on the association between functional measures of feeding, such as the organization of oral motor skills, as they relate to the modulation of crying during feeding interactions (Ferguson, Bier, Cucca, Andreozzi, & Lester, 1996). Miller-Loncar, Bigsby, High, Wallach, and Lester (2004) provided evidence of feeding-related problems in four areas for a clinic-referred sample of infants with colic. Compared with infants without colic, these infants demonstrated:

1. More evidence of reflux
2. More sucking and feeding problems on the Neonatal Oral-Motor Assessment Scale (NOMAS) and Clinical Feeding Evaluation as evidenced by arrhythmic jaw movements and difficulty coordinating sucking, swallowing, and breathing

3. Less responsiveness during feeding interactions
4. More episodes of feeding discomfort

It is not known whether feeding problems contribute to colic, if colic contributes to feeding problems, or if the two often coexist. Only about 5–10% of colic is due to organic disturbances such as gastrointestinal disorders (Barr & Rappaport, 1999). Popular remedies containing simethicone are ineffective in alleviating crying associated with colic (Garrison & Christakis, 2000; Lucassen et al., 1998; Metcalf, Irons, Sher, & Young, 1994).

A study of children who had been referred for clinical treatment of colic during infancy demonstrated difficulties with sensory processing, emotional reactivity, and inattention at 3–8 years of age (DeSantis, Coster, Bigsby, & Lester, 2004). These data, as well as other investigations, suggest an underlying dysregulation in children who present with clinical levels of colic:

- The preprandial and postprandial plasma levels of cholecystokinin are lower in colicky infants, resulting in the possible predisposition to excessive crying in the absence of the calming effect of cholecystokinin (Huhtala, Lehtonen, Uvnas-Moberg, & Korvenranta, 2003).
- A vagal tone imbalance has been suggested as a theory for underlying colic symptoms.
- Cortisol (White, Gunnar, Larson, Donzella, & Barr, 2000) and melatonin (Weissbluth, 1994) have both been studied as contributors in the larger hormonal and neural balance that may contribute to excessive crying through the biochemical effects of inherent or induced imbalances in these substances.

Excessive crying may also indicate underlying pathology with a history and physical examination in order when an infant presents with a chief complaint of crying, irritability, fussiness, or screaming.

Urinary tract infections should be ruled out (Freedman, Al-Harthy, & Thull-Freedman, 2009). Physical abuse/shaken infant syndrome is a serious medical consequence of early unremitted infant crying.

It is important to address colic because Howard, Lanphear, Lanphear, Eberly, and Lawrence (2006) found that mothers of infants with a physician diagnosis of colic experienced a shorter breastfeeding duration, as did mothers whose breastfeeding did not provide an effective means of comforting. Thus, excessive infant crying as defined by a physician diagnosis of colic independently shortened the duration of breastfeeding, possibly because infants with colic are less likely to be comforted by breastfeeding compared with crying infants without such a diagnosis. Mothers who rated breastfeeding as a highly effective means of comforting their crying infant breastfed for longer durations.

There are myriad strategies for coping with colic that include rocking, holding, use of a sling, breastfeeding, craniosacral osteopathic manipulation, acupuncture for both mother and infant, infant massage, crib vibrator, sucrose, gripe water, prone positioning across an adult arm, car rides, and car-ride simulators. Numerous pharmaceutical interventions have been suggested such as simethicone, dicyclomine, and methylscopolamine, which may be ineffective and/or hazardous (Joanna Briggs Institute, 2008). There is evidence that a sucrose solution can effectively treat colic in breastfed infants. In two trials, colicky infants responded positively to sucrose. The first trial found that positive effects were seen in 89% of infants receiving sucrose compared with 32% of infants receiving the placebo. In the second trial a controlled environment measured the effects of sucrose on colicky and noncolicky infants. This trial found that both groups responded positively to sucrose. However, sucrose appears to be effective for only a short time as the infants' response only lasted, on average, between 3 and 30 minutes (Garrison & Christakis, 2000). Minimal acupuncture has been shown to be an effective intervention in reducing crying and pain-related behavior in colicky infants (Landgren, Kvorning, & Hallstrom, 2010) by reducing intestinal peristaltic movements (Reinthal et al., 2008).

Cakmak (2011) has theorized that increased levels of cytokine tumor necrosis factor alpha (TNFα) in the breastmilk of some mothers might influence the metabolism of melatonin and serotonin in the infant, contributing to the pathophysiology of colic. Melatonin can reduce smooth muscle contraction in the gastrointestinal tract as well as reduce abdominal pain. Peak levels of serotonin can cause intestinal cramps associated with colic, as serotonin increases intestinal smooth muscle contractions. Elevated levels of TNFα in breastmilk could contribute to colic because increased circulating levels of TNFα suppress melatonin production and increase serotonin levels. Thus, TNFα that is repeated transferred to the infant through breastmilk could potentially downregulate the production of melatonin and upregulate serotonin levels, triggering colic in the infant. While it has been shown that applying acupuncture to the colicky infant can reduce colic symptoms, the use of acupuncture in the mother can result in reduced levels of TNFα in the breastmilk, which can help overcome the suppression of melatonin secretion in the infant and normalize the elevated serotonin levels (Cakmak, 2011). A reasonable intervention for colic might be to provide acupuncture treatments for infant and mother. Laughter in the mother has been shown to elevate melatonin levels in breastmilk (Kimata, 2007). Mothers might try viewing a humorous DVD to help raise melatonin levels in their milk.

GER and GER Disease

Gastroesophageal reflux (GER), the involuntary passage or backwash of gastric contents into the esophagus, occurs in approximately half of all infants 1–3 months of age, peaks around 4 months, and diminishes between 8 and 10 months of age (Nelson et al., 1997) after physiological maturation of the lower esophageal sphincter and lengthening of the intra-abdominal esophagus. It is common in infants with persistent crying and frequent regurgitation (Heine, Jordan, Lubitz, Meehan, & Catto-Smith, 2006). GER manifestations vary between infants fed breastmilk and infants fed formula (Campanozzi et al., 2009). Breastfed infants demonstrate GER episodes of significantly shorter duration than formula-fed infants, possibly due to the lower pH value in breastfed infants, which stimulates peristalsis and limits the duration of reflux (Heacock, Jeffery, Baker, & Page, 1992). Transient lower esophageal sphincter relaxation is the predominant mechanism of GER in healthy infants. However, symptomatic infants with GER and complications of the condition are said to have gastroesophageal reflux disease (GERD).

GERD is much less common than GER, affecting 1 in 300 infants (Jung, 2001). Infants with GERD typically have more episodes of transient lower esophageal sphincter relaxation with acid reflux (Omari et al., 2002), which can contribute to persistent symptoms. Clinical manifestations of GERD include vomiting, poor weight gain, dysphagia, abdominal or substernal pain, esophagitis, and respiratory disorders. GERD is common in children with neurological impairments, in preterm infants, and in infants with anomalies of the gastrointestinal tract and the lower and upper airways. GER/GERD is associated with and can be induced by cow's milk allergy (Salvatore & Vandenplas, 2002). It may occur secondary to a number of genetic syndromes, chromosomal anomalies, and birth defects. GERD can result from certain external factors such as supine positioning and medical interventions and procedures, including:

- Exposure to tobacco smoke (Alaswad, Toubas, & Grunow, 1996)
- Administration of medications such as caffeine and theophylline (Vandenplas, De Wolf, & Sacre, 1986)
- Use of antenatal steroids such as betamethasone and dexamethasone (Chin, Brodsky, & Bhandari, 2003)
- Use of nasogastric tubes for feeding premature infants (Peter, Wiechers, Bohnhorst, Silny, & Poets, 2002)

GERD can contribute to ongoing feeding problems during and beyond infancy. In a study of 700 children referred to a tertiary care institution for severe feeding problems, 33% were diagnosed with GERD (Rommel, De Meyer, Feenstra, & Veereman-Wauters, 2003). Infants with GERD ranging in age from 5–7 months showed significantly more feeding problems affecting swallowing, behavior, food intake, and mother–child interactions compared with control infants (Mathisen, Worrall, Masel, Wall, & Shepherd, 1999). Coughing, stridor, and an inflamed throat may be present, even in the absence of spitting up or vomiting. GERD is capable of contributing to severe events such as pneumonia, asthma, apnea, and bradycardia (Jadcherla, 2002). Infants with GERD may have alterations in their sleeping patterns with less daytime sleep and increased night awakenings (Ghaem et al., 1998). Swallowing dysfunction may be present with laryngeal edema or laryngomalacia from the acid reflux (Mercado-Deane et al., 2001). Pathological regurgitation, as opposed to frequent spitting up, is characterized by actual vomiting, frequent wet burps, problems with weight gain or weight loss, abdominal pain, and gagging or choking at the end of a feeding (Mason, 2000; Rudolph et al., 2001). The following are not benign symptoms, nor are they indicative of GER or GERD: projectile vomiting, bile-stained (green or yellow) vomiting or blood in the vomit, regurgitation beyond 1 year of age, growth faltering, or marked distress that has increased. Whenever such symptoms are present, immediate follow-up by the infant's physician is required.

At the extreme end of the GERD spectrum are a number of more severe complications such as esophagitis, hematemesis, Sandifer syndrome (torticollis of the head and arching of the body; (De Ybarrondo & Mazur, 2000), Barrett esophagus (changes in the epithelial lining of the esophagus leading to malignancy), and adenocarcinoma (American Society for Gastrointestinal Endoscopy, 1999; Ault & Schmidt, 1998). Even though symptoms may improve over time for many infants, histology from esophageal biopsy may remain abnormal, raising the possibility of ongoing esophageal insult and predisposing the individual to GERD-related complications (Gold, 2006; Orenstein, Shalaby, Kelsey, & Frankel, 2006).

Breastfeeding Management

A progression of management therapies ranges from positioning and feeding modifications to pharmacological and/or surgical intervention (Henry, 2004).

Positioning Modifications. Positioning is the first and most fundamental intervention for GER and GERD. Traditionally, the prone and elevated prone positions were used for infants with GERD. This has been modified due to the supine sleeping recommendations of the AAP Task Force on Infant Positioning and SIDS (2000), which recommends prone positioning only in special circumstances (Rudolph et al., 2001). Some parents use prone positioning during the daytime when the infant can be continuously observed. Placing preterm infants in the prone or left lateral position after eating has been shown to limit GER and esophageal acid exposure (Corvaglia et al., 2007). Infants can be seated in an upright position supported in an infant seat with about 90 degrees of hip flexion. They should not be slouched where the abdomen can be compressed such as in an infant seat, car seat, sling, or umbrella stroller. Infants can be carried in a front pack carrier, keeping them fully upright. A left lateral sleeping position is also used by some parents because it decreases reflux (Ewer, James, & Tobin, 1999; Tobin, McCloud, & Cameron, 1997). Positioning for breastfeeding should be between a 45-degree and a 60-degree angle with no abdominal compression (Wolf & Glass, 1992). Positioning changes may be needed if the infant cries during feedings, arches from the breast, or pulls off the breasts before completing the feeding. If other feeding positions do not provide relief, such as the ventral or prone position, then the mother can try feeding the infant while standing upright. The infant should be kept in an upright position after feedings.

Thickened Feedings. Thickening the feeding liquid with rice cereal has long been used and thought to keep the stomach contents heavy enough to resist rising into the esophagus. This practice is controversial with mixed results. Although it may reduce the frequency and volume of regurgitation, acid reflux remains unaffected, with as much or more exposure of the esophagus to acidic backwash (Bailey, Andres, Danek, & Pineiro-Carrero, 1987). Some parents feed their infant 1–2 tablespoons of rice cereal by spoon first and then breastfeed if they see decreased episodes of spitting up by doing so. However, there is little evidence that feed thickening affects the actual acid backwash or the course of the condition (Carroll, Garrison, & Christakis, 2002; Huang, Forbes, & Davies, 2003). Introducing solid foods has the potential to disrupt the gut microbiome, leading to alterations in immune programming and gut closure. Thickened feedings are also used with preterm infants to reduce spitting up or with infants and children with swallowing problems. One brand of thickening agent (SimplyThick) has been implicated in the sickening with necrotizing enterocolitis (NEC) of 22 infants, 7 of whom died (Beal, Silverman, Bellant, Young, & Klontz, 2012). The thickening agent was added to expressed breastmilk or infant formula products. Twenty-one of the infants were premature and 1 was a term infant. The Food and Drug Administration (FDA; 2012) has issued a warning to clinicians to cease using this product in infants under 37 weeks of age. Thickening breastmilk can increase its osmolality, which may worsen GERD.

Small, Frequent Feedings. Smaller and more frequent feedings have been associated with decreased reflux episodes (Orenstein, 1999).

Prolonged Feeding Durations. Jadcherla and colleagues (2012) reported that in preterm infants, prolonged feeding durations and slower flow rate and milk intake were associated with a decreased frequency of GER. This information might be extrapolated to the breastfeeding situation such that infants with GER could be put to breast after the letdown reflex or after some breastmilk had been expressed to slow the flow rate of the milk. A nipple shield might also slow the flow rate.

Drug Therapy. Gastric acidity inhibitors and proton pump inhibitors are used for GERD treatment. However, gastric acid is a disease-protective factor because it limits the survival of microorganisms ingested by the infant. Canani and colleagues (2006) demonstrated that the use of gastric acidity inhibitors was associated with an increased risk of acute gastroenteritis and community-acquired pneumonia. Sodium alginate (Gaviscon) has been suggested for use in breastfed infants for 1–2 weeks if marked distress is present and continues despite positional changes and other nonpharmaceutical interventions (Davies, Burman-Roy, & Murphy, 2014).

Chiropractic Therapy. Alcantara and Anderson (2008) described improvement in GERD symptoms in a 3-month-old infant using chiropractic manipulation and craniosacral therapy.

Colitis/Proctocolitis

Inflammation of the colon (colitis) and/or rectum (proctocolitis) with mild rectal bleeding is occasionally seen in a breastfed infant, even one fed exclusively on breastmilk. The dietary-induced inflammatory reaction is usually caused by allergy to cow's milk protein transferred to the infant from the maternal milk (Anvenden-Hertzberg, Finkel, Sandstedt, & Karpe, 1996; Lake, Whittington, & Hamilton, 1982; Odze, Bines, Leichtner, Whitington, & Hamilton, 1993; Patenaude, Bernard, Schreiber, & Sunsky, 2000). Infants usually present with mild to moderate diarrhea or grossly blood-streaked stool with mucus. Onset is between 1 week and 5 months of age, with the infant in apparently very good health other than the bleeding. Onset in the first week of life may be due to intrauterine sensitization.

Specific diagnostic criteria are lacking, but Hwang and colleagues (2007) suggested that certain endoscopic and histopathological findings are effective in a differential diagnosis. Smehilova and colleagues (2008) reported that infants with allergic colitis had significantly lower counts of bifidobacteria in their intestines compared with infants without colitis. It is not known whether this contributes to the onset of colitis or is the result of the condition. Other differences in the microbiota of infants with allergic colitis include lower levels of fecal secretory immunoglobulin A (sIgA), indicating a less mature intestinal microbiota. Such infants may also have less exposure to microbes in the environment due to hygienic practices in the hospital and at home (Kumagai et al., 2012).

Generally, eliminating cow's milk protein from the maternal diet alleviates the bleeding, often within 72–96 hours (Pumberger, Pomberger, & Geissler, 2001). Most infants experience a benign course of the condition, with many showing gradual resolution even when there are no changes in the maternal diet, suggesting that this may be a self-limiting situation (Machida, Catto-Smith, Gall, Trevenen, & Scott, 1994). Mothers should be reminded to check food labels for all forms of cow's milk such as casein, whey, and other ingredients derived from cow's milk. Sometimes, eliminating all forms of cow's milk products from the maternal diet fails to completely resolve the bleeding and mothers may be asked to eliminate soy protein, eggs, corn, nuts, fish, shellfish, wheat, and chocolate from their diet, because these foods may cause a similar reaction either as the sole allergen or in combination with the cow's milk (Choi et al., 2005; Machida et al., 1994). Rechallenge with the offending protein within the first 6 months may provoke recurrence of the rectal bleeding within 72 hours (Atanaskovic-Markovic, 2014).

If infants do not respond to the elimination of cow's milk protein, it might be due to cross-reactivity between human milk proteins and cow's milk proteins. Some similarities between cow's milk and human milk amino acid structures may provoke allergic symptoms in cow's milk–allergic infants when they ingest human milk (Bernard et al., 2000; Restani et al., 2000). Mothers may also need to eliminate beef from their diet. Casein hydrolysate formulas (Nutramigen, Pregestimil, or elemental amino acid formulas) are sometimes given temporarily to the infant if the bleeding remains or intensifies during the time of the maternal elimination diet, with breastfeeding resuming after the bleeding ceases. If this more extreme measure is taken, the mother should pump her milk and freeze it. That milk can be given to the infant when he or she is a little older and has outgrown the problem. Although this intervention may resolve rectal bleeding, it deprives infants and mothers of the advantages of breastfeeding. If a maternal elimination diet does not improve the condition, some infants may have multiple food allergies (Lucarelli et al., 2011). If rectal bleeding persists in spite of maternal dietary restrictions, there may be other sources of the allergen in the diet or perhaps an allergen that has not been identified

Finding blood in the stool of their infant is quite alarming to parents. Many ask why and how this could happen in an exclusively breastfed infant and in a family with no history of such occurrences. The clinician should ask if the infant received a bottle of cow's milk–based formula in the hospital before discharge. Supplementation of breastfed infants is common and many times done without the knowledge or permission of the mother. In a susceptible infant, one bottle can sensitize the infant, with subsequent exposure to cow's milk through the maternal diet resulting in allergic symptoms. Only small amounts of bovine beta-lactalbumin (i.e., 1 ng [a billionth of a gram]) are necessary to create the sensitizing event. Although human milk contains 0.5–32 ng/L of bovine beta-lactalbumin, a 40-mL feeding of cow's milk–based formula contains the equivalent amount of beta-lactalbumin that a breastfed infant would receive from 21 years of breastfeeding (Businco, Bruno, & Giampietro, 1999)! While beta-lactoglobulin is an allergenic cow's milk protein, its presence alone may not explain the development of cow's milk allergy in breastfed infants. Bovine alpha-S1-casein is also considered a major cow's milk allergen and is readily secreted into human milk, making it another possible cause of sensitization in an exclusively breastfed infant (Orru et al., 2013).

A treatment regimen has been developed that may reduce the colic symptoms, eliminate or decrease the bloody stools, facilitate breastfeeding, and avoid the use of hypoallergenic formulas. It is based on the maternal use of Pancrease, a medication that contains digestive enzymes that break down fats, proteins, and carbohydrates in the mother's diet before they circulate and enter her milk (Repucci, 1999). The three-part regimen (Schach & Haight, 2002) allows mothers to continue breastfeeding and includes the maternal elimination of dairy products, soy, nuts, strawberries, and chocolate, and further eliminating wheat, eggs, and corn if this does not resolve the infant's symptoms. The mother also takes two Pancrease MT-4-strength tablets with each meal and one with each snack.

Clinicians report an amazing variety of foods that have been traced back as sources for colitis. Some recommend that the mother eat foods that she has never before had in her diet as a mechanism to completely eliminate the offending food or family of foods from her system. Breastfeeding should not be abandoned except in the most severe of cases, because the infant most often simply outgrows the problem. Mothers can express their milk during the time it takes for the infant to outgrow the problem.

The Academy of Breastfeeding Medicine (2011) has published a clinical protocol for the management of allergic proctocolitis in the exclusively breastfed infant. Severe symptoms such as vomiting, excessive diarrhea, or abdominal distention are very rare and may indicate the necessity for referral to a specialist for discovery of other allergic disorders.

Pyloric Stenosis

Hypertrophic pyloric stenosis is the narrowing of the pyloric orifice that connects the stomach to the duodenum due to excessive thickening of the pyloric sphincter or hypertrophy (excessive growth) of the mucosa or submucosa of the pylorus. The enlarged pyloric musculature obstructs the gastric outlet, resulting in the classic symptom of projectile vomiting following feedings. Pyloric stenosis:

- Affects 0.5–3.0 infants per 1,000 live births (Applegate & Druschel, 1995; Persson, Ekborn, Granath, & Nordenskjold, 2001).
- Is the most common condition requiring surgery in the early months of life (Chung, 2008).
- May have a familial or genetic component in its etiology (Everett et al., 2008; Mitchell & Risch, 1991).
- Is more common among first-born children (Dodge, 1975; Jedd et al., 1986; Webb, Lari, & Dodge, 1983) and less common in African American infants (Wang, Waller, Hwang, Taylor, & Canfield, 2008).
- Occurs in a preponderance of male infants (Habbick, Khanna, & To, 1989; Lammer & Edmonds, 1987; Webb et al., 1983), affecting males four times more frequently than females (Everett et al., 2008).
- Is generally not congenital, because infants who eventually develop pyloric stenosis have structurally normal pylori at birth.
- Usually develops between the 2nd and 6th weeks of life with intermittent vomiting at first, progressing to include vomiting that is often forceful or projectile after each feeding. The infant remains hungry, continues to feed eagerly, but weight loss and dehydration, decreased urine and stool output, irritability, and weakness could eventually result in an electrolyte imbalance and the need for corrective surgery.
- May occur in an early form during the first 2 weeks of life. Demian, Nguyen, and Emil (2009) found a genetic predisposition to the early form of pyloric stenosis. The early form may be confused with reflux, making a diagnosis difficult during the first 14 days.

The etiology of pyloric stenosis shows a strong postnatal influence on its development. A number of causal factors have been linked to or associated with the occurrence of pyloric stenosis:

- Maternal smoking. Maternal smoking has been shown to be a risk factor for pyloric stenosis, with infants of smokers being twice as likely to develop the condition. It is not known whether the association is caused by maternal prenatal smoking, exposure to second-hand smoke after birth, or exposure through breastmilk (Sorensen, Norgard, Pedersen, Larsen, & Johnsen, 2002).
- *Helicobacter pylori*. This bacterium is commonly found in the human stomach, and its epidemiological and clinical features are very similar to pyloric stenosis, suggesting that some pyloric stenosis may have an infectious etiology (Paulozzi, 2000).
- Abnormalities in pyloric innervation. Some abnormalities in the intramuscular innervation of the pyloric muscle have been reported, suggesting that the reduced production of neurotrophins (nerve growth factors) may be responsible for the delay in the functional and structural maturation of pyloric innervation, leading to the abnormalities in growth (Guarino, Yoneda, Shima, & Puri, 2001).

- Early postnatal exposure to erythromycin. Young infants who received erythromycin antibiotics have shown a significantly increased incidence of pyloric stenosis (Hauben & Amsden, 2002), especially when the drug was prescribed systemically (not ophthalmically) for the infant during the first 2 weeks of life (Mahon, Rosenman, & Kleinman, 2001). Exposure to erythromycin through breastmilk also significantly increases the risk (13-fold increased risk) and occurrence of pyloric stenosis in breastfed infants between 0 and 90 days of age, depending on the period of postnatal exposure (Sorensen et al., 2003; Stang, 1986).
- Early postnatal exposure to azithromycin. Exposure to azithromycin during the first 2 weeks of life leads to an 8-fold increase in the odds of developing pyloric stenosis; this risk may persist, albeit to a lesser extent, when infants are exposed to the drug between 15 and 42 days of age (Eberly, Eide, Thompson, & Nylund, 2015). Such infants who receive azithromycin should be monitored for pyloric stenosis for 6 weeks following this treatment.
- Lack of breastfeeding. Infants with pyloric stenosis are less likely to have been breastfed during the first week of life (Pisacane et al., 1996). Although other studies are not consistent with feeding-type effects on pyloric stenosis, Pisacane and colleagues (1996) showed that 35% of the cases of pyloric stenosis in their study of 102 infants with surgically confirmed pyloric stenosis could be associated with the lack of exclusive breastfeeding during the early neonatal period. They speculated on the possible protective effects that breastmilk may have on the development of this condition, including the presence of high levels of hormones such as vasoactive intestinal peptide, which favors pyloric relaxation, or the increased plasma gastrin levels seen in formula-fed infants or supplemented breastfed infants (Marchini, Simoni, Bartolini, & Uvnas-Moberg, 1994), which could be associated with spasm of the pylorus, pyloric hypertrophy, and the consequent damage to peptide-containing nerve fibers. Results from a large population-based cohort study performed by Krogh and colleagues (2012), showed that bottle-fed infants experienced a 4.6-fold higher risk of pyloric stenosis compared with infants who were not bottle-fed. A possible explanation for this might be that bottle-fed infants consume a larger volume of formula in less time than it takes to breastfeed. Formula remains in the stomach for a longer period of time. The side effect of this type of overfeeding may challenge the pylorus muscle and lead to its hypertrophy. Breastmilk contains high levels of endogenous vasoactive intestinal peptide, which may help to mediate pyloric relaxation and facilitate gastric emptying, whereas infants fed by bottle have higher serum gastrin levels, which can be associated with pylorospasm.

  One study showed that the association between bottle-feeding and pyloric stenosis is more pronounced in children of older and multiparous mothers. One explanation for this pattern is that higher estrogen levels in utero in older and multiparous mothers could "prime" the fetus's pyloric muscle via a decrease in nitric oxide–mediated relaxation, making it more susceptible to the effects of bottle-feeding after birth (McAteer, Ledbetter, & Goldin, 2013).

Surgical intervention (pyloromyotomy) may be performed with correction of dehydration and electrolyte imbalance. Either an open or a laparoscopic procedure may be performed, with earlier full feedings and decreased length of hospitalization seen with laparoscopic pyloromyotomy (Fugimoto, Lane,

Segawa, Esaki, & Miyano, 1999). After an uncomplicated procedure, infants can usually begin ad lib breastfeeding once they have recovered from the anesthesia, decreasing the time spent in the hospital and reducing the stress of surgery on the family (Carpenter et al., 1999; Garza, Morash, Dzakovic, Mondschein, & Jaksic, 2002; Puapong, Kahng, Ko, & Applebaum, 2002). Mothers may need to pump their milk during the surgical period.

Breastfeeding Management

Breastfeeding management during the early course of this condition (often before it is diagnosed) usually consists of frequent feedings, often with refeeding right after the infant has spit up. As the spitting up becomes more frequent and forceful, mothers need to keep track of diaper counts, and more frequent weight checks may be in order. If weight stasis or loss becomes evident, hindmilk refeeds can be tried, but surgery may be necessary if weight loss and electrolyte imbalance become problematic. Clinicians may wish to refrain from prescribing erythromycin and azithromycin to lactating mothers and young infants and to explain that smoking increases the risk for this condition.

METABOLIC DISORDERS

Abnormalities in the newborn's body chemistry that affect how food is built up or broken down are typically referred to as inborn errors of metabolism. These may take the form of amino acid disorders, fatty acid oxidation disorders, organic acid disorders, and urea cycle disorders. Most metabolic disorders are inherited as autosomal recessive traits (two copies of the defective gene are needed for the disorder to be expressed, one from each parent).

All U.S. states screen newborns for two disorders: phenylketonuria (PKU) and congenital hypothyroidism. Most states also screen newborns for some other disorders, such as galactosemia, hemoglobin abnormalities, maple syrup urine disease, homocystinuria, biotinidase deficiency, congenital adrenal hyperplasia, and medium-chain Acyl-CoA dehydrogenase deficiency. Although the AAP Newborn Screening Task Force (2000) has recommended that all states screen for 30 specific disorders, screening varies from state to state and what is screened is inconsistent. In 2005 the AAP Newborn Screening Authoring Committee (2008) endorsed a report from the American College of Medical Genetics (2006), which recommended that all states screen newborn infants for a core panel of 29 treatable congenital conditions and an additional 25 conditions that may be detected by screening. Clinicians should check with their own state for screening information. Information on the screening panels for each state can be found at http://www.babysfirsttest.org/newborn-screening/states. General clinical guidelines for screened conditions can be found at https://www.acmg.net/ACMG/Publications/ACT_Sheets_and_Confirmatory_Algorithms/NBS_ACT_Sheets_and_Algorithm_Table/ACMG/Publications/ACT_Sheets_and_Confirmatory_Algorithms/NBS_ACT_Sheets_and_Algorithms_Table.aspx?hkey=e2c16055-8cdc-4b22-a53b-b863622007c0.

Breastfeeding is quite possible with many inherited metabolic disorders, including not only PKU but also organic acidemias (Huner, Baykal, Demir, & Demirkol, 2005; MacDonald et al., 2006). Gokcay, Baykal, Gokdemir, and Demirkol (2006) reported that breastfed infants with organic acidemias experienced a decreased frequency of infections, acute metabolic episodes, and hospital admissions compared with infants with organic acidemias who were not breastfed. However, close monitoring of clinical parameters such as growth, development, and biochemistry is imperative. Mothers should be closely supported to ensure an abundant milk supply, especially if breastfeeding gets off to a slow start or there are interruptions in the infant feeding directly at the breast.

Blood specimens for newborn screening in the United States are usually obtained during the first 24–48 hours of life, prior to hospital discharge. A study by Santoro, Martinez, Ricco, and Jorge (2010) showed that the amount of colostrum ingested by exclusively breastfeeding infants prior to screening can be quite low, with such a small amount of protein in some cases leading to an abnormal screening result. In other words, the dietary intake of protein may not be enough for PKU screening, and result in false-negative screening results (Porta, Mussa, & Ponzone, 2010). Infants may need follow-up, and additional blood specimens obtained when they are seen at their first pediatric appointment.

Phenylketonuria

Phenylketonuria (PKU) is an inherited autosomal recessive trait affecting 1 in 10,000–15,000 newborns in the United States each year. It is caused by a deficiency in the hepatic enzyme phenylalanine hydroxylase (PAH), which is required for the metabolism of the essential amino acid phenylalanine (PHE) into tyrosine. PKU has a variable presentation and severity depending on the different mutations in the gene-encoding PAH enzyme. Four different phenotypes are distinguished—classical PKU, moderate PKU, mild PKU, and mild hyperphenylalaninemia—based on the amount of residual activity of the PAH enzyme. When this enzyme deficiency goes untreated, PHE accumulates in the tissues and brain where it can interfere with brain development, eventually causing mental retardation as well as a host of bizarre behaviors and failure to thrive. PKU is treated by dietary management, providing enough PHE for normal growth and development while preventing excessive amounts from accumulating.

Breastmilk is extremely important for infants with PKU, especially during the time before diagnosis and institution of dietary interventions. Riva and colleagues (1996) found that infants breastfed for 20–40 days during the prediagnostic stage showed improved neurodevelopment, with a 12.9-point IQ advantage over infants fed formula during the same period. Breastfeeding can successfully continue (Motzfeldt, Lilje, & Nylander, 1999) once a diagnosis has been made and is done in combination with a PHE-free formula. Blood levels of PHE are monitored, with dietary adjustments as needed to keep PHE serum concentrations between 120 and 360 |mmol/L (Medical Research Council Working Party on Phenylketonuria, 1993).

Because human milk is lower in PHE than commercial formulas, 40 mg/dL versus 70–85 mg/dL (McCabe, Leonard, Medici, Seashore, & Weiss, 1992), infants with PKU can continue to receive significant amounts of human milk in their diet. Infants fed 362 mL (1st month) to 464 mL (4th month) of breastmilk daily in addition to PHE-free formula showed a lower PHE intake than infants fed exclusively with a low-PHE formula during the first 6 months of life. These infants demonstrated normal weight, length, head circumference, and hematological indices (McCabe et al., 1989). Banta-Wright, Shelton, Lowe, Knafl, and Houck (2012) showed that more breastfed infants with PKU in their study had PHE levels within the normal range and were less likely to have low PHE levels than formula-fed infants with PKU. Mothers in this study were quite able to both breastfeed successfully and manage their infant's special needs. Breastmilk is the optimal base feeding for infants with PKU and should be encouraged and supported (Feillet & Agostoni, 2010).

Breastfeeding Management

A number of feeding protocols have been used to incorporate breastfeeding into the dietary management of this condition using breastmilk as the PHE source (Kanufre et al., 2007). For instance, during the first few days after diagnosis, especially with high serum PHE levels, the infant is given limited amounts of breastmilk or only PHE-free formula to normalize serum PHE levels quickly while the mother pumps her milk during this time to maintain her supply. When serum PHE levels normalize, breastfeeding is begun, with each feeding consisting of a measured amount of PHE-free formula first (10–30 mL; Clark, 1992) followed by breastfeeding. Breastfeeding times are adjusted depending on the results of weekly blood tests (Purnell, 2001). PHE-free formula can be given by bottle, alternative feeding method, or by supplementer at the breast, but should not be offered after a breastfeeding. Over half of the infant's diet can be breastmilk.

Breastfeeding can alternate with PHE-free formula feeds. At each feeding, the infant feeds until satiety on either the PHE-free formula or at the breast. The number of feedings at the breast is adapted to the plasma PHE concentrations. Compared with a regimen where both bottle and breast are offered at each feeding, this approach may be more convenient for parents, and the infant can fully drain the breasts to receive the full complement of fat-rich milk available as the breasts drain (van Rijn et al., 2003).

The first 2 weeks following an infant's diagnosis with PKU are very important in maintaining adequate milk production over time. Mothers should be advised to secure a multiuser electric breast pump and utilize a combination of breastfeeding and pumping 8–10 times each 24 hours. Many of these breastfeeding sessions can occur after feeding the PHE-free medical beverage (Banta-Wright, Kodadek, Steiner, & Houck, 2015).

Published estimates of volume and energy of daily human milk consumption are used to calculate how much PHE-free formula to include in a 24-hour period of time. Starting with the weight of the infant, the total volume of milk needed in a 24-hour period is calculated along with the maximal amount of PHE allowed (25–45 mg/kg/day), the maximum allowable amount of human milk (based on 0.41 mg/mL of PHE in human milk), and the amount of PHE-free formula for the infant to consume such that he or she does not exceed the maximum amount of breastmilk allowed in the diet. The PHE-free formula is divided into equal amounts to be given either before each breastfeeding or during each breastfeeding with a supplementer device (Greve, Wheeler, Green-Burgeson, & Zorn, 1994). Mothers can weigh the infant before and after feeding from the breast to determine the amount of breastmilk consumed, and the next feeding can consist of an appropriately measured amount of PHE-free formula (Yannicelli, Ernest, Heifert, & McCabe, 1988). This is a cumbersome but fairly accurate method of determining breastmilk intake.

The infant's intake at the breast also can be correlated with a time measurement. The infant is weighed before and after each breastfeeding over a 48-hour time period, along with recording the number of minutes the infant nurses at each feeding. These numbers are used to calculate an average of minutes per ounce consumed. The PHE recommendations are converted to the number of minutes of feeding from the breast that is allowed in a 24-hour period. Infants feed from the breast until the total time specified has been met for the day and PHE-free formula is given for the rest of the feedings. This method usually requires more frequent monitoring of serum levels of PHE because it is a less accurate method for determining the true PHE intake (Duncan & Elder, 1997).

The treatment plan for an infant is individualized and managed by a physician and dietitian specializing in metabolic disorders. Each state has one or more medical centers capable of providing consultation and treatment for metabolic defects. The clinician should be aware of each facility that has this capability and be prepared to work as part of a team to optimize the dietary management of infants with PKU. Clinicians should remind parents to avoid giving their infant any product containing aspartame. Aspartame is an artificial sweetener made from PHE and is found in foods, drinks, and medicines, in addition to products designed as sugar substitutes. Because infants with PKU are more susceptible to thrush, mothers should be vigilant for signs of Candida overgrowth in the infant as well as on their nipples and areolae (Lawrence & Lawrence, 2016).

Breastfeeding an infant with PKU can be challenging due to the increased work involved in monitoring feedings and blood levels of PHE, pumping milk, and making constant adjustments in the feeding regimen. Many mothers of infants with PKU initiate breastfeeding, but breastfeeding rates then drop off rapidly due to the ongoing demands of managing their infant's therapy, which include performing heelstick blood sampling once or twice per week and sending the dried, blood-soaked filter paper to a laboratory for PHE analysis (Banta-Wright, Press, Knafl, Steiner, & Houck, 2014). Mothers report challenges with breastmilk supply, pumping, and nipple confusion. Infants' tolerance changes weekly, with mothers being able to breastfeed at varying times each day; this inconsistency necessitates sudden changes in breastfeeding frequency, from many times per day to fewer times per day, and back again. Breastmilk should remain the base feeding for infants with PKU, but mothers often find it difficult to find information on how to breastfeed an infant with this disorder (Banta-Wright, Kodadek, Houck, Steiner, & Knafl, 2015).

Cystic Fibrosis

Cystic fibrosis (CF) is a genetic disease. In 2013, 651 infants were born and diagnosed with cystic fibrosis in the United States. The CF gene defect causes abnormalities in the cells that line the airways, biliary tree, pancreatic ducts, vas deferens, sweat ducts, and intestines, accounting for the multiple systems and organs involved in the condition. Secretions from all these sites become thickened to the point of obstructing the hepatic ducts, blocking the flow of pancreatic digestive enzymes, and interfering with the movement of cilia in the lungs. Thick secretions from the lungs place the child at high risk for pulmonary complications due to persistent respiratory infections. Symptoms vary from person to person due in part to the more than 1,000 mutations of the CF gene. Newborns may present with meconium ileus, which is a surgical emergency, or may already have pancreatic insufficiency. Parents may remark that the infant's skin and sweat taste salty, which is a classic symptom. Weight gain can be a problem because fat and nutrient absorption is usually impaired, even though the infant may feed frequently and vigorously. The median age of survival for a person with CF is about 33 years, with many female infants with CF growing up and having infants of their own.

Breastfeeding is highly beneficial to infants with CF due to the protective factors in human milk that lower the risk of respiratory infections. Breastfeeding exclusively for 6 months is associated with a decreased need for intravenous antibiotic use, confirming a decreased incidence and severity of infections in infants with CF (Parker, O'Sullivan, Shea, Regan, & Freedman, 2004). Breastfeeding helps protect children against decline in pulmonary function and decreases the number of infections in the first 3 years of life (Colombo et al., 2007).

Cystic fibrosis has been associated with altered microbial colonization of the intestinal and respiratory tracts. Exposure to breastmilk increases the diversity of the gut microbiota—a factor that is associated with prolonged periods of health and delay in the time to initial *Pseudomonas aeruginosa* colonization in the lungs and the first CF exacerbation (Hoen et al., 2015). The gut microbiome in the early life of an infant with cystic fibrosis is a determinant of respiratory and systemic disease progression, making it extremely important that infants with CF be breastfed and receive as much breastmilk as possible.

Not all infants with CF are diagnosed at birth, but most infants are identified by the time they reach 12 months. Failure to gain an appropriate amount of weight may persist, respiratory problems may increase, and when solid foods are introduced, the stool may turn bulky, foul smelling, and greasy. Jadin and colleagues (2011) showed that exclusive breastfeeding for the first 2 months was associated with adequate growth and protected against *Pseudomonas aeruginosa* infections during the first 2 years of life in CF infants who have pancreatic insufficiency. Infants who also have meconium ileus tend to need supplements to maintain adequate growth during breastfeeding.

Mothers of infants diagnosed with CF have higher levels of anxiety and depression than mothers whose infants were diagnosed with congenital hypothyroidism, infants identified as CF carriers, or infants with normal newborn screening results (Tluczek, Clark, McKechnie, Orland, & Brown, 2010).

Tluczek and colleagues (2010) observed that bottle-feeding mothers were more highly task oriented than breastfeeding mothers. They also more often engaged in behaviors that were insensitive to the infant and resulted in feeding dysregulation than did breastfeeding mothers. There was a favorable relationship between breastfeeding and the quality of mother–infant interactions, which may help prevent future feeding problems as the infant grows.

Breastfeeding Management

Breastfeeding should proceed as usual, because children with CF who were exclusively breastfed were found to be heavier and taller than those exclusively bottle-fed (Holliday et al., 1991). Most CF centers recommend exclusive breastfeeding, the use of pancreatic enzymes, and/or hydrolyzed formula if needed (Luder, Kattan, Tanzer-Torres, & Bonforte, 1990). Breastmilk contains lipase, an enzyme that helps digest fats, which is beneficial in working to improve fat absorption from the diet. Because about half of even asymptomatic infants show pancreatic insufficiency and nutritional deficits at diagnosis, breastmilk may be augmented with extra calories, a pancreatic replacement enzyme, and fat-soluble vitamins (Koletzko & Reinhardt, 2001). Replacement enzymes along with exclusive breastfeeding improve nutrient tolerance and weight gain, reducing or eliminating the need to use or wean to infant formula (Cannella, Bowser, Guyer, & Borum, 1993). Young children with CF can require 120% of the normal dietary recommendation for calories to maintain normal growth. Thus, mothers are usually very concerned about making sure that their infant consumes adequate calories and may engage in behaviors that are counterproductive to increasing caloric intake. Mothers can optimize caloric intake at the breast through the use of alternate massage, good drainage of the breasts at each feeding, and frequent feedings. Fat-rich hindmilk can also be used for calorie supplementation either through a bottle or a tube-feeding system at the breast. If mothers have an abundant milk supply, they can fractionate the milk using creamatocrit measurements to provide high caloric density breastmilk as a supplement (as is done with feeding preterm infants).

Galactosemia

Galactosemia is a hereditary autosomal recessive disorder of carbohydrate metabolism, occurring in about 1 in every 60,000 live births. **Figure 7-1** demonstrates that an infant who inherits two normal genes would neither be affected nor would he or she be a carrier. A carrier of classic galactosemia inherits one normal gene and one galactosemia gene, resulting in enzyme activity that is less than normal but neither requiring dietary management nor showing apparent medical complications. If an infant inherited both galactosemia genes, he or she would have classic galactosemia.

Galactosemia is an autosomal recessive disorder and a general term referring to a category of metabolic defects in which an enzyme deficiency disrupts the normal metabolism of the sugar galactose. Normally, galactose is metabolized by the body into glucose in a step-wise fashion by three specific enzyme reactions. Galactose is composed of half lactose, the sugar found in milk, and half glucose. When this metabolic process is interrupted, high levels of galactose-1-phosphate accumulate in the body, causing damage to the liver, kidney, brain, and eyes. More than 230 GALT gene mutations have been detected globally. Most positive newborn screening tests are due to the Duarte variant condition or just a false positive (Berry, 2012). Although there are more than 100 heritable mutations that can cause galactosemia, the three most common are:

1. Galactose-1-phosphate uridyl transferase deficiency, the classic and most severe form, which causes the complete loss of the ability to process galactose
2. Galactokinase deficiency
3. Uridyl diphosphate galactose-4-empiridase deficiency

Diagnosis is usually made during the 1st week of life through blood analysis from a newborn screening test. Symptoms typically start about the 3rd day of life and include jaundice, enlarged liver, vomiting,

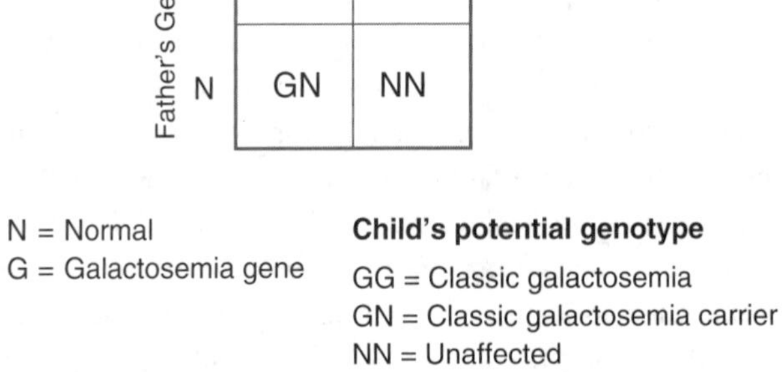

Figure 7-1 Genotypes involving classic galactosemia.

Data from www.galactosemia.org. Accessed September 19, 2005.

poor feeding, poor weight gain, lethargy, irritability, convulsions, and cataracts. When parents receive notice that the screening test indicates possible galactosemia, breastmilk feeding is stopped and replaced with a lactose-free formula. However, mothers should continue to pump and store their milk until a confirming test is done to determine if the infant has the classic form or a variant of galactosemia called Duarte galactosemia.

Duarte Galactosemia

Duarte galactosemia is a variant of the classic galactosemia, and infants with this form may have varying levels of enzyme activity depending on their genotype (Beutler, Baluda, Sturgeon, & Day, 1965). The child with Duarte galactosemia inherits a gene for classic galactosemia from one parent and a Duarte variant gene from the other parent. The possible variations include the following: A carrier of Duarte galactosemia may have approximately 75% enzyme activity, a homozygous carrier of Duarte would have about 50% enzyme activity, and a person with Duarte galactosemia may have about 25–50% enzyme activity.

Depending on the levels of galactose-1-phosphate (Gal-1-P) in the blood, some infants with the Duarte form of galactosemia may be able to partially or totally breastfeed. Mothers may be able to breastfeed every other feeding, alternating with a lactose-free formula. Such enzyme levels should be confirmed before abandoning breastfeeding and ceasing breastmilk expression. A typical recommendation would be to continue breastfeeding and check the RBC Gal-1-P levels monthly. If the Gal-1-P level is above the normal range, continue breastfeeding but consider substituting 1–2 feedings per day with a soy-based formula. Recheck the Gal-1-P level every 2–6 weeks and make diet adjustments thereafter.

Treatment of Duarte galactosemia varies, as there are conflicting recommendations about the best approach. Options range from complete removal of galactose from the diet, to avoidance of breastmilk for 4 months, to unrestricted breastfeeding (Schmidt, Beebe, & Berg-Drazin, 2013).

CONGENITAL HEART DISEASE

Congenital heart disease (CHD) refers to any functional or structural defect in the heart or major blood vessels that is present at birth. Between 4.05 and 10.2 infants per 1,000 live births experience some form of CHD, with an overall incidence of about 1% (Botto, 2000; Hoffman, 1990). An estimated 40,000 infants are affected by CHD each year in the United States. Of these, an approximate 25%, or 2.4 per 1,000 live births, require invasive treatment in the first year of life (Moller, 1998).

Women at high risk of having an infant with CHD include mothers with diabetes, a family history of CHD, exposure to certain medications such as indomethacin (Indocin), 1st-trimester exposure to rubella, and residing at high altitudes, which increases the incidence of patent ductus arteriosus (Allan, 1996; Mahoney, 1993). A study of infants born with heart defects unrelated to genetic syndromes who were included in the National Birth Defects Prevention Study found that women who reported smoking in the month before becoming pregnant or in the 1st trimester were more likely to give birth to a child with a septal defect. Compared with the infants of mothers who did not smoke during pregnancy, infants of mothers who were heavy smokers (> 25 cigarettes daily) were twice as likely to have a septal defect (Malik et al., 2008).

CHD is also part of many congenital birth defects and syndromes such as CHARGE, Down syndrome, fetal alcohol syndrome, Goldenhar syndrome, Turner syndrome, Rubinstein-Taybi syndrome, and velocardiofacial syndrome (Frommelt, 2004). Two classification systems describe CHDs based on their cyanotic or acyanotic characteristics and based on their hemodynamic characteristics (**Box 7-1**).

Infants with cyanotic CHD receive more interventions, experience significant delays in the time it takes to feed orally, and spend more time in the hospital compared with infants who are acyanotic. After

Box 7-1 Most Common Types of Congenital Heart Disease

Acyanotic

Increased Pulmonary Blood Flow

- Atrial septal defect: A hole in the wall between the atria (the two entry chambers of the heart)
- Ventricular septal defect: A hole in the wall between the ventricles (the pumping chambers of the heart); this is the most common CHD, accounting for 20–25% of CHD (Kenner, Brueggemeyer, & Porter-Gunderson, 1993)
- Patent ductus arteriosus: Persistence of the connection between the pulmonary artery and the aorta (failure to close) after birth
- Atrioventricular canal: Combination of atrial septal defect, ventricular septal defect, and common atrioventricular valve

Obstruction to Blood Flow From Ventricles

- Coarctation of the aorta: Narrowing of the aorta
- Aortic stenosis: Impairment of blood flow from left ventricle to the aorta due to aortic valve disease or obstruction
- Pulmonic stenosis: Narrowing of the opening into the pulmonary artery from the right ventricle

Cyanotic

Decreased Pulmonary Blood Flow

- Tetralogy of Fallot: A combination of four defects consisting of pulmonary stenosis, interventricular septal defect, dextraposed aorta that receives blood from both ventricles, and hypertrophy of the right ventricle
- Tricuspid atresia: Narrowing of the opening to the tricuspid valve

Mixed Blood Flow

- Transposition of the great arteries: The aorta arises from the right ventricle and the pulmonary artery arises from the left ventricle (the exact opposite of where they should be located)
- Total anomalous pulmonary venous return
- Truncus arteriosus
- Hypoplastic left heart syndrome: Underdevelopment of the left ventricle

Data from Coffey, P. M. (1997). Breastfeeding the infant with congenital heart disease. In D. Dowling, S. C. Danner, & P. M. Coffey (Eds.), *Breastfeeding the infant with special needs*. March of Dimes Nursing Modules. White Plains, NY: March of Dimes Birth Defects Foundation.

the surgical correction of some forms of CHD, infants may experience feeding challenges such as dysphagia, vocal cord injury, aspiration, or laryngeal nerve injury. Infants with CHD are also at risk for central nervous system injury such as bleeds or stroke (Jadcherla, Vijayapal, & Leuthner, 2009).

Congestive heart failure is a syndrome associated with most CHD. Depending on the defect, the extent of involvement, and the existence of other problems, symptoms may manifest shortly after birth or weeks after discharge from the hospital. Symptoms may include eager sucking for only a few minutes followed by frequent pauses or rests, short sucking bursts, lethargy, fatigue, poor appetite, sweating while feeding, poor suck, uncoordinated suck–swallow–breathe patterns, weak suck, cyanosis, tachypnea (rapid breathing), heart murmur, and poor weight gain in older infants (Coffey, 1997). Although some infants may not become cyanotic, their coloring turns dusky. This is not to be confused with acrocyanosis, the normal bluish coloring of a newborn's hands and feet due to delayed capillary opening. Some infants may also demonstrate circumoral cyanosis (bluish coloring around the lips) when feeding.

Parents are sometimes discouraged from nursing their infant because of misconceptions regarding breastfeeding and human milk (Lambert & Watters, 1998). Some believe that breastfeeding is harder or more work for the infant than bottle-feeding. However, cardiorespiratory efforts during breastfeeding are less strenuous and more physiological than during bottle-feeding. Oxygen saturation levels during breastfeeding in infants with CHD are maintained at higher and less variable levels compared with feeding from a bottle (Marino, O'Brien, & LoRe, 1995). Data from oxygenation studies on preterm and full-term infants have shown that during bottle-feeding, transcutaneous oxygen pressure levels decrease and, for some infants, continue to drop for up to 10 minutes after feedings (Hammerman & Kaplan, 1995; Koenig, Davies, & Thach, 1990; Meier, 1988). In infants with cyanotic lesions, it is extremely important to maintain their oxygen saturation as high as possible, and therefore it may be necessary to breastfeed to ensure this happens (Wheat, 2002).

Others believe that breastfeeding burns more calories, human milk has fewer calories, infants will have inadequate caloric intake, and infants will not be able to consume sufficient calories at the breast to meet increased metabolic and energy demands. Infants with CHD can suffer growth impairments due to anorexia, early satiety, mild gastrointestinal abnormalities, excess protein loss, fluid restriction, or frequent respiratory infections. After accounting for these and other effects on energy needs, infants with CHD may have only half as much energy available for growth as healthy infants (Weintraub & Menahem, 1993). However, it has been shown in a comparison between breastfed and formula-fed infants with CHD that breastfed infants gained weight more quickly and had shorter hospital stays than bottle-fed infants and that the severity of the cardiac defect was not predictive of the infant's ability to breastfeed or of breastfeeding duration (Combs & Marino, 1993). The higher concentrations of anti-infective factors in human milk are especially beneficial for infants with CHD, because these infants are more vulnerable to respiratory illness. These infants benefit from the incorporation into body tissues of components such as nucleotides that result in improved recovery after body injuries and surgery (Carver, 1999). Owens (2002) described an infant experiencing a heart transplant who successfully breastfed after transplantation, gained weight, showed no signs of organ rejection, and breastfed until 13 months of age.

CHD infants who require additional calories:

- May receive higher caloric content feedings at breast when the mother uses alternate massage, when there are short intervals between feedings, and when the breasts have been well drained

- May receive expressed hindmilk through a supplementer device at the breast
- May have high-energy supplements added to breastmilk
- May be on fluid restrictions and benefit from fractionated human milk that delivers 28–30 calories per ounce
- May be gavage fed supplements (hindmilk or high-energy formula) after feedings at the breast
- May be breastfed during the day and placed on a continuous feeding pump at night

Mothers may experience a number of obstacles to breastfeeding an infant with CHD, including separations during procedures or surgeries, fasting protocols that interrupt breastfeeding, anxiety regarding feedings, difficulty establishing lactation, inconsistent or apathetic support from healthcare providers (Barbas & Kelleher, 2004), and lack of access to breast pumps and privacy for pumping (Lambert & Watters, 1998). Mothers also describe difficulty distinguishing the infant's satiation cues (when an infant stops breastfeeding because he or she is full) from fatigue (when an infant stops breastfeeding due to exhaustion; Lobo, 1992).

Breastfeeding Management

Feeding plans must be individualized to the needs and conditions of both infant and mother. CHD does not preclude breastfeeding, and feedings at breast can begin at birth with modifications as needed. During the preoperative period for infants who require surgery, mothers may wish to put the infant to breast for the purpose of imprinting and practicing sucking and swallowing skills. Behavioral sensitization prior to surgery may enhance breastfeeding abilities during the recovery period of time (Jadcherla et al., 2009).

Positioning

Positioning the infant at the breast may be more comfortable and efficient for the infant in an upright position because GERD is more common in infants with cardiac problems. Infants should be positioned such that the rib cage can fully expand and the head is just slightly extended to open the airway. Some infants feed better in a side-lying position that avoids pressure on the abdomen.

Latch and Sucking

Many infants have a weak suck and fatigue easily at the breast. Alternate massage helps increase the caloric content of the feeding and assists the infant to sustain sucking. Some infants are capable of feeding on only one breast per feeding and others benefit from use of a nipple shield. Mothers may find that the Dancer hand position helps support the infant and improve sucking.

Shorter and More Frequent Feedings

This pattern may meet the needs and limitations of many infants as well as increase the fat content of the milk. The feeding should be interrupted if the infant becomes tachypneic, short of breath, blue around the lips, pale, or fatigued. The infant may not wake spontaneously for feedings.

Mothers may need to pump their milk after feedings to provide milk that the infant is unable to extract as well as to maintain an abundant milk supply. The cream layer from this stored milk can be used as a high-calorie supplement. Mothers will also express milk during the times surrounding surgery.

Preoperative and Postoperative Fasting Times

These times vary considerably from one institution to another (American Society of Anesthesiologists, 1999). The Academy of Breastfeeding Medicine (2012) recommends:

- If the procedure is minor and does not require sedation or general anesthesia, then infants should be fed normally.
- If the procedure is a surgery or diagnostic examination under anesthesia, then infants can breastfeed up until 4 hours prior to the procedure, followed by clear liquids up until 2 hours prior to the procedure.
- During the perioperative period, mothers should be provided with:
  - A private, quiet place to pump milk
  - A multiuser electric breast pump
  - Sink, soap, and dishwashing liquid to wash hands and pump parts
  - Refrigeration for storing pumped milk (or she can use a cooler with blue ice brought from home)
  - Nutritious food and water
  - Unequivocal support for breastfeeding and pumping milk
  - A place to rest and lie down; rooming-in accommodations

Families of infants with complex congenital heart disease struggle with a myriad of problems, with feeding issues being a prime stressor for parents (Hartman & Medoff-Cooper, 2012). Daily milk intake and weight gain are a constant struggle for many parents. However, mothers of infants with complex congenital heart disease are able to successfully initiate lactation, express adequate amounts of milk, and produce a volume of milk similar to mothers of healthy infants when properly supported.

The period directly before the birth and immediately following delivery are two important periods of time in supporting breastfeeding for these infants. Immediate and continued follow-up on expressing milk and milk production, provision of needed resources, and referral to an IBCLC helps establish the maternal milk supply (Torowicz, Seelhorst, Froh, & Spatz, 2015). If other obligations preclude the mother from rooming-in or spending long periods of time with the infant, arrangements should be made for her pumped milk to be brought to the hospital and given to her infant.

NEUROLOGICAL DISEASES, DEFICITS, IMPAIRMENTS, AND DISORDERS

Neurological deficits, disorders, diseases, or impairments can affect breastfeeding to either a greater or a lesser extent. Some infants can feed well in spite of the problem or can learn over time, depending on the severity. Some neurological impairment occurs as a nervous system insult and may be temporary, such as with asphyxia, cranial bleeds, sepsis, birth trauma, or the effect of maternal medications or drugs. The central nervous system could be abnormally developed or damaged during the prenatal or peripartum period, resulting in feeding difficulties either immediately after birth or gradually over a period of time. McBride and Danner (1987) divided sucking abnormalities related to neurological involvement into three categories:

1. Depressed sucking reflex (prematurity, Down syndrome [trisomy 21], trisomy 18, Prader-Willi syndrome, asphyxia, hypothyroidism)

2. Weak sucking reflex (Down syndrome, medullary lesions, congenital myasthenia gravis, muscle abnormalities)
3. Incoordinated sucking (cerebral bleeds, asphyxia, Arnold-Chiari malformation)

Other conditions such as neonatal/perinatal stroke, cerebral palsy, and neural tube defects can also contribute to ongoing feeding problems. Many of these conditions have common breastfeeding suggestions.

Down Syndrome

Down syndrome is a congenital condition caused by the duplication (a third copy) of chromosome 21. The chance of having an infant with Down syndrome is 1 in 1,000 births for mothers in their 20s, 1 in every 350 births for mothers over age 35, and 1 in 100 for women over 40 years of age. Many of these infants also have congenital heart defects, anomalies of the gastrointestinal tract, a large-appearing tongue with flaccid tone, and some degree of developmental delay. Mothers can be informed that breastfeeding is important to infants with Down syndrome to help reduce many infections and bowel problems and promote brain growth and development. Breastfeeding helps strengthen the infant's jaw and facial muscles, which provides a foundation for speech and language development. Skin-to-skin contact provided by breastfeeding is a form of sensory stimulation that facilitates neural connections important to future learning.

A number of characteristics of the infant with Down syndrome present challenges to breastfeeding (Lewis & Kritzinger, 2004):

- Generalized hypotonia that impacts the amount of body and head support needed to position and stabilize the infant at the breast.
- Hypotonia of the perioral muscles, lips, and masseter muscle; milk may leak out the sides of the mouth because an adequate seal is not achieved. Colon and colleagues (2009) found that poor sucking was the major reason why mothers of infants with Down syndrome discontinued breastfeeding.
- Passively or actively protruding tongue that may not form a central groove. A study on bottle-fed infants with Down syndrome showed that the tongue lacked the normal peristaltic movements and tended to fall to the back of the mouth, impairing the sucking motion (Mizuno & Ueda, 2001).
- Weak suck that may improve with time.
- The hard palate may be highly arched, narrow, and stair-like with acutely aligned palatine plates. The high palatal height is associated with a constricted palate that contributes to the commonly seen tongue projection and a smaller volume of the oral cavity (Bhagyalakshmi Renukarya, & Rajangam, 2007).
- Cardiac defects that, depending on the type and severity, contribute to excessive perspiring, fatigue during feeding, tachypnea, inadequate intake, long feeding sessions, and slow weight gain.
- Mid-face hypoplasia. The shape of the mid-face may narrow the nose passages, sinuses, middle and inner ear, and throat. Any congestion in the nasal passages makes breastfeeding more difficult as they are easily obstructed with mucus.

Breastfeeding Management

Pacifiers (and bottles if possible) should be avoided because pacifiers may mask hunger cues. Artificial nipples reinforce the narrowing of the palate, to which infants with Down syndrome are already prone. Sucking on artificial nipples can weaken the masseter muscles. Some infants may not suck long enough or effectively enough to trigger the letdown reflex. Mothers may wish to cause the milk to let down before placing the infant at the breast. Some infants with Down syndrome may have significant cardiac, gastrointestinal, and/or renal complications that may require additional nutrients to increase the caloric density or protein content of breastmilk (Thomas, Marinelli, Hennessy, & Academy of Breastfeeding Medicine Protocol Committee, 2007).

Oral Stimulation. Oral stimulation before feedings may decrease dysfunctional sucking movements and patterns, ease mouth opening, and stimulate central grooving of the tongue (Genna, 2013).

Positioning. Positioning the infant should involve complete body support such that no part of the infant falls into extension, pulling down on the shoulder girdle and causing the infant to exert muscles in the neck or mouth to stay attached to the breast. Some of these infants do best when held in a nearly horizontal fashion with their hips almost at the same level as their head when in a cradle or cross-cradle position (Danner, 1992b). Flexing the infant's thighs and knees increases resting muscle tone throughout the body and reduces the tendency to hyperextension (Saenz, 2004). Some infants may feed better in a ventral position. Swaddling may help some infants who either arch or who are very floppy to maintain better tone.

Supporting the Jaw. Use of the Dancer hand position provides jaw stability, decreases intraoral space, supports flaccid cheeks, and may assist the infant in generating and maintaining sufficient negative pressure to sustain milk transfer (Einarsson-Backes, Deitz, Price, Glass, & Hays, 1994).

Latch and Sucking. Use of alternate massage, a supplementer device, and/or a nipple shield may improve milk transfer and overall intake at each feeding. If a nipple shield is used, mothers can be instructed to make sure that they employ alternate massage to keep the shield teat full of milk. The supplementer tubing can be placed under a nipple shield to deliver supplements while feeding at the breast. Use of an asymmetrical latch while bringing the infant to the breast chin first may help achieve a deeper latch. Sucking pressures usually improve over time and breastfeeding can help strengthen hypotonic oral structures. Tremors of the jaw and tongue may be observed during the beginning of the feeding and remain frequent and persistent (Genna, 2013).

Tongue Protrusion. The infant's head should be brought into a neutral position to prevent neck extension from leading to an overly protruded tongue during latch attempts. Firm downward pressure, tapping with a finger to the midline of the tongue, and moving from tongue tip to tongue base may improve tone and central grooving (Wolf & Glass, 1992).

Referrals. Children with Down syndrome and any number of other conditions that significantly affect the capacity for oral feeding may need to be referred to specialists such as an occupational therapist, a physical therapist, or a speech-and-language pathologist for a more thorough evaluation of feeding impediments and an individualized therapeutic plan. Random orofacial exercises may not have the desired effects in solving breastfeeding problems unless tailored to the particular deficits and needs of the individual infant (Bovey, Noble, & Noble, 1999).

Permanent brain alterations originate during fetal life in infants affected by Down syndrome. Research is investigating the possibility of prenatal therapy for the fetus with Down syndrome. Animal studies have shown that prenatal treatment with certain neuroprotective peptides may prevent or reverse some of the developmental delays and learning deficits associated with Down syndrome (Incerti et al., 2012). Pharmacotherapy, neural stem cell implantation, and molecular interventions have been studied in animal models, with many of these interventions producing therapeutic effects that persisted into adulthood (Geudj, Bianchi, & Delabar, 2014).

Cerebral Palsy

Cerebral palsy describes a group of chronic conditions affecting motor control and postural abnormalities. It is caused by damage to differing areas of the brain, often occurring during fetal development as well as during the perinatal period (such as umbilical cord accidents) or postnatal period. It is nonprogressive in nature, but clinical manifestations generally change over time. The estimated prevalence is 1.5 to 2.5 per 1,000 live births. Low-birth-weight infants comprise about 25% of all cases of cerebral palsy.

Spastic cerebral palsy, which is the most common type, is seen in 70–80% of affected individuals. It is characterized by stiff or permanently contracted muscles. A newborn with this type of cerebral palsy might have tremors or uncontrollable shaking limited to one side of the body. Athetoid (dyskinetic) cerebral palsy is seen in 10–20% of affected individuals. A newborn may drool or appear to be frowning, and there may be a slow, uncontrolled writhing of the arms, hands, feet, and legs. Symptoms tend to disappear when the infant is sleeping. Motor dysfunction becomes more evident as the infant matures. Weak sucking, difficulty swallowing, head lag, and hypotonia may be apparent at first with the infant displaying hypertonia 2–3 months later. Involvement ranges from mild to severe, but all children with cerebral palsy have a primary problem with the control of motor function (McMurray, Jones, & Khan, 2002).

Cerebral palsy is often not diagnosed until after 1 year of age, but feeding difficulties have already manifested themselves and may vary over time. Poor sucking can impact weight gain and growth and may be an early sign of problems to come. Motion, Northstone, Emond, Stucke, and Golding (2002) reported that feeding problems at 4 weeks of age that included weak sucking, choking, and fatigue while breastfeeding as well as persistent feeding problems at 6 months were associated with the diagnosis of cerebral palsy. While these indicators may also be present in other infants such as preterm infants, clinicians may wish to follow these babies more closely to assure adequate growth and pick up potential neurodevelopmental problems early. Breastfeeding or the provision of breastmilk is important to this population of infants. Sacker, Quigley, and Kelly (2006) demonstrated that in a population of healthy term infants, those who were never breastfed had at least a 40% greater likelihood of fine motor delay than infants who were given breastmilk for a prolonged period. Any advantage that could improve motor activities of these infants is important to consider.

Breastfeeding Management

Many parents gradually become aware that there is something wrong with the infant with cerebral palsy. As developmental milestones fail to be achieved, difficulty with feeding may be one of a number of concerns that parents express.

Positioning for breastfeeding is especially important to handle both hypotonia and hypertonia, which may both manifest at different ages in the same infant. Parents may wish to carry the infant in a sling between feedings to help reinforce a flexed position, especially if the infant tends to arch his or her back. Infants with tone abnormalities can take longer to establish a pattern of effective breastfeeding, with initiation and maintenance of maternal milk supply being a significant challenge. They may favor one side of their body, making positioning at breast a trial and error effort. The infant's tongue may be fixed toward the roof of the mouth, making latch difficult to achieve. Some infants may have excessively wide jaw excursions that continually disrupt the seal on the breast. A hypertonic infant may exhibit jaw clenching with short jaw excursions and a flattened, anterior tongue and a bunched posterior tongue. Jaw and cheek support may be required for infants with hypotonic facial muscles and wide jaw excursions. It may be necessary to stroke the infant's tongue down and forward prior to latching.

Clinicians need to follow mothers closely to ensure that milk production is maintained under circumstances that include weak sucking, separation, and potential inadequate weight gain in the infant. Mothers may need to pump milk after or in between feedings to provide breastmilk supplements, preferably through a tube-feeding device at the breast. Feeding (and supplementing) at the breast provides opportunities for low-tone infants to stimulate their oral-facial muscles, helping with proper muscular development in preparation for handling solid foods and speech.

Rubinstein-Taybi Syndrome

Rubinstein-Taybi syndrome affects about 1 in 300,000 individuals and is similar to other syndromes and neurological disorders that have low muscle tone as a predominant characteristic. In addition to the distinctive hand and facial features, these infants also present with a small mouth, high arched palate, low muscle tone in the face and jaw, and GERD (Holland, 1996). Moe, Holland, and Johnson (1998) surveyed the breastfeeding practices of mothers whose infants had Rubinstein-Taybi syndrome and reported that breastfeeding problems included poor sucking, inadequate weight gain, poor nipple grasp, failure to thrive, swallowing difficulties, infant fatigue, and GER—similar problems to those seen in many situations involving neurological conditions in infants. Most children experience poor weight gain in early life primarily due to feeding problems, including vomiting and swallowing difficulties. Frequent ear infections are seen in about half of children, with mild degrees of hearing loss being seen in 25% of infants. Recurrent upper respiratory infections are also common in infancy and childhood, making breastmilk an important contributor to reducing complications.

Breastfeeding Management

Small, frequent feedings may reduce vomiting and improve weight gain. Critical to maintaining lactation in situations where infants experience low tone is to ensure that mothers express their milk to stimulate their breasts in compensation for infants who cannot. Positioning infants with Rubinstein-Taybi syndrome is similar to that for infants with Down syndrome. Gartner (1996) recommended placing the infant on a nearly level plane across the mother's lap or swaddled in a flexed position with the chin down and spine rounded. Weak sucking may also be compensated for by using alternate massage, supplementation of pumped milk with a tube-feeding device at the breast, use of a nipple shield, and use of the Dancer hand position.

Neural Tube Defects

Neural tube defects are congenital deformities involving the coverings of the nervous system. They vary in severity and location; occur early in embryogenesis, usually by 23–28 days' gestation; and may be caused by aberrant expression of a gene or family of genes, with the primary defect in all neural tube defects being the failure of the neural tube to close. Carbamazepine (Tegretol) and valproic acid (Depakote) are anticonvulsants that, when taken during pregnancy, have been definitively identified as acting as a teratogen for neural tube defects. A woman taking valproic acid has a 1–2% risk of having a child with a neural tube defect; therefore, women taking antiepileptic medications during pregnancy often undergo prenatal screening tests such as alpha-fetoprotein. The mildest form is spina bifida aperta, and a very common form is spina bifida cystica or myelomeningocele. This defect involves a saclike casing filled with cerebrospinal fluid, spinal cord, and nerve roots that have herniated through a defect in the vertebral arches and dura. Certain neurological anomalies such as hydrocephalus and Chiari II malformation also accompany myelomeningoceles. Chiari II malformation is a herniation of the brainstem below the foramen magnum that can pose a life-threatening situation if it requires decompression. Symptomatic Chiari II is a neurosurgical emergency and may begin with such signs as stridor, poor suck, swallowing difficulties, central apnea, aspiration, and hypotonia. Spina bifida occulta involves the lesion being covered by skin without herniation through a bony defect. A skin lesion may be present such as a hairy patch, dermal sinus tract, dimple, hemangioma, or lipoma in the thoracic, lumbar, or sacral regions. If the brainstem is involved, feeding at the breast may not be possible.

There has been a dramatic reduction in the occurrence of neural tube defects due to the recommendation for women of childbearing age to consume 0.4 mg of folic acid per day. Surgical repair is sometimes accomplished in utero but usually within 24–72 hours after birth. Up to 50% of children with myelomeningocele may be latex sensitive, requiring clinicians to use latex-free products when working with these children. Infants benefit from breastfeeding, which reduces overweight and obesity, improves pain management, reduces infection rates, decreases incidence of allergy, and improves cognitive development (Hurtekant & Spatz, 2007).

Breastfeeding Management

Most of these infants can be breastfed (unless the brainstem is significantly compromised), but mothers may encounter problems with reduced motor control and an infant who gags easily. Weakness may be present in the upper extremities. Most problems revolve around positioning the infant for feedings at the breast after surgery. Flexion of the spine may not be possible, and the infant is usually placed prone, flat on his or her back, or on his or her side for a number of days. The mother can lie on her side next to the infant to feed, slide the infant on pillows into the mother's lap, or, if the infant is supine (after a shunt placement for hydrocephalus), the mother can lean over the infant, bringing the breast to the infant rather than the infant to the breast (Merewood & Philipp, 2001). It is important that the clinician support the mother in her efforts to breastfeed her special infant because mothers have described hospital staff as another barrier to breastfeeding (Rivera, Davilla Torres, Parilla Rodriguez, de Longo, & Gorrin Peralta, 2008).

SUMMARY: THE DESIGN IN NATURE

A number of challenges are present when breastfeeding infants with major congenital malformations that include separation during the 1st week of life, surgeries, low-birth-weight, type of malformation (especially infants with digestive system malformations), suction and swallowing difficulties, inadequate weight gain, and real or perceived insufficient milk production (Rendon-Macias, Castaneda-Mucino, Cruz, Mejia-Aranguré, & Villasis-Keever, 2002). All these issues should be addressed by clinicians working with affected families. Mothers are often in shock and emotionally upset or grieving when their infant is diagnosed with a congenital disorder of any kind. Establishing a nursing relationship may be fundamental to working through parenting the special child (Mojab, 2002).

REFERENCES

Academy of Breastfeeding Medicine. (2011). ABM clinical protocol #24: Allergic proctocolitis in the exclusively breastfed infant. *Breastfeeding Medicine, 6,* 435–440.

Academy of Breastfeeding Medicine. (2012). ABM clinical protocol #25: Recommendations for preprocedural fasting for the breastfed infant: "NPO" guidelines. *Breastfeeding Medicine, 7,* 197–202.

Academy of Breastfeeding Medicine, Protocol Committee, Ballard, J., Chantry, C., & Howard, C. R. (2004). *Clinical protocol #11. Guidelines for the evaluation and management of neonatal ankyloglossia and its complications in the breastfeeding dyad.* Under revision.

Alaswad, B., Toubas, P. L., & Grunow, J. E. (1996). Environmental tobacco smoke exposure and gastroesophageal reflux in infants with apparent life-threatening events. *Journal of the Oklahoma State Medical Association, 89,* 233–237.

Alcantara, J., & Anderson, R. (2008). Chiropractic care of a pediatric patient with symptoms associated with gastroesophageal reflux disease, fuss–cry–irritability with sleep disorder syndrome and irritable infant syndrome of musculoskeletal origin. *Journal of the Canadian Chiropractic Association, 52,* 248–255.

Allan, L. D. (1996). Fetal cardiology. *Current Opinion in Obstetrics and Gynecology, 8,* 142–147.

American Academy of Pediatrics (AAP), Newborn Screening Authoring Committee. (2008). Newborn screening expands: Recommendations for pediatricians and medical homes—implications for the system. *Pediatrics, 121,* 192–217.

American Academy of Pediatrics (AAP), Newborn Screening Task Force. (2000). Newborn screening: A blueprint for the future—a call for a national agenda on state newborn screening programs. *Pediatrics, 106,* 389–422.

American Academy of Pediatrics (AAP), Task Force on Infant Positioning and SIDS. (2000). Changing concepts of sudden infant death syndrome: Implications for infant sleeping environment and sleep position. *Pediatrics, 32,* 45–49.

American College of Medical Genetics. (2006). Newborn screening: Toward a uniform screening panel and system. *Genetics and Medicine, 8*(suppl), 1S–252S.

American Society for Gastrointestinal Endoscopy. (1999). The role of endoscopy in the management of GERD: Guidelines for clinical application. *Gastrointestinal Endoscopy, 49,* 834–835.

American Society of Anesthesiologists. (1999). Practice guidelines for preoperative fasting and the use of pharmacologic agents to reduce the risk of pulmonary aspiration: Application to healthy patients undergoing elective procedures—a report by the American Society of Anesthesiologists task force on preoperative fasting. *Anesthesiology, 90,* 896–905.

Amir, L. H., James, J. P., & Donath, S. M. (2006). Reliability of the Hazelbaker assessment tool for lingual frenulum function. *International Breastfeeding Journal, 1,* 3.

Aniansson, G., Svensson, H., Becker, M., & Ingvarsson, L. (2002). Otitis media and feeding with breast milk of children with cleft palate. *Scandinavian Journal of Plastic and Reconstructive Surgery and Hand Surgery, 36,* 9–15.

Anonymous. (1986). Milk fat, diarrhoea and the ileal brake. *Lancet, 1,* 658.

Anvenden-Hertzberg, L., Finkel, Y., Sandstedt, B., & Karpe, B. (1996). Proctocolitis in exclusively breastfed infants. *European Journal of Paediatrics, 155,* 464–467.

Applegate, M. S., & Druschel, C. M. (1995). The epidemiology of infantile hypertrophic pyloric stenosis in New York State, 1983 to 1990. *Archives of Pediatrics and Adolescent Medicine, 149,* 1123–1129.

Argiris, K., Vasani, S., Wong, G., Stimpson, P., Gunning, E., & Caufield, H. (2011). Audit of tongue-tie division in neonates with breastfeeding difficulties: How we do it. *Clinical Otolaryngology, 36,* 256–260.

Asnes, R. S., & Mones, R. L. (1982). Infantile colic: A review. *Journal of Developmental and Behavioral Pediatrics, 4,* 57–62.

Atanaskovic-Markoviv, M. (2014). Refractory proctocolitis in the exclusively breastfed infants. *Endocrine, Metabolic, & Immune Disorders—Drug Targets, 14,* 63–66.

Auer, C., & Gromada, K. K. (1998). A case report of breastfeeding quadruplets: Factors perceived as affecting breastfeeding. *Journal of Human Lactation, 14,* 135–141.

Ault, D. L., & Schmidt, D. (1998). Diagnosis and management of gastroesophageal reflux in infants and children. *Nurse Practitioner, 23,* 78, 82, 88–89, 94, 99–100.

Avelino, M. A. G., Liriano, R. Y. G., Fujita, R., Pignatari, S., & Weckx, L. L. M. (2005). Management of laryngomalacia: Experience with 22 cases. *Revista Brasileira de Otorrinolaringologia, 71,* 330–334.

Axelsson, I., Jakobsson, I., Lindberg, T., & Benediktsson, B. (1986). Bovine beta-lactoglobulin in the human milk: A longitudinal study during the whole lactation period. *Acta Paediatrica Scandinavica, 75,* 702–707.

Ayari, S., Aubertin, G., Girschig, T., Van den Abbeele, T., & Mondain, M. (2012). Pathophysiology and diagnostic approach to laryngomalacia in infants. *European Annals of Otorhinolaryngology, Head and Neck Diseases, 129,* 257–263.

Bailey, D. J., Andres, J. M., Danek, G. D., & Pineiro-Carrero, V. M. (1987). Lack of efficacy of thickened feeding as treatment for gastroesophageal reflux. *Journal of Pediatrics, 110,* 187–189.

Ballard, J. L., Auer, C. E., & Khoury, J. C. (2002). Ankyloglossia: Assessment, incidence, and effect of frenuloplasty on the breastfeeding dyad. *Pediatrics, 110,* e63.

Banta-Wright, S. A., Kodadek, S. M., Houck, G. M., Steiner, R. D., & Knafl, K. A. (2015). Commitment to breastfeeding in the context of phenylketonuria. *Journal of Obstetric, Gynecologic, and Neonatal Nursing, 44,* 726–736.

Banta-Wright, S. A., Kodadek, S. M., Steiner, R. D., & Houck, G. M. (2015). Challenges to breastfeeding infants with phenylketonuria. *Journal of Pediatric Nursing, 30,* 219–226.

Banta-Wright, S. A., Press, N., Knafl, K. A., Steiner, R. D., & Houck, G. M. (2014). Breastfeeding infants with phenylketonuria in the United States and Canada. *Breastfeeding Medicine, 9,* 142–148.

Banta-Wright, S. A., Shelton, K. C., Lowe, N. D., Knafl, K. A., & Houck, G. M. (2012). Breastfeeding success among infants with phenylketonuria. *Journal of Pediatric Nursing, 27,* 319–327.

Barbas, K. H., & Kelleher, D. K. (2004). Breastfeeding success among infants with congenital heart disease. *Pediatric Nursing, 30,* 285–289.

Barr, R. G. (1996). Colic. In W. A. Walker, P. Durie, J. Hamilton, J. A. Walker-Smith, & J. B. Watkins (Eds.), *Pediatric gastrointestinal disease: Pathophysiology, diagnosis, and management* (2nd ed.). St. Louis, MO: Mosby-Year Book.

Barr, R. G., & Rappaport, L. (1999). Infant colic and childhood recurrent abdominal pain syndromes: Is there a relationship? *Journal of Developmental and Behavioral Pediatrics, 20,* 315–317.

Beal, J., Silverman, B., Bellant, J., Young, T. E., & Klontz, K. (2012). Late onset necrotizing enterocolitis in infants following use of a xanthan gum–containing thickening agent. *Journal of Pediatrics, 161,* 354–356.

Belmont, J. R., & Grundfast, K. (1984). Congenital laryngeal stridor (laryngomalacia): Etiologic factors and associated disorders. *Annals of Otology, Rhinology, and Laryngology, 93,* 430–437.

Berg, K. L. (1990a). Two cases of tongue-tie and breastfeeding. *Journal of Human Lactation, 6,* 124–126.

Berg, K. L. (1990b). Tongue-tie (ankyloglossia) and breastfeeding: A review. *Journal of Human Lactation, 6,* 109–112.

Berkowitz, D., Naveh, Y., & Berant, M. (1997). "Infantile colic" as the sole manifestation of gastroesophageal reflux. *Journal of Pediatric Gastroenterology and Nutrition, 24,* 231–233.

Berlin, C. M., Jr. (2007). "Exclusive" breastfeeding of quadruplets. *Breastfeeding Medicine, 2,* 125–126.

Bernard, H., Negroni, L., Chatel, J. M., Clement, G., Adel-Patient, K., Peltre, G., . . . Wal, J. M. (2000). Molecular basis of IgE cross-reactivity between human beta-casein and bovine beta-casein, a major allergen of milk. *Molecular Immunology, 37,* 161–167.

Berry, G. T. (2012). Galactosemia: When is it a newborn emergency? *Molecular Genetics and Metabolism, 106,* 7–11.

Berry J., Griffins, M., & Westcott, C. (2012). A double-blind, randomized, controlled trial of tongue-tie division and its immediate effect on breastfeeding. *Breastfeeding Medicine, 7,* 189–193.

Beutler, E., Baluda, M. C., Sturgeon, P., & Day, R. (1965). A new genetic abnormality resulting in galactose-1-phosphate uridyltransferase (GALT) deficiency. *Lancet, 1,* 353–354.

Bhagyalakshmi, G., Renukarya, A. J., & Rajangam, S. (2007). Metric analysis of the hard palate in children with Down syndrome: A comparative study. *Down Syndrome Research and Practice, 12,* 55–59.

Biancuzzo, M. (1994). Breastfeeding preterm twins: A case report. *Birth, 21,* 96–100.

Biancuzzo, M. (1998). Yes! Infants with clefts can breastfeed. *AWHONN Lifelines, 2,* 45–49.

Bibi, H., Khvolis, E., Shoseyov, D., Ohaly, M., Ben Dor, D., London, D., & Ater, D. (2001). The prevalence of gastroesophageal reflux in children with tracheomalacia and laryngomalacia. *Chest, 119,* 409–413.

Blenkinsop, A. (2003). A measure of success: Audit of frenulotomy for infant feeding problems associated with tongue-tie. *MIDIRS Midwifery Digest, 13,* 389–392.

Botto, L. (2000). Occurrence of congenital heart defects in relation to maternal multivitamin use. *American Journal of Epidemiology, 151,* 878–884.

Bovey, A, Noble, R., & Noble, M. (1999). Orofacial exercises for babies with breastfeeding problems? *Breastfeeding Review, 7,* 23–28.

Bowers, N. A., & Gromada, K. K. (2003). *Nursing management of multiple gestation: Preconception to postpartum* [Nursing module]. White Plains, NY: March of Dimes.

Bowley, D. M., & Arul, G. S. (2014). Fifteen-minute consultation on the infant with a tongue-tie. *Archives of Disease in Children Education—Practice Edition, 99,* 127–129.

Brown, J. E., & Carlson, M. (2000). Nutrition and multifetal pregnancy. *Journal of the American Dietetic Association, 100,* 343–348.

Buckley, M. (2000). Some new and important clues to the causes of colic. *British Journal of Community Nursing, 5,* 462–465.

Buryk, M., Bloom, D., & Shope, T. (2011). Efficacy of neonatal release of ankyloglossia: A randomized trial. *Pediatrics, 128,* 280–288.

Businco, L., Bruno, G., & Giampietro, P. G. (1999). Prevention and management of food allergy. *Acta Paediatrica Supplement, 88*(430), 104–109.

Byrnes, A. L., Berk, N. W., Cooper, M. E., & Marazita, M. L. (2003). Parental evaluation of informing interviews for cleft lip and/or palate. *Pediatrics, 112,* 308–313.

Cakmak, Y. O. (2011). Infantile colic: Exploring the potential role of maternal acupuncture. *Acupuncture Medicine, 29,* 295–297.

Campanozzi, A., Boccia, G., Pensabene, L., Panetta, F., Marseglia, A., Strisciuglio, P., . . . Staiano, A. (2009). Prevalence and natural history of gastroesophageal reflux: Pediatric prospective survey. *Pediatrics, 123,* 779–783.

Canani, R. B., Cirillo, P., Roggero, P., Romano, C., Malamisura, B., Terrin, G., . . . Guarino, A. (2006). Therapy with gastric acidity inhibitors increases the risk of acute gastroenteritis and community-acquired pneumonia in children. *Pediatrics, 117,* e817–e820.

Canivet, C., Jackobsson, I., & Hagander, B. (2002). Colicky infants according to maternal reports in telephone interviews and diaries: A large Scandinavian study. *Journal of Developmental and Behavioral Pediatrics, 23,* 1–8.

Canivet, C. A., Ostergren, P. O., Jakobsson, I. L., Dejin-Karlsson, E., & Hagander, B. M. (2008). Infantile colic, maternal smoking and infant feeding at 5 weeks of age. *Scandinavian Journal of Public Health, 36,* 284–291.

Cannella, P. C., Bowser, E. K., Guyer, L. K., & Borum, P. R. (1993). Feeding practices and nutrition recommendations for infants with cystic fibrosis. *Journal of the American Dietetic Association, 93,* 297–300.

Cant, A., Marsden, R. A., & Kilshaw, P. J. (1985). Egg and cow's milk hypersensitivity in exclusively breastfed infants with eczema, and detection of egg protein in breast milk. *British Medical Journal (Clinical Research Edition), 291,* 932–935.

Carpenter, R. O., Schaffer, R. L., Maeso, C. E., Sasan, F., Nuchtern, J. G., Jaksic, T., . . . Brandt, M. L. (1999). Postoperative ad lib feeding for hypertrophic pyloric stenosis. *Journal of Pediatric Surgery, 34,* 959–961.

Carroll, A. E., Garrison, M. M., & Christakis, D. A. (2002). A systematic review of nonpharmacological and nonsurgical therapies for gastroesophageal reflux in infants. *Archives of Pediatrics and Adolescent Medicine, 156,* 109–113.

Carver, J. (1999). Dietary nucleotides: Effects on the immune and gastrointestinal systems. *Acta Paediatrica, 88*(suppl), 83–88.

Chen, D. C., Nommsen-Rivers, L., Dewey, K. G., & Lonnerdal, B. (1998). Stress during labor and delivery and early lactation performance. *American Journal of Clinical Nutrition, 68,* 335–344.

Chin, S. S., Brodsky, N. L., & Bhandari, V. (2003). Antenatal steroid use is associated with increased gastroesophageal reflux in neonates. *American Journal of Perinatology, 20,* 205–213.

Choi, B. H., Kleinheinz, J., Joos, U., & Komposch, G. (1991). Sucking efficiency of early orthopaedic plate and teats in infants with cleft lip and palate. *International Journal of Oral and Maxillofacial Surgery, 20,* 167–169.

Choi, S. Y., Park, M. H., Choi, W. J., Kang, U., Oh, H. K., Kam, S., & Hwang, J. B. (2005). Clinical features and the natural history of dietary protein induced proctocolitis: A study on the elimination of offending foods from the maternal diet. *Korean Journal of Pediatric Gastroenterology and Nutrition, 8,* 21–30.

Chung, E. (2008). Infantile hypertrophic pyloric stenosis: Genes and environment. *Archives of Disease in Childhood, 93,* 1003–1004.

Clark, B. J. (1992). After a positive Guthrie—what next? Dietary management for the child with phenylketonuria. *European Journal of Clinical Nutrition, 46*(Suppl. I), S33.

Clark, D. (1999). Esophageal atresia and tracheoesophageal fistula. *American Family Physician, 59,* 910–916.

Clarren, S. K., Anderson, B., & Wolf, L. S. (1987). Feeding infants with cleft lip, cleft palate, or cleft lip and palate. *Cleft Palate Journal, 24,* 244–249.

Clifford, T. J., Campbell, M. K., Speechley, K. N., & Gorodzinsky, F. (2002). Sequelae of infant colic: Evidence of transient infant distress and absence of lasting effects on maternal mental health. *Archives of Pediatrics and Adolescent Medicine, 156,* 1183–1188.

Coffey, P. M. (1997). Breastfeeding the infant with congenital heart disease. In D. Dowling, S. C. Danner, & P. M. Coffey (Eds.), *Breastfeeding the infant with special needs.* March of Dimes Nursing Modules. White Plains, NY: March of Dimes Birth Defects Foundation.

Cohen, M., Marschall, M. A., & Schafer, M. E. (1992). Immediate unrestricted feeding of infants following cleft lip and palate repair. *Journal of Craniofacial Surgery, 3,* 30–32.

Cohen, M. M., & Bankier, A. (1991). Syndrome delineation involving orofacial clefting. *Cleft Palate–Craniofacial Journal, 28,* 119–120.

Cohen Engler, A., Hadash, A., Shehadeh, N., & Pillar, G. (2012). Breastfeeding may improve nocturnal sleep and reduce infantile colic: Potential role of breast milk melatonin. *European Journal of Pediatrics, 171,* 729–732.

Colombo, C., Costantini, D., Zazzeron, L., Faelli, N., Russo, M. C., Ghisleni, D., . . . Agostoni, C. (2007). Benefits of breastfeeding in cystic fibrosis: A single-centre follow-up survey. *Acta Paediatrica, 96,* 1228–1232.

Colon, E., Davila-Torres, R. R., Parrilla-Rodriguez, A. M., Toledo, A., Gorrin-Peralta, J. J., & Reyes-Ortiz, V. E. (2009). Exploratory study: Barriers for initiation and/or discontinuation of breastfeeding in mothers of children with Down syndrome. *Puerto Rico Health Sciences Journal, 28,* 340–344.

Combs, V. L., & Marino, B. L. (1993). A comparison of growth patterns in breast and bottle fed infants with congenital heart disease. *Pediatric Nursing, 19,* 175–179.

Conforti, A., Valfre, L., Falbo, M., Bagolan, P., & Cerchiari, A. (2015). Feeding and swallowing disorders in esophageal atresia patients: A review of a critical issue. *European Journal of Pediatric Surgery, 25,* 318–325.

Cooper-Brown, L., Copeland, S., Dailey, S., Downey, D., Petersen, M. C., Stimson, C., & Van Dyke, D. C. (2008). Feeding and swallowing dysfunction in genetic syndromes. *Developmental Disabilities Research Reviews, 14,* 147–157.

Corvaglia, L., Rotatori, R., Ferlini, M., Aceti, A., Ancora, G., & Faldella, G. (2007). The effect of body positioning on gastroesophageal reflux in premature infants: Evaluation by combined impedance and pH monitoring. *Journal of Pediatrics, 151,* 591–596.

Coryllos, E., Genna, C. W., & Salloum, A. C. (2004). Congenital tongue-tie and its impact on breastfeeding. In American Academy of Pediatrics, *Breastfeeding: Best for baby and mother.* Retrieved from http://www2.aap.org/breastfeeding/files/pdf/bbm-8-27%20Newsletter.pdf

Coryllos, E. V., Genna, C. W., & Fram, J. L. (2013). Minimally invasive treatment for posterior tongue-tie (the hidden tongue-tie). In C. W. Genna, (Ed.), *Supporting sucking skills in breastfeeding infants* (2nd ed.). Burlington, MA: Jones & Bartlett Learning.

Coy, K., Speltz, M. L., & Jones, K. (2002). Facial appearance and attachment in infants with orofacial clefts: A replication. *Cleft Palate–Craniofacial Journal, 39,* 66–71.

Crossman, K. (1998). Breastfeeding a baby with a cleft palate: A case report. *Journal of Human Lactation, 14,* 47–50.

Curtin, G. (1990). The infant with cleft lip or palate: More than a surgical problem. *Journal of Perinatal and Neonatal Nursing, 3,* 80–89.

Damato, E. G., Dowling, D. A., Madigan, E. A., & Thanattherakul, C. (2005). Duration of breastfeeding for mothers of twins. *Journal of Obstetric, Gynecologic, and Neonatal Nursing, 34,* 201–209.

Damato, E. G., Dowling, D. A., Standing, T. S., & Schuster, S. D. (2005). Explanation for cessation of breastfeeding in mothers of twins. *Journal of Human Lactation, 21,* 296–304.

Danner, S. C. (1992a). Breastfeeding the infant with a cleft defect. *NAACOG's Clinical Issues in Perinatal and Women's Health Nursing: Breastfeeding, 3,* 634–639.

Danner, S. C. (1992b). Breastfeeding the neurologically impaired infant. *NAACOG's Clinical Issues in Perinatal and Women's Health Nursing: Breastfeeding, 3,* 640–646.

Danner, S. C. (1997). Breastfeeding infants with cleft defects. In D. Dowling, S. C. Danner, & P. M. Coffey (Eds.), *Breastfeeding the infant with special needs.* March of Dimes Nursing Modules. White Plains, NY: March of Dimes Birth Defects Foundation.

Darzi, M. A., Chowdri, N. A., & Bhat, A. N. (1996). Breastfeeding or spoon feeding after cleft lip repair: A prospective, randomised study. *British Journal of Plastic Surgery, 49,* 24–26.

Davies, I., Burman-Roy, S., & Murphy, M. S., on behalf of Guideline Development Group. (2014). Gastro-oesophageal reflux disease in children: NICE guidance. *BMJ, 350,* g7703.

De Ybarrondo, L., & Mazur, L. J. (2000). Sandifer's syndrome in a child with asthma and cerebral palsy. *Southern Medicine Journal, 93,* 1019–1021.

Dellert, S. F., Hyams, J. S., Treem, W. R., & Geertsma, M. A. (1993). Feeding resistance and gastroesophageal reflux in infancy. *Journal of Pediatric Gastroenterology and Nutrition, 17,* 66–71.

Demian, M., Nguyen, S., & Emil, S. (2009). Early pyloric stenosis: A case control study. *Pediatric Surgery International, 25,* 1053–1057.

Denk, M. J. (1998). Advances in neonatal surgery. *Pediatric Clinics of North America, 45,* 1479–1506.

DeSantis, A., Coster, W, Bigsby, R., & Lester, B. M. (2004). Colic and fussing in infancy and sensory processing at 3–8 years of age. *Infant Mental Health Journal, 25,* 522–539.

Dewey, K. G. (2001). Maternal and fetal stress are associated with impaired lactogenesis in humans. *Journal of Nutrition, 131,* 3012S–3015S.

Dewey, K. G., Nommsen-Rivers, L., Heinig, M. J., & Cohen, R. J. (2003). Risk factors for suboptimal infant breastfeeding behavior, delayed onset of lactation, and excess neonatal weight loss. *Pediatrics, 112,* 607–619.

Dobbelsteyn, C., Marche, D. M., Blake, K., & Rashid, M. (2005). Early oral sensory experiences and feeding development in children with CHARGE syndrome: A report of five cases. *Dysphagia, 20,* 89–100.

Dobbelsteyn, C., Peacocke, S. D., Blake, K., Crist, W., & Rashid, M. (2008). Feeding difficulties in children with CHARGE syndrome: Prevalence, risk factors, and prognosis. *Dysphagia, 23,* 127–135.

Dodge, J. A. (1975). Infantile hypertrophic pyloric stenosis in Belfast, 1957–1969. *Archives of Disease in Childhood, 50,* 171–178.

Dollberg, S., Botzer, E., Grunis, E., & Mimouni, F. B. (2006). Immediate nipple pain relief after frenotomy in breastfed infants with ankyloglossia: A randomized, prospective study. *Journal of Pediatric Surgery, 41,* 1598–1600.

Dollberg, S., Marom, R., & Botzer, E. (2014). Lingual frenotomy for breastfeeding difficulties: A prospective follow-up study. *Breastfeeding Medicine, 9,* 286–289.

Dombrowski, M., Anderson, G. C., Santori, C., Roller, C. G., Pagliotti, F., & Dowling, D. A. (2000). Kangaroo skin-to-skin care for premature twins and their adolescent parents. *MCN: The American Journal of Maternal/Child Nursing, 25,* 92–94.

Donati-Bourne, J., Batool, Z., Hendrickse, C., & Bowley, D. (2015). Tongue-tie assessment and division: A time-critical intervention to optimize breastfeeding. *Journal of Neonatal Surgery, 4,* 3.

Donovan, K. (2012). Breastfeeding the infant with cleft lip and palate. *ICAN: Infant, Child, and Adolescent Nutrition, 4,* 194–198.

Duncan, L. L., & Elder, S. B. (1997). Breastfeeding the infant with PKU. *Journal of Human Lactation, 13,* 231–235.

Eberly, M. D., Eide, M. B., Thompson, J. L., & Nylund, C. M. (2015). Azithromycin in early infancy and pyloric stenosis. *Pediatrics, 135,* 483–488.

Edmondson, R., & Reinhartsen, D. (1998). The young child with cleft lip and palate: Intervention needs in the first three years. *Infants and Young Children, 11,* 12–20.

Edmunds, J., Hazelbaker, A., Murphy, J. G., & Philipp, B. L. (2012). Tongue-tie. *Journal of Human Lactation, 28,* 14–17.

Edmunds, J. E., Fulbrook, P., & Miles, S. (2013). Understanding the experiences of mothers who are breastfeeding an infant with tongue-tie: A phenomenological study. *Journal of Human Lactation, 29,* 190–195.

Einarsson-Backes, L. M., Deitz, J., Price, R., Glass, R., & Hays, R. (1994). The effect of oral support on sucking efficiency in preterm infants. *American Journal of Occupational Therapy, 48,* 490–498.

El Amm, C. A., & Denny, A. (2008). Hyoid bone abnormalities in Pierre Robin patients. *Journal of Craniofacial Surgery, 19,* 259–263.

Emmanouil-Nikoloussi, E. N., & Kerameos-Foroglou, C. (1992a). Developmental malformations of human tongue and associated syndromes [Review]. *Bulletin du Groupement International Pour la Recherche Scientifique en Stomatologie & Odontologie, 35,* 5–12.

Emmanouil-Nikoloussi, E. N., & Kerameos-Foroglou, C. (1992b). Congenital syndromes connected with tongue malformations. *Bulletin de l'Association des Anatomies, 76,* 67–72.

Erkkila, A. T., Isotalo, E., Pulkkinen, J., & Haapanen, M. L. (2005). Association between school performance, breast milk intake and fatty acid profile of serum lipids in ten-year-old cleft children. *Journal of Craniofacial Surgery, 16,* 764–769.

Everett, K. V., Capon, F., Georgoula, C., Chioza, B. A., Reece, A., Jaswon, M., . . . Chung, E. M. (2008). Linkage of monogenic infantile hypertrophic pyloric stenosis to chromosome 16q24. *European Journal of Human Genetics, 16,* 1151–1154.

Ewer, A. K., James, M. E., & Tobin, J. M. (1999). Prone and left lateral positioning reduce gastro-oesophageal reflux in preterm infants. *Archives of Disease in Childhood—Fetal and Neonatal Edition, 81,* F201–F205.

Feillet, F., & Agostoni, C. (2010). Nutritional issues in treating phenylketonuria. *Journal of Inherited Metabolic Disease, 33,* 659–664.

Feranchak, A. P., Orenstein, S. R., & Cohn, J. F. (1994). Behaviors associated with the onset of gastroesophageal reflux episodes in infants: Prospective study using split screen video and pH probe. *Clinical Pediatrics, 33,* 654–662.

Ferguson, A., Bier, J. B., Cucca, J., Andreozzi, L., & Lester, B. (1996). The quality of sucking in infants with colic. *Infant Mental Health, 17,* 161–169.

Fernando, C. (1998). *Tongue-tie: From confusion to clarity.* Sydney, Australia: Tandem Publications.

Finnegan, L. P. (1982). Substance abuse: Implication for the newborn. *Perinatology and Neonatology, 6,* 17–24.

Fleiss, P. M., Burger, M., Ramkumar, H., & Carrington P. (1990). Ankyloglossia: A cause of breastfeeding problems? *Journal of Human Lactation, 6,* 128–129.

Fletcher, S. G., & Meldrum, J. R. (1968). Lingual function and relative length of the lingual frenulum. *Journal of Speech, Language, and Hearing Research, 2,* 382–390.

Flidel-Rimon, O., & Shinwell, E. S. (2002). Breastfeeding multiples. *Seminars in Neonatology, 7,* 231–239.

Flidel-Romin, O., & Shinwell, E. S. (2006). Breastfeeding twins and high multiples. *Archives of Disease in Childhood—Fetal and Neonatal Edition, 91,* F377–F380.

Food and Drug Administration (FDA). (2012). FDA expands caution about SimplyThick. Retrieved from http://www.fda.gov/ForConsumers/ConsumerUpdates/ucm256250.htm

Forlenza, G. P., Black, N. M. P., McNamara, E. G., & Sullivan, S. E. (2010). Ankyloglossia, exclusive breastfeeding, and failure to thrive. *Pediatrics, 125,* e1500–e1504.

Forrester, M. B., & Merz, D. (2004). Descriptive epidemiology of oral clefts in a multiethnic population, Hawaii, 1986–2000. *Cleft Palate–Craniofacial Journal, 41,* 622–628.

Freedman, S. B., Al-Harthy, N., & Thull-Freedman, J. (2009). The crying infant: Diagnostic testing and frequency of serious underlying disease. *Pediatrics, 123,* 841–848.

Friedman, S., Flidel-Rimon, O., Lavie, E., & Shinwell, E. S. (2004). The effect of prenatal consultation with a neonatologist on human milk feeding in preterm infants. *Acta Paediatrica, 93,* 775–778.

Frommelt, M. A. (2004). Differential diagnosis and approach to a heart murmur in term infants. *Pediatric Clinics of North America, 51,* 1023–1032.

Fuentes, A., & Goldkrand, J. W. (1987). Angiotensin-converting enzyme activity in hypertensive subjects after magnesium sulfate therapy. *American Journal of Obstetrics and Gynecology, 156,* 1375–1379.

Fugimoto, T., Lane, G. J., Segawa, O., Esaki, S., & Miyano, T. (1999). Laparoscopic extramucosal pyloromyotomy versus open pyloromyotomy for infantile hypertrophic pyloric stenosis: Which is better? *Journal of Pediatric Surgery, 34,* 370–372.

Garbin, C. P., Sakalidis, V. S., Chadwick, L. M., Whan, E., Hartmann, P. E., & Geddes, D. T. (2013). Evidence of improved milk intake after frenotomy: A case report. *Pediatrics, 132,* e1413–e1417.

Garcez, L. W., & Giugliani, E. R. (2005). Population-based study on the practice of breastfeeding in children born with cleft lip and palate. *Cleft Palate-Craniofacial Journal, 42,* 687–693.

Garrison, M., & Christakis, A. (2000). A systematic review of treatments for infantile colic. *Pediatrics, 106,* 184–190.

Gartner, S. L. (1996). Breastfeeding the infant with physical and developmental needs. *Nutrition Focus,* 1–8.

Garza, J. J., Morash, D., Dzakovic, A., Mondschein, J. K., & Jaksic, T. (2002). Ad libitum feeding decreases hospital stay for neonates after pyloromyotomy. *Journal of Pediatric Surgery, 37,* 493–495.

Geddes, D. T., Kent, J. C., McClellan, H. L., Garbin, C. P., Chadwick, L. M., & Hartmann, P. E. (2010). Sucking characteristics of successfully breastfeeding infants with ankyloglossia: A case series. *Acta Paediatrica, 99,* 301–303.

Geddes, D. T., Langton, D. B., Gollow, I., Jacobs, L. A., Hartmann, P. E., & Simmer, K. (2008). Frenulotomy for breastfeeding infants with ankyloglossia: Effect on milk removal and sucking mechanism as imaged by ultrasound. *Pediatrics, 122,* e188–e194.

Genna, C. W. (2013). *Supporting sucking skills in breastfeeding infants* (2nd ed.). Burlington, MA: Jones & Bartlett Learning.

Geraghty, S. R., Khoury, J. C., & Kalkwarf, H. J. (2004). Comparison of feeding among multiple birth infants. *Twin Research, 7,* 542–547.

Geraghty, S. R., Khoury, J. C., & Kalkwarf, H. J. (2005). Human milk pumping rates of mothers of singletons and mothers of multiples. *Journal of Human Lactation, 21,* 413–420.

Geraghty, S. R., Pinney, S. M., Sethuraman, G., Roy-Chaudhury, A., & Kalkwarf, H. J. (2004). Breast milk feeding rates of mothers of multiples compared to mothers of singletons. *Ambulatory Pediatrics, 4,* 226–231.

Ghaem, M., Armstrong, K. L., Trocki, O., Cleghorn, G. J., Patrick, M. K., & Shepherd, R. W. (1998). The sleep patterns of infants and young children with gastroesophageal reflux. *Journal of Pediatric Child Health, 34,* 160–163.

Gibson, S. E. (2004). Laryngomalacia and its management: When to worry about the squeaky baby. *Medicine and Health, Rhode Island, 87,* 304–306.

Glass, R. P., & Wolf, L. S. (1994). Incoordination of sucking, swallowing, and breathing as an etiology for breastfeeding difficulty. *Journal of Human Lactation, 10,* 185–189.

Glass, R. P., & Wolf, L. S. (1999). Feeding management of infants with cleft lip and palate and micrognathia. *Infant and Young Children, 12,* 70–81.

Gokcay, G., Baykal, T., Gokdemir, Y., & Demirkol, M. (2006). Breastfeeding in organic acidemias. *Journal of Inherited Metabolic Disease, 29,* 304–310.

Gold, B. D. (2006). Is gastroesophageal reflux disease really a life-long disease: Do babies who regurgitate grow up to be adults with GERD complications? *American Journal of Gastroenterology, 101,* 641–644.

Golonka, N. R., & Hayashi, A. H. (2008). Early "sham" feeding of neonates promotes oral feeding after delayed primary repair of major congenital esophageal anomalies. *American Journal of Surgery, 195,* 659–662.

Goyal, M., Chopra, R., Bansal, K., & Marwaha, M. (2014). Role of obturators and other feeding interventions in patients with cleft lip and palate: A review. *European Archives of Paediatric Dentistry, 15,* 1–9.

Grady, E. (1977). Breastfeeding the baby with a cleft of the soft palate. *Clinical Pediatrics, 16,* 182–184.

Greve, L. C., Wheeler, M. D., Green-Burgeson, D. K., & Zorn, E. M. (1994). Breastfeeding in the management of the newborn with phenylketonuria: A practical approach to dietary therapy. *Journal of the American Dietetic Association, 94,* 305–309.

Griffiths, D. M. (2004). Do tongue ties affect breastfeeding? *Journal of Human Lactation, 20,* 409–414.

Gromada, K. (1981). Maternal–infant attachment: The first step toward individualizing twins. *Maternal–Child Nursing Journal, 6,* 129–134.

Gromada, K. K. (1992). Breastfeeding more than one: Multiples and tandem breastfeeding. *NAACOG's Clinical Issues in Perinatal and Women's Health Nursing: Breastfeeding, 3,* 656–666.

Gromada, K. K. (1999). *Mothering multiples: Breastfeeding and caring for twins or more!!* Schaumburg, IL: La Leche League International.

Gromada, K. K., & Spangler, A. K. (1998). Breastfeeding twins and higher-order multiples. *Journal of Obstetric, Gynecologic, and Neonatal Nursing, 27,* 441–449.

Guarino, N., Yoneda, A., Shima, H., & Puri, P. (2001). Selective neurotrophin deficiency in infantile hypertrophic pyloric stenosis. *Journal of Pediatric Surgery, 36,* 1280–1284.

Guedj, F., Bianchi, D. W., & Delabar, J. M. (2014). Prenatal treatment of Down syndrome: A reality? *Current Opinions in Obstetrics and Gynecology, 26,* 92–103.

Habbick, B. F., Khanna, C., & To, T. (1989). Infantile hypertrophic pyloric stenosis: A study of feeding practices and other possible causes. *Canadian Medical Association Journal, 140,* 401–404.

Haberman, M. (1988). A mother of invention. *Nursing Times, 84,* 52–53.

Haldeman, W. (1993). Can magnesium sulfate therapy impact lactogenesis? *Journal of Human Lactation, 9,* 249–252.

Hale, T. W. (2012). *Medications and mothers' milk* (15th ed.). Amarillo, TX: Hale Publishing.

Hale, T. W., & Ilett, K. F. (2002). *Drug therapy and breastfeeding: From theory to clinical practice.* New York, NY: Parthenon.

Hammerman, C., & Kaplan, M. (1995). Oxygen saturation during and after feeding in healthy term infants. *Biology of the Neonate, 67,* 94–99.

Harris, E. F., Friend, G. W., & Tolley, E. A. (1992). Enhanced prevalence of ankyloglossia with maternal cocaine abuse. *Cleft Palate–Craniofacial Journal, 29,* 72–76.

Hartman, D. M., & Medoff-Cooper, B. (2012). Transition to home after neonatal surgery for congenital heart disease. *MCN: American Journal of Maternal Child Nursing, 37,* 95–100.

Hattori, R., & Hattori, H. (1999). Breastfeeding twins: Guidelines for success. *Birth, 26,* 37–42.

Hauben, M., & Amsden, G. W. (2002). The association of erythromycin and infantile hypertrophic pyloric stenosis: Causal or coincidental? *Drug Safety, 25,* 929–942.

Hazelbaker, A. K. (1993). *The assessment tool for lingual frenulum function* (Unpublished master's thesis). Pacific Oaks College, Pasadena, CA.

Heacock, H. J., Jeffery, H. E., Baker, J. L., & Page, M. (1992). Influence of breast versus formula milk on physiological gastroesophageal reflux in healthy, newborn infants. *Journal of Pediatric Gastroenterology and Nutrition, 14,* 41–46.

Heine, R. G., Jordan, B., Lubitz, L., Meehan, M., & Catto-Smith, A. G. (2006). Clinical predictors of pathological gastroesophageal reflux in infants with persistent distress. *Journal of Paediatrics and Child Health, 42,* 134–139.

Henly, S. J., Anderson, C. M., Avery, M. D., Hills-Bonczyk, S. G., Potter, S., & Duckett, L. J. (1995). Anemia and insufficient milk in first-time mothers. *Birth, 22,* 86–92.

Henry, L., & Hayman, R. (2014). Ankyloglossia and its impact on breastfeeding. *Nursing for Women's Health, 18,* 122–129.

Henry, S. M. (2004). Discerning differences: Gastroesophageal reflux and gastroesophageal reflux disease in infants. *Advances in Neonatal Care, 4,* 235–247.

Hiimae, K. M., & Palmer, J. B. (2003). Tongue movements in feeding and speech. *Critical Reviews in Oral Biology and Medicine, 14,* 413–429.

Hill, D. J., Hudson, I. L., Sheffield, L. J., Shelton, M. J., Menahem, S., & Hosking, C. S. (1995). A low allergen diet is a significant intervention in infantile colic: Results of a community-based study. *Journal of Allergy and Clinical Immunology, 96,* 886–892.

Hill, D. J., Roy, N., Heine, R. G., Hosking, C. S., Francis, D. E., Brown, J., . . . Carlin, J. B. (2005). Effect of a low-allergen maternal diet on colic among breastfed infants: A randomized, controlled trial. *Pediatrics, 116,* e709–e715.

Hill, P., Aldag, J., & Chatterton, R. (2001). Initiation and frequency of pumping and milk production in mothers of non-nursing preterm infants. *Journal of Human Lactation, 17,* 9–13.

Hoen, A. G., Li, J., Moulton, L. A., O'Toole, G. A., Housman, M. L., Koestler, D. C., . . . Madan, J. C. (2015). Associations between gut microbial colonization in early life and respiratory outcomes in cystic fibrosis. *Journal of Pediatrics, 167,* 138–147.

Hoffman, J. (1990). Congenital heart disease: Incidence and inheritance. *Pediatric Clinics of North America, 37,* 25–43.

Hogan, M., Westcott, C., & Griffiths, M. (2005). Randomized, controlled trial of division of tongue-tie in infants with feeding problems. *Journal of Paediatrics and Child Health, 41,* 246–250.

Holland, M. (1996). Rubenstein-Taybi syndrome. *Nutrition Focus, 11,* 1–4.

Holliday, K. E., Allen, J. R., Waters, D. L., Gruca, M. A., Thompson, S. M., & Gaskin, K. J. (1991). Growth of human milk–fed and formula-fed infants with cystic fibrosis. *Journal of Pediatrics, 118,* 77–79.

Hong, P., Lago, D., Seargeant, J., Pellman, L., Magit, A. E., & Pransky, S. M. (2010). Defining ankyloglossia: A case series of anterior and posterior tongue ties. *International Journal of Pediatric Otorhinolaryngology, 74,* 1003–1006.

Howard, C. R., Lanphear, N., Lanphear, B. P., Eberly, S., & Lawrence, R. A. (2006). Parental responses to infant crying and colic: The effect on breastfeeding duration. *Breastfeeding Medicine, 1,* 146–155.

Huang, R.-C., Forbes, D. A., & Davies, M. W. (2003). Feed thickener for newborn infants with gastroesophageal reflux (Cochrane Review*). Cochrane Library (Issue 2).* Oxford, UK: Update Software.

Huggins, K. (1990). Ankyloglossia: One lactation consultant's personal experience. *Journal of Human Lactation, 6,* 123–124.

Huhtala, V., Lehtonen, L., Uvnas-Moberg, K., & Korvenranta, H. (2003). Low plasma cholecystokinin levels in colicky infants. *Journal of Pediatric Gastroenterology and Nutrition, 37,* 42–46.

Humenczuk, M. (1998). *Feeding assistance for infants with cleft lip and palate.* Presented at the annual meeting of the American Dietetic Association, October 10, Kansas City, MO.

Huner, G., Baykal, T., Demir, F., & Demirkol, M. (2005). Breastfeeding experience in inborn errors of metabolism other than phenylketonuria. *Journal of Inherited Metabolic Disease, 28,* 457–465.

Hurtekant, K. M., & Spatz, D. L. (2007). Special considerations for breastfeeding the infant with spina bifida. *Journal of Perinatal and Neonatal Nursing, 21,* 69–75.

Hwang, J.-B., Park, M. H., Kang, Y. N., Kim, S. P., Suh, S. I., & Kam, S. (2007). Advanced criteria for clinicopathological diagnosis of food protein–induced proctocolitis. *Journal of Korean Medical Science, 22,* 213–217.

Incerti, M., Horowitz, K., Roberson, R., Abebe, D., Toso, L., Calallero, M., & Spomg, C. Y. (2012). Prenatal treatment prevents learning deficit in Down syndrome model. *PLoS One, 7*(11), e50724.

Ingram, J., Johnson, D., Copeland, M., Churchill, C., Taylor, H., & Emond, A. (2015). The development of a tongue assessment tool to assist with tongue-tie identification. *Archives of Disease in Children—Fetal Neonatal Edition, 100,* F344–F348.

International Affiliation of Tongue-Tie Professionals. (2014). Definition of tongue-tie. Retrieved from http://tonguetieprofessionals.org/about/assessment/definition-of-tongue-tie/

Ize-Iyamu, I. N., & Saheeb, B. D. (2011). Feeding intervention in cleft lip and palate babies: A practical approach to feeding efficiency and weight gain. *International Journal of Oral and Maxillofacial Surgery, 40,* 916–919.

Jadcherla, S. R. (2002). Gastroesophageal reflux in the neonate. *Recent Advances in Neonatal Gastroenterology, 29,* 135–158.

Jadcherla, S. R., Chan, C. Y., Moore, R., Malkar, M., Timan, C. J., & Valentine, C. J. (2012). Impact of feeding strategies on the frequency and clearance of acid and nonacid gastroesophageal reflux events in dysphagic neonates. *Journal of Parenteral and Enteral Nutrition, 36,* 449–455.

Jadcherla, S. R., Vijayapal, A. S., & Leuthner, S. (2009). Feeding abilities in neonates with congenital heart disease: A retrospective study. *Journal of Perinatology, 29,* 112–118.

Jadin, S. A., Wu, G. S., Zhang, Z., Shoff, S. M., Tippets, B. M., Farrell, P. M., . . . Lai, H. J. (2011). Growth and pulmonary outcomes during the first 2 y of life of breastfed and formula-fed infants diagnosed with cystic fibrosis through the Wisconsin Routine Newborn Screening Program. *American Journal of Clinical Nutrition, 93,* 1038–1047.

Jain, E. (1995). Tongue-tie: Its impact on breastfeeding. *AARN News Letter, 51,* 18.

Jain, E. (1996). Tongue-tie: Impact on breastfeeding. Retrieved from http://www.drjain.com

Jakobsson, I., Borulf, S., Lindberg, T., & Benediktsson B. (1983). Partial hydrolysis of cow's milk proteins by human trypsins and elastases in vitro. *Journal of Pediatric Gastroenterology and Nutrition, 2,* 613–616.

Jakobsson, I., & Lindberg, T. (1978). Cow's milk as a cause of infantile colic in breastfed infants. *Lancet, 312,* 437–439.

Jakobsson, I., & Lindberg, T. (1983). Cow's milk proteins cause infantile colic in breastfed infants: A double-blind crossover study. *Pediatrics, 71,* 268–271.

Jedd, M. B., Melton, L. J., Griffin, M. R., Kaufman, B., Hoffman, A. D., Broughton, D., & O'Brien, P. C. (1986). Factors associated with infantile hypertrophic pyloric stenosis. *American Journal of Diseases of Children, 142,* 334–337.

Joanna Briggs Institute. (2008). The effectiveness of interventions for infant colic. *Best Practice: Evidence-Based Practice Information Sheets for Health Professionals, 12,* 1–4.

Jocelyn, L. J., Penko, M. A., & Rode, H. L. (1996). Cognition, communication, and hearing in young children with cleft lip and palate and in control children: A longitudinal study. *Pediatrics, 97,* 529–534.

Jones, E., Dimmock, P. W., & Spencer, S. A. (2001). A randomised controlled trial to compare methods of milk expression after preterm delivery. *Archives of Disease in Childhood—Fetal and Neonatal Edition, 85,* F91–F95.

Jung, A. D. (2001). Gastroesophageal reflux in infants and children. *American Family Physician, 64,* 1853–1860.

Kanufre, V., Starling, A. L. P., Leao, E., Aguiar, M. J., Santos, J. S., Soares, R. D., & Silveira, A. M. (2007). Breastfeeding in the treatment of children with phenylketonuria. *Journal of Pediatrics, 83,* 447–452.

Karabulut, R., Sonmez, K., Turkyilmaz, Z., Demirogullari, B., Ozen, I. O., Bagbanci, B., . . . Baçaklar, A. C. (2008). Ankyloglossia and effects on breastfeeding, speech problems and mechanical/social issues in children. *B-ENT, 4,* 81–85.

Kaye, A., Thaeta, K., Snell, A., Chesser, C., Goldak, C., & Huff, H. (2016). Initial nutritional assessment of infants with cleft lip and/or palate: Interventions and return to birth weight. *Cleft Palate Craniofacial Journal.* [Epub ahead of print].

Kenner, C., Brueggemeyer, A., & Porter-Gunderson, L. (1993). *Comprehensive neonatal nursing: A physiologic perspective.* Philadelphia, PA: W. B. Saunders.

Khoo, A. K., Dabbas, N., Sudhakaran, N., Ade-Ajayi, N., & Patel, S. (2009). Nipple pain at presentation predicts success of tongue-tie division for breastfeeding problems. *European Journal of Pediatric Surgery, 19,* 370–373.

Kilshaw, P. J., & Cant, A. J. (1984). The passage of maternal dietary proteins into human breast milk. *International Archives of Allergy and Immunology, 75,* 8–15.

Kimata, H. (2007). Laughter elevates the levels of breastmilk melatonin. *Journal of Psychosomatic Research, 62,* 699–702.

Kleinman, R. E. (Ed.). (2013). Formula feeding of term infants. In: *American Academy of Pediatrics pediatric nutrition handbook* (7th ed.). Elk Grove Village, IL: American Academy of Pediatrics.

Knox, I. (2010). Tongue tie and frenotomy in the breastfeeding newborn. *NeoReviews, 11,* c513–c519.

Koenig, J. S., Davies, A. M., & Thach, B. T. (1990). Coordination of breathing, sucking and swallowing during bottle feedings in human infants. *Journal of Applied Physiology, 69,* 1623–1629.

Kogo, M., Okada, G., Ishii, S., Shikata, M., Iida, S., & Matsuya, T. (1997). Breastfeeding for cleft lip and palate patients using the Hotz-type plate. *Cleft Palate–Craniofacial Journal, 34,* 351–353.

Koletzko, S., & Reinhardt, D. (2001). Nutritional challenges of infants with cystic fibrosis. *Early Human Development, 65*(suppl), S53–S61.

Kotlow, L. (2011). Infant reflux and aerophagia associated with the maxillary lip-tie and ankyloglossia (tongue-tie). *Clinical Lactation, 2,* 25–29.

Kotlow, L. A. (1999). Ankyloglossia (tongue-tie): A diagnostic quandary. *Quintessence International, 30,* 259–262.

Kotlow, L. A. (2004a). Oral diagnosis of abnormal frenum attachments in neonates and infants: Evaluation and treatment of the maxillary and lingual frenum using the erbium: YAG laser. *Journal of Pediatric Dental Care, 10.* Retrieved from http://www.kiddsteeth.com/articles/finasltfrenarticleoct2004.pdf

Kotlow, L. A. (2004b). Using the erbium: YAG laser to correct an abnormal lingual frenum attachment in newborns. *Journal of the Academy of Laser Dentistry, 12,* 22–23.

Kotlow, L. A. (2013). Diagnosing and understanding the maxillary lip-tie (superior labial, the maxillary labial frenum) as it relates to breastfeeding. *Journal of Human Lactation, 29,* 458–464.

Kramer, G. J. C., Hoeksma, J. B., & Prahl-Andersen, B. (1994). Palatal changes after lip surgery in different types of cleft lip and palate. *Cleft Palate–Craniofacial Journal, 31,* 376–384.

Krogh, C., Biggar, R. J., Fischer, T. K., Lindholm, M., Wholfahrt, J., & Melbye, M. (2012). Bottle-feeding and the risk of pyloric stenosis. *Pediatrics, 130,* e943–e949.

Kumagai, H., Maisawa, S-i., Tanaka, M., Takahashi, M., Takasago, Y., Nishijima, A., & Watanabe, S. (2012). Intestinal microbiota and secretory immunoglobulin A in feces of exclusively breastfed infants with blood-streaked stools. *Microbiology Immunology, 56,* 657–663.

Kumar, M., & Kalke, E. (2012). Tongue-tie, breastfeeding difficulties and the role of frenotomy. *Acta Paediatrica, 101,* 687–689.

Kwong, K. M. (2015). Current updates on choanal atresia. *Frontiers in Pediatrics, 3,* 52.

LaFleur, E., & Niesen, K. (1996). Breastfeeding conjoined twins. *Journal of Obstetric, Gynecologic, and Neonatal Nursing, 25,* 241–244.

Lake, A. M., Whitington, P. F., & Hamilton, S. R. (1982). Dietary protein–induced colitis in breastfed infants. *Journal of Pediatrics, 101,* 906–910.

Lalakea, M. L., & Messner, A. H. (2002). Frenotomy and frenuloplasty: If, when, and how. *Op Tech Otolaryngology, 13,* 96.

Lalakea, M. L., & Messner, A. H. (2003a). Ankyloglossia: Does it matter? *Pediatric Clinics of North America, 50,* 381–397.

Lalakea, M. L., & Messner, A. H. (2003b). Ankyloglossia: The adolescent and adult perspective. *Otolaryngology—Head and Neck Surgery, 128,* 746–752.

Lambert, J. M., & Watters, N. E. (1998). Breastfeeding the infant/child with a cardiac defect: An informal survey. *Journal of Human Lactation, 14,* 151–155.

Lammer, E. J., & Edmonds, L. D. (1987). Trends in pyloric stenosis incidence, Atlanta, 1968 to 1982. *Journal of Medical Genetics, 24,* 482–487.

Landgren, K., Kvorning, N., & Hallstrom, I. (2010). Acupuncture reduces crying in infants with infantile colic: A randomised, controlled, blind clinical study. *Acupuncture Medicine, 28,* 174–179.

Lawlor-Smith, C., & Lawlor-Smith, L. (1998). Lactose intolerance. *Breastfeeding Review, 6,* 29–30.

Lawrence, R. A., & Lawrence, R. M. (2016). *Breastfeeding: A guide for the medical profession* (8th ed.). St. Louis, MO: Mosby.

Leonard, L. G. (1982). Twin pregnancy: Maternal–fetal nutrition. *Journal of Obstetric, Gynecologic, and Neonatal Nursing, 11,* 139–145.

Leonard, L. G. (2000). Breastfeeding triplets: The at-home experience. *Public Health Nursing, 17,* 211–221.

Leonard, L. G. (2002). Breastfeeding higher order multiples: Enhancing support during the postpartum hospitalization period. *Journal of Human Lactation, 18,* 386–392.

Leonard, L. G. (2003). Breastfeeding rights of multiple birth families and guidelines for health professionals. *Twin Research, 6,* 34–45.

Lewanda, A. F., & Jabs, E. W. (1994). Genetics of craniofacial disorders. *Current Opinion in Pediatrics, 6,* 690–697.

Lewis, E., & Kritzinger, A. (2004). Parental experiences of feeding problems in their infants with Down syndrome. *Down's Syndrome Research and Practice, 9,* 45–52.

Liang, R., Gunn, A. J., & Gunn, T. R. (1997). Can preterm twins breastfeed successfully? *New Zealand Medical Journal, 110,* 209–212.

Lindberg, N., & Berglund, A. L. (2014). Mothers' experiences of feeding babies born with cleft lip and palate. *Scandinavian Journal of Caring Science, 28,* 66–73.

Lobo, M. (1992). Parent–infant interaction during feeding when the infant has congenital heart disease. *Journal of Pediatric Nursing, 7,* 97–105.

Loffredo, C. A., Wilson, P. D., & Ferencz, C. (2001). Maternal diabetes: An independent risk factor for major cardiovascular malformations with increased mortality of affected infants. *Teratology, 64,* 98–106.

Losee, J. E., Mason, A. C., Dudas, J., Hua, L. B., & Mooney, M. P. (2007). Nonsynostotic occipital plagiocephaly: Factors impacting onset, treatment, and outcomes. *Plastic and Reconstructive Surgery, 119,* 1866–1873.

Lothe, L., & Lindberg, T. (1989). Cow's milk whey protein elicits symptoms of infantile colic in colicky formula-fed infants: A double-blind crossover study. *Pediatrics, 83,* 262–266.

Lothe, L., Lindberg, T., & Jakobsson, I. (1982). Cow's milk formula as a cause of infantile colic: A double blind study. *Pediatrics, 70,* 7–10.

Lucarelli, S., Di Nardo, G., Lastrucci, G., D'Alfonso, Y., Marcheggiano, A., Federici, T., . . . Cucchiara, S. (2011). Allergic proctocolitis refractory to maternal hypoallergenic diet in exclusively breastfed infants: A clinical observation. *BMC Gastroenterology, 11,* 82.

Lucassen, P. (2010). Colic in infants. *BMJ Clinical Evidence, 2010,* 0309. Retrieved from http://www.ncbi.nlm.nih.gov/pmc/articles/PMC2907620/pdf/2010-0309.pdf

Lucassen, P. L., Assendelft, W. J., van Eijk, J. T., Gubbels, J., Douwes, A., & van Geldrop, W. J. (2001). Systematic review of the occurrence of infantile colic in the community. *Archives of Disease in Childhood, 84,* 398–403.

Lucassen, P. L. B. J., Assendelft, W. J. J., Gubbels, J. W., van Eijk, J. T. M., van Geldrop, W. J., & Knuistingh Neven, A. (1998). Effectiveness of treatments for infantile colic: Systematic review. *BMJ, 317,* 1563–1569.

Luder, E., Kattan, M., Tanzer-Torres, G., & Bonforte, R. J. (1990). Current recommendations for breastfeeding in cystic fibrosis centers. *American Journal of Diseases of Children, 144,* 1153–1156.

Luke, B., Hediger, M. L., Nugent, C., Newman, R. B., Mauldin, J. G., Witter, F. R., & O'Sullivan, M. J. (2003). Body mass index: Specific weight gains associated with optimal birth weights in twin pregnancies. *Journal of Reproductive Medicine, 48,* 217–224.

MacDonald, A., Depondt, E., Evans, S., Daly, A., Hendriksz, C., Chakrapani, A. A., & Saudubray, J. M. (2006). Breastfeeding in IMD. *Journal of Inherited Metabolic Disease, 29,* 299–303.

Machida, H. M., Catto-Smith, A. G., Gall, D. G., Trevenen, C., & Scott, R. B. (1994). Allergic colitis in infancy: Clinical and pathological aspects. *Journal of Pediatric Gastroenterology and Nutrition, 19,* 22–26.

Madlon-Kay, D. J., Ricke, L. A., Baker, N. J., & DeFor, T. A. (2008). Case series of 148 tongue-tied newborn babies evaluated with the assessment tool for lingual frenulum function. *Midwifery, 24,* 353–357.

Mahon, B. E., Rosenman, M. B., & Kleinman, M. B. (2001). Maternal and infant use of erythromycin and other macrolide antibiotics as risk factors for infantile hypertrophic pyloric stenosis. *Journal of Pediatrics, 139,* 380–384.

Mahoney, L. T. (1993). Acyanotic congenital heart disease. Atrial and ventricular septal defects, atrioventricular canal, patent ductus arteriosus, pulmonic stenosis. *Cardiology Clinics, 11,* 603–616.

Mair, E. A., & Parsons, D. S. (1992). Pediatric tracheobronchomalacia and major airway collapse. *Annals of Otology, Rhinology, and Laryngology, 101,* 300–309.

Malik, S., Cleves, M. A., Honein, M. A., Romitti, P. A., Botto, L. D., Yang, S., & Hobbs, C. A. (2008). Maternal smoking and congenital heart defects. *Pediatrics, 121,* e810–e816.

Marcellus, L. (2001). The infant with Pierre Robin sequence: Review and implications for nursing practice. *Journal of Pediatric Nursing, 15,* 23–33.

Marchini, G., Simoni, M. R., Bartolini, F., & Uvnas-Moberg, K. (1994). Plasma gastrin and somatostatin levels in newborn infants receiving supplementary formula feeding. *Acta Paediatrica, 83,* 374–377.

Marino, B. L., O'Brien, P., & LoRe, H. (1995). Oxygen saturations during breast and bottle feedings in infants with congenital heart disease. *Journal of Pediatric Nursing, 10,* 360–364.

Marmet, C., Shell, E., & Marmet, R. (1990). Neonatal frenotomy may be necessary to correct breastfeeding problems. *Journal of Human Lactation, 6,* 117–121.

Marques, I. L., de Sousa, T. V., Carneiro, A. F., Barbieri, M. A., Bettiol, H., & Gutierrez, M. R. (2001). Clinical experience with infants with Robin sequence: A prospective study. *Cleft Palate–Craniofacial Journal, 38,* 171–178.

Martin, J. A., Hamilton, B. E., Sutton, P. D., Ventura, S. J., Menacker, F., & Munson, M. L. (2003). *Births: Final data for 2002. National Vital Statistics Reports, 52.* Hyattsville, MD: National Center for Health Statistics.

Martin, J. A., Hamilton, B. E., Osterman, M. J. K., Curtin, S. C., & Mathews, T. J. (2015). *Births: Final data for 2013. National Vital Statistics Reports, 64*(1), Hyattsville, MD, National Center for Health Statistics.

Martinelli, R. L. de C., Marchesan, I. Q., & Berretin-Feliz, G. (2012). Lingual frenulum protocol with scores for infants. *International Journal of Orofacial Myology, 38,* 104–112.

Martinelli, R. L. de C., Marchesan, I. Q., Gusmao, R. J., Honorio, H. M., & Berretin-Felix, G. (2015). The effects of frenotomy on breastfeeding. *Journal of Applied Oral Science, 23,* 153–157.

Masaitis, N. S., & Kaempf, J. W. (1996). Developing a frenotomy policy at one medical center: A case study approach. *Journal of Human Lactation, 12,* 229–232.

Masarei, A. G., Sell, D., Habel, A., Mars, M., Sommerlad, B. C., & Wade, A. (2007). The nature of feeding in infants with unrepaired cleft lip and/or palate compared with healthy noncleft infants. *Cleft Palate–Craniofacial Journal, 44,* 321–328.

Mason, D. (2000). Gastroesophageal reflux in children: A guide for the advanced practice nurse. *Nursing Clinics of North America, 35,* 15–36.

Masters, I. B., Chang, A. B., Patterson, L., Wainwright, C., Buntain, H., Dean, B. W., & Francis, P. W. (2002). Series of laryngomalacia, tracheomalacia, and bronchomalacia disorders and their associations with other conditions in children. *Pediatric Pulmonology, 34,* 189–195.

Mathisen, B., Worrall, L., Masel, J., Wall, C., & Shepherd, R. W. (1999). Feeding problems in infants with gastro-oesophageal reflux disease: A case controlled study. *Journal of Paediatrics and Child Health, 35,* 163–169.

McAteer, J. P., Ledbetter, D. J., & Goldin, A. B. (2013). Role of bottle feeding in the etiology of hypertrophic pyloric stenosis. *JAMA Pediatrics, 167,* 1143–1149.

McBride, M. C., & Danner, S. C. (1987). Sucking disorders in neurologically impaired infants. *Clinics in Perinatology, 14,* 109–130.

McCabe, E., Leonard, C. O., Medici, F. N., Seashore, M. R., & Weiss, L. (1992). Issues in newborn screening. *Pediatrics, 89,* 345–349.

McCabe, L., Ernest, A. E., Neifert, M. R., Yannicelli, S., Nord, A. M., Garry, P. J., & McCabe, E. R. (1989). The management of breastfeeding among infants with phenylketonuria. *Journal of Inherited Metabolic Disease, 12,* 467–474.

McMurray, J. L., Jones, M. W., & Khan, J. H. (2002). Cerebral palsy and the NICU graduate. *Neonatal Network, 21,* 53–57.

Mead, L. J., Chuffo, R., Lawlor-Klean, P., & Meier, P. P. (1992). Breastfeeding success with preterm quadruplets. *Journal of Obstetric, Gynecologic, and Neonatal Nursing, 21,* 221–227.

Medical Research Council Working Party on Phenylketonuria. (1993). Recommendations on the dietary management of phenylketonuria. *Archives of Disease in Childhood, 68,* 426–427.

Meier, P. (1988). Bottle and breastfeeding: Effect of transcutaneous oxygen pressure and temperature in premature infants. *Nursing Research, 37,* 36–41.

Mercado-Deane, M., Burton, E. M., Harlow, S. A., Glover, A. S., Deane, D. A., Guill, M. F., & Hudson, V. (2001). Swallowing dysfunction in infants less than 1 year of age. *Pediatric Radiology, 31,* 423–428.

Merewood, A., & Philipp, B. L. (2001). *Breastfeeding: Conditions and diseases. A reference guide.* Amarillo, TX: Pharmasoft.

Merritt, L. (2005a). Part 1. Understanding the embryology and genetics of cleft lip and palate. *Advances in Neonatal Care, 5,* 64–71.

Merritt, L. (2005b). Part 2. Physical assessment of the infant with cleft lip and/or palate. *Advances in Neonatal Care, 5,* 125–134.

Messner, A. H., & Lalakea, M. L. (2000). Ankyloglossia: Controversies in management. *International Journal of Pediatric Otorhinolaryngology, 54,* 123–131.

Messner, A. H., & Lalakea, M. L. (2002). The effect of ankyloglossia on speech in children. *Otolaryngology—Head and Neck Surgery, 127,* 539–545.

Messner, A. H., Lalakea, L., Aby, J., Macmahon, J., & Bair, E. (2000). Ankyloglossia: Incidence and associated feeding difficulties. *Archives of Otolaryngology—Head and Neck Surgery, 126,* 36–39.

Metcalf, T. J., Irons, T. G., Sher, L. D., & Young, P. C. (1994). Simethicone in the treatment of infant colic: A randomized, placebo-controlled, multicenter trial. *Pediatrics, 94,* 29–34.

Michaels, A. M., & Wanner, H. (2013). Breastfeeding twins after mastectomy. *Journal of Human Lactation, 29,* 20–22.

Milczuk, H. A., & Johnson, S. M. (2000). Effect on families and caregivers of caring for a child with laryngomalacia. *Annals of Otology, Rhinology, and Laryngology, 109,* 348–354.

Milidou, I., Henriksen, T. B., Jensen, M. S., Olsen, J., & Sondergaard, C. (2012). Nicotine replacement therapy during pregnancy and infantile colic in the offspring. *Pediatrics, 129,* e652–e658.

Miller, J. H. (1998). *The controversial issue of breastfeeding cleft-affected infants.* Innisfail, Alberta, Canada: InfoMed.

Miller-Loncar, C., Bigsby, R., High, P., Wallach, M., & Lester, B. (2004). Infant colic and feeding difficulties. *Archives of Disease in Childhood, 89,* 908–912.

Mitchell, L. E., & Risch, N. (1991). The genetics of infantile hypertrophic pyloric stenosis: A reanalysis. *American Journal of Diseases of Children, 147,* 1203–1211.

Mizuno, K., & Ueda, A. (2001). Development of sucking behavior in infants with Down's syndrome. *Acta Paediatrica, 90,* 1384–1388.

Moe, J. K., Holland, M. D., & Johnson, R. K. (1998). Breastfeeding practices of infants with Rubinstein-Taybi syndrome. *Journal of Human Lactation, 14,* 311–315.

Mojab, C. G. (2002). *Congenital disorders in the nursling.* Unit 5/Lactation Consultant Series Two. Schaumburg, IL: La Leche League International.

Moller, J. (1998). Prevalence and incidence of cardiac malformation. In J. H. Moller (Ed.), *Perspectives in pediatric cardiology: Surgery of congenital heart disease: Pediatric Cardiac Care Consortium, 1984–1995* (pp. 19–26). Armonk, NY: Futura Publishing.

Moravej, H., Imanieh, M. H., Kashef, S., Handjani, F., & Eghterdari, F. (2010). Predictive value of the cow's milk skin prick test in infantile colic. *Annals of Saudi Medicine, 30,* 468–470.

Morton, J., Hall, J. Y., Wong, R. J., Thairu, L., Benitz, W. E., & Rhine, W. D. (2009). Combining hand techniques with electric pumping increases milk production in mothers of preterm infants. *Journal of Perinatology, 29,* 757–764.

Motion, S., Northstone, K., Emond, A., Stucke, S., & Golding, J. (2002). Early feeding problems in children with cerebral palsy: Weight and neurodevelopmental outcomes. *Developmental Medicine and Child Neurology, 44,* 40–43.

Motzfeldt, K., Lilje, R., & Nylander, G. (1999). Breastfeeding in phenylketonuria. *Acta Paediatrica Supplement, 88,* 25–27.

Moxley, S., & Haddon, L. (1999). Teaching breastfeeding to parents expecting multiple births. *International Journal of Childbirth Education, 14,* 22–27.

Mukai, S., Mukai, C., & Asaoka, K. (1991). Ankyloglossia with deviation of the epiglottis and larynx. *Annals of Otology, Rhinology, and Laryngology, 100,* 3–20.

Murphy, J. (2009). *Ankyloglossia and its significance for breastfeeding.* Presented at International Lactation Consultant Association Conference, Orlando, FL.

Naimer, S. A., Biton, A., Vardy, D., & Zvulunov, A. (2003). Office treatment of congenital ankyloglossia. *Medical Science Monitor, 9,* CR432–CR435.

National Institute for Health and Clinical Excellence. (2005). Interventional procedure guidance 149. *Division of ankyloglossia (tongue-tie) for breastfeeding.* London, UK: NICE.

Nelson, S. P., Chen, E. H., Syniar, G. M., & Christoffel, K. K. (1997). Prevalence of symptoms of gastroesophageal reflux during infancy: A pediatric office based survey. *Archives of Pediatrics and Adolescent Medicine, 151,* 569–572.

Noble, R., & Bovey, A. (1997). Therapeutic teat use for babies who breastfeed poorly. *Breastfeeding Review, 5,* 37–42.

Notestine, G. E. (1990). The importance of the identification of ankyloglossia (short lingual frenulum) as a cause of breastfeeding problems. *Journal of Human Lactation, 6,* 113–115.

Nyqvist, K. H. (2002). Breastfeeding in preterm twins: Development of feeding behavior and milk intake during hospital stay and related caregiving practices. *Journal of Pediatric Nursing, 17,* 246–256.

Nyqvist, K. H., & Lutes, L. M. (1998). Co-bedding twins: A developmentally supportive care strategy. *Journal of Obstetric, Gynecologic, and Neonatal Nursing, 27,* 450–456.

Ochi, J. W. (2014). Treating tongue-tie. *Clinical Lactation, 5,* 20–27.

Odze, R. D., Bines, J., Leichtner, A. M., Whitington, P. F., & Hamilton (1993). Allergic proctocolitis in infants: A prospective clinicopathologic biopsy study. *Human Pathology, 24,* 668–674.

Oliver, R. G., & Jones, G. (1997). Neonatal feeding of infants born with cleft lip and/or palate: Parental perceptions of their experience in South Wales. *Cleft Palate–Craniofacial Journal, 34,* 526–532.

Omari, T. I., Barnett, C. P., Benninga, M. A., Lontis, R., Goodchild, L., Haslam, R. R., . . . Davidson, G. P. (2002). Mechanisms of gastro-oesophageal reflux in preterm and term infants with reflux disease. *Gut, 51,* 475–479.

Orenstein, S. R. (1999). Gastroesophageal reflux. *Pediatric Review, 20,* 24–28.

Orenstein, S. R., Shalaby, T. M., Kelsey, S. F., & Frankel, E. (2006). Natural history of infant reflux esophagitis: Symptoms and morphometric histology during one year without pharmacotherapy. *American Journal of Gastroenterology, 101,* 628–640.

Orru, S., Di Nicola, P., Giuliani, F., Fabris, C., Conti, A., Coscia, A., & Bertibo, E. (2013). Detection of bovine alpha-S1-casein in term and preterm human colostrum with proteomic techniques. *International Journal of Immunopathology and Pharmacology, 26,* 435–444.

Osuji, O. O. (1995). Preparation of feeding obturators for infants with cleft lip and palate. *Journal of Clinical Pediatric Dentistry, 19,* 211–214.

Owens, B. (2002). Breastfeeding an infant after heart transplant surgery. *Journal of Human Lactation, 18,* 53–55.

Palmer, B. (2001). Frenum presentation. Retrieved from www.brianpalmerdds.com/frenum.htm

Palmer, B. (2003). Breastfeeding and frenulums. Retrieved from www.brianpalmerdds.com/bfeed_frenulums.htm

Paradise, J. L., Elster, B. A., & Tan, L. (1994). Evidence in infants with cleft palate that breast milk protects against otitis media. *Pediatrics, 94,* 853–860.

Parker, E. M., O'Sullivan, B. P., Shea, J. C., Regan, M. M., & Freedman, S. D. (2004). Survey of breastfeeding practices and outcomes in the cystic fibrosis population. *Pediatric Pulmonology, 37,* 362–367.

Parker, S. E., Mai, C. T., Canfield, M. A., Rickard, R., Wang, Y., Meyer, R. E., . . . Correa, A.; National Birth Defects Prevention Network. (2010). Updated national birth prevalence estimates for selected birth defects in the United States, 2004–2006. *Birth Defects Research: Part A, Clinical and Molecular Teratology, 88,* 1008–1016.

Patenaude, Y., Bernard, C., Schreiber, R., & Sunsky, A. B. (2000). Cow's-milk–induced allergic colitis in an exclusively breastfed infant: Diagnosed with ultrasound. *Pediatric Radiology, 30,* 379–382.

Paulozzi, L. J. (2000). Is *Helicobacter pylori* a cause of infantile hypertrophic pyloric stenosis? *Medical Hypotheses, 55,* 119–125.

Perkins, J. A., Sie, K. C. Y., Milczuk, H., & Richardson, M. A. (1997). Airway management in children with craniofacial anomalies. *Cleft Palate–Craniofacial Journal, 34,* 135–140.

Persson, S., Ekborn, A., Granath, F., & Nordenskjold, A. (2001). Parallel incidences of sudden infant death syndrome and infantile hypertrophic pyloric stenosis: A common cause? *Pediatrics, 108,* 379–381.

Peter, C. S., Wiechers, C., Bohnhorst, B., Silny, J., & Poets, C. F. (2002). Influence of nasogastric tubes on gastroesophageal reflux in preterm infants: A multiple intraluminal impedance study. *Journal of Pediatrics, 141,* 277–279.

Pineda, R. (2011). Direct breastfeeding in the neonatal intensive care unit: Is it important? *Journal of Perinatology, 31,* 540–545.

Pinheiro, P. F. M., Simoes e Silva, A. C., & Pereira, R. M. (2012). Current knowledge on esophageal atresia. *World Journal of Gastroenterology, 18,* 3662–3672.

Pisacane, A., de Luca, U., Criscuolo, L., Vaccaro, F., Valiante, A., Inglese, A., . . . Pinto, L. (1996). Breastfeeding and hypertrophic pyloric stenosis: Population based case-control study. *BMJ, 312,* 745–746.

Porta, F., Mussa, A., & Ponzone, A. (2010). Breastfeeding effects on newborn screening. *Journal of Pediatrics, 156,* 1033; author reply 1033–1034.

Praborini, A., Purnamasari, H., Munandar, A., & Wulandari, R. A. (2015). Early frenotomy improves breastfeeding outcomes. *Clinical Lactation, 6,* 9–15.

Practice Committee of the American Society for Reproductive Medicine, & Practice Committee of Society for Assisted Reproductive Technology. (2009). Guidelines on number of embryos transferred. *Fertility and Sterility, 92,* 1518–1519.

Pransky, S. M., Lago, A. D., & Hong, P. (2015). Breastfeeding difficulties and oral cavity anomalies: The influence of posterior ankyloglossia and upper lip ties. *International Journal of Pediatric Otorhinolaryngology, 79,* 1714–1717.

Prows, C. A., & Bender, P. L. (1999). Beyond Pierre Robin sequence. *Neonatal Network, 18,* 13–19.

Puapong, D., Kahng, D., Ko, A., & Applebaum, H. (2002). Ad libitum feeding: Safely improving the cost-effectiveness of pyloromyotomy. *Journal of Pediatric Surgery, 37,* 1667–1668.

Puapornpong, P., Raungrongmorakot, K., Mahasitthiwat, V., & Ketsuwan, S. (2014). Comparisons of the latching on between newborns with tongue-tie and normal newborns. *Journal of the Medical Association of Thailand, 97,* 255–259.

Pumberger, W., Pomberger, G., & Geissler, W. (2001). Proctocolitis in breastfed infants: A contribution to differential diagnosis of haematochezia in early childhood. *Postgraduate Medical Journal, 77,* 252–254.

Purnell, H. (2001). Phenylketonuria and maternal phenylketonuria. *Breastfeeding Review, 9,* 19–21.

Radhakrishnan, J., & Sharma, A. (2011). Feeding plate for a neonate with Pierre Robin sequence. *Journal of the Indian Society of Pedodontics and Preventive Dentistry, 29,* 239–243.

Rawashdeh, M. A., & Jawdat Abu-Hawas, B. (2008). Congenital associated malformations in a sample of Jordanian patients with cleft lip and palate. *Journal of Oral and Maxillofacial Surgery, 66,* 2035–2041.

Redford-Badwal, D. A., Mabry, K., & Frassinelli, J. D. (2003). Impact of cleft lip and/or palate on nutritional health and oral–motor development. *Dental Clinics of North America, 47,* 305–317.

Reid, J. (2004). A review of feeding interventions for infants with cleft palate. *Cleft Palate–Craniofacial Journal, 41,* 268–278.

Reid, J., Kilpatrick, N., & Reilly, S. (2006). A prospective, longitudinal study of feeding skills in a cohort of babies with cleft conditions. *Cleft Palate–Craniofacial Journal, 43,* 702–709.

Reid, J., Reilly, S., & Kilpatrick, N. (2007). Sucking performance of babies with cleft conditions. *Cleft Palate–Craniofacial Journal, 44,* 312–320.

Reijneveld, S. A., Brugman, E., & Hirasing, R. A. (2000). Infantile colic: Maternal smoking as potential risk factor. *Archives of Disease in Childhood, 83,* 302–303.

Reilly, S., Reid, J., Skeat, J., Cahir, P., Mei, C., Bunik, M., & Academy of Breastfeeding Medicine. (2013). ABM clinical protocol #18: Guidelines for breastfeeding infants with cleft lip, cleft palate, or cleft lip and palate. Revised 2013. *Breastfeeding Medicine, 8,* 349–353.

Reinthal, M., Andersson, S., Gustafsson, M., Plos, K., Lund, I., Lundeberg, T., & Gustaf Rosén, K. (2008). Effects of minimal acupuncture in children with infantile colic: A prospective, quasi-randomised single blind controlled trial. *Acupuncture and Medicine, 26,* 171–182.

Rendon-Macias, M. E., Castaneda-Mucino, G., Cruz, J. J., Mejia-Aranguré, J. M., & Villasis-Keever, M. A. (2002). Breastfeeding among patients with congenital malformations. *Archives of Medical Research, 33,* 269–275.

Repucci, A. (1999). Resolution of stool blood in breastfed infants with maternal ingestion of pancreatic enzymes. *Journal of Pediatric Gastroenterology and Nutrition, 29,* 500A.

Restani, P., Gaiaschi, A., Plebani, A., Beretta, B., Velonà, T., Cavagni, G., . . . Galli, C. L. (2000). Evaluation of the presence of bovine proteins in human milk as a possible cause of allergic symptoms in breastfed children. *Annals of Allergy, Asthma, and Immunology, 84,* 353–360.

Riaz, M., Porat, R., Brodsky, N. L., & Hurt, H. (1998). The effects of maternal magnesium sulfate treatment on newborns: A prospective controlled study. *Journal of Perinatology, 18,* 449–454.

Richard, M. E. (1991). Feeding the newborn with cleft lip and/or palate: The enlargement, stimulate, swallow, rest (ESSR) method. *Journal of Pediatric Nursing, 6,* 317–321.

Ricke, L. A., Baker, N. J., Madlon-Kay, D. J., & DeFor, T. A. (2005). Newborn tongue-tie: Prevalence and effect on breastfeeding. *Journal of the American Board of Family Practice, 18,* 1–7.

Riva, E., Agostoni, C., Biasucci, G., Trojan, S., Luotti, D., Fiori, L., & Giovannini, M. (1996). Early breastfeeding is linked to higher intelligence quotient scores in dietary treated phenylketonuric children. *Acta Paediatrica, 85,* 56–58.

Rivera, A. F., Davilla Torres, R. R., Parilla Rodriguez, A. M., de Longo, I. M., & Gorrin Peralta, J. J. (2008). Exploratory study: Knowledge about the benefits of breastfeeding and barriers for initiation in mothers of children with spina bifida. *Maternal and Child Health Journal, 12,* 734–738.

Roem, K. (2003). Nutritional management of multiple pregnancies. *Twin Research, 6,* 514–519.

Rommel, N., De Meyer, A.-M., Feenstra, L., & Veereman-Wauters, G. (2003). The complexity of feeding problems in 700 infants and young children presenting to a tertiary care institution. *Journal of Pediatric Gastroenterology and Nutrition, 37,* 75–84.

Ross, K. (2012). MOST medical birth survey. Retrieved from http://www.raisingmultiples.org/page/2/?s=breastfeeding

Rudolph, C. D., Mazur, L. J., Liptak, G. S., Baker, R. D., Boyle, J. T., Colletti, R. B., . . . Werlin, S. L. (2001). Pediatric GE reflux clinical practice guidelines. *Journal of Pediatric Gastroenterology and Nutrition, 32*(suppl 2), S1–S31.

Ryckman, F. C., & Balistreri, W. F. (2002). Upper gastrointestinal disorders. In A. A. Fanaroff & R. J. Martin (Eds.), *Neonatal-perinatal medicine: Diseases of the fetus and infant* (7th ed.). St. Louis, MO: Mosby.

Sacker, A., Quigley, M. A., & Kelly, Y. J. (2006). Breastfeeding and developmental delay: Findings from the Millennium Cohort Study. *Pediatrics, 118,* e682–e689.

Saenz, R. B. (2004). *Helping a mother breastfeed her baby with Down syndrome.* Unit 9 Lactation Consultant Series Two. Schaumburg, IL: La Leche League International.

Saint, L., Maggiore, P., & Hartmann, P. E. (1986). Yield and nutrient content of milk in eight women breastfeeding twins and one woman breastfeeding triplets. *British Journal of Nutrition, 56,* 49–58.

Salvatore, S., & Vandenplas, Y. (2002). Gastroesophageal reflux and cow milk allergy: Is there a link? *Pediatrics, 110,* 972–984.

Santoro, W., Martinez, F. E., Ricco, R. G., & Jorge, S. M. (2010). Colostrum ingested during the first day of life by exclusively breastfed healthy infants. *Journal of Pediatrics, 156,* 29–32.

Savino, F., Bailo, E., Oggero, R., Tullio, V., Roana, J., Carlone, N., . . . Silvestro, L. (2005). Bacterial counts of intestinal *Lactobacillus* species in infants with colic. *Pediatric Allergy and Immunology, 16,* 72–75.

Savino, F., Cresi, F., Castagno, E., Silvestro, L., & Oggero, R. (2005). A randomized double-blind placebo-controlled trial of a standardized extract of *Matricariae recutita, Foeniculum vulgare* and *Melissa officinalis* (ColiMil) in the treatment of breastfed colicky infants. *Phytotherapy Research, 19,* 335–340.

Savino, F., Cresi, F., Pautasso, S., Palumeri, E., Tullio, V., Roana, J., . . . Oggero, R. (2004). Intestinal microflora in breastfed colicky and non-colicky infants. *Acta Paediatrica, 93,* 825–829.

Savino, F., Pelle, E., Palumeri, E., Oggero, R., & Miniero, R. (2007). *Lactobacillus reuteri* (American Type Culture Strain 55730) versus simethicone in the treatment of infantile colic: A prospective randomized study. *Pediatrics, 119,* e124–e130.

Schach, B., & Haight, M. (2002). Colic and food allergy in the breastfed infant: Is it possible for an exclusively breastfed infant to suffer from food allergy? *Journal of Human Lactation, 18,* 50–52.

Schmidt, D., Beebe, R., & Berg-Drazin, P. (2013). Galactosemia and the continuation of breastfeeding with variant form. *Clinical Lactation, 4,* 148–153.

Schwartz, K., d'Arcy, H., Gillespie, B., Bobo, J., Longeway, M., & Foxman, B. (2002). Factors associated with weaning in the first 3 months postpartum. *Journal of Family Practice, 51,* 439–444.

Segal, L. M., Stephenson, R., Dawes, M., & Feldman, P. (2007). Prevalence, diagnosis, and treatment of ankyloglossia. *Canadian Family Physician, 53,* 1027–1033.

Sethi, N., Smith, D., Kortequee, S., Ward, V. M., & Clarke, S. (2013). Benefits of frenulotomy in infants with ankyloglossia. *International Journal of Pediatric Otorhinolaryngology, 77,* 762–765.

Sharma, S. D., & Jayaraj, S. (2015). Tongue-tie division to treat breastfeeding difficulties: Our experience. *Journal of Laryngology & Otology, 129,* 986–989.

Shaw, G. M., Lammer, E. F., Wasserman, C. R., O'Malley, C. D., & Tolarova, M. M. (1995). Risks of orofacial clefts in children born to women using multivitamins containing folic acid periconceptually. *Lancet, 346,* 393–396.

Shaw, W. C., Bannister, R. P., & Roberts, C. T. (1999). Assisted feeding is more reliable for infants with clefts: A randomized trial. *Cleft Palate–Craniofacial Journal, 36,* 262–268.

Sheffield, L. J., Reiss, J. A., Strohm, K., & Gilding, M. (1987). A genetic follow-up study of 64 patients with the Pierre Robin complex. *American Journal of Medical Genetics, 28,* 25–36.

Shenassa, E. D., & Brown, M.-J. (2004). Maternal smoking and infantile gastrointestinal dysregulation: The case of colic. *Pediatrics, 114,* e497–e505.

Smedegaard, L., Marxen, D., Moes, J., Glassou, E. N., & Scientsan, C. (2008). Hospitalization, breastmilk feeding, and growth in infants with cleft palate and cleft lip born in Denmark. *Cleft Palate–Craniofacial Journal, 45,* 628–632.

Smehilova, M., Vlkova, E., Nevoral, J., Flajsmanova, K., Killer, J., & Rada, V. (2008). Comparison of intestinal microflora in healthy infants and infants with allergic colitis. *Folia Microbiologica, 53,* 255–258.

Sollid, D. T., Evans, B. T., McClowry, S. G., & Garrett, A. (1989). Breastfeeding multiples. *Journal of Perinatal and Neonatal Nursing, 3,* 46–65.

Solomons, N. B., & Prescot, C. A. J. (1987). Laryngomalacia: A review and the surgical management for severe cases. *International Journal of Pediatric Otorhinolaryngology, 13,* 31–39.

Sondergaard, C., Henriksen, T. B., Obel, C., & Wisborg, K. (2001). Smoking during pregnancy and infantile colic. *Pediatrics, 108,* 342–346.

Sorensen, H. T., Norgard, B., Pedersen, L., Larsen, H., & Johnsen, S. P. (2002). Maternal smoking and risk of hypertrophic infantile pyloric stenosis: 10 year population based cohort study. *BMJ, 325,* 1011–1012.

Sorensen, H. T., Skriver, M. V., Pedersen, L., Larsen, H., Ebbesen, F., & Schønheyder, H. C. (2003). Risk of hypertrophic pyloric stenosis after maternal postnatal use of macrolides. *Scandinavian Journal of Infectious Disease, 35,* 104–106.

Spoon, J. M. (2003). VATER association. *Neonatal Network, 22,* 71–75.

Sprintzen, R. F., Siegel-Sadewitz, V. L., Amato, J., & Goldberg, R. B. (1985). Anomalies associated with cleft lip, cleft palate, or both. *American Journal of Medical Genetics, 20,* 585–595.

Srinivasan, A., Dobrich, C., Mitnick, H., & Feldman, P. (2006). Ankyloglossia in breastfeeding infants: The effect of frenotomy on maternal nipple pain and latch. *Breastfeeding and Medicine, 1,* 216–224.

Stang, H. (1986). Pyloric stenosis associated with erythromycin ingested through breastmilk. *Minnesota Medicine, 69,* 669–670, 682.

Steehler, M. W., Steehler, M. K., & Harley, E. H. (2012). A retrospective review of frenotomy in neonates and infants with feeding difficulties. *International Journal of Pediatric Otorhinolaryngology, 76,* 1236–1240.

Stockdale, H. J. (2000). Long-term expressing of breastmilk. *Breastfeeding Review, 8,* 19–22.

Storr, G. (1989). Breastfeeding premature triplets: One woman's experience. *Journal of Human Lactation, 5,* 74–77.

Stuart, C. A., Twiselton, R., Nicholas, M. K., & Hide, D. W. (1984). Passage of cow's milk protein in breast milk. *Clinical Allergy, 14,* 533–535.

Styer, G. W., & Freeh, K. (1981). Feeding infants with cleft lip and/or palate. *Journal of Obstetric, Gynecologic, and Neonatal Nursing, 10,* 329–332.

Summers, J., Ludwig, J., & Kanze, D. (2014). Pierre Robin sequence in a neonate with sucking difficulty and weight loss. *Journal of the American Osteopathic Association, 114,* 727–731.

Sung, V., Collett, S., de Grooyer, T., Hiscock, H., Tang, M., & Wake, M. (2013). Probiotics to prevent or treat excessive infant crying: Systematic review and meta-analysis. *JAMA Pediatrics, 167,* 1150–1157.

Szucs, K. A., Axline, S. E., & Rosenman, M. B. (2009). Quintuplets and a mother's determination to provide human milk: It takes a village to raise a baby—how about five? *Journal of Human Lactation, 25,* 79–84.

Thomas, J., Marinelli, K. A., Hennessy, M., & Academy of Breastfeeding Medicine Protocol Committee. (2007). ABM clinical protocol #16: Breastfeeding the hypotonic infant. *Breastfeeding Medicine, 2,* 112–118.

Tluczek, A., Clark, R., McKechnie, A. C., Orland, K. M., & Brown, R. L. (2010). Task-oriented and bottle feeding adversely affect the quality of mother–infant interactions following abnormal newborn screens. *Journal of Developmental and Behavioral Pediatrics, 31,* 414–426.

Tobin, J. M., McCloud, P., & Cameron, D. J. S. (1997). Posture and gastroesophageal reflux: A case for left lateral positioning. *Archives of Disease in Childhood, 7,* 254–258.

Tolarova, M., & Harris, J. (1995). Reduced recurrence of orofacial clefts after periconceptional supplementation with high-dose folic acid and multivitamins. *Teratology, 51,* 71–78.

Torowicz, D. L., Seelhorst, A., Froh, E. B., & Spatz, D. L. (2015). Human milk and breastfeeding outcomes in infants with congenital heart disease. *Breastfeeding Medicine, 10,* 31–37.

Trenouth, M. J., & Campbell, A. N. (1996). Questionnaire evaluation of feeding methods for cleft lip and palate neonates. *International Journal of Paediatric Dentistry, 6,* 241–244.

Turner, L., Jacobsen, C., Humenczuk, M., Singhal, V. K., Moore, D., & Bell, H. (2001). The effects of lactation education and a prosthetic obturator appliance on feeding efficiency in infants with cleft lip and palate. *Cleft Palate-Craniofacial Journal, 38,* 519–524.

Turner, L., & Moore, D. (1995). *Use of feeding aids for cleft lip and palate infants.* Presented at the International Lactation Consultant Association, Phoenix, AZ.

van Rijn, M., Bekhof, J., Dijkstra T., Smit, P. G., Moddermam, P., & van Spronsen, F. J. (2003). A different approach to breastfeeding of the infant with phenylketonuria. *European Journal of Paediatrics, 162,* 323–326.

Vandenplas, Y., De Wolf, D., & Sacre, L. (1986). Influence of xanthines on gastroesophageal reflux in infants at risk for sudden infant death syndrome. *Pediatrics, 77,* 807–810.

Walker, M. (1989). Management of selected early breastfeeding problems seen in clinical practice. *Birth, 16,* 148–157.

Wang, J., Waller, D. K., Hwang, L. Y., Taylor, L. G., & Canfield, M. A. (2008). Prevalence of infantile hypertrophic pyloric stenosis in Texas, 1999–2002. *Birth Defects Research: Part A, Clinical and Molecular Teratology, 82,* 763–767.

Ward, N. (1990). Ankyloglossia: A case study in which clipping was not necessary. *Journal of Human Lactation, 6,* 126–127.

Weatherly-White, R. C. A., Kuehn, D. P., Mirrett, P., Gilman, J. I., & Weatherley-White, C. C. (1987). Early repair and breastfeeding for infants with cleft lip. *Plastic and Reconstructive Surgery, 79,* 879–885.

Webb, A. R., Lari, J., & Dodge, J. A. (1983). Infantile hypertrophic pyloric stenosis in South Glamorgan 1970–9. *Archives of Disease in Childhood, 58,* 586–590.

Weintraub, R. G., & Menahem, G. (1993). Growth and congenital heart disease. *Journal of Paediatrics and Child Health, 29,* 95–98.

Weissbluth, M. (1994). Melatonin increases cyclic guanosine monophosphate: Biochemical effects mediated by porphyrins, calcium and nitric oxide. Relationship to infant colic and the sudden infant death syndrome. *Medical Hypotheses, 42,* 390–392.

Wessel, M. A., Cogg, J. C., Jackson, E. B., Harris, G. S., Jr., & Detwiler, A. C. (1954). Paroxysmal fussing in infancy, sometimes called "colic." *Pediatrics, 14,* 421–434.

Wheat, J. C. (2002). Nutritional management of children with congenital heart disease. *Nutrition Bytes, 8*(2). Retrieved from http://repositories.cdlib.org/uclabiolchem/nutritionbytes/vol8/iss2/art5

White, B. P., Gunnar, M. R., Larson, M. C., Donzella, B., & Barr, R. G. (2000). Behavioral and physiological responsivity, sleep, and patterns of daily cortisol production in infants with or without colic. *Child Development, 71,* 862–877.

White, D. R., Giambra, B. K., Hopkin, R. J., Daines, C. L., & Rutter, M. J. (2005). Aspiration in children with CHARGE syndrome. *International Journal of Pediatric Otorhinolaryngology, 69,* 1205–1209.

Willis, C. E., & Livingstone, V. (1995). Infant insufficient milk syndrome associated with maternal postpartum hemorrhage. *Journal of Human Lactation, 11,* 123–126.

Wilson, A. C., Moore, D. J., Moore, M. H., Martin, A. J., Staugas, R. E., & Kennedy, J. D. (2000). Late presentation of upper airway obstruction in Pierre Robin sequence. *Archives of Disease in Childhood, 83,* 435–438.

Wilton, J. M. (1990). Sore nipples and slow weight gain related to a short frenulum. *Journal of Human Lactation, 6,* 122–123.

Wolf, L. S., & Glass, R. P. (1992). *Feeding and swallowing disorders in infancy.* Tucson, AZ: Therapy Skill Builders.

Wood, R. E. (1984). Spelunking in the pediatric airway: Exploration with the flexible fiberoptic bronchoscope. *Pediatric Clinics of North America, 31,* 785–799.

Woolridge, M. W., & Fisher, C. (1988). Colic, "overfeeding," and symptoms of lactose malabsorption in the breastfed baby: A possible artifact of feed management. *Lancet, 2,* 382–384.

Wright, J. E. (1995). Tongue-tie. *Journal of Paediatrics and Child Health, 31,* 276–278.

Yannicelli, S., Ernest, A., Heifert, M., & McCabe, E. (1988, October). *Guide to breastfeeding the infant with PKU* (2nd ed., publication no. HRS-M-CH88-12). Washington, DC: Department of Health and Human Services.

Young, J. L., O'Riordan, M., Goldstein, J. A., & Robin, N. H. (2001). What information do parents of newborns with cleft lip, palate, or both want to know? *Cleft Palate–Craniofacial Journal, 38,* 55–58.

Yousefi, J., Namini, F. T., Raisolsadat, S. M. A., Gillies, R., Ashkezari, A., & Meara, J. G. (2015). Tongue-tie repair: Z-plasty vs simple release. *Iranian Journal of Otorhinolaryngology, 27,* 127–135.

Zucchero, T. M., Cooper, M. E., Maher, B. S., Daack-Hirsch, S., Nepomuceno, B., . . . Murray, J. C. (2004). Interferon regulatory factor 6 (IRF6) gene variants and the risk of isolated cleft lip or palate. *New England Journal of Medicine, 351,* 769–780.

ADDITIONAL READING AND RESOURCES

Genna, C. W. (2013). *Supporting sucking skills in breastfeeding infants* (2nd ed.). Burlington, MA: Jones & Bartlett Learning.

Twins and Higher Order Multiples

Center for the Study of Multiple Birth
http://www.multiplebirth.com

Mothers of Supertwins (Raising Multiples, a MOST Community)
http://www.mostonline.org

Multiple Births Canada
http://multiplebirthscanada.org/index.php/education/publications/booklets

National Organization of Mothers of Twins Clubs (Multiples of America)
http://www.nomotc.org

Twins Magazine
http://www.twinsmagazine.com/twins-magazine

Ankyloglossia (Tongue-Tie)

Dr. Brian Palmer, DDS
http://www.brianpalmerdds.com/bfeed_frenulums.htm

Frenotomy video
http://www.drjaintonguetie.com/New-Video.html

Genna, C. W., & Coryllos, E. V. (2009). Breastfeeding and tongue-tie. *Journal of Human Lactation, 25,* 111–112.

Hazelbaker, A. K. (2010). *Tongue-tie: morphogenesis, impact, assessment and treatment.* Columbus, OH: Aidan and Eva Press.
http://www.alisonhazelbaker.com/tongue-tie-book

International Affiliation of Tongue-tie Professionals
http://tonguetieprofessionals.org/

Tongue Tie: from confusion to clarity
http://www.tonguetie.net/index.php?option=com_frontpage&Itemid=1

Gastroesophageal Reflux Disease (GERD)

Gastroesophageal Reflux Disease and the Breastfeeding Baby
Susan Boekel, RD, CSP, LD, IBCLC
Independent Study Module
International Lactation Consultant Association
http://www.ilca.org

Breastfeeding Special Needs Infants

Dowling, D., & McCain, G. C. (2006). *Breastfeeding the infant with special needs* (2nd ed.). White Plains, NY: March of Dimes.

McCrea, N., & Meredith, S.H. (2015). Welcoming a newborn with Down syndrome: A new parent's guide to the first month. Retrieved from http://downsyndromepregnancy.org/book/welcoming-a-newborn-with-down-syndrome

Mojab, C. G. (2002). *Congenital disorders in the nursling.* Unit 5/Lactation consultant series two. Schaumburg, IL: La Leche League International.

Redstone, F. (2014). *Effective SLP interventions for children with cerebral palsy.* San Diego, CA: Plural Publishing.

III

Maternal-Related Challenges to Breastfeeding

Chapter 8

Maternal Pathology: Breast and Nipple Issues

INTRODUCTION

Breast and nipple problems are the bane of nursing mothers and have been reported in the medical literature since the 1500s (Fildes, 1986). Some of these problems may be related to underlying anatomic variations in a woman's breast, areola, and nipple. Problems may occur early or late in lactation, with some having a significant impact on the duration of exclusive breastfeeding and contributing to premature weaning. In this chapter we address maternal breastfeeding problems and issues related to the breast, areola, and nipple and inappropriate or ineffective breastfeeding guidelines.

NIPPLE TYPES

The following are common nipple descriptors:

- Inverted. This nipple type results from the failure of the mammary pit to elevate during embryonic development as a result of the lack of mesenchymal proliferation (Bland & Romnell, 1991). These are also referred to as tied, invaginated, or tethered.
- Retracted. These are described as occurring from adhesions at the base of the nipple.
- Nonprotractile. A type occurring from an anatomic fault that has been ascribed to short lactiferous ducts that tether the nipple and prevent it from projecting (McGeorge, 1994).
- Pseudoinverted. Also referred to as umbilicated (Terrill & Stapleton, 1991), these nipples appear inverted, but when the areola around them is compressed they evert. The connective tissue is thought to be deficient, but the length of the underlying ductwork is normal, and an adequately suckling infant will sufficiently elongate the nipple for proper latch.

Plastic surgeons have graded inverted nipples through evaluation and surgical confirmation relative to the degree of fibrosis (replacement of normal cells with connective tissue, similar to scar tissue; Han & Hong, 1999):

- Grade I. The nipple is easily pulled out manually, maintains its protrusion or projection, and contains minimal fibrosis.

- Grade II. The nipple can be manually pulled out but does not maintain its protrusion, retreating back into the areola, and thought to have moderate fibrosis beneath the nipple.
- Grade III. The nipple can barely be manually pulled out, with severe fibrotic bands and less soft tissue underlying the nipple.

Inverted or nonprotractile nipples have been reported to occur in 7–10% of pregnant women who wish to breastfeed (Alexander, 1991; Hytten & Baird, 1958). Dewey, Nommsen-Rivers, Heinig, and Cohen (2003) reported a 9% incidence of flat or inverted nipples on the day the infant was born and a 7% incidence 7 days later. Although flat nipples are usually unable to be visually assessed, some inverted or dimpled nipples are easily seen during the prenatal period. A dimpled nipple folds back in on itself, with moist tissues adhering and setting the stage for skin breakdown after breastfeeding begins. The "pinch test," or compressing the areola, can reveal flat or retracted nipples because there is little protrusion and lack of definition between where the nipple ends and the areolar tissue begins. Nipples typically gain elasticity throughout the pregnancy, and the degree of inversion decreases with subsequent pregnancies.

Early data failed to find an association between an infant's ability to breastfeed successfully and the extent of maternal nipple protrusion (Inch, 1989). However, in a review of five infants admitted to the hospital with severe dehydration and hypernatremia, three of the mothers had inverted nipples and experienced problems with their infants attaining a proper latch (Cooper, Atherton, Kahana, & Kotagal, 1995). Dewey and colleagues (2003) showed that suboptimal infant breastfeeding behavior (defined as scoring less than or equal to 10 on the Infant Breastfeeding Assessment Tool) and delayed onset of lactation were significantly related to the presence of flat or inverted nipples on days 1, 3, and 7 postpartum. They specifically recommended that women with flat or inverted nipples be given special breastfeeding assistance until the infant is able to latch effectively.

Breastfeeding Recommendations Based on Nipple Type

Maternal nipples elongate two to three times their resting length when drawn into the infant's mouth (Smith, Erenberg, & Nowak, 1988) and present an expected and strong physical sucking signal to the infant when the teat reaches deep into the oral cavity. However, a nipple that retreats when stimulated may present a challenge for the infant who is unable to sufficiently elongate a nonprotractile nipple into a teat (composed of the nipple plus the underlying areola). Gunther (1955) described infants as becoming "apathetic" to the breast when flat or inverted nipples were present. She speculated that breastfeeding would be interrupted if the infant did not receive the proper physical signal (an elastic protrusive nipple/areola) to set an innate behavior in motion.

Antenatal Nipple Preparations

Three methods of antenatal nipple preparation were taught to women for decades in the belief that prenatal preparation would correct the defect and contribute to problem-free initiation of breastfeeding (Cadwell, 1981; Otte, 1975):

1. Nipple rolling involves pulling out the nipple to its outermost position and either holding it or rolling it, repeated 10 times twice a day to increase elasticity of the tissue (Applebaum, 1969).

2. In Hoffman's (1953) technique the thumbs are positioned to each side of the nipple and the areola is stretched sideways and then up and down.
3. Breast shells are a two-piece plastic system consisting of a flat disk with a hole in the center through which the nipple protrudes. The disk is covered by a vented dome and placed under the bra to exert pressure on the base of the nipple "to gradually stretch and loosen its attachment to the deep structures of the breast" (Waller, 1946).

Two randomized trials comparing the use of Hoffman's exercises and breast shells showed little change in nipple anatomy from the use of either treatment and no increase in the duration of breastfeeding (Alexander, Grant, & Campbell, 1992; MAIN Trial Collaborative Group, 1994). A more recent study looked at the use of breast shells in mothers whose nipples were defined as being short (less than 7.0 mm), but not inverted. Compared to a control group of mothers with normal-length nipples, the short nipples on which mothers wore breast shells 8 hours per day showed a significant increase in length (Chanprapaph, Luttarapakul, Siribariruck, & Boonyawanichkul, 2013).

The application of suction prenatally has been suggested as a nonsurgical method of everting nipples (Gangal & Gangal, 1978). A device called the Niplette (Avent) uses the concept of tissue expansion through continuous long-term suction, derived from the disciplines of plastic and aesthetic surgery (McGeorge, 1994). This device consists of a transparent, thimble-like nipple mold with a syringe port. The mold is placed over the flat nipple, air is evacuated from the mold by the connected syringe, and the nipple is slowly drawn out to the mother's comfort level and held in place while the device is worn. The device is worn 8 or more hours a day during the first 6 months of the pregnancy. Successful breastfeeding has been reported in a small number of mothers with the use of the device, but it has the potential for pain and nipple bleeding if too much suction is applied. It can be used briefly before each feeding in the first few days after birth, but the presence of milk in the mold impairs the device's suction.

In situations of severe inversion, minimally invasive surgical techniques may offer resolution to the problem without destroying the chances of successful breastfeeding. A gradual traction technique has been described that everts the nipple over a 4- to 6-month period without interfering with breastfeeding function or nipple sensation (Mu, Luan, Mu, & Xin, 2012). A telescoping surgical procedure that pulls out the nipple and tightens the nipple base has been reported that may also preserve breastfeeding function (Shiau, Chin, Lin, & Hsiao, 2011).

After the infant is born, the flat or inverted nipple can be temporarily everted before each feeding such that enough nipple–areolar tissue is presented to the infant to enable latch. The application of a breast pump has been recommended and used for this purpose. However, a pump distributes vacuum over a relatively large area and has the potential to increase interstitial fluid pressure (Cotterman, 2004), causing nipple swelling (Wilson-Clay & Hoover, 2002): This creates another layer of fluid within the areola under the pump flange area that thickens the superficial areolar tissue and further impedes the infant's ability to latch (Cotterman, 2003). A simpler and less expensive tool can be fashioned from a 10-mL disposable plastic syringe. Kesaree, Banapurmath, Banapurmath, and Shamanur (1993) modified the syringe by removing the plunger, cutting off the end of the syringe ¼ inch above where a needle would attach, and inserting the plunger through the end that was cut. The mother then places the smooth end of the syringe directly over her nipple and pulls back gently on the plunger to her comfort for 30 seconds to 1 minute before each feeding. This allows the nipple itself to be drawn out from the surrounding areola (Thorley, 1997). A commercial version of this device, called the Evert-It Nipple Enhancer, is also available.

Some nipples may appear flat but are actually enveloped by an edematous areola after labor and delivery. Large amounts of intravenous fluids, use of Pitocin, or excessive water retention such as in preeclampsia (Cotterman, 2004; Miller & Riordan, 2004) may contribute to an areola that is so swollen it obliterates the nipple, erasing the definition or boundary between the nipple itself and the external areola. This may remove the normally expected tactile stimulation that the infant's sensitive lips seek at latch-on, leading to a difficult or painful latching process.

Breastfeeding Management

A severely inverted or dimpled nipple may be obvious during pregnancy. A flat nipple may be apparent when the areola is gently squeezed (pinch test) and the nipple is seen flattening to the level of the areola. Nipple rolling and the Hoffman technique have not been shown to improve the elasticity or lengthen the nipple. If the nipple is less than 7 mm in length, however, breast shells worn prenatally have been shown to elongate these nipples, making it potentially easier for an infant to latch on. The Niplette has been shown to evert nipples in a small number of women and can be worn during the first 2 trimesters of pregnancy. Many flat-appearing nipples may resolve by the end of the pregnancy and require no prenatal manipulation. Another product called Supple Cups uses the concept of mechanical stretching. These are small thimble-size silicone cups available in four sizes that are designed to lengthen and evert the nipple through gentle suction. They are worn for up to 4 hours each day during late pregnancy and can also be used following delivery between and/or prior to feedings. In a small sample of 12 women, Bouchet-Horwitz (2011) reported that 83% (10 of the 12 women) were able to successfully latch and breastfeed their infants after using the Supple Cups.

After the birth, to shape the nipple the mother can place a cold compress on the nipple, gently pull and roll it before feedings, or place her thumb and index finger above and below the nipple, pressing inward and together to help "pop" out the nipple. In addition, a modified syringe or the Evert-It Nipple Enhancer can be applied for 30 seconds to a minute before each feeding, or Supple Cups can be applied for 10 minutes prior to feeds. Areolar compression can be done before latch attempts on an edematous areola (Miller & Riordan, 2004). The mother applies pressure with both thumbs and index fingers into the areola directly behind the nipple. Indentations are created as interstitial fluid is displaced and the fingers are then placed above and below the initial indentations, working their way up to the margins of the areola. The mother rotates her fingers to a new position behind the nipple and works her way to the outer margin of the areola again until the nipple becomes pliable and easily everted, at which point the infant is brought to the breast.

Reverse pressure softening has a number of variations (Cotterman, 2004) using the mother's fingertips to create pits around the circumference of the nipple. The mother uses three or four fingertips of both hands encircling the base of the nipple and pushing inward for about 1–3 minutes firmly enough to form six to eight pits. This exposes the nipple and presents a better tactile stimulus for latching. A nipple shield can be applied either before or after areolar compression or reverse pressure softening if there appears no other way to effect a latch.

The "teacup" hold may be tried with a nonengorged breast and nonedematous areola. This involves shaping the nipple–areolar complex into a wedge whose long axis matches the long axis of the open mouth of the infant. The mother or clinician uses a thumb and index finger to grasp the areola directly above the nipple plus some of the breast tissue above it to form as much tissue as possible into a wedge, placing it as deep as possible into the infant's mouth. It is held in place until the infant is latched correctly and sucking well (Wilson-Clay & Hoover, 2002).

Caution should be exercised in placing a breast pump on swollen tissues. Hand expression may also aggravate an edematous areola.

Some mothers find that wearing breast shells under their bra between feedings everts flat nipples. This may result from the displacement of fluid from the continuous pressure exerted by the rim of the nipple opening. However, when the shells are worn for prolonged periods of time and there is significant areolar edema, potential for exacerbating edema and damaging underlying tissues exists from the strangulation of capillary circulation.

Both areolar compression and reverse pressure softening may have an added benefit, which is the stimulation of the milk-ejection reflex. Compression directly on the center or core of the areola at the base of the nipple can have the effect of triggering milk letdown within a minute or 2, either from stimulation of the nerves converging in the center of the areola or as a reflex contraction of the myoepithelial cells caused by the pressure alone (Cotterman, 2004).

SORE NIPPLES

Because the concept of soreness or pain is subjective and studies on nipple pain vary in their methodology, reports in the literature of the incidence of sore nipples range from none at 6 days after delivery (Humenick & van Steenkiste, 1983) to 96% of breastfeeding mothers at some time during the first 6 weeks postpartum (Ziemer, Paone, Schupay, & Cole, 1990). Sore nipples are a frequent reason for early termination of breastfeeding (Neifert & Seacat, 1986; West, 1980; Yeung, Pennell, Leung, & Hall, 1981). Nipple pain (of any definition) has been reported to occur from the 2nd to the 15th postpartum day, continuing in some mothers through 90 days (Drewett, Kahn, Parkhurst, & Whiteley, 1987). It peaks in intensity from day 2 or 3 (Hewat & Ellis, 1987; Newton, 1952) to days 4 through 7 (Ziemer et al., 1990). There are also reported differences and many aspects of nipple pain, such as transient latch-on pain, sustained pain during a feeding, persistent nipple pain over a prolonged period of time, pain between feedings, burning pain, and degrees of pain, from mild sensitivity to excruciating. Nipple pain not only affects the process of breastfeeding itself but can negatively affect the mother's general activities, mood, and sleep (McClellan, Hepworth, Garbin, et al., 2012).

In a study of the nipple pain experiences of 69 women, Heads and Higgins (1995) reported that about 75% of the mothers had pain at the outset of breastfeeding that declined sharply to 22% after letdown and the establishment of breastfeeding. Hill and Humenick (1993) described the daily occurrence of latch-on pain for the first 14 days in 155 first- and second-time breastfeeding mothers as well as the occurrence of pain severe enough to disrupt breastfeeding over the course of the first 6 weeks. Virtually all mothers experienced some level of discomfort when the infant first latched on (as also noted by L'Esperance, 1980). The maximum level of latch-on pain was reached by day 5 in 73.8% of mothers.

Nipple pain is not just commonly reported, but can last for many weeks. In one study, 79% of mothers reported nipple pain before hospital discharge. At the end of the 8-week study, 20% of women were still experiencing nipple pain (Buck, Amir, Cullinane, & Donath for the CASTLE Study Team, 2014).

Latch-on pain and breast engorgement were positively correlated, showing that mothers experiencing more engorgement experienced more latch-on pain. The incidence of mothers experiencing nipple pain severe enough to interfere with breastfeeding ranged from 42.3% at week 1 to 12.4% at week 6. The experience of nipple pain severe enough to interfere with mothers' desire to continue breastfeeding was significantly associated with latch-on pain at weeks 1 and 2. Up to one-third of mothers experiencing nipple pain and trauma may change to alternate feeding methods within the first 6 weeks postpartum (Briggs, 2003). Mothers who experience nipple pain can also suffer from high levels of psychological distress (Amir, Dennerstein, Garland, Fisher, & Farish, 1997), confirming that clinical support to improve nipple pain is important during the early days and weeks postpartum if breastfeeding is to continue. Pain or the anticipation of pain can delay or disrupt the milk-ejection reflex, which can set in motion a cascade of undesirable side effects leading to ineffective milk transfer, residual milk buildup, and more or extended engorgement, coming full circle to more nipple pain (Newton & Newton, 1948).

McClellan, Hepworth, Kent, and colleagues (2012) investigated whether or not mothers with persistent nipple pain produced less milk. In spite of the potential for pain to negatively affect the letdown reflex, mothers in this study with persistent nipple pain achieved full milk production. In this study, the only predictor of lower milk production was feedings that lasted longer than 33 minutes. Such protracted feeding times can be an indicator of faulty sucking and poor milk transfer. Clinicians would need to observe feedings in this situation to determine and correct problematic sucking mechanics.

Ziemer and Pigeon (1993) described nipple skin changes in 20 breastfeeding mothers during the first week of lactation. Changes and damage to the nipple skin were confined to the face or tip of the nipple, suggesting that normal changes and actual damage were due to suction. Ninety percent of the women experienced pain. Magnified photographs of the nipple tip in all women studied showed visible skin changes during the study period. The tip of the nipple before the start of breastfeeding was light pink and typically showed a papillar (small bumps) appearance with small lines and crevices uniquely distributed over the surface. Ten changes were observed over time:

1. Erythema (reddening or inflamed areas): peaking on day 3
2. Edema (swelling) of the nipple and papillar bumps: occurred in all women and peaked on day 5
3. Fissures: for 65% of the mothers, some of the fissures widened and became raw, peaking on day 5
4. Blisters: 80% of the mothers had small blisters that could have been papillae that filled with fluid; occurred on day 3
5. Eschar (scabs)
6. White patches
7. Peeling
8. Dark patches
9. Pus
10. Ecchymosis (bruising or bleeding under the skin)

Positioning or proper nipple–areolar placement in the infant's mouth was not evaluated in this study; however, nipple skin changes were seen to occur right from the start of breastfeeding. These normal changes may be responsible for the common complaints of mothers describing some amount of nipple sensitivity or discomfort, whereas severe nipple pain may represent an exaggeration or extension of these changes.

Positioning: Proper Nipple–Areolar Placement

Gunther (1945) was one of the earliest authors to associate severe nipple pain and damage with the position of the infant at the breast: She described two common types of damage as erosive (petechial) and ulcerative (fissure). Woolridge (1986) described frictional trauma and suction lesions as the two main physical sources of nipple pain (as opposed to dermatological or infective causes). Frictional trauma is thought to be caused by inadequate amounts of breast tissue being drawn into the infant's mouth, resulting in poor milk transfer and distortion of the nipple. Rather than being compressed and extending to twice its resting length, the nipple–areolar complex is not formed into a teat, and the nipple skin can become abraded or pinched into a compression stripe. A nipple that is creased in a horizontal, vertical, or oblique manner has the potential for significant pain and skin breakdown (contributed by compression and suction concentrated on the distorted area).

Trauma from suction has been related to the application of continuous suction that is not relieved by periodic swallowing. Righard (1996) provided further insight into the effect of faulty sucking on nipple pain. Of the 52 mother–infant pairs referred for breastfeeding problems, 94% had a pattern of superficial nipple sucking where the infant sucked only on the nipple tip, failing to draw the nipple–areolar complex deep into the mouth. Of the 94% of mother–infant pairs with the superficial sucking pattern, 33% of the mothers complained of sore nipples. An interesting finding in this study was that infants using pacifiers more often had a superficial sucking pattern at the breast than nonusers of pacifiers.

Nipple pain from faulty mechanics of infant sucking, either poor latch or failure to form a teat (Righard, 1998; Widström & Thingstrom-Paulsson, 1993), can occur quickly, with mothers experiencing nipple pain and damage before discharge from the hospital. Blair, Cadwell, Turner-Maffei, and Brimdyr (2003) studied 95 mothers reporting nipple pain within 10 days of giving birth. Their results showed that nipple pain was related to positioning and latching errors but that no single isolated part of the positioning and latch sequence was more related to pain than another. Clinicians therefore need to assess all elements of the positioning, latching, and sucking processes. Six specific types of nipple trauma were distributed among the mothers in this study: (1) 64.4% presented with fissures, (2) 53.3% with erythema, (3) 51.1% with crusting/scabs, (4) 32.2% with swelling, (5) 4.4% with blisters or blebs, and (6) 1.1% with exudate (oozing of fluid). It is interesting to note that Ziemer and Pigeon (1993) also reported a 65% rate of fissures in their description of causes of nipple pain. It could be speculated that faulty positioning, latching, and sucking mechanics could place enough stress on the normal anatomic features of the nipple (papillae and fissures on the face of the nipple) to cause erosion or a break in the skin integrity. The disruption of the skin surface by suction or friction, concomitant stretching or rupturing of the skin within the fissures, and destruction of the underlying skin layers may move the mother on a continuum from minor discomfort to macerated and bleeding nipple wounds if interventions do not rectify the problem.

After study infants painlessly drew the nipple/areola into their mouths, Jacobs, Dickinson, Hart, Doherty, and Faulkner (2007) measured by ultrasound the distance between the tip of the nipple and the junction of the hard and soft palates. Only 25% of correctly latched infants drew in the nipple as far as the hard–soft palate junction. The median distance between the tip of the nipple and this junction was 5 mm, and the nipple showed a range of movement during breastfeeding of 4.0 ± 1.3 mm. Nipple positioning and movements outside these ranges may be predictive of nipple pain.

Ankyloglossia (tongue-tie) can restrict the movement of the tongue, potentially inhibiting the nipple/areola from being drawn far enough into the mouth to prevent pain and promote optimal milk transfer. Geddes and colleagues (2008) reported that release of the frenulum altered tongue movement as imaged by ultrasound during breastfeeding. Infants with ankyloglossia showed two types of sucking dynamics. One type pinched the nipple tip, placing it a large distance from the junction of the hard and soft palates. The other type of sucking pinched the nipple at its base, placing the nipple tip in close proximity to the hard–soft palate junction. Frenotomy reduced the extent of nipple distortion and significantly relieved nipple pain experienced by mothers. This is in agreement with Dollberg, Botzer, Grunis, and Mimouni (2006) and Srinivasan, Dobrich, Mitnick, and Feldman (2006), who detailed the immediate relief from nipple pain after frenotomy.

A retrospective cross-sectional analysis of 653 breastfeeding mothers with nipple trauma explored the potential risk factors for experiencing nipple damage (Thompson et al., 2016). Nipple trauma was found to be associated with the cross cradle hold, manipulating the breast and nipple, and non-symmetrical contact with the breast of the infant's nose, chin, and cheeks. The odds of having nipple trauma in this study were more than four times greater with the use of the cross cradle hold. This may be related not to the technique itself but to how mothers apply the technique. Holding the infant's head, neck, and mid-shoulders with a pincer-like grasp may restrict the movement of the cervical spine and interfere with the nuchal ligament which stabilizes the head. The infant's head may be unable to rotate and tilt for an optimal latch onto the breast leading to nipple soreness. If the clinician suspects that this position is restricting the infant's head and body movements, the ventral or laid back position could be substituted.

Although most nipple pain may be relieved by correcting positioning and attachment at the breast, assessment and correction of technique may not always relieve all nipple pain (Cadwell, Turner-Maffei, Blair, Brimdyr, & McInerney, 2004; Henderson, Stamp, & Pincombe, 2001). McClellan and colleagues (2008) demonstrated that despite help with positioning and attachment, the infants of mothers with persistent nipple pain applied significantly stronger vacuums and transferred less milk than infants not causing pain. Their data revealed that infants causing pain exerted vacuums that were more than 50% stronger during active sucking and more than double during pausing when compared with infants not causing pain. In a group of breastfeeding mothers experiencing persistent nipple pain, abnormal infant tongue movements and nipple expansion were observed under ultrasound in association with high intraoral vacuum and reduced milk transfer. The tongue movements that limited the expansion of the nipple could contribute to not only pain but also slower milk transfer by occluding the ducts within the nipple and areola, which could not expand when the jaw was lowered (McClellan, Kent, Hepworth, Hartmann, & Geddes, 2015). Interventions to reduce these strong vacuums are unknown, but techniques of more frequent feeding to reduce strong sucking due to hunger or changes in positioning such as to ventral positioning could be tried.

Because there are numerous causes of nipple pain or combinations of causes, nipple pain may actually be the end product of a cascade of events. Positioning and attachment may need to be assessed several times during the first weeks after birth and interventions to correct any problems may need to be repeated (Kent et al., 2015).

Nipple pain can be a complex issue. Using a clinical reasoning model (**Figure 8-1**), nipple pain may be classified into three categories: local stimulation, external influences, and central modulation (Amir, Jones, & Buck, 2015). Local stimulation includes mechanical stressors such as nipple compression as well as inflammatory and infective states; collectively, these factors contribute to nociception. A nociceptor

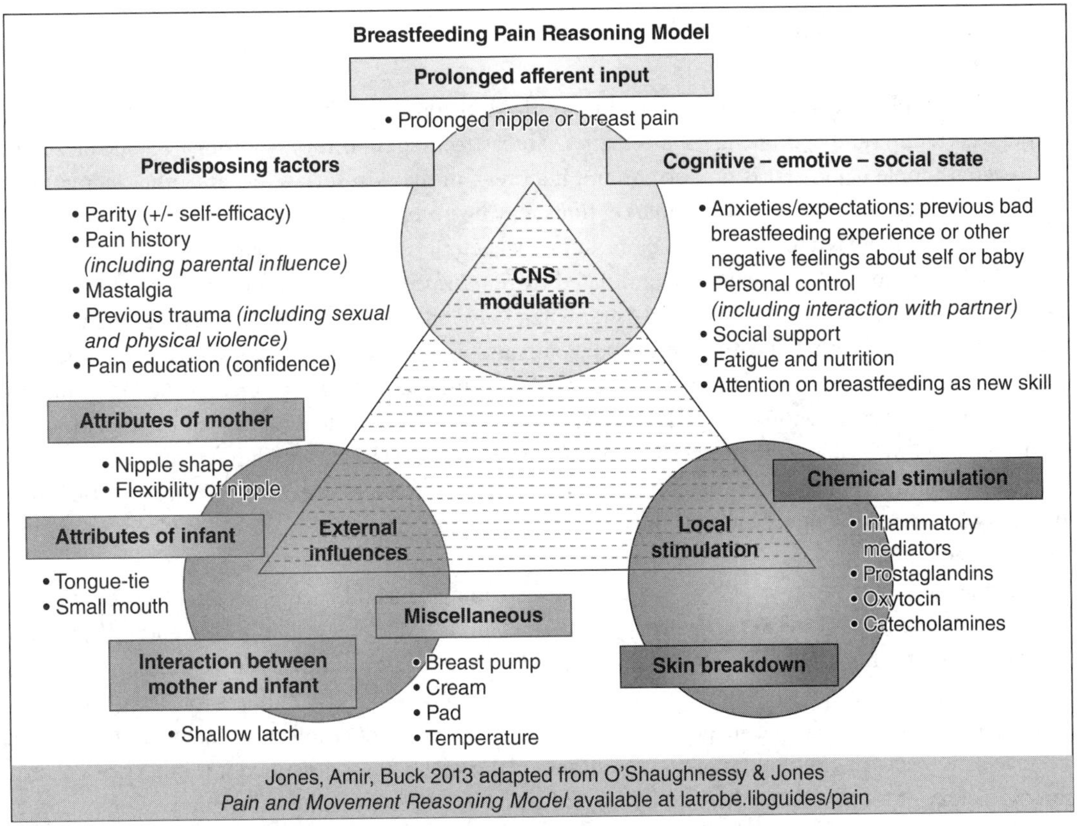

Figure 8-1 Breastfeeding pain reasoning model.

Reproduced with permission from the Royal Australian College of General Practitioners: Amir, L. H., Jones, L. E., & Buck, M. L. (2015). Nipple pain associated with breastfeeding: Incorporating current neurophysiology into clinical reasoning. *Australian Family Physician, 44*, 127–132. Retrieved from http://www.racgp.org.au/afp/2015/march/nipple-pain-associated-with-breastfeeding-incorporating-current-neurophysiology-into-clinical-reasoning.

is a sensory neuron (nerve cell) that responds to potentially damaging stimuli by sending signals to the spinal cord and brain. This process of nociception usually contributes to the perception of pain. When the damaging stimulation is strong and frequent enough to break down the skin, cytokines are released, the inflammatory response is activated, and an inflammatory exudate (discharge) may be produced that further activates the nociceptors. If pathogenic bacteria colonize the broken skin, they may not only trigger an inflammatory response but also activate nociceptors directly. External influences include attributes of the mother, such as the shape and elasticity of the nipple, as well as attributes of the infant, such as alterations in the oral anatomy and movement of the tongue and jaw. Central modulation refers to the effect of other sources of pain, increased pain response due to genetic predisposition, or increased pain sensitivity from issues such as sleep deprivation and social distress. This multifaceted model allows the clinician to explore the range of influences on nipple pain in a mother, identify the predominant contributors to nipple pain, and increase the number of potential management strategies.

When Extensive Interventions May Be Necessary

Bacterial Infection

Most early nipple discomfort and pain is due to physical forces on the nipple that can be remedied through correcting and optimizing the mechanics of breastfeeding (Renfrew, Woolridge, & McGill, 2000). However, if nipple pain persists or worsens and if a break in the skin surface occurs, other factors may become involved and more extensive interventions may be necessary. Once the integrity of the skin has been disrupted, there is a tendency for colonization by bacterial and fungal species.

Nipple wounds are frequently contaminated by *Staphylococcus aureus*, a common bacterial resident of the skin. Livingstone, Willis, and Berkowitz (1996) showed that mothers with infants younger than 1 month who presented with severe nipple pain and damage (cracks, fissures, ulcers, or exudates) had a 64% chance of having a positive bacterial skin culture and a 54% chance of having *S. aureus* impetigo vulgaris colonization. Impetigo vulgaris is a bacterial skin infection caused by staphylococci or streptococci with yellow to red weeping and crusted or pustular lesions, with the term *vulgaris* referring to the common form of this infection. Repetitive trauma to the nipple skin is thought to overcome the natural barriers to infection, and once bacterial contamination has occurred, a delay in wound healing may follow.

Livingstone and Stringer (1999) described a cascade of possible sequelae once a break in the integumentum occurs (**Box 8-1**). Eglash, Plane, and Mundt (2006) described a collection of physical and laboratory findings in a population of mothers with deep breast aching or pain, tender breasts upon palpation, and nipple lesions. Half of the mothers' nipples showed positive cultures for pathogenic bacteria. These symptoms may be suggestive of a bacterial lactiferous duct infection that responded to an average of 5 weeks of antibiotic treatment. Eglash and Proctor (2007) described a mother with a prolonged history of nipple cracks, dull throbbing of the breasts, sharp shooting pains, pain on palpation of the breasts, and redness and swelling of the left breast. Laboratory findings of the cultured milk showed *Viridans streptococcus* and coagulase-negative *Staphylococcus*. The authors postulated that the clinical and laboratory findings were descriptive of infections caused by small colony variants (SCV) of staphylococci. SCVs cause low-grade, persistent, antibiotic-resistant, chronic, and recurrent infections that take many weeks of antibiotics to clear. This type of infection may respond better to macrolides for 4–8 weeks.

Box 8-1 Cascade of Sequelae From *Staphylococcus aureus* Colonization and Infection of the Nipple Skin

- A break in the skin facilitates a secondary infection due to bacterial or fungal contamination, delaying wound healing.
- Cracks, fissures, and ulcerations have a high risk of contamination.
- Strains of *S. aureus* can penetrate the superficial layers of the skin at the site of minor skin trauma.
- The toxins they produce can cause inflammation, skin separation, and the formation of blisters.
- The blisters break down, leaving erosions in the skin that become covered with a yellow, crusted exudate.
- An ascending lactiferous duct infection can contribute to mastitis and abscess.

If a nipple infection persists after topical and/or systemic antibiotic therapy, clinicians may wish to have laboratory testing done for small colony variants.

Cascade of Sequelae From S. aureus *Colonization and Infection of the Nipple Skin*

Clinicians should be on the lookout for an ascending infection when a mother presents with severe nipple pain or a break of any sort in the nipple skin because there is a significantly increased risk for mastitis in the presence of cracked nipples (Kinlay, O'Connell, & Kinlay, 2001). In a study of 28 mothers with nipple pain (Graves, Wright, Harman, & Bailey, 2003), 57% had nipple swabs positive for *S. aureus* and 48% had positive milk specimens, indicative of ascending infection of the lactiferous ducts. Mothers complaining of deep breast pain are frequently treated for fungal infections; however, Thomassen, Johansson, Wassberg, and Petrini (1998) found that bacteria were often found both on the nipple and in the milk of mothers who described deep breast pain during or after breastfeeding. Betzold (2012) discusses that SCV and organisms found in biofilms can contribute to deep breast pain, low rates of positive cultures, low-grade symptoms, and the lengthy treatment courses necessary to eradicate the infection. Some mothers may have mixed-colony biofilms consisting of both *Candida* and *S. aureus*. In Betzold's meta-analysis of nonrandomized trials, women with deep breast pain or similar symptoms had higher rates of microbes in their milk, contributing to the theory that deep or burning breast pain is an infection of the duct with both *Candida* and/or other bacterial species as the likely pathogens.

For women with chronic breast pain in whom conservative therapy fails to improve the problem, oral antibiotic therapy may be needed to resolve the pain. Antibiotics matched by bacterial sensitivity on breastmilk culture have been shown to significantly decrease breast pain after a 14-day course of treatment (Witt, Burgess, Hawn, & Zyzanski, 2014). Persistence or worsening of nipple pain requires careful history taking and direct observation to identify the etiology (Walker & Driscoll, 1989).

Eczema and Psoriasis

Mothers with a history of atopic dermatitis and other underlying dermatological conditions are more prone to experience nipple dermatitis during breastfeeding and develop secondary fungal and bacterial infections. Nursing mothers with a history of psoriasis may experience a flare-up of psoriasis during lactation. They are also more likely to develop new plaques of psoriasis in areas of skin injury due to abrasion from infant sucking (Heller, Fullerton-Stone, & Murase, 2012). Eczema can be present on the nipple itself or can extend onto and beyond the areola (Barankin & Gross, 2004). The clinical appearance can include erythema, papules, vesicles (fluid-filled blisters), oozing (Rago, 1988), crusts, lichenification (thickening and hardening of the skin), skin erosion, fissures, excoriations, and scaling (Ward & Burton, 1997). Burning and/or itching are typical symptoms of eczema (Bracket, 1988). Differentially, itching is not prominent in candidal infections.

Eczema is a general term for several types of dermatitis, including atopic, seborrheic, irritant contact, and allergic contact. These types usually respond to removing the irritant or allergen and/or the application of topical corticosteroids (Amir, 1993). In many instances atopic dermatitis is accompanied by high colony counts of *S. aureus*, necessitating treatment with a topical antibiotic also (Lever, Hadley, Downey, & Mackie, 1988). Both nipples are commonly involved. When eczema appears on just one nipple, the clinician should consider physician referral to rule out the presence of Paget disease (cancer), which has the appearance of a steadily progressing eczema.

Herpes Infection

Numerous discrete lesions at the junction of the nipple and areola and/or farther back on the areola can be a herpes simplex infection (Amir, 2004). Herpes simplex may appear as miniature vesicles on a reddened base and can be quite tender (Heller et al., 2012). The mother usually has extreme pain, and cultures of the lesions generally show herpes simplex type 1. Herpes in the neonate can be serious or fatal and transmitted through direct contact with active lesions (Sullivan-Bolyai, Fife, Jacobs, Miller, & Corey, 1983). The mother can continue to breastfeed on the nonaffected side, resuming on the infected side when the lesions have fully healed. Herpes can infect intact skin (Dekio, Kawasaki, & Jidoi, 1986) and originate in the infant's mouth from gingivostomatitis (Sealander & Kerr, 1989), a condition peaking in children between 6 months and 3 years of age. Older infants and toddlers with sores in the anterior portion of the mouth and refusal to eat should be checked for this condition. Mothers should take extra care in washing their hands.

Raynaud Phenomenon of the Nipple

Raynaud phenomenon was first described in 1862 as intermittent ischemia typically affecting the fingers and toes, but it can involve other parts of the body, including blood vessels supplying the heart, gastrointestinal system, genitourinary system, and placental vasculature. It is more common in women than men, affecting up to 20% of women aged 21–50 years (Olsen & Nielson, 1978). In a series of events in susceptible people, a precipitating event such as exposure to cold temperatures causes vasospasms of arterioles and intermittent ischemia to the affected body part. Clinically, this is seen as pallor or blanching, followed by a cyanotic coloring as oxygen is cut off from the venous blood, ending with erythema (redness) as reflex vasodilation occurs. These color changes may involve all three changes (triphasic) or just two changes (biphasic).

It is felt as a sensation of pain (O'Sullivan & Keith, 2011), burning, numbness, prickling, or stinging. Gunther (1970) described this type of vasospasm in the nipple but attributed it to psychosomatic causes. Coates (1992) described bilateral nipple vasospasms in a mother who complained of intense pain, biphasic color changes, and partial relief from heat applications to the nipples. Because heat provided some relief and the symptoms were bilateral, it was suggested that this particular set of conditions could be a variant of Raynaud phenomenon. Blanching of the nipples can occur not only during or just after a feeding but also between feedings, with or without a history of Raynaud phenomenon in other parts of the body and in conjunction with nipple trauma such as ulceration, cracking, or blistering (Lawlor-Smith & Lawlor-Smith, 1997). The pain associated with nipple vasospasm can be so throbbing and severe that some women may completely abandon breastfeeding. It can also occur with subsequent pregnancies.

Other causes of nipple blanching and pain arise from inappropriate positioning, faulty latching, and variations of infant sucking that cause mechanical trauma from biting the nipple. A diagnosis of Raynaud phenomenon requires that other factors be present, such as the biphasic or triphasic color changes and precipitation by a stimulus such as cold temperatures. Raynaud phenomenon has been misdiagnosed as it may mimic some of the symptoms of mastitis. Differentiation of Raynaud's from mastitis has been demonstrated by culturing milk samples, with milk from breasts with mastitis showing higher levels of bacteria (Delgado et al., 2009). Because of the nature of the pain, Raynaud phenomenon of the nipples may be misidentified as a *Candida albicans* infection and treated with medications that provide no relief from the symptoms (Morino & Winn, 2007; Wu, Chason, & Wong, 2012). If mothers have been treated for *Candida* and experience no relief from nipple pain, then clinicians may wish to explore the possibility of Raynaud's. Raynaud phenomenon of the nipple has been reported as a side effect of the use of labetalol, an antihypertensive beta blocker (McGuinness & Cording, 2013). Given that this drug is associated with peripheral vasoconstriction and is commonly prescribed for hypertension during pregnancy, clinicians may wish to determine if mothers have a history of peripheral vascular disease or if use of the medication was associated with nipple vasospasm during the pregnancy.

Many of the options for treating this condition are extrapolated from interventions used for Raynaud phenomenon occurring in other parts of the body. The provision of warmth and the avoidance of cold stress are the first-line management options for Raynaud phenomenon of the nipples (Lawlor-Smith & Lawlor-Smith, 1996). Mothers may need to keep their entire body warm, use a heating pad over the breasts, wear warm clothing, wear warm coverings over the breasts, sleep under an electric blanket, or have warm packs available for application to the breast not being nursed on. If vasospasms occur between feedings, some mothers find relief by immersing the breasts in warm water. Mothers should avoid vasoconstricting drugs such as caffeine and nicotine. Mothers experiencing this acute pain during lactation require immediate relief if breastfeeding is to continue.

Nifedipine, a calcium channel blocker with vasodilating effects, has been used successfully to treat Raynaud phenomenon of the nipples (Anderson, Held, & Wright, 2004; Barrett, Heller, Fullerton-Stone, & Murase, 2013a; Page & McKenna, 2006). Only small amounts are measurable in breastmilk (Ehrenkranz, Ackerman, & Hulse, 1989; Hale, 2008), and the American Academy of Pediatrics (2001) identified the drug as usually compatible with breastfeeding. Nifedipine can be prescribed for dosing of 5 mg three times per day or as 30–60 mg per day in slow-release formulations. Usually, one 2-week course eliminates the symptoms, but some mothers may require two or three courses of treatment for complete resolution.

Nipple dermatitis can be multifactorial. A mother may have a combination of conditions simultaneously, such as eczematous dermatitis compounded by a bacterial infection, and periodic Raynaud phenomenon. In such a case, the woman may need to be referred to a dermatologist to identify and treat each condition (Barrett, Heller, Stone, & Murase, 2013b).

Nipple Bleb

A nipple bleb typically represents a nipple pore that is blocked by milk seeping under the epidermis, causing a raised, opaque, shiny white bump on the tip of the nipple. The mother usually complains of extreme pinpoint pain when the infant feeds. The incidence is unknown, and speculation on its cause has mentioned a tendency in some people for epithelial overgrowth or the encouragement of epithelial growth by the epithelial growth factor in the mother's milk (Noble, 1991). If this tissue overgrowth obstructs milk flow from a nipple pore that drains a larger area of the breast, the possibility exists for milk stasis, a plugged duct farther back in the breast, or mastitis.

If the bleb does not open spontaneously, some mothers soften the skin with warm saline soaks and gently rub with a towel or scrape with sterilized tweezers. If these efforts are unsuccessful, the mother's healthcare provider can open it with a sterile needle and express out any material that has accumulated behind it. Some of this material may be thick and stringy, representing milk that has thickened as the water in it is reabsorbed by the body. Many mothers who experience continuous nipple blebs learn to open them at home.

In a study by O'Hara (2012), nipple bleb histology showed the lack of bacteria or fungi and the presence of immune cells, when the rubbery white nipple pore blockages were removed and studied microscopically. Blebs resistant to conventional treatments were removed by O'Hara using a punch biopsy tool, which resolved the pain and symptoms. The presence of immune cells indicated a tissue reaction to milk that had leaked from the nipple pore and infiltrated into the surrounding tissue. Based on these findings, O'Hara recommended a short daily course of a very thin layer of a mid-potency steroid under an occlusive dressing to enhance penetration of the steroid into the inflamed and fibrotic tissue. Nipple blebs appeared to be an inflammatory response to nipple trauma in some women. They have been treated with topical lecithin (Lawrence & Lawrence, 2016). Lecithin acts as an emulsifier when added to foods, preventing "sticking." Topical lecithin can be rubbed into the nipple after each feeding or a lecithin supplement can be taken orally (1 or 2 1200-mg capsules 3 or 4 times per day).

Whereas a nipple bleb presents on the face of the nipple, a sebaceous cyst has been reported on the shaft or side of the nipple, with relief obtained when the oily material was removed (Wilson-Clay & Hoover, 2002).

Obstructed Glands of Montgomery

Because the glands of Montgomery have a secretory apparatus and capacity, they have the potential to become obstructed. The ductal system of the areola can also become infected (Al-Qattan & Robertson, 1990). A mother can experience a painful inflamed or infected Montgomery gland, appearing as a reddened raised bump or fluid-filled blister farther back on the areola. Although the condition is usually self-limiting, it can occasionally require interventions such as the application of warm compresses, the use of antibiotics (topical or systemic), and gentle squeezing to remove infected material. Mothers should be aware of equipment or irritants that could precipitate or aggravate Montgomery glands to the point of actual obstruction or damage. Use of pump flanges, breast shells, or nipple shields that could abrade these glands or the application of topical preparations that block the openings of the Montgomery glands should be investigated when mothers present with painful conditions on the areola rather than the nipple.

Nipple pain may originate from preparations applied to the nipples, misuse of breastfeeding equipment, allergies or sensitivity to chemicals or irritants, or other conditions such as psoriasis. Nipples may also swell during pumping. Clinicians should ask if the mother is pumping milk and make sure that she is correctly using a high-quality pump with the appropriate size flange.

Fungal Colonization

In addition to mechanical trauma of the nipple and bacterial infection, the fungal pathogen *Candida albicans* can contribute to nipple and breast pain in lactating women. Although the terms candidiasis, mammary candidosis, and thrush are used interchangeably, the old term monilia for moniliasis is not interchangeable because it refers to a different genus. *C. albicans* is an opportunistic, commensal, normally harmless organism residing on the skin and in the gastrointestinal and genitourinary tracts. Dry, healthy, intact skin and the presence of normal competing flora typically allow *C. albicans* to exist in harmony with its host. Stratified squamous epithelial cells lining the gastrointestinal and genitourinary tracts are easily colonized by *C. albicans*. Portions of the lining of the lactiferous ducts are also composed of layered squamous epithelial cells, posing the possibility that under the right circumstances these too could be vulnerable to fungal invasion (Heinig, Francis, & Pappagianis, 1999).

Laboratory evidence confirming the presence of *C. albicans* in the mammary ducts of humans is sparse (Amir, Garland, Dennerstein, & Farish, 1996; Thomassen et al., 1998), whereas ductal infections in dairy cattle and goats have been reported (Moretti, Pasquali, Mencaroni, Boncio, & Piergili Fioretti, 1998; Singh, Sood, Gupta, Jand, & Banga, 1998). *C. albicans* has also been isolated from milk samples of dairy cows with mastitis and subclinical mastitis (dos Santos & Marin, 2005). This invites speculation that ductal colonization or infection in humans may be facilitated when the breast becomes susceptible through subclinical mastitis. Subclinical mastitis may render the ducts an easy target if they have become inflamed through a local adverse immune response to milk proteins that have remained in prolonged contact with them (Michie, Lockie, & Lynn, 2003). Opening of the tight junctions between luminal epithelial cells from milk stasis may increase the areas for colonization by pathogenic organisms.

Ultrasound imaging of the breasts has shown dilatation of the milk ducts by the milk-ejection reflex, followed by a decrease in ductal diameter and a backflow of the milk that is not removed (Ramsay, Kent, Owens, & Hartmann, 2004). It could be speculated that the backward flow of milk away from the nipple and into the smaller collecting ducts and ductules could carry pathogens deeper into the breast. Hale, Bateman, Finkelman, and Berens (2009) evaluated the presence of *C. albicans* in the milk of breastfeeding women with and without breast pain suggestive of a clinical diagnosis of a fungal infection. An assay for beta-glucan, the presence of which is reflective of an active candidal infection, was performed on milk samples from mothers with and without symptoms. There was no significant difference in beta-glucan levels between the two groups, indicating that *Candida* was not present in the ductal system of the breasts.

C. albicans exists in at least three different morphologies (forms): yeast, pseudohyphae, and hyphae. By activating appropriate sets of genes, it can alter its form to adapt to its changing environment and increase its virulence, allowing it to colonize or infect virtually all body sites (Staib, Kretschmar, Nichterlein, Hof, & Morschhäuser, 2000). *C. albicans* may appear as spherical yeast cells on the skin, and although they can change into filamentous forms that readily penetrate tissues, the organism has many other mechanisms to circumvent and take advantage of changing host conditions. The filamentous forms of hyphae and pseudohyphae adhere better to epithelial cells than spherical yeast cells. Their projections can follow surface discontinuities and penetrate through breaks in tissue, such as those occurring in nipple fissures (Odds, 1994). They can secrete enzymes that digest epidermal keratin, the tough top layer of skin, assisting hyphal filaments in their invasive process and inducing an inflammatory response.

A number of risk factors for mammary candidiasis have been put forward:

- Between 22% (Cotch, Hillier, Gibbs, & Eschenbach, 1998) and 33% (Vidotto et al., 1992) of pregnant women test positive for vaginal candidiasis by the end of their pregnancy, with the majority (95%) caused by *C. albicans* (Odds, 1994).
- Use of antibiotics during the peripartum period or while breastfeeding increases the risk factor (Amir et al., 1996; Chetwynd, Ives, Payne, & Edens-Bartholomew, 2002; Dinsmoor, Viloria, Lief, & Elder, 2005; Tanquay, McBean, & Jain, 1994).
- Sore or damaged nipples provide a route of entry for pathogens (Amir, 1991; Amir et al., 1996; Amir & Hoover, 2003; Livingstone et al., 1996; Tanquay et al., 1994).
- Colonization and development of oral thrush in infants occurs from the birth process (Remington & Klein, 1983) and other vectors, such as healthcare workers (Pfaller, 1994), as the infant gets older. Approximately 40–60% of infants carry the organism in their mouths, with 10–24% developing oral thrush within the first 18 months (Darwazeh & al-Bashir, 1995). Morrill, Heinig, Pappagianis, and Dewey (2005) reported oral colonization in 20% of infants studied, of whom 75% developed oral thrush by 9 weeks of age.
- Use of pacifiers in infants (Brook & Gober, 1997; Darwazeh & al-Bashir, 1995; Mattos-Graner, de Moraes, Rontani, & Birman, 2001) may facilitate oral colonization and contribute to persistence of candidal presence in the mouth (Manning, Coughlin, & Poskitt, 1985).
- The use of bottles has been demonstrated to be a key risk factor for *C. albicans* colonization in both mothers and infants. Morrill, Heinig, Pappagianis, and Dewey (2005) reported that of 52 mother–infant dyads that used bottles in the first 2 weeks postpartum, 44% of the mothers and 38% of the infants tested positive for *C. albicans*. They suggest that it may not be bottle use alone but the fluid contained in the bottle that provides the growth medium for facilitating *C. albicans* colonization. Infant formula contains large amounts of iron, and iron is known to increase growth of *C. albicans* in vitro (Andersson, Lindquist, Lagerqvust, & Hernell, 2000). Lactoferrin in human milk typically keeps *C. albicans* in check. However, the absence of lactoferrin in artificial infant milk plus its relatively heavy load of iron may combine to augment yeast proliferation in the infant's mouth. *C. albicans*' adherence to epithelial surfaces can also be encouraged by the presence of sucrose or fructose (Pizzo, Giuliana, Milici, & Giangreco, 2000), as seen in soy-based infant formulas. Some soy-based formulas can contain as much as 10% sucrose (table sugar).

The exact prevalence of *C. albicans* colonization in mothers in not known. Twenty-six percent of breastfeeding women referred to a clinic for nipple and breast pain fulfilled the clinical diagnosis for nipple candidiasis (Tanquay et al., 1994). Thomassen and colleagues (1998) reported that 50% of women with superficial nipple pain and 20% of women with deep breast pain had positive cultures for *C. albicans*. Thus deep breast pain or shooting breast pain by itself may not be indicative of candidal infection within the breast (Carmichael & Dixon, 2002). In a healthy population of lactating women, Morrill and colleagues (2005) found 23% were colonized by *Candida* species on the nipple/areola or in their milk. The occurrence of mammary candidiasis, defined as colonization plus symptoms, was 20% between 2 and 9 weeks postpartum. In the Morrill study, the rate of weaning by 9 weeks for this painful condition was 2.2 times higher in women who developed mammary candidiasis. *C. albicans* was found more frequently in mothers who reported breastfeeding-associated pain (Andrews et al., 2007), possibly due to nipple alterations that predispose to candidal overgrowth.

Detecting *C. albicans* and diagnosing mammary candidiasis can be difficult (Wiener, 2006). Accurate detection of candidal species in human milk is complicated by the action of lactoferrin. The lactoferrin in human milk inhibits yeast growth in vitro (Soukka, Tenovuo, & Lenander-Lumikari, 1992), often resulting in false-negative test results when the milk is cultured. Skin scrapings of the nipple/areola can be placed under a microscope in a 10% potassium hydroxide wet mount to identify the presence of yeast, yet few clinicians order any type of laboratory testing to identify and diagnose mammary candidiasis (Brent, 2001). A laboratory technique that uses the addition of iron to counteract the action of lactoferrin has been shown to reduce the likelihood of false-negative test results and provide a more accurate means of confirming the presence of *Candida* in human milk (Morrill, Pappagianis, Heinig, Lonnerdall, & Dewey, 2003). Accurate laboratory testing still takes about 3 days, leaving the mother in pain and validating the need for a more rapid means of determining when and how to treat the symptoms.

Mammary candidiasis is most often diagnosed presumptively by signs and symptoms that are subjective, can be indicative of other problems, and are rarely confirmed by laboratory findings (Amir & Pakula, 1991; Johnstone & Marcinak, 1990). Signs include a nipple and/or areola that is red, shiny, or flaky, and symptoms include burning pain of the nipple/areola and deep, shooting, burning, or stabbing pain in the breast. In an effort to better delineate the signs and symptoms, clinicians could use to determine treatment, Morrill, Heinig, Pappagianis, & Dewey, (2004) used the measure of positive predictive value (PPV) for each sign and symptom. PPV was chosen as a measure because a PPV above 70% is considered to be of clinical value (Grimes & Schulz, 2002). The PPV was 50% or less for each of the signs and symptoms when they occurred individually. However, when the following combinations of signs and symptoms occurred, the PPV rose to over 70%, indicating that there was a high probability that the mother had *Candida*:

- When the signs of shiny and flaky skin of the nipple/areola occurred together
- When either of the skin symptoms occurred together with nonstabbing or stabbing breast pain
- When combinations of three or more signs and symptoms occurred simultaneously, especially when the combination included either shiny or flaky skin of the nipple/areola

Candida species are associated with burning nipple and breast pain, independent of the presence of nipple damage or *S. aureus*. Nipple damage itself has been associated with burning nipple and radiating breast pain, so caution should be exercised about asserting that fungal infection is the cause of this pain (Amir et al., 2013).

Treatments for Sore Nipples

Candida can be difficult to eradicate (Hanna & Cruz, 2011). Treatment approaches should begin by assessing and correcting mechanical causes of nipple pain, including assessing for Raynaud phenomenon of the nipples (Amir, 2003), because sore nipples alone may not be indicative of *Candida*. If nipple pain persists after correction of breastfeeding techniques, bacterial infection may be present and can be treated with a topical antibiotic such as mupirocin (Bactroban). However, if the nipple pain worsens or is described as burning, a combined bacterial and fungal infection may be present to which a topical antifungal such as miconazole 2% can be added. Gentian violet, a strong purple dye that kills yeast on contact, can be painted on the nipples and areolae using a 0.5–1.0% strength aqueous solution for 4–7 days. At a higher concentration or used for a prolonged period of time, gentian violet has the potential for toxicity (Piatt & Bergeson, 1992). Therefore a dilution of 0.25–0.5% can be used in the infant's mouth once or twice daily for 3–7 days to avoid oral mucosal ulceration (Utter, 1990, 1992).

If signs and symptoms occur in any of the previous combinations or these treatments fail to address the problem, Newman's all-purpose nipple ointment (APNO; Newman, 2005) can be compounded in the following proportions:

- Mupirocin 2% ointment (15 g)
- Betamethasone 0.1% ointment (15 g)
- Miconazole powder is added so that the final concentration is 2% miconazole

APNO ointment should be applied sparingly after each feeding until the mother is pain free and then decreased over a week or 2 until the pain stops. If this topical treatment provides no pain relief in 3–4 days or is needed longer than 2–3 weeks to keep pain free, then the nipple–areolar skin and the milk should be tested.

Fluconazole (Diflucan) is a systemic agent that may be used when the previous treatments fail or when laboratory results confirm the presence of *Candida* in the milk. The loading dose is usually 400 mg followed by 100 mg twice daily for 2 weeks, until the mother is pain free for a week. It should be used in combination with Newman's topical nipple ointment because fluconazole can take several days to start working. If there is no relief after 14–21 days of fluconazole treatment, the deep breast pain may have a different cause such as a bacterial infection. Some persistent or mismanaged cases of candidiasis may require a longer course of fluconazole, not only for the mother (Bodley & Powers, 1997) but also for the infant (Chetwynd et al., 2002). Both mother and infant should be treated simultaneously, even if thrush is not visible in the infant's mouth. There is a high correlation between oral and diaper candidiasis among infants of mothers with nipple candidiasis (Tanquay et al., 1994). Mothers with deep breast pain may also benefit from anti-inflammatory pain medications such as ibuprofen.

Nystatin has long been used on the nipples of the mother and the oral mucosa of the infant. However, its effective clinical cure rate for oral candidiasis has been reported to be only 54% in infants compared with a 99% cure rate when using miconazole (Hoppe & Hahn, 1996). Its effectiveness has been reduced over time because almost 45% of *Candida* strains are resistant to nystatin (Hale & Berens, 2002). *C. albicans* persistently adheres to buccal mucosa and is less affected by nystatin than other *Candida* species (Ellepola, Panagoda, & Samaranayake, 1999). Nystatin is more fungistatic than fungicidal; thus it may reduce symptoms in some mothers and infants but can be ineffective in eradicating the infection.

Some mothers take acidophilus supplements (one tablet daily containing 40 million to 1 billion viable units) to help restore a balance of microorganisms in the body. Mothers may question if milk they expressed during a yeast infection can be given to the infant later. Under susceptible conditions, this milk may have the potential to infect or reinfect because freezing does not kill yeast (Rosa, Novak, Almeida, Hagler, & Hagler, 1990), although lactoferrin may keep yeast levels low.

Panjaitan, Amir, Costs, Rudland, and Tabrizi (2008) demonstrated an association between *Candida* infection and nipple pain but identified other fungal species on sore nipples. This raised the possibility that nipple pain/thrush could be due to the presence of fungal organisms other than *C. albicans*.

Optimizing the mechanics of breastfeeding (positioning, latch, suck) continues to function as the first-line intervention for the prevention of sore and damaged nipples (Morland-Schultz & Hill, 2005). Repetitive trauma from uncorrected faulty breastfeeding patterns may set the stage for breaks in skin integrity, which even when corrected may leave nipples in poor condition for healing.

Nipples that have been traumatized with breaks in skin integrity are easily colonized with bacterial and fungal species, are slow to heal, represent significant pain to the mother, and may lead to partial or total discontinuation of breastfeeding if therapeutic interventions do not provide quick relief. Topical antibiotics may be needed for rapid and effective resolution of pain and prevention of possible ascending infection into the breast itself. Because of the link between severe nipple soreness and colonization and infection of the nipple by *S. aureus* (Livingstone et al., 1996), careful washing of the nipple with soap and water and the application of mupirocin 2% ointment (Bactroban) may be effective in the early stages of the infection. Bacteria have the ability to grow in colonies and protect the colony with a coating called a biofilm. Biofilms may potentially be stimulated by saliva, such as when an infant feeds at the breast (Stewart & Costerton, 2001). To disrupt this protective biofilm, washing the nipple wound with soap and water once a day followed by a coating of mupirocin may penetrate the biofilm, promote wound healing, and prevent progression to an infection (Ryan, 2007). Because much nipple pain may stem from inflammation, topical application of low- to medium-strength steroids may provide welcome relief. No adverse effects have been reported when these types of preparations are used sparingly as thin coats to the nipples (Huggins & Billion, 1993). Systemic antibiotics may need to be added to the treatment regime if exudate is seen, erythema increases, or dry-scab formation is absent. Persistent sore nipples may be due to a combination of yeast and bacterial infection, causing difficulty in differentiating the offending organism. Some clinicians use miconazole 2% (Monistat) as the antifungal preparation in combination with the mupirocin and a topical steroid to ensure the best results (Porter & Schach, 2004). Tracing the source of infection when it persists or recurs may involve treating the infant with nasal mupirocin ointment if he or she is found to harbor the offending organism in the oropharynx (Livingstone & Stringer, 1999). Use of topical preparations on the nipple is consistent with the principles of moist wound healing.

Dry wound healing (air drying, sunlight, sun lamp, hair dryer, heat from a light bulb) has been advocated for many years. It was thought that continued tissue destruction and slower wound healing would occur if the nipples remained wet and that rapid drying would prevent this. However, close observation of damaged nipples usually reveals fissuring, which results from an insufficient amount of moisture in the stratum corneum (uppermost layer of the skin) and/or friction damage from the infant's sucking.

Treatment of nipple fissures is consistent with treating other types of skin fissures, which is to increase the moisture content of the skin and reduce further drying by applying an emollient to the damaged area (Sharp, 1992). An emollient is soothing and provides a moisture barrier that slows the evaporation of moisture naturally present in the skin, eliminating further drying and cracking. Scab formation does not occur when using moist wound healing. Rapid drying causes the stratum corneum to shrink in an irregular manner, placing tension on a layer of fragile tissue. The use of an emollient such as USP-modified anhydrous lanolin allows the contours of the stratum corneum to return to normal, enhancing the movement of cells across the wound as it heals. Sharp (1992) delineated a difference between surface skin moisture and internal moisture, stating that although a mother may pat the nipple area with a clean cloth to remove surface wetness, rapid drying can deplete the skin of internal moisture. He compared this with the act of licking dry chapped lips, which sets up a rapid wet-to-dry process that worsens the original condition.

When observing treatment methods for wound healing on other parts of the body, occlusive or semi-occlusive dressings are frequently used to cover the wound, maintain moisture, inhibit scab or crust formation, reduce pain, and enhance epithelial migration for wound repair (Ziemer, Cooper, & Pigeon, 1995). Ziemer and colleagues (1995) studied the prophylactic use of a polyethylene film dressing (BlisterFilm, Sherwood Medical) with an adhesive border on the occurrence of nipple skin damage during the 1st week of breastfeeding. Although significantly reducing pain, this dressing did not prevent skin changes and damage. A high dropout rate was seen due to skin pain and damage from the adhesive backing when the dressing was removed. No special breastfeeding instructions or corrections of feeding mechanics were provided for the mothers.

Building on the approach of using occlusive wound dressings for healing damaged nipples, Brent, Rudy, Redd, Rudy, and Roth (1998) randomized 42 mothers to receive a hydrogel wound dressing or a combination of breast shells and lanolin. The hydrogel dressing (Elasto-Gel, Southwest Technologies, Inc.) used was glycerin based, highly absorbent, and nonadhesive with cooling properties. Breastfeeding technique was controlled for and help was provided when needed. Mothers using the breast shells and lanolin experienced fewer breast infections and less pain than the group using the glycerin-based dressing. Cable, Stewart, and Davis (1997) used a water-based hydrogel dressing (ClearSite, New Dimensions in Medicine/ConMed) to avoid potential problems with breast infections associated with glycerin-based products. Mothers in their study experienced significant pain relief when the dressing was worn between feedings. The sheet was changed every 1–3 days until the nipple wound healed. Dodd and Chalmers (2003) compared the prophylactic use of lanolin with the water-based hydrogel dressing Maternimates (Tyco Healthcare Group; currently marketed as Ameda ComfortGel Pads, Ameda, Inc.). Mothers reported significantly lower pain scores when using the hydrogel dressing as a preventive measure, with no breast infections (vs. eight cases of mastitis in the lanolin group). Cadwell (2001) studied the use of a glycerin-based hydrogel dressing (Soothies, Puronyx, Inc. [now Lansinoh Laboratories]) compared with lanolin application/breast-shell use in mothers presenting with established nipple pain and damage. Rates of healing between the two groups were similar, but the mothers using the hydrogel pads experienced markedly more relief from pain than the lanolin/shell group.

The moist wound-healing options of lanolin and hydrogel dressings have been used both prophylactically to prevent nipple pain and damage and therapeutically as remedies. Lanolin may be a reasonable choice for sore or abraded nipples, whereas a hydrogel dressing may prove helpful for open sores or cracks with exudate. The dressing absorbs wound discharge and prevents the skin from adhering to the mother's bra. Lanolin use, however, has been associated with a longer healing time in mothers with sore nipples compared with the use of breastmilk (Mohammadzadeh, Farhat, & Esmaeily, 2005). The best defense against *C. albicans* is healthy, intact skin and a robust immune system. Efforts should be made to ensure correct latch by the infant and assessment of any nipple pain reported by the mother. The longer incorrect sucking patterns persist, the greater the chance for both bacterial and fungal overgrowth of damaged nipple tissue. Pacifiers and bottles containing infant formulas should be avoided. Persistent nipple soreness, fissured nipples that are slow to heal, and nipples with obvious dermatological abnormalities must be addressed immediately. Clinicians may consider avoiding the use of nystatin because it often prolongs the amount of time until the mother finds relief from the pain of a candidal infection. Unresolved nipple pain may cause untimely weaning (Schwartz et al., 2002). Both mother and infant should be treated if one or the other shows signs of candidiasis.

Light-emitting diode (LED) phototherapy has been used to heal nipple trauma in breastfeeding mothers. Chaves, Araujo, Santos, Pinotti, and Oliveira (2012) used LED phototherapy treatment on an experimental group of mothers with nipple lesions compared with a control group of mothers who were provided with standard information on nipple care and breastfeeding techniques. Mothers in the LED-treated group enjoyed more rapid healing of their nipple lesions and a significant reduction in pain intensity compared with the untreated group.

No single agent has been shown to be clearly superior to any other agent in treating nipple pain or trauma (Morland-Schultz & Hill, 2005). **Table 8-1** provides selected studies that compare various topical agents to each other, with some yielding better results than others.

A number of other plant extracts and therapies have been used topically for wound healing and share a common component. They produce what are called flavonoid compounds with phytochemicals, or highly reactive compounds that neutralize free radicals.

- Green tea contains catechins that facilitate natural wound healing (Hsu, 2005). The application of green tea bags to sore nipples has a soothing effect.
- Olive oil has been shown to possess antioxidant and anti-inflammatory properties that help in healing as well as squalene, which serves as an antioxidant and emollient. One study looked at patient satisfaction with the use of olive oil versus lanolin on nipples relative to nipple pain. Mothers significantly preferred olive oil to lanolin in the reduction of nipple pain (Gungor et al., 2013). In another study, 56 mothers prophylactically applied extra virgin olive oil to one nipple and lanolin to the other nipple after nursing. The results showed that 89% of the mothers were more satisfied with olive oil. Sore nipples were observed in 33.9% of the lanolin group and 7.1% of the olive oil group. No nipple pain was described in 66.1% of the olive oil group and 46.4% in the lanolin group (Oguz, Isik, Gungor, Seker, & Ogretmen, 2014). Olive oil that has been treated with gaseous ozone produces a product to which bacteria cannot become resistant. Ozonated olive oil is available commercially, but no studies have been found on its use in breastfeeding mothers.
- Peppermint water has been used as a prophylactic measure. Prevention of sore, abraded, or cracked nipples is always preferable to treating the condition after the fact. Sayyah-Melli, Rashidi, Delazar, and colleagues (2007) randomized 196 primiparous mothers to use either peppermint water or expressed breastmilk prophylactically on their nipples after feedings for the first 14 days

Table 8-1 Comparison of Selected Topical Sore Nipple Treatments

Agent	Positive Results	Equivalent Results	Negative Results
Expressed mother's milk (EMM)	Superior to lanolin (Mohammadzadeh, Farhat, & Esmaeily, 2005)	Equivalent to lanolin (Hewat & Ellis, 1987)	Inferior to warm water compresses (Buchko et al., 1994; Pugh et al., 1996) Inferior to keeping nipples dry and clean (Akkuzu & Taskin, 2000) Inferior to lanolin (Coca & Abrao, 2008) Inferior to peppermint water (Sayyah-Melli et al., 2007a) Inferior to silver cups (Marrazzu et al., 2015) Inferior to extra virgin olive oil (Cordero, Villar., Barrilao, Cortes, & Lopez, 2015)
Tea bag compress		Equivalent to lanolin in neither preventing nor reducing soreness (Riordan, 1985) Equivalent to warm water compress (Lavergne, 1997)	Inferior to warm water compresses (Buchko et al., 1994)
Warm water compress	Superior to tea bags or EMM (Buchko et al., 1994) Superior to lanolin and EMM (Pugh et al., 1996)	Equivalent to tea bags (Lavergne, 1997)	Inferior to keeping nipples dry and clean (Akkuzu & Taskin, 2000)
Lanolin	Superior to no treatment after 5 days (Spangler & Hildebrandt, 1993) Superior to EMM (Coca & Abrao, 2008)	Equivalent to EMM (Hewat & Ellis, 1987) Equivalent to tea bags in neither preventing nor reducing soreness (Riordan, 1985) Equivalent to peppermint and dexpanthenol (a B complex vitamin) (Shanazi et al, 2015)	Inferior to warm water compresses (Pugh et al., 1996) Inferior to hydrogel dressings (Dodd & Chalmers, 2003) Inferior to EMM (Mohammadzadeh et al., 2005) Inferior to peppermint gel (Seyyah-Melli et al., 2007b) Inferior to olive oil (Gungor et al., 2013; Oguz et al., 2014)

Hydrogel dressing	Superior to lanolin (Dodd & Chalmers, 2003)	
Peppermint gel	Superior to lanolin (Manizheh et al., 2007b)	Equivalent to lanolin and dexpanthenol (Shanazi et al, 2015)
Peppermint water	Superior to EMM (Manizheh et al., 2007a)	
Menthol essence	Superior to mothers' own breastmilk (Akbari, Alamolhoda, Baghban, & Mirabi, 2014)	
All-purpose nipple ointment (APNO)		Not more effective than lanolin in relation to nipple pain, breastfeeding duration and exclusivity rates, mastitis, yeast symptoms, healing time, side effects, and satisfaction with treatment (Dennis, Schottle, Hodnett, & McQueen, 2012)
LED phototherapy	Superior to standard nipple care and adequate breastfeeding techniques (Chaves et al., 2012)	
Olive oil	Superior to lanolin in reducing pain (Gungor et al., 2013; Oguz et al., 2014) Superior to expressed mother's milk (Cordero et al, 2015)	
Silver cups	Superior to mother's own milk in reducing fissures, bleeding, and pain in mothers with cracked nipples (Marrazzu et al., 2015)	
Dexpanthenol (vitamin B complex family)		Equivalent to lanolin and peppermint gel (Shanazi et al, 2015)

Data from Lochner, J. E., Livingston, C. J., & Judlins, D. Z. (2009). Which interventions are best for alleviating nipple pain in nursing mothers? *Journal of Family Practice, 58,* 612a–612c; Walker, M. (2010). *The nipple and areola in breastfeeding and lactation: Anatomy, physiology, problems, and solutions.* Amarillo, TX: Hale Publishing.

after delivery. Nipple pain and damage were much less likely in the group of mothers using peppermint water compared with the group who used breastmilk, with peppermint water being three times more effective than expressed breastmilk.

- Peppermint gel has also been used as a treatment for sore nipples. In a study of this therapy, Sayyah-Melli, Rashidi, Nokhoodchi, and colleagues (2007) randomized 163 primiparous mothers into three groups, one using purified lanolin, one using a peppermint gel, and one using a placebo gel after each feeding. The group using the peppermint gel had the lowest rates of nipple cracks; use of the peppermint gel was more effective than the use of peppermint water or any other of the interventions studied. Peppermint (*Mentha piperita*) has a calming and numbing effect and has been used to relieve skin irritations (Blumenthal, Goldberg, & Brinckmann, 2000). Peppermint also has antibacterial activity, increasing tissue flexibility and making tissue resistant to cracks (Schelz, Molnar, & Hohmann, 2006).
- Menthol essence has been used in a study to treat nipple cracks in breastfeeding mothers 3 days postpartum. Mothers in the study with cracked nipples were asked to place 4 drops of menthol essence on the nipple and areola after each feeding. The mothers in the control group with cracked nipples were instructed to apply 4 drops of their own milk to the nipple after each feeding. Mothers in the menthol group showed significant improvement in pain intensity scores and skin damage severity compared with the control group (Akbari, Alamolhoda, Baghban, & Mirabi, 2014).
- Virgin coconut oil (VCO) is more effective against *S. aureus* than olive oil and VCO-treated wounds heal much faster, as indicated by a decreased time of complete epithelization and higher levels of various skin components. Studies are lacking regarding the use of coconut oil on sore nipples, but lactation consultants anecdotally report good outcomes.
- Medihoney is a commercial product made with honey that has been irradiated to eliminate the presence of botulism spores. Medihoney exerts antimicrobial action against a broad spectrum of fungi and bacteria, including antibiotic-resistant bacteria such as methicillin-resistant *S. aureus*, multidrug-resistant Gram-negative organisms, and vancomycin-resistant enterococci. Honey has been used successfully as a dressing for wounds, including burns, ulcers, infected surgical wounds, necrotizing soft-tissue infections, meningococcal wounds, and abdominal wound dehiscence. It is bactericidal against multiple strains of bacteria and has the ability to penetrate biofilm formation on bacterial colonies. Breast pads containing honey are available from Manuka Health (http://www.honeywoundcare.com).
- Emu oil is a skin-hydrating vehicle with anti-inflammatory properties. Prophylactic application of emu oil following feedings at breast showed a significant improvement in the level of stratum corneum hydration in the areola (Zanardo, Giarrizzo, Maiolo, & Straface, 2016). Reducing the nipple's and areola's susceptibility to cracking by improving hydration while delivering potent anti-inflammatory agents to the nipple–areolar complex might help improve skin barrier function.
- Dexpanthenol, which belongs to the family of B complex vitamins, has been shown to be effective in reducing nipple cracking. It functions as a moisturizer by reducing water loss through the skin and contributing to its elasticity (Shanazi et al., 2015).

- Silver cups are shaped like a nipple shield but made of high-grade silver with no holes in the tip. They are designed to be worn under the bra between feedings and removed prior to breastfeeding. Silver is a natural antibacterial and healing agent to which bacteria is not resistant. In a study of 40 mothers with nipple cracks and fissures, 20 were assigned to an experimental group, which used the silver cups, and 20 to the control group, which applied their own breastmilk to nipples following feedings. Mothers in the silver cup group showed more rapid disappearance of symptoms (pain, bleeding, and fissures) and more rapid healing than mothers in the control group (Marrazzu et al., 2015).

Mothers with sore or damaged nipples will benefit from specific feeding plans that serve to promptly resolve the pain they are feeling. **Box 8-2** provides sample intervention plans for clinicians to use or modify in helping mothers to rectify problems with painful or traumatized nipples.

Box 8-2 Sample Plans for Preventing and Resolving Nipple Pain and Trauma

Preventive Strategies

- Assess latch, suck, and swallowing and correct positioning if necessary.
- Use a modified syringe, nipple rolling, or teacup hold to evert nipples and assist with latch if nipples are flat.
- Place infant in ventral position (prone) for gravity assistance, optimal ventilation, and advantageous use of primitive neonatal reflexes to provide physical environment for optimal latch (Colson, Meek, & Hawdon, 2008).
- Check to make sure the infant's mouth is open to 160 degrees, with lips flared outward and neck slightly extended.
- Use reverse pressure softening if areola is edematous.
- If pumping, assure the flange is large enough to prevent nipple strangulation in flange tunnel. If nipple does not move during pumping, switch to larger flange.
- Provide relief from engorgement.
- Avoid pacifiers until breastfeeding is well established.
- Correct ankyloglossia if present.
- Apply peppermint water or peppermint gel to nipples after each early feeding.

When Nipples Are Already Sore

In addition to the preventative measures, the following preparations may be tried for soothing, pain relief, and healing:

- Warm water compresses
- Saline soaks
- Warm green tea bag compresses
- Peppermint water or gel
- Olive oil (virgin)—antibacterial properties

- Coconut oil (virgin)—antibacterial properties
- Medihoney—antibacterial properties
- Commercial nipple creams with a 0-2 rating on the Environmental Working Group's cosmetic safety database (check at http://www.ewg.org/skindeep/browse.php?category=nipplecream)
- Nipple shield—if nothing else is working and the mother verbalizes her desire to stop breastfeeding

When Nipples Are Cracked or Damaged

If there is a break in the nipple skin:

- Wash nipple with soap and water once each day to disrupt biofilm formation
- Apply topical mupirocin
- Avoid pacifier use or wash pacifiers thoroughly with soap and water
- Apply topical low-strength steroids for inflammation
- Take systemic anti-inflammatory such as ibuprofen

If exudate (pus) is seen, erythema increases, or dry scab is present:

- Add systemic antibiotics
- If *Candida albicans* is suspected, add 2% miconazole

If infection is recurrent or persistent:

- Treat infant with nasal mupirocin
- Test for small colony variant (SCV) bacteria; ask for culture and sensitivity laboratory testing

If SCV bacteria are present, switch to macrolide therapy and:

- Use hydrogel dressing for comfort and moist wound healing
- Be watchful for an ascending infection (mastitis)
- Correct anemia

Data from Walker, M. (2010). *The nipple and areola in breastfeeding and lactation: Anatomy, physiology, problems, and solutions.* Amarillo, TX: Hale Publishing.

ENGORGEMENT

Engorgement is a well-known but poorly researched aspect of lactation. Medical dictionaries define engorgement as congestion and/or distention with fluid. General lactation literature refers to engorgement as the physiological condition characterized by the painful swelling of the breasts associated with the sudden increase in milk volume, lymphatic and vascular congestion, and interstitial edema during the first 2 weeks after birth. Engorgement is a normal physiological process with a progression of changes, without trauma or injury to tissues. When milk production increases rapidly, the volume of milk in the breast can exceed the capacity of the alveoli to store it. If the milk is not removed, overdistention of the alveoli can cause the milk-secreting cells to become flattened, drawn out, and even to rupture. The distention can partly or completely occlude the capillary blood circulation surrounding the alveolar cells, further decreasing cellular activity (Dawson, 1935). Congested blood vessels leak fluid into the surrounding tissue space, contributing to edema. Pressure and congestion obstruct lymphatic drainage of the breasts, stagnating the system that rids the breasts of toxins, bacteria, and cast-off cell parts, thereby predisposing the breast to mastitis (both inflammation and infection). In addition, a protein called the feedback inhibitor of lactation accumulates in the mammary gland during milk stasis, further reducing milk production (Prentice, Addey, & Wilde, 1989).

Accumulation of milk and the resulting engorgement are major triggers of apoptosis (programmed cell death) that causes involution of the milk-secreting gland, milk resorption, collapse of the alveolar structures, and the cessation of milk production (Marti, Feng, Altermatt, & Jaggi, 1997). A clinical sign of possible glandular involution may relate to descriptions of exceptionally thick or stringy milk being expressed from an engorged breast (Glover, 1998). This may represent milk inspissation (increased thickness or decreased fluidity) secondary to fluid resorption and an accumulation of fat cells in the gland (Weichert, 1980).

Engorgement has also been classified as involving only the areola, only the body of the breast, or both. Areolar engorgement involves clinical observations of a swollen areola with tight, shiny skin, probably involving overfull lactiferous ducts. A puffy areola is thought to be tissue edema, possibly contributed by large amounts of intravenous fluids received by some mothers during labor.

Some degree of breast engorgement is normal. Minimal or no engorgement in the first week postpartum has been associated with insufficient milk (Neifert et al., 1990; Newton & Newton, 1951), early supplementation, and a higher percentage of breastfeeding decline in the early weeks (Humenick, Hill, & Anderson, 1994). Delayed onset of copious milk production, judged by mothers as breast fullness or engorgement, is of equal importance as the overfull breast. Excess infant weight loss was shown to be 7.1 times greater if the mother experienced delayed onset of lactation (Dewey et al., 2003). Rates of delayed engorgement (over 72 hours after birth) range between 22% (Dewey et al., 2003) and 31% (Chapman & Perez-Escamilla, 1999) of breastfeeding mothers. Risk factors for this delay include primiparity (Chapman & Perez-Escamilla, 1999), cesarean section (Chapman & Perez-Escamilla, 1999; Vestermark, Hogdall, Birch, Plenov, & Toftager-Larsen, 1991), stress during labor and delivery (Chen, Nommsen-Rivers, Dewey, & Lonnerdal, 1998; Dewey, 2001), maternal diabetes (Hartmann & Cregan, 2001), and high maternal body mass index (Dewey et al., 2003; Rasmussen, Hilson, & Kjolhede, 2001). Presence of these risk factors should initiate intensive provision of lactation care and services to ensure adequate infant weight gain and the preservation of breastfeeding.

Also of concern are the moderate to severe degrees of engorgement because painful breasts are concerns of new mothers (Hill, Humenick, & West, 1994). Objective methods to measure engorgement have appeared in the literature and include measurements of chest circumference changes (Newton & Newton, 1951), thermography (Menczer & Eskin, 1969), use of a pressure gauge to measure skin tension (Ferris, 1990, 1996; Geissler, 1967; Riedel, 1991), and mothers' self-ratings (Hill & Humenick, 1994; Moon & Humenick, 1989). None of these however have become clinically useful (Academy of Breastfeeding Medicine, 2009). A four-level scale to assess breast edema was developed that grades pain, enlargement, and edema from minimal to extreme on a continuum from 1 (minimal) to 4 (extreme) (Robson, 1990). Edema in the breast could be graded similar to the manner in which peripheral edema is described (1+ to 4+) when pressing a finger into edematous tissue and determining the depth of the dent or pit, its duration, and the time it takes for the tissue to rebound. Palpation is probably a more accurate means than visualization for determining what is happening in the underlying breast tissue.

Rates of engorgement between 20% and 85% have been reported in the literature, encompassing numerous definitions and usually limited to the first few days postpartum. Such reports described engorgement as peaking between days 3 and 6 and declining thereafter. However, data from two unpublished master's theses suggested that mothers actually experience more than one peak of engorgement (Csar, 1991) and that engorgement may continue for as long as 10 days or more (Riedel, 1991).

Four patterns of engorgement have been described: 1) firm, tender breasts followed by a resolution of symptoms; 2) multiple peaks of engorgement followed by resolution; 3) intense and painful engorgement lasting up to 14 days; and 4) minimal breast changes. These demonstrate that the experience of engorgement is not the same for all mothers (Humenick et al., 1994).

Predicting an individual mother's risk for and course of engorgement is difficult. In one study of women who suffered severe postpartum engorgement, 90% also reported intense breast engorgement during the luteal phase of their menstrual cycle (Alekseev, Vladimir, & Nadezhda, 2015). More intense colostrum expression in addition to infant suckling may help remove the higher-viscosity colostrum from the milk ducts, clearing the way for better transitional milk drainage. If colostrum and transitional milk cannot flow, the fluid portion of the milk may seep through ductal walls into the surrounding space, causing edema in the surrounding tissues.

Some general principles may be of help in anticipating situations that predispose to a higher risk for engorgement:

- A failure to prevent or resolve milk stasis resulting from infrequent or inadequate drainage of the breasts. The higher the cumulative number of minutes of sucking during the early days postpartum, the less pain from engorgement mothers describe (Evans, Evans, & Simmer, 1995; Moon & Humenick, 1989).
- Mothers with small breasts (other than hypoplastic and tubular). Although small breast size does not limit milk production, it can influence storage capacity and feeding patterns. Mothers with small breasts may need to engage in a greater number of breastfeedings over 24 hours than women with a larger milk-storage capacity (Daly & Hartmann, 1995). Robson (1990) described a similar observation in engorged women who wore a significantly smaller bra cup size (34%) than women who did not become engorged (12.5%).
- Previous breastfeeding experience. Second-time breastfeeding mothers experience greater levels of engorgement sooner with faster resolution than do first-time breastfeeding mothers. Breast engorgement for multiparous mothers breastfeeding for the first time was similar to primiparous breastfeeding mothers (Hill & Humenick, 1994). Robson (1990) found that mothers in a non-engorged group were more likely to have never experienced engorgement after previous births than mothers in the engorged group. McLachlan, Milne, Lumley, and Walker (1993) found that 70% of multiparous mothers experiencing engorgement in a current lactation had also experienced engorgement with previous infants.
- Mothers with high rates of milk synthesis (hyperlactation; Livingstone, 1996) or large amounts of milk. Mothers of multiples may see milk stasis magnified if infants consume less milk, if less milk is pumped, or whenever milk volume significantly exceeds milk removal.

- Limited mother–infant contact in the early days. Shiau (1997) demonstrated significantly less engorgement on day 3 in mothers who participated in skin-to-skin care of their full-term infants rather than standard nursery care.
- Maternal IV fluids during the peripartum period. Upon breast palpation, mothers in one study who had received IV fluids during labor had significantly more severe breast edema than mothers who had received no IV fluids (Kujawa-Myles, Noel-Weiss, Dunn, Peterson, & Cotterman, 2015). In addition, as many as 53% of mothers who received IV fluids had moderate to deep breast edema as late as days 8 and 9 postpartum, suggesting that this type of edema does not resolve within a day or two of birth and that expressing milk does not resolve this type of engorgement. Identifying breast edema as lactogenesis II may provide misleading information regarding the onset of copious milk production.

Numerous strategies to reduce or prevent engorgement have been seen over the years. Mothers experience less severe forms of engorgement with early frequent feedings (Newton & Newton, 1951), self-demand feedings (Illingworth & Stone, 1952), unlimited sucking times (Slaven & Harvey, 1981), thorough breast drainage (Evans et al., 1995), and with infants who demonstrate correct suckling techniques (Righard & Alade, 1992). Short, frequent feeds were shown to increase engorgement in one study (Moon & Humenick, 1989), probably because abbreviated feeds for as short as 2 minutes did not allow sufficient drainage of the breasts to prevent milk accumulation.

A more effective technique called alternate breast massage has been shown to significantly reduce the incidence and severity of engorgement while simultaneously increasing milk intake, increasing the fat content of the milk, and increasing infant weight gain (Bowles, Stutte, & Hensley, 1987; Iffrig, 1968; Stutte, Bowles, & Morman, 1988). Alternate massage is a simple technique of massaging and compressing the breast during the infant's pause between sucking bursts. The technique alternates with the infant's sucking and is continued throughout the feeding on both breasts.

Treatment Modalities for Engorgement: Fact Versus Fiction

A plethora of treatment modalities for engorgement has been put forward, both anecdotally and in lactation literature. Some of the most commonly proposed treatments follow.

Heat Therapy

Heat application in the form of hot compresses, hot showers, or hot soaks is poorly researched and has usually been more of a comfort measure to activate the milk-ejection reflex rather than a treatment for edema. Some mothers complain that heat exacerbates the engorgement and causes throbbing and an increased feeling of fullness (Robson, 1990).

Cold Therapy

Cold applications in the form of ice packs, gel packs, frozen bags of vegetables, frozen wet towels, and the like have been studied under various application conditions. Cold application triggers a cycle of vasoconstriction during the first 9–16 minutes in which blood flow is reduced, local edema decreases, and lymphatic drainage is enhanced (Hocutt, Jaffe, Rylander, & Beebe, 1982). This is followed by a deep-tissue vasodilation phase lasting 4–6 minutes that prevents thermal injury (Barnes, 1979). Robson (1990) discussed that the application of cold for 20 minutes would have a minimal vasoconstriction effect in the deeper breast tissue and that venous and lymphatic drainage would be enhanced in the deeper tissues due to the accelerated circulation to and from the superficial tissues. Sandberg (1998) reported on the application of cold packs for 20 minutes before each feeding on a small sample of women. Mothers reported increased comfort (compared with heat), decreased chest circumference, and no adverse effect on milk ejection or milk transfer. Cold therapy may not be appropriate for postpartum women in Chinese cultures as exposure to cold is typically discouraged during the month following delivery.

Ultrasound

Thermal (continuous) ultrasound treatments of engorged breasts have not been shown to have objective beneficial effects on engorgement (McLachlan et al., 1993); however, mothers have found ultrasound to be comforting (Fetherston, 1997).

Lymphatic Breast Drainage Therapy

This is a gentle massage of the lymphatic drainage channels in the breast. Lymphatic drainage is thought to improve the movement of the stagnated fluid, to reduce edema, and to improve cellular function (Chikly, 1999; Upledger Institute, n.d.). Wilson-Clay and Hoover (2002) reported the relief of discomfort and better subsequent milk yields during pumping of three women with unrelieved severe engorgement after manual lymphatic drainage therapy. No data could be found regarding the remote possibility of moving cancer cells into lymphatic circulation by massaging the breast toward the axilla.

Combination of Hand Techniques

A combination of hand techniques may be helpful in reducing engorgement (Bolman, Saju, Oganesyan, Kondrashova, & Witt, 2013). With the mother reclined, massage the areola with reverse pressure softening followed by general breast massage toward the axillae. This may help fluid drain down and away from the areola. As some of the swelling is reduced, the infant can be put to the breast or the mother can pump. Therapeutic breast massage has been shown to significantly reduce engorgement severity and its associated pain (Witt, Bolman, Kredit, & Vanic, 2016). This can be performed by the clinician or the mother as the technique provides both immediate and longer term relief.

Chilled Cabbage Leaves

Rosier (1988) anecdotally described the use of chilled cabbage leaves applied to engorged breasts and changed every 2 hours in a small sample of women as having a rapid effect on reducing edema and increasing milk flow. Nikodem, Danziger, Gebka, Gulmezoglu, and Hofmeyr (1993) showed a nonsignificant trend in reduced engorgement in mothers using cabbage leaves. Roberts (1995) compared chilled cabbage leaves and gel packs, showing similar significant reduction in pain with both methods, with two-thirds of the mothers preferring the cabbage due to a stronger, more immediate effect. Roberts, Reiter, and Schuster (1998) studied the use of cabbage extract cream applied to the breasts and found no more effect than the placebo cream.

Expressing Milk

Refraining from expressing milk because the mother will "just make more milk" cannot be justified. Hand expressing or pumping to comfort reduces the buildup of feedback inhibitor of lactation; decreases the mechanical stress on the alveoli, preventing the cell death process; prevents blood circulation changes; alleviates the impedance to lymph and fluid drainage; decreases the risk of mastitis and compromised milk production; and feels good to the mother. It is not known what degree of engorgement or duration of milk stasis poses an unrecoverable situation. The milk production in the alveoli not experiencing engorgement continues normally. The breast is capable of compensating to a point; future research will delineate this further.

Gua-Sha Therapy

Gua-sha or scraping therapy is widely used in Asia by traditional practitioners. Its purpose is to promote normal circulation by moving blood and metabolic waste that congest in surface tissues, resulting in the resolution of fluid and blood stasis. Chiu and colleagues (2010) applied short and soft scraping therapy to the engorged breasts of the intervention sample of mothers and compared this with hot compresses and massage in the control group. The Gua-sha group showed significantly higher improvements in lowered body and breast temperature, breast engorgement, and pain and discomfort scales at both 5 and 30 minutes following the intervention. This is somewhat analogous to the anecdotal recommendation of using a comb to gently stroke the engorged breast to improve circulation and reduce congestion.

Breastfeeding Management

A Cochrane review of engorgement treatments (Mangesi & Dowswell, 2010) indicated that the overall quality of the studies needs substantial improvement and that there is no one particular intervention that is the best for relieving engorgement. Unrestricted, frequent, and effective breastfeedings contribute to the occurrence of lactogenesis II by 72 hours postpartum. Physiological engorgement is part of a continuum for abundant milk production. Efforts to relieve excessive congestion in the breast should not be delayed. Anti-inflammatory medication (the enzyme serrapeptase) has been shown to relieve some of the discomfort and symptoms of engorgement (Kee, Tan, & Salmon, 1989; Snowden, Renfrew, & Woolridge, 2001).

An overfull breast with flattening of the areola may make latching difficult and painful. Mothers may need to hand express or pump milk before placing the infant at the breast. Pumping or hand expressing milk following feedings may also help relieve pressure inside the breast. An edematous areola benefits from reverse pressure softening for easier latch. Most mothers find relief from the use of cold compresses, frequent milk removal, and anti-inflammatory medication for discomfort.

PLUGGED DUCTS

Many breastfeeding women encounter tender small lumps in their breasts, usually related to the blockage of a milk duct. The lump may also have reddened skin over it and be warm to the touch. The exact cause is unknown. Clinicians have speculated that a large milk supply or pressure on the outside of the breasts, such as from purse straps, backpack straps, or an ill-fitting bra, could result in a physical obstruction of milk flow and a local collection of milk products that are too large to move down the small ductwork. Fetherston (1998) identified breastmilk that appeared thicker than normal as a predictor for blocked ducts in multiparous women. Eglash (1998) described a mother with repeatedly plugged ducts who routinely experienced a long delay in the milk-ejection reflex at each feeding. Poor milk flow may subsequently ensue from the area of the breasts experiencing the blockage, contributing to milk stasis behind the plug. This focal area of engorgement used to be referred to as a caked breast.

Focal engorgement from a blocked duct may cause a segment of the breast to become swollen, firm, and tender. Milk secretions that remain blocked from exiting the breast may become inspissated (thickened by absorption of fluid). Milk expressed from the breast experiencing plugged ducts may contain the displaced material from the plug that is often of a fatty composition. Strings that resemble spaghetti or lengths of fatty-looking material have been described (Minchin, 1985). Ductal blockage from this material may account for the sometimes ropy texture of the breast upon palpation over the obstructed area. The observation of fatty material from the blockage has led clinicians to recommend the addition of lecithin to the maternal diet (Lawrence & Lawrence, 2016). Lecithin is a phospholipid; it is used by the food industry as an emulsifier. An emulsifier keeps fat dispersed and suspended in water rather than aggregated in a fatty mass. One tablespoon per day of oral granular lecithin has been reported to relieve plugged ducts and to prevent their recurrence (Eglash, 1998; Lawrence & Lawrence, 2016).

Breastfeeding Management

Plugged ducts may also respond well to the use of a warm compress and direct massage over the lump while the infant is sucking. Studies of ultrasound treatment have shown mixed results (Campbell & Smillie, 2003; Snowden et al., 2001). Massage over and/or behind the blockage has been a traditional recommendation to reduce and disperse the material obstructing the duct. A different approach has been recommended whereby the mother massages in front of the lump toward the nipple (Smillie, 2004). The mother begins the massage close to the nipple, then repositions the massage farther back until she is massaging directly in front of the blockage (Campbell, 2006). This is thought to help clear the way through convoluted ductwork that may not be in straight alignment to the nipple. Plugged ducts require prompt attention because they can start a cascade of events that leads to breast inflammation and breast infection (Kinlay et al., 2001).

A six-step recanalization manual therapy intervention has been discussed as a massage technique for resolving plugged ducts (Zhao et al., 2014). This process involves nipple and breast manipulation to dilate the milk ducts first, followed by manipulation of the obstructing material down the widened milk ducts and out through the nipple. A successful multimodal approach to the treatment of block milk ducts includes the use of heat, ultrasound, specific manual techniques, and patient education (Cooper & Kowalsky, 2015). Twenty-nine of thirty breastfeeding mothers who were unable to clear the blocked ducts themselves with heat and massage and were referred to physical therapy showed resolution with this multimodal treatment that included ultrasound. In most mothers, the blocked ducts cleared quickly with one or two visits.

MASTITIS

Mastitis is an inflammatory condition of the breast that may eventually or concurrently involve an infection (Walker, 2004). Confusion can arise in defining mastitis because the words "mastitis" and "infection" are often used interchangeably. Mastitis the inflammation is often treated as if it were an infection. Thomsen, Espersen, and Maigaard (1984) microscopically examined milk to differentiate between milk stasis, inflammation, and infection. The diagnosis of an infection was made by observing and counting (not culturing) leukocytes and bacteria in milk samples to identify three clinical states, recommending antibiotics for the last classification only:

1. Milk stasis: $<10^6$ leukocytes and $<10^3$ bacteria/mL of milk
2. Noninfectious inflammation: $>10^6$ leukocytes and $<10^3$ bacteria/mL of milk
3. Infectious mastitis: $>10^6$ leukocytes and $>10^3$ bacteria/mL of milk

Hunt and colleagues (2012) have shown that in addition to increased sodium concentrations, mastitis is also associated with three inflammatory markers: increased somatic (immune) cells, increased concentration of IL-8, and increased free fatty acid concentrations. Alkaline phosphatase (ALP) is detectable in the lactocytes and serves as a specific indicator of disease states. In a study that measured ALP in colostrum, it was found that ALP was an early predictive marker for lactational mastitis. The mean level of colostrum ALP activity from the affected breasts was significantly higher when compared with ALP activity from the contralateral asymptomatic as well as "healthy" breasts (Bjelakovic et al., 2012). Most clinicians do not microscopically observe milk or use laboratory results, but rely on a cluster of signs and symptoms to diagnose mastitis the infection (Freed, Landers, & Schanler, 1991; Lawrence & Lawrence, 2016; Niebyl, Spence, & Parmley, 1978):

- Fever of 38.4°C (101°F)
- Flu-like aching
- Nausea
- Chills
- Pain or swelling at the site
- Red, tender, hot area, often wedge shaped
- Red streaks extending toward the axilla (inflammation of the lymphatics may indicate a more generalized infection of the breast)
- Increased pulse rate
- Increased sodium levels in the milk; seen as the infant possibly rejecting the affected side due to the salty taste of the milk

Sometimes, signs and symptoms of breast complaints such as engorgement, plugged ducts, noninfectious mastitis, and infectious mastitis overlap, with each process having some element related to obstructed milk flow, making differential diagnosis difficult (Betzold, 2007). When drainage of breastmilk is blocked, paracellular pathways open, allowing for the leakage of cytokines that can induce fever, chills, muscle aches, and general malaise. This state can provide the clinical impression of an infective process whether or not an infection is actually present. Not all fevers in breastfeeding mothers indicate a breast infection. In the absence of a cluster of the listed symptoms, the origin of the fever should be investigated (infected cesarean incision, urinary tract infection, endometritis).

The incidence of mastitis (of any definition) ranges between 1% and 33% (Inch, 1997), depending on the duration of the study. Studies that contained data up to 3 months postpartum showed the incidence of mastitis ranging from 2.9% to 24% (Evans & Heads, 1995; Hesseltine, Freundlich, & Hite, 1948;

Jonsson & Pulkkinen, 1994; Kaufmann & Foxman, 1991; Nicholson & Yuen, 1995). Riordan and Nichols (1990) reported a 33% incidence of mastitis in a retrospective study that spanned the entire lactation period of the mothers, including durations exceeding 12 months.

Breast infections are the most common breast-related complaint seen by physicians during pregnancy and the postpartum period (Scott-Conner & Schorr, 1995). The highest occurrence of mastitis is generally at 2–3 weeks postpartum (Inch, 1997), with the bulk of cases developing within the first 12 weeks of breastfeeding (Riordan & Nichols, 1990). However, mastitis can occur at any time during the course of lactation, frequently occurring during the winter months (Evans & Heads, 1995). Bilateral mastitis occurs much less frequently than unilateral infection, ranging from 3–12% of cases (Evans & Heads, 1995; Inch & Fisher, 1995; Moon & Gilbert, 1935; Riordan, 1983; Riordan & Nichols, 1990). Although most cases of mastitis involve *S. aureus* as the causative organism (Osterman & Rahm, 2000), other organisms, such *as S. epidermis* and beta-hemolytic *Streptococcus*, may also be involved. Kenny (1977) described a case of recurrent group B beta-hemolytic streptococcal infection in an infant whose mother also presented with bilateral mastitis positive for group B beta-hemolytic streptococci. Because bilateral mastitis is relatively rare, clinicians may wish to culture the milk from both breasts should this condition occur.

Human milk is not sterile (Carroll, Osman, Davies, & McNeish, 1979); the areolae, breast skin, and milk ducts are also not sterile. Bacterial counts of pathological and nonpathological bacteria have been noted to be indistinguishable between the mastitic and nonmastitic breast in women with unilateral mastitis (Matheson, Aursnes, Horgen, Aabø, & Melby, 1988). The presence of bacteria does not necessarily indicate or precipitate a breast infection. Kvist, Larsson, Hall-Lord, Steen, and Schalen (2008) demonstrated that many healthy mothers have potentially pathogenic bacteria in their breastmilk and do not go on to develop mastitis. There generally needs to be some other condition or risk factor present for developing either a breast inflammation or infection. The following are some precipitating factors:

- Nipple damage/cracked nipple.
- Infant is a nasal carrier of *S. aureus* (Amir, Garland, & Lumley, 2006).
- Plugged milk ducts.
- Milk stasis.
- Blocked nipple pore.
- Hyperlactation or a high rate of milk synthesis.
- Insulin-dependent diabetes mellitus (IDDM). Neubauer, Ferris, and Hinckley (1990) studied milk from 67 breasts of mothers with IDDM and 114 breasts of non-IDDM lactating mothers. Mastitis was categorized according to leukocyte and bacteria counts according to the parameters established by Thomsen and colleagues (1984). Although the incidence of infectious mastitis was similar, significantly more mothers with IDDM (20.9% vs. 1.8%) tested positive for noninfectious inflammation. This may serve to remind the clinician that mothers with IDDM need to breastfeed frequently with no delays in initiation of breastfeeding and usually require closer monitoring for correct breastfeeding management and techniques.
- Nipple piercing. In the months after this procedure, infection, mastitis, and abscess formation have been reported to be as high as 10–20%, with healing of the wound channel taking 6–12 months (Jacobs, Golombeck, Jonat, & Kiechle, 2003). Because some nipple piercings take

up to 18 months to heal, the potential for scar tissue development could interfere with milk transfer, cause sore nipples, or contribute to plugged ducts and mastitis. Clinicians are reminded to check pierced nipples for numbness, discharge, hypersensitivity, healing, and scar tissue (Martin, 2004). Some mothers regret the piercing and seek to reverse it. A surgical procedure that excises the epithelial tunnel core can be performed with minimal damage to the surrounding tissue (Sadove & Clayman, 2008).

- Reduced concentration of secretory IgA. Secretory IgA is a defense component within the breast and has been shown to increase in concentration during mastitis (Fetherston, Lai, & Hartmann, 2006). Low levels of secretory IgA have been found in the milk of mothers with recurrent mastitis as well as in mothers with recurrent plugged ducts (Fetherston, 2001; Fetherston et al., 2006; Lawrence & Lawrence, 2010).
- Stress. Wockel, Beggel, Rucke, Abou-Dakn, and Arck (2010) observed that higher maternal age, an increase in postpartum maternal stress perception, and a low number of leucocytes in the postpartum blood count were associated with a higher incidence of inflammatory breast conditions.

Other factors appear to be associated with mastitis rather than being causative, such as full-time employment (Kaufmann & Foxman, 1991), maternal stress or fatigue (Riordan & Nichols, 1990), poor nutrition, anemia (Dever, 1992), tight bra (Fetherston, 1998) or restrictive clothing, and use of nipple creams (Jonsson & Pulkkinen, 1994).

Subclinical Mastitis

Subclinical mastitis is usually described as an elevated milk sodium-to-potassium ratio that rises from 5–6 mmol/L of sodium in normal human milk to 12–20 mmol/L of sodium, often in association with the presence of inflammatory cytokines. Studies of subclinical mastitis in human mothers have shown that even though there may be no apparent clinical symptoms, biochemical changes occur in the milk. Increased sodium levels are also seen in colostrum, during weaning, in mastitis the infection, and in preterm mother's milk. Milk stasis may contribute to subclinical mastitis by promoting inflammation if there is a local adverse immune response to milk proteins left in contact with breast epithelium for prolonged periods of time (Michie et al., 2003). After that, changes might occur in the tight junctions between luminal epithelial cells, with a resultant leak of sodium, inflammatory cells, and other mediators into the milk.

The mammary gland has protective capabilities to modulate inflammation in the mammary alveoli (Semba, Kumwenda, Taha, Hoover, et al., 1999) and uses the natural defense mechanisms of nipple skin integrity and the flushing action of milk flow during the milk-ejection reflex. However, bacteria may be able to resist or overcome these mechanisms by adhering to damaged epithelial cells lining the ducts and nipple pores, perhaps through trauma or the conditions presented by milk stasis (Fetherston, 2001). With ultrasound imaging of the lactating breast showing a reverse flow of breastmilk within the ducts after the end of a milk-ejection reflex (Ramsay et al., 2004), backward milk flow (away from the nipple) into the smaller collecting ducts could possibly carry bacteria with it.

Subclinical mastitis has been associated with decreased milk production, slow infant weight gain (Filteau, Rice, et al., 1999; Morton, 1994), mixed feeding (breastmilk and formula; Willumsen et al., 2000), and increased cell counts. In HIV-infected mothers, this increases the risk of elevated milk viral loads, a risk factor for vertical transmission of HIV (Semba, Kumwenda, Hoover, et al., 1999; Semba, Kumwenda, Taha, Quinn, et al., 1999; Willumsen et al., 2000). There appears to be a spectrum or continuum of pathology from mild changes initiated by milk stasis, which, if left unchecked or improperly treated, progresses through subclinical mastitis, clinically evident mastitis the inflammation, mastitis the infection, and, at its worst, abscess formation (Walker, 2004).

Interventions to prevent or manage subclinical mastitis have been shown to significantly reduce the occurrence of elevated sodium-to-potassium ratios.

- Basic lactation counseling on exclusive breastfeeding for 4–6 months, correct position and latch, feeding on cue, and early breastfeeding after delivery resulted in a 14% decrease in sodium-to-potassium elevations in a group of 60 women counseled on simple lactation practices compared with a control group of 66 women who did not receive early breastfeeding counseling (Flores & Filteau, 2002). Optimal breastfeeding management would appear to be the correct approach to preventing or managing a condition that lacks easily recognizable clinical signs in the mother (Baeza, 2016a).
- Because antioxidant micronutrient status in dairy cattle has been related to mastitis, studies have examined if supplementing human mothers with antioxidants might prevent subclinical mastitis. Supplementation with retinol and beta-carotene did not reduce inflammation (Filteau, Rice, et al., 1999), but supplementation with sunflower oil, a potent source of vitamin E, reduced the incidence of mastitis among women in a study from Tanzania (Filteau, Lietz, et al., 1999).
- Although most attempts at vaccination against mastitis have met with little to no success, a vaccine based on newer technology has suggested some protection for those mothers at risk for recurrent mastitis (Shinefield et al., 2002).
- Antisecretory factor (AF) can be produced in the mammary gland and seems to have an anti-inflammatory effect by reducing fluid secretion (Hanson, 2004). AF has been found in samples of milk from mothers in developing countries, possibly because the mother herself was challenged with enterotoxin-producing bacteria (Hanson, Lonnroth, Lange, Bjersing, & Dahlgren, 2000). A preliminary study showed a significant reduction in the prevalence of mastitis in Swedish women that resulted when AF was induced in their milk through the ingestion of a specially treated cereal (Svensson, Lange, Lonnroth, Widström, & Hanson, 2004). Eventually, if AF can be shown to reliably prevent subclinical mastitis, it may be used to reduce the risk of transfer of HIV-1 from mother to infant via breastfeeding.

Recurrent Mastitis

Mastitis most frequently recurs when the bacteria are resistant or not sensitive to the prescribed antibiotic, when antibiotics are not continued long enough, when an incorrect antibiotic is prescribed, when the mother stopped nursing on the affected side, or when the initial cause of the mastitis was not addressed (such as milk stasis). *Staphylococcus epidermidis* is also a prevalent staphylococcal species isolated from breastmilk of women with mastitis, where it is present at a concentration notably higher than that present in milk of healthy women (Delgado, Arroyo, Martin, & Rodriguez, 2008). The percentage of strains showing biofilm production ability and resistance to mupirocin, erythromycin, clindamycin, and/or methicillin was significantly higher among those obtained from women with lactational mastitis than among those isolated from healthy women (Delgado et al., 2009). The resistance to many antibiotics and its propensity to form protective bio films may help explain chronic or recurrent episodes of mastitis when this organism is present. Clinicians usually recommend that the mother continues to feed (or pump) on the affected side, that she rest, that she take a full 10- to 14-day course of antibiotics, and that the cause or precipitating factors be identified and remedied. If mastitis recurs, Lawrence and Lawrence (2016) recommend milk culture and sensitivity testing as well as cultures of the infant's nasopharynx and oropharynx to determine the offending organism and to what antibiotic it is sensitive. Milk cultures should be taken if the mastitis is unresponsive to antibiotics after 2 days (Spencer, 2008) because organisms can be resistant to multiple medications (Betzold, 2005). Other family members may sometimes need to be cultured to determine the vector for transmission to keep it from reinfecting the mother. Infants who are nasal carriers of *S. aureus* should be identified and can be treated with mupirocin 2% (Bactroban nasal ointment; Amir, 2002). If the infection seems to be chronic, low-dose antibiotics can be instituted for the duration of the lactation (erythromycin 500 mg/day; Lawrence & Lawrence, 2016). If the locus of the infection occurs more than two or three times in the same location, a closer follow-up and evaluation must be done to rule out an underlying mass (Academy of Breastfeeding Medicine, 2014).

Identifying and treating the underlying cause of inflammatory signs and symptoms in the breast may halt the progression to an infection. If the mother has a low-grade fever, aching, red splotches, and a painful area in the breast, she may find relief from use of a nonsteroidal anti-inflammatory drug such as ibuprofen. Underlying causes should be explored and remedied (see **Appendix 8-1**). If there is no improvement within 8–24 hours, if the mother continues to run a fever, if the fever suddenly rises or spikes, if she develops flu-like symptoms, if she feels ill, or if she has obvious signs of a bacterial infection such as discharge of pus from the nipple, then she needs to call her care provider, who will usually prescribe a 10- to 14-day course of antibiotics.

Bacterial Pathogens

Because *S. aureus* is the most common organism associated with mastitis, penicillinase-resistant penicillins or cephalosporins are usually the initial drugs of choice. Antibiotic selection may include dicloxacillin (for non-methicillin-resistant *S. aureus*), clindamycin (for community-acquired methicillin-resistant *S. aureus* [MRSA]), erythromycin and azithromycin for penicillin-allergic mothers, trimethoprim–sulfamethoxazole for some community-acquired MRSA, and cephalexin for methicillin-susceptible *S. aureus*. Mothers should take the antibiotic for the full course prescribed even if they start feeling better within 24 hours. Improvement in the mother's condition may be due to the antibiotics but not necessarily because they are eliminating an infection. Antibiotics are effective anti-inflammatory drugs (even though they are not used for that purpose). Mothers who are treated with antibiotics when they do not have a laboratory-confirmed infection may experience improvement in their situation, but the underlying cause of the inflammatory process must be addressed because it will return if left unresolved. Repeated treatments with antibiotics of mastitis the inflammation can lead to bacterial resistance to antibiotics.

More recently, community-acquired MRSA has emerged as an increasingly common pathogen in cases of mastitis and abscesses (Reddy, Qi, Zembower, Noskin, & Bolon, 2007; Saiman et al., 2003). Clinicians caring for mothers with mastitis need to be aware of MRSA and prepared to treat it appropriately

(Schoenfeld & McKay, 2010). Delayed nipple wound healing, stress, chronic engorgement, persistent breast pain, difficulty breastfeeding in-hospital and for employed mothers (Branch-Elliman et al., 2012), and breast masses with or without fever predispose mothers to mastitis and abscesses, making them easy prey to more virulent pathogens. Increased risk for hospital-acquired MRSA is seen in mothers who had a cesarean delivery, were administered antibiotics in the peripartum period, had multiple gestation, and have experienced in vitro fertilization (Behari, Englund, Alcasid, Garcia-Houchins, & Weber, 2004; Gastelum, Dassey, Mascola, & Yasuda, 2005; Morel et al., 2002). Delay in antibiotic therapy for mastitis, incorrect antibiotic choice, inadequate courses of antibiotics, and lack of culture and sensitivity testing of milk cultures and infant nasal swabs raise the risk of complications of mastitis such as abscesses (Wilson-Clay, 2008).

Milk production in the affected breast may decrease during the few days of florid symptoms (Wambach, 2003) and for a period of days beyond that time (Matheson et al., 1988). This may be due to the infant rejecting that breast or from a drop in lactose and problems with milk synthesis from alveolar tissue damage (Fetherston, 2001). Infants can consume milk from the mastitic breast because it contains the same anti-inflammatory components and characteristics found in normal milk. Elevations occur in certain factors that protect the infant from developing clinical illness due to consuming mastitic milk (Buescher & Hair, 2001).

Breasts that have undergone augmentation can also demonstrate signs of inflammatory or infective processes, such as swelling, tenderness, or induration around the prosthesis itself (Johnson & Hanson, 1996). *S. aureus* infections tend to be more localized and invasive. *Streptococcus* infections are often more diffuse with abscess formation in advanced stages (Sabate et al., 2007).

Breastfeeding Management

General breastfeeding guidelines during mastitis involve bedrest and increased fluids for the mother. Pain medication such as ibuprofen can be used because it also acts as an anti-inflammatory in conjunction with antibiotics. If antibiotics are prescribed, they should be taken for a full 10–14 days. Shorter courses or courses that are stopped by the mother because she feels better may lead to recurrence. Some mothers find that hot compresses before feedings feel good and help elicit the milk-ejection reflex. Mothers should continue breastfeeding on both sides, starting on the affected side and using alternate massage. If pain affects the letdown, the mother can start on the unaffected side to achieve milk ejection, then switch to and thoroughly drain the affected side. If the infant is unable or unwilling to feed from the affected side, then the infected breast should be pumped.

Complementary and alternative therapies have been anecdotally recommended:

- Hot castor oil packs. Preheat a heating pad. A washcloth that has been dampened with hot water is placed on a sheet of plastic wrap. A tablespoonful of castor oil is poured on the cloth and spread around. This preparation is placed over the affected area of the breast with the heating pad over it while the mother lies down and rests for at least 20 minutes. The oil should be washed off of the nipple before the next feeding.
- Homeopathics. Phytolacca 30C every 3–4 hours; belladonna 30C every 3–4 hours; other homeopathic options include Heparsulphuris and Bellisperennis (Barbosa-Cesnik, Schwartz, & Foxman, 2003).

- Acupuncture has been suggested as a potential remedy, as has the use of oxytocin nasal spray to enhance the milk-ejection reflex, which may be less effective due to distended milk ducts (Kvist, Hall-Lord, & Larsson, 2007).
- Jimenez and colleagues (2008) treated mothers with mastitis with probiotics as an alternative. Two strains of *Lactobacillus* (*L. salivarius and L. gasseri*) were shown to improve clinical symptoms of mastitis, which disappeared by day 7. The probiotic *L. fermentum* was shown to reduce the bacterial load of *S, aureus* in the breastmilk of mothers with breast pain symptoms suggestive of subacute mastitis (Maldonado-Lobon et al., 2015). The oral administration of both *L. salivarius* and *L. fermentum* appeared to be an effective alternative to commonly prescribed antibiotics for the treatment of infectious mastitis (Arroyo et al., 2010). However, while lactobacilli are common low level residents in breastmilk, might artificially raising their levels through the administration of oral probiotics disrupt the microbiome of the mother's milk (Baeza, 2016b)?
- The topical application of curcumin to the breast has been shown to be effective in reducing the inflammation and pain associated with noninfectious mastitis within 72 hours (Afshariani, Farhadi, Ghaffarpasand, & Roozbeh, 2014). Curcuminoids are derived from the yellow-pigmented fraction of turmeric and have strong anti-inflammatory properties.

Cracked nipples are frequently reported to accompany mastitis, as either causative or coexisting (Amir, Forster, Lumley, & McLachlan, 2007; Kvist et al., 2007; Scott, Robertson, Fitzpatrick, Knight, & Mulholland, 2008), making it imperative that clinicians endeavor to provide guidance in their prevention or offer effective interventions for their timely resolution. Strong (2011) reported inadequate and non-evidence-based management of breast- and nipple-related sources of pain in a mid-South obstetric and gynecologic practice. It is extremely important that clinicians engage in best practices when breastfeeding mothers experience any type of breast or nipple pain. Infections that do not improve rapidly require further investigation for breast abscess and nonlactational causes of inflammation, including the rare cause of inflammatory breast cancer.

BREAST ABSCESS

A breast abscess can be an infrequent complication of mastitis resulting from untreated, delayed, inadequate, or incorrect treatment of mastitis. An abscess is a walled-off, localized collection of pus that lacks an outlet for the material from the affected area. Once encapsulated, it requires surgical drainage. Risk factors also include prior episodes of mastitis, avoiding breastfeeding on the affected side, or acute weaning. Estimates of the incidence of breast abscess among lactating women range from 0.04% (Waller, 1946) to 11% (Devereux, 1970). Calculation of the actual incidence is complicated by the varied definitions used for mastitis; however, in laboratory-confirmed cases of mastitis the infection, 2.8% of mothers with mastitis went on to develop an abscess (Thomsen et al., 1984). More current statistics indicate that 10–20% of women with mastitis will develop an abscess (Berens, Swaim, & Peterson, 2010).

In an Australian study of women with mastitis, 3% of women were estimated to develop an abscess (Amir, Forster, McLachlan, & Lumley, 2004). Primiparous women appear to be at a greater risk for abscess as well as mothers over the age of 30 and those who give birth after term (Kvist & Rydhstroem, 2005).

Benson and Goodman (1970) classified abscesses as subareolar (superficial and near the nipple)—23%, intramammary unilocular (a single area of pus deep in the breast and away from the nipple)—12%, and intramammary multilocular (having multiple sites of pus within the abscess)—65%. The most common offending organism is *S. aureus* (World Health Organization, 2000), although other organisms are occasionally cultured from an abscess, such as *Pseudomonas aeruginosa* (Bertrand & Rosenblood, 1991; Dixon, 1988; Karstrup et al., 1993).

Of abscesses containing *S. aureus*, over 50% can be MRSA, with trimethoprim–sulfamethoxazole (Proloprim) often being the antibiotic of choice (Berens, Swaim, & Peterson, 2010; Moazzez et al., 2007). Lawrence and Lawrence (2016) remind clinicians that any abscess drainage should be cultured and antibiotic sensitivities determined due to the increasing number of oxacillin-resistant *S. aureus* and MRSA infections occurring in hospitals. An infection with oxacillin-resistant *S. aureus* and MRSA may require the use of vancomycin, clindamycin, or rifampin therapy and may start as an inflammation of the lymphatics in the breast.

Delay in seeking treatment for a breast infection is consistently associated with poor lactation outcomes (Bertrand & Rosenblood, 1991; Devereux, 1970; Matheson et al., 1988; Thomsen et al., 1984; Walsh, 1949) and increases the risk of late-diagnosed abscesses (Martic & Vasilj, 2012). However, antibiotic treatment of mastitis does not always prevent abscess formation (Rench & Baker, 1989).

It is not always possible to confirm the existence of an abscess by clinical examination or mammography. An abscess may have overlying skin necrosis or a palpable, reddened lump close to the surface of the skin (Cusack & Brennan, 2011). Ultrasound is typically used to diagnose the presence of an abscess and to mark the site for either surgical drainage (Hayes, Michell, & Nunnerley, 1991) or needle or catheter aspiration and drainage. Surgical drainage of an abscess has been mostly replaced by needle drainage and appropriate antibiotics in abscesses less than 3 cm in diameter (Dener & Inan, 2003; Dixon, 1988; Hook & Ikeda, 1999; Karstrup et al., 1993; O'Hara, Dexter, & Fox, 1996) and catheter placement and drainage in abscesses 3 cm or larger (Ulitzsch, Nyman, & Carlson, 2004). Ultrasound-guided needle aspiration is not dependent on the size of the abscess, and repeated aspiration, if needed, can circumvent the need for surgical intervention in many mothers (Giess, Golshan, Flaherty, & Birdwell, 2014). Needle aspiration yields better cosmetic results. Moreover, needle or catheter placement has the advantage that mothers and infants are not separated because the condition is treated on an outpatient basis.

Abscess treatment and resolution should be followed closely because breast masses and inflammatory breast cancer can also masquerade as an abscess. Clinical signs that increase the likelihood that an abscess is present include fever that does not decrease within 48–72 hours of antibiotic therapy for mastitis and development of a fluctuant palpable breast mass. Mothers are more vulnerable to abscess formation during the first month of lactation and at weaning. During the early stages, the infection tends to be confined to a single segment of the breast; in the later stages of the process, however, it may extend to other segments of the breast (Kataria, Srivastava, & Dhar, 2013).

A breast abscess is a painful and highly disruptive outcome of mastitis. In addition, the stress and burden of this condition often lead to the abandonment of breastfeeding, especially if the condition requires multiple treatments or inpatient readmission and treatment with IV antibiotics (Branch-Elliman et al., 2013).

Breastfeeding Management

Breastfeeding can and should continue during and after the period of treatment (Cantile, 1988; Dixon, 1988; Karstrup et al., 1993) because it promotes drainage of the affected segment and helps resolve the infection. Weaning or inhibiting lactation may actually hinder the rapid resolution of the abscess by contributing to the production of increasingly viscid fluid that tends to promote rather than reduce breast engorgement (Benson, 1989). Breastfeeding should continue from the affected side unless the abscess is so close to the areola that the infant's mouth would cover it during feeding. If the infant will not feed from the affected side, the breast should be pumped. Changes in protein, carbohydrate, and electrolyte concentrations from an affected breast may decrease the level of lactose and cause a rise in sodium and chloride concentrations (Connor, 1979; Prosser & Hartmann, 1983), making the milk taste salty. The onset of mastitis can be rapid, with many negative emotions elicited surrounding the continuation of breastfeeding (Amir & Lumley, 2006). Mothers need close ongoing support for the resolution of mastitis and the prevention of its recurrence.

ADDITIONAL BREAST-RELATED CONDITIONS

A number of other breast- and nipple-related conditions may occur as a result of, or concurrently with, lactation.

Galactoceles and Other Breast Lumps

Most lumps or palpable lesions in the breast during pregnancy and lactation are benign, but 3% of breast cancers are diagnosed in this population. All breast masses should be evaluated, especially any that remain persistent. Galactoceles are localized collections of milk formed as a result of ductal obstruction (Stevens, Burrell, Evans, & Sibbering, 1997; Winkler, 1964). These tend to be smooth, mobile, tender masses that during and shortly after lactation are filled with milk. As time passes, the water portion of the milk is reabsorbed by the body, leaving thickened, cheesy material that can be aspirated. Several aspirations may be required because the cysts tend to refill with milk. The cysts form as a result of duct dilatation and may be surrounded by a fibrous capsule that can be associated with inflammation. Rare infections of the galactocele are possible. Surgical removal is seldom necessary.

Galactoceles can be painful but do not preclude breastfeeding. Bevin and Persok (1993) described a case study of a mother with a long-standing galactocele behind the left areola. This mother experienced multiple episodes of plugged ducts, mastitis, and ultimately an abscess, with antibiotics at one time causing temporary disappearance of the galactocele. Vuolo, Suhrland, Madan, and Oktay (2009) speculate that in lactating women, preexisting benign breast lesions may interfere with milk flow, causing milk stasis and retention contributing to the formation of a galactocele. Squeezing or compressing the galactocele can cause milk release from the nipple but does not completely evacuate the cyst. Clinicians need to be vigilant when a mother presents with breast lumps, ensuring they are benign in nature and helping the mother create a breastfeeding pattern that works for her.

A number of benign lesions in the breasts can occur during pregnancy and lactation. These include lipomas, lactating adenoma (a painless mass, usually in the upper outer quadrant composed of densely packed masses of acini or lobules), fibroadenoma or fibroid, and breast hamartoma (an overgrowth of many types of normal tissues). Lactating adenoma, fibroadenoma, and galactoceles account for greater than 80% of pregnancy- and lactation-associated breast masses. The likelihood of these breast masses being malignant in these mothers is 10%. Differentiating one from another and benign from malignant can be challenging, with fine-needle aspiration used as a quick, safe, and simple method of diagnosis. More extensive evaluations in the lactating breast by either core biopsy or excisional biopsy carry the potential side effect of the formation of a milk fistula. Fibrocystic disease or fibrocystic changes involve proliferations of the alveolar system and may have a range of signs and symptoms from mild tenderness to pain, along with thickened areas of the breasts or nodules of various sizes. Depending on the size and location of the mass, milk flow may be obstructed due to compression of adjacent milk ducts and alveoli (Geddes, 2009). This may predispose the area to inflammation or infection. Women with type 1 diabetes are also prone to benign breast lumps, referred to as diabetic mastopathy or sclerosing lymphocytic lobulitis (Kudva, O'Brien, & Oberg, 2002). Although none are contraindications to breastfeeding, clinicians can help the mother remain observant that areas around, beneath, or behind these lesions are well drained of milk. Milk production within each breast is usually not affected.

The failure of one breast to produce abundant amounts of milk, along with the infant refusing to feed from that breast, and/or the presence of a mass indicates a need for further evaluation. Unilateral failure of lactation in a symptomatic breast may be associated with a malignancy (Makanjuola, 1998). Infant rejection of only one breast (as opposed to a nursing strike on both breasts or breast preference), either sudden or with no apparent reason, has been described as a possible indicator of breast carcinoma (Goldsmith, 1974; Makanjuola, 1998; Saber, 1996). Not all infants will reject the cancerous breast (Petok, 1995), but there are usually other signs and symptoms that would prompt an immediate referral to the mother's physician:

- A breast mass that shows no improvement within 72 hours of treatment
- Unilateral lactation failure combined with either infant rejection of the breast and/or a palpable mass
- Plugged duct or an area of milk stasis that repeatedly occurs in the same location
- Symptoms of mastitis unaccompanied by a fever that do not resolve after antibiotic treatment

The last of these indicators may serve as a cautionary flag for clinicians to further explore and to rule out inflammatory breast cancer that can mimic mastitis in its early stages.

Inflammatory breast cancer may initially present with pain, tenderness, firmness, and an increase in breast size. This is followed in a few weeks by the skin becoming warm, pink or red in color, raised, heavy, hard, and edematous. The edema is sometimes described as a roughening or thickening of the skin with little pits (peau d'orange). The skin thickening is caused by direct tumor invasion along the subdermal lymphatics, resulting in a cutaneous lymphedema. The nipple may become flattened, red, and crusted over time. Mammography is generally supportive of a diagnosis, but fine-needle aspiration and cytology are needed to confirm the presence or absence of malignant cells (Dahlbeck, Donnelly, & Theriault, 1995).

Nipple Discharge

Both human milk and other types of nipple secretions and discharges are seen in a rainbow of colors. Colostrum may be light yellow to bright orange. Mother's milk may have a bluish tint when first expressed and when stored will have a thick white or yellow layer of cream on the top. Layered milk may take on colors from food that the mother consumes, such as a green layer of milk from the consumption of green vegetables. The most common cause of nipple discharge is a benign papilloma followed by duct ectasia (Hussain, Policarpio, & Vincent, 2006). Other common nipple discharges include the following:

- Green, yellow, brown, reddish brown, or gray discharges may be associated with manipulation of the nipple at the end of a pregnancy or in early lactation (O'Callaghan, 1981).
- Purulent (pus) discharge may be seen with mastitis or an abscess.
- Duct ectasia may produce a sticky discharge of various colors. Dilatation of the terminal ducts during pregnancy may start a process of the formation of an irritating lipid resulting in an inflammatory response and the resulting nipple discharge. Most often, the discharge is dark green or black, appearing to be blood but actually testing guaiac negative (Falkenberry, 2002). The discharge is more commonly multiductal, bilateral, and colored. Smoking may be associated with duct ectasia (Rahal, deFreitas-Junior, & Paulinelli, 2005). The nipple and areola may also be painful, burn, itch, and swell. Clinicians should be watchful for plugging of the nipple pores and the development of a mass in the breast.
- Approximately 15% of asymptomatic lactating mothers have blood in their early milk when cytologically tested (Lafreniere, 1990). Delicate capillary networks that are traumatized during the rapid cellular proliferation that takes place during pregnancy may result in early milk that is blood tinged (Kline & Lash, 1962). Bloody, brown (Cizmeci, Kanburoglu, Akelma, & Tatli, 2013), or serosanguinous nipple discharge may be seen in some women at the onset of lactation (or sometimes during pregnancy) as painless, spontaneous, and self-limiting. Popularly termed "rusty pipe syndrome," this discoloration generally clears up within the first week postpartum (Virdi, Goraya, & Khadwal, 2001). It may be unilateral or bilateral, may begin in one breast first, and can frighten mothers when present. This syndrome may be recognized when the mother expresses milk or the infant vomits blood that tests positive for adult hemoglobin (Thota, Machiraju, & Jampana, 2013). No treatment is necessary, and breastfeeding should continue without interruption. Further evaluation is recommended if the discharge persists for more than 7–10 days (Silva, Carvalho, Maia, Osorio, & Barbosa, 2014).

Intraductal papilloma is a common cause of blood in the milk. This is a tiny growth from the lining of the duct that protrudes into the lumen or duct channel and can bleed when disrupted by breastfeeding or breast pumping. Most women are not aware of these growths unless they see blood in their pumped milk or if their infant vomits blood-tinged milk. The bleeding usually stops spontaneously. If an infant vomits blood-tinged milk, clinicians need to determine the source of the blood. Testing for fetal or adult hemoglobin determines the origin of the blood. If the infant tolerates the milk, he or she can continue breastfeeding from the affected side. If the infant cannot tolerate the blood because it acts as an emetic, the mother can pump her breast until the milk is clear of blood, usually from 3 to 7 days. Parents also need to know that they may see black flecks in the infant's stool, or the stool may at times be black or tarry as the blood passes through the infant's intestines. Bloody nipple discharge that persists must be evaluated by the mother's physician.

ADDITIONAL REASONS FOR BREAST PAIN (MASTALGIA)

Breast discomfort or pain is one of the most common reasons that women seek urgent breast care (Givens & Luszczak, 2002). Clinicians may wish to explore these other sources of pain when breastfeeding mothers describe deep or shooting pains in their breasts:

- A source external to the breast such as costochondritis may cause breast pain. This inflammation of the joints where the ribs attach to the sternum is treated with a nonsteroidal anti-inflammatory agent.
- Breast discomfort may be felt with capsular contracture or if an implant ruptures. Along with pain, the clinician may observe breast deformity or skin changes (Brown, Todd, Cope, & Sachs, 2006).
- Postfeed breast pain or interfeeding deep breast pain has been reported and ascribed to pulling or tugging on the nipple by the infant (Ellis, 1993) and "internal injury" to the nipple during feeding (Hopkinson, 1992). Deep breast pain may relate to the relative diameter of the milk ducts. Peters, Diemer, Meeks, and Behnken (2003) described the positive relationship between breast pain and the width of milk ducts. The wider the milk ducts, the more severe the pain, with women correlating the site of the duct dilatation as seen on ultrasound with the site of the pain. Duct dilatation in these nonlactating women with noncyclical pain was similar to the duct dilatation seen in lactating women (Ramsay et al., 2004) following the milk-ejection reflex. Extra-wide ducts may provide a partial explanation of why some breastfeeding mothers describe such intense pain with milk letdown and increasing breast discomfort between feedings.
- Thoracic muscle constriction (i.e., upper thoracic muscle tension) has been described as a contributing factor to breast pain of unknown etiology (Kernerman & Park, 2014). The pectoralis muscles may experience tension from poor posture, underdevelopment, or repetitive positioning that is felt as mastalgia. Kernerman and Park (2014) suggest pectoral muscle stretching and massage as both prevention and treatment.

SUMMARY: THE DESIGN IN NATURE

Nature provides an almost infinite variety of breasts and infants, each with their unique shape, size, and set of concerns and problems. Almost any breast and infant can be paired up to produce and receive human milk. However, it is the clinician's knowledge, skills, and empathy that facilitate optimal outcomes—whether the infant feeds directly from the breast or receives his or her mother's milk in another manner. Many breastfeeding problems can be chronic and discouraging to new mothers; clinicians should remember that the best therapeutic tool they can offer is themselves.

REFERENCES

Academy of Breastfeeding Medicine. (2009). ABM clinical protocol #20: Engorgement. *Breastfeeding Medicine, 4,* 111–113.

Academy of Breastfeeding Medicine. (2014). ABM clinical protocol # 4: Mastitis, Revised March 2014. *Breastfeeding Medicine, 9,* 239–243.

Afshariani, R., Farhadi, P., Ghaffarpasand, F., & Roozbeh, J. (2014). Effectiveness of topical cucumin for treatment of mastitis in breastfeeding women: A randomized double-blind, placebo-controlled trial. *Oman Medical Journal, 29,* 330–334.

Akbari, S. A. A., Alamolhoda, S. H., Baghban, A. A., & Mirabi, P. (2014). Effects of menthol essence and breast milk on the improvement of nipple fissures in breastfeeding women. *Journal of Research in Medical Sciences, 19,* 629–633.

Akkuzu, G., & Taskin, L. (2000). Impacts of breast-care techniques on prevention of possible postpartum nipple problems. *Professional Care of Mother and Child, 10,* 38–41.

Al-Qattan, M. M., & Robertson, G. A. (1990). Bilateral chronic infection of the lactosebaceous glands of Montgomery. *Annals of Plastic Surgery, 25,* 491–493.

Alekseev, N. P., Vladimir, I. I., & Nadezhda, T. E. (2015). Pathological postpartum breast engorgement: Prediction, prevention, and resolution. *Breastfeeding Medicine, 10,* 203–208.

Alexander, J. M. (1991). *The prevalence and management of inverted and non-protractile nipples in antenatal women who intend to breastfeed* (Unpublished doctoral dissertation). University of Southampton, Southampton, UK.

Alexander, J. M., Grant, A. M., & Campbell, M. J. (1992). Randomised controlled trial of breast shells and Hoffman's exercises for inverted and non-protractile nipples. *BMJ, 304,* 1030–1032.

American Academy of Pediatrics. (2001). The transfer of drugs and other chemicals into human milk. *Pediatrics, 108,* 776–789.

Amir, L. (1993). Eczema of the nipple and breast: A case report. *Journal of Human Lactation, 9,* 173–175.

Amir, L. (2002). Breastfeeding and *Staphylococcus aureus*: Three case reports. *Breastfeeding Review, 10,* 15–18.

Amir, L. (2004). Nipple pain in breastfeeding. *Australian Family Physician, 33,* 44–45.

Amir, L., & Hoover, K. (2003). *Candidiasis and breastfeeding.* Lactation Consultant Series 2. Schaumburg, IL: La Leche League International.

Amir, L. H. (1991). *Candida* and the lactating breast: Predisposing factors. *Journal of Human Lactation, 7,* 177–181.

Amir, L. H. (2003). Breast pain in lactating women: Mastitis or something else? *Australian Family Physician, 32,* 392–397.

Amir, L. H., Dennerstein, L., Garland, S. M., Fisher, J., & Farish, S. J. (1997). Psychological aspects of nipple pain in lactating women. *Breastfeeding Review, 5,* 29–32.

Amir, L. H., Donath, S. M., Garland, S. M., Tabrizi, S. N., Bennett, C. M., Cullinane, M., & Payne, M. S. (2013). Does *Candida* and/or *Staphylococcus* play a role in nipple and breast pain in lactation? A cohort study in Melbourne, Australia. *BMJ Open, 3,* e002351.

Amir, L. H., Forster, D., McLachlan, H., & Lumley, J. (2004). Incidence of breast abscess in lactating women: Report from an Australian cohort. BJOG: An *International Journal of Obstetrics and Gynaecology, 111,* 1378–1381.

Amir, L. H., Forster, D. A., Lumley, J., & McLachlan, H. (2007). A descriptive study of mastitis in Australian breastfeeding women: Incidence and determinants. *BMC Public Health, 7,* 62.

Amir, L. H., Garland, S., Dennerstein, L., & Farish, S. (1996). *Candida albicans*: Is it associated with nipple pain in lactating women? *Gynecologic and Obstetric Investigation, 41,* 30–34.

Amir, L. H., Garland, S. M., & Lumley, J. (2006). A case-control study of mastitis: Nasal carriage of *Staphylococcus aureus. BMC Family Practice, 7,* 57.

Amir, L. H., Jones, L. E., & Buck, M. L. (2015). Nipple pain associated with breastfeeding: Incorporating current neurophysiology into clinical reasoning. *Australian Family Physician, 44,* 127–132.

Amir, L. H., & Lumley, J. (2006). Women's experience of lactational mastitis. *Australian Family Physician, 35,* 745–747.

Amir, L. H., & Pakula, S. (1991). Nipple pain, mastalgia and candidiasis in the lactating breast. *Australian and New Zealand Journal of Obstetrics and Gynaecology, 31,* 378–380.

Anderson, J. E., Held, N., & Wright, K. (2004). Raynaud's phenomenon of the nipple: A treatable cause of painful breastfeeding. *Pediatrics, 113,* e360–e364.

Andersson, Y., Lindquist, S., Lagerqvust, C., & Hernell, O. (2000). Lactoferrin is responsible for fungistatic effect of human milk. *Early Human Development, 59,* 95–105.

Andrews, J. I., Fleener, D. K., Messer, S. A., Hansen, W. F., Pfaller, M. A., & Diekema, D. J. (2007). The yeast connection: Is *Candida* linked to breastfeeding associated pain? *American Journal of Obstetrics and Gynecology, 197,* 424.e1–424.e4.

Applebaum, R. M. (1969). *Abreast of the times.* Miami: RM Applebaum.

Arroyo, R., Martin, V., Maldonado, A., Jimenez, E., Fernandez, L., & Rodriguez, J. M. (2010). Treatment of infectious mastitis during lactation: Antibiotics versus oral administration of lactobacilli isolated from breast milk. *Clinical Infectious Diseases, 50,* 1551–1558.

Baeza, C. (2016a). Acute, subclinical, and subacute mastitis: Definitions, etiology, and clinical management. *Clinical Lactation, 7,* 7–10.

Baeza, C. (2016b). Chronic mastitis, mastalgia, and breast pain: A narrative review of definitions, bacteriological findings, and clinical management. *Clinical Lactation, 7,* 11–17.

Barankin, B., & Gross, M. S. (2004). Nipple and areolar eczema in the breastfeeding woman. *Journal of Cutaneous Medicine and Surgery, 8,* 126–130.

Barbosa-Cesnik, C., Schwartz, K., & Foxman, B. (2003). Lactation mastitis. *Journal of the American Medical Association, 289,* 1609–1612.

Barnes, L. (1979). Cryotherapy: Putting injury on ice. *The Physician and Sports Medicine, 7,* 130–136.

Barrett, M. E., Heller, M. M., Fullerton-Stone, H., & Murase, J. E. (2013a). Raynaud phenomenon of the nipple in breastfeeding mothers: An underdiagnosed cause of nipple pain. *JAMA Dermatology, 149,* 300–306.

Barrett, M. E., Heller, M. M., Stone, H. F., & Murase, J. E. (2013b). Dermatoses of the breast in lactation. *Dermatologic Therapy, 26,* 331–336.

Behari, P., Englund, J., Alcasid, G., Garcia-Houchins, S., & Weber, S. (2004). Transmission of methicillin-resistant *Staphylococcus aureus* to preterm infants through breast milk. *Infection Control and Hospital Epidemiology, 25,* 778–780.

Benson, E. A. (1989). Management of breast abscesses. *World Journal of Surgery, 13,* 753–756.

Benson, E. A., & Goodman, M. A. (1970). Incision with primary suture in the treatment of acute puerperal breast abscess. *British Journal of Surgery, 57,* 55–58.

Berens, P., Swaim, L., & Peterson, B. (2010). Incidence of methicillin-resistant *Staphylococcus aureus* in postpartum breast abscesses. *Breastfeeding Medicine, 5,* 113–115.

Bertrand, H., & Rosenblood, L. K. (1991). Stripping out pus in lactational mastitis: A means of preventing breast abscess. *Canadian Medical Association Journal, 145,* 299–306.

Betzold, C. M. (2005). Infections of the mammary ducts in the breastfeeding mother. *Journal for Nurse Practitioners, 1,* 15–21.

Betzold, C. M. (2007). An update on the recognition and management of lactational breast inflammation. *Journal of Midwifery and Women's Health, 52,* 595–605.

Betzold, C. M. (2012). Results of microbial testing exploring the etiology of deep breast pain during lactation: A systematic review and meta-analysis of nonrandomized trials. *Journal of Midwifery and Women's Health, 57,* 353–364.

Bevin, T. H., & Persok, C. K. (1993). Breastfeeding difficulties and a breast abscess associated with a galactocele: A case report. *Journal of Human Lactation, 9,* 177–178.

Bjelakovic, L., Kocic, G., Bjelakovic, B., Zivkovic, N., Stojanovic, D., Sokolovic, D., . . . Sokolovic, D. (2012). Alkaline phosphatase activity in human colostrum as a valuable predictive biomarker for lactational mastitis in nursing mothers. *Biomarkers in Medicine, 6,* 553–558.

Blair, A., Cadwell, K., Turner-Maffei, C., & Brimdyr, K. (2003). The relationship between positioning, the breastfeeding dynamic, the latching process and pain in breastfeeding mothers with sore nipples. *Breastfeeding Review, 11,* 5–10.

Bland, K. I., & Romnell, L. J. (1991). Congenital and acquired disturbances of breast development and growth. In K. I. Bland & E. M. Copeland III (Eds.), *The breast: Comprehensive management of benign and malignant diseases.* Philadelphia, PA: Saunders.

Blumenthal, M., Goldberg, A., & Brinckmann, J. (2000). *Herbal medicine: Expanded Commission E monographs* (pp. 297–303). Newton, MA: Integrative Medicine Communications.

Bodley, V., & Powers, D. (1997). Long-term treatment of a breastfeeding mother with fluconazole-resolved nipple pain caused by yeast: A case study. *Journal of Human Lactation, 13,* 307–311.

Bolman, M., Saju, L., Oganesyan, K., Kondrashova, T., & Witt, A. M. (2013). Recapturing the art of therapeutic breast massage during breastfeeding. *Journal of Human Lactation, 29,* 328–331.

Bouchet-Horwitz, J. (2011). The use of supple cups for flat, retracting, and inverted nipples. *Clinical Lactation, 2,* 30–33.

Bowles, B. C., Stutte, P. C., & Hensley, J. (1987). Alternate breast massage: New benefits from an old technique. *Genesis, 9,* 5–9.

Bracket, V. H. (1988). Eczema of the nipple/areola area. *Journal of Human Lactation, 4,* 167–169.

Branch-Elliman, W., Golen, T. H., Gold, H. S., Yassa, D. S., Baldini, L. M., & Wright, S. B. (2012). Risk factors for *Staphylococcus aureus* postpartum breast abscess. *Clinical Infectious Diseases, 54,* 71–77.

Branch-Elliman, W., Lee, G. M., Golen, T. H., Gold, H. S., Baldini, L. M., & Wright, S. B. (2013). Health and economic burden of post-partum *Staphylococcus aureus* breast abscess. *PLoS One, 8*(9), e73155.

Brent, N., Rudy, S. J., Redd, B., Rudy, T. E., & Roth, L. A. (1998). Sore nipples in breastfeeding women: A clinical trial of wound dressings vs conventional care. *Archives of Pediatrics and Adolescent Medicine, 152,* 1077–1082.

Brent, N. B. (2001). Thrush in the breastfeeding dyad: Results of a survey on diagnosis and treatment. *Clinical Pediatrics, 40,* 503–506.

Briggs, J. (2003). The management of nipple pain and/or trauma associated with breastfeeding. *Best Practice, 7*(3), 1–6.

Brook, I., & Gober, A. E. (1997). Bacterial colonization of pacifiers of infants with acute otitis media. *Journal of Laryngology and Otology, 111,* 614–615.

Brown, S. L., Todd, J. F., Cope, J. U., & Sachs, H. C. (2006). Breast implant surveillance reports to the US Food and Drug Administration: Maternal–child health problems. *Journal of Long Term Effects of Medical Implants, 16,* 281–290.

Buchko, B. L., Pugh, L. C., Bishop, B. A., Cochran, J. F., Smith, L. R., & Lerew, D. J. (1994). Comfort measures in breastfeeding, primiparous women. *Journal of Obstetric, Gynecologic, and Neonatal Nursing, 23,* 46–52.

Buck, M. L., Amir, L. H., Cullinane, M., & Donath, S. M., for the CASTLE Study Team. (2014). Nipple pain, damage, and vasospasm in the first 8 weeks postpartum. *Breastfeeding Medicine, 9,* 56–62.

Buescher, E. S., & Hair, P. S. (2001). Human milk anti-inflammatory components during acute mastitis. *Cell Immunology, 210,* 87–95.

Cable, B., Stewart, M., & Davis, J. (1997). Nipple wound care: A new approach to an old problem. *Journal of Human Lactation, 13,* 313–318.

Cadwell, K. (1981, July–August). Improving nipple graspability for success at breastfeeding. *Journal of Obstetric, Gynecologic, and Neonatal Nursing, 10,* 277–279.

Cadwell, K. (2001). Preliminary results: A comparison of treatment for sore nipples in nursing mothers: The use of Soothies glycerine gel therapy and the use of breast shells with Lansinoh lanolin cream. Retrieved from http://www.puronyx.com/html/soothies/latvia.html

Cadwell, K., Turner-Maffei, C., Blair, A., Brimdyr, K., & McInerney, Z. (2004). Pain reduction and treatment of sore nipples in nursing mothers. *Journal of Perinatal Medicine, 13,* 29–35.

Campbell, S. H. (2006). Recurrent plugged ducts. *Journal of Human Lactation, 22,* 340–343.

Campbell, S. H., & Smillie, C. M. (2003, August). *Recurrent plugged ducts: The effect of traditional therapy versus ultrasound therapy.* Proceedings of the Conference and Annual Meeting of the International Lactation Consultant Association, Sydney, Australia.

Cantile, H. B. (1988). Treatment of acute puerperal mastitis and breast abscess. *Canadian Family Physician, 34,* 2221–2227.

Carmichael, A. R., & Dixon, J. M. (2002). Is lactation mastitis and shooting breast pain experienced by women during lactation caused by *Candida albicans*? *Breast, 11,* 88–90.

Carroll, L., Osman, M., Davies, D. P., & McNeish, A. S. (1979). Bacteriologic criteria for feeding raw breast milk to babies on neonatal units. *Lancet, 2*(8145), 732–733.

Chanprapaph, P., Luttarapakul, J., Siribariruck, S., & Boonyawanichkul, S. (2013). Outcome of non-protractile nipple correction with breast cups in pregnant women: A randomized controlled trial. *Breastfeeding Medicine, 8,* 408–412.

Chapman, D. J., & Perez-Escamilla, R. (1999). Identification of risk factors for delayed onset of lactation. *Journal of the American Dietetic Association, 99,* 450–454.

Chaves, M. E., Araujo, A. R., Santos, S. F., Pinotti, M., & Oliveira, L. S. (2012). LED phototherapy improves healing of nipple trauma: A pilot study. *Photomedicine and Laser Surgery, 30,* 172–178.

Chen, D. C., Nommsen-Rivers, L., Dewey, K. G., & Lonnerdal, B. (1998). Stress during labor and delivery and early lactation performance. *American Journal of Clinical Nutrition, 68,* 335–344.

Chetwynd, E. M., Ives, T. J., Payne, P. M., & Edens-Bartholomew, N. (2002). Fluconazole for postpartum candidal mastitis and infant thrush. *Journal of Human Lactation, 18,* 168–171.

Chikly, B. (1999, August 2). *Lymph drainage therapy: Treatment for engorgement.* Presented at International Lactation Consultant Association Conference, Scottsdale, AZ.

Chiu, J.-Y., Gau, M.-L., Kuo, S.-Y., Chang, Y.-H., Kuo, S.-C., & Tu, H.-C. (2010). Effects of Gua-sha therapy on breast engorgement: A randomized controlled trial. *Journal of Nursing Research, 18,* 1–9.

Cizmeci, M. N., Kanburoglu, M. K., Akelma, A. Z., & Tatli, M. M. (2013). Rusty-pipe syndrome: A rare cause of change in the color of breastmilk. *Breastfeeding Medicine, 8,* 340–341.

Coates, M.-M. (1992). Nipple pain related to vasospasm in the nipple? *Journal of Human Lactation, 8,* 153.

Coca, K. P., & Abrao, A. C. F. V. (2008). An evaluation of the effect of lanolin in healing nipple injuries. *Acta Paulista de Enfermagen, 21,* 11–16.

Colson, S. D., Meek, J. H., & Hawdon, J. M. (2008). Optimal positions for the release of primitive neonatal reflexes stimulating breastfeeding. *Early Human Development, 84,* 441–449.

Connor, A. E. (1979). Elevated levels of sodium and chloride in milk from mastitic breasts. *Pediatrics, 63,* 910–911.

Cooper, B. B., & Kowalsky, D. (2015). Physical therapy intervention for treatment of blocked milk ducts in lactating women. *Journal of Women's Health Physical Therapy, 39,* 115–126.

Cooper, W. O., Atherton, H. D., Kahana, M., & Kotagal, U. R. (1995). Increased incidence of severe breastfeeding malnutrition and hypernatremia in a metropolitan area. *Pediatrics, 96,* 957–960.

Cordero, M. J., Villar N. M., Barrilao, R. G., Cortes, M. E., & Lopez, A. M. (2015). Application of extra virgin olive oil to prevent nipple cracking in lactating women. *Worldviews on Evidence Based Nursing, 12,* 364–369.

Cotch, M. F., Hillier, S. L., Gibbs, R. S., & Eschenbach, D. A. (1998). Epidemiology and outcomes associated with moderate to heavy *Candida* colonization during pregnancy. *American Journal of Obstetrics and Gynecology, 178,* 374–380.

Cotterman, K. J. (2003, April/May). Too swollen to latch on? Try reverse pressure softening first. *Leaven,* 38–40.

Cotterman, K. J. (2004). Reverse pressure softening: A simple tool to prepare areola for easier latching during engorgement. *Journal of Human Lactation, 20,* 227–237.

Csar, N. (1991). *Breast engorgement: What is the incidence and pattern?* (Unpublished master's thesis). University of Illinois, Chicago, IL.

Cusack, L., & Brennan, M. (2011). Lactational mastitis and breast abscess. *Australian Family Physician, 40,* 976–979.

Dahlbeck, S. W., Donnelly, J. F., & Theriault, R. L. (1995). Differentiating inflammatory breast cancer from acute mastitis. *American Family Physician, 52,* 929–934.

Daly, S. E. J., & Hartmann, P. E. (1995). Infant demand and milk supply. Part 2: The short-term control of milk synthesis in lactating women. *Journal of Human Lactation, 11,* 27–37.

Darwazeh, A. M., & al-Bashir, A. (1995). Oral candidal flora in healthy infants. *Journal of Oral Pathology and Medicine, 24,* 361–364.

Dawson, E. K. (1935). Histological study of normal mamma in relation to tumour growth: Mature gland in lactation and pregnancy. *Edinburgh Medical Journal, 42,* 569.

Dekio, S., Kawasaki, Y., & Jidoi, J. (1986). Herpes simplex on nipples inoculated from herpes gingivostomatitis of a baby. *Clinical and Experimental Dermatology, 11,* 664–666.

Delgado, S., Arroyo, R., Jimenez, E., Marín, M. L., del Campo, R., Fernández, L., & Rodríguez, J. M. (2009). *Staphylococcus epidermidis* strains isolated from breast milk of women suffering infectious mastitis: Potential virulence traits and resistance to antibiotics. *BMC Microbiology, 9,* 82.

Delgado, S., Arroyo, R., Martin, R., & Rodriguez, J. M. (2008). PCR-DGGE assessment of the bacterial diversity of breast milk in women with lactational infectious mastitis. *BMC Infectious Diseases, 8,* 51.

Dener, C., & Inan, A. (2003). Breast abscesses in lactating women. *World Journal of Surgery, 27,* 130–133.

Dennis, C.-L., Schottle, N., Hodnett, E., & McQueen, K. (2012). An all-purpose nipple ointment versus lanolin in treating painful damaged nipples in breastfeeding women: A randomized controlled trial. *Breastfeeding Medicine, 7*(6), 473–479.

Dever, J. (1992). Mastitis: Positive interventions. *Midwifery Today, 22,* 22–25.

Devereux, W. P. (1970). Acute puerperal mastitis: Evaluation of its management. *American Journal of Obstetrics and Gynecology, 108,* 78–81.

Dewey, K. (2001). Maternal and fetal stress are associated with impaired lactogenesis in humans. *Journal of Nutrition, 131,* 3012S–3015S.

Dewey, K. G., Nommsen-Rivers, L. A., Heinig, M. J., & Cohen, R. J. (2003). Risk factors for suboptimal infant breastfeeding behavior, delayed onset of lactation, and excess neonatal weight loss. *Pediatrics, 112,* 607–619.

Dinsmoor, M. J., Viloria, R., Lief, L., & Elder, S. (2005). Use of intrapartum antibiotics and the incidence of postnatal maternal and neonatal yeast infections. *Obstetrics and Gynecology, 106,* 19–22.

Dixon, J. M. (1988). Repeated aspiration of breast abscesses in lactating women. *BMJ, 297,* 1517–1518.

dos Santos, R. de C., & Marin, J. M. (2005). Isolation of Candida spp. from mastitic bovine milk in Brazil. *Mycopathologia, 159,* 251–253.

Dodd, V., & Chalmers, C. (2003). Comparing the use of hydrogel dressings to lanolin ointment with lactating mothers. *Journal of Obstetric, Gynecologic, and Neonatal Nursing, 32,* 486–494.

Dollberg, S., Botzer, E., Grunis, E., & Mimouni, F. B. (2006). Immediate nipple pain relief after frenotomy in breastfed infants with ankyloglossia: A randomized, prospective study. *Journal of Pediatric Surgery, 41,* 1598–1600.

Drewett, R., Kahn, H., Parkhurst, S., & Whiteley, S. (1987). Pain during breastfeeding: The first three months. *Journal of Reproductive and Infant Psychology, 5,* 183–186.

Eglash, A. (1998). Delayed milk ejection reflex and plugged ducts: Lecithin therapy. *ABM News and Views, 1,* 4.

Eglash, A., Plane, M. B., & Mundt, M. (2006). History, physical and laboratory findings, and clinical outcomes of lactating women treated with antibiotics for chronic breast and/or nipple pain. *Journal of Human Lactation, 22,* 429–433.

Eglash, A., & Proctor, R. (2007). Case report: A breastfeeding mother with chronic breast pain. *Breastfeeding Medicine, 2,* 99–104.

Ehrenkranz, R., Ackerman, B., & Hulse, J. (1989). Nifedipine transfer into human milk. *Journal of Pediatrics, 114,* 478–480.

Ellepola, A. N., Panagoda, G. J., & Samaranayake, L. P. (1999). Adhesion of oral *Candida* species to human buccal epithelial cells following brief exposure to nystatin. *Oral Microbiology and Immunology, 14,* 358–363.

Ellis, D. (1993). Post-feed breast pain: A case report. *Journal of Human Lactation, 9,* 182.

Evans, K., Evans, R., & Simmer, K. (1995). Effect of the method of breastfeeding on breast engorgement, mastitis, and infantile colic. *Acta Paediatrica, 84,* 849–852.

Evans, M., & Heads, J. (1995). Mastitis: Incidence, prevalence and cost. *Breastfeeding Review, 3,* 65–72.

Falkenberry, S. S. (2002). Nipple discharge. *Obstetrics and Gynecology Clinics of North America, 29,* 21–29.

Ferris, C. D. (1990). Instrumentation system for breast engorgement evaluation. *Biomedical Instrumentation and Technology, 90,* 227–229.

Ferris, C. D. (1996). Hand-held instrument for evaluation of breast engorgement. *Biomedical Instrumentation and Technology, 96,* 299–304.

Fetherston, C. (1997). Management of lactation mastitis in a Western Australian cohort. *Breastfeeding Review, 5,* 13–19.

Fetherston, C. (1998). Risk factors for lactation mastitis. *Journal of Human Lactation, 14,* 101–109.

Fetherston, C. (2001). Mastitis in lactating women: Physiology or pathology. *Breastfeeding Review, 9,* 5–12.

Fetherston, C., Lai, C., & Hartmann, P. (2006). Relationships between symptoms and changes in breast physiology during lactation mastitis. *Breastfeeding Medicine, 1,* 136–145.

Fildes, V. (1986*). Breasts, bottles, and babies: A history of infant feeding.* Edinburgh, UK: Edinburgh University Press.

Filteau, S. M., Lietz, G., Mulokozi, G., Mulokozi, G., Bilotta, S., Henry, C. J., & Tomkins, A. M. (1999). Milk cytokines and subclinical breast inflammation in Tanzanian women: Effects of dietary red palm oil or sunflower oil supplementation. *Immunology, 97,* 595–600.

Filteau, S. M., Rice, A. L., Ball, J. J., Chakraborty, J., Stoltzfus, R., de Francisco, A., & Willumsen, J. F. (1999). Breast milk immune factors in Bangladeshi women supplemented postpartum with retinol or beta-carotene. *American Journal of Clinical Nutrition, 69,* 953–958.

Flores, M., & Filteau, S. (2002). Effect of lactation counseling on subclinical mastitis among Bangladeshi women. *Annals of Tropical Paediatrics, 22,* 85–88.

Freed, G. L., Landers, S., & Schanler, R. J. (1991). A practical guide to successful breastfeeding management. *American Journal of Diseases of Children, 145,* 917–921.

Gangal, H. T., & Gangal, M. H. (1978). Suction method for correcting flat nipples or inverted nipples. *Plastic and Reconstructive Surgery, 61,* 294–296.

Gastelum, D. T., Dassey, D., Mascola, L., & Yasuda, L. M. (2005). Transmission of community-associated methicillin-resistant *Staphylococcus aureus* from breast milk in the neonatal intensive care unit. *Pediatric Infectious Disease Journal, 24,* 1122–1124.

Geddes, D. T. (2009). Ultrasound imaging of the lactating breast: Methodology and application. *International Breastfeeding Journal, 4,* 4.

Geddes, D. T., Langton, D. B., Gollow, I., Jacobs, L. A., Hartmann, P. E., & Simmer, K. (2008). Frenulotomy for breastfeeding infants with ankyloglossia: Effect on milk removal and sucking mechanism as imaged by ultrasound. *Pediatrics, 122,* e188–e194.

Geissler, N. (1967). An instrument used to measure breast engorgement. *Nursing Research, 16,* 130–136.

Giess, C. S., Golshan, M., Flaherty, K., & Birdwell, R. L. (2014). Clinical experience with aspiration of breast abscesses based on size and etiology at an academic medical center. *Journal of Clinical Ultrasound, 42,* 513–521.

Givens, M. L., & Luszczak, M. (2002). Breast disorders: A review for emergency physicians. *Journal of Emergency Medicine, 22,* 59–65.

Glover, R. (1998). The engorgement enigma. *Breastfeeding Review, 6,* 31–34.

Goldsmith, H. S. (1974). Milk rejection sign of breast cancer. *American Journal of Surgery, 1*(27), 280–281.

Graves, S., Wright, W., Harman, R., & Bailey, S. (2003). Painful nipples in nursing mothers: Fungal or staphylococcal? *Australian Family Physician, 32,* 570–571.

Grimes, D. A., & Schulz, K. F. (2002). Uses and abuses of screening tests. *Lancet, 359,* 881–884.

Gungor, A. N. C., Oguz, S., Vurur, G., Gencer, M., Uysal, A., Hacivelioglu, S., . . . Cosar, E. (2013). Comparison of olive oil and lanolin in the prevention of sore nipples in nursing mothers. *Breastfeeding Medicine, 8,* 334–335.

Gunther, M. (1945). Sore nipples: Causes and prevention. *Lancet, 2,* 590–593.

Gunther, M. (1955). Instinct and the nursing couple. *Lancet, 1,* 575–578.

Gunther, M. (1970). *Infant feeding.* London, UK: Metheun.

Hale, T. W. (2008). *Medications and mother's milk* (13th ed.). Amarillo, TX: Hale Publishing.

Hale, T. W., Bateman, T. L., Finkelman, M. A., & Berens, P. D. (2009). The absence of *Candida albicans* in milk samples of women with clinical symptoms of ductal candidiasis. *Breastfeeding Medicine, 4,* 57–61.

Hale, T. W., & Berens, P. (2002). *Clinical therapy in breastfeeding patients* (2nd ed.). Amarillo, TX: Pharmasoft Publishing.

Han, S., & Hong, Y. G. (1999). The inverted nipple: Its grading and surgical correction. *Plastic and Reconstructive Surgery, 104,* 389–395.

Hanna, L., & Cruz, S. A. (2011). *Candida* mastitis: A case report. *Permanente Journal, 15,* 62–64.

Hanson, L. A. (2004). *Immunobiology of human milk: How breastfeeding protects babies.* Amarillo, TX: Pharmasoft Publishing.

Hanson, L. A., Lonnroth, I., Lange, S., Bjersing, J., & Dahlgren, U. I. (2000). Nutrition resistance to viral propagation. *Nutrition Review, 58,* S31–S37.

Hartmann, P., & Cregan, M. (2001). Lactogenesis and the effects of insulin-dependent diabetes mellitus and prematurity. *Journal of Nutrition, 131,* 3016S–3020S.

Hayes, R., Michell, M., & Nunnerley, H. B. (1991). Acute inflammation of the breast: Role of breast ultrasound in diagnosis and management. *Clinical Radiology, 44,* 253–256.

Heads, J., & Higgins, L. C. (1995). Perceptions and correlates of nipple pain. *Breastfeeding Review, 3,* 59–64.

Heinig, M. J., Francis, J., & Pappagianis, D. (1999). Mammary candidosis in lactating women. *Journal of Human Lactation, 15,* 281–288.

Heller, M. M., Fullerton-Stone, H., & Murase, J. E. (2012). Caring for new mothers: Diagnosis, management and treatment of nipple dermatitis in breastfeeding mothers. *International Journal of Dermatology, 51,* 1149–1161.

Henderson, A., Stamp, G., & Pincombe, J. (2001). Postpartum positioning and attachment education for increasing breastfeeding: A randomized trial. *Birth, 28,* 236–242.

Hesseltine, H. C., Freudlich, C. G., & Hite, K. E. (1948). Acute puerperal mastitis: Clinical and bacteriological studies in relation to penicillin therapy. *American Journal of Obstetrics and Gynecology, 55,* 778–788.

Hewat, R., & Ellis, D. (1987). A comparison of the effectiveness of two methods of nipple care. *Birth, 14,* 41–45.

Hill, P. D., & Humenick, S. S. (1993). Nipple pain during breastfeeding: The first two weeks and beyond. *Journal of Perinatal Education, 2,* 21–35.

Hill, P. D., & Humenick, S. S. (1994). The occurrence of breast engorgement. *Journal of Human Lactation, 10,* 79–86.

Hill, P. D., Humenick, S. S., & West, B. (1994). Concerns of breastfeeding mothers: The first six weeks postpartum. *Journal of Perinatal Education, 3,* 47–58.

Hocutt, J. E., Jaffe, R., Rylander, C. R., & Beebe, J. K. (1982). Cryotherapy in ankle sprains. *American Journal of Sports Medicine, 10,* 317–319.

Hoffman, J. B. (1953). A suggested treatment for inverted nipples. *American Journal of Obstetrics and Gynecology, 66,* 346.

Hook, G. W., & Ikeda, D. M. (1999). Treatment of breast abscesses with US-guided percutaneous needle drainage without indwelling catheter placement. *Radiology, 213,* 579–582.

Hopkinson, J. (1992). Interfeeding breast pain: A case report. *Journal of Human Lactation, 8,* 149–151.

Hoppe, J. E., & Hahn, H. (1996). Randomized comparison of two nystatin oral gels with miconazole oral gel for treatment of oral thrush in infants. *Infection, 24,* 136–139.

Hsu, S. (2005). Green tea and the skin. *Journal of the American Academy of Dermatology, 52,* 1049–1059.

Huggins, K. E., & Billion, S. F. (1993). Twenty cases of persistent sore nipples: Collaboration between lactation consultant and dermatologist. *Journal of Human Lactation, 9,* 155–160.

Humenick, S., & van Steenkiste, S. (1983). Early indicators of breastfeeding progress. *Issues in Comprehensive Pediatric Nursing, 6,* 205–215.

Humenick, S. S., Hill, P. D., & Anderson, M. A. (1994). Breast engorgement: Patterns and selected outcomes. *Journal of Human Lactation, 10,* 87–93.

Hunt, K. M., Williams, J. E., Shafii, B., Hunt, M. K., Behre, R., Ting, R., . . . McGuire, M. A. (2012). Mastitis is associated with increased free fatty acids, somatic cell count, and interleukin-8 concentrations in human milk. *Breastfeeding Medicine, 8,* 105–110.

Hussain, A. N., Policarpio, C., & Vincent, M. T. (2006). Evaluating nipple discharge. *Obstetrical and Gynecological Survey, 61,* 278–283.

Hytten, F. E., & Baird, D. (1958). The development of the nipple in pregnancy. *Lancet, 1*(7032), 1201–1204.

Iffrig, M. C. (1968). Nursing care and success in breastfeeding. *Nursing Clinics of North America, 3,* 345–354.

Illingworth, R., & Stone, D. (1952). Self-demand feeding in a maternity unit. *Lancet, 1,* 683–687.

Inch, S. (1989). Antenatal preparation for breastfeeding. In I. Chalmers, M. Enkin, & M. J. N. C. Keirse (Eds.), *Effective care in pregnancy and childbirth.* Oxford, UK: Oxford University Press.

Inch, S. (1997). *Mastitis: A literature review.* Geneva, Switzerland: World Health Organization, Division of Child Health & Development.

Inch, S., & Fisher, C. (1995). Mastitis: Infection or inflammation. *Practitioner, 239,* 472–476.

Jacobs, L. A., Dickinson, J. E., Hart, P. D., Doherty, D. A., & Faulkner, S. J. (2007). Normal nipple position in term infants measured on breastfeeding ultrasound. *Journal of Human Lactation, 23,* 52–59.

Jacobs, V. R., Golombeck, K., Jonat, W., & Kiechle, M. (2003). Mastitis nonpuerperalis after nipple piercing: Time to act. *International Journal of Fertility and Women's Medicine, 48,* 226–231.

Jamali, F., Ricci, A., & Deckers, P. (1996). Paget's disease of the nipple–areola complex. *Surgical Clinics of North America, 76,* 365–381.

Jimenez, E., Fernandez, L., Maldonado, A., Martín, R., Olivares, M., Xaus, J., & Rodriguez, J. M. (2008). Oral administration of *Lactobacillus* strains isolated from breast milk as an alternative for the treatment of infectious mastitis during lactation. *Applied and Environmental Microbiology, 74,* 4650–4655.

Johnson, P. E., & Hanson, K. D. (1996). Acute puerperal mastitis in the augmented breast. *Plastic and Reconstructive Surgery, 98,* 723–725.

Johnstone, H. A., & Marcinak, J. F. (1990). Candidiasis in the breastfeeding mother and infant. *Journal of Obstetric, Gynecologic, and Neonatal Nursing, 19,* 171–173.

Jonsson, S., & Pulkkinen, M. O. (1994). Mastitis today: Incidence, prevention and treatment. *Annales Chirurgiae et Gynaecologiae Supplementum, 208,* 84–87.

Karstrup, S., Solvig, J., Nolsøe, C. P., Nilsson, P., Khattar S., Loren I., . . . Court-Payen, M. (1993). Acute puerperal breast abscess: US-guided drainage. *Radiology, 188,* 807–809.

Kataria, K., Srivastava, A., & Dhar, A. (2013). Management of lactational mastitis and breast abscesses: Review of current knowledge and practice. *Indian Journal of Surgery, 75,* 430–435.

Kaufmann, R., & Foxman, B. (1991). Mastitis among lactating women: Occurrence and risk factors. *Social Science Medicine, 33,* 701–705.

Kee, W. H., Tan, S. L., & Salmon, Y. M. (1989). The treatment of breast engorgement with serrapeptase (Danzen): A double-blind controlled trial. *Singapore Medical Journal, 30,* 48–54.

Kenny, J. F. (1977). Recurrent group B streptococcal disease in an infant associated with the ingestion of infected mother's milk. *Journal of Pediatrics, 91,* 158.

Kent, J. C., Ashton, E., Hardwick, C. M., Rowan, M. K., Chia, E. S., Fairclough, K. A., . . . Geddes, D. T. (2015). Nipple pain in breastfeeding mothers: Incidence, causes and treatments. *International Journal of Environmental Research and Public Health, 12,* 12247–12263.

Kernerman, E., & Park, E. (2014). Severe breast pain resolved with pectoral muscle massage. *Journal of Human Lactation, 30,* 287–291.

Kesaree, N., Banapurmath, C. R., Banapurmath, S., & Shamanur, K. (1993). Treatment of inverted nipples using a disposable syringe. *Journal of Human Lactation, 9,* 27–29.

Kinlay, J. R., O'Connell, D. L., & Kinlay, S. (2001). Risk factors for mastitis in breastfeeding women: Results of a prospective cohort study. *Australian and New Zealand Journal of Public Health, 25,* 115–120.

Kline, T. S., & Lash, S. R. (1962). Nipple secretion in pregnancy: A cytologic and histologic study. *American Journal of Clinical Pathology, 37,* 626.

Kudva, Y. C., O'Brien, T., & Oberg, A. L. (2002). "Diabetic mastopathy," or sclerosing lymphocytic lobulitis, is strongly associated with type 1 diabetes. *Diabetes Care, 25,* 121–126.

Kujawa-Myles, S., Noel-Weiss, J., Dunn, S., Peterson, W. E., & Cotterman, K. J. (2015). Maternal intravenous fluids and postpartum breast changes: A pilot observational study. *International Breastfeeding Journal, 10,* 18.

Kvist, L. J., Hall-Lord, M. L., & Larsson, B. W. (2007). A descriptive study of Swedish women with symptoms of breast inflammation during lactation and their perceptions of the quality of care given at a breastfeeding clinic. *International Breastfeeding Journal, 2,* 2.

Kvist, L. J., Larsson, B. W., Hall-Lord, M. L., Steen, A., & Schalen, C. (2008). The role of bacteria in lactational mastitis and some considerations of the use of antibiotic treatment. *International Breastfeeding Journal, 3,* 6.

Kvist, L. J., & Rydhstroem, H. (2005). Factors related to breast abscess after delivery: A population-based study. *BJOG: An International Journal of Obstetrics and Gynaecology, 112,* 1070–1074.

Lafreniere, R. (1990). Bloody nipple discharge during pregnancy: A rationale for conservative treatment. *Journal of Surgical Oncology, 43,* 228.

Lavergne, N. A. (1997). Does application of tea bags to sore nipples while breastfeeding provide effective relief? *Journal of Obstetric, Gynecologic, and Neonatal Nursing, 26,* 53–58.

Lawlor-Smith, L., & Lawlor-Smith, C. (1996). Nipple vasospasm in the breastfeeding woman. *Breastfeeding Review, 4,* 37–39.

Lawlor-Smith, L., & Lawlor-Smith, C. (1997). Vasospasm of the nipple: A manifestation of Raynaud's phenomenon: Case reports. *BMJ, 314,* 844–845.

Lawrence, R. A., & Lawrence, R. M. (2016). *Breastfeeding: A guide for the medical profession* (8th ed.). Philadelphia, PA: Elsevier Mosby.

L'Esperance, C. (1980). Pain or pleasure: The dilemma of early breastfeeding. *Birth, 7,* 21–26.

Lever, R., Hadley, K., Downey, D., & Mackie R. (1988). Staphylococcal colonization in atopic dermatitis and the effect of topical mupirocin therapy. *British Journal of Dermatology, 119,* 189–198.

Livingstone, V. (1996). Too much of a good thing: Maternal and infant hyperlactation syndromes. *Canadian Family Physician, 42,* 89–99.

Livingstone, V., & Stringer, L. J. (1999). The treatment of *Staphylococcus aureus* infected sore nipples: A randomized comparative study. *Journal of Human Lactation, 15,* 241–246.

Livingstone, V. H., Willis, C. E., & Berkowitz, J. (1996). *Staphylococcus aureus* and sore nipples. *Canadian Family Physician, 42,* 654–659.

Lochner, J. E., Livingston, C. J., & Judlins, D. Z. (2009). Which interventions are best for alleviating nipple pain in nursing mothers? *Journal of Family Practice, 58,* 612a–612c.

MAIN Trial Collaborative Group. (1994). Preparing for breastfeeding: Treatment of inverted and non-protractile nipples in pregnancy. *Midwifery, 10,* 200–214.

Makanjuola, D. (1998). A clinico-radiological correlation of breast diseases during lactation and the significance of unilateral failure of lactation. *West African Journal of Medicine, 17,* 217–223.

Mangesi, L., & Dowswell, T. (2010). Treatments for breast engorgement during lactation. *Cochrane Database of Systematic Reviews*, CDS006946. doi: 10.1002/14651858.CD006946.pub2

Manning, D. J., Coughlin, R. P., & Poskitt, E. M. E. (1985). *Candida* in mouth or on dummy? *Archives of Disease in Childhood, 60,* 381–382.

Marrazzu, A., Sanna, M. G., Dessole, F., Capobianco, G., Piga, M. D., & Dessole, S. (2015). Evaluation of the effectiveness of a silver-impregnated medical cap for topical treatment of nipple fissure of breastfeeding mothers. *Breastfeeding Medicine, 10,* 232–238.

Marti, A., Feng, H. J., Altermatt, H. J., & Jaggi, R. (1997). Milk accumulation triggers apoptosis of mammary epithelial cells. *European Journal of Cell Biology, 73,* 158–165.

Martic, K., & Vasilj, O. (2012). Extremely large breast abscess in a breastfeeding mother. *Journal of Human Lactation, 28,* 460–463.

Martin, J. (2004). Is nipple piercing compatible with breastfeeding? *Journal of Human Lactation, 20,* 319–321.

Matheson, I., Aursnes, I., Horgen, M., Aabø, O., & Melby, K. (1988). Bacteriological findings and clinical symptoms in relation to clinical outcome in puerperal mastitis. *Acta Obstetrica et Gynecologica Scandinavica, 67,* 23–726.

Mattos-Graner, R. O., de Moraes, A. B., Rontani, R. M., & Birman, E. G. (2001). Relation of oral yeast infection in Brazilian infants and the use of a pacifier. *ASDC Journal of Dentistry for Children, 68,* 33–36.

McClellan, H. L., Geddes, D. T., Kent, J. C., Garbin, C. P., Mitoulas, L. R., & Hartmann, P. E. (2008). Infants of mothers with persistent nipple pain exert strong sucking vacuums. *Acta Paediatrica, 97,* 1205–1209.

McClellan, H. L., Hepworth, A. R., Garbin, C. P., Rowan, M. K., Deacon, J., Hartmann, P. E., & Geddes, D. T. (2012). Nipple pain during breastfeeding with or without visible trauma. *Journal of Human Lactation, 28*(4), 511–521.

McClellan, H. L., Hepworth, A. R., Kent, J. C., Garbin, C. P., Williams, T. M., Hartmann, P. E., & Geddes, D. T. (2012). Breastfeeding frequency, milk volume, and duration in mother–infant dyads with persistent nipple pain. *Breastfeeding Medicine, 7,* 275–281.

McClellan, H. L., Kent, J. C., Hepworth, A. R., Hartmann, P. E., & Geddes, D. T. (2015). Persistent nipple pain in breastfeeding mothers associated with abnormal infant tongue movement. *International Journal of Environmental Research and Public Health, 12,* 10833–10845.

McGeorge, D. D. (1994). The "niplette": An instrument for the non-surgical correction of inverted nipples. *British Journal of Plastic Surgery, 47,* 46–49.

McGuiness, N., & Cording, V. (2013). Raynaud's phenomenon of the nipple associated with labetalol use. *Journal of Human Lactation, 29,* 17–19.

McLachlan, Z., Milne, E. J., Lumley, J., & Walker, B. L. (1993, May). Ultrasound treatment for breast engorgement: A randomized double-blind trial. *Breastfeeding Review*, 316–321.

Menczer, J., & Eskin, B. (1969). Evaluation of postpartum breast engorgement by thermography. *Obstetrics and Gynecology, 33,* 260–263.

Michie, C., Lockie, F., & Lynn, W. (2003). The challenge of mastitis. *Archives of Disease in Childhood, 88,* 818–821.

Miller, V., & Riordan, J. (2004). Treating postpartum breast edema with areolar compression. *Journal of Human Lactation, 20,* 223–226.

Minchin, M. (1985). *Breastfeeding matters: What we need to know about infant feeding.* Victoria, Australia: Alma Publications & George Allen & Unwin Australia Pty Ltd.

Moazzez, A., Kelso, R. L., Towfigh, S., Sohn, H., Berne, T. V., & Mason, R. J. (2007). Breast abscess bacteriologic findings in the era of community-acquired methicillin-resistant *Staphylococcus aureus* epidemics. *Archives of Surgery, 142,* 881–884.

Mohammadzadeh, A., Farhat, A., & Esmaeily, H. (2005). The effect of breast milk and lanolin on sore nipples. *Saudi Medicine Journal, 26,* 1231–1234.

Maldonado-Lobon, J. A., Diaz-Lopez, M. A., Carputo, R., Duarte, P., Diaz-Ropero, M. P., Valero, A. D., . . . Martin, M. O. (2015). *Lactobacillus fermentum* CECT 5716 reduced *Staphylococcus* load in the breastmilk of lactating mothers suffering breast pain: A randomized controlled trial. *Breastfeeding Medicine, 10,* 425–431.

Moon, A. A., & Gilbert, B. (1935). A study of acute mastitis of the puerperim. *Journal of Obstetrics and Gynaecology of the British Commonwealth, 42,* 268–282.

Moon, J. L., & Humenick, S. S. (1989). Breast engorgement: Contributing variables and variables amenable to nursing intervention. *Journal of Obstetric, Gynecologic, and Neonatal Nursing, 18,* 309–315.

Morel, A., Wu, F., Dell-Latta, P., Cronquist, A., Rubenstein, D., & Saiman, L. (2002). Nosocomial transmission of methicillin-resistant *Staphylococcus aureus* from a mother to her preterm quadruplet infants. *American Journal of Infection Control, 30,* 170–173.

Moretti, A., Pasquali, P., Mencaroni, G., Boncio, L., & Piergili Fioretti, D. (1998). Relationship between cell counts in bovine milk and the presence of mastitis pathogens (yeasts and bacteria*). Zentralblatt fur Veterinarmedizin, 45,* 129–132.

Morino, C., & Winn, S. M. (2007). Raynaud's phenomenon of the nipples: An elusive diagnosis. *Journal of Human Lactation, 23,* 191–193.

Morland-Schultz, K., & Hill, P. D. (2005). Prevention of and therapies for nipple pain: A systematic review. *Journal of Obstetric, Gynecologic, and Neonatal Nursing, 34,* 428–437.

Morrill, J. F., Heinig, M. J., Pappagianis, D., & Dewey, K. G. (2004). Diagnostic value of signs and symptoms of mammary candidosis among lactating women. *Journal of Human Lactation, 20,* 288–295.

Morrill, J. F., Heinig, M. J., Pappagianis, D., & Dewey, K. G. (2005). Risk factors for mammary candidosis among lactating women. *Journal of Obstetric, Gynecologic, and Neonatal Nursing, 34,* 37–45.

Morrill, J. M., Pappagianis, D., Heinig, M. J., Lonnerdall, B., & Dewey, K. G. (2003). Detecting *Candida albicans* in human milk. *Journal of Clinical Microbiology, 41,* 475–478.

Morton, J. A. (1994). The clinical usefulness of breast milk sodium in the assessment of lactogenesis. *Pediatrics, 93,* 802–806.

Mu, D., Luan, J., Mu, L., & Xin, M. (2012). A minimally invasive gradual traction technique for inverted nipple correction. *Aesthetic Plastic Surgery, 36,* 1151–1154.

Neifert, M., DeMarzo, S., Seacat, J., Young, D., Leff, M., & Orleans M. (1990). The influence of breast surgery, breast appearance, and pregnancy-induced breast changes on lactation sufficiency as measured by infant weight gain. *Birth, 17,* 31–38.

Neifert, M., & Seacat, J. (1986). Medical management of successful breastfeeding. *Pediatric Clinics of North America, 33,* 743–762.

Neubauer, S. H., Ferris, A. M., & Hinckley, L. (1990). The effect of mastitis on breast milk composition in insulin dependent diabetic and non-diabetic women. *FASEB Journal, 4,* A915.

Newman, J. (2005). *Candida* protocol. Retrieved from http://www.breastfeedinginc.ca/content.php?pagename=doc-CP

Newton, N. (1952). Nipple pain and nipple damage. *Journal of Pediatrics, 41,* 411–423.

Newton, M., & Newton, N. (1951). Postpartum engorgement of the breast. *American Journal of Obstetrics and Gynecology, 61,* 664–667

Newton, M., & Newton, N. R. (1948). The let-down reflex in human lactation. *Journal of Pediatrics, 33,* 698.

Nicholson, W., & Yuen, H. P. (1995). A study of breastfeeding rates at a large Australian obstetric hospital. *Australian and New Zealand Journal of Obstetrics and Gynaecology, 35,* 393–397.

Niebyl, J. R., Spence, M. R., & Parmley, T. H. (1978). Sporadic (non-epidemic) puerperal mastitis. *Journal of Reproductive Medicine, 20,* 97–100.

Nikodem, V. C., Danziger, D., Gebka, N., Gulmezoglu, A. M., & Hofmeyr, G. J. (1993). Do cabbage leaves prevent breast engorgement? A randomized controlled study. *Birth, 20,* 61–64.

Noble, R. (1991). Milk under the skin (milk blister): A simple problem causing other breast conditions. *Breastfeeding Review, 2,* 118–119.

O'Callaghan, M. A. (1981). Atypical discharge from the breast during pregnancy and/or lactation. *Australian and New Zealand Journal of Obstetrics and Gynaecology, 21,* 214–216.

Odds, F. C. (1994). *Candida* species and virulence. *American Society for Microbiology News, 60,* 313–318.

Oguz, S., Isik, S., Gungor, A. N. C., Seker, M., & Ogretmen, Z. (2014). Protective efficacy of olive oil for sore nipples during nursing. *Journal of Family Medicine Community Health, 1,* 1021.

O'Hara, M. A. (2012). Bleb histology reveals inflammatory infiltrate that regresses with topical steroids: A case series. *Breastfeeding Medicine, 7*(suppl 1), S-2.

O'Hara, R. J., Dexter, S. P., & Fox, J. N. (1996). Conservative management of infective mastitis and breast abscesses after ultrasonographic assessment. *British Journal of Surgery, 83,* 1413–1414.

Olsen, N., & Nielson, S. L. (1978). Prevalence of primary Raynaud's phenomenon in young females. *Scandinavian Journal of Clinical and Laboratory Investigation, 37,* 761–776.

Osterman, K. L., & Rahm, V. A. (2000). Lactation mastitis: Bacterial cultivation of breast milk, symptoms, treatment, and outcome. *Journal of Human Lactation, 16,* 297–302.

Osther, P., Balslev, E., & Blichert-Toft, M. (1990). Paget's disease of the nipple: A continuing enigma. *Acta Chirurgiae Scandinavica, 156,* 343-352.

O'Sullivan, S., & Keith, M. P. (2011). Raynaud phenomenon of the nipple: A rare finding in rheumatology clinic. *Journal of Clinical Rheumatology, 17,* 371–372.

Otte, M, J. (1975). Correcting inverted nipples: An aid to breastfeeding. *MCN: The American Journal of Maternal/Child Nursing, 75,* 454–456.

Page, S. M., & McKenna, D. S. (2006). Vasospasm of the nipple presenting as painful lactation. *Obstetrics and Gynecology, 108,* 806–808.

Panjaitan, M., Amir, L. H., Costs, A.-M., Rudland, E., & Tabrizi, S. (2008). Polymerase chain reaction in detection of *Candida albicans* for confirmation of clinical diagnosis of nipple thrush [Letter]. *Breastfeeding Medicine, 3,* 185–187.

Peters, F., Diemer, P., Meeks, O., & Behnken, L. J. (2003). Severity of mastalgia in relation to milk duct dilatation. *Obstetrics and Gynecology, 101,* 54–60.

Petok, E. S. (1995). Breast cancer and breastfeeding: Five cases. *Journal of Human Lactation, 11,* 205–209.

Pfaller, M. A. (1994). Epidemiology and control of fungal infections. *Clinical Infectious Diseases, 19*(Suppl. 1), S8–S13.

Piatt, J. P., & Bergeson, P. S. (1992). Gentian violet toxicity. *Clinical Pediatrics, 31,* 756–757.

Pizzo, G., Giuliana, G., Milici, M. E., & Giangreco, R. (2000). Effects of dietary carbohydrate on the in vitro epithelial adhesion of *Candida albicans, Candida tropicalis,* and *Candida krusei. New Microbiology, 23,* 63–71.

Porter, J., & Schach, B. (2004). Treating sore, possibly infected nipples. *Journal of Human Lactation, 20,* 221–222.

Prentice, A., Addey, C. V. P., & Wilde, C. J. (1989). Evidence for local feedback control of human milk secretion. *Biochemical Society Transactions, 15,* 122.

Prosser, C. G., & Hartmann, P. E. (1983). Comparison of mammary gland function during the ovulatory menstrual cycle and acute breast inflammation in women. *Australian Journal of Experimental and Biological Medical Science, 61,* 277–286.

Pugh, L. C., Buchko, B. L., Bishop, B. A., Cochran, J. F., Smith, L. R., & Lerew, D. J. (1996). A comparison of topical agents to relieve nipple pain and enhance breastfeeding. *Birth, 23,* 88–93.

Rago, J. L. (1988). Weeping areolar eczema. *Journal of Human Lactation, 4,* 166–167.

Rahal, R. M., deFreitas-Junior, R., & Paulinelli, R. R. (2005). Risk factors for duct ectasia. *Breast Journal, 11,* 262–265.

Ramsay, D. T., Kent, J. C., Owens, R. A., & Hartmann, P. E. (2004). Ultrasound imaging of milk ejection in the breast of lactating women. *Pediatrics, 113,* 361–367.

Rasmussen, K. M., Hilson, J. A., & Kjolhede, C. L. (2001). Obesity may impair lactogenesis II. *Journal of Nutrition, 131,* 3009S–3011S.

Reddy, P., Qi, C., Zembower, T., Noskin, G. A., & Bolon, M. (2007). Postpartum mastitis and community-acquired methicillin-resistant *Staphylococcus aureus*. *Emerging Infectious Diseases, 13,* 298–301.

Remington, J. S., & Klein, J. O. (1983). *Infectious diseases of the fetus and newborn.* Philadelphia, PA: WB Saunders.

Rench, M. A., & Baker, C. J. (1989). Group B streptococcal breast abscess in a mother and mastitis in her infant. *Obstetrics and Gynecology, 73,* 875–877.

Renfrew, M. J., Woolridge, M. W., & McGill, H. R. (2000). *Enabling women to breastfeed: A review of practices which promote or inhibit breastfeeding—with evidence-based guidance for practice.* London, UK: Stationary Office.

Riedel, L. J. (1991*). Breast engorgement: Subjective and objective measurements and patterns of occurrence in primiparous mothers.* Master's thesis. Laramie, WY: Department of Nursing, University of Wyoming.

Righard, L. (1996). Early enhancement of successful breastfeeding. *World Health Forum, 17,* 92–97.

Righard, L. (1998). Are breastfeeding problems related to incorrect breastfeeding technique and the use of pacifiers and bottles? *Birth, 25,* 40–44.

Righard, L., & Alade, M. O. (1992). Sucking technique and its effect on success of breastfeeding. *Birth, 19,* 185–189.

Riordan, J. (1983). *A practical guide to breastfeeding.* St. Louis, MO: Mosby.

Riordan, J. (1985). The effectiveness of topical agents in reducing nipple soreness of breastfeeding mothers. *Journal of Human Lactation, 1,* 36–41.

Riordan, J. M., & Nichols, F. H. (1990). A descriptive study of lactation mastitis in long-term breastfeeding women. *Journal of Human Lactation, 6,* 53–58.

Roberts, K. L. (1995). A comparison of chilled cabbage leaves and chilled gelpaks in reducing breast engorgement. *Journal of Human Lactation, 11,* 17–20.

Roberts, K. L., Reiter, M., & Schuster, D. (1998). Effects of cabbage leaf extract on breast engorgement. *Journal of Human Lactation, 14,* 231–236.

Robson, B. A. (1990). *Breast engorgement in breastfeeding women.* PhD dissertation. Cleveland, OH: Case Western Reserve University.

Rosa, C., Novak, F. R., Almeida, J. A. G., Hagler, L. C., & Hagler, A. N. (1990). Yeasts from human milk collected in Rio de Janeiro, Brazil. *Reviews in Microbiology, 21,* 361–363.

Rosier, W. (1988). Cool cabbage compresses. *Breastfeeding Review, 12,* 28–31.

Ryan, T. J. (2007). Infection following soft tissue injury: Its role in wound healing. *Current Opinion in Infectious Disease, 20,* 124–128.

Sabate, J. M., Clotet, M., Torrubia, S., Gomez, A., Guerrero, R., de Las Heras, P., & Lerma, E. (2007). Radiologic evaluation of breast disorders related to pregnancy and lactation. *RadioGraphics, 27,* S101–S124.

Saber, A. (1996). The milk rejection sign: A natural tumor marker. *American Surgeon, 62,* 998–999.

Sadove, R., & Clayman, M. A. (2008). Surgical procedure for reversal of nipple piercing. *Aesthetic Plastic Surgery, 32,* 563–565.

Saiman, L., O'Keefe, M., Graham, P. L., 3rd, Saïd-Salim, B., Kreiswirth, B., LaSala, A., . . . Della-Latta, P. (2003). Hospital transmission of community-acquired methicillin-resistant *Staphylococcus aureus* among postpartum women. *Clinical Infectious Diseases, 37,* 1313–1319.

Sandberg, C. A. (1998). *Cold therapy for breast engorgement in new mothers who are breastfeeding* (Unpublished master's thesis). College of St. Catherine, St. Paul, MN.

Sayyah-Melli, M., Rashidi, M. R., Delazar, A., Madarek, E., Kargar Maher, M. H., Ghasemzadeh, A., . . . Tahmasebi, Z. (2007a). Effect of peppermint water on prevention of nipple cracks in lactating primiparous women: A randomized controlled trial. *International Breastfeeding Journal, 2,* 7.

Sayyah-Melli, M. S., Rashidi, M. R., Nokhoodchi, A., Tagavi, S., Farzadi, L., Sadaghat, K., . . . Sheshvan, M. K. (2007b). A randomized trial of peppermint gel, lanolin ointment, and placebo gel to prevent nipple crack in primiparous breastfeeding women. *Medical Science Monitor, 13,* CR406–CR411.

Schelz, Z., Molnar, J., & Hohmann, J. (2006). Antimicrobial and antiplasmid activities of essential oils. *Fitoterapia, 77,* 279–285.

Schoenfeld, E. M., & McKay, M. P. (2010). Mastitis and methicillin-resistant *Staphylococcus aureus* (MRSA): The calm before the storm? *Journal Emergency Medicine, 38,* e31–e34.

Schwartz, K., D'Arcy, H. J., Gillespie, B., Bobo, J., Longeway, M., & Foxman, B. (2002). Factors associated with weaning in the first 3 months postpartum. *Journal of Family Practice, 51,* 439–444.

Scott, J. A., Robertson, M., Fitzpatrick, J., Knight, C., & Mulholland, S. (2008). Occurrence of lactational mastitis and medical management: A prospective cohort study in Glasgow. *International Breastfeeding Journal, 3,* 21.

Scott-Conner, C. E., & Schorr, S. J. (1995). The diagnosis and management of breast problems during pregnancy and lactation. *American Journal of Surgery, 170,* 401–405.

Sealander, J. Y., & Kerr, C. P. (1989). Herpes simplex of the nipple: Infant-to-mother transmission. *American Family Physician, 39,* 111–113.

Semba, R. D., Kumwenda, N., Hoover, D. R., Taha, T. E., Quinn, T. C., Mtimavalye, L., . . . Chiphangwi, J. D. (1999). Human immunodeficiency virus load in breast milk, mastitis, and mother-to-child transmission of human immunodeficiency virus type 1. *Journal of Infectious Disease, 180,* 93–98.

Semba, R. D., Kumwenda, N., Taha, T., Hoover, D. R., Lan, Y., Eisinger, W., . . . Chiphangwi, J. D. (1999). Mastitis and immunological factors in breast milk of lactating women in Malawi. *Clinical and Diagnostic Laboratory Immunology, 6,* 671–674.

Semba, R. D., Kumwenda, N., Taha, T. E., Quinn, T. C., Lan, Y., Mtimavalye, L., . . . Chiphangwi, J. D. (1999). Mastitis and immunological factors in breast milk of human immunodeficiency virus–infected women. *Journal of Human Lactation, 15,* 301–306.

Shanazi, M., Khalili, A.F., Kamalifard, M., Jafarabadi, M.A., Masoudin, K., & Esmaeli, F. (2015). Comparison of the effects of lanolin, peppermint, and dexpanthenol creams on treatment of traumatic nipples in breastfeeding mothers. *Journal of Caring Sciences, 4,* 297–307.

Sharp, D. A. (1992). Moist wound healing for sore or cracked nipples. *Breastfeeding Abstracts, 12*(2), 19.

Shiau, J. P., Chin, C. C., Lin, M. H., & Hsiao, C. W. (2011). Correction of severely inverted nipple with telescope method. *Aesthetic Plastic Surgery, 35,* 1137–1142.

Shiau, S.-H. H. (1997*). Randomized controlled trial of kangaroo care with full term infants: Effects on maternal anxiety, breast milk maturation, breast engorgement, and breastfeeding status* (Unpublished doctoral dissertation). Case Western Reserve University, Cleveland, OH.

Shinefield, H., Black, S., Fattom, A., Horwith, G., Rasgon, S., Ordonez, J., . . . Naso, R. (2002). Use of a *Staphylococcus aureus* conjugate vaccine in patients receiving hemodialysis. *New England Journal of Medicine, 346,* 491–496.

Silva, J. R., Carvalho, R., Maia, C., Osorio, M., & Barbosa, M. (2014). Rusty pipe syndrome, a cause of bloody nipple discharge: Case report. *Breastfeeding Medicine, 9,* 411–412.

Singh, P., Sood, P. P., Gupta, S. K., Jand, S. K., & Banga, H. S. (1998). Experimental candidal mastitis in goats: Clinical, haematological, biochemical and sequential pathological studies. *Mycopathologia, 140,* 89–97.

Slaven, S., & Harvey, D. (1981). Unlimited suckling time improves breastfeeding. *Lancet, 1,* 392–393.

Smillie, C. M. (2004). *The prevention and treatment of plugged ducts.* Clinical handout. Stratford, CT: Breast-feeding Resources.

Smith, W., Erenberg, A., & Nowak, A. (1988). Imaging evaluation of the human nipple during breastfeeding. *American Journal of Diseases of Children, 142,* 76–78.

Snowden, H. M., Renfrew, M. J., & Woolridge, M. W. (2001). Treatments for breast engorgement during lactation. *Cochrane Database of Systematic Reviews, 2,* CD000046.

Soukka, T., Tenovuo, J., & Lenander-Lumikari, M. (1992). Fungicidal effect of human lactoferrin against *Candida albicans. FEMS Microbiology Letters, 69,* 223–228.

Spangler, A., & Hildebrandt, E. (1993). The effect of modified lanolin on nipple pain/damage during the first ten days of breastfeeding. *International Journal of Childbirth Education, 8,* 15–19.

Spencer, J. P. (2008). Management of mastitis in breastfeeding women. *American Family Physician, 78,* 727–731.

Srinivasan, A., Dobrich, C., Mitnick, H., & Feldman, P. (2006). Ankyloglossia in breastfeeding infants: The effect of frenotomy on maternal nipple pain and latch. *Breastfeeding Medicine, 1,* 216–224.

Staib, P., Kretschmar, M., Nichterlein, T., Hof, H., & Morschhäuser, J. (2000). Differential activation of a *Candida albicans* virulence gene family during infection. *Proceedings of the National Academy of Science USA, 97,* 6102–6107.

Stevens, K., Burrell, H. C., Evans, A. J., & Sibbering, D. M. (1997). The ultrasound appearances of galactoceles. *British Journal of Radiology, 70,* 239–241.

Stewart, P. S., & Costerton, J. W. (2001). Antibiotic resistance of bacteria in biofilms. *Lancet, 358*(9276), 135–138.

Strong, G. D. (2011). Provider management and support for breastfeeding pain. *Journal of Obstetric, Gynecologic, and Neonatal Nursing, 40,* 753–764.

Stutte, P. C., Bowles, B. C., & Morman, G. Y. (1988). The effects of breast massage on volume and fat content of human milk. *Genesis, 10,* 22–25.

Sullivan-Bolyai, J. Z., Fife, K. H., Jacobs, R. F., Miller, Z., & Corey, L. (1983). Disseminated neonatal herpes simplex virus type 1 from a maternal breast lesion. *Pediatrics, 71,* 455–457.

Svensson, K., Lange, S., Lonnroth, I., Widström, A. M., & Hanson, L. A. (2004). Induction of anti-secretory factor in human milk may prevent mastitis. *Acta Paediatrica, 93,* 1228–1231.

Tanquay, K., McBean, M., & Jain, E. (1994). Nipple candidosis among breastfeeding mothers: A case control study of predisposing factors. *Canadian Family Physician, 40,* 1407–1413.

Terrill, P. J., & Stapleton, M. J. (1991). The inverted nipple: To cut the ducts or not? *British Journal of Plastic Surgery, 44,* 372–377.

Thomassen, P., Johansson, V. A., Wassberg, C., & Petrini, B. (1998). Breastfeeding, pain and infection. *Gynecologic and Obstetric Investigation, 46,* 73–74.

Thompson, R., Kruske, S., Barclay, L., Linden, K, Gao, Y., & Kildea, S. (2016). Potential predictors of nipple trauma from an in-home breastfeeding programme: A cross-sectional study. *Women and Birth,* [Epub ahead of print], doi: 10.1016/j.wombi.2016.01.002.

Thomsen, A. C., Espersen, T., & Maigaard, S. (1984). Course and treatment of milk stasis, noninfectious inflammation of the breast, and infectious mastitis in nursing women. *American Journal of Obstetrics and Gynecology, 149,* 492–495.

Thorley, V. (1997). Inverted nipple with fatty plaques on areola and nipple. *Breastfeeding Review, 5,* 43–44.

Thota, U., Machiraju, V. M., & Jampana, V. R. (2013). Rusty pipe syndrome: A case report. *Health, 5,* 157–158.

Ulitzsch, D., Nyman, M. K., & Carlson, R. A. (2004). Breast abscess in lactating women: US-guided treatment. *Radiology, 232,* 904–909.

Upledger Institute, Inc. (n.d.). International Alliance of Healthcare Educators. Retrieved from http://www.iahe.com

Utter, A. R. (1990). Gentian violet treatment for thrush: Can its use cause breastfeeding problems? *Journal of Human Lactation, 6,* 178–180.

Utter, A. R. (1992). Gentian violet and thrush. *Journal of Human Lactation, 8,* 6.

Vestermark, V., Hogdall, C. K., Birch, M., Plenov, G., & Toftager-Larsen, K. (1991). Influence of the mode of delivery on initiation of breastfeeding. *European Journal of Obstetrics, Gynecology, and Reproductive Biology, 38,* 33–38.

Vidotto, B., Guevara-Ochoa, L., Ponce, L. M., Tello, G. M., Prada, G. R., & Bruatto, M. (1992). Vaginal yeast flora of pregnant women in the Cusco region of Peru. *Mycoses, 35,* 229–234.

Virdi, V. S., Goraya, J. S., & Khadwal, A. (2001). Rusty-pipe syndrome. *Indian Pediatrics, 38,* 931–932.

Vuolo, M., Suhrland, M. J., Madan, R., & Oktay, M. H. (2009). Discrepant cytologic and radiographic findings in adjacent galactocele and fibroadenoma. *Acta Cytologica, 53,* 211–214.

Walker, M. (2004). *Mastitis in lactating women.* Unit 2/Lactation Consultant Series Two. Schaumburg, IL: La Leche League International.

Walker, M. (2010). *The nipple and areola in breastfeeding and lactation: Anatomy, physiology, problems, and solutions.* Amarillo, TX: Hale Publishing.

Walker, M., & Driscoll, J. W. (1989). Sore nipples: The new mother's nemesis. *MCN: The American Journal of Maternal/Child Nursing, 14,* 260–265.

Waller, H. (1946). The early failure of breastfeeding: A clinical study of its causes and their prevention. *Archives of Disease in Childhood, 21,* 1–12.

Walsh, A. (1949). Acute mastitis. *Lancet, 2,* 635–639.

Wambach, K. A. (2003). Lactation mastitis: A descriptive study of the experience. *Journal of Human Lactation, 19,* 24–34.

Ward, K. A., & Burton, J. L. (1997). Dermatologic diseases of the breast in young women. *Clinics in Dermatology, 15,* 45–52.

Weichert, C. E. (1980). Prolactin cycling and the management of breastfeeding failure. *Advances in Pediatrics, 27,* 391–407.

West, C. (1980). Factors influencing the duration of breastfeeding. *Journal of Biosocial Science, 12,* 325–331.

Widström, A. M., & Thingstrom-Paulsson, J. (1993). The position of the tongue during rooting reflexes elicited in newborn infants before the first suckle. *Acta Paediatrica Scandinavia, 82,* 281–283.

Wiener, S. (2006). Diagnosis and management of *Candida* of the nipple and breast. *Journal of Midwifery and Women's Health, 51,* 125–128.

Willumsen, J. F., Filteau, S. M., Coutsoudis, A., Uebel, K. E., Newell, M. L., & Tomkins, A. M. (2000). Subclinical mastitis as a risk factor for mother–infant HIV transmission. *Advances in Experimental Medicine and Biology, 478,* 211–223.

Wilson-Clay, B. (2008). Case report of methicillin-resistant *Staphylococcus aureus* (MRSA) mastitis with abscess formation in a breastfeeding woman. *Journal of Human Lactation, 24,* 326–329.

Wilson-Clay, B., & Hoover, K. (2002). *The breastfeeding atlas* (2nd ed.). Austin, TX: LactNews Press.

Wilson-Clay, B., & Hoover, K. (2008). *The breastfeeding atlas* (4th ed.). Austin, TX: LactNews Press.

Winkler, J. M. (1964). Galactocele of the breast. *American Journal of Surgery, 108,* 357–360.

Witt, A. M., Bolman, M., Kredit, S., & Vanic, A. (2016). Therapeutic breast massage in lactation for the management of engorgement, plugged ducts, and mastitis. *Journal of Human Lactation, 32,* 123–131.

Witt, A. M., Burgess, K., Hawn, T. R., & Zyzanski, S. (2014). Role of oral antibiotics in treatment of breastfeeding women with chronic breast pain who fail conservative therapy. *Breastfeeding Medicine, 9,* 63–72.

Wockel, A., Beggel, A., Rucke, M., Abou-Dakn, M., & Arck, P. (2010). Predictors of inflammatory breast diseases during lactation: Results of a cohort study. *American Journal of Reproductive Immunology, 63,* 28–37.

Woolridge, M. W. (1986). Aetiology of sore nipples. *Midwifery, 2,* 172–176.

World Health Organization. (2000). *Mastitis: Causes and management.* Geneva, Switzerland: Author.

Wu, M., Chason, R., & Wong, M. (2012). Raynaud's phenomenon of the nipple. *Obstetrics and Gynecology, 119,* 447–449.

Yeung, D., Pennell, M., Leung, M., & Hall, J. (1981). Breastfeeding: Prevalence and influencing factors. *Canadian Journal of Public Health, 72,* 323–330.

Zanardo, V., Giarrizzo, D., Maiolo, L., & Straface, G. (2016). Efficacy of topical application of emu oil on areola skin barrier in breastfeeding women. *Journal of Evidence-Based Complementary & Alternative Medicine, 21,* 10–13.

Zhao, C., Tang, R., Wang, J., Guan, X., Zheng, J., Hu, J., . . . Song, C. (2014). Six-step recanalization manual therapy: A novel method for treating plugged ducts in lactating women. *Journal of Human Lactation, 30,* 324–330.

Ziemer, M., Paone, J., Schupay, J., & Cole, E. (1990). Methods to prevent and manage nipple pain in breastfeeding women. *Western Journal of Nursing Research, 12,* 732–744.

Ziemer, M. M., Cooper, D. M., & Pigeon, J. G. (1995). Evaluation of a dressing to reduce nipple pain and improve nipple skin condition in breastfeeding women. *Nursing Research, 44,* 347–351.

Ziemer, M. M., & Pigeon, J. G. (1993). Skin changes and pain in the nipple during the 1st week of lactation. *Journal of Obstetric, Gynecologic, and Neonatal Nursing, 22,* 247–256.

ADDITIONAL READING AND RESOURCES

Academy of Breastfeeding Medicine

Protocol #4: Mastitis

Protocol #11: Neonatal Ankyloglossia

Protocol #20: Engorgement

http://www.bfmed.org

Walker, M. (2010). *The nipple and areola in breastfeeding and lactation: Anatomy, physiology, problems, and solutions.* Amarillo, TX: Hale Publishing.

Appendix 8-1

Summary Questions for Breastfeeding Troubleshooting and Observation

Questions for troubleshooting the underlying cause of inflammatory or infective processes in the breast:

- Have there been skipped or hurried feedings that leave large amounts of residual milk in the breast?
- Is there a time limitation placed on the first breast so the infant will take the other side?
- Is an older infant sleeping longer at night?
- Are there restrictions on the number of times the infant is fed each 24 hours?
- Is the mother unable to express milk at her place of employment?
- Is there a plugged milk duct or blocked nipple pore?
- Are the nipples sore, cracked, or bleeding?
- Has the infant been given bottles or pacifiers?
- Has the infant started solid foods (either at the appropriate age of about 6 months or in a younger infant to urge him or her to sleep longer)?
- Does the mother use nipple shields?
- Is the infant an effective feeder and gaining weight appropriately?
- Has the mother been attending or hosting holiday or family functions?
- Has the mother been ill, stressed, or extremely fatigued?
- Does the mother have preexisting breast lesions such as fibroadenomas?
- Does the mother smoke?
- Has the mother previously had mastitis?

Checkpoints for feeding observation at the breast:

- Is the infant positioned and latched correctly?
- Is there milk transfer verified by audible swallowing or pre- and postfeed weight checks?
- Have all areas of the breast been drained after the feeding or can areas of stasis be felt upon palpation?
- Is there nipple pain during the feeding?
- Is the nipple creased, compressed, distorted, or in spasm when the infant comes off the breast?
- Does the infant suck in a weak or uncoordinated manner that leaves large milk residuals in the breast?

Chapter 9

Physical, Medical, Emotional, and Environmental Challenges to the Breastfeeding Mother

INTRODUCTION

A mother may encounter a variety of challenges to breastfeeding depending on her own health and the environment in which she lives. With support and good clinical management, most mothers are capable of breastfeeding or providing breastmilk in spite of these difficulties or conditions.

PHYSICALLY CHALLENGED MOTHERS

There are approximately 4.1 million (6.2%) parents with disabilities who have children under age 18 living at home with them (Kaye, 2012). Physical challenges to mothers may include many types of impairments, including spinal cord injury, loss of limbs or loss of the use of limbs from accidents or disease, and visual or hearing impairments. Breastfeeding is usually possible and should be encouraged for both the empowerment of the mothers and the close mother–baby relationship it engenders. Breastfeeding is often more convenient, time-saving, economical, and safer than mixing bottles of formula, especially if a mother is visually impaired or has physical difficulty in mixing, measuring, and pouring. Holding a bottle for prolonged periods of time may be difficult with arm, wrist, or hand impairment or loss.

Spinal Cord Injury or Involvement

The course of lactation for mothers with spinal cord injury depends on the location and extent of the injury. The spinal column consists of 33 vertebrae: 7 cervical (neck), 12 thoracic (trunk), 5 lumbar (back), 5 sacral (lower back), and 4 coccygeal (tailbone). Thirty-one pairs of spinal nerves exit the spinal cord and surrounding vertebrae and innervate the trunk and limbs. Complete spinal cord injury means that there is loss of sensory and motor function at and below the level of injury, whereas an incomplete injury results in some sensory or motor function at and below the level of injury. Injury to the cervical area (C-1–3) results in the inability to breathe independently, whereas injury at C-6–8 allows good upper extremity use; injury at T-1 results in paraplegia. For a breastfeeding woman, injury at the T-6 level and above may affect milk production because disruption occurs in the communication between the nipple, myoepithelial cells, and pituitary gland. A T-6 level injury or above may result in diminished milk production by 6 weeks postpartum due to disrupted sympathetic nervous system feedback (Craig, 1990) and cessation of lactation by 3 months or so from the concomitant lack of nipple stimulation (Sipski, 1991). Nipple stimulation is not effective in the feedback loop unless the injury is at or below the point of origin for the fourth, fifth, and sixth intercostal nerves (T-4–6) that innervate the breast and nipple (Cesario, 2002; Halbert, 1998). Sucking-induced afferent stimuli are absent in women with spinal cord injury above T-4 and reduced if the injury is between T-4 and T-6. A spinal cord injury at the T-6 level or higher places the mother at risk for autonomic dysreflexia, a condition caused by noxious stimuli below the level of injury that can result in headaches, severe high blood pressure, stroke, coma, or death. Mothers with a T-6 or higher injury usually receive an epidural during labor to avoid this. Although rare, breastfeeding has been reported as an unusual and unexpected cause of autonomic dysreflexia (Dakhil-Jerew, Brook, & Derry, 2008).

Mothers with an incomplete spinal cord lesion, such as Brown-Sequard-plus syndrome, may be able to breastfeed at least partially. This syndrome may range from mild to severe, such that one side of the body may suffer loss of sensation, pain, and tone. Mothers with Brown-Sequard-plus syndrome should certainly be encouraged to breastfeed, but the breast on the affected side may fail to produce much milk. Not only motor and sensory dysfunction may be absent, but the autonomic control that would contribute to asymmetric lactation may be lacking. In a case study of a mother with Brown-Sequard-plus syndrome, milk production in the breast on the affected side was reduced by 83% (Liu & Krassioukov, 2013). Even though supplementation may be necessary, mothers with this condition may be able to partially breastfeed and enjoy the experience, and their infants will benefit from any amount of breastmilk that can be provided. There may be a sufficient volume of milk available in the early weeks to help program the infant's immune system, which is a definite benefit.

Breastfeeding Management

Positioning considerations depend on the level and extent of the injury. Nursing bras should be chosen with elastic or Velcro closures if the mother's arms are affected. Some mothers set up a "nursing nest" on the floor where feedings as well as diapering and other caretaking activities are done to avoid issues with lifting and transferring the infant. Breastfeeding guidelines should be directed toward maximizing milk production and even pumping and freezing surplus milk to extend the period of time for full breastmilk feeding. In a mother with lesions at T-6 or higher, every effort should be made to avoid sore, cracked, or damaged nipples because this can be a trigger for autonomic dysreflexia. Positioning, latch, and proper sucking are important right from the start and should be immediately corrected if causing sore nipples. If nipple pain becomes a significant problem at each feeding, the mother may need medications for autonomic dysreflexia or may need to pump or hand express breastmilk until the nipples are healed.

Weight gain should be watched closely in infants of mothers with spinal cord injury; occasionally, some mothers may not experience the milk-ejection reflex when the infant is at the breast. Oxytocin nasal spray can be prescribed and obtained from a compounding pharmacy for use before each feeding. Some mothers find that mental imaging and relaxation techniques combined with oxytocin nasal spray help maintain long-term breastfeeding (Cowley, 2005).

Limb Deficiencies, Abnormalities, or Absence

Limb abnormalities may be congenital or occur as a result of disease or injury. Limited use of arms may also occur as a result of a cerebral vascular accident or stroke. A major problem for the breastfeeding mother with an above- or below-the-elbow limb absence is positioning the infant at the breast. Some mothers may use a prosthesis, whereas others may find it more difficult to position a wiggling infant and control the prosthesis simultaneously. The father of the infant and/or other helpers can be shown how to assist the infant to the breast. Mothers usually develop their own systems for positioning the infant at the breast. Although mothers are usually advised to bring the infant to the breast, a mother with a limb abnormality sometimes finds it more efficient to bring the breast to the infant. Thomson (1995) described a mother with the absence of her left forearm sitting upright, using a pillow on her lap, shaping the breast, and placing it in the infant's mouth by leaning forward. The infant can also be positioned straddled across the thigh. The infant could be seated and supported in an infant seat with the mother bringing each breast to the infant. Mothers with good leg flexibility can sit in bed, on the floor, or on a couch with their knees bent and the infant placed in their lap, facing the breasts. Some mothers find that a sling is easier for them to use for both feeding and transporting the infant. Breastfeeding for mothers with physical challenges provides a unique connection between the mother and infant. This helps avoid maternal–child distancing that could occur if someone else fed the infant by bottle (Dunne & Fuerst, 1995).

Limb function can also be disrupted by a cerebral vascular accident, either occurring before the birth of the infant or during the peripartum period. The occurrence of stroke has been estimated to be between 8.1 per 100,000 pregnancies (Kittner et al., 1996) and 26 per 100,000 deliveries (Jaigobin & Silver, 2000). The risk for stroke seems greatest during the postpartum period, possibly due to the large decrease in blood volume or rapid changes in hormonal status (Kittner & Adams, 1996). The presence of hypercoagulability, preeclampsia, eclampsia, cocaine use, HELLP (hemolysis, elevated liver enzymes, low platelet count) syndrome (Kidner & Flanders-Stepans, 2004), and/or sickle cell disease (Kittner & Adams, 1996) adds to the risk.

Differing effects on sensory capacity and motor function may manifest themselves depending on the type of stroke and the location of the affected area within the brain. A stroke in the left hemisphere of the brain affects the right side of the body, with right-sided weakness or paralysis, right-sided visual problems, speech difficulty, emotional lability, possible attention difficulties, intellectual deficits, and poor judgment. A stroke on the right side of the brain can result in left-sided weakness or paralysis and left-sided visual deficits. Lactation itself should remain intact as long as the function of the hypothalamus and pituitary gland has not been compromised. Sensory interruption to either areola may remove the afferent arc necessary for the release of prolactin from areolar stimulation. However, because the nature of a stroke permits normal functioning on one side, complete function of one breast and its associated sensory pathways may remain intact (Halbert, 1998).

A number of medications, such as those used immediately during a stroke, antihypertensives, and anticoagulants, may remain compatible with breastfeeding. Poststroke medications such as low-dose aspirin should also be safe for the infant. Early interventions may separate the mother and infant, necessitating the possibility of pumping milk when the mother is stabilized. Positioning for breastfeeding requires a creative look at what works best. Mothers may lie on the affected side while using the unaffected arm for support and positioning the infant. A nursing pillow, sling, or other supportive piece of equipment may be needed for the mother to safely hold the infant while breastfeeding. Oxytocin release may be beneficial to the mother with a stroke because it lowers blood pressure and exerts a calming effect. Close attention should also center on infant weight gain and adequacy of the milk supply if one breast does not produce an abundant amount of milk. Clinicians need to assess any deficits in the mother's field of vision because she may be unable to see the infant in certain nursing positions.

EPILEPSY

Seizure disorders affect approximately 1.1 million women of reproductive age in the United States (Pschirrer, 2004), with about 20,000 of these women giving birth each year. Although most women with epilepsy can conceive and bear normal, healthy children, their pregnancies present a greater risk for complications. One-fourth to one-half of women with epilepsy may experience an exacerbation of their seizures during pregnancy, mostly toward the end of the pregnancy, with about 31% experiencing this increase during their first trimester (Yerby, Kaplan, & Tran, 2004). This is frequently due to the decline in plasma concentrations of antiepileptic medications, even with correct or increasing doses. Maternal seizures increase the risk of injury, miscarriage, and epilepsy and developmental delay in the children.

Many medications are used either singly or in combination to control the numerous types of seizures, with specific medications used for specific seizure types. First-generation antiepileptic drugs include carbamazepine (Tegretol), ethosuximide (Zarontin), phenobarbital (Liminal), phenytoin (Dilantin), primidone (Myidone), and valproic acid (Depakene, Depakote). Seizure activity during pregnancy and some antiepileptic medications place infants at risk for a number of complications. Infants of mothers with epilepsy are at increased risk for congenital malformations (orofacial clefts and congenital heart disease) and anomalies (dysmorphic facial features), neural tube defects, neonatal hemorrhage, low-birth-weight, developmental delay, and childhood epilepsy. Antiepileptic medication monotherapy causes fewer birth defects compared with therapy that involves the use of more than one medication. The risk for infant birth defects is increased with each additional drug included in the regimen (Ozdemir, Sari, Kurt, Sakar, & Atalay, 2015).

Several clinical syndromes have been described in infants of mothers with epilepsy, with learning and behavioral disturbances prominent aspects of these syndromes (Moore et al., 2000). The medication primidone (Myidone), especially when used in combination with other drugs, is associated with lower intelligence scores in school-aged children (Koch et al., 1999). Lower cognitive scores have also been seen in children whose mothers took valproate (Meador et al., 2009). This makes it extremely important that infants of mothers with epilepsy are breastfed or provided with as much mother's milk as possible. Meador and colleagues (2008) demonstrated that children of mothers with epilepsy who had been breastfed had better cognitive scores than those who were bottle-fed. Meador and colleagues (2010) studied the effects on IQ in children whose breastfeeding mothers took carbamazepine, lamotrigine, phenytoin, or valproate. Results showed no deleterious effects on cognitive outcomes when mothers were receiving a single antiepileptic drug during pregnancy and lactation. IQ in children at 6 years of age was enhanced when breastfed as an infant by a mother with epilepsy. At age 6 months, infants who were exposed to antiepileptic medications prenatally had a higher risk of impaired fine motor skills and social skills. Breastfeeding was associated with less impaired development at 6 months and 18 months compared with those infants who breastfed less than 6 months or did not breastfeed at all (Veiby, Engelsen, & Gilhus, 2013).

There are no medical contraindications to breastfeeding when a mother has epilepsy (Crawford, 2009). A number of newer or second-generation antiepileptic drugs with limited data on their safety have been marketed in the United States since 1993, including gabapentin (Neurontin), felbamate (Felbatol), lamotrigine (Lamictal), levetiracetam (Keppra), oxcarbazepine (Trileptal), tiagabine (Gabitril), topiramate (Topamax), and zonisamide (Zonegran). Breastfeeding mothers taking phenobarbital or primidone may have infants who are sedated by the medications and should be monitored for adequate intake and weight gain. Infants whose mothers are taking lamotrigine should be monitored, as some infants display significant plasma levels of this medication. This is probably due to genetic variations among infants in their drug-metabolizing capabilities (Chen, Liu, Yoshida, & Kaneko, 2010). Taking antiepileptic medications is not considered a contraindication to breastfeeding (Delgado-Escueta & Janz, 1992; Veiby, Bjørk, Engelsen, & Gilhus, 2015), with infant reactions to maternal medications usually far outweighed by the benefits of breastfeeding and human milk (Ito, Moretti, Liau, & Koren, 1995). In fact, breastfeeding may reverse the cognitive impairment associated with prenatal exposure to antiepileptic drugs such as valproate (Meador et al., 2010). Breastfeeding should be encouraged by all members of the healthcare team, including neurologists (Geller, Yagil, Biriotto, & Neufeld, 2013; Meador et al., 2014).

Lack of sleep and missed medications in the postpartum period increase the risk for seizures. If mothers experience increased seizure activity due to sleep deprivation they can express extra milk during the day and have it fed to their infant at night to avoid sleep disruption. Mothers with epilepsy (especially if the mother experiences no aura or warning of an impending seizure) may wish to have helpers during the early weeks to assure safety of both mother and infant should a seizure occur during infant caretaking activities (Klein, 2012).

MATERNAL VISUAL OR HEARING IMPAIRMENT

Visual or hearing impairment is not a contraindication to breastfeeding. Mothers with limited or no sight or with limited or no hearing use their intact senses to interact with their infant. The senses of touch, taste, and smell as well as the mother's intuitive sensitivity contribute to facilitate breastfeeding (Martin Cookson, 1992). For visually impaired mothers, breastfeeding avoids the problems of preparing and cleaning bottles of formula. Feeding cues are recognized easily when a mother carries her infant in a sling or front pack carrier. Breastfeeding consultation can be accomplished in sign language for hearing-impaired mothers (Bowles, 1991). While deaf mothers may have limited access to audio materials, several support mechanisms can be accessed, such as fellow deaf community mothers, healthcare providers who are fluent in American Sign Language, YouTube videos, Facebook sharing, and the use of sign language interpreters (Chin et al., 2013). Materials written in Braille are available from La Leche League International for mothers who have limited or no sight. Not all mothers with visual or hearing impairment are totally blind or totally deaf. If a mother appears to have trouble understanding what is being said to her, ask if she has a visual or hearing impairment. Some mothers are embarrassed or find it difficult to ask for help.

INSUFFICIENT MILK SUPPLY

There are no specific diagnostic tests for lactation sufficiency. Insufficient milk supply, either real or perceived, remains the most frequent reason for the abandonment of breastfeeding (Ahluwalia, Morrow, & Hsia, 2005; Gatti, 2008; Li, Fein, Chen, & Grummer-Strawn, 2008; Segura-Millan, Dewey, & Perez-Escamilla, 1994; Verronen, 1982).

The perception of insufficient milk may begin within the first 48 hours after delivery when clinicians and mothers are unaware of the normal amounts of colostrum available to the infant as well as the infant's small stomach capacity. Attempts at pumping the breasts at this time often yield only drops of colostrum, further reinforcing the appearance of insufficient milk. Mothers' perceptions of insufficient milk commonly encompass the lack of fullness in the breasts, increased frequency of infant feeding, and an infant who continues to fuss after a feeding or does not settle between feeds. Measurement of infant intake and weight gain during the times of these perceptions (transient lactation crisis) revealed both parameters to be normal variations in infant appetite and behavior (Hillervik-Lindquist, 1991; Hillervik-Lindquist, Hofvander, & Sjolin, 1991). Mothers who describe insufficient milk supply most frequently do so because their infant was not satisfied after a feeding and, as a result, offer a bottle of formula as a complement after a breastfeeding (Hill & Aldag, 1991).

Although mothers most commonly report infant crying as the cue used to determine insufficient milk (Huang, Lee, Huang, & Gau, 2009), actual milk production is seldom assessed nor is the infant's efficiency at milk removal observed. Once crying is perceived as hunger, mothers and healthcare providers often turn to formula supplementation as a remedy to stop the crying and to fill up the infant (Sacco, Caulfield, Gittelsohn, & Martinez, 2006). Supplementing with bottles of formula has the potential to depress milk production and result in a real milk-supply problem. Maternal descriptions of insufficient milk are not only based on a perception of too little milk being produced for appropriate infant weight gain and for infant satisfaction (Hill & Humenick, 1989), but also as doubts in maternal self-efficacy (McCarter-Spaulding & Kearney, 2001).

Overlapping etiologies exist for the development of real or perceived insufficient milk. The most common overarching contributors are mismanagement of breastfeeding (Powers, 1999) and lack of information (Hill, 1991). A number of factors may contribute to insufficient milk, either real or perceived:

- Breastfeeding mismanagement may include a limited number of feedings, short times at the breast, scheduled feedings that do not coincide with the infant's behavioral feeding-readiness cues, poor latch, failure to assess for swallowing, inappropriate formula supplementation, unrelieved severe engorgement, and use of artificial nipples and pacifiers.
- Maternal conditions may include overweight/obesity and diabetes (Neubauer et al., 1993) that delay lactogenesis II, history of breast surgery or breast reduction (Hill, Wilhelm, Aldag, & Chatterton, 2004; Hughes & Owen, 1993), retained placental fragments, breast hypoplasia (Neifert et al., 1990; Neifert, Seacat, & Jobe, 1985), use of certain medications such as pseudoephedrine (Sudafed; Aljazaf et al., 2003) or ergot alkaloids, maternal smoking (Hopkinson, Schanler, Fraley, & Garza, 1992), oral contraceptives (Kennedy, Short, & Tully, 1997), inverted nipples, Sheehan syndrome (Sert, Tetiker, Kirim, & Kocak, 2003) or maternal postpartum

hemorrhage (Willis & Livingstone, 1995), anemia (Henly et al., 1995), and endocrine problems such as hypothyroidism or polycystic ovary syndrome (Marasco, Marmet, & Shell, 2000).

- Situations where the mother must initiate lactation in the absence of the infant at the breast such as prematurity can place the mother at a 2.8 times increased risk for insufficient milk (Hill, Aldag, Chatterton, & Zinaman, 2005). Milk output during the first 6 weeks predicts feeding method at week 12 (Hill, Aldag, Zinaman, & Chatterton, 2007). Other contributors to insufficient milk production include infant conditions and diseases that preclude direct feeding from the breast or result in ineffective feedings, long-term pumping situations such as a hospitalized infant or a mother returning to employment, use of a poor breast pump or a poorly fitted flange on a breast pump, not enough pumping, exposure to acute or long-term stressors (Hill, Chatterton, & Aldag, 2003), and stressful labor and delivery (Chen, Nommsen-Rivers, Dewey, & Lonnerdal, 1998).
- Genetic variables may play a part in mothers with insufficient milk production that does not respond to typical interventions or to medications or other galactagogues. Mutation of the protein ZnT2, which transports zinc in specific body tissues, may result in not only decreased zinc levels in the milk but also functional problems in the development of the breast itself, leading to insufficient milk production (Lee, Hennigar, Alam, Nishida, & Kelleher, 2015). Genetic variations in ZnT2 may modify milk production and the Zn level in breastmilk could serve as a biomarker of breast function during lactation (Alam, Hennigar, Gallagher, Soybel, & Kelleher, 2015). While abnormalities in breastmilk Zn levels do not automatically imply a milk production problem, testing breastmilk Zn levels in mothers at high risk for insufficient milk production, or when this condition exists, may help isolate a potential cause of this problem. Women diagnosed with low milk supply were shown to be significantly more likely to have had diabetes in pregnancy compared with other mothers who experienced any type of lactation difficulty (Riddle & Nommsen-Rivers, 2016). Women with decreased insulin sensitivity may experience a slower and less robust increase in milk output as a result of overexpression of protein tyrosine phosphatase receptor type F (PTPRF) in the mammary gland (Lemay et al., 2013). These genetic alterations are not always readily apparent and may occasionally preclude the development of full milk production.

Indicators or signs and symptoms of insufficient milk may not be clearly evident. Assumptions of insufficient milk are often made if the infant loses more than 7% of birth weight and fails to regain birth weight by 2 weeks. However, this may also indicate an infant with poor breastfeeding skills who is unable to transfer milk even when there is an abundant supply. Weight gain of less than 5 oz per week; concentrated urine in the diapers; passing of dry, hard stools; lethargy; and dry mucous membranes signal a potential problem with either milk transfer or milk supply and require assessment and intervention (Amir, 2006). Infants who sleep excessively or who feed for longer than 45 minutes at a feed or appear to want to nurse continuously signal the need for a feeding observation. Mothers who have been pumping regularly and report a drop in the amount of milk pumped may be experiencing transient fluctuation in milk output, especially if their hospitalized infant's condition has deteriorated. This can happen early in lactation during the establishment of optimal milk production or later in lactation as a pump motor wears out.

Breastfeeding Management

Clinicians should first assess the infant during a breastfeeding to ascertain the status and amount of milk transfer. Pre- and postfeed weights can verify the amount of milk transfer following a single feeding. Twenty-four-hour pre- and postfeed weights provide a more accurate measurement of actual milk production (Kent, Prime, & Garbin, 2012). Faulty sucking skills, oral anomalies, and poor positioning may be recognized and remedied at this time.

Management options depend on the cause of the milk insufficiency. Clinicians could select options or combinations of options that best fit the etiology of the problem:

- Extra feedings (Decarvalho, Robertson, Friedman, & Klaus, 1983), extra pumpings, pumping after a feeding, improving infant positioning (Morton, 1992), and assisting milk transfer of the infant by using alternate massage (Lau & Hurst, 1999; Yokoyama, Ueda, Irahara, & Aono, 1994) can be used.
- Mothers can use alternate massage on each breast at each feeding to increase milk transfer and milk production. Breast massage should also be used while pumping.
- Mothers can use a tube-feeding device at the breast to deliver milk to the infant while the infant stimulates the breast.
- Mothers of preterm infants should be encouraged to engage in skin-to-skin care while their infant is hospitalized because this has been shown to improve milk output (Hurst, Valentine, Renfro, Burns, & Ferlic, 1997). They can also pump next to their infant's bed while looking at or touching their infant.
- The increased use of an effective, electric, hospital-grade breast pump with double collection kit and properly fitted breast flange should be considered. Mothers may need flange sizes greater than 24 mm. Prime, Geddes, Spatz, Trengove, and Hartmann (2010) showed that mothers with high intraglandular fat removed the highest percentage of available milk with larger flanges (> 30 mm). Most of the mothers in their study of flange sizes and milk removal removed their highest percentage of available milk with flanges larger than 24 mm. Check the vacuum with a vacuum gauge to ensure the pump is operating efficiently.
- Have the mother warm the pump flange prior to placing it on her breast to improve the efficiency of milk removal (Kent, Geddes, Hepworth, & Hartmann, 2011). Warm compresses on the breast may also be helpful.
- Consider the use of relaxation techniques such as listening to a guided-imagery audio recording (Feher, Berger, Johnson, & Wilde, 1989).
- Mothers who smoke should be encouraged to quit or reduce the number of cigarettes smoked per day. Smoking should not occur directly before a feeding as it may inhibit the letdown reflex.
- Medications have been used to improve milk production (Gabay, 2002); however, many studies on the use of metoclopramide and other medical galactagogues suffer from poor methodology and conflicting results, with some finding that pharmaceutical galactagogues made no difference in lactation success (Anderson & Valdes, 2007). Parity may also influence the effectiveness of these medications. Brown, Fernandes, Grant, Hutsul, & McCoshen (2000) administered single doses of two strengths of metoclopramide and a single dose of domperidone to

nonpregnant women. Nulliparous women had the highest prolactin secretion with the 10-mg metoclopramide dose and multiparous women had prolactin secretion patterns that were equivalent between the medications. Medications could be selected for mothers who do not respond to other interventions:

- Metoclopramide (Reglan), a dopamine antagonist (dopamine is a physiological inhibitor of prolactin), has been shown to stimulate basal prolactin levels, leading to increased milk production at doses of 30–45 mg/day (Budd, Erdman, Long, Trombley, & Udall, 1993; Ehrenkranz & Ackerman, 1986; Gupta & Gupta, 1985; Kauppila et al., 1983). Metoclopramide is dose dependent, with some mothers not responding, especially if their prolactin levels are normal (Kauppila et al., 1983). Fife and colleagues (2011) gave preterm mothers a 10-mg dose of metoclopramide 3 times daily for 8 days starting within 36 hours of birth compared with a control group who received a placebo. They reported no significant difference in milk production between the 2 groups at the end of 8 days. This outcome could have resulted from a dose that was too low or the fact that none of the mothers was already experiencing milk production problems. It may be wise to do plasma prolactin levels on mothers prior to recommending metoclopramide therapy to assess the potential response to the medication. Maternal side effects of metoclopramide include gastric cramping, diarrhea, and depression with longer term use (more than 4 weeks), but no untoward effects have been reported in infants (Hale, 2012). Metoclopramide may not be the best choice for mothers who are experiencing depression. Abrupt discontinuation of the medication can result in a precipitous drop in milk production; tapering the dosage by decreasing it 10 mg/week is recommended. The Food and Drug Administration (FDA) issued a black box warning for use of metoclopramide due to its association with tardive dyskinesia (involuntary, repetitive body movements) when used for more than 3 months.
- Domperidone (Motilium) is a peripheral dopamine antagonist similar to metoclopramide. However, unlike metoclopramide it does not cross the blood–brain barrier as it is less soluble, has a higher molecular weight, and binds to plasma protein more strongly. These features reduce the likelihood of central nervous system side effects such as depression as seen in some mothers using metoclopramide. This also reduces adverse extrapyramidal effects (such as tardive dyskinesia), making domperidone a good alternative to metoclopramide (Zuppa et al., 2010). Domperidone produces significant increases in prolactin levels (Newman, 1998) and stimulates milk production at doses of 10–20 mg three to four times daily without maternal gastric side effects. Not all mothers respond to the use of domperidone, but for those who do, there is somewhat of a dose–response relationship, with higher doses resulting in more milk production (Wan et al., 2008). Knoppert and colleagues (2013) compared the effect of 2 different doses of domperidone on milk supply over a 6-week period (10 mg 3 times daily and 20 mg 3 times daily). Daily milk volumes were more than 300 mL higher in the 20-mg dosing group. There have been no reported effects on the infant and it is considered a better choice as a galactagogue (Brouwers, Assies, Wiersinga, Huizing, & Tytgat, 1980; Brown et al., 2000; da Silva, Knoppert, Angelini, & Forret, 2001; Hofmeyr & van Iddekinge, 1983; Hofmeyr, van Iddekinge, & Blott, 1985;

Petraglia et al., 1985). Domperidone has been shown to significantly increase milk volume in full-term mothers who have experienced a cesarean delivery (Jantarasaengaram & Sreewapa, 2012). Osadchy, Moretti, and Koren (2012) found that in a meta-analysis of high-quality studies on domperidone, an increase of 74.72% was seen in daily milk production in mothers treated with this medication compared with placebo-treated mothers. This outcome was deemed as clinically meaningful in that there was a consistency in positive outcomes within the high quality of evidence studied. Domperidone has been shown to be slightly more effective in increasing milk production compared to metoclopramide (Ingram, Taylor, Churchill, Pike, & Greenwood, 2012).

A systematic review of domperidone showed that the safety profile of the drug for both mother and infant was mostly positive (Paul et al., 2015). However, domperidone is contraindicated if the mother is taking other medications with anticholinergic properties because these may antagonize the effects on the gastrointestinal tract. Domperidone should not be prescribed if the mother is taking medications that could alter the metabolism of domperidone such as antacids, histamine antagonists, proton pump inhibitors, anifungal medications, macrolide antibiotics, and monoamine oxidase inhibitors. Mothers with cardiac disease or conditions should avoid this drug as it has been associated with cardiac arrhythmias. Domperidone should not be administered to mothers with preexisting QT prolongation, with electrolyte abnormalities, or with other risk factors for QT prolongation (Doggrell & Hancox, 2014).

It is recommended that once milk production is satisfactory, mothers should taper off domperidone slowly rather than stopping its use abruptly, so as not to depress milk production. It is also important to slowly taper off the medication after long-term use to avoid withdrawal symptoms (Papstergiou, Abdallah, Tran, & Folkins, 2013).

The galactagogue effects of domperidone may not be seen for 3–4 days, with the maximum effect taking up to 2–3 weeks (Henderson, 2003a). Most mothers take the medication for 3–8 weeks. Domperidone prescribed as a galactagogue is an off-label use of the drug. Although not available in the United States, some compounding pharmacies may still be able to formulate domperidone with a physician's prescription. In countries where domperidone is readily available, its use has increased, sometimes before other nonpharmacological interventions have been exhausted (Grzeskowiak, Lim, Thomas, Ritchie, & Gordon, 2013). There are no consistent guidelines as to when to start domperidone therapy in either primiparous or multiparous mothers. Preterm birth and neonatal hospitalization are strong factors associated with receiving domperidone (Grzeskowiak, Dalton, & Fielder, 2015).

Haase, Taylor, Mauldin, Johnson, & Wagner (2016) have created a domperidone treatment protocol for pump-dependent mothers of preterm infants that includes a set of standing orders, a consent for treatment, and an information handout. These documents will be helpful for clinicians wishing to include the use of domperidone in their practice.

- Human growth hormone has been used to successfully increase milk production in mothers of term and preterm infants, with (Gunn et al., 1996; Milsom, Rabone, Gunn, & Gluckman, 1998) and without (Breier et al., 1993; Milsom et al., 1992) lactation insufficiency.

Results are dose dependent with no maternal or infant side effects reported over a 7-day study period.

- Oxytocin, although normally used to elicit the milk-ejection reflex, has also been shown to improve milk production in older studies (Ruis, Rolland, Doesburg, Broeders, & Corbey, 1981). An appropriate dose of sublingual or buccal (not nasal) oxytocin may help improve milk output, especially in pump-dependent mothers, but should not replace proper breastfeeding and pumping guidelines (Renfrew, Lang, & Woolridge, 2000).
- Thyrotropin-releasing hormone has been minimally studied and shown to significantly improve milk production in mothers with lactation insufficiency, with little effect on normally lactating mothers (Tyson, Perez, & Zanartu, 1976).
- Recombinant human prolactin was studied in non-postpartum women and showed expressible galactorrhea over a 7-day study period as a viable option for short-term lactation augmentation (Page-Wilson, Smith, & Welt, 2007). Powe and colleagues (2010) demonstrated that twice-daily doses of recombinant human prolactin significantly increased milk volume in mothers with prolactin deficiency and in preterm mothers with lactation insufficiency. Powe and colleagues (2011) showed that treatment of mothers with lactation insufficiency and prolactin deficiency with recombinant prolactin increased baseline and peak prolactin levels to those seen during normal lactogenesis. Treatment increased milk volume as well as lactose and calcium concentrations in the milk. Sodium levels fell and all were within normal limits. Treatment was associated with milk composition changes that match those in mothers with normal lactogenesis during the first 2–10 days following delivery. Treatment with recombinant prolactin also increased oligosaccharide levels, potentially improving the immune properties of the milk. Mothers and infants experienced no side effects. This is a promising treatment, especially for mothers of preterm infants who will benefit from both the increased volume of milk and the enhanced ability of the milk to provide immune protection to the infant.

- Acupuncture is an ancient and effective treatment used in China for insufficient milk (Zhao & Guo, 2006). Clavey (1996) discussed the procedure and reported a more than 90% effectiveness rate when acupuncture was initiated within 20 days of birth but less than an 85% success rate after 20 days postpartum. The earlier postpartum the treatment is begun, the quicker the results and the more likely that milk production will significantly improve. Wei, Wang, Han, and Li (2008) described the very effective use of electro-acupuncture at Shaoze (SI 1) in 46 mothers with insufficient milk. Acupuncture delivered for 3 weeks postpartum in a small group of mothers was significantly more effective in preserving exclusive breastfeeding for 3 months than in a control group who received no acupuncture treatments (Neri et al., 2011).
- Acupressure is a form of Chinese traditional medicine that involves placing pressure on specific acupoints in various places on the body. In a randomized clinical trial, acupressure was shown to be an effective noninvasive means of improving milk production (Esfahani, Berenji-Sooghe, Valiani, & Ehsanpour, 2015). The acupoints used were GB20 (in a depression between the upper portion of the sternocleidomastoid muscle and the trapezius on the same level with GV16), acupoint LI4 (on the dorsum of the hand, between the first and second metacarpal bones), and

acupoint SI1 (1 cm posterior to the corner of the nail on the upper side of the little finger). The mothers were educated to press the acupoints on both sides of the body 3 times per day, each time for 2–5 minutes, and for 12 sequential days. The level of pressure was sufficient to cause the nail of the pressing thumb to become pale. Significantly more milk was produced in the group that received the acupressure intervention compared with a control group who did not utilize acupressure.

- Herbal and botanical preparations have been used since antiquity to stimulate milk production. Although there is little science behind the use of most of these preparations or their effectiveness, many herbs and herbal preparation are widely used for improving milk output. This is in spite of the lack of high-quality clinical trials and evidence supporting the safety of their use (Amer, Cipriano, Venci, & Gandhi, 2015). While some healthcare providers recommend the use of herbal galactagogues, most mothers use herbal remedies based on recommendations from family members and friends (Sim, Sherriff, Hattingh, Parsons, & Tee, 2013). Many mothers have a high comfort level with the use of herbal preparations and feel empowered and confident when taking these preparations. Herbal supplements may also have a psychological effect on breastfeeding mothers, boosting their self-efficacy, which in turn may contribute to improved breastfeeding outcomes (Sim, Hattingh, Sherriff, & Tee, 2015).

  In the United States, herbs are classified as nutritional supplements and do not require FDA approval, nor do they need to demonstrate evidence of safety or efficacy. Nice (2011) reminds clinicians that because there is little oversight regarding herbals, active ingredients may be present in more or less amounts than the package label states and that strengths of the ingredients may vary depending on the particular plant used or the parts of the plant that are contained in the package. It is estimated that at least 15% of breastfeeding women use herbal galactagogues at some point (National Children's Study, 2003). Some herbals include fenugreek, milk thistle, raspberry leaf, and nettle; however, a number are unsafe for lactating women (Low Dog & Micozzi, 2005). Other herbal galactagogues frequently seen are goat's rue, fennel seed, chaste tree seed, fireweed, anise seed, blessed thistle, stinging nettle, and cotton root (Bingel & Farnsworth, 1994). Many of these herbs are combined in commercial galactagogue preparations such as Mother's Milk herbal blend tea (red raspberry leaf, fennel seed, nettle leaf, alfalfa leaf, blessed thistle, dandelion leaf, and fenugreek seed powder), More Milk Plus by Motherlove (a tincture blend of fenugreek, blessed thistle, nettle, and fennel), and Mother's Lactaflow (a tincture blend of fennel, blessed thistle, goat's rue, and fenugreek).

  - Fenugreek (*Trigonella foenum-graecum*) is probably the most widely used herbal galactagogue. Fenugreek has been shown to have antianxiety effects, which may contribute to the herb's anecdotal effectiveness (Abascal & Yarnell, 2008). Turkyilmaz and colleagues (2011) showed that mothers who drank fenugreek tea during the early days following birth had increased milk production and infants who lost significantly less weight than controls. A study of 26 mothers of preterm infants who pumped 5 to 7 times each 24 hours and took 1,725 mg of fenugreek daily for 21 days showed no difference in milk production compared to a placebo-controlled group who did not consume fenugreek. Prolactin levels were similar between the two groups (Reeder, LeGrand, & O'Connor-Von, 2013). The dosage of fenugreek is usually one 1,200-mg capsule taken 2–3 times daily.

- Goat's rue (*Galega officinalis*) is a common galactagogue (Weiss, 2001) used historically not only for insufficient milk but also for symptoms of noninsulin-resistant diabetes. Several of the plant's constituents (guanidine and galegine) have been studied as antidiabetic agents, with metformin being a synthetic chemical based on galegine. Goat's rue is dosed as 1 teaspoon of dried herb steeped in 1 cup of water twice daily or 1–2 mL of tincture 3 times daily.
- Fennel seed (*Foeniculum vulgare*) is used to increase milk production at a dose of 5–7 g of seed (as a tea) per day.
- Chaste tree seed (*Vitex adnus-castus*) is used at a dosage of 1 teaspoon of the berries steeped in 1 cup of water 3 times daily or 2.5 mL of tincture 3 times daily.
- Shatavari (*Asparagus racemosus*) has been shown to improve milk production at doses of 60 mg/kg/day (Gupta & Shaw, 2011).
- Milk thistle (*Silybum marianum*) was studied in a micronized 420-mg dose form in women with marginal milk production (Di Pierro, Callegari, Carotenuto, & Tapia, 2008). Fifty mothers (half in the experimental group and half in the placebo group) were treated for 63 days, with an increase of 85.94% of the daily milk production in the treatment group and a 32.09% increase in milk production in the placebo group. It is interesting to note that the herb was micronized before being administered, which improves its poor bioavailability.
- *Moringa oleifera* has been shown to produce a significant improvement in breastmilk volume on day 7 as well as an improvement in infant weight gain (Raguindin, Dans, & King, 2014). This effect may be due to improved prolactin production in the mother's anterior pituitary gland.

Many authors disagree or provide completely contradictory information on the use of various preparations (Humphrey, 2003). Zapantis, Steinberg, and Schilit (2012) caution that there is scare evidence on the safety and effectiveness of many of the herbals associated with improving milk production. Systematic reviews of herbal galactagogues generally acknowledge that it is difficult to develop accurate information on the safety and efficacy of specific herbs taken by breastfeeding mothers (Budzynska, Gardner, Low Dog, & Gardner, 2013; Mortel & Mehta, 2013). This is especially true in the United States, where there are no regulatory guidelines or protocols to determine the safety and efficacy of herbal use during lactation (Budzynska, Gardner, Dugoua, Low Dog, & Gardiner, 2012). Other "remedies" such as beer (hops) and brewer's yeast (vitamin B complex) are sometimes recommended rather than addressing the underlying cause of milk insufficiency. Although herbal and botanical preparations are commonly used, they require caution: Clinicians can refer to the German Commission E Monographs for safety profiles of botanicals (Blumenthal & Busse, 1998), to the American Herbal Products Association (http://www.ahpa.org) for information on manufacturing and labeling standards, and to the American Botanical Council (http://www.herbalgram.org) for information on the quality of herbal products. Some herbals that contain pyrrolizidine alkaloids such as comfrey leaf (*Symphytum officinalis*) and borage leaf (*Borago officinalis*) are well avoided as they have the potential to cause liver damage and cross into breastmilk (Panter & James, 1990).

Medications or herbal preparations should not replace breastfeeding management guidelines tailored to each mother's situation. Any use of a galactagogue requires close follow-up by the clinician of both mother and infant (Academy of Breastfeeding Medicine, 2011).

HYPERLACTATION

Until the breasts calibrate the amount of milk to synthesize based on infant intake, it is possible for a mother to make amounts of milk far in excess of what the infant needs to consume. Milk production late in the first week of lactation ranges from 200–900 mL/day, with a milk synthesis rate of 11–58 mL/hour. When mothers have a high rate of milk synthesis, 60 mL/hour or more, a spectrum of breast and infant signs and symptoms may become apparent (**Box 9-1**), indicating hyperlactation and the need for clinical intervention (Livingstone, 1996).

This particular cluster of signs and symptoms in the infant, as listed in Box 9-1, may mimic lactose intolerance or an infant with uncoordinated sucking. Although lactose intolerance is unlikely, the high-volume, low-fat meals may experience a rapid transit through the gut, causing the green stools as mentioned in Box 9-1. Much of the gas may be the result of both fermentation of lactose and swallowed air from gulping during the fast flow of milk. Choking and sputtering at the breast are usually the result of an infant who is unable to swallow fast enough to accommodate a high flow of fluid into the throat. Mothers may describe the necessity of frequently burping the infant during each feeding as well as removing the infant from the breast several times during the feeding to allow the infant to breathe between periods of rapid milk flow. Oversupply can also mask real problems with sucking coordination, so clinicians should always look for improvement in the condition over time.

Box 9-1 Signs and Symptoms of Hyperlactation

Maternal Breast

- Breasts that never feel comfortable or drained and that refill very quickly
- Shooting pain deep in the breast
- Firm, lumpy, or tender areas
- Chronic plugged ducts or mastitis
- Intense pain with first milk ejection
- Forceful letdown
- Constant leaking between feedings
- Leaking milk prenatally

Infant

- Gulping, choking, or coughing while at the breast
- Milk leaking from the mouth
- Arching back off of the breast, thrashing, difficulty remaining latched to the breast
- Spitting up
- Excessive gas
- Green, frothy, explosive stools that may cause irritating diaper rash
- Excessive infant weight gain
- Poor weight gain or initial good weight gain with slow weight gain later

Galactorrhea can also have nonbreastfeeding etiologies (Pena & Rosenfeld, 2001) that, although rare, should be considered:

- Neoplastic processes (prolactinoma)
- Hypothalamic–pituitary disorders
- Systemic diseases (hypothyroidism, hyperthyroidism, Cushing disease)
- Medications (antidepressants, selective serotonin reuptake inhibitors [SSRIs], antihypertensives)
- Chest wall irritation (ill-fitting clothing or bra, herpes zoster, atopic dermatitis, esophageal reflux)

Thyroid function tests may be in order if other interventions fail to reduce milk production (Trimeloni & Spencer, 2016). Other causes of hyperlactation such as excessive pumping or overuse of galactogogues should be ruled out.

Breastfeeding Management

A number of options and combinations of interventions can be used to form individual feeding plans:

1. Reduce the rate of milk synthesis:
   - Offer one breast per feeding that the infant thoroughly drains (Smillie, Campbell, & Iwinski, 2005). If the infant wishes to return to the breast within an hour or so, the mother can use the same breast. Infants who are switched to the second breast before finishing the first may ingest a high volume of low-fat milk (Woolridge & Fischer, 1988).
   - If the other breast becomes uncomfortable, the mother should express just enough milk to soften the breast.
   - Decrease the frequency of feedings by allowing the infant to become satiated on the fat-rich milk available at the end of the feeding, which is assisted in its availability by the use of alternate massage.
   - Block feeding divides the day into equal time blocks starting with a 3-hour time block, where the same breast is offered for each feeding during the time block. At the start of the next time block, the other breast is offered for each feeding. Time blocks can be gradually lengthened if necessary if the condition does not improve after the first few time blocks. van Veldhuizen-Staas (2007) recommended a protocol of full breast drainage and block feedings where the breasts are as fully drained as possible by pumping before the block feedings begin. They are fully drained/pumped again if they become overfull despite the block feedings.
   - Use of pseudoephedrine (Sudafed) (Aljazaf et al., 2003) can decrease but not eliminate milk production.
   - Herbal treatment includes the use of sage (Bisset, 1994).
   - Some mothers find that drinking peppermint tea lowers their milk output.
   - Cabbage leaves placed inside the bra for extended periods of time have been anecdotally reported to diminish milk production.
   - As a last resort when mothers have not responded to any other treatments or if mothers are attempting to wean without success, cabergoline could be chosen as it inhibits prolactin

secretion by the pituitary (Eglash, 2014). In carefully administered doses, it is possible to lower the prolactin levels to safe ranges, while allowing prolactin levels to remain high enough to facilitate lactation.

2. Management of feedings:
   - Have the mother place the infant in a semiprone position directly facing her breast with the mother leaning back or reclining.
   - The mother can express her milk until after the first milk-ejection reflex, reducing the gush of milk and the forceful flow into the infant's mouth.
   - The mother may need to burp the infant frequently and pace the feeding by allowing the infant to rest between periods of strong milk flow.
   - The mother needs to make sure that any plugged milk ducts or areas of the breast that are not draining well are massaged during the feeding.

INDUCED LACTATION AND RELACTATION

Induced lactation is the initiation of milk production in a woman who has never been pregnant. Women who wish to induce lactation may be infertile, may be adopting an infant, or may be the intended mother of a surrogate pregnancy. Clinicians can help such mothers understand that they may be unable to produce all the milk necessary to meet the infant's needs without supplementation, but they will certainly meet the goal of a wonderful and unique nurturing experience (Wittig & Spatz, 2008). Numerous breast-preparation techniques are used with varying amounts of milk being produced (L. Goldfarb & J. Newman, unpublished data, 2002; Newman & Pittman, 2000). Newman and Goldfarb (2010) have several protocols for inducing lactation, which are varying combinations of medications, pumping, and herbs.

Adopting mothers typically start preparation several months ahead of the scheduled time for receiving the infant by using nipple stimulation (hand or breast pump) and a galactagogue such as metoclopramide (Cheales-Siebenaler, 1999). Szucs, Axline, and Rosenman (2010) report on a mother of adopted twins who successfully induced lactation through a combination of oral contraceptive pills, pumping, domperidone, fenugreek, and blessed thistle. Oxytocin nasal spray is sometimes used before each pumping and breastfeeding session to enhance the milk-ejection reflex and to stimulate milk flow. Protocols for induced lactation typically encourage nipple stimulation, estrogen and progesterone preparations to induce structural changes in the breast (as would happen during pregnancy), use of a dopamine antagonist to increase prolactin levels, and frequent breastfeeding when the infant is available (Bryant, 2006). If the mother is adopting an infant and has a long lead time or is the intended mother of a surrogate pregnancy, she may find the protocol in **Box 9-2** helpful.

However, sometimes adopting mothers are given such short notice of the infant's arrival that neither partial nor full lactation is established and the process proceeds with the infant providing breast stimulation if he or she will latch. Often in this situation, mothers use a tube-feeding system to provide formula supplementation while the infant suckles at the breast. They may follow this with frequent breast pumping and/or the use of galactagogues. Mothers may find that power pumping helps increase milk production. Breastfeeding after a surrogate pregnancy allows a longer period of preparation time to induce lactation before the infant arrives (Biervliet, Maguiness, Hay, Killick, & Atkin, 2001). The composition of milk from an induced lactation is similar to and quite adequate for normal infant growth (Lawrence & Lawrence, 2016).

Box 9-2 Selected Interventions from the Newman Goldfarb Protocols for Induced Lactation®

Time Frame	Intervention
6 months before due date	Take one active birth control pill/day + 10 mg domperidone 4 times/day for 1 week. Increase dosage to 20 mg 4 times/day.
6 weeks before due date	Stop the birth control pill and continue the domperidone and begin breast pumping approximately 8 times/day. Add blessed thistle herb (390 mg/capsule) and fenugreek seed (610 mg/capsule). Take 3 capsules of each 3 times per day with meals.
After birth of infant	Breastfeed as often as possible, continue domperidone, maintain herbal intake, and pump after feedings.

Complete protocols for inducing lactation with long and short lead times and for menopausal women can be found at http://www.asklenore.info/breastfeeding/induced_lactation/gn_protocols.shtml. Reprinted by permission from Jack Newman, MD, FRCPC and Lenore Goldfarb, PhD, CCC, IBCLC, ALC.

Relactation is a process of reestablishing lactation some time after it has ended. Mothers may choose to relactate if they change their mind about infant feeding, if they have an infant who cannot tolerate infant formula, if they have a preterm or ill infant and decide to breastfeed during the course of the infant's hospitalization (Thompson, 1996), or if they had experienced a life crisis that has been resolved. Because the mother has experienced a pregnancy and lactogenesis II, establishing significant milk production may occur much sooner than in induced lactation. Mothers may find that using a tube feeding device at the breast for each feeding (Kayhan-Tetik, Baydar-Artantas, Bozcuk-Guzeldemirci, Ustu, & Yilmaz, 2013) and pumping several times each day may start the relactation process.

In a small study of mothers who relactated, it was found that many of the infants were described as colicky, were difficult to feed, cried excessively, and had difficulty latching to the breast. Mothers described feelings of failure and lack of readiness for breastfeeding challenges (Lommen, Brown, & Hollist, 2015).

Not all mothers will be able to recover a full milk supply depending on the length of time since the last breastfeeding and other factors contributing to the original abandonment of breastfeeding. Nevertheless, mothers who recover even a partial milk supply will be able to enjoy the breastfeeding relationship and reinforce their feelings of empowerment and success. Infants in a relactation or induced lactation situation should be monitored closely for normal weight gain and their mothers closely supported and praised for their hard work and dedication to their infant's health and well-being (World Health Organization, 1998).

OVERWEIGHT AND OBESE MOTHERS

The prevalence of obesity in the United States has continued to rise in women over 18 years of age, from 25.4% in 1994 to 33.4% in 2000 (Flegal, Carroll, Ogden, & Johnson, 2002) and up again to 56.6% in 2011 (Kaiser Family Foundation, 2011). Analysis of 2003–2004 National Health and Nutrition Examination Survey (NHANES) data showed 51.7% of nonpregnant women aged 20–39 years were overweight or obese (body mass index [BMI] = 25 kg/m^2), 28.9% were obese (BMI = 30 kg/m^2), and 8.0% were extremely obese (BMI = 40 kg/m^2; Ogden et al., 2006). Obesity can have numerous effects on health and reproduction, including an increased risk of diabetes mellitus, gestational diabetes, osteoarthritis, cardiovascular disease, miscarriage, hypertension in pregnancy, and cesarean delivery (Norman & Clark, 1998). Cesarean delivery risk is increased by 50% in overweight women and is more than double for obese women compared with women with a normal BMI (Poobalan, Aucott, Gurung, Smith, & Bhattacharya, 2009). Cesarean section increases the risk of delayed lactogenesis and low milk supply (Rowe-Murray & Fisher, 2002). Infants born to obese mothers have an increased risk of neural tube defects such as spina bifida, a higher rate of birth injuries, an increased incidence of low Apgar scores, and more admissions to neonatal intensive care units. Infants of overweight mothers have greater body fat mass in the neonatal period compared with infants of lean mothers, suggesting that maternal overweight may predispose fetal metabolism to favor fat storage (Andres, Shankar, & Badger, 2012). McClure and colleagues (2011) found that until menopause, mothers who did not breastfeed all of their children for at least 3 months exhibit significantly greater amounts of metabolically active visceral fat than mothers who had breastfed all of their children for 3 months or longer. Wiklund and colleagues (2012) showed that a short duration of breastfeeding induced weight retention and fat mass accumulation, which resulted in an increased risk for cardiometabolic disorders 16 to 20 years after their last pregnancy. Ten months or more of lactation has been shown to result in a better maternal metabolic profile and a reduced waist-to-hip ratio that persists for many years following the cessation of breastfeeding (Thrris et al., 2013). This points out the importance of breastfeeding for lifelong health.

Maternal obesity is an adverse determinant for breastfeeding success (Turcksin, Bel, Galjaard, & Devlieger, 2014; Wojcicki, 2011). Excessive body weight and obesity can negatively influence the initiation and duration of breastfeeding (Donath & Amir, 2000; Li, Jewell, & Grummer-Strawn, 2003), with a higher BMI related to decreased initiation (Hilson, Rasmussen, & Kjolhede, 1997; Manios et al., 2009) and duration (Donath & Amir, 2008; Oddy, Landsborough, Kendall, Henderson, & Downie, 2006; Rutishauser & Carlin, 1992) of breastfeeding. The risk of early termination of any breastfeeding rises progressively with increasing BMI—the greater the prepregnancy BMI, the earlier the termination of breastfeeding (Baker, Michaelsen, Sorensen, & Rasmussen, 2007). Perceived insufficient milk production, slow infant weight gain, and embarrassment to breastfeed in public have been reported to result in decreased exclusive breastfeeding rates in obese mothers (Mok et al., 2008). Kitsantas, Gaffney, and Kornides (2011) examined socioeconomic status (SES) and racial/ethnic differences within the context of prepregnancy weight. Their study revealed specific groups of mothers with low rates of breastfeeding initiation and duration. Normal BMI Hispanic women of low SES demonstrated higher rates of breastfeeding initiation (74%) compared to other groups. Overweight/obese black women of low SES had lower rates of breastfeeding initiation. Overweight/obese Hispanic women of middle SES were significantly less likely to continue breastfeeding up to 4 months compared to their white counterparts. Among women who initiated breastfeeding, overweight/obese white women of low SES had the highest rate of stopping within 2 months of giving birth (66.7%). Women with high prepregnant BMI have been reported to have a lack of comfort and confidence in their body that may contribute to the reduced initiation and duration of any breastfeeding (Hauff & Demerath, 2012).

Animal studies found that the timing of the onset of obesity affects lactation, with early-onset obesity (before menarche) resulting in lower milk production in Holstein heifers (Zanton & Heinrichs, 2005). Onset of obesity (before development of the breasts) has not been studied in humans relative to milk-production effectiveness. Psychological, behavioral, and cultural influences also have a role in reduced lactation in overweight and obese women (Amir & Donath, 2007). Obese mothers may experience lower SES (a group less likely to breastfeed), may be less likely to participate in preventive health behaviors, or may be embarrassed to breastfeed in public due to their discomfort with their body image.

Excessive body weight and obesity have been shown to be a risk factor for delayed lactogenesis II (Chapman & Perez-Escamilla, 1999b; Lepe, Bacardi Gascon, Castaneda-Gonzalez, Perez Morales, & Jimenez Cruz, 2011), with low milk transfer at 60 hours postpartum seen in obese women (Chapman & Perez-Escamilla, 2000). Part of this delay has been attributed to the tendency of overweight/obese mothers to have large areolas with flat nipples, contributing to a difficult latch, sore nipples, and resulting limited milk transfer.

For each 1-unit (1 kg/m^2) increase in prepregnant BMI, a 0.5-hour delay in onset of lactogenesis II has been calculated (Hilson, Rasmussen, & Kjolhede, 2004). Thus, the difference in the onset of copious milk production can be up to 10 hours later in a mother with a BMI of 40 kg/m^2 compared with a mother with a BMI of 20 kg/m^2. This delay occurs at a time when the mother has been discharged from the hospital and is concerned about the delay in the onset of a copious milk supply. It is interesting to note that although increasing the frequency of breastfeeding in the early postpartum period is associated with an earlier onset of lactogenesis II in nonobese mothers, among obese women, no benefit was seen from increasing breastfeeding frequency (Chapman & Perez-Escamilla, 1999a).

Animal models have also shown impaired lactogenesis in the presence of obesity. In the murine model, lipid accumulation in the secretory epithelial cells of obese mice was indicative of the absence of copious milk secretion, with the addition of marked abnormalities in the alveolar development of the mammary gland itself (Flint, Travers, Barber, Binart, & Kelly, 2005). Kamikawa and colleagues (2009) showed that obesity disrupts mammary ductal development in mice, with less dense distribution of ducts, reduced branching, and ducts that were incompletely lined with myoepithelium. Obese mice have been shown to exhibit prolactin resistance in mammary tissue and the hypothalamus resulting in reduced lactation performance (Buonfiglio et al., 2016). Maternal systematic inflammation in a mouse model was associated with breastfeeding failure due to premature mammary involution and cellular degradation (Hennigar, Velasquez, & Kelleher, 2015). It is not known if such breast changes and effects are associated with obesity in women.

The negative effect on breastfeeding of being overweight or obese is multifactorial, with hormonal alterations linked to lactation difficulties. Obesity may facilitate alterations in the hypothalamic–pituitary–gonadal axis and in fat metabolism that affects milk production and composition (Bray, 1997; Rasmussen, Hilson, & Kjolhede, 2001). Research has shown that overweight/obese women have a lower prolactin response to suckling during the early days when prolactin is more important to milk production than it is later in lactation (Hilson et al., 2004; Rasmussen & Kjolhede, 2004). At 48 hours postpartum, obese mothers compared with nonobese mothers showed a 45-ng/mL decrease in prolactin response to suckling that persisted over the first week. At 7 days postpartum, excess body weight/obesity was associated with a reduction in the prolactin response to suckling of almost 100 ng/mL. The delay in lactogenesis II and the blunted prolactin response to suckling during the first 7 days may be contributors to the high proportion of obese mothers who abandon breastfeeding during this important period of time (Hilson et al., 1997). A proinflammatory diet during pregnancy has been associated with a lower likelihood of breastfeeding beyond one month (Sen et al., 2016). The dietary inflammatory index determines the inflammatory potential of a person's diet. A high dietary inflammatory index during pregnancy might be predictive or serve as a marker for the potential for an abbreviated course of lactation. Obesity has been associated with postpartum depression. One study found that self-reported moderate or greater postpartum depressive symptoms was 30.8% in a sample of 3,439 women compared to 22.8% in normal weight women (Lacoursiere, Baksh, Bloebaum, & Varner, 2006). Obese mothers may be quite self-conscious about their weight or require special bariatric beds and chairs if their BMI exceeds 40 kg/m^2. Obese mothers may appreciate extra attention to their concerns for modesty and may benefit from care that provides privacy during breast exposure (Anstey & Jevitt, 2011).

With surgical management of obesity available for people with a BMI of 40 or more (or a BMI of 35–40 with other health problems), many women who were infertile as a result of extreme obesity can become pregnant and deliver healthy infants. Breastfeeding is certainly recommended for overweight/obese mothers and also for mothers who have undergone gastric bypass or bariatric surgery. Breastfeeding may help with maternal weight control and may contribute to the prevention of overweight/obesity in their children. Breastfeeding has been shown to reduce postpartum weight retention in all but the heaviest of women (Baker et al., 2008).

Mothers who have undergone bariatric surgery, however, should be closely followed postpartum. After gastric bypass surgery, mothers may have difficulty absorbing vitamin B_{12}, with consequently lower milk levels. Vitamin B_{12} deficiencies in breastfeeding infants of mothers who have undergone bariatric surgery have been reported, manifesting as slow growth, developmental delays, apathy, hypotonia, hyperreflexivity, and slow head growth (Granger & Finlay, 1994; Wardinsky et al., 1995). Mothers may be given monthly B_{12} injections and infants may be placed on supplemental vitamins to avoid adverse outcomes. Following bariatric surgery, some mothers may manifest dermatological signs and symptoms of malabsorption such as eczema, skin lesions, hair loss, or depigmentation of hair, with these conditions often reflecting low levels of vitamin A or zinc or other nutrients. Clinicians must be aware of such manifestations not only to assure better health of the mother, but also to avoid nutrient deficiencies in her breastmilk (Monshi et al., 2015).

A retrospective chart review of 21 mothers who had undergone bariatric surgery showed that of the 26 infants born to these mothers, 96% were given formula supplementation at an average age of 5 days. The average birth weight of the infants was 5.9 pounds, 48% were born before term, and 33% of infants required admission to the special care nursery (Caplinger et al., 2015). Continued weight loss or poor weight gain may have contributed to formula supplementation if lactogenesis II was delayed. Low-birth-weight, birth before term, and admission into a special care nursery all negatively impact the start of breastfeeding. Insufficient milk seems to be a common theme in the maternal population with obesity (O'Sullivan, Perrine, & Rasmussen, 2015).

Following the loss of a large amount of adipose tissue in the breasts, they may demonstrate ptosis, or excessive sagging. This may make it difficult for the mother to visualize the nipple and areola and cause latch difficulties. The breasts may feel very soft and billowy with glandular tissue hard to access (Lamb, 2011). Because of the loose skin in the breast following fat loss, mothers may have difficulty using a breast pump, as the surrounding breast tissue may stretch to the point of being drawn into the pump flange along with the nipple and areola. Changing the standard flange sizes may not help. Mothers may instead need to use a flange that exerts compression on the nipple/areola rather than just vacuum, or may need to pad a standard flange to prevent excess breast skin from entering the flange tunnel.

Breastfeeding Management

Although it has been shown that obese women are at an increased risk of delay in establishing lactation and for lactation failure, many clinicians do not manage obese mothers differently from normal weight women (Rasmussen, Lee, Ledkovsky, & Kjolhede, 2006). This could be a contributing factor to the less than optimal initiation and duration rates seen in obese mothers. Clinicians, however, may observe that obese mothers experience more challenges to breastfeeding than nonobese mothers—for example, difficulty positioning the infant, impaired mobility of the mother, and large pendulous breasts with flat nipples that make latching difficult—and may note that caring for obese women is more physically challenging to the clinician (Garner, Ratcliff, Devine, Thornburg, & Rasmussen, 2014). If obese mothers experience a delay in lactogenesis, then the infant will be presented with a prolonged colostral phase, during which time increased numbers of feedings are necessary to offset the low availability of a copious milk supply. Mothers should be encouraged to breastfeed about 10–12 times each day until lactogenesis II has been confirmed and the infant is gaining weight well. Increased numbers of feedings may not contribute to earlier lactogenesis II but will help keep the infant well hydrated, prevent weight loss, and avoid the need to supplement with infant formula. The infant should be monitored closely for sufficient weight gain.

Positioning for breastfeeding should include support for large breasts, such as a rolled-up towel or receiving blanket under the breast for support. If the infant is fed in a clutch or football position, care should be taken that the heavy breast does not rest on the infant's chest. Excess adipose tissue within the breast may stretch the areola and flatten out the nipple, making latch difficult for the infant (Anstey & Jevitt, 2011). If the nipples are flat, a modified syringe can be used to pull them out before each feeding. If a mother needs to use a breast pump, the clinician should make sure that the flange is properly fitted to the mother's breast and is not so small that the nipple strangulates in the flange's nipple tunnel. Both mother and infant may be supplemented with vitamin B_{12} if the mother has undergone gastric bypass surgery, especially if the mother's milk levels are very low. Intertrigo (inflammation of skinfolds due to skin-to-skin contact or friction from clothing) is commonly seen in obese breasts. Mothers should clean and dry breast skinfolds daily to prevent progression from the itching, burning, and pain to an infection (Jevitt, Hernandez, & Groer, 2007).

PERIPARTUM MOOD, DEPRESSIVE, AND ANXIETY DISORDERS

Lifetime rates of depression in women range between 10% and 25% (Kessler et al., 1994), with the onset of depression peaking between the ages of 25 and 44, the prime childbearing years. Overall postpartum depression (PPD) prevalence has been estimated to be 13% (one in eight women; O'Hara & Swain, 1996). However, Gavin and colleagues (2005) reported that as many as 19.2% of women have a depressive episode during the first 3 months postpartum. This may mean that older reports of PPD prevalence were underestimates. Many mood and anxiety disorders can occur before, during, or after a pregnancy, such as major depression, bipolar disorders, panic disorder, obsessive–compulsive disorder, general anxiety disorder, posttraumatic stress disorder, and PPD. Highly anxious mothers are less likely to exclusively breastfeed or breastfeed after delivery (Britton, 2007). Bogen, Hanusa, Moses-Kolko, and Wisner (2010) showed that use of selective serotonin reuptake inhibitors (SSRIs) during pregnancy negatively affects initiation of breastfeeding and continuation of breastfeeding to 12 weeks. Mothers with high postnatal depression scores immediately after delivery are more likely to be bottle-feeding at 3 months (Gagliardi,

Petrozzi, & Rusconi, 2012). Stuebe, Grewen, Pedersen, Propper, and Meltzer-Brody (2012) hypothesize that failed lactation and perinatal depression overlap in clinical settings and that shared neuroendocrine mechanisms may underlie both disorders. Watkins, Meltzer-Brody, Zolnoun, and Stuebe (2011) reported that negative early breastfeeding experiences, such as severe breastfeeding pain during the first 2 weeks, were associated with depressive symptoms at 2 months postpartum. This alerts the clinician to screen mothers with breastfeeding problems for depressive symptoms and to strive to remedy early problems as quickly as possible. Childbearing may coincide with the onset of a mood or anxiety disorder or the exacerbation of a preexisting one due to the synergistic effects of reproductive hormones, brain neurotransmitters, and stress (Driscoll, 2005). Sharma and Corpse (2008) described a case study of a mother who experienced three episodes of major depression, each of which closely followed the cessation of breastfeeding.

Birth-related trauma can be a trigger for posttraumatic stress disorder or posttraumatic stress symptoms, which in turn can complicate the breastfeeding relationship (Kendall-Tackett, 2014). Mothers who experienced birth interventions such as epidurals, other pain medications, and postpartum surgery appear to be more prone to develop depressive symptoms than mothers who do not experience these interventions (Kendall-Tackett, Cong, & Hale, 2015). Higher doses of synthetic oxytocin during labor have been associated with greater depressive, anxious, and physical symptoms at 2 months postpartum (Gu et al., 2016). Traumatic births can delay lactogenesis II by as much as several days (Grajeda & Perez-Escamilla, 2002).

Depressed mothers may experience anxiety, fatigue, lack of concentration, insomnia, and a loss of interest in their usual activities. Infants of untreated depressed mothers may experience delayed psychomotor development as well as negative effects on cognitive and emotional development. Pregnant women should be screened for depressive symptoms early, but a number of barriers exist for appropriate treatment, including concerns regarding the effect of medications on the fetus and newborn (Fitelson, Kim, Baker, & Leight, 2011).

Maternal state anxiety during the postpartum hospitalization period is much more common than depression among breastfeeding mothers. A positive screen for state anxiety in the hospital is significantly associated with reduced breastfeeding duration in primiparous but not multiparous mothers (Paul, Downs, Schaefer, Beiler, & Weisman, 2013). Highly anxious mothers are more likely to supplement their infant with formula, further increasing the risk of early abandonment of breastfeeding (Gagnon, Leduc, Waghorn, Yang, & Platt, 2005).

Holistic care for childbearing women with mood and anxiety disorders usually includes a number of modalities (psychotherapy, meditation, stress reduction, dietary interventions) constructed and based on the unique aspects of each woman's needs (Sichel & Driscoll, 1999). Breastfeeding can be very important in the realm of mood disorders. Breastfeeding women have lower depression, fatigue, anxiety and dysphoric moods, less perception of stress, and more positive life events than formula-feeding mothers (Groer, 2005). Breastfeeding mothers have an up-regulated inflammatory response system that helps protect them from infectious disease (Groer et al., 2005), a stressor that is certainly not welcome during the postpartum period. Formula-feeding mothers appear to have diminished cellular immunity when experiencing stress, placing them at higher risk for certain illnesses (Groer & Davis, 2006).

Postpartum Depression

PPD is the most common mood disorder after childbirth that emerges within several weeks of delivery. Rates of PPD can be as high as 26% among adolescent mothers (Troutman & Cutrona, 1990) and 38.2% among low-income, first-time mothers (Hobfoll, Ritter, Lavin, Hulsizer, & Cameron, 1995). In the United States, 14.5% of women develop a new episode of depression during pregnancy (Gaynes et al., 2005). PPD affects maternal–infant interactions, with descriptions that depressed mothers may be less affectionate and withdrawn or intrusive and hostile, and their infants may demonstrate behavior that is avoidant, discontent, and withdrawn (Horowitz & Goodman, 2005). PPD can affect the entire family, including exerting negative influences on fathers' mental health (Goodman, 2004a). Although PPD often remits within the first few months postpartum, depressive symptoms can continue for an extensive time beyond the postpartum period and well into the second year after childbirth (Goodman, 2004b).

Infant temperament has been linked to stable breastfeeding patterns in mothers with depressive symptoms; infants who demonstrate highly reactive temperaments generally had less stable breastfeeding relationships (Jones, McFall, & Diego, 2004). Affective and physiological dysregulation in infants of depressed mothers may already be present when the clinician encounters such mother–infant pairs for breastfeeding interventions. Breastfeeding difficulties experienced by mothers with PPD have been described that include PPD's effects on mothers' high expectations for breastfeeding success, their difficulty in dealing with breastfeeding problems, problems with seeking professional lactation care and services, difficulties coping, and feelings of guilt (Shakespeare, Blake, & Garcia, 2004). Although depression during pregnancy may not affect the initiation of breastfeeding, depressed breastfeeding mothers have a greater risk of early abandonment of breastfeeding before 4 weeks than do nondepressed new mothers (Akman et al., 2008; Henderson, 2003b; Pippins, Brawarsky, Jackson, Fuentes-Afflick, & Haas, 2006). Depressed mothers report more breastfeeding worries and difficulties, are more unsatisfied with their infant-feeding method, and have decreased levels of breastfeeding confidence (Dennis & McQueen, 2007, 2009).

Exclusive breastfeeding is lower in depressed mothers than in nondepressed mothers (Hasselmann, Werneck, & Silva, 2008; McCarter-Spaulding & Horowitz, 2007). Some mothers with PPD (either the mild "infant blues" or those with more intense symptoms) may self-medicate with botanical preparations such as St. John's wort. St. John's wort is no more effective in treating major depression than a placebo (Shelton et al., 2001) and should not be relied on if a mother is severely depressed or is suffering from postpartum psychosis. Studies on the efficacy of this herb for PPD are lacking, and there are no standardizations of the preparation. In a published case report of a mother taking 300 mg 3 times a day of a standardized extract of St. John's wort, low levels were detected in her milk and none in the infant's plasma (Klier, Schaefer, Schmid-Siegel, Lenz, & Mannel, 2002).

Depressed mothers are in psychic pain, and they and their family require much support. Depressed mothers may feel lonely and isolated, may be unable to sleep or concentrate, may experience few positive emotions, may suffer from anxiety, and may describe experiencing an overwhelming loss of control (Beck, 1992, 1993). Many mothers with postpartum blues or mild PPD benefit from talking with a therapist and becoming involved in postpartum support groups. Mothers with severe PPD are generally medicated and engage in psychotherapeutic sessions with a psychiatrist, a psychologist, or an advanced practice clinical nurse specialist. Mothers who express irrational ideas, experience hallucinations, or threaten to harm themselves or the infant need immediate referral to a mental health specialist. If the mother is hospitalized, some psychiatric hospitals or psychiatric units within a hospital may also admit the infant but most will not.

Pharmacological Interventions

Pharmacological interventions are often used to normalize the brain chemistry based on the type of disorder present. An estimated 90,000 (2.8%) pregnant women each year are prescribed SSRIs (Reefhuis, Rasmussen, & Friedman, 2006). Depressed breastfeeding mothers often have concerns about taking antidepressant medications due to their potential effects on the infant. Breastfeeding mothers who take antidepressants often have more severe symptoms, greater functional impairment, and more extensive psychiatric histories (Battle et al., 2008). Depressive disorders are usually treated with SSRIs such as fluoxetine (Prozac), sertraline (Zoloft), and paroxetine (Paxil). Other antidepressants include bupropion (Wellbutrin), escitalopram (Lexapro, which can cause sleepiness in the infant), and venlafaxine (Effexor). Tricyclic antidepressants such as nortriptyline (Aventyl), amitriptyline (Elavil), and desipramine (Pertofrane) are older and still used but tend to have a greater number of side effects. Medications for mood swing (bipolar) disorders include mood stabilizers such as lithium (Lithobid), valproic acid (Depakene), divalproex, lamotrigine (Lamictal), and carbamazepine (Tegretol). Anxiety disorders are often treated with benzodiazepines such as lorazepam (Ativan), diazepam (Valium), and clonazepam (Klonopin). Although many, but not all, of these medications are safe for use during pregnancy and lactation, a number of possible side effects are relevant to breastfeeding, of which the clinician should be aware.

Side Effects

Neonatal withdrawal syndrome may occur in some infants exposed to paroxetine (Paxil) in utero, which includes jitteriness, vomiting, irritability, hypoglycemia, and necrotizing enterocolitis (Stiskal, Kulin, Koren, Ho, & Ito, 2001). Difficulty has been described in differentiating whether these symptoms are due to withdrawal or actual toxicity from the drug (Isbister et al., 2001). The extent of side effects in newborns from maternal use of a number of different SSRIs is linked to third trimester use of the medications. Fetal exposure to SSRIs during the third trimester has been reported to cause a number of symptoms in newborns such as irritability, constant crying, increased tone, shivering, feeding and sleeping difficulties, hypotonia, convulsions, and respiratory distress (Laine, Heikkinen, Ekblad, & Kero, 2003; Moses-Kolko et al., 2005; Nordeng, Lindemann, Perminov, & Reikvam, 2001; Oberlander et al., 2004). These are generally considered as symptoms of poor adaptation. Although these symptoms may be transient, self-limiting, and resolve within 2 weeks, they pose a problem for early breastfeeding.

Lithium toxicity in a breastfed infant can cause floppiness and an infant who is unresponsive. Lithium use must be closely monitored, and often the medication is changed if possible to one less likely to cause side effects in the infant. However, reassessment of the use of lithium in monotherapy has been considered, as serum lithium levels in infants of mothers with bipolar disorders have been reported as being low, and no significant clinical or behavioral effects have been seen in these infants (Davanzo, Copertino, De Cunto, Minen, & Amaddeo, 2011; Viguera et al., 2007). Sit and colleagues (2011) did not find an association between cord–maternal concentration ratios of SSRIs or maternal depression and adverse perinatal events.

Clinicians should also be aware that benzodiazepine medications tend to have a long half-life and can be sedating in a breastfed infant if the mother is medicated over a long period of time. Shorter acting drugs from this family, such as lorazepam (Ativan), are sometimes substituted if their use is intermittent, short term, low dose, and after the 1st week of life (Maitra & Menkes, 1996).

Some selected side effects include the following:

- Anecdotal reports of reduced milk supply in mothers taking Wellbutrin have been reported (Hale, 2012).
- Several side effects in infants of mothers receiving fluoxetine (Prozac) have been reported and include severe colic, fussiness, crying (Lester, Cucca, Andreozzi, Flanagan, & Oh, 1993), seizures (Brent & Wisner, 1998), and growth deficits (Chambers et al., 1999).
- Fluoxetine has been reported to induce a state of anesthesia in the vagina and nipples (Michael & Mayer, 2000). If this is so, anesthetized nipples may be unable to transmit signals for the milk-ejection reflex, coming full circle to the reports of weight gain deficits in some infants.
- Berle and Spigset (2011) recommend that women undergoing antidepressant treatment be encouraged to breastfeed and that paroxetine and sertraline be considered first. Fluoxetine and citalopram are excreted in breastmilk in higher amounts.
- Salisbury and colleagues (2011) found that newborn behavioral patterns differed between infants whose mothers had a major depressive disorder and received SSRI treatment compared to those infants whose mothers had a major depressive disorder but did not receive these medications. Full-term infants exposed to a maternal major depressive disorder treated with SSRIs had a lower gestation age, lower quality of movement, and more central nervous system stress signs than infants whose mothers had a major depressive disorder but were not treated with these drugs. Clinicians may wish to more carefully watch infants prenatally exposed to SSRIs, as neurobehavioral alterations may have the potential to adversely affect breastfeeding in the early weeks.

Nonpharmacological Interventions

Research has found that inflammation plays a role in the etiology of depression (Kendall-Tackett, 2008). A function of cortisol is to keep inflammation in check, but depression down-regulates cortisol, with abnormally low levels of cortisol seen in depressed women (Groer & Morgan, 2007). The immune system under psychological stress releases cytokines, but when levels are very high they increase the risk of depression (Maes, 2001). Many nonpharmacological interventions for depression are used for their anti-inflammatory properties, such as the fatty acids eicosapentaenoic acid and docosahexaenoic acid, bright light therapy, exercise, social support, psychotherapy, and St. John's wort (which can interact with antidepressants and should not be taken if the mother is also being treated with prescription antidepressants; Kendall-Tackett, 2008). Vagal stimulation and massage therapy have also been noted to reduce depression (Field, 2008).

Other nonpharmacological treatments are available for mothers who have experienced childbirth-related trauma and posttraumatic stress disorder, such as psychotherapy, cognitive-behavioral therapy, eye movement desensitization and reprocessing, acupuncture, mindfulness, and expressive writing (Kendall-Tackett, 2014). Sometimes just listening to mothers and letting them know that their symptoms are treatable and that many mothers experience some of these same feelings may be enough to relieve their anxiety.

Breastfeeding Management

Early feeding problems, hypotonia, irritability, high tone (extensor reflexes are stronger than flexion), and the other side effects seen in some newborns of mothers who have taken prenatal SSRIs may mimic behaviors seen with other newborn conditions. The therapeutic intervention of skin-to-skin care may help the infant modulate and regain state control. Skin-to-skin care has also been reported to lessen postpartum blues in the mother by reengaging a blunted hypothalamic–pituitary–adrenal axis to its normal nonpregnant state (Dombrowski, Anderson, Santori, & Burkhammer, 2001). Every effort should be made to keep the mother and infant together to encourage a strong attachment between them. Breastfeeding has been shown to be protective against maternal neglect, with the odds for maternal maltreatment for nonbreastfed children being 2.6 times higher than for children whose mothers breastfeed (Strathearn, Mamun, Najman, & O'Callaghan, 2009).

Infants of mothers taking psychotropic medications should be monitored closely for appropriate weight gain (Hendrick, Smith, Hwang, Altshuler, & Haynes, 2003), sufficient nurturing, alterations in behavior or activity level, and achievement of developmental milestones (Burt et al., 2001). Infants who are irritable or not readily comforted can increase the stress in an already difficult situation. Restoring some control to the situation by suggesting the use of a sling, frequent suckling opportunities, and planned rest periods may reduce feelings of being overwhelmed. Mothers who are severely depressed and cannot handle placing the infant to the breast or fear they will harm the infant may be able to pump their milk and have it fed to the infant by the father or another caretaker. If a breastfeeding mother is hospitalized, she may or may not be able to pump her milk during the separation. Many mothers experience this depressed time as a period of "just trying to survive." The preservation of milk production may be an accomplishment that the mother appreciates once she is feeling better, helping her to experience one less loss.

ENDOCRINE, METABOLIC, AND AUTOIMMUNE CONDITIONS

Diabetes

Nearly 26 million Americans have diabetes. In addition, an estimated 79 million U.S. adults have prediabetes, a condition in which blood sugar levels are higher than normal, but not high enough to be diagnosed as diabetes. Prediabetes raises a person's risk of type 2 diabetes, heart disease, and stroke (Centers for Disease Control and Prevention, 2011). A number of forms of diabetes can occur in childbearing women:

- Insulin-dependent diabetes mellitus, or type 1 diabetes, is a polygenic autoimmune disorder resulting from destruction of the insulin-producing beta cells in the pancreas. It is thought to have a genetic component that is triggered by an environmental insult or event such as the early introduction of cow's milk protein, viral infections, or exposure to toxins.

- Non-insulin-dependent diabetes mellitus, or type 2 diabetes, is typically associated with a metabolic syndrome that includes obesity and hypertension and is usually seen in adults (although with the rising rates of childhood overweight and obesity, it is now seen at an increased rate in children). Insulin is produced in the pancreas, but the cells' insulin receptors do not respond to it. Some mothers may be taking oral hypoglycemic agents such as glipizide (Glucotrol) or glyburide (Micronase) and should be encouraged to breastfeed because these medications are safe during lactation (Feig, Briggs, & Koren, 2007; Glatstein, Djokanovic, Garcia-Bournissen, Finkelstein, & Koren, 2009).
- Gestational diabetes mellitus (GDM) manifests itself as impaired glucose tolerance during pregnancy. The rates of GDM have risen from 1% to 2.5% in 1976 to 4% in 2000, and 7% of all pregnancies being complicated by GDM in 2004 (American Diabetes Association, 2004). New diagnostic criteria for gestational diabetes will increase the proportion of women diagnosed with gestational diabetes. Using these new diagnostic criteria, an international, multicenter study of gestational diabetes found that 18% of the pregnancies were affected by gestational diabetes (International Association of Diabetes and Pregnancy Study Groups Consensus Panel, 2010). This is primarily due to the increase in maternal overweight and obesity. Women with GDM are at increased risk for the development of diabetes, usually type 2, after pregnancy (Albareda et al., 2003; Schaefer-Graf, Buchanan, Xiang, Peters, & Kjos, 2002). Obesity enhances the risk of developing type 2 diabetes after GDM (American Diabetes Association, 2004). The recurrence rates for GDM in subsequent pregnancies range from 35% in predominantly white populations to greater than 50% in nonwhite populations (MacNeill, Dodds, Hamilton, Armson, & VandenHof, 2001). Women who experience GDM and do not breastfeed the infant from that pregnancy are twice as likely to develop type 2 diabetes (Kjos, Henry, Lee, Buchanan, & Mishell, 1993). In a study of 959 mothers with gestational diabetes, it was found that 113 (nearly 12%) went on to develop type 2 diabetes. Those who breastfed cut their risk by half, and the longer they breastfed and the more heavily they relied on their breastmilk rather than formula, the more they lowered their risk. Those who breastfed for more than 10 months cut their risk of a diabetes diagnosis by almost 60% in the 2 years they were followed. Of the 205 women who only breastfed and used no formula for the first 2 months of the baby's life, 17 (3.9%) developed diabetes, compared with 27 women (8.79%) of the 153 mothers who did not breastfeed and only used formula (Gunderson et al., 2015).
- O'Reilly, Avalos, Dennedy, O'Sullivan, and Dunne (2011) reported that persistent hyperglycemia was significantly lower in women who had breastfed compared to mothers who had bottle-fed when given a postpartum 75-g oral glucose tolerance test. Intensity of breastfeeding in mothers with gestational diabetes is predictive of glucose metabolism and insulin sensitivity. Compared with exclusive or mostly formula feeding (> 17 oz formula per 24 hours), exclusive breastfeeding and mostly exclusive breastfeeding (< 6 oz formula per 24 hours) groups of mothers with GDM had lower fasting plasma glucose levels and much more favorable effects on insulin sensitivity (Gunderson et al., 2012). The dose–response relationship between increasing intensity of lactation and decreasing fasting plasma glucose levels is very important to diabetic women, as the diversion of glucose and lipids into breastmilk production helps unload the pancreatic B-cells and preserve long-term insulin production in mothers (Gunderson et al., 2012).

Lifestyle modifications such as breastfeeding are an important intervention in efforts to prevent type 2 diabetes in women with a history of gestational diabetes (Bentley-Lewis, Levkoff, Stuebe, & Seely, 2008; Feig, 2012). Mothers whose weight is 190 lbs or more at the start of the subsequent pregnancy are 70% more likely to have a recurrence of GDM, reinforcing the importance of breastfeeding as a potential contributor to reducing weight between pregnancies and helping lessen insulin resistance.

The type of diabetes can be a significant predictor of breastfeeding intention and initiation. Soltani and Arden (2009) found that women with type 1 diabetes breastfed in lower proportions than other women with diabetes. Women with GDM were more likely to breastfeed than those with type 1 and type 2 diabetes. The type of first feed was also significant in this study, as mothers who breastfed as the first feeding were more likely to be breastfeeding at 6 weeks compared with mothers who used formula for the first feeding. Liu, Jorn, and Banks (2010) showed that compared with nulliparous women, mothers who do not breastfeed have approximately a 50% increased risk of type 2 diabetes in later life. Schwarz and colleagues (2010) reported similar findings among a cohort of women aged 40–78 years. The risk of type 2 diabetes increased when term pregnancy was followed by less than 1 month of breastfeeding, independent of physical activity and BMI in later life. Breastfeeding has been reported to be less frequent and of a shorter duration in mothers with type 1 diabetes (Hummel et al., 2007). However, with optimal breastfeeding support, mothers with type 1 diabetes are quite capable of breastfeeding for prolonged periods of time, similar to mothers without diabetes (Schoen, Sichert-Hellert, Hummel, Ziegler, & Kersting, 2008). Breastfeeding can function as an important therapeutic intervention in the face of any type of diabetes (Taylor, Kacmar, Nothnagle, & Lawrence, 2005). Women with any type of diabetes should be actively encouraged to breastfeed (Gunderson, 2007; Metzger et al., 2007). Body fat accumulation after pregnancy is associated with alterations in insulin secretion; however, breastfeeding has a long-lasting protective effect on the insulin response (Diniz & da Costa, 2004).

Fasting blood glucose levels are significantly lower in type 1 diabetic mothers during the exclusively breastfeeding period compared with women with type 1 diabetes who stop breastfeeding or who have never breastfed (Ferris et al., 1988; Ferris et al., 1993). Milk production could be limited in the presence of too much or too little insulin. Too much insulin causing hypoglycemia can potentially cause epinephrine to be released from the adrenal glands, inhibiting the release of milk (Asselin & Lawrence, 1987). After an initial episode of hypoglycemia after delivery, the ongoing metabolism of glucose into galactose and lactose during milk synthesis reduces the amount of insulin needed by a lactating mother. While glucose uptake into the breast can lower maternal serum glucose levels, infant sucking reduces maternal glucose levels but is not a contributor to maternal hypoglycemia (Achong, McIntyre, Callaway, & Duncan, 2015). Mothers may find that insulin requirements are reduced between 27% (Davies, Clark, Dalton, & Edwards, 1989) and 50% (Asselin & Lawrence, 1987) while they are breastfeeding. Insulin dosages will need to be adjusted during the early days of lactation. Riviello, Mello, and Jovanovic (2009) recommended that total daily basal insulin dosage for type 1 diabetic women who breastfeed be calculated as 0.21 units times their weight in kilograms per day. Once insulin dosage and diet are in balance, diabetic mothers are quite capable of synthesizing abundant amounts of milk and lactating successfully (Benz, 1992).

Women with type 1 diabetes have a 5–10% incidence of hyper- or hypothyroidism, with goiter and Hashimoto thyroiditis being common. Mothers with type 1 diabetes have three times the risk of developing postpartum thyroiditis (Gallas, Stolk, Bakker, Endert, & Wiersinga, 2002). In women with type 2 diabetes where obesity is common, the clinician should be vigilant for the possibility of hypothyroidism (Jovanovic, 2000). This issue should be kept in mind if a diabetic mother reports problems with milk insufficiency.

Infants of diabetic mothers are at an increased risk for a number of conditions that can pose barriers to their breastfeeding such as prematurity, respiratory distress syndrome, congenital anomalies, hypoglycemia, large for gestational age (Cordero, Treuer, Landon, & Gabbe, 1998), hyperbilirubinemia (Sirota, Ferrera, Lerer, & Dulitzky, 1992), hypocalcemia (Metcalfe & Baum, 1992), and being born by cesarean section. Many of these conditions result in separation of mother and infant during the important early time when breastfeeding is becoming established (Nigro et al., 1985). Breastfeeding within 2 hours of birth can be reduced in diabetic mothers, a situation that contributes to decreased breastfeeding at discharge and out to 6 months postpartum (Sparud-Lundin, Wennergren, Elfvin, & Berg, 2011). Delaying breastfeeding as the first feed reduces the chances of an infant being breastfed on discharge (Simmons, Conroy, & Thompson, 2005). Postponing the first feeding at the breast, lack of breast stimulation, and use of large amounts of formula contribute to cessation of breastfeeding by 7 days postpartum (Ferris et al., 1988). Further complicating the early days is a 15- to 28-hour delay in lactogenesis II typically accompanying maternal diabetes, which can result in low milk intake by the infant during the first few days of life (Arthur, Kent, & Hartmann, 1994; Bitman et al., 1989; Hartmann & Cregan, 2001; Miyake, Tahara, Koike, & Tanizawa, 1989; Murtaugh, Ferris, Capacchione, & Reece, 1998; Ostrom & Ferris, 1993). Delayed lactogenesis seems more likely to occur in mothers with poor metabolic control (Neubauer et al., 1993), but good metabolic control (Whichelow & Doddridge, 1983) and intense breastfeeding support (Webster, Moore, & McMullan, 1995) work together to mitigate many potentially adverse effects on breastfeeding.

Because diabetic mothers can possibly have colostrum for 2–3 days longer than nondiabetic mothers, they may become discouraged if they feel unable to satisfy the hunger needs of their infants (Hutt, 1989). Clinicians may need to make extra efforts to ensure adequate infant intake in the early days and that optimal milk production takes place to avoid having the mother give her infant cow's milk–based infant formula supplements or cereal to satisfy the infant's hunger. The relative risk of developing diabetes can be as much as 13 times higher when a genetically susceptible infant receives cow's milk–based formula during the first 3–4 months of life (Perez-Bravo et al., 1996), putting cow's milk–associated diabetes risk in the same range as the link between cigarette smoking and lung cancer, with a relative risk of approximately 10 (Hammond-McKibben & Dosch, 1997). Early introduction of cereal before 4 months of age also increases the infant's risk of developing type 1 diabetes (Norris et al., 2003; Ziegler, Schmid, Huber, Hummel, & Bonifacio, 2003).

Breastfeeding Management

Anticipating certain situations common to diabetic mothers and their infants in the immediate postpartum helps to avoid ongoing problems. The number of feedings in the first 24 hours has been shown to be a positive predictor for long-term breastfeeding in women with type 2 diabetes (Herskin et al., 2015). For this reason, it is very important to encourage diabetic mothers to feed frequently as soon as they give birth, and that this behavior be encouraged rather than offering bottles of supplemental formula as a routine intervention for breastfeeding infants of diabetic mothers.

Infant Hypoglycemia

The incidence of hypoglycemia in the infant of a diabetic mother is 25–40% (Reece & Homko, 1994), usually occurring within 1–2 hours of birth. This is usually transient with spontaneous improvement. Persistent or recurrent hypoglycemia may require intravenous glucose infusions or pharmacological management. In asymptomatic infants who have blood glucose levels of 40 mg/dL or less, feeding practices should include the following (California Diabetes and Pregnancy Program, 2002):

- Breastfeed by 1 hour of age, followed by hourly for three or four feedings until the blood glucose is stable, and then every 2–3 hours until 12 hours of age (stable is 40 mg/dL or more). Mothers may wish to use alternate breast massage to help transfer as much colostrum as possible when the infant is latched.
- Help from a lactation consultant may be necessary due to the infant's feeding difficulties, with supplementation to be considered if the infant is unable to feed directly at the breast.
- Glucose water should not be given due to its rapid absorption and resulting stimulation of insulin release.
- Some institutions use buccal administered 40% glucose gel to raise blood sugar levels. This has been shown to have a similar absorption rate as IV administered glucose and be more effective than feeding alone (Harris, Weston, Signal, Chase, & Harding, 2013). This procedure does not require NICU admission, is easy to administer and is not associated with any adverse effects such as rebound hypoglycemia. A protocol and algorithm outlining the use of a weight-based dosing of oral glucose gel resulted in a 73% reduction in NICU admissions for hypoglycemia that avoids the separation of mother and infant, reduces the use of bottles of formula, and facilitates exclusive breastfeeding (Bennett, Fagan, Chaharbakhshi, Zamfirova, & Flicker, 2016).

Plans should be in place for how and what to feed an infant of a diabetic mother if he or she is placed in a special care nursery or is unable to transfer milk from the breast. Expressed colostrum should be the first choice. Mothers may express colostrum prenatally, freeze it, and bring it to the hospital for use if the infant is unable to breastfeed during the early hours. They can also hand express colostrum into a spoon and spoon-feed it to the infant if the infant is unable to feed directly from the breast. If the infant cannot tolerate oral feeds, the expressed colostrum can be refrigerated for use when the infant's condition has improved. Finally, banked human milk may be ordered before the birth by the infant's physician and kept frozen on the unit until needed.

Cow's milk–based infant formula should be avoided because of its potential for further sensitizing a susceptible infant to diabetes. If infant formula becomes temporarily necessary, a hydrolyzed formula can be used because it is less diabetogenic (Karges et al., 1997; Knip & Akerblom, 1998). Mothers and infants should be kept in skin-to-skin contact as much as possible to keep the infant's blood sugar levels from dropping due to separation, thermal stress, or crying. This is especially important because it allows the mother to immediately respond to the infant's behavioral feeding cues, which can be difficult if an infant is near-term with state-control difficulties.

Delayed Lactogenesis II

Delayed onset of lactation is common in mothers with GDM, with one-third of mothers in one study experiencing the delayed arrival of copious milk production, especially with increasing severity of

GDM as evidenced by insulin treatment during pregnancy (Matias, Dewey, Quesenberry, & Gunderson, 2014). In a small sample of 27 women with diabetes, more than 25% experienced delayed lactogenesis II, reporting that copious milk production did not occur until 5 or more days postpartum (Jagiello & Chertok, 2015). These mothers also experienced other lactation challenges, including reduced milk supply following lactogenesis II, concern for the infant's health especially in regard to hypoglycemia, and separation.

In anticipation of an extended colostral phase, infants of diabetic mothers should be breastfed 10–12 times each 24 hours during the first 4 days following birth or until the mother experiences the onset of copious milk production. If the infant is unable to feed this frequently, mothers should pump their breasts. The mother should use a double electric pump and should massage and compress each breast while pumping to maximize output. Because only colostrum is available at this stage, it may not flow in appreciable amounts at first or may stick to the sides of the flange and collection bottle. Mothers may find that they extract more colostrum by hand expression than with the use of an electric breast pump. Mothers can also add alternate massage to each breastfeeding session, whereby they massage and compress the breast during the pauses between sucking bursts on each side at each feeding. This may help the infant transfer as much colostrum and transitional milk as possible.

Milk production should be monitored during the first 2 weeks postpartum; diaper output in infants should be monitored as well as signs of jaundice and appropriate infant weight gain. If the infant was large at birth, positioning at the breast may need to be adapted to any birth injuries from shoulder dystocia such as a fractured clavicle, Erb's palsy, phrenic nerve palsy, temporomandibular joint misalignment, or latch problems from vacuum extraction.

Maternal Hypoglycemia

Mothers with type 1 diabetes may experience erratic blood glucose patterns. Hypoglycemia is most likely to occur within an hour after breastfeeding, making this an important time to measure blood glucose. Mothers should eat a snack containing carbohydrates and protein before or during nursing to avoid this problem rather than frequently changing insulin dosages. Nocturnal hypoglycemia is a common occurrence and can be avoided by addressing the nighttime insulin dose or eating a high-protein snack before sleep. Some mothers keep a nonperishable snack in locations where they breastfeed as well as glucose tablets or fast-acting sugars in case of a hypoglycemic emergency.

Mothers with type 2 diabetes who are unable to maintain normal glucose levels through exercise and diet may need to continue on insulin during the time they are lactating. Mothers with GDM may be transitioned from insulin over the first month of lactation to an oral hypoglycemic agent. Diabetic mothers should exercise caution in the use of herbal products because many have the potential to affect blood glucose levels.

Mastitis, Candidosis, Nipple Trauma

Every effort should be made to prevent or intervene promptly if a diabetic mother develops signs and symptoms of mastitis, candidosis, or nipple trauma that could lead to bacterial and yeast overgrowth of the damaged skin. Infections can raise blood glucose levels, and diabetic mothers are sometimes reported to be more susceptible to mastitis if blood sugars are not well controlled (Ferris et al., 1988; Gagne, Leff, & Jefferis, 1992).

Diabetic Mastopathy

This is a less common complication seen in premenopausal long-term type 1 or 2 diabetic women. The breast lesions consist of one or more hard lumps with irregular edges that are moveable and painless (Mak, Chou, Chen, Lee, & Chang, 2003). It is a benign dense fibrous condition that can be easily confused with breast carcinoma. Surgical excision may be necessary to confirm the absence of malignancy (Boullu et al., 1998). Some long-standing diabetic mothers may have had biopsies or surgical incisions to remove small lumps. Any palpable lumps in the breasts of diabetic women should always be closely followed because the number and size of diabetic fibrous masses tend to increase with age.

Polycystic Ovary Syndrome

Insulin resistance and type 2 diabetes can be present in up to 12.6% of women with polycystic ovary syndrome (PCOS; Talbott, Zborowski, & Boudreaux, 2004), with an even higher prevalence in obese women with PCOS. The prevalence of PCOS among women with type 2 diabetes is estimated to be from 21% (Conn, Jacobs, & Conway, 2000) to 26.7% (Peppard, Marfori, Iuorno, & Nestler, 2001). The clinician working with type 2 diabetic mothers should be aware that PCOS could affect approximately one-fourth of these women and may need to consider PCOS when diabetic mothers report perceived or real insufficient milk supplies or an infant with poor weight gain (Marasco et al., 2000).

PCOS, formerly known as Stein-Leventhal syndrome, is a complex syndrome of ovarian, metabolic, and endocrine dysfunction of unknown cause. Its clinical manifestations usually include menstrual irregularities, signs of androgen excess (hirsutism—growth of dark body hair), and obesity. Diagnostic criteria have recently been revised (**Box 9-3**), with no single diagnostic criterion being sufficient for a clinical diagnosis.

Women with PCOS may exhibit combinations of clinical and laboratory manifestations (**Box 9-4**) that may have started developing during adolescence. These women form the largest group of women at risk for the development of cardiovascular disease and diabetes (Polycystic Ovary Syndrome Writing Committee, 2005). PCOS occurs in 10% of reproductive-aged women, constituting the most common metabolic abnormality in young women (Azziz et al., 2004; Hart, Hickey, & Franks, 2004). Carlsen, Jacobsen, and Vanky (2010) measured maternal androgen levels at 25 weeks' gestation and found that high maternal androgen levels in mid-pregnancy were negatively associated with breastfeeding. Vanky

Box 9-3 Revised Diagnostic Criteria for Polycystic Ovary Syndrome

Two of the following three criteria need to be present for a diagnosis of PCOS:

- Oligoovulation and/or anovulation
- Clinical and/or biochemical signs of hyperandrogenism
- Polycystic ovaries and the exclusion of other etiologies such as congenital adrenal hyperplasias, androgen-secreting tumors, or Cushing syndrome

The Rotterdam ESHRE/ASRM-sponsored PCOS Consensus Workshop Group. Revised 2003 consensus on diagnostic criteria and long-term health risks related to polycystic ovary syndrome (PCOS). *Human Reproduction 2004, 19,* 41–47, by permission of Oxford University Press.

Box 9-4 Clinical and Laboratory Manifestations of Polycystic Ovary Syndrome

- Excessive body hair growth, alopecia, balding
- Persistent acne, seborrhea, acanthosis nigricans (dark velvety plaques of thickened skin under the arms, in the groin, and at the nape of neck usually associated with insulin excess)
- Obesity, elevated waist-to-hip ratio
- Reversed ratio of luteinizing hormone to follicle-stimulating hormone
- Elevated free androgen index, elevated testosterone levels
- Elevated fasting insulin levels, insulin resistance
- Menstrual disturbances:
    - Amenorrhea (lack of menstruation)
    - Oligomenorrhea (scanty or infrequent menstrual flow)
    - Anovulation (menstrual cycle in which ovulation is absent)
- Ovaries with increased cystic structures or increased ovarian volume
- History of infertility
- High triglycerides, low levels of high-density lipoprotein cholesterol, increased blood pressure

and colleagues (2012) found that women with no increased breast size during pregnancy seemed to be more metabolically challenged and breastfed less than those mothers who experienced breast size enlargement during pregnancy. Mothers with PCOS and no breast size change during pregnancy had higher blood pressure, higher fasting insulin and triglyceride levels, and were more obese than mothers whose breasts enlarged during pregnancy. The mothers with no breast enlargement seemed to experience more metabolic abnormalities than women who reported breast enlargement during pregnancy. Many women with PCOS experience quality-of-life issues that involve depression, anxiety, and low self-esteem, especially regarding their weight (McCook, Reame, & Thatcher, 2005). Galactorrhea with high serum prolactin levels has been reported in some women with PCOS (Isik, Gulekli, Zorlu, Ergin, & Gokmen, 1997), but it is insufficient milk supply that has brought PCOS to the attention of clinicians working with breastfeeding mothers. Hormonal aberrations are speculated to be associated with milk-supply problems (**Box 9-5**), but the exact mechanism is not known.

Although there is a typical set of clinical manifestation of PCOS (obesity, skin and hair alterations, and menstrual or infertility issues), not all women share all the many variations of the condition. Some mothers with less extensive hormonal alterations may produce abundant amounts of milk, whereas others may experience any number of symptoms (e.g., a combination of hypothyroidism, hypoplastic breasts, and insulin resistance) that collectively result in diminished milk production. Multiparous mothers may produce more milk under the same hormonal conditions due to an increase in prolactin receptors from the previous pregnancy (Zuppa et al., 1988). Hormonal medications that improve breast morphology such as progesterone therapy have been reported to improve lactation in infertile women (Bodley & Powers, 1999). Metformin (Glucophage) is a medication used to improve insulin sensitivity and reduce glucose levels in non-insulin-dependent diabetics while not altering glucose concentrations in healthy people. This property often influences it to be a preferred choice for use in breastfeeding

Box 9-5 Hormonal Aberrations and Milk-Supply Problems

- High levels of androgens (testosterone and androstenedione) may down-regulate estrogen and prolactin receptors (Marasco et al., 2000).
- Elevated estrogen levels in obese women with PCOS postpartum may suppress prolactin.
- Insulin resistance may disrupt lactogenesis.
- Low progesterone levels may disrupt ductile and lobuloalveolar development in the breast, resulting in asymmetrical or hypoplastic breasts.
- Low estrogen levels or limited estrogen receptors may predispose the woman to poor breast tissue development.
- Low prolactin or decreased prolactin receptors may interfere with breast growth during pregnancy and with lactogenesis after delivery.

women (Hale, Kristensen, Hackett, Kohan, & Ilett, 2002). Metformin appears to have no adverse effects on the nursing infant (Glueck & Wang, 2007). Metformin has been used to increase milk production in mothers with insulin resistance (such as in PCOS) with mixed results (Gabbay & Kelly, 2003). Gabbay and Kelly described episodes of engorgement after dosage increases and a limited increase in milk output, but speculated that starting the medication after lactation compromise has become apparent may be too late. However, even combinations of progesterone, metformin, domperidone (Motilium), or metoclopramide (Reglan) or additions of herbal galactagogues may be ineffective in increasing milk production with severe breast hypoplasia.

Breastfeeding Management

Mothers who present with a diagnosis of PCOS or delayed lactogenesis II and signs and symptoms associated with PCOS should be guided by the usual efforts to improve and increase milk production. Frequent feedings, use of alternate massage, additional milk expression, galactagogues, and whatever other medications their physician has placed them on for PCOS treatment may or may not result in adequate milk production. Infant weight must be monitored closely, and some mothers will need to supplement their infant with formula if they are unable to produce sufficient quantities of milk. Supplementation can be done at the breast with tube-feeding systems.

Mothers should be tested for hypothyroidism. Women need to be screened for depression before the use of metoclopramide, and herbal galactagogues that alter blood glucose levels should be used with caution in the presence of insulin resistance or diabetes. Mothers with PCOS should be encouraged to breastfeed, especially because this may help improve the chances for increased milk production with subsequent pregnancies. Many women with PCOS have difficulty conceiving or carrying a pregnancy to term and can be heavily invested in the health and care of the infant. Mothers should be helped to develop a feeding plan right from the start to maximize milk production. Clinicians should praise the mother for any amount of milk produced and help her understand that supplementation does not represent failure or inadequacy on her part.

Hyperreactio Luteinalis

Although more common in pregnancies complicated by hydatidiform mole, fetal hydrops, and multiple pregnancies (Bakri, Bakhashwain, & Hugosson, 1994), hyperreactio luteinalis (theca lutein cysts) can occasionally occur in normal pregnancies. These types of cysts result in ovaries that are enlarged by multiple cysts, producing high levels of testosterone. Mothers may notice hirsutism and limited breast growth during pregnancy. As with PCOS, this hormonal alteration has the potential to disrupt lactogenesis II and delay the establishment of a full milk supply. As the cysts resolve postpartum and the testosterone levels drop, milk production usually increases, leading to full lactation in most situations, but this can take up to a month to happen (Betzold, Hoover, & Snyder, 2004). The normal female adult value of testosterone is 62 ng/dL or less. Case reports in the literature have reported values up to 711 ng/dL, with mothers describing their milk coming in when levels fell to approximately 300 ng/dL (Hoover, Barbalinardo, & Platia, 2002).

Breastfeeding Management

If the presence of theca lutein cysts has been confirmed prenatally, breastfeeding mothers should be encouraged to breastfeed their infant often and monitor the infant's weight closely until the infant is gaining adequately and consistently. Clinicians should schedule frequent weight checks and may need to recommend supplementation with either pumped breastmilk or infant formula until testosterone levels fall and the mother's milk production rebounds. Any needed supplementation should be done at the breast. If undiagnosed in the prenatal period, theca lutein cysts may present postpartum as delayed lactogenesis II, limited milk production, infant weight-gain problems, and lack of breast changes in the prenatal period. In the presence of these conditions, the clinician might wish to ask the mother if she has experienced excess body hair growth or other signs of virilization during her pregnancy. If so, the clinician may wish to have testosterone levels measured and pelvic ultrasound to confirm the presence of theca lutein cysts.

Thyroid Disorders

The thyroid gland is a butterfly-shaped endocrine gland located in the lower front of the neck whose hormones are actively involved in controlling metabolic functions, energy use, heat generation, and the activity of the brain, heart, muscles, and other organs. The thyroid gland produces the hormones thyroxine (T_4), triiodothyronine (T_3), and calcitonin.

Thyroid disease is more common in women than in men, with about 2–3% of Americans having pronounced hypothyroidism and about 10–15% having subclinical or mild hypothyroidism. A breastfeeding mother can present with one of several types of thyroid diseases: hypothyroidism, hyperthyroidism, or postpartum thyroiditis.

Hypothyroidism

Hypothyroidism is an underactive thyroid gland resulting from a number of causes, including Hashimoto disease or Hashimoto thyroiditis. This is an autoimmune thyroiditis in which the immune system's attack on the thyroid causes a goiter (swelling) and possibly results in hypothyroidism. Disruptions in communication with the pituitary gland, which directs the thyroid in how much hormone to produce, could lead to low thyroid levels with a resulting diminished milk supply. In the dairy cow, low thyroid levels have been associated with low fat content of the milk, low prolactin levels, and decreased milk production and poor weight gain in the calves (Thrift et al., 1999), further implicating a thyroid–pituitary axis involvement. Because the thyroid is responsible for cellular activity, diminished milk production could also result from a slowdown in milk-secreting cell activity.

Undiagnosed and/or untreated hypothyroidism during the first trimester of pregnancy places the fetus at increased risk for intellectual impairment, abnormal neuropsychological development, and impaired psychomotor functioning (Berbel et al., 2009; Morreale, Obregon, & Escobar, 2000; Pop et al., 1999), and as much as a 10-point lower IQ in the presence of autoimmune thyroiditis (Muller, Drexhage, & Berghout, 2001). Many common symptoms of hypothyroidism mimic those of the normal postpartum period, such as fatigue, sleepiness, decreased energy, hair loss, poor concentration, weight gain, carpal tunnel syndrome, muscle aches, constipation, and dry skin. If low milk production is also present, the clinician may wish to have the mother's thyroid function tested (Shames & Youngkin, 2002). Many people with low thyroid levels also complain of being cold and demonstrate periorbital edema and hoarseness. Hypothyroidism is generally treated with synthetic thyroxine or levothyroxine (Synthroid, Levothyroid, Thyroid, Unithyroid, Levoxyl), including during pregnancy and lactation. Oral levothyroxine transfer into milk is extremely low (Hale, 2012).

Hyperthyroidism

Hyperthyroidism, commonly called Graves disease, is the production of excess thyroid hormone. It is characterized by weight loss despite increased appetite, nervousness, sweating, heat intolerance, heart palpitations, and possibly bulging eyes and goiter. Poorly controlled hyperthyroidism during pregnancy has been reported to be followed by an early and dramatic onset of lactogenesis II, failure of the milk-ejection reflex, and painful engorgement from milk stasis, followed by mastitis (Marasco, 2014). Although suppression of the milk-ejection reflex is not seen in all mothers with hyperthyroidism, it should be assessed and monitored in women with this thyroid disease.

A large concern during lactation is the safety of the medications used to treat the mother. Medications may be used to treat both the symptoms of the disease and the high thyroid levels. Propranolol (Inderal) is a beta-blocker and may be used to treat hypertension and cardiac arrhythmias. Propylthiouracil is usually the drug of choice in breastfeeding mothers to suppress maternal thyroid function (Hale & Berens, 2002). Many endocrinologists still do not recommend breastfeeding during propylthiouracil therapy (Lee et al., 2000), even though the American Academy of Pediatrics, Committee on Drugs (2001) has classified this drug as usually compatible with breastfeeding and has done so for many years. Methimazole (Tapazole) has also been shown safe to use during lactation with no adverse outcomes reported in infants, including changes in thyroid function or physical or intellectual development (Azizi, Khoshniat, Bahrainian, & Hedayati, 2000).

Mothers should be aware that their infant's thyroid may be monitored periodically to ensure adequate functioning. The use of radioactive diagnostic material such as technetium-99m pertechnetate is compatible with breastfeeding with a 12- to 24-hour interruption of nursing until the material is cleared, but radioactive ablation of the thyroid gland with iodine-131 requires cessation of breastfeeding (Hale, 2012). The breast tissue itself acts as a repository for almost 40% of the iodine-131 dose, which may increase the risk of breast cancer. For maximal protection of the mother, Hale and Berens (2002) recommended that the mother cease breastfeeding several weeks before the ablation procedure to reduce deposition of iodine-131 material into the breast tissue. Hale (2012) states that radioactivity decays at a set rate, so breastmilk that is pumped and stored in a freezer during treatment for at least 8–10 half-lives can be fed to the infant with no problem. All of the radioactivity will be gone by then.

Postpartum Thyroiditis

Postpartum thyroiditis occurs in approximately 5–10% of women. Inflammation of the thyroid gland is not uncommon in the postpartum woman. The risk is greater in women with autoimmune disorders, positive antithyroid antibodies, or a history of previous thyroid dysfunction, with 20% of women having a recurrence of thyroiditis with subsequent pregnancies. Thyroiditis includes two phases: initial thyrotoxicosis (high thyroid hormone levels), occurring 1–3 months after delivery, followed by a hypothyroid phase, occurring 4–8 months after delivery and lasting up to 1 year. Not all women experience both phases. Treatment of the thyrotoxicosis phase is usually with beta-blockers to reduce the palpitations, tremors, and shakes, not antithyroid medication, because this phase is transient. The hypothyroid phase is treated with thyroid hormone replacement and gradually tapered off because 80% of mothers regain normal thyroid function.

Although primary thyroid dysfunction is associated with mood disorders (Harris, 1999), PPD has been shown to be associated with positive thyroid antibody status and an increase in depressive symptoms in antibody-positive mothers (Harris et al., 1992). Clinicians may wish to ask mothers with thyroid dysfunction or mothers encountering lactation problems thought to occur in association with thyroid problems if they are experiencing "infant blues" or new-onset depression. Symptoms of thyroid dysfunction can mimic normal postpartum adjustment and fatigue and should be distinguished from these so that treatment may commence (Pereira & Brown, 2008). Lawrence and Lawrence (2016) recommended screening for thyroid disease before prescribing antidepressants. In addition, mothers should be asked if they are self-medicating with herbal products, such as St. John's wort, which could mask the thyroid disease.

Breastfeeding Management

Good initial breastfeeding guidelines are always important. Mothers with milk-production problems, infants who experience weight-gain difficulties, and mothers with a predisposing history for thyroid problems should be followed closely. Hypothyroid mothers have been shown to produce significantly less milk during the first 6 days postpartum (Miyake et al., 1989). Lactation deficiency has been reported in association with infant weight-gain problems due to reduced milk production (Buckshee, Kriplani, Kapil, Bhargava, & Takkar, 1992; Stein, 2002). Animal studies in rats revealed a reduction in circulating oxytocin in hypothyroid mothers resulting in less milk release, poor milk transfer, and reduced litter growth (Hapon, Simoncini, Via, & Jahn, 2003). Similar problems have been reported in both animal and human mothers who are hyperthyroid.

When lactogenesis has occurred yet there seems to be little milk transfer and other explanations have been ruled out, hyperthyroid should be considered as a possibility (Marasco, 2006). Insufficient milk supplies that do not improve by standard corrective measures should alert the clinician to a possible endocrine problem and recommend diagnostic testing. Diminished milk output between 4 and 8 months postpartum, although certainly related to other issues, may also have an endocrine origin, with the clinician wishing to possibly check thyroid hormone levels at this time. Breastfeeding should not be interrupted unless radioactive diagnostic procedures are needed nor abandoned unless ablation of the thyroid gland is indicated. It is especially important for mothers with a history of thyroid problems to continue breastfeeding because lack of breastfeeding has been associated with an increased risk for thyroid cancer (Mack, Preston-Martin, Bernstein, Qian, & Xiang, 1999).

Both hypothyroidism and hyperthyroidism seem to impair milk release, not milk synthesis. Without adequate milk removal, milk production decreases, placing the infant at a higher risk for insufficient weight gain. Efforts to improve milk release include the use of oxytocin nasal spray to induce milk ejection, use of alternate massage/breast compressions, reverse-pressure softening, and stimulation of the nipple–areolar complex.

Fibromyalgia

Fibromyalgia affects as many as 8 million people in the United States, occurring mainly in women of childbearing age. Symptoms usually arise between the ages of 20 and 55 years, but the condition also may be diagnosed in childhood. Symptoms of fibromyalgia typically include:

- Feeling of pain, burning, aching, and soreness in the body
- Headaches, tenderness of the scalp, pain in the back of the skull
- Pain in the neck, shoulder, shoulder blades, and elbows
- Pain in hips, top of buttocks, outside the lower hip, below buttocks, and the pelvis
- Pain in the knees and kneecap area
- Fatigue, unrefreshing sleep, waking up tired, morning stiffness
- Insomnia, frequent waking, difficulty falling asleep, or falling asleep immediately
- Raynaud's phenomenon
- Irritable bowel syndrome, diarrhea and constipation, bloating, cramping
- Balance problems
- Neurally mediated hypotension; balance problems
- Restless leg syndrome
- Sense of tissues feeling swollen
- Numbness, tingling, and feeling of cold in the hands and feet
- Chest pain, palpitations
- Shortness of breath
- Anxiety, depression, and "fibrofog"—term used to describe the confusion and forgetfulness, inability to concentrate and difficulty recalling simple words and numbers, and transposing words and numbers

Fibromyalgia can negatively affect breastfeeding by making it very difficult to stay in one position for very long during breastfeeding sessions. Mothers may experience extreme pain or stiffness when holding their infant for extended periods of time in the same position. Breastfeeding mothers with fibromyalgia may experience sore nipples, insufficient milk supply, and depression (Schaefer, 2004).

Breastfeeding Management

Mothers need help in finding comfortable nursing positions and may need to switch positions several times during each breastfeeding session. Lying down while breastfeeding and semireclining with ventral positioning of the infant are relaxing positions. Mothers may find that the use of a sling or breastfeeding pillow reduces strain on muscles. Adaptive infant care equipment may be needed in severe situations (see Physically Challenged Mothers, near the beginning of this chapter). Clinicians need to remain vigilant regarding sore nipples, Raynaud's phenomenon of the nipples, and milk production. Warm compresses or heating pads may be helpful for sore neck and back muscles.

Cystic Fibrosis

Cystic fibrosis (CF) is an autosomal recessive disease involving multiple body organs and systems including the lungs, pancreas, urogenital system, skeleton, and skin. CF is the most common genetic disease among whites. It affects about 30,000 children and adults in the United States and about 70,000 people worldwide. Although CF is more commonly found in the white population, the disease affects all racial groups. CF occurs in about 1 in every 3,500 white births, 1 in every 17,000 black births, and 1 in every 90,000 Asian births. About 12 million people (about 1 in 30 people) in the United States carry one CF gene mutation. Dysfunction in exocrine glands and chronic lung problems are typical manifestations of the condition. With improved diagnostic and therapeutic interventions, many young women with CF bear children and breastfeed, whereas in the past, few people with CF lived to adulthood. The median age of survival is 35 years (Cystic Fibrosis Foundation, n.d.).

Some mothers with CF choose or are advised not to breastfeed due to real or perceived concerns for maternal health or fear of potential harm to the infant from maternal medications. Breastfeeding decisions should be based on the overall health and wishes of the mother (Edenborough et al., 2008). Possible side effects of medications are a common reason among women's decisions not to breastfeed (Gilljam et al., 2000), but most medications needed for the treatment of CF are safe to take while breastfeeding. Festini and colleagues (2006) reported a mother who underwent intravenous tobramycin (Tobrex) therapy while breastfeeding with no detectable medication found in her milk. An increasing number of women with CF are choosing to breastfeed (Luder, Kaltan, Tanzer-Torres, & Bonforte, 1990), with breastmilk composition quite capable of adequately nourishing their infants (Michel & Mueller, 1994), even if the fat content is slightly lower than normal (Bitman, Hamosh, Wood, Freed, & Hamosh, 1987). Shiffman, Seale, Flux, Rennert, and Swender (1989) reported that concentrations of milk macronutrients were decreased during exacerbations of the pulmonary aspect of CF and that mothers and infants should be monitored more closely during these times.

As long as the mother remains healthy, maintaining her weight and respiratory status, breastfeeding benefits both her and her infant. Breastfeeding increases maternal nutritional requirements for energy, calcium, and many other vitamins and minerals. Mothers with CF may or may not be able to sustain exclusive breastfeeding for the recommended period of time but should be encouraged to continue for as long as possible (Odegaard et al., 2002). Breastfeeding after transplantation is possible with needed medications reviewed by the CF and transplant teams. Infants of breastfeeding mothers with CF are protected against many of the pathogens that the mother chronically carries, reducing the incidence and severity of illness in the infant (Parker, O'Sullivan, Shea, Regan, & Freedman, 2004).

Breastfeeding Management

Clinicians should monitor the caloric requirements of both the mother and infant, ensuring that each partner maintains adequate weight under conditions of increased need. Mothers with mild CF usually do quite well with breastfeeding but should receive close support during the establishment of lactation. Maternal diabetes and gestational diabetes are common in women with CF during pregnancy, so close monitoring for infant hypoglycemia and hyperglycemia is important. Infants may need to be weighed more frequently, especially during times of maternal disease exacerbations. The most common complication for the infant born to a mother with CF is prematurity, with about 25% of these infants born preterm. Some clinicians occasionally monitor the mother's milk for sodium, chloride, and total fat, and routinely do so when the mother experiences pulmonary infections or disease flare-ups.

Phenylketonuria

Phenylketonuria (PKU) is an autosomal recessive inherited metabolic disorder arising from a defect in the enzyme phenylalanine hydroxylase that converts phenylalanine (PHE) to tyrosine. Women with PKU can breastfeed quite successfully, produce milk with normal levels of components, and should maintain their special PKU diet throughout their lifetime (Matalon, Michals, & Gleason, 1986). It is vital that nonpregnant women and mothers with PKU be on their special diet before conception and throughout the entire pregnancy (Lee, Ridout, Walter, & Cockburn, 2005; Maillot, Lilburn, Baudin, Morley, & Lee, 2008). High levels of PHE can be present in the fetus from very early in the pregnancy (Purnell, 2001). High PHE levels during pregnancy can result in maternal PKU effects on the developing fetus that include facial dysmorphism, microcephaly, intrauterine growth retardation, developmental delays, and congenital heart disease. The longer it takes to achieve metabolic control during pregnancy, the lower developmental scores are in the infant (Waisbren et al., 2000). High serum and milk levels of PHE in mothers with PKU do not result in abnormal PHE levels in their non-PKU breastfeeding infants (Fox-Bacon, McCamman, Therou, Moore, & Kipp, 1997). Breastfeeding mothers with PKU usually remain on a modified diet during breastfeeding, avoiding aspartame, an artificial sweetener made from PHE. A neurological assessment of the infant is usually done at 4 and 8 weeks and an echocardiogram should be done for infants conceived off diet (Maillot, Cook, Lilburn, & Lee, 2007).

Breastfeeding Management

Good breastfeeding management practices are important as usual. After the infant is born, he or she is no longer at risk for side effects from high maternal PHE levels. Infants of mothers with PKU should be breastfed and should be tested for PKU during their routine newborn screening. It is important to breastfeed right from the start because even if this infant eventually tests positive for PKU, breastfeeding during the early days until dietary intervention begins has been linked to higher intelligence quotient scores in dietary-treated phenylketonuric children (Riva et al., 1996).

Multiple Sclerosis

Multiple sclerosis (MS) is a progressive autoimmune demyelinating disease of the central nervous system. It is one of the most common causes of neurological disability in young adults, affecting females two to three times more frequently than males, with onset between the ages of 20 and 40 years. Approximately 70%

of those with MS are women. The prevalence of MS has been reported as 46 per 100,000 in the United States and 90 per 100,000 in Canada (Pugliatti, Sotgiu, & Rosati, 2002). The condition is unpredictable, has periods of exacerbations and remissions, has no cure, and has an unknown cause. Having been breastfed for over 4 months is associated with a lower risk of developing MS (Conradi et al., 2013). Symptoms may be erratic and progressive, and include numbness and tingling, urinary tract problems, difficulty walking, visual disturbances, weakness, profound fatigue, vertigo, loss of balance, incoordination, speech difficulties, and paralysis. Women may experience relief from relapses of the condition during pregnancy followed by an increased relapse rate after delivery (Lorenzi & Ford, 2002), especially during the first 3 months postpartum (Worthington, Jones, Crawford, & Forti, 1994).

Breastfeeding does not adversely affect the health of mothers with MS (Birk & Rudick, 1986), does not cause an increase in relapse rate postpartum (Nelson, Franklin, & Jones, 1988), and has been shown to promote their health by decreasing MS relapse rates by between 10% and 50% during the first 6 months postpartum (Confavreux, Hutchinson, Hours, Cortinovis-Tourniaire, & Moreau, 1998; Gulick & Halper, 2002; Hellwig et al., 2015). Exclusive breastfeeding is extremely important because women with MS who breastfeed exclusively during the first 2 months are approximately five times less likely to relapse in the first year postpartum than women who did not breastfeed or began supplemental formula feedings during that time (Langer-Gould et al., 2009). Hellwig, Haghikia, Rockhoff, and Gold (2012) showed that women who breastfed exclusively had lower disease activity during the first 3 months postpartum than women who only partially breastfed or who did not breastfeed at all. These authors speculate that high prolactin levels may be responsible for reducing relapses because in experimental situations, high prolactin levels were shown to promote remyelination (Gregg et al., 2007). Breastfeeding the infant of a mother with MS is very important because human-milk feeding appears to decrease the risk of developing MS (Conradi et al., 2013; Houtchens & Kolb, 2013; Pisacane et al., 1994). Breastfed infants of mothers with MS experience reduced rates of otitis media, lower respiratory illness, constipation, milk intolerance, and allergy during the first year of life (Gulick & Johnson, 2004), sparing a fatigued mother the further burden of caring for a sick infant.

Women with MS have numerous concerns regarding their own health as well as that of the fetus and newborn. These include the fear of transmitting MS to their infant, relapses in the postpartum period and how to handle an infant during those times, effects of medications on the infant while breastfeeding, effects of profound fatigue on child care and lactation (Eggum, 2001; Halbert, 1998), and concern that breastfeeding would be more exhausting than preparing bottles of formula. Many mothers receive conflicting advice from healthcare providers regarding breastfeeding in the presence of MS and become confused by differing opinions of the specialists caring for them (Coyle et al., 2004; Smeltzer, 1994). MS is not transmitted through breastmilk but may have a familial tendency. The lifetime risk of MS developing in a child whose mother has MS is 0.5–3%, compared with the general population risk of 0.1%. The nature of the condition creates uncertainty regarding if and when relapses will occur and if the symptoms will abate without treatment. This results in a high level of emotional distress (Kroencke & Denney, 1999). Mothers are particularly distressed by fatigue, limb weakness, balance problems, vision disturbances, tingling and numbness, and urinary incontinence (Gulick & Kim, 2004), which without appropriate interventions could lead to depression (Harrison & Stuifbergen, 2002).

Numerous medications may be prescribed for the mother, such as glatiramer (Copaxone), a mixture of polymers of four amino acids that is similar to myelin basic protein; adrenocorticotropic hormone;

and interferon beta-1A (Avonex) and interferon beta-1B (Betaseron), which are immunomodulators and appear to be moderately safe, with transport into human milk being limited (Hale, 2012). Methylprednisolone (Solu-Medrol, Medrol) or other corticosteroids are used to treat a number of MS symptoms but can be prescribed in high-dose courses either intravenously or orally over a period of up to 2 weeks. High doses and prolonged administration of these types of medications could affect an infant when exposed through breastmilk. Hale (2012) recommended a brief period of pumping and discarding milk (8–24 hours) after intravenous administration of methylprednisolone at doses up to 1 g. Given that the amount of drug transferred into breastmilk appears to be less than the dose given to neonates who require this medication, and if the maternal treatment with methylprednisolone is very brief, mothers could continue to breastfeed without interruption. To further limit infant exposure, the mother could wait 2–4 hours after IV administration of methylprednisolone before breastfeeding her infant, which would significantly limit the amount of drug in the milk (Cooper, Felkins, Baker, & Hale, 2015). At least 17 medications may be prescribed for women with MS; however, not all are compatible with breastfeeding. Almas, Vance, Baker, & Hale (2016) review these drugs in the context of breastfeeding.

Breastfeeding Management

It is most helpful for the clinician to meet with the mother before the birth of her infant to determine the extent of the MS progression and begin preparations for social and lactation support postpartum. Prenatal preparation can include the following:

- A plan should be developed for household help and help with the care of the infant and other children.
- Family and friends who provide care and support should be educated about why breastfeeding is important to both the mother and infant. Caregivers should understand that breastfeeding does not exacerbate the disease. They should not take over complete care of the infant, especially the feeding of the infant, so that the mother can rest (Siebenaler, 2002). Helpers can bring the infant to the mother and help her assume a comfortable, supported position for breastfeeding.
- Mothers should purchase or rent a high-grade electric breast pump with a double collection kit (Jacobson, 1998). Mothers use the pump to express milk during disease remission periods and store it for use if necessary during times when exacerbations occur and/or breastfeeding must be interrupted for drug therapy. Mothers also may need to pump during interruptions in breastfeeding to ensure an abundant milk supply once the infant is back on the breast.
- Mothers may desire a special nursing pillow, a sling, and a small footstool. These can be used if needed for help with positioning.
- If the mother is in a wheelchair, the home should be arranged for unobstructed access to the infant and an area set up where the mother can comfortably nurse the infant.
- Resting and sleeping arrangements can be prepared before delivery. Mothers may find it easier to breastfeed if the infant is kept within arm's reach next to the bed in a small crib designed to attach to the adult bed.
- Arrangements should be made for community support services as well as lactation support for the postpartum period.

In-hospital support during the initial stay after birth should center on the creation of an individualized breastfeeding plan for both the time spent in the hospital and for feedings after discharge. Many suggestions are designed to minimize the fatigue associated with MS. For instance, positioning for breastfeeding may need to be modified depending on the extent of the MS progression. Before hospital discharge, mothers should be documented as being able to position their infant for breastfeeding or a helper should be documented as capable to assist for proper positioning. Mothers breastfeeding in the sitting position may benefit from strategically placed pillows or the use of a pillow designed for breastfeeding to provide support for both the infant and the mother's arms (**Figure 9-1**).

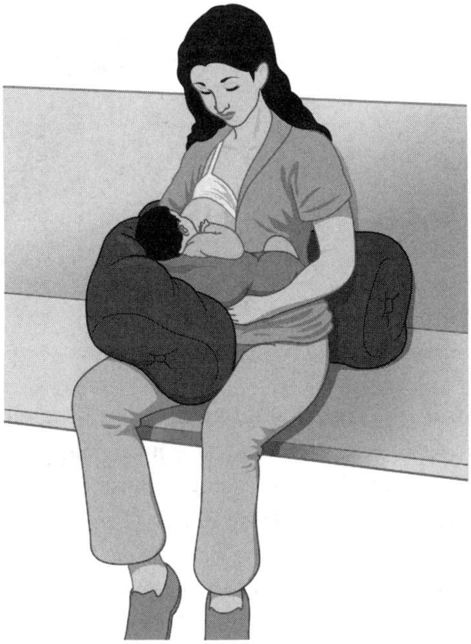

Figure 9-1 Multiple pillows: supportive positioning for mothers with MS.

Some mothers find that use of a sling helps stabilize and support the weight of the infant if the mother's arms have muscular weakness, lack coordination, or are painful (**Figure 9-2**). In addition, a mother who uses a wheelchair will need to use pillows or a tray across her lap (**Figure 9-3**).

Mothers should be taught how to breastfeed while lying down. Mothers who nurse in the reclining position have reported fewer fatigue-related symptoms after nursing in the side-lying position as opposed to the sitting position (Milligan, Flenniken, & Pugh, 1996). An alternative position might be reclining the mother to a 30-degree angle with the infant placed in a ventral or biological nurturing position that avoids strain from gravity when seated upright.

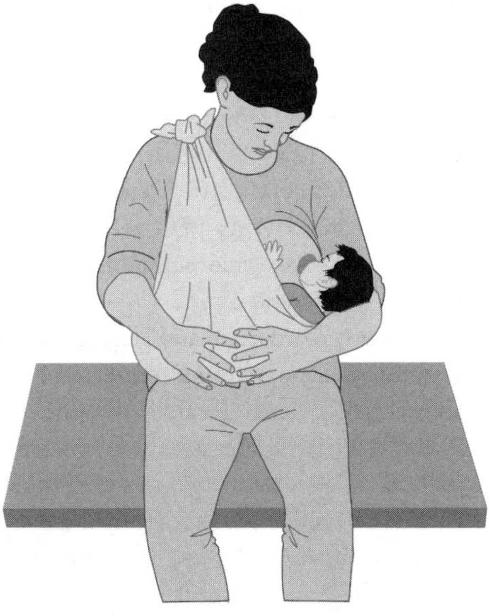

Figure 9-2 A baby sling: support suggestions for mothers with muscular weakness.

Systemic Lupus Erythematosus

Systemic lupus erythematosus (SLE) is a chronic autoimmune inflammatory disease distinguished by the presence of non–organ-specific autoantibodies. SLE can affect almost any part of the body, including the joints, kidneys, skin, heart, lungs, brain, and blood vessels. It most often affects young adults under 40 years of age and has a 3 times higher incidence in African Americans and African Caribbeans. Approximately 85% of people

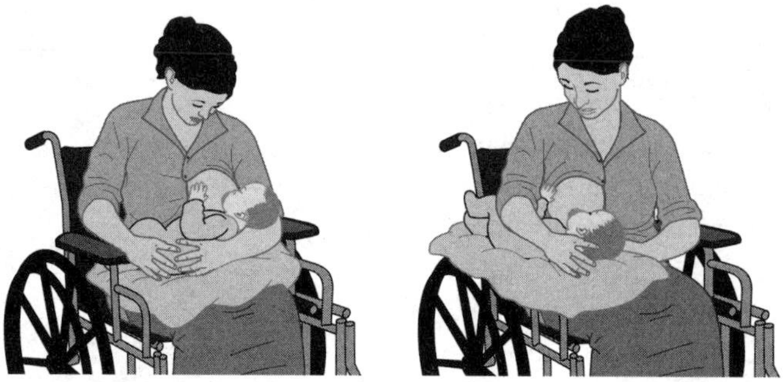

Figure 9-3 Pillows and tray: support suggestions for mothers who use wheelchairs.

with SLE are women, and SLE may be familial (Lupus Foundation of America, 2013). This makes it especially important that all women, and especially if there is a family history of SLE, are encouraged and assisted with breastfeeding because breastfeeding is associated with a decreased risk of developing SLE (Cooper, Dooley, Treadwell, St. Clair, & Gilkeson, 2002). There are little data regarding disease flares during lactation. One case study (Mok, Wong, & Lau, 1998) reported a disease flare with hyperprolactinemia during breastfeeding, but because other hormones were not assayed, it remains important for mothers to understand that breastfeeding will not exacerbate their disease.

Of the different types of lupus, SLE is the most common, with varying signs and symptoms that alternate between remissions and flares. More frequently seen symptoms include a butterfly-like rash across the nose and cheeks, skin rashes on body parts exposed to the sun, sores in the mouth or nose, painful or swollen joints, fatigue, chest pain during deep breathing, Raynaud's phenomenon, kidney inflammations, depression, headaches, memory and thinking problems, strokes, and blood clots.

Preeclampsia, prematurity, and intrauterine growth retardation are more common in mothers with SLE. A number of medications are used to treat SLE depending on the extent of organ involvement and frequency and types of disease flares. Aspirin, subcutaneous heparin, nonsteroidal anti-inflammatory drugs (NSAIDs), and corticosteroids may be used during the pregnancy to improve the chances of carrying the infant to term and for reducing joint and muscle pain and inflammation. Antimalarial medications such as hydroxychloroquine (Plaquenil) and chloroquine (Aralen) are sometimes used to treat joint pain, skin rashes, and ulcers.

High doses of aspirin and NSAIDs are generally avoided in the last weeks of pregnancy to avoid any unwanted effects on uterine contraction, platelet function, or closure of the ductus arteriosus. Medication use during lactation can involve the use of aspirin but not in large doses. Most but not all NSAIDs are compatible with breastfeeding; however, NSAIDs can displace bilirubin and are contraindicated in jaundiced infants. Small amounts of corticosteroids can be found in breastmilk. When the dose exceeds 20 mg/day, some clinicians recommend that mothers wait at least 4 hours before nursing to reduce infant exposure (Ost, Wettrell, Bjorkhem, & Rane, 1985). Tacrolimus (Prograf, Protopic) has recently been used for steroid-resistant SLE and appears safe for breastfed newborns, with low blood concentration levels of this drug being seen in the infant (Izumi, Miyashita, & Migita, 2014).

Immunosuppressive agents/chemotherapy medications are used in serious cases of SLE when major organs are losing their ability to function (Mok & Wong, 2001). Azathioprine (Imuran) and cyclosporin

A are not teratogenic and may be considered in situations of severe lupus, whereas cyclophosphamide (Cytoxan) is a teratogen in humans and is not used during pregnancy.

About 3% of infants born to mothers with lupus have neonatal lupus. This lupus consists of a temporary rash and abnormal blood counts. Neonatal lupus usually disappears by the time the infant is 3–6 months old and does not recur. About one-half of infants with neonatal lupus are born with a heart condition. This condition is permanent but can be treated with a pacemaker.

Breastfeeding Management

Mothers with SLE may also experience chronic fatigue syndrome and fibromyalgia, compounding the major problem of fatigue. Because most mothers with SLE are taking some type of medication or multiple medications, the clinician should be aware of and ensure the safety of all drugs taken during lactation. Anecdotal reports of insufficient milk supply in breastfeeding mothers with SLE may alert the clinician to ensuring a good start to breastfeeding with steps taken to maximize milk production. It is not known whether the SLE itself, high blood pressure/preeclampsia, or some combination of medications inhibits sufficient milk production. The infant should be closely monitored for normal weight gain and any possible side effects from maternal medications. Planned rest periods and breastfeeding in the side-lying or ventral position may help with SLE-related fatigue. Because people with SLE may experience Raynaud's phenomenon, breastfeeding mothers and their healthcare providers should be vigilant for this condition in the nipple. Some infants of mothers with SLE are preterm, intrauterine growth retarded, or separated from their mother during the early days of life. If the infant is not available to be put directly to the breast, mothers need to begin pumping as soon as possible after delivery. Breastfeeding management guidelines should be incorporated into an individualized feeding plan for this mother.

Rheumatoid Arthritis

Rheumatoid arthritis (RA) is a chronic inflammatory condition with autoimmune, genetic predisposition and familial clustering properties. Some researchers are uncertain if RA is just one disease or several different diseases with common features. Prevalence estimates range from 0.3–1.5% in North America (Silman & Pearson, 2002), with prevalence increasing with age and 2.5 times higher in women than in men. Researchers believe that female reproductive hormones may have an influence on the greater incidence of RA seen in women. Evidence regarding reproductive hormones, pregnancy, and breastfeeding as risk factors for RA is conflicting. Because RA has both genetic and familial clustering trends, mothers who have a family history of RA should be encouraged and supported to breastfeed. Karlson, Mandl, Hankinson, and Grodstein (2004) showed that women who breastfed for 13–23 months had a 20% reduction in risk for development of RA, whereas those breastfeeding for at least 24 months during their childbearing years increased their risk reduction to 50%.

Many women with RA enjoy a remission in their condition during pregnancy, when levels of the proinflammatory hormone prolactin are reduced, but experience flares postpartum, especially in the presence of breastfeeding (Barrett, Brennan, Fiddler, & Silman, 2000). However, the onset of RA and flares of the condition postpartum in susceptible mothers (Hampl & Papa, 2001) may also be related to limited durations of breastfeeding as well as the cumulative effects of the number of total months spent breastfeeding. Brennan and Silman (1994) looked at 187 women who had developed RA within 12 months of a pregnancy.

Eighty-eight women (47%) with RA developed it after their first pregnancy, and 71 of these 88 mothers had breastfed. However, breastfeeding by the third pregnancy posed no increased risk of developing RA.

The duration of breastfeeding has been shown to be inversely related to the risk of RA, with the protective effect of longer breastfeeding remaining significant even after adjustment for other environmental influences (Liao, Alfredsson, & Karlson, 2009; Pikwer et al., 2009). Cortisol levels are increased during lactation, with a long-term association seen between the cumulative duration of breastfeeding and elevated cortisol playing protective roles in the acquisition of certain autoimmune diseases such as RA long after the childbearing years (Lankarani-Fard, Kritz-Silverterin, Barrett-Connor, & Goodman-Gruen, 2001). Other confounding factors could also place first-time mothers at an increased risk for development of RA, including irregular menstrual cycles (Karlson et al., 2004). Such subfertility may be a marker for women at increased risk for development of RA, as could states of hyperprolactinemia or abnormal responses to prolactin. It is known that pregnant women with SLE have significantly elevated prolactin levels (Jara, Lavelle, & Espinoza, 1992), as do patients with RA, osteoarthritis, and fibromyalgia. Problems with the pituitary regulation of prolactin may contribute to RA in susceptible populations, whereas a high cumulative duration or "dose" of breastfeeding is related to a decreased risk of RA, perhaps because lactation provides a regulatory mechanism.

Drug therapy usually involves a combination of medications depending on the extent of the disease, exacerbations, and tolerance. Some drugs are safe for use during lactation, some are not, and some have effects that are simply unknown. The main categories of drugs used to treat RA are as follows:

- NSAIDs are used to reduce inflammation and relieve pain. These may include aspirin, ibuprofen (Advil, Motrin), acetaminophen (Tylenol, Paracetamol), flurbiprofen (Ansaid, Froben), diclofenac (Cataflam, Voltaren), indomethacin (Indocin), and piroxicam (Feldene). NSAIDs have many gastrointestinal side effects and should not be used in the presence of a jaundiced infant. Their use requires closer monitoring of the infant for potential side effects.
- Analgesic drugs used to relieve pain but not inflammation include acetaminophen, propoxyphene (Darvocet N, Darvon), and ketorolac (Toradol).
- Glucocorticoids or prednisone are used in low doses to prevent joint damage.
- Disease-modifying antirheumatic drugs, used along with NSAIDs and/or prednisone, slow joint destruction over time. Examples include methotrexate (Folex, Rheumatrex), injectable gold (Myochrysine, Solganal), penicillamine (Cuprimine, Depen), azathioprine (Imuran), chloroquine (Aralen, Novo-chloroquine), hydroxychloroquine (Plaquenil), sulfasalazine (Azulfidine), and oral gold (Ridaura). Hydroxychloroquine has been safely used, but methotrexate can be stored in the mucosal cells of the gastrointestinal tract in infants and could be problematic. Gold has a very long half-life and would expose an infant for long periods of time to a very toxic product. These drugs can suppress the immune system, so it is important to practice good breastfeeding management to prevent infections such as mastitis.
- Biological response modifiers directly modify the immune system by inhibiting cytokines that contribute to inflammation. These include etanercept (Enbrel), infliximab (Remicade), adalimumab (Humira), anakinra (Kineret), abatacept (Orencia), and rituximab (Rituxan).
- Protein-A immunoadsorption therapy is a process that filters the blood to remove antibodies and immune complexes that promote inflammation.
- Steroids such as triamcinolone (Aristocort) can be directly injected into affected joints.

Breastfeeding Management

Prenatal preparation for breastfeeding should include the promotion of breastfeeding for women with RA and plans for handling any relapse or flares after delivery. Medications are often given in combination and should be chosen based on their safety profile and urgency of need. Along with good breastfeeding management guidelines, special attention may need to be directed to help the mother with RA assume a comfortable position for breastfeeding depending on which joints are affected. Any adaptive equipment or special household arrangements should be made at this time. Mothers should ensure that any forms of anemia are corrected and that they will follow good nutritional guidelines to prevent anemia from interfering with the establishment and maintenance of an abundant milk supply.

Cervical Spine

A mother with pain, stiffness, or a limited range of motion in the neck may be unable to look down for any length of time while placing her infant to the breast or while using a breast pump. A heating pad or application of warm compresses to the neck before breastfeeding or pumping may be soothing. The mother may find that breastfeeding in front of a mirror (Drazin, 1995) provides a mechanism to visualize positioning, latch, suck, and swallowing of the infant and allows the proper placement and use of a breast pump. Some mothers may find the side-lying position or ventral positioning of the infant to be effective and comfortable.

Spinal Column

Mothers with back pain usually need to experiment with positions and supporting pillows to see what feels best for them. Some mothers find that placing their feet on a small footstool when in a seated position removes strain from the lower back and tips the infant slightly toward the mother's body. With the infant tipped toward the mother, she will not need to provide as much support with her arm, lessening the strain on the shoulder girdle and upper back. Reclining at a 30-degree angle with ventral positioning of the infant may ease back strain.

Wrist, Hand, and Fingers

Some mothers with RA find a nursing pillow that allows the infant to maintain a position that does not require extended use of the wrist can be helpful. The side-lying positioning eases strain on the wrist and hands and can reduce the need to reposition the infant if the mother shifts her position to present the upper breast to the infant while still lying on her side. A small, rolled towel can be placed under the breast if a large breast requires support throughout the feeding.

If a mother requires the use of a breast pump, the clinician should consider the use of an electric pump with a double collection kit. Use of a cylinder pump, especially with the wrist pronated, can provoke or exacerbate lateral epicondylitis (tennis elbow) and strain on the wrist (Williams, Auerbach, & Jacobi, 1989). Use of a manual pump with a squeeze handle places considerable stress on the wrist, as will any pump that requires repetitive hand motion. Even holding the collection kits of an electric pump in place may strain painful joints. Mothers can consider the use of a nursing bra with special openings constructed to hold pump flanges in place for hands-free pumping. She may also consider using a hands-free pump that fits under each bra cup.

Fatigue remains a primary problem for women with RA or any chronic pain and can be quite overwhelming to a mother (Carty, Connie, & Wood-Johnson, 1986). Planned rest periods along with braces or splints may help reduce fatigue and improve joint mobility (Carty, Connie, & Hall, 1990).

MATERNAL EMPLOYMENT

In 2011, the labor force participation rate of mothers with children under 6 years old was 63.9%. The participation rate of mothers with infants under a year old was 55.8% (U.S. Bureau of Labor Statistics, 2012). Employment outside the home is associated with a shorter duration of breastfeeding, with intention to work full time significantly related to lower rates of breastfeeding initiation and shorter duration (Fein & Roe, 1998). Prenatal plans for employment focus on how a mother intends to feed her infant in the early weeks postpartum. In one study, mothers who planned to return to work within 12 weeks of delivery or planned to work full time were less likely to plan and engage in exclusive breastfeeding during the early weeks postpartum (Mirkovic, Perrine, Scanlon, & Grummer-Strawn, 2014). Mothers who exclusively breastfed in the hospital have been found to plan to breastfeed more months into the future than mothers who use mixed feeding (Thomas-Jackson, Bentley, Keyton, Reifman, Boylan, & Hart, 2015).

The clinician should assess the mother's employment intentions and probe how that may affect her long-term breastfeeding goals, using this information to create a breastfeeding plan specifically suited to her needs. Low-income women are more likely to return to work earlier than higher income earners and are more likely to be employed in jobs that present numerous challenges to the continuation of breastfeeding (Lindberg, 1996). Mothers who believe that breastfeeding while employed cannot be done without a considerable amount of additional work and stress may not even consider breastfeeding (Stewart-Glenn, 2008). Mothers with professional jobs are similar to stay-at-home mothers in terms of breastfeeding duration (Kimbro, 2006). Changes in federal welfare policy that require work by women with young infants has contributed significantly to lower national breastfeeding rates. Women in the Special Supplemental Nutrition Program for Women, Infants, and Children (WIC) living in states with the most stringent work laws showed a reduced breastfeeding rate of 22% relative to imposing no work requirements on new mothers. Estimates for all mothers (not just WIC participants) imply that if welfare reform had not been enacted, national breastfeeding rates 6 months after birth would have been 5.5% higher than they were in 2000 (Haider, Jacknowitz, & Schoeni, 2003).

Employment and workplace constraints exact a heavy toll on breastfeeding for African American mothers, as these women are more likely to hold jobs with little maternity leave, have less flexible working hours, have less social support for breastfeeding, and may return to work much earlier than women from other racial and ethnic groups (Johnson, Kirk, & Muzik, 2015). African American women are disproportionately employed in low-income jobs with high workplace stress and few options available to alter their work environment to pump breastmilk. Many need to rely on public transportation to travel to and from work and their childcare provider; may experience a high level of stress, poverty, and uncertainty regarding their safety; and live in a more communal home environment where breastfeeding itself may be difficult. Clinicians will need to engage women to find creative solutions to these issues, as each mother's situation may require individualized interventions.

The duration of work leave contributes significantly to the duration of breastfeeding, with each week of work leave increasing breastfeeding duration by approximately half a week (Roe, Whittington, Fein, & Teisl, 1999). Returning to work within the first 12 weeks after birth is related to the greatest decrease in breastfeeding duration. Guendelman and colleagues (2009) found that a maternity leave of less than or equal to 6 weeks and from 6 to 12 weeks after delivery were associated, respectively, with fourfold and twofold higher odds of failure to establish breastfeeding and an increased probability of cessation after successful establishment, relative to women not returning to work, after adjusting for covariates. The impact of short postpartum leave on breastfeeding cessation was stronger among nonmanagers, women with inflexible jobs, and with high psychosocial distress. However, for low-income women, a long maternity leave is usually not an option, especially if welfare benefits are tied to work requirements. The greater the number of hours worked each day, the fewer breastmilk feedings an infant receives, placing infants whose mothers return to work within 4–6 weeks of birth at high risk of partial or no breastmilk intake. Employment is significantly associated with breastfeeding cessation as early as 2–3 months postpartum, with working no more than 20 hours per week protective for continued breastfeeding (Gielen, Faden, O'Campo, Brown, & Paige, 1991).

Many mothers continue to experience childbirth-related symptoms at 5 weeks postpartum, such as fatigue, low hemoglobin levels, pain, breast symptoms in lactating mothers, role limitations, and incomplete recovery, especially mothers who delivered by cesarean section (McGovern et al., 2006). Mothers may wish to use intermittent rather than straight-time leave under the Family and Medical Leave Act, which allows a gradual, part-time return to work over a longer period of time. Physicians must certify mothers for intermittent leave under Family and Medical Leave Act regulations (McGovern et al., 2006). Many mothers cannot afford to take uncompensated maternity leave or may have a short-term disability policy that provides a partial salary for 4 to 6 weeks.

In addition to work-leave issues, employed breastfeeding mothers face a number of conflicts (Cardenas & Major, 2005) and challenges from the worksite itself, including lack of flexibility in work schedules or alternative work options, difficulty arranging breaks for pumping, breaks that are too short or lactation rooms that are located too far from the mother's area of work, inappropriate or no locations for pumping, and lack of support from coworkers and supervisors (Bar-Yam, 1998; Johnston & Esposito, 2007; Rojjanasrirat, 2004). Employers may believe that breastfeeding is a personal choice and not a matter of employer responsibility (Dunn, Zavela, Cline, & Cost, 2004), with little understanding how the health benefits of breastfeeding (Bridges, Frank, & Curtin, 1997) translate into employer cost savings (Cohen & Mrtek, 1994; Cohen, Mrtek, & Mrtek, 1995). Coworkers may believe that breastfeeding accommodation is unfair (Seijts, 2004), even though monetary costs for the employer to put in place such accommodations tend to be minimal (Prince, 2002). Working mothers who do not breastfeed have higher absentee rates and health costs than those who do. Employers may be unaware that lactation support can be a relatively inexpensive boost to the company's bottom line (Tyler, 1999), especially as a $15-per-hour employee who is absent for just 1 day costs a company $160 (Faught, 1994). Employee retention is less costly than hiring new employees and a supportive work environment strengthens employee commitment to the company (Bond, Galinsky, & Swanberg, 1998).

A major reason companies with lactation support programs continue to offer such accommodation is that mothers remain with the company, even through two or more births (Ortiz, McGilligan, & Kelly, 2004). Lactation accommodation by an employer can have a positive effect on the employee recruitment process, with potential employees being more likely to submit a resume and accept a job offer (Seijts, 2002). Employee lactation programs work effectively to aid mothers in meeting their breastfeeding goals and result in increasing the initiation, duration, and exclusivity of breastfeeding among employees (Spatz, Kim, & Froh, 2014). Mothers can express their milk two to three times per day, spending less than an hour total, often coinciding with their already allotted break time (Slusser, Lange, Dickson, Hawkes, & Cohen, 2004).

Lack of time to pump milk and the resulting diminishing milk supply are common causes of premature weaning (Arthur, Saenz, & Replogle, 2003). A hostile work environment that forces mothers to secretly breastfeed or to experience negative feedback from coworkers and management may result in untimely weaning (Gatrell, 2007). Poor or expensive childcare options reduce breastfeeding success. Some child-care providers sabotage breastfeeding by feeding formula when mothers are away at work or are uneasy handling breastmilk. When child care is onsite or nearby, working mothers report increased breastfeeding success (Thompson & Bell, 1997).

Until the 2010 Patient Protection and Affordable Care Act was passed, no United States federal legislation dealt directly with breastfeeding among employed women. In March 2010, breastfeeding mothers were granted worksite support from the U.S. federal government through Section 4207 of the Patient Protection and Affordable Care Act, which states that employers shall provide breastfeeding employees with "reasonable break time" and a private, nonbathroom place to express breastmilk during the workday, up until the child's first birthday. This section amends the Fair Labor Standards Act (FLSA), which applies to approximately 130 million workers. The employers included in the FLSA are subject to this law. Companies with less than 50 workers must also comply, unless they can demonstrate that complying with the law would cause "an undue hardship." The law, however, does not apply to all employed breastfeeding mothers because the law is an amendment to existing federal minimum wage and overtime laws. This means that it only covers the workers subject to those laws, who are the "nonexempt employees." This term usually means hourly workers—for example, those who work in retail sales, assembly-line or factory workers, restaurant workers such as waitresses, and any other employees who work on an hourly basis. They are subject to overtime laws and are paid when they work overtime. "Exempt" workers are those on a salary and are exempt from having to be paid when they work overtime.

On November 20, 2015, the Supporting Working Moms Act of 2015 (SWMA) was introduced in both houses of the U.S. Congress. This bipartisan legislation would protect and expand working mothers' right to breastfeed by extending the existing federal law to ensure that executive, administrative, and professional employees, including elementary and secondary school teachers, have break time and a private place to pump in the workplace.

Clinicians can educate mothers regarding the federal breastfeeding law, and on breastfeeding laws in their state, to ensure that they understand their rights and receive the greatest amount of protection. Many states have laws covering employed breastfeeding mothers, some of which may be stronger than the federal law.

Breastfeeding Management

Preparation in advance is most important to the continuation of breastfeeding after the return to work (Meek, 2001). Unanticipated fatigue, anxiety, role conflict/overload, competing demands, household chores, and childcare issues challenge the new mother and should be addressed before a mother returns to work (Nichols & Roux, 2004). Clinicians should help mothers address the following issues:

- Length of maternity leave, options for full-time work, flex time, use of earned time, job sharing, phased-back work schedule, part-time work, compressed work week, telecommuting, and on-site or near-site child care (Bar-Yam, 1998). Use of these options may allow the mother to spend more time with her infant, increasing the amount of breastfeeding and breastmilk feedings per day. Fein, Mandal, and Roe (2008) found that feeding the infant from the breast during the workday is the most effective strategy for combining breastfeeding and work. Ways to enable direct feeding include onsite child care, telecommuting, keeping the infant at work, allowing the mother to leave work to go to the infant, and having the infant brought to the worksite.

- What options exist for expressing milk at the workplace. Discuss with the employer the use of break times, a location for pumping, coworker and supervisor support, and how pumped milk will be stored.

Based on the age of the infant when the mother returns to work, the clinician and mother can create a breastfeeding plan for the times before and after resumption of employment (Biagioli, 2003). For instance, mothers returning to work at 6 months postpartum may find that expressing milk twice each workday is sufficient to keep up with the infant's needs because the infant is likely to start solid foods around this age. Mothers with a 3-month maternity leave should plan to have breastfeeding well established, address any early breastfeeding problems, have an infant gaining weight adequately, and consider pumping milk several times per week to have a supply in the freezer for times of fluctuating milk supply. Mothers should secure a high-quality, personal-use electric pump with a double collection kit, a small cooler or insulated bag, "blue ice" to keep the milk cool during storage and transport, and bottles or bags in which to store the milk. Expressed milk is safe and stable when stored for 24 hours in a little cooler case at 15°C (59°F) (Hamosh, Ellis, Pollock, Henderson, & Hamosh, 1996).

Mothers generally need to pump two to three times each day, depending on the length of their workday. Mothers can plan how the infant will be fed in their absence. Infants at this age can be given a bottle; however, some breastfed infants may refuse a bottle. Starting infants on a bottle in the early days does not guarantee that an infant will take one at 3 months and can interfere with breastfeeding and milk production. An infant can be started on a bottle about 7–10 days before the return to work at the times when the mother is usually gone. Many mothers begin a gradual introduction of the infant to the bottle and childcare environment at this time, such that a bottle is given by someone other than the mother in the location where such feedings will take place. Infants who refuse a bottle can be fed with a small cup or a child's sippy cup with a spout. Some mothers in this situation use a reverse-cycle feeding technique whereby the infant's sleep patterns are encouraged to change to longer sleep periods during the time the mother is at work, minimizing milk intake, and then remaining awake for longer periods in the evening for clustered feeds at the breast.

Mothers with a 4- to 6-week maternity leave can experience a more difficult course, especially if any early breastfeeding problems continue unresolved. Faltering milk production is often the most pressing problem once a mother starts back to work at this early time. Using the model of initiating and maintaining abundant milk production in the preterm mother, mothers returning to work this early can follow a plan to maximize milk output by the 6-week mark through 10–12 feedings each 24 hours for the first 14 days. After this time (or during the first 2 weeks if the mother has a large supply or if the infant is not effectively stimulating the supply), mothers can pump milk after each feeding such that the breasts calibrate to a 50% oversupply of milk to be stored in the freezer. This oversupply compensates for the natural falloff in milk production when a mother returns to work and ensures that breastmilk is available for growth spurts, supply fluctuations, missed pumping sessions, or other unforeseen circumstances. **Box 9-6** provides a sample plan for a mother returning to work soon after the birth of the baby.

Box 9-6 Sample Plan for a Mother Returning to Work or School 2–6 Weeks Postpartum

- During the first 3 days after delivery, aim to breastfeed the infant approximately 8 times each 24 hours. Hand express milk five times each day, making sure to massage and compress each quadrant of the breast during the expressing process.
- After the first 3 days and during the time prior to returning to work or school, hand express or pump milk following as many breastfeedings as possible. If a pump is used, massage and compress each quadrant of each breast during each pumping session. For mothers returning to work at 6 weeks, even starting to pump at 4 weeks in most situations should be sufficient to preserve an abundant milk supply unless any breastfeeding problems remain unresolved. The goal is to create about a 50% oversupply to ensure a sufficient supply and account for a possible falloff in milk production after the return to work.
- Store the expressed milk in the freezer, labeling it with the date it was expressed, so the oldest can be used first.
- Pump or hand express milk once during any long gaps between the infant's feedings.
- Aim to drain the breasts as thoroughly as possible.
- A bottle can be introduced at 7 days if returning to work or school at 2 weeks; at 3 weeks if returning to work or school at 4 weeks; and at 5 weeks if returning to work or school at 6 weeks.

Mothers should be encouraged to breastfeed right before dropping off the infant at child care or just before leaving for work and to breastfeed again at the childcare setting or immediately upon arrival at home, frequently during the evening, and frequently on her days off.

To avoid faltering milk production, it is not only important to calibrate the breasts to an initial very high milk volume but also to express milk on a thorough and regular basis with a high-quality personal-use or multiuser breast pump with a double collection kit. Mothers prefer high-quality electric pumps over nonelectrical pumps that take longer to express milk and use up short pumping times (Stevens & Janke, 2003). Some employers provide a multiuser pump that is shared among the breastfeeding employees who each use their own collection kit. Some employers give their breastfeeding employees a personal collection kit as an employee benefit. Some mothers have jobs that leave little to no time for pumping and find that other types of pumps might work better in their situation. This might include pumps that are battery operated, worn under the bra, and leave the hands free for work activities.

Some mothers find it difficult to pump under time constraints and may experience a delayed letdown reflex or minimal volumes of milk per pumping session. Mothers can be encouraged to elicit the milk-ejection reflex first, before applying the pump, by looking at a picture of the infant or by massaging and hand expressing until milk spurts or sprays. If this is ineffective, oxytocin nasal spray can be used to hasten the letdown reflex. The pump flanges should then be put in place and the mother can continue to massage and compress each breast while pumping to maximize output, minimize pumping time, and avoid leaving milk residuals that can contribute to diminished milk production, focal engorgement, and mastitis. Mothers can hold the flanges in place with one arm placed across the collection kits or use a bra that is specially made with openings to secure the flanges in place for hands-free pumping.

Clinicians may wish to help employed mothers by writing a letter to the employer detailing the importance of accommodations in the workplace (Angeletti, 2009) or may wish to work with employers to create an onsite lactation program (Click, 2006). Physicians and advanced practice nurses may write a prescription for breastmilk that mothers can show to employers. Many states have legislation regarding workplace accommodation for breastfeeding mothers with which clinicians should be familiar. Mothers should be encouraged to ask for breastfeeding accommodation, because one reason for the lack of such employer support is the absence of employee demand. Clinicians should be vocal proponents of paid maternity leave (Calnen, 2007).

Not all employed mothers work in office buildings—or even buildings at all. Some mothers work outdoors, drive a bus or patrol in a police cruiser, or are in the military. Breastfeeding can work for these mothers as well, with some planning and creativity. Shared space with other businesses and mobile (**Figure 9-4**) or flexible (**Figure 9-5**) pumping areas are some of the many options for breastfeeding locales

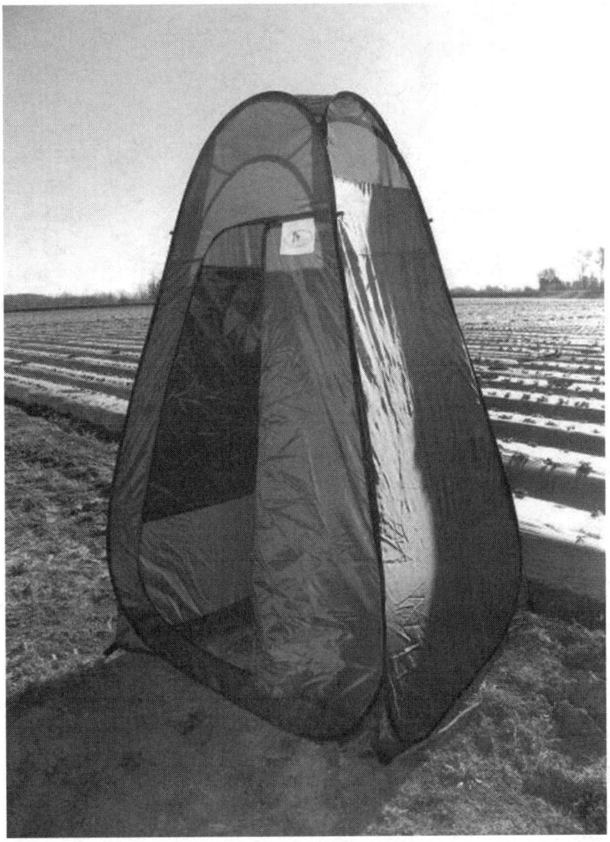

Figure 9-4 Pop-up tent for indoor or outdoor spaces.

Office on Women's Health, U.S. Department of Health and Human Services. http://www.womenshealth.gov/breastfeeding/employer-solutions/common-solutions/outdoor-mobile.html

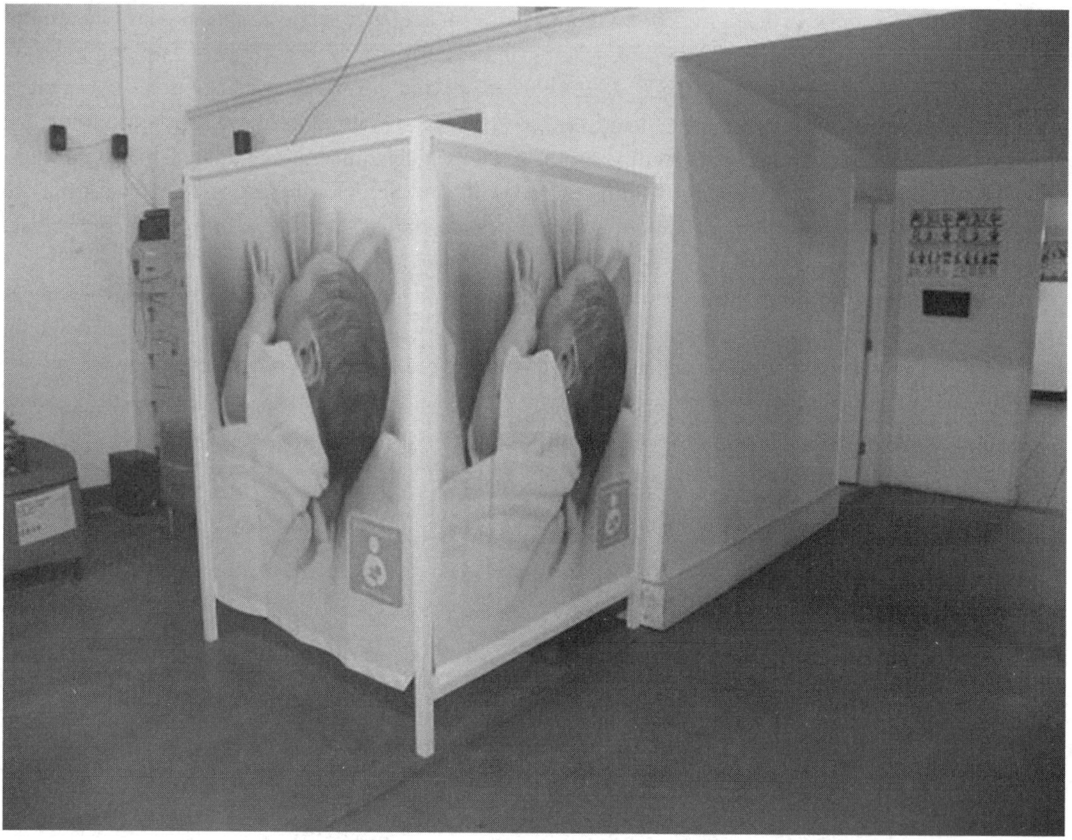

Figure 9-5 Movable screen for partitioned area.

Office on Women's Health, U.S. Department of Health and Human Services. http://www.womenshealth.gov/breastfeeding/employer-solutions/common-solutions/flexible-space.html.

that can be found at the Office of Women's Health of the Department of Health and Human Services (http://www.womenshealth.gov/breastfeeding/employer-solutions/common-solutions/outdoor-mobile.html).

SUMMARY: THE DESIGN IN NATURE

Except under the most extraordinary circumstances, mothers should be encouraged and supported to breastfeed or provide expressed milk for their infants.

REFERENCES

Abascal, K., & Yarnell, E. (2008). Botanical galactagogues. *Alternative and Complementary Therapy, 14,* 288–294.

Academy of Breastfeeding Medicine. (2011). Clinical protocol number 9: Use of galactogogues in initiating or augmenting the rate of maternal milk secretion. *Breastfeeding Medicine, 6,* 41–49.

Achong, N., McIntyre, H. D., Callaway, L., & Duncan, E. L. (2015). Glycaemic behaviour during breastfeeding in women with type I diabetes. *Diabetic Medicine,* [Epub ahead of print]. doi: 10.1111/dme.12993

Ahluwalia, I. B., Morrow, B., & Hsia, J. (2005). Why do women stop breastfeeding? Findings from the Pregnancy Risk Assessment and Monitoring System. *Pediatrics, 116,* 1408–1412.

Akman, I., Kuscu, M. K., Yurdakul, Z., Ozdemir, N., Solakoglu, M., Orhon, L., . . . Ozek, E. (2008). Breastfeeding duration and postpartum psychological adjustment: Role of maternal attachment styles. *Journal of Pediatric Child Health, 44,* 369–373.

Alam, S., Hennigar, S. R., Gallagher, C., Soybel, D. I., & Kelleher, S. L. (2015). Exome sequencing of SLC30A2 identifies novel loss- and gain-of-function variants associated with breast cell dysfunction. *Journal of Mammary Gland Biology and Neoplasia, 20,* 159–172.

Albareda, M., Caballero, A., Badell, G., Piquer, S., Ortiz, A., de Leiva, A., & Corcoy, R. (2003). Diabetes and abnormal glucose tolerance in women with previous gestational diabetes. *Diabetes Care, 26,* 1199–1205.

Aljazaf, K., Hale, T. W., Ilett, K. F., Hartmann, P. E., Mitoulas, L. R., Kristensen, J. H., & Hackett, L. P. (2003). Pseudoephedrine: Effects on milk production in women and estimation of infant exposure via breastmilk. *British Journal of Clinical Pharmacology, 56,* 18–24.

Almas, S., Vance, J., Baker, T., & Hale, T. (2016). Management of multiple sclerosis in the breastfeeding mother. Multiple Sclerosis International, [Epub ahead of print], doi: 10.1155/2016/6527458.

Amer, M. R., Cipriano, G. C., Venci, J. V., & Gandhi, M. A. (2015). Safety of popular herbal supplements in lactating women. *Journal of Human Lactation, 31,* 348–353.

American Academy of Pediatrics, Committee on Drugs. (2001). The transfer of drugs and other chemicals into human milk. *Pediatrics, 108,* 776–788.

American Diabetes Association. (2004). Gestational diabetes mellitus. Position statement. *Diabetes Care, 27*(suppl 1), S88–S90.

Amir, L. H. (2006). Breastfeeding: Managing supply difficulties. *Australian Family Physician, 35,* 686–689.

Amir, L. H., & Donath, S. (2007). A systematic review of maternal obesity and breastfeeding intention, initiation, and duration. *BMC Pregnancy and Childbirth, 7,* 9.

Anderson, P. O., & Valdes, V. (2007). A critical review of pharmaceutical galactagogues. *Breastfeeding Medicine, 2,* 229–242.

Andres, A., Shankar, K., & Badger, T. M. (2012). Body fat mass of exclusively breastfed infants born to overweight mothers. *Journal of the Academy of Nutrition and Dietetics, 112,* 991–995.

Angeletti, M. A. (2009). Breastfeeding mothers returning to work: Possibilities for information, anticipatory guidance and support from US health care professionals. *Journal of Human Lactation, 25,* 226–232.

Anstey, E. H., & Jevitt, C. (2011). Maternal obesity and breastfeeding. *Clinical Lactation, 2,* 11–16.

Arthur, C., Saenz, R. B., & Replogle, W. H. (2003). The employment-related breastfeeding decisions of physician mothers. *Journal of the Mississippi State Medical Association, 44,* 383–387.

Arthur, P. G., Kent, J. C., & Hartmann, P. E. (1994). Metabolites of lactose synthesis in milk from diabetic and nondiabetic women during lactogenesis II. *Journal of Pediatric Gastroenterology and Nutrition, 19,* 100–108.

Asselin, B. L., & Lawrence, R. A. (1987). Maternal disease as a consideration in lactation management. *Clinics in Perinatology, 14,* 71–87.

Azizi, F., Khoshniat, M., Bahrainian, M., & Hedayati, M. (2000). Thyroid function and intellectual development of infants nursed by mothers taking methimazole. *Journal of Clinical Endocrinology and Metabolism, 85,* 3233–3238.

Azziz, R., Woods, K. S., Reyna, R., Key, T. J., Knochenhauer E. S., & Yildiz, B. O. (2004). The prevalence and features of the polycystic ovary syndrome in an unselected population. *Journal of Clinical Endocrinology and Metabolism, 89,* 2745–2749.

Baker, J. L., Gamborg, M., Heitmann, B. L., Lissner, L., Sorenses, T. I., & Rasmussen, K. M. (2008). Breastfeeding reduces postpartum weight retention. *American Journal of Clinical Nutrition, 88,* 1543–1551.

Baker, J. L., Michaelsen, K. F., Sorensen, T. I., & Rasmussen, K. M. (2007). High prepregnant body mass index is associated with early termination of full and any breastfeeding in Danish women. *American Journal of Clinical Nutrition, 86,* 404–411.

Bakri, Y. N., Bakhashwain, M., & Hugosson, C. (1994). Massive theca-lutein cysts, virilization, and hypothyroidism associated with normal pregnancy. *Acta Obstetricia et Gynecologica Scandinavica, 73,* 153–155.

Bar-Yam, N. B. (1998). Workplace lactation support, part 1: A return-to-work breastfeeding assessment tool. *Journal of Human Lactation, 14,* 249–254.

Barrett, J. H., Brennan, P., Fiddler, M., & Silman, A. (2000). Breastfeeding and postpartum relapse in women with rheumatoid arthritis. *Arthritis and Rheumatism, 43,* 1010–1015.

Battle, C. L., Ziotnick, C., Pearlstein, T., Miller, I. W., Howard, M., Salisbury, A., & Stroud, L. (2008). Depression and breastfeeding: Which postpartum patients take antidepressant medications? *Depression and Anxiety, 25,* 888–891.

Beck, C. T. (1992). The lived experience of postpartum depression: A phenomenological study. *Nursing Research, 41,* 166–170.

Beck, C. T. (1993). Teetering on the edge: A substantive theory of postpartum depression. *Nursing Research, 42,* 42–48.

Bennett, C., Fagan, E., Chaharbakhshi, E., Zamfirova, I., & Flicker, J. (2016). Implementing a protocol using glucose gel to treat neonatal hypoglycemia. *Nursing and Womens Health, 20,* 64–74.

Bentley-Lewis, R., Levkoff, S., Stuebe, A., & Seely, E. W. (2008). Gestational diabetes mellitus: Postpartum opportunities for the diagnosis and prevention of type 2 diabetes mellitus. *National Clinical Practice: Endocrinology and Metabolism, 4,* 552–558.

Benz, J. (1992). Antidiabetic agents and lactation. *Journal of Human Lactation, 8,* 27–28.

Berbel, P., Mestre, J. L., Santamaria A., Palazon, I., Franco, A., Graells, M., . . . de Escobar, G. M. (2009). Delayed neurobehavioral development in children born to pregnant women with milk hypothyroxinemia during the first month of gestation: The importance of early iodine supplementation. *Thyroid, 19,* 511–519.

Berle, J. O., & Spigset, O. (2011). Antidepressant use during breastfeeding. *Current Women's Health Reviews, 7,* 28–34.

Betzold, C. M., Hoover, K. L., & Snyder, C. L. (2004). Delayed lactogenesis II: A comparison of four cases. *Journal of Midwifery and Women's Health, 49,* 132–137.

Biagioli, F. (2003). Returning to work while breastfeeding. *American Family Physician, 68,* 2201–2208, 2215–2217.

Biervliet, F. P., Maguiness, S. D., Hay, D. M., Killick, S. R., & Atkin, S. L. (2001). Induction of lactation in the intended mother of a surrogate pregnancy. *Human Reproduction, 16,* 581–583.

Bingel, A. S., & Farnsworth, N. R. (1994). Higher plants as potential sources of galactagogues. *Economic and Medical Plant Research, 6,* 1–54.

Birk, K., & Rudick, R. (1986). Pregnancy and multiple sclerosis. *Archives of Neurology, 43,* 719–726.

Bisset, N. G. (1994). *Herbal drugs and phytopharmaceuticals.* London, UK: CRC Press.

Bitman, J., Hamosh, M., Hamosh, P., Lutes, V., Neville, M. C., Seacat, J., & Wood, D. L. (1989). Milk composition and volume during the onset of lactation in a diabetic mother. *American Journal of Clinical Nutrition, 50,* 1364–1369.

Bitman, J., Hamosh, M., Wood, D. L., Freed, L. M., & Hamosh, P. (1987). Lipid composition of milk from mothers with cystic fibrosis. *Pediatrics, 80,* 927–932.

Blumenthal, M., & Busse, W. R. (Eds.). (1998). *The complete German commission E monographs: Therapeutic guide to herbal medicine* (trans. S. Klein & R. S. Rister). Austin, TX: American Botanical Council.

Bodley, V., & Powers, D. (1999). Patient with insufficient glandular tissue experiences milk supply increase attributed to progesterone treatment for luteal phase defect. *Journal of Human Lactation, 15,* 339–343.

Bogen, D. L., Hanusa, B. H., Moses-Kolko, E., & Wisner, K. L. (2010). Are maternal depression or symptom severity associated with breastfeeding intention or outcomes? *Journal of Clinical Psychiatry, 71,* 1069–1078.

Bond, J., Galinsky, E., & Swanberg, J. (1998). *The 1997 national study of the changing workforce.* New York, NY: Families and Work Institute.

Boullu, S., Andrac, L., Piana, L., Darmon, P., Dutour, A., & Oliver, C. (1998). Diabetic mastopathy, complication of type 1 diabetes mellitus: Report of two cases and a review of the literature. *Diabetes and Metabolism, 24,* 448–454.

Bowles, B. C. (1991). Breastfeeding consultation in sign language. *Journal of Human Lactation, 7,* 21.

Bray, G. A. (1997). Obesity and reproduction. *Human Reproduction, 12*(suppl 1), 26–32.

Breier, B. H., Milsom, S. R., Blum, W. F., Schwander, J., Gallaher, B. W., & Gluckman, P. D. (1993). Insulinlike growth factors and their binding proteins in plasma and milk after growth hormone–stimulated galactopoiesis in normally lactating women. *Acta Endocrinologica, 129,* 427–435.

Brennan, P., & Silman, A. (1994). Breastfeeding and the onset of rheumatoid arthritis. *Arthritis and Rheumatism, 37,* 808–813.

Brent, N. B., & Wisner, K. L. (1998). Fluoxetine and carbamazepine concentrations in a nursing mother/infant pair. *Clinical Pediatrics, 37,* 41–44.

Bridges, C. B., Frank, D. I., & Curtin, J. (1997). Employer attitudes toward breastfeeding in the workplace. *Journal of Human Lactation, 13,* 215–219.

Britton, J. R. (2007). Postpartum anxiety and breastfeeding. *Journal of Reproductive Medicine, 52,* 689–695.

Brouwers, J. R., Assies, J., Wiersinga, W. M., Huizing, G., & Tytgat, G. N. (1980). Plasma prolactin levels after acute and subchronic oral administration of domperidone and of metoclopramide: A crossover study in healthy volunteers. *Clinical Endocrinology, 12,* 435–440.

Brown, T. E., Fernandes, P. A., Grant, L. J., Hutsul, J. A., & McCoshen, J. A. (2000). Effect of parity on pituitary prolactin response to metoclopramide and domperidone: Implications for the enhancement of lactation. *Journal of the Society for Gynecologic Investigation, 7,* 65–69.

Bryant, C. A. (2006). Nursing the adopted infant. *Journal of the American Board of Family Medicine, 19,* 374–379.

Buckshee, K., Kriplani, A., Kapil, A., Bhargava, V. L., & Takkar, D. (1992). Hypothyroidism complicating pregnancy. *Australian and New Zealand Journal of Obstetrics and Gynaecology, 32,* 240–242.

Budd, S. C., Erdman, S. H., Long, D. M., Trombley, S. K., & Udall, J. N., Jr. (1993). Improved lactation with metoclopramide: A case report. *Clinical Pediatrics, 32,* 53–57.

Budzynska, K., Gardner Z. E., Dugoua, J-J., Low Dog, T., & Gardiner, P. (2012). Systematic review of breastfeeding and herbs. *Breastfeeding Medicine, 7,* 489–501.

Budzynska, K., Gardner, Z. E., Low Dog, T., & Gardner, P. (2013). Complementary, holistic, and integrative medicine: Advice for clinicians on herbs and breastfeeding. *Pediatrics in Review, 34,* 343–353.

Buonfiglio, D. C., Ramos-Lobo, A. M., Freitas, V. M., Zampieri, T. T., Nagaishi, V. S., Magalhaes, M. . . . Donato Jr, J. (2016). Obesity impairs lactation performance in mice by inducing prolactin resistance. *Scientific Reports, 6,* 22421.

Burt, V. K., Suri, R., Altshuler, L., Stowe, Z., Hendrick, V. C., & Muntean, E. (2001). The use of psychotropic medications during breastfeeding. *American Journal of Psychiatry, 158,* 1001–1009.

California Diabetes and Pregnancy Program. (2002*). Guidelines for care: Sweet success express.* Sacramento, CA: Maternal and Child Health Branch, Department of Health Services.

Calnen, G. (2007). Paid maternity leave and its impact on breastfeeding in the United States: An historic, economic, political, and social perspective. *Breastfeeding Medicine, 2,* 34–44.

Caplinger, P., Cooney, A. T., Bledsoe, C., Hagan, P., Smith, A., Whitfield, P., . . . Tipton, P. H. (2015). Breastfeeding outcomes following bariatric surgery. *Clinical Lactation, 6,* 144–152.

Cardenas, R. A., & Major, D. A. (2005). Combining employment and breastfeeding: Utilizing a work–family conflict framework to understand obstacles and solutions. *Journal of Business Psychology, 20,* 31–51.

Carlsen, S. M., Jacobsen, G., & Vanky, E. (2010). Mid-pregnancy androgen levels are negatively associated with breastfeeding. *Acta Obstetricia et Gynecologica Scandinavica, 89,* 87–94.

Carty, E., Connie, T. A., & Hall, L. (1990). Comprehensive health promotion for the pregnant woman who is disabled. *Journal of Nurse-Midwifery, 35,* 133–142.

Carty, E., Connie, T. A., & Wood-Johnson, F. (1986). Rheumatoid arthritis and pregnancy: Helping women to meet their needs. *Midwives Chronicles, 99,* 254–257.

Centers for Disease Control and Prevention. (2011). *National diabetes fact sheet: National estimates and general information on diabetes and prediabetes in the United States, 2011.* Atlanta, GA: U.S. Department of Health and Human Services, Centers for Disease Control and Prevention. Retrieved from http://www.cdc.gov/diabetes/pubs/pdf/ndfs_2011.pdf

Cesario, S. K. (2002). Spinal cord injuries. *AWHONN Lifelines, 6,* 225–232.

Chambers, C. D., Anderson, P. O., Thomas, R. G., Dick, L. M., Felix, R. J., Johnson, K. A., & Jones, K. L. (1999). Weight gain in infants breastfed by mothers who take fluoxetine. *Pediatrics, 104*(5), e61.

Chapman, D., & Perez-Escamilla, R. (1999a). *Maternal perception of delayed onset of lactogenesis (OL): A useful marker of delayed onset of lactogenesis stage II (OLII).* Presented at the 9th International Conference of the International Society of Research in Human Milk and Lactation, October, Irsee, Germany.

Chapman, D. J., & Perez-Escamilla, R. (1999b). Identification of risk factors for delayed onset of lactation. *Journal of the American Dietetics Association, 99,* 450–454.

Chapman, D. J., & Perez-Escamilla, R. (2000). Maternal perception of the onset of lactation is a valid, public health indicator of lactogenesis stage II. *Journal of Nutrition, 130,* 2972–2980.

Cheales-Siebenaler, N. J. (1999). Induced lactation in an adoptive mother. *Journal of Human Lactation, 15,* 421–423.

Chen, D. C., Nommsen-Rivers, L., Dewey, K. G., & Lonnerdal, B. (1998). Stress during labor and delivery and early lactation performance. *American Journal of Clinical Nutrition, 68,* 335–344.

Chen, L., Liu, F., Yoshida, S., & Kaneko, S. (2010). Is breastfeeding of infants advisable for epileptic mothers taking antiepileptic drugs? *Psychiatry and Clinical Neuroscience, 64,* 460–468.

Chin, N. P., Cuculick, J., Starr, M., Panko, T., Widanka, H., & Dozier, A. (2013). Deaf mothers and breastfeeding: Do unique features of Deaf culture and language support breastfeeding success? *Journal of Human Lactation, 29,* 564–571.

Clavey, S. (1996). The use of acupuncture for the treatment of insufficient lactation (Que Ru). *American Journal of Acupuncture, 24,* 35–46.

Click, E. R. (2006). Developing a worksite lactation program. *MCN: The American Journal of Maternal/Child Nursing, 31,* 313–317.

Cohen, R., & Mrtek, M. B. (1994). The impact of two corporate lactation programs on the incidence and duration of breastfeeding by employed mothers. *American Journal of Health Promotion, 8,* 436–441.

Cohen, R., Mrtek, M. B., & Mrtek, R. G. (1995). Comparison of maternal absenteeism and infant illness rates among breastfeeding and formula-feeding women in two corporations. *American Journal of Health Promotion, 10,* 148–153.

Confavreux, C., Hutchinson, M., Hours, M. M., Cortinovis-Tourniaire, P., & Moreau, T. (1998). Rate of pregnancy-related relapse in multiple sclerosis. *New England Journal of Medicine, 339,* 285–291.

Conn, J. J., Jacobs, H. S., & Conway, G. S. (2000). The prevalence of polycystic ovaries in women with type 2 diabetes mellitus. *Clinical Endocrinology, 52,* 81–86.

Conradi, S., Malzahn, U., Paul, F., Quill, S., Harms, L., Then Bergh, F., . . . Rosche, B. (2013). Breastfeeding is associated with lower risk for multiple sclerosis. *Multiple Sclerosis, 19,* 553–558.

Cooper, G. S., Dooley, M. A., Treadwell, E. L., St. Clair, E. W., & Gilkeson, G. S. (2002). Hormonal and reproductive risk factors for development of systemic lupus erythematosus. *Arthritis and Rheumatism, 46,* 1830–1839.

Cooper, S. D., Felkins, K., Baker, T. E., & Hale, T. W. (2015). Transfer of methylprednisolone into breast milk in a mother with multiple sclerosis. *Journal of Human Lactation, 31,* 237–239.

Cordero, L., Treuer, S. H., Landon, M. B., & Gabbe, S. G. (1998). Management of infants of diabetic mothers. *Archives of Adolescent Medicine, 152,* 249–254.

Cowley, K. C. (2005). Psychogenic and pharmacologic induction of the let-down reflex can facilitate breastfeeding by tetraplegic women: A report of 3 cases. *Archives of Physical Medicine and Rehabilitation, 86,* 1261–1264.

Coyle, P. K., Christie, S., Fodor, P., Fuchs, K., Giesser, B., Gutierrez, A., . . . Pardo, L. (2004). Multiple sclerosis gender issues: Clinical practices of women neurologists. *Multiple Sclerosis, 10,* 582–588.

Craig, D. (1990). The adaptation to pregnancy of spinal cord injured women. *Rehabilitation Nursing, 15,* 6–9.

Crawford, P. M. (2009). Managing epilepsy in women of childbearing age. *Drug Safety, 32,* 293–307.

Cystic Fibrosis Foundation. (n.d.). Home. Retrieved from http://www.cff.org

da Silva, O. P., Knoppert, D. C., Angelini, M. M., & Forret, P. A. (2001). Effect of domperidone on milk production in mothers of premature newborns: A randomized, double-blind, placebo-controlled trial. *Canadian Medical Association Journal, 164,* 17–21.

Dakhil-Jerew, F., Brook, S., & Derry, F. (2008). Autonomic dysreflexia triggered by breastfeeding in a tetraplegic mother. *Journal of Rehabilitation Medicine, 40,* 780–782.

Davanzo, R., Copertino, M., De Cunto, A., Minen, F., & Amaddeo, A. (2011). Antidepressant drugs and breastfeeding: A review of the literature. *Breastfeeding Medicine, 6,* 89–98.

Davies, H. A., Clark, J. D. A., Dalton, K. J., & Edwards, O. M. (1989). Insulin requirements of diabetic women who breastfeed. *British Medical Journal, 298,* 1357–1358.

DeCarvalho, M., Robertson, S., Friedman, A., & Klaus, M. (1983). Effect of frequent breastfeeding on early milk production and infant weight gain. *Pediatrics, 72,* 307.

Delgado-Escueta, A. V., & Janz, D. (1992). Consensus guidelines: Preconception counseling, management, and care of the pregnant women with epilepsy. *Neurology, 42*(suppl 5), 149–160.

Dennis, C. L., & McQueen, K. (2007). Does maternal postpartum depressive symptomatology influence infant feeding outcomes? *Acta Paediatrica, 96,* 590–594.

Dennis, C. L., & McQueen, K. (2009). The relationship between infant-feeding outcomes and postpartum depression: A qualitative systematic review. *Pediatrics, 123,* e736–e751.

Di Pierro, F., Callegari, A., Carotenuto, D., & Tapia, M. M. (2008). Clinical efficacy, safety and tolerability of BIO-C (micronized Silymarin) as a galactagogue. *Acta Biomedica, 79,* 205–210.

Diniz, J. M., & da Costa, T. H. (2004). Independent of body adiposity, breastfeeding has a protective effect on glucose metabolism in young adult women. *British Journal of Nutrition, 92,* 905–912.

Doggrell, S. A., & Hancox, J. C. (2014). Cardiac safety concerns for domperidone, an antiemetic and prokinetic, and galactagogue medicine. *Expert Opinion on Drug Safety, 13,* 131–138.

Dombrowski, M. A., Anderson, G. C., Santori, C., & Burkhammer, M. (2001). Kangaroo (skin-to-skin) care with a postpartum woman who felt depressed. *MCN: The American Journal of Maternal/Child Nursing, 26,* 214–216.

Donath, S., & Amir, L. (2000). Does maternal obesity adversely affect breastfeeding initiation and duration? *Journal of Paediatrics and Child Health, 36,* 482–486.

Donath, S. M., & Amir, L. H. (2008). Maternal obesity and initiation and duration of breastfeeding: Data from the longitudinal study of Australian children. *Maternal and Child Nutrition, 4,* 163–170.

Drazin, P. (1995). Use of a mirror to assist breast pumping. *Journal of Human Lactation, 11,* 219.

Driscoll, J. W. (2005). Recognizing women's common mental health problems: The earthquake assessment model. *Journal of Obstetric, Gynecologic, and Neonatal Nursing, 34,* 246–254.

Dunn, B. F., Zavela, K. J., Cline, A. D., & Cost, P. A. (2004). Breastfeeding practices in Colorado businesses. *Journal of Human Lactation, 20,* 170–177.

Dunne, G., & Fuerst, K. (1995). Breastfeeding by a mother who is a triple amputee: A case report. *Journal of Human Lactation, 11,* 217–218.

Edenborough, F. P., Borgo, G., Knoop, C., Lannefors, L., Mackenzie, W. E., Madge S., . . . Johannesson, M. (2008). Guidelines for the management of pregnancy in women with cystic fibrosis. *Journal of Cystic Fibrosis, 7,* S2–S32.

Eggum, M. (2001). Breastfeeding with multiple sclerosis: Helping women confront their fears. *AWHONN Lifelines, 5,* 36–40.

Eglash, A. (2014). Treatment of maternal hypergalactia. *Breastfeeding Medicine, 9,* 423–425.

Ehrenkranz, R. A., & Ackerman, B. A. (1986). Metoclopramide effect on faltering milk production by mothers of premature infants. *Pediatrics, 78,* 614–620.

Esfahani, M. S., Berenji-Sooghe, S., Valiani, M., & Ehsanpour, S. (2015). Effect of acupressure on milk volume of breastfeeding mothers referring to selected health care centers in Tehran. *Iranian Journal of Nurse Midwifery Research, 20,* 7–11.

Faught, L. (1994, September/October). Lactation programs benefit the family and the corporation. *Journal of Compensation Benefits,* 44–47.

Feher, D. K., Berger, L. R., Johnson, D., & Wilde, J. B. (1989). Increasing breast milk production for preterm infants with a relaxation/imagery audiotape. *Pediatrics, 83,* 57.

Feig, D. S. (2012). Avoiding the slippery slope: Preventing the development of diabetes in women with a history of gestational diabetes. *Diabetes/Metabolism Research and Reviews, 28,* 317–320.

Feig, D. S., Briggs, G. G., & Koren, G. (2007). Oral antidiabetic agents in pregnancy and lactation: A paradigm shift? *Annals of Pharmacotherapy, 41,* 1174–1180.

Fein, S. B., Mandal, B., & Roe, B. E. (2008). Success of strategies for combining employment and breastfeeding. *Pediatrics, 122*(Suppl. 2), S56–S62.

Fein, S. B., & Roe, B. (1998). The effect of work status on initiation and duration of breastfeeding. *American Journal of Public Health, 88,* 1042–1046.

Ferris, A. M., Dalidowitz, C. K., Ingardia, C. M., Reece, E. A., Fumia, F. D., Jensen R. G., & Allen, L. H. (1988). Lactation outcome in insulin-dependent diabetic women. *Journal of the American Dietetics Association, 88,* 317–322.

Ferris, A. M., Neubauer, S. H., Bendel, R. R., Green, K. W., Ingardia, C. J., & Reece, E. A. (1993). Perinatal lactation protocol and outcome in mothers with and without insulin-dependent diabetes mellitus. *American Journal of Clinical Nutrition, 58,* 43–48.

Festini, F., Ciuti, R., Taccetti, G., Repetto, T., Campana, S., & De Martino, M. (2006). Breastfeeding in a woman with cystic fibrosis undergoing antibiotic intravenous treatment. *Journal of Maternal–Fetal and Neonatal Medicine, 19,* 375–376.

Field, T. (2008). Breastfeeding and antidepressants. *Infant Behavior and Development, 31,* 481–487.

Fife, S., Gill, P., Hopkins, M., Angello, C., Boswell, S., & Nelson, K. M. (2011). Metoclopramide to augment lactation, does it work? A randomized trial. *Journal of Maternal–Fetal and Neonatal Medicine, 24,* 1317–1320.

Fitelson, E., Kim, S., Baker, A. S., & Leight, K. (2011). Treatment of postpartum depression: Clinical, psychological and pharmacological options. *International Journal of Women's Health, 3,* 1–14.

Flegal, K. M., Carroll, M. D., Ogden, C. L., & Johnson, C. L. (2002). Prevalence and trends in obesity among U.S. adults, 1999–2000. *Journal of the American Medical Association, 288,* 1723–1727.

Flint, D. J., Travers, M. T., Barber, M. C., Binart, N., & Kelly, P. A. (2005). Diet-induced obesity impairs mammary development and lactogenesis in murine mammary gland. *American Journal of Physiology—Endocrinology and Metabolism, 288*(6), E1179–E1187.

Fox-Bacon, C., McCamman, S., Therou, L., Moore, W., & Kipp, D. E. (1997). Maternal PKU and breastfeeding: Case report of identical twin mothers. *Clinical Pediatrics, 36,* 539–542.

Gabay, M. P. (2002). Galactagogues: Medications that induce lactation. *Journal of Human Lactation, 18,* 274–279.

Gabbay, M., & Kelly, H. (2003). Use of metformin to increase breastmilk production in women with insulin resistance: A case series. *ABM News and Views, 9,* 20–21.

Gagliardi, L., Petrozzi, A., & Rusconi, F. (2012). Symptoms of maternal depression immediately after delivery predict unsuccessful breastfeeding. *Archives of Disease in Childhood, 97,* 355–357.

Gagne, M. G., Leff, E. W., & Jefferis, S. C. (1992). The breastfeeding experience of women with type 1 diabetes. *Health Care for Women International, 13,* 249–260.

Gagnon, A. J., Leduc, G., Waghorn, K., Yang, H., & Platt, R. W. (2005). In-hospital formula supplementation of healthy breastfeeding newborns. *Journal of Human Lactation, 21,* 397–405.

Gallas, P. R., Stolk, R. P., Bakker, K., Endert, E., & Wiersinga, W. M. (2002). Thyroid dysfunction during pregnancy and in the first postpartum year in women with diabetes mellitus type 1. *European Journal of Endocrinology, 147,* 443–451.

Garner, C. D., Ratcliff, S. L., Devine, C. M., Thornburg, L. L., & Rasmussen, K. M. (2014). Health professionals' experiences providing breastfeeding-related care for obese women. *Breastfeeding Medicine, 9,* 503–509.

Gatrell, C. J. (2007). Secrets and lies: Breastfeeding and professional paid work. *Social Science and Medicine, 65,* 393–404.

Gatti, L. (2008). Maternal perceptions of insufficient milk supply in breastfeeding. *Journal of Nursing Scholarship, 40,* 355–363.

Gavin, N. I., Gaynes, B. N., Lohr, K. N., Meltzer-Brody, S., Gartlehner, G., & Swinson, T. (2005). Perinatal depression: A systematic review of prevalence and incidence. *Obstetrics and Gynecology, 106,* 1071–1083.

Gaynes, B. N., Gavin, N., Meltzer-Brody, S., Lohr, K. N., Swinson, T., Gartlehner, G., . . . Miller, W. C. (2005). *Perinatal depression: Prevalence, screening accuracy, and screening outcomes* (Evidence Report Technology Assessment No. 119). Rockville, MD: Agency for Healthcare Research and Quality.

Geller, S., Yagil, Y., Biriotti, S., & Neufeld, M. Y. (2013). Breastfeeding with epilepsy: Mothers' experiences and the role of professionals, family, and friends. *Breastfeeding Medicine, 8,* 424–425.

Gielen, A. C., Faden, R. R., O'Campo, P., Brown, C. H., & Paige, D. M. (1991). Maternal employment during the early postpartum period: Effects on initiation and continuation of breastfeeding. *Pediatrics, 87,* 298–305.

Gilljam, M., Antoniou, M., Shin J., Dupuis A., Corey, M., & Tullis, D. E. (2000). Pregnancy in cystic fibrosis: Fetal and maternal outcome. *Chest, 118,* 85–91.

Glatstein, M. M., Djokanovic, N., Garcia-Bournissen, F., Finkelstein, Y., & Koren, G. (2009). Use of hypoglycemic drugs during lactation. *Canadian Family Physician, 55,* 371–373.

Glueck, C. J., & Wang, P. (2007). Metformin before and during pregnancy and lactation in polycystic ovary syndrome. *Expert Opinion on Drug Safety, 6,* 191–198.

Goodman, J. H. (2004a). Paternal postpartum depression, its relationship to maternal depression, and implications for family health. *Journal of Advanced Nursing, 45,* 26–35.

Goodman, J. H. (2004b). Postpartum depression beyond the early postpartum period. *Journal of Obstetric, Gynecologic, and Neonatal Nursing, 33,* 410–420.

Grajeda, R., & Perez-Escamilla, R. (2002). Stress during labor and delivery is associated with delayed onset of lactation among urban Guatemalan women. *Journal of Nutrition, 132,* 3055–3060.

Granger, D. K., & Finlay, J. L. (1994). Nutritional vitamin B_{12} deficiency in a breastfed infant following maternal gastric bypass. *Journal of Pediatric Hematology/Oncology, 11,* 311–318.

Gregg, C., Shikar, V., Larsen, P., Mak, G., Chojnacki, A., Yong, V., & Weiss, S. (2007). White matter plasticity and enhanced remyelination in the maternal CNS. *Journal of Neuroscience, 27,* 1812–1823.

Groer, M. (2005). Relationships among naturalistic stress, mood, lactational status, and endocrine variables. *Biological Research for Nursing, 7,* 106–117.

Groer, M. W., Davis, M., Casey, K., Smith, K., Kramer, V., & Bukovsky, E. (2005). Immunity and infection: Differences between breastfeeders, formula feeders and controls. *American Journal of Reproductive Immunology, 54,* 222–231.

Groer, M. W., & Davis, M. W. (2006). Cytokines, infections, stress, and dysphoric moods in breastfeeders and formula feeders. *Journal of Obstetric, Gynecologic, and Neonatal Nursing, 35,* 599–607.

Groer, M. W., & Morgan, K. (2007). Immune, health and endocrine characteristics of depressed postpartum mothers. *Psychoneuroendocrinology, 32,* 133–139.

Grzeskowiak, L. E., Dalton, J. A., & Fielder, A. L. (2015). Factors associated with domperidone use as a galactagogue at an Australian tertiary teaching hospital. *Journal of Human Lactation, 31,* 249–253.

Grzeskowiak, L. E., Lim, S. W., Thomas, A. E., Ritchie, U., & Gordon, A. L. (2013). Audit of domperidone use as a galactogogue at an Australian tertiary teaching hospital. *Journal of Human Lactation, 29*(1), 32–37.

Gu, V., Feeley, N., Gold, I., Hayton, B., Robins, S., Mackinnon, A., . . . Zelkowitz, P. (2016). Intrapartum synthetic oxytocin and its effects on maternal well-being at 2 months postpartum. *Birth, 43,* 28–35.

Guendelman, S., Kosa, J. L., Pearl, M., Graham, S., Goodman, J., & Kharrazi, M. (2009). Juggling work and breastfeeding: Effects of maternity leave and occupational characteristics. *Pediatrics, 123,* e38–e46.

Gulick, E. E., & Halper, J. (2002). Influence of infant feeding method on postpartum relapse of mothers with multiple sclerosis. *International Journal of Multiple Sclerosis Care, 4,* 183–191.

Gulick, E. E., & Johnson, S. (2004). Infant health of mothers with multiple sclerosis. *Western Journal of Nursing Research, 26,* 632–649.

Gulick, E. E., & Kim, S. (2004). Postpartum emotional distress in mothers with multiple sclerosis. *Journal of Obstetric, Gynecologic, and Neonatal Nursing, 33,* 729–738.

Gunderson, E. P. (2007). Breastfeeding after gestational diabetes pregnancy: Subsequent obesity and type 2 diabetes in women and their offspring. *Diabetes Care, 30*(suppl 2), S161–S168.

Gunderson, E. P., Hedderson, M. M., Chiang, V., Crites, Y., Walton, D., Azevedo, R. A., . . . Selby, J. V. (2012). Lactation intensity and postpartum maternal glucose tolerance and insulin resistance in women with recent GDM: The SWIFT cohort. *Diabetes Care, 35,* 50–56.

Gunderson, E. P., Hurston, S. R., Ning, X., Lo, J. C., Crites, Y., Walton, D., . . . Quesenberry, C. P. (2015). Lactation and progression to type 2 diabetes mellitus after gestational diabetes mellitus: a prospective cohort study. *Annals of Internal Medicine, 163,* 889–898.

Gunn, A. J., Gunn, T. R., Rabone, D. L., Breier, B. H., Blum, W. F., & Gluckman, P. D. (1996). Growth hormone increases breast milk volumes in mothers of preterm infants. *Pediatrics, 98,* 279–282.

Gupta, A. P., & Gupta, P. K. (1985). Metoclopramide as a lactogogue. *Clinical Pediatrics, 24,* 269–272.

Gupta, M., & Shaw, B. (2011). A double-blind randomized clinical trial for evaluation of galactogogue activity of *Asparagus racemosus* wild. *Iranian Journal of Pharmaceutical Research, 10,* 167–172.

Haase, B., Taylor, S. N., Mauldin, J., Johnson, & Wagner, C. L. (2016). Domperidone for treatment of low milk supply in breast pump-dependent mothers of hospitalized premature infants: A clinical protocol. *Journal of Human Lactation*, [Epub ahead of print]. pii: 0890334416630539.

Haider, S. J., Jacknowitz, A., & Schoeni, R. F. (2003). Welfare work requirements and child well-being: Evidence from the effects on breastfeeding. *Demography, 40,* 479–497.

Halbert, L.-A. (1998). Breastfeeding in the woman with a compromised nervous system. *Journal of Human Lactation, 14,* 327–331.

Hale, T. W. (2012). *Medications and mothers' milk* (15th ed.). Amarillo, TX: Hale Publishing.

Hale, T. W., & Berens, P. (2002). *Clinical therapy in breastfeeding patients.* Amarillo, TX: Pharmasoft Publishing.

Hale, T. W., Kristensen, J. H., Hackett, L. P., Kohan, R., & Ilett, K. F. (2002). Transfer of metformin into human milk. *Diabetologia, 45,* 1509–1514.

Hammond-McKibben, D., & Dosch, H.-M. (1997). Cow milk, BSA and IDDM: Can we settle the controversies? *Diabetes Care, 20,* 897–901.

Hampl, J. S., & Papa, D. J. (2001). Breastfeeding-related onset, flare, and relapse of rheumatoid arthritis. *Nutrition Reviews, 59,* 264–268.

Hamosh, M., Ellis, L. A., Pollock, D. R., Henderson, T. R., & Hamosh, P. (1996). Breastfeeding and the working mother: Effect of time and temperature of short-term storage on proteolysis, lipolysis, and bacterial growth in milk. *Pediatrics, 97,* 492–498.

Hapon, M., Simoncini, M., Via, G., & Jahn, G. A. (2003). Effect of hypothyroidism on hormone profiles in virgin, pregnant and lactating rats, and on lactation. *Reproduction, 126,* 371–382.

Harris, B. (1999). Postpartum depression and thyroid antibody status. *Thyroid, 9,* 699–703.

Harris, B., Othman, S., Davies, J. A., Weppner, G. J., Richards, C. J., Newcombe, R. G., & Phillips, D. I. (1992). Association between postpartum thyroid dysfunction and thyroid antibodies and depression. *British Medical Journal, 305,* 152–156.

Harris, D. L., Weston, P. J., Signal, M., Chase, J. G., & Harding, J. E. (2013). Dextrose gel for neonatal hypoglycemia (the Sugar Babies Study): A randomised, double-blind, placebo-controlled trial. *Lancet, 382,* 2077–2083.

Harrison, T., & Stuifbergen, A. (2002). Disability, social support, and concern for children: Depression in mothers with multiple sclerosis. *Journal of Obstetric, Gynecologic, and Neonatal Nursing, 31,* 444–453.

Hart, R., Hickey, M., & Franks, S. (2004). Definitions, prevalence and symptoms of polycystic ovaries and polycystic ovary syndrome. *Best Practice and Research Clinical Obstetrics and Gynaecology, 18,* 671–683.

Hartmann, P., & Cregan, M. (2001). Lactogenesis and the effects of insulin-dependent diabetes mellitus and prematurity. *Journal of Nutrition, 131,* 3016S–3020S.

Hasselmann, M. H., Werneck, G. L., & Silva, C. V. (2008). Symptoms of postpartum depression and early interruption of exclusive breastfeeding in the first two months of life. *Cadernos de Saude Publica, 24*(suppl 2), S341–S352.

Hauff, L. E., & Demerath, A. W. (2012). Body image concerns and reduced breastfeeding duration in primiparous overweight and obese women. *American Journal of Human Biology, 24,* 339–349.

Hellwig, K., Haghikia, A., Rockhoff, M., & Gold, R. (2012). Multiple sclerosis and pregnancy: Experience from a nationwide database in Germany. *Therapeutic Advances in Neurologic Disorders, 5,* 247–253.

Hellwig, K., Rockhoff, M., Herbstritt, S., Borisow, N., Haghikia, A., Elias-Hamp, B., . . . Langer-Gould, A. (2015). Exclusive breastfeeding and the effect on postpartum multiple sclerosis relapses. *JAMA Neurology, 72,* 1132–1138.

Henderson, A. (2003a). Domperidone: Discovering new choices for lactating mothers. *AWHONN Lifelines, 7,* 55–60.

Henderson, J. (2003b). Impact of postnatal depression on breastfeeding duration. *Birth, 30,* 175–180.

Hendrick, V., Smith, L. M., Hwang, S., Altshuler, L. L., & Haynes, D. (2003). Weight gain in breastfed infants of mothers taking antidepressant medications. *Journal of Clinical Psychiatry, 64,* 401–412.

Henly, S., Anderson, C., Avery, M., Hills-Bonczyk, S. G., Potter, S., & Duckett, L. J. (1995). Anemia and insufficient milk in first-time mothers. *Birth, 22,* 87–92.

Hennigar, S. R., Velasquez, V., & Kelleher, S. I. (2015). Obesity-induced inflammation is associated with alterations in subcellular zinc pools and premature mammary gland involution in lactating mice. *Journal of Nutrition, 145,* 1999–2005.

Herskin, C. W., Stage, E., Barfred, C., Emmersen, P., Ladefoged Nichum, V., Damm, P., & Mathiesen, E. R. (2015). Low prevalence of long-term breastfeeding among women with type 2 diabetes. *Journal of Maternal Fetal Neonatal Medicine.* [Epub ahead of print]. doi:10.3109/14767058.2015.1092138.

Hill, P. D. (1991). The enigma of insufficient milk supply. *MCN: The American Journal of Maternal/Child Nursing, 16,* 31–316.

Hill, P. D., & Aldag, J. (1991). Potential indicators of insufficient milk supply syndrome. *Research in Nursing and Health, 14,* 11–19.

Hill, P. D., Aldag, J. C., Chatterton, R. T., & Zinaman, M. (2005). Comparison of milk output between mothers of preterm and term infants: The first 6 weeks after birth. *Journal of Human Lactation, 21,* 22–30.

Hill, P. D., Aldag, J. C., Zinaman, M., & Chatterton, R. T. (2007). Predictors of preterm infant feeding methods and perceived insufficient milk supply at week 12 postpartum. *Journal of Human Lactation, 23,* 32–38.

Hill, P. D., Chatterton, R. T., Jr., & Aldag, J. C. (2003). Neuroendocrine responses to stressors in lactating and nonlactating mammals: A literature review. *Biological Research for Nursing, 5,* 79–86.

Hill, P. D., & Humenick, S. S. (1989). Insufficient milk supply. *Journal of Nursing Scholarship, 21,* 145–148.

Hill, P. D., Wilhelm, P. A., Aldag, J. C., & Chatterton, R. T. Jr. (2004). Breast augmentation and lactation outcome: A case report. *MCN: The American Journal of Maternal/Child Nursing, 29,* 238–242.

Hillervik-Lindquist, C. (1991). Studies on perceived breast milk insufficiency. *Acta Paediatrica Scandinavica, 80*(suppl 376), 6–27.

Hillervik-Lindquist, C., Hofvander, Y., & Sjolin, S. (1991). Studies on perceived breast milk insufficiency. *Acta Paediatrica Scandinavica, 80,* 297–303.

Hilson, J. A., Rasmussen, K. M., & Kjolhede, C. L. (1997). Maternal obesity and breastfeeding success in a local population of Caucasian women. *American Journal of Clinical Nutrition, 66,* 1371–1378.

Hilson, J. A., Rasmussen, K. M., & Kjolhede, C. L. (2004). High prepregnant body mass index is associated with poor lactation outcomes among white, rural women independent of psychosocial and demographic correlates. *Journal of Human Lactation, 20,* 18–29.

Hobfoll, S. E., Ritter, C., Lavin, J., Hulsizer, M. R., & Cameron, R. P. (1995). Depression prevalence and incidence among inner-city pregnant and postpartum women. *Journal of Consulting and Clinical Psychology, 63,* 445–453.

Hofmeyr, G. J., & van Iddekinge, B. (1983). Domperidone and lactation. *Lancet, 1*(8325), 647.

Hofmeyr, G. J., van Iddekinge, B., & Blott, J. A. (1985). Domperidone: Secretion in breast milk and effect on puerperal prolactin levels. *British Journal of Obstetrics and Gynaecology, 92,* 141–144.

Hoover, K. L., Barbalinardo, L. H., & Platia, M. P. (2002). Delayed lactogenesis II secondary to gestational ovarian theca lutein cysts in two normal singleton pregnancies. *Journal of Human Lactation, 18,* 264–268.

Hopkinson, J., Schanler, R., Fraley, J., & Garza, C. (1992). Milk production by mothers of premature infants: Influence of cigarette smoking. *Pediatrics, 90,* 934–938.

Horowitz, J. A., & Goodman, J. H. (2005). Identifying and treating postpartum depression. *Journal of Obstetric, Gynecologic, and Neonatal Nursing, 34,* 264–273.

Houtchens, M. K., & Kolb, C. M. (2013). Multiple sclerosis and pregnancy: Therapeutic considerations. *Journal of Neurology, 260,* 1202–1214.

Huang, Y. Y., Lee, J. T., Huang, C. M., & Gau, M. L. (2009). Factors related to maternal perception of milk supply while in the hospital. *Journal of Nursing Research, 17,* 179–188.

Hughes, V., & Owen, J. (1993). Is breastfeeding possible after breast surgery? *MCN: The American Journal of Maternal/Child Nursing, 18,* 213–217.

Hummel, S., Winkler, C., Schoen, S., Knopff, A., Marienfeld, S., Bonifacio, E., & Ziegler, A. G. (2007). Breastfeeding habits in families with type 1 diabetes. *Diabetes and Medicine, 24,* 671–676.

Humphrey, S. (2003). *The nursing mother's herbal.* Minneapolis, MN: Fairview Press.

Hurst, N. M., Valentine, C. J., Renfro, L., Burns, P., & Ferlic, L. (1997). Skin-to-skin holding in the neonatal intensive care unit influences maternal milk volume. *Journal of Perinatology, 17,* 213.

Hutt, P. (1989). The effect of diabetes on lactation. *Breastfeeding Review, 14,* 21–25.

Ingram, J., Taylor, H., Churchill, C., Pike, A., & Greenwood, R. (2012). Metoclopramide or domperidone for increasing maternal breast milk output: A randomized controlled trial. *Archives of Disease in Children—Fetal and Neonatal Edition, 97,* F241–F245.

International Association of Diabetes and Pregnancy Study Groups Consensus Panel. (2010). International Association of Diabetes and Pregnancy Study Groups recommendations on the diagnosis and classification of hyperglycemia in pregnancy. *Diabetes Care, 33,* 676–682.

Isbister, G. K., Dawson, A., Whyte, I. M., Prior, F., Clancy, C., Smith, A., . . . Ito, S. (2001). Neonatal paroxetine withdrawal syndrome or actually serotonin syndrome? *Archives of Disease in Childhood—Fetal and Neonatal Edition, 85,* F147–F148.

Isik, A. Z., Gulekli, B., Zorlu, C. G., Ergin, T., & Gokmen, O. (1997). Endocrinological and clinical analysis of hyperprolactinemic patients with and without ultrasonically diagnosed polycystic ovary syndrome. *Gynecologic and Obstetric Investigation, 43,* 183–185.

Ito, S., Moretti, M., Liau, M., & Koren, G. (1995). Initiation and duration of breastfeeding in women receiving antiepileptics. *American Journal of Obstetrics and Gynecology, 173,* 881–886.

Izumi, Y., Miyashita, T., & Migita, K. (2014). Safety of tacrolimus treatment during pregnancy and lactation in systemic lupus erythematosus: A report of two patients. *Tohoku Journal of Experimental Medicine, 234,* 51–56.

Jacobson, P. M. (1998). Multiple sclerosis: A supportive approach for breastfeeding. *Mother and Baby Journal, 3,* 13–17.

Jagiello, K. P., & Chertok, I. R. A. (2015). Women's experiences with early breastfeeding after gestational diabetes. *Journal of Obstetric, Gynecologic, and Neonatal Nursing, 44,* 500–509.

Jaigobin, C., & Silver, F. L. (2000). Stroke and pregnancy. *Stroke, 31,* 2948–2951.

Jantarasaengaram, S., & Sreewapa, P. (2012). Effects of domperidone on augmentation of lactation following cesarean delivery at full term. *International Journal of Gynaecology and Obstetrics, 116,* 240–243.

Jara, L. J., Lavelle, C., & Espinoza, L. R. (1992). Does prolactin have a role in the pathogenesis of systemic lupus erythematosus? *Journal of Rheumatology, 19,* 1333.

Jevitt, C., Hernandez, I., & Groer, M. (2007). Lactation complicated by overweight and obesity: Supporting the mother and newborn. *Journal of Midwifery and Women's Health, 52,* 606–613.

Johnson, A. M., Kirk, R., & Muzik, M. (2015). Overcoming workplace barriers: A focus group study exploring African American mothers' needs for workplace breastfeeding support. *Journal of Human Lactation, 31,* 425–433.

Johnston, M. L., & Esposito, N. (2007). Barriers and facilitators for breastfeeding among working women in the United States. *Journal of Obstetric, Gynecologic, and Neonatal Nursing, 36,* 9–20.

Jones, N. A., McFall, B. A., & Diego, M. A. (2004). Patterns of brain electrical activity in infants of depressed mothers who breastfeed and bottle feed: The mediating role of infant temperament. *Biological Psychology, 67,* 103–124.

Jovanovic, L. (Ed.). (2000). *Medical management of pregnancy complicated by diabetes* (3rd ed.). Alexandria, VA: American Diabetes Association.

Kaiser Family Foundation. (2011). Overweight and obesity rates for adults by gender, 2011. Retrieved from http://www.statehealthfacts.kff.org/comparebar.jsp?ind=90&cat=2

Kamikawa, A., Ichii, O., Yamaji, D., Imao, T., Suzuki, C., Okamatsu-Ogura, Y., . . . Kimura, K. (2009). Diet-induced obesity disrupts ductal development in the mammary glands of nonpregnant mice. *Developmental Dynamics, 238,* 1092–1099.

Karges, W., Hammond-McKibben, D., Cheung, R. K., Visconti, M., Shibuya, N., Kemp, D., & Dosch, H. M. (1997). Immunological aspects of nutritional diabetes prevention in NOD mice: A pilot study for the cow's milk based IDDM prevention trial. *Diabetes, 46,* 557–564.

Karlson, E. W., Mandl, L. A., Hankinson, S. E., & Grodstein, F. (2004). Do breastfeeding and other reproductive factors influence future risk of rheumatoid arthritis? Results from the Nurses' Health Study. *Arthritis and Rheumatism, 50,* 3458–3467.

Kauppila, A., Arvela, P., Koivisto, M., Kivinen, S., Ylikorkala, O., & Pelkonen, O. (1983). Metoclopramide and breast feeding: Transfer into milk and the newborn. *European Journal of Clinical Pharmacology, 25,* 819–823.

Kaye, H. S. (2012). Current demographics of parents with disabilities in the U.S. Retrieved from http://www.lookingglass.org/services/national-services/220-research/126-current-demographics-of-parents-with-disabilities-in-the-us

Kayhan-Tetik, B., Baydar-Artantas, A., Bozcuk-Güzeldemirci, G., Ustu, Y., & Yilmaz, G., (2013). A case report of successful relactation. *Turkish Journal of Pediatrics, 55,* 641–644.

Kendall-Tackett, K. (2008). *Non-pharmacologic treatments for depression in new mothers.* Amarillo, TX: Hale Publishing.

Kendall-Tackett, K. (2014a). Childbirth-related posttraumatic stress disorder. *Clinical Lactation, 5,* 51–55.

Kendall-Tackett, K. (2014b). Intervention for mothers who have experienced childbirth-related trauma and post-traumatic stress disorder. *Clinical Lactation, 5,* 56–61.

Kendall-Tackett, K., Cong, Z., & Hale, T. W. (2015). Birth interventions related to lower rates of exclusive breastfeeding and increased risk of postpartum depression in a large sample. *Clinical Lactation, 6,* 87–97.

Kennedy, K. I., Short, R. V., & Tully, M. R. (1997). Premature introduction of progestin-only contraceptive methods during lactation. *Contraception, 55,* 347–350.

Kent, J. C., Geddes, D. T., Hepworth, A. R., & Hartmann, P. E. (2011). Effect of warm breastshields on breast milk pumping. *Journal of Human Lactation, 27,* 331–338.

Kent, J. C., Prime, D. K., & Garbin, C. P. (2012). Principles for maintaining or increasing breast milk production. *Journal of Obstetric, Gynecologic, and Neonatal Nursing, 41,* 114–121.

Kessler, R. C., McGonagle, K. A., Zhao, S., Nelson, C. B., Hughes, M., Eshleman, S., . . . Kendler, K. S. (1994). Lifetime and 12 month prevalence of *DSM-IVR* psychiatric disorders in the United States: Results from the National Comorbidity Survey. *Archives of General Psychiatry, 51,* 8–19.

Kidner, M. C., & Flanders-Stepans, M. B. (2004). A model for the HELLP syndrome: The maternal experience. *Journal of Obstetric, Gynecologic, and Neonatal Nursing, 33,* 44–53.

Kimbro, R. T. (2006). On-the-job moms: Work and breastfeeding initiation and duration for a sample of low-income women. *Maternal and Child Health Journal, 10,* 19–26.

Kitsantas, P., Gaffney, K. F., & Kornides, M. L. (2011). Prepregnancy body mass index, socioeconomic status, race/ethnicity and breastfeeding practices. *Journal of Perinatal Medicine, 40,* 77–83.

Kittner, S., & Adams, R. (1996). Stroke in children and young adults. *Current Opinion in Neurology, 9,* 53–56.

Kittner, S. J., Stern, B. J., Feeser, B. R., Hebel, J. R., Nagey, D. A., Buchholz, D. W., . . . Wozniak, M. A. (1996). Pregnancy and the risk of stroke. *New England Journal of Medicine, 335,* 768–774.

Kjos, S. L., Henry, O., Lee, R. M., Buchanan, T. A., & Mishell, D. R., Jr. (1993). The effect of lactation on glucose and lipid metabolism in women with recent gestational diabetes. *Obstetrics and Gynecology, 82,* 451–455.

Klein, A. (2012). The postpartum period in women with epilepsy. *Neurologic Clinics, 30,* 867–875.

Klier, C. M., Schaefer, M. R., Schmid-Siegel, B., Lenz, G., & Mannel, M. (2002). St. John's wort (*Hypericum perforatum*): Is it safe during breastfeeding? *Pharmacopsychiatry, 35,* 29–30.

Knip, M., & Akerblom, H. K. (1998). IDDM prevention trials in progress: A critical assessment. *Journal of Pediatric Endocrinology and Metabolism, 11,* 371.

Knoppert, D. C., Page, A., Warren, J., Seabrook, J. A., Carr, M., Angelini, M., . . . daSilva, O. P. (2013). The effect of two different domperidone doses on maternal milk production. *Journal of Human Lactation, 29*(1), 38–44.

Koch, S., Titze, K., Zimmermann, R. B., Schröder, M., Lehmkuhl, U., & Rauh, H. (1999). Long-term neuropsychological consequences of maternal epilepsy and anticonvulsant treatment during pregnancy for school age children and adolescents. *Epilepsia, 40,* 1237–1243.

Kroencke, D. C., & Denney, D. R. (1999). Stress and coping in multiple sclerosis: Exacerbation, remission and chronic subgroups. *Multiple Sclerosis, 5,* 89–93.

Lacoursiere, D. Y., Baksh, L., Bloebaum, L., & Varner, M. W. (2006). Maternal body mass index and self-reported postpartum depressive symptoms. *Maternal and Child Health Journal, 10*(4), 385–390.

Laine, K., Heikkinen, T., Ekblad, U., & Kero, P. (2003). Effects of exposure to selective serotonin reuptake inhibitors during pregnancy on serotonergic symptoms in newborns and cord blood monoamine and prolactin concentrations. *Archives of General Psychiatry, 60,* 720–726.

Lamb, M. (2011). Weight-loss surgery and breastfeeding. *Clinical Lactation, 2,* 17–21.

Langer-Gould, A., Huang, S. M, Gupta, R., Leimpeter, A. D., Greenwood, E., Albers, K. B., . . . Nelson, L. M. (2009). Exclusive breastfeeding and the risk of postpartum relapses in women with multiple sclerosis. *Archives of Neurology, 66*(8), 958–963.

Lankarani-Fard, A., Kritz-Silverterin, D., Barrett-Connor, E., & Goodman-Gruen, D. (2001). Cumulative duration of breastfeeding influences cortisol levels in postmenopausal women. *Journal of Women's Health and Gender-Based Medicine, 10,* 681–687.

Lau, C., & Hurst, N. (1999). Oral feeding in infants. *Current Problems in Pediatrics, 29,* 101.

Lawrence, R. A., & Lawrence, R. M. (2016). *Breastfeeding: A guide for the medical profession* (8th ed.). Philadelphia: Elsevier Mosby.

Lee, A., Moretti, M. E., Collantes, A., Chong, D., Mazzotta, P., Koren, G., . . . Ito, S. (2000). Choice of breastfeeding and physicians' advice: A cohort study of women receiving propylthiouracil. *Pediatrics, 106,* 27–30.

Lee, P. J., Ridout, D., Walter, J. H., & Cockburn, F. (2005). Maternal phenylketonuria: Report from the United Kingdom Registry 1978–97. *Archives of Disease in Childhood, 90,* 143–146.

Lee, S., Hennigar, S. R., Alam, S., Nishida, K., & Kelleher, S. L. (2015). Essential role for zinc transporter 2 (ZnT2)–mediated zinc transport in mammary gland development and function during lactation. *Journal of Biological Chemistry, 22,* 13064–13078.

Lemay, D. G., Ballard, O. A., Highes, M. A., Morrow, A. L., Horseman, N. D., & Nommsen-Rivers, L. A. (2013). RNA sequencing of the human milk fat layer transcriptome reveals distinct gene expression profiles at three stages of lactation. *PLoS One, 8,* e67531.

Lepe, M., Bacardi Gascon, M., Castaneda-Gonzalez, L. M., Perez Morales, M. E., & Jimenez Cruz, A. (2011). Effect of maternal obesity on lactation: Systematic review. *Nutrición Hospitalaria, 26,* 1266–1269.

Lester, B. M., Cucca, J., Andreozzi, L., Flanagan, P., & Oh, W. (1993). Possible association between fluoxetine hydrochloride and colic in an infant. *Journal of the American Academy of Child and Adolescent Psychiatry, 32,* 1253–1255.

Li, R., Fein, S. B., Chen, J., & Grummer-Strawn, L. M. (2008). Why mothers stop breastfeeding: Mothers' self-reported reasons for stopping during the first year. *Pediatrics, 122*(suppl 2), S69–S76.

Li, R., Jewell, S., & Grummer-Strawn, L. (2003). Maternal obesity and breastfeeding practices. *American Journal of Clinical Nutrition, 77,* 931–936.

Liao, K. P., Alfredsson, L., & Karlson, E. W. (2009). Environmental influences on risk for rheumatoid arthritis. *Current Opinion in Rheumatology, 21,* 279–283.

Lindberg, L. D. (1996). Trends in the relationship between breastfeeding and postpartum employment in the United States. *Social Biology, 43,* 191–202.

Liu, B., Jorn, L., & Banks, E. (2010). Parity, breastfeeding, and the subsequent risk of maternal type 2 diabetes. *Diabetes Care, 33,* 1239–1241.

Liu, N., & Krassioukov, A. V. (2013). Postpartum hypogalactia in a woman with Brown-Sequard-plus syndrome: A case report. *Spinal Cord, 51,* 794–796.

Livingstone, V. (1996). Too much of a good thing: Maternal and infant hyperlactation syndromes. *Canadian Family Physician, 42,* 89–99.

Lommen, A., Brown, B., & Hollist, D. (2015). Experiential perceptions of relactation: A phenomenological study. *Journal of Human Lactation, 31,* 498–503.

Lorenzi, A. R., & Ford, H. L. (2002). Multiple sclerosis and pregnancy. *Postgraduate Medical Journal, 78,* 460–464.

Low Dog, T., & Micozzi, M. S. (2005). *Women's health in complementary and integrative medicine: A clinical guide.* St. Louis, MO: Elsevier.

Luder, E., Kaltan, M., Tanzer-Torres, G., & Bonforte, R. J. (1990). Current recommendations for breastfeeding in cystic fibrosis centers. *American Journal of Diseases of Children, 144,* 1153.

Lupus Foundation of America. (2013). Homepage. Retrieved from http://www.lupus.org

Mack, W. J., Preston-Martin, S., Bernstein, L., Qian, D., & Xiang, M. (1999). Reproductive and hormonal risk factors for thyroid cancer in Los Angeles County females. *Cancer Epidemiology, Biomarkers and Prevention, 8,* 991–997.

MacNeill, S., Dodds, L., Hamilton, D. C., Armson, B. A., & VandenHof, M. (2001). Rates and risk factors for recurrence of gestational diabetes. *Diabetes Care, 24,* 659–662.

Maes, M., (Ed.). (2001). Psychological stress and the inflammatory response system. *Clinical Science. 101,* 193–194.

Maillot, F., Cook, P., Lilburn, M., & Lee, P. J. (2007). A practical approach to maternal phenylketonuria management. *Journal of Inherited Metabolic Disease, 30,* 198–201.

Maillot, F., Lilburn, M., Baudin, J., Morley, D. W., & Lee, P. J. (2008). Factors influencing outcomes in the offspring of mothers with phenylketonuria during pregnancy: The importance of variation in maternal blood phenylalanine. *American Journal of Clinical Nutrition, 88,* 700–705.

Maitra, R., & Menkes, D. B. (1996). Psychotropic drugs and lactation. *New Zealand Medical Journal, 109,* 217–218.

Mak, C. W., Chou, C. K., Chen, S. Y., Lee, P. S., & Chang, J. M. (2003). Case report: Diabetic mastopathy. *British Journal of Radiology, 76,* 192–194.

Manios, Y., Grammatikaki, E., Kondaki, K., Ioannou, E., Anastasiadou, A., & Birbilis, M. (2009). The effect of maternal obesity on initiation and duration of breastfeeding in Greece: The GENESIS study. *Public Health and Nutrition, 12,* 517–524.

Marasco, L. (2006). The impact of thyroid dysfunction on lactation. *Breastfeeding Abstracts, 25,* 9–12.

Marasco, L., Marmet, C., & Shell, E. (2000). Polycystic ovary syndrome: A connection to insufficient milk supply? *Journal of Human Lactation, 16,* 143–148.

Marasco, L. A. (2014). Unsolved mysteries of the human mammary gland: Defining and redefining the critical questions from the lactation consultant's perspective. *Journal of Mammary Gland Biology Neoplasia, 19,* 271–288.

Martin Cookson, D. (1992). La Leche League and the mother who is blind. *Leaven, 5,* 67–68.

Matalon, R., Michals, K., & Gleason, L. (1986). PKU: Strategies for dietary treatment and monitoring compliance. *Annals of the New York Academy of Sciences, 477,* 223.

Matias, S. L., Dewey, K. G., Quesenberry, C. P., & Gunderson, E. P. (2014). Maternal prepregnancy obesity and insulin treatment during pregnancy are independently associated with delayed lactogenesis in women with recent gestational diabetes mellitus. *American Journal of Clinical Nutrition, 99,* 115–121.

McCarter-Spaulding, D., & Horowitz, J. A. (2007). How does postpartum depression affect breastfeeding? *MCN American Journal of Maternal Child Nursing, 32,* 10–17.

McCarter-Spaulding, D. E., & Kearney, M. H. (2001). Parenting self-efficacy and perception of insufficient breast milk. *Journal of Obstetric, Gynecologic, and Neonatal Nursing, 30,* 515–522.

McClure, C. K., Schwarz, E. B., Conroy, M. B., Tepper, P. G., Janssen, I., & Sutton-Tyrrell, K. C. (2011). Breastfeeding and subsequent maternal visceral adiposity. *Obesity, 19,* 2205–2213.

McCook, J. G., Reame, N. E., & Thatcher, S. S. (2005). Health-related quality of life issues in women with polycystic ovary syndrome. *Journal of Obstetric, Gynecologic, and Neonatal Nursing, 34,* 12–20.

McGovern, P., Dowd, B., Gjerdingen, D., Gross, C. R. Kenney, S., Ukestad, L., & Lundberg, U. (2006). Post partum health of employed mothers 5 weeks after childbirth. *Annals of Family Medicine, 4,* 159–167.

Meador K., Baker, G. A., Browning, N., Clayton-Smith, J., Combs-Cantrell, D. T., Cohen, M., . . . Loring, D. W. (2008). *Effects of breastfeeding in women taking antiepileptic drugs on their children's cognitive outcomes* (Abstract S45.001). Paper presented at the annual meeting of the American Academy of Neurology. Summary retrieved from http://www.medpagetoday.com/MeetingCoverage/AAN/9183

Meador, K. J., Baker, G. A., Browning, N., Clayton-Smith, J., Combs-Cantrell, D. T., Cohen, M., . . . Loring, D. W. (2009). Cognitive function at 3 years of age after fetal exposure to antiepileptic drugs. *New England Journal of Medicine, 360,* 1597–1605.

Meador, K. J., Baker, G. A., Browning, N., Clayton-Smith, J., Combs-Cantrell, D. T., Cohen, M., . . . Loring, D. W. (2010). Effects of breastfeeding in children of women taking antiepileptic drugs. *Neurology, 75,* 1954–1960.

Meador, K. J., Baker, G. A., Browning, N., Cohen, M. J., Bromley, R. L., Clayton-Smith, J., . . . Loring, D. W. (2014). Breastfeeding in children of women taking antiepileptic drugs: Cognitive outcome at 6 years. *JAMA Pediatrics, 168,* 729–736.

Meek, J. Y. (2001). Breastfeeding in the workplace. *Pediatric Clinics of North America, 48,* 461–474.

Metcalfe, M. A., & Baum, J. D. (1992). Family characteristics and insulin dependent diabetes. *Archives of Disease in Childhood, 67,* 731.

Metzger, B. E., Buchanan, T. A., Coustan, D. R., de Leiva, A., Dunger, D. B., Hadden, D. R., . . . Zoupas, C. (2007). Summary and recommendations of the Fifth International Workshop-Conference on Gestational Diabetes Mellitus. *Diabetes Care, 30*(suppl 2), S251–S260.

Michael, A., & Mayer, C. (2000). Fluoxetine-induced anesthesia of vagina and nipples. *British Journal of Psychiatry, 176,* 299.

Michel, S. H., & Mueller, D. H. (1994). Impact of lactation on women with cystic fibrosis and their infants: A review of five cases. *Journal of the American Dietetics Association, 94,* 159–165.

Milligan, R. A., Flenniken, P. M., & Pugh, L. C. (1996). Positioning intervention to minimize fatigue in breastfeeding women. *Applied Nursing Research, 9,* 67–70.

Milsom, S. R., Breier, B. H., Gallaher, B. W., Cox, V. A., Gunn, A. J., & Gluckman, P. D. (1992). Growth hormone stimulates galactopoiesis in healthy lactating women. *Acta Endocrinologica, 127,* 337–343.

Milsom, S. R., Rabone, D. L., Gunn, A. J., & Gluckman, P. D. (1998). Potential role for growth hormone in human lactation insufficiency. *Hormone Research, 50,* 147–150.

Mirkovic, K. R., Perrine, C. G., Scanlon, K. S., & Grummer-Strawn, L. M. (2014). Maternity leave duration and full-time/part-time work status are associated with US mothers' ability to meet breastfeeding intentions. *Journal of Human Lactation, 30,* 416–419.

Miyake, A., Tahara, M., Koike, K., & Tanizawa, O. (1989). Decrease in neonatal suckled milk volume in diabetic women. *European Journal of Gynecology and Reproductive Biology, 33,* 49–53.

Mok, C. C., & Wong, R. W. S. (2001). Pregnancy in systemic lupus erythematosus. *Postgraduate Medical Journal, 77,* 157–165.

Mok, C. C., Wong, R. W. S., & Lau, C. S. (1998). Systemic lupus erythematosus exacerbated by breastfeeding. *Lupus, 7,* 569–570.

Mok, E., Multon, C., Piguel, L., Barroso, E., Goua, V., Christin, P., . . . Hankard, R. (2008). Decreased full breastfeeding, altered practices, perceptions, and infant weight change of prepregnant obese women: A need for extra support. *Pediatrics, 121,* e1319–e1324.

Monshi, B., Stockinger, T., Vigl, K., Richter, L., Weihsengruber, F., & Rappersberger, K. (2015). Phrynoderma and acquired acrodermatitis enteropathica in breastfeeding women after bariatric surgery. *Journal der Deutschen Dermatologischen Gesellschaft, 13,* 1147–1154.

Moore, S. J., Turnpenny, P., Quinn, A., Glover, S., Lloyd, D. J., Montgomery, T., & Dean, J. C. (2000). A clinical study of 57 children with fetal anticonvulsant syndromes. *Journal of Medical Genetics, 37,* 489–497.

Morreale, D. E., Obregon, M. J., & Escobar, D. R. (2000). Is neuropsychological development related to maternal hypothyroidism or to maternal hypothroxinemia? *Journal of Clinical Endocrinology and Metabolism, 85,* 3975–3987.

Mortel, M., & Mehta, S. D. (2013). Systematic review of the efficacy of herbal galactagogues. *Journal of Human Lactation, 29,* 154–162.

Morton, J. A. (1992). Ineffective suckling: A possible consequence of obstructive positioning. *Journal of Human Lactation, 8,* 83–85.

Moses-Kolko, E. L., Bogen, D., Perel, J., Bregar, A., Uhl, K., Levin, B., & Wisner, K. L. (2005). Neonatal signs after late in utero exposure to serotonin reuptake inhibitors: Literature review and implications for clinical applications. *Journal of the American Medical Association, 293,* 2372–2383.

Muller, A. F., Drexhage, H. A., & Berghout, A. (2001). Postpartum thyroiditis and autoimmune thyroiditis in women of childbearing age: Recent insights and consequences for antenatal and postnatal care. *Endocrine Reviews, 22,* 605–630.

Murtaugh, M. A., Ferris, A. M., Capacchione, C. M., & Reece, E. A. (1998). Energy intake and glycemia in lactating women with type 1 diabetes. *Journal of the American Dietetics Association, 98,* 642–648.

National Children's Study. (2003, December 16). Use of herbal products in pregnancy, breastfeeding, and childhood workshop. Retrieved from http://www.nationalchildrensstudy.gov/about/organization/advisorycommittee/2004Mar/Pages/workshop_herbals_032004.aspx

Neifert, M., DeMarzo, S., Seacat J., Young, D., Leff, M., & Orleans, M. (1990). The influence of breast surgery, breast appearance, and pregnancy-induced breast changes on lactation sufficiency as measured by infant weight gain. *Birth, 17,* 31–38.

Neifert, M. R., Seacat, J. M., & Jobe, W. E. (1985). Lactation failure due to insufficient glandular development of the breast. *Pediatrics, 76,* 823 -828.

Nelson, L. M., Franklin, G. M., & Jones, M. C. (1988). Risk of multiple sclerosis exacerbation during pregnancy and breastfeeding. *Journal of the American Medical Association, 259,* 3441–3443.

Neri, I., Allais, G., Vaccaro, V., Minniti, S., Airola, G., Schiapparelli, P., . . . Facchinetti, F. (2011). Acupuncture treatment as breastfeeding support: Preliminary data. *Journal of Alternative and Complementary Medicine, 17,* 133–137.

Neubauer, S. H., Ferris, A. M., Chase, C. G., Fanelli, J., Thompson, C. A., Lammi-Keefe, C. J., . . . Green, K. W. (1993). Delayed lactogenesis in women with and without insulin-dependent diabetes mellitus. *American Journal of Clinical Nutrition, 58,* 54–60.

Newman, J. (1998, January). Domperidone. Retrieved from http://www.breastfeedinginc.ca/content.php?pagename=doc-DGS

Newman, J., & Goldfarb, L. (2010). The protocols for induced lactation: A guide for maximizing breastmilk production. Retrieved from http://www.asklenore.info/breastfeeding/induced_lactation/regular_protocol.shtml

Newman, J., & Pittman, T. (2000). *The ultimate breastfeeding book of answers.* Roseville, CA: Prima Publishing.

Nice, F. J. (2011). Common herbs and foods used as galactogogues. *ICAN: Infant, Child, and Adolescent Nutrition, 3,* 129–132.

Nichols, M. R., & Roux, G. M. (2004). Maternal perspectives on postpartum return to the workplace. *Journal of Obstetric, Gynecologic, and Neonatal Nursing, 33,* 463–471.

Nigro, G., Campea, L., DeNovellis, A., Recker, B., Weyman-Daum, M., Pugliese, M., & Lifshitz, F. (1985). Breastfeeding and insulin-dependent diabetes mellitus. *Lancet, 1,* 467.

Nordeng, H., Lindemann, R., Perminov, K. V., & Reikvam, A. (2001). Neonatal withdrawal syndrome after in utero exposure to selective serotonin reuptake inhibitors. *Acta Paediatrica, 90,* 288–291.

Norman, R., & Clark, A. (1998). Obesity and reproductive disorders: A review. *Reproduction, Fertility, and Development, 10,* 55–63.

Norris, J. M., Barriga, K., Klingensmith, G., Hoffman, M., Eisenbarth, G. S., Erlich, H. A., & Rewers, M. (2003). Timing of initial cereal exposure in infancy and risk of islet autoimmunity. *Journal of the American Medical Association, 290,* 1713–1720.

Oberlander, T. F., Misri, S., Fitzgerald, C. E., Kostaras, X., Rurak, D., & Riggs, W. (2004). Pharmacologic factors associated with transient neonatal symptoms following prenatal psychotropic medication exposure. *Journal of Clinical Psychiatry, 65,* 230–237.

Oddy, W. H., Landsborough, L., Kendall, G. E., Henderson, S., & Downie, J. (2006). The association of maternal overweight and obesity with breastfeeding duration. *Journal of Pediatrics, 149,* 185–191.

Odegaard, I., Stray-Pedersen, B., Hallberg, K., Haanaes, O. C., Storrosten, O. T., & Johannesson, M. (2002). Maternal and fetal morbidity in pregnancies of Norwegian and Swedish women with cystic fibrosis. *Acta Obstetrica Gynecologica Scandinavica, 81,* 698–705.

Ogden, C. L., Carroll, M. D., Curtin, L. R., McDowell, M. A., Tabak, C. J., & Flegal, K. M. (2006). Prevalence of overweight and obesity in the United States, 1999–2004. *Journal of the American Medical Association, 295,* 1549–1555.

O'Hara, M. W., & Swain, A. M. (1996). Rates and risk of postpartum depression: A meta-analysis. *International Review of Psychiatry, 8,* 37–54.

O'Reilly, M. W., Avalos, G., Dennedy, M. C., O'Sullivan, E. P., & Dunne, F. (2011). Atlantic DIP: High prevalence of abnormal glucose tolerance postpartum is reduced by breastfeeding in women with prior gestational diabetes mellitus. *European Journal of Endocrinology, 165,* 953–959.

Ortiz, J., McGilligan, K., & Kelly, P. (2004). Duration of breast milk expression among working mothers enrolled in an employer-sponsored lactation program. *Pediatric Nursing, 30,* 111–119.

Osadchy, A., Moretti, M. E., & Koren, G. (2012). Effect of domperidone on insufficient lactation in puerperal women: A systematic review and meta-analysis of randomized controlled trials. *Obstetrics and Gynecology International, 2012,* 642893.

Ost, L., Wettrell, G., Bjorkhem, I., & Rane, A. (1985). Prednisone excretion in human milk. *Journal of Pediatrics, 106,* 1008–1011.

Ostrom, K. M., & Ferris, A. M. (1993). Prolactin concentrations in serum and milk of mothers with and without insulin-dependent diabetes mellitus. *American Journal of Clinical Nutrition, 58,* 49–53.

O'Sullivan, E. J., Perrine, C. G., & Rasmussen, K. M. (2015). Early breastfeeding problems mediate the negative association between maternal obesity and exclusive breastfeeding at 1 and 2 months postpartum. *Journal of Nutrition, 145,* 2369–2378.

Ozdemir, O., Sari, M. E., Kurt, A., Sakar, V. S., & Atalay, C. R. (2015). Pregnancy outcome of 149 pregnancies in women with epilepsy: Experience from a tertiary care hospital. *Interventional Medicine & Applied Science, 7,* 108–113.

Page-Wilson, G., Smith, P. C., & Welt, C. K. (2007). Short-term prolactin administration causes expressible galactorrhea but does not affect bone turnover: Pilot data for a new lactation agent. *International Breastfeeding Journal, 2,* 10.

Panter, K. E., & James, L. F. (1990). Natural plant toxicants in milk: a review. *Journal of Animal Science, 68,* 892–904.

Papastergiou, J., Abdallah, M., Tran, A., & Folkins, C. (2013). Domperidone withdrawal in a breastfeeding woman. *Canadian Pharmacists Journal, 146,* 210–212.

Parker, E. M., O'Sullivan, B. P., Shea, J. C., Regan, M. M., & Freedman, S. D. (2004). Survey of breastfeeding practices and outcomes in the cystic fibrosis population. *Pediatric Pulmonology, 37,* 362–367.

Paul, C., Zenut, M., Dorcut, A., Coudore, M-A., Vein, J., Cardot, J-M., & Balayssac, D. (2015). Use of domperidone as a galactagogue drug: A systematic review of the benefit–risk ratio. *Journal of Human Lactation, 31,* 57–63.

Paul, I. M., Downs, D. S., Schaefer, E. W., Beiler, J. S., & Weisman, C. S. (2013). Postpartum anxiety and maternal–infant health outcomes. *Pediatrics, 131,* e1218–1284.

Pena, K. S., & Rosenfeld, J. A. (2001). Evaluation and treatment of galactorrhea. *American Family Physician, 63,* 1763–1770, 1775.

Peppard, H. R., Marfori, J., Iuorno, M. J., & Nestler, J. E. (2001). Prevalence of polycystic ovary syndrome among premenopausal women with type 2 diabetes. *Diabetes Care, 24,* 1050–1052.

Pereira, K., & Brown, A. (2008). Postpartum thyroiditis: Not just a worn out mom. *Journal of Nurse Practitioner, 4,* 175–182.

Perez-Bravo, F., Carrasco, E., Gutierrez-Lopez, M. D., Martinez, M. T., Lopez, G., & de los Rios, M. G. (1996). Genetic predisposition and environmental factors leading to the development of insulin dependent diabetes mellitus in Chilean children. *Journal of Molecular Medicine, 74,* 105–109.

Petraglia, F., De Leo, V., Sardelli, S., Pieroni, M. L., D'Antona, N., & Genazzani, A. R. (1985). Domperidone in defective and insufficient lactation. *European Journal of Obstetrics and Gynecology and Reproductive Biology, 19,* 281–287.

Pikwer, M., Bergstrom, U., Nilsson, J. A., Jacobsson, L., Berglund, G., & Turesson, C. (2009). Breastfeeding, but not use of oral contraceptives, is associated with a reduced risk of rheumatoid arthritis. *Annals of the Rheumatic Diseases, 68,* 526–530.

Pippins, J. R., Brawarsky, P., Jackson, R. A., Fuentes-Afflick, E., & Haas, J. S. (2006). Association of breastfeeding with maternal depressive symptoms. *Journal of Women's Health, 15*(6), 754–762.

Pisacane, A., Impagliazzo, N., Russon, M., Valiani, R., Mandarini, A., Florio, C., & Vivo, P. (1994). Breastfeeding and multiple sclerosis. *British Medical Journal, 308,* 1411–1412.

Polycystic Ovary Syndrome Writing Committee. (2005). American Association of Clinical Endocrinologists position statement on metabolic and cardiovascular consequences of polycystic ovary syndrome. *Endocrine Practice, 11,* 126–134.

Poobalan, A. S., Aucott, L. S., Gurung, T., Smith, W. C., & Bhattacharya, S. (2009). Obesity as an independent risk factor for elective and emergency cesarean delivery in nulliparous women: Systematic review and meta-analysis of cohort studies. *Obesity Reviews, 10,* 28–35.

Pop, V. J., Kuijpens, J. L., van Barr, A., Verkerk, G., van Son, M. M., de Vijlder, J. J., . . . Vader, H. L. (1999). Low maternal free thyroxine concentrations during early pregnancy are associated with impaired psychomotor development in infancy. *Clinical Endocrinology, 50,* 149–155.

Powe, C. E., Allen, M., Puopolo, K. M., Merewood, A., Worden, S., Johnson, L. C., . . . Welt, C. K. (2010). Recombinant human prolactin for the treatment of lactation insufficiency. *Clinical Endocrinology, 73,* 645–653.

Powe, C. E., Puopolo, K. M., Newburg, D. S., Lonnerdal, B., Chen, C., Allen, M., . . . Welt, C. K. (2011). Effects of recombinant human prolactin on breast milk composition. *Pediatrics, 127,* e359–e366.

Powers, N. G. (1999). Slow weight gain and low milk supply in the breastfeeding dyad. *Clinics in Perinatology, 26,* 399–430.

Prime, D. K., Geddes, D. T., Spatz, D. L., Trengove, N. J., & Hartmann, P. E. (2010). The effect of breast-shield size and anatomy on milk removal in women. *Journal of Human Lactation, 26,* 433.

Prince, M. (2002, April 22). More employers are offering lactation rooms for new moms. *Business Insurance,* p. 6.

Pschirrer, E. R. (2004). Seizure disorders in pregnancy. *Obstetrics and Gynecology Clinics of North America, 31,* 373–384.

Pugliatti, M., Sotgiu, S., & Rosati, G. (2002). The worldwide prevalence of multiple sclerosis. *Clinical Neurology and Neurosurgery, 104,* 182–191.

Purnell, H. (2001). Phenylketonuria and maternal phenylketonuria. *Breastfeeding Review, 9,* 19–21.

Raguindin, P. F. N., Dans, L. F., & King, J. F. (2014). *Moringa oleifera* as a galactagogue. *Breastfeeding Medicine, 9,* 323–324.

Rasmussen, K. M., Hilson, J. A., & Kjolhede, C. L. (2001). Obesity may impair lactogenesis II. *Journal of Nutrition, 131,* 3009S–3011S.

Rasmussen, K. M., & Kjolhede, C. L. (2004). Prepregnant overweight and obesity diminish the prolactin response to suckling in the first week postpartum. *Pediatrics, 113,* e465–e471.

Rasmussen, K. M., Lee, V. E., Ledkovsky, T. B., & Kjolhede, C. L. (2006). A description of lactation counseling practices that are used with obese mothers. *Journal of Human Lactation, 22,* 322–327.

Reece, E. A., & Homko, C. J. (1994). Infant of the diabetic mother. *Seminars in Perinatology, 18,* 459–469.

Reeder, C., LeGrand, A., & O'Connor-Von, S.K. (2013). The effect of fenugreek on milk production and prolactin levels in mothers of preterm infants. *Clinical Lactation, 4,* 159–165.

Reefhuis, J., Rasmussen, S. A., & Friedman, J. M. (2006). Selective serotonin reuptake inhibitors and persistent pulmonary hypertension of the newborn [Comment]. *New England Journal of Medicine, 340,* 2188–2190.

Renfrew, M. F., Lang, S., & Woolridge, M. (2000). Oxytocin for promoting successful lactation. *Cochrane Database of Systematic Reviews, 2,* CD000156.

Riddle, S. W., & Nommsen-Rivers, L. A. (2016). A case control study of diabetes during pregnancy and low milk supply. *Breastfeeding Medicine, 11,* 80–85.

Riva, E., Agostini, C., Biasucci, G., Trojan, S., Luotti, D., Fiori, L., & Giovannini, M. (1996). Early breastfeeding is linked to higher intelligence quotient scores in dietary treated phenylketonuric children. *Acta Paediatrica, 85,* 56–58.

Riviello, C., Mello, G., & Jovanovic, L. G. (2009). Breastfeeding and the basal insulin requirement in type 1 diabetic women. *Endocrine Practice, 15,* 187–193.

Roe, B., Whittington, L. A., Fein, S. B., & Teisl, M. F. (1999). Is there competition between breastfeeding and maternal employment? *Demography, 36,* 157–171.

Rojjanasrirat, W. (2004). Working women's breastfeeding experiences. *MCN: The American Journal of Maternal/Child Nursing, 29,* 222–227.

The Rotterdam ESHRE/ASRM-sponsored PCOS Consensus Workshop Group. (2004). Revised 2003 consensus on diagnostic criteria and long-term health risks related to polycystic ovary syndrome (PCOS). *Human Reproduction, 19,* 41–47.

Rowe-Murray, H. J., & Fisher, J. R. (2002). Baby friendly hospital practices: Cesarean section is a persistent barrier to early initiation of breastfeeding. *Birth, 29,* 124–131.

Ruis, H., Rolland, R., Doesburg, W., Broeders, G., & Corbey, R. (1981). Oxytocin enhances onset of lactation among mothers delivering prematurely. *British Medical Journal, 283,* 340–342.

Rutishauser, I. H. E., & Carlin, J. B. (1992). Body mass index and duration of breastfeeding: A survival analysis during the first six months of life. *Journal of Epidemiology and Community Health, 46,* 559–565.

Sacco, L. M., Caulfield, L. E., Gittelsohn, J., & Martinez, H. (2006). The conceptualization of perceived insufficient milk among Mexican mothers. *Journal of Human Lactation, 22,* 277–286.

Salisbury, A. L., Wisner, K. L., Pearlstein, T., Battle, C. L., Stroud, L., & Lester, B. M. (2011). Newborn neurobehavioral patterns are differentially related to prenatal major depressive disorder and serotonin reuptake inhibitor treatment. *Depression and Anxiety, 28,* 1008–1019.

Schaefer, K. M. (2004). Breastfeeding in chronic illness: The voices of women with fibromyalgia. *MCN: The American Journal of Maternal/Child Nursing, 29,* 248–253.

Schaefer-Graf, U. M., Buchanan, T. A., Xiang, A. H., Peters, R. K., & Kjos, S. L. (2002). Clinical predictors for a high risk for the development of diabetes mellitus in the early puerperium in women with recent gestational diabetes mellitus. *American Journal of Obstetrics and Gynecology, 186,* 751–756.

Schoen, S., Sichert-Hellert, W., Hummel, S., Ziegler, A. G., & Kersting, M. (2008). Breastfeeding duration in families with type 1 diabetes compared to non-affected families: Results from BABYDIAB and DONALD studies in Germany. *Breastfeeding Medicine, 3,* 171–165.

Schwarz, E. B., Brown, J. S., Creasman, J. M., Stuebe, A., McClure, C. K., van den Eeden, S. K., & Thom, D. (2010). Lactation and maternal risk of type-2 diabetes: A population-based study. *American Journal of Medicine, 123,* 863. 863.el–e6.

Segura-Millan, S., Dewey, K. G., & Perez-Escamilla, R. (1994). Factors associated with perceived insufficient milk in a low-income urban population in Mexico. *Journal of Nutrition, 124,* 202–212.

Seijts, G. H. (2002). Milking the organization? The effect of breastfeeding accommodation on perceived fairness and organizational attractiveness. *Journal of Business Ethics, 40,* 1–13.

Seijts, G. H. (2004). Coworker perceptions of outcome fairness of breastfeeding accommodation in the workplace. *Employee Responsibility and Rights Journal, 16,* 149–166.

Sen, S., Rifas-Shiman, S. L., Shivappa, N., Wirth, M. D., Hebert, J. R., Gold, D. R. . ..Oken, E. (2016). Dietary inflammatory potential during pregnancy is associated with lower fetal growth and breastfeeding failure: Results from Project Viva. *Journal of Nutrition,* [Epub ahead of print], doi: 10.3945/jn.115.225581.

Sert, M., Tetiker, T., Kirim, S., & Kocak, M. (2003). Clinical report of 28 patients with Sheehan's syndrome. *Endocrine Journal, 50,* 297–301.

Shakespeare, J., Blake, F., & Garcia, J. (2004). Breastfeeding difficulties experienced by women taking part in a qualitative interview study of postnatal depression. *Midwifery, 20,* 251–260.

Shames, K. H., & Youngkin, E. Q. (2002). The thyroid dance: Nursing approaches to autoimmune low thyroid. *AWHONN Lifelines, 6,* 53–59.

Sharma, V., & Corpse, C. S. (2008). Case study revisiting the association between breastfeeding and postpartum depression. *Journal of Human Lactation, 24,* 77–79.

Shelton, R. C., Keller, M. B., Gelenberg, A., Dunner, D. L., Hirschfeld, R., Thase, M. E., . . . Halbreich, U. (2001). Effectiveness of St. John's wort in major depression: A randomized controlled trial. *Journal of the American Medical Association, 285,* 1978–1986.

Shiffman, M. L., Seale, T. W., Flux, M., Rennert, O. R., & Swender, P. T. (1989). Breast milk composition in women with cystic fibrosis: Report of two cases and a review of the literature. *American Journal of Clinical Nutrition, 49,* 612–617.

Sichel, D. A., & Driscoll, J. W. (1999). *Women's moods: What every woman must know about the hormones, the brain, and emotional health.* New York, NY: William Morrow.

Siebenaler, N. (2002). Maternal physical impairments. In M. Walker (Ed.), *Core curriculum for lactation consultant practice.* Sudbury, MA: Jones and Bartlett.

Silman, A. J., & Pearson, J. E. (2002). Epidemiology and genetics of rheumatoid arthritis. *Arthritis Research, 9*(suppl 3), S265–S272.

Sim, T. F., Hattingh, H. L., Sherriff, J., & Tee, L. B. G. (2015). The use, perceived effectiveness and safety of herbal galactagogues during breastfeeding: A qualitative study. *International Journal of Environmental Research and Public Health, 12,* 11050–11071.

Sim, T. F., Sherriff, J., Hattingh, H. L., Parsons, R., & Tee, L. B. G. (2013). The use of herbal medicines during breastfeeding: A population-based survey in Western Australia. *BMC Complementary and Alternative Medicine, 13,* 317.

Simmons, D., Conroy, C., & Thompson, C. F. (2005). In-hospital breastfeeding rates among women with gestational diabetes and pregestational type 2 diabetes in *South Auckland. Diabetes Medicine, 22,* 177–181.

Sipski, M. L. (1991). The impact of spinal cord injury on female sexuality, menstruation, and pregnancy: A review of the literature. *Journal of American Paraplegia Society, 14,* 122–126.

Sirota, L., Ferrera, M., Lerer, N., & Dulitzky, F. (1992). Beta glucuronidase and hyperbilirubinemia in breastfed infants of diabetic mothers. *Archives of Disease in Childhood, 67,* 120.

Sit, D., Perel, J. M., Wisniewski, S. R., Helsel, J. C., Luther, J. F., & Wisner, K. L. (2011). Mother–infant antidepressant levels, maternal depression and perinatal events. *Journal of Clinical Psychiatry, 72,* 994–1001.

Slusser, W. M., Lange, L., Dickson, V., Hawkes, C., & Cohen, R. (2004). Breast milk expression in the workplace: A look at frequency and time. *Journal of Human Lactation, 20,* 164–169.

Smeltzer, S. (1994). The concerns of pregnant women with multiple sclerosis. *Quality of Health Research, 4,* 480–502.

Smillie, C. M., Campbell, S. H., & Iwinski, S. (2005). Hyperlactation: How left-brained "rules" for breastfeeding can wreak havoc with a natural process. *Newborn and Infant Nursing Reviews, 5,* 49–58.

Soltani, H., & Arden, M. (2009). Factors associated with breastfeeding up to 6 months postpartum in mothers with diabetes. *Journal of Obstetric, Gynecologic, and Neonatal Nursing, 38,* 586–594.

Sparud-Lundin, C., Wennergren, M., Elfvin, A., & Berg, M. (2011). Breastfeeding in women with type 1 diabetes. *Diabetes Care, 34,* 296–301.

Spatz, D. L., Kim, G. S., & Froh, E. B. (2014). Outcomes of a hospital-based employee lactation program. *Breastfeeding Medicine, 9,* 510–514.

Stein, M. (2002). Failure to thrive in a four-month-old nursing infant. *Journal of Developmental and Behavioral Pediatrics, 23,* S69–S73.

Stevens, K. V., & Janke, J. (2003). Breastfeeding experiences of active duty military women. *Military Medicine, 168,* 380–384.

Stewart-Glenn, J. (2008). Knowledge, perceptions, and attitudes of managers, coworkers, and employed breastfeeding mothers. *AAOHN Journal, 56,* 423–429.

Stiskal, J. A., Kulin, N., Koren, G., Ho, T., & Ito, S. (2001). Neonatal paroxetine withdrawal syndrome. *Archives of Disease in Childhood—Fetal and Neonatal Edition, 84,* F134–F135.

Strathearn, L., Mamun, A. A., Najman, J. M., & O'Callaghan, M. J. (2009). Does breastfeeding protect against substantiated child abuse and neglect? A 15-year cohort study. *Pediatrics, 123,* 483–493.

Stuebe, A. M., Grewen, K., Pedersen, C. A., Propper, C., & Meltzer-Brody, S. (2012). Failed lactation and perinatal depression: Common problems with shared neuroendocrine mechanisms? *Journal of Women's Health, 21,* 264–272.

Szucs, K. A., Axline, S. E., & Rosenman, M. B. (2010). Induced lactation and exclusive breast milk feeding of adopted premature twins. *Journal of Human Lactation, 26,* 309–313.

Talbott, E. O., Zborowski, J. V., & Boudreaux, M. Y. (2004). Do women with polycystic ovary syndrome have an increased risk of cardiovascular disease? Review of the evidence. *Minerva Ginecologica, 56,* 27–39.

Taylor, J. S., Kacmar, J. E., Nothnagle, M., & Lawrence, R. A. (2005). A systematic review of the literature associating breastfeeding with type 2 diabetes and gestational diabetes. *Journal of the American College of Nutrition, 24,* 320–326.

Thomas-Jackson, S. C., Bentley, G. E., Keyton, K., Reifman, A., Boylan, M., & Hart, S. L. (2015). In-hospital breastfeeding intention to return to work influence mothers' breastfeeding intentions. *Journal of Human Lactation.* [Epub ahead of print]. pii: 0890334415597636.

Thompson, N. M. (1996). Relactation in a newborn intensive care setting. *Journal of Human Lactation, 12,* 233–235.

Thompson, P., & Bell, P. (1997). Breastfeeding in the workplace: How to succeed. *Issues in Comprehensive Pediatric Nursing, 20,* 1–9.

Thomson, V. M. (1995). Breastfeeding and mothering one-handed. *Journal of Human Lactation, 11,* 211–215.

Thrift, T. A., Bernal, A., Lewis, A. L., Neuendorff, D. A., Willard, C. C., & Randel, R. D. (1999). Effects of induced hypothyroidism on weight gains, lactation and reproductive performance of primiparous Brahman cows. *Journal of Animal Science, 77,* 1844–1850.

Thrris, C., Thune, I., Emaus, A., Finstad, S. E., Bye, A., Furberg, A.-S., . . . Hjartaker, A. (2013). Duration of lactation, maternal metabolic profile, and body composition in the Norwegian EBBA I-study. *Breastfeeding Medicine, 8,* 8–15.

Trimeloni, L., & Spencer, J. (2016). Diagnosis and management of breastmilk oversupply. *Journal of the American Board of Family Medicine, 29,* 139–142.

Troutman, B., & Cutrona, C. (1990). Nonpsychotic postpartum depression among adolescent mothers. *Journal of Abnormal Psychology, 99,* 69–78.

Turcksin, R., Bel, S., Galjaard, S., & Devlieger, R. (2014). Maternal obesity and breastfeeding intention, initiation, intensity and duration: A systematic review. *Maternal and Child Nutrition, 10,* 166–183.

Turkyilmaz, C., Onal, E., Hirfanoglu, I. M., Turan, O., Koc, E., Ergenekon, E., & Atalay, Y. (2011). The effect of galactagogue herbal tea on breast milk production and short-term catch-up of birth weight in the first week of life. *Journal of Alternative and Complementary Medicine, 17,* 139–142.

Tyler, K. (1999). Got milk? *HR Magazine, 44*(3), 68–73.

Tyson, J. E., Perez, A., & Zanartu, J. (1976). Human lactational response to oral thyrotropin releasing hormone. *Journal of Clinical Endocrinology and Metabolism, 43,* 760–768.

U.S. Bureau of Labor Statistics. (2012, April). Employment characteristics of families in 2011 (News release USDL-12-0771). Retrieved from http://www.bls.gov/news.release/pdf/famee.pdf

van Veldhuizen-Staas, C. G. A. (2007). Overabundant milk supply: An alternative way to intervene by full drainage and block feeding. *International Breastfeeding Journal, 2,* 11.

Vanky, E., Nordskar, J. J., Leithe, H., Hjorth-Hansen, A. K., Martinussen, M., & Carlsen, S. M. (2012). Breast size increment during pregnancy and breastfeeding in mothers with polycystic ovary syndrome: A follow-up study of a randomized controlled trial on metformin versus placebo. *BJOG: An International Journal of Obstetrics and Gynecology, 119,* 1403–1409.

Veiby, G., Bjørk, M., Engelsen, B. A., & Gilhus, N. E. (2015). Epilepsy and recommendations for breastfeeding. *Seizure, 28,* 57–65.

Veiby, G., Engelsen, B. A., & Gilhus, N. E. (2013). Early child development and exposure to antiepileptic drugs prenatally and through breastfeeding: A prospective cohort study on children of women with epilepsy. *JAMA Neurology, 70,* 1367–1374.

Verronen, P. (1982). Breastfeeding: Reasons for giving up and transient lactational crises. *Acta Paediatrica Scandinavica, 71,* 447–450.

Viguera, A. C., Newport, D. J., Ritchie, J., Stowe, Z., Whitfield, T., Mogielnicki, J., . . . Cohen, L. S. (2007). Lithium in breast milk and nursing infants: Clinical implications. *American Journal of Psychiatry, 164,* 342–345.

Waisbren, S. E., Hanley, W., Levy, H. L., Shifrin, H., Allred, E., Azen, C., . . . Koch, R. (2000). Outcome at age 4 years in offspring of women with maternal phenylketonuria: The Maternal PKU Collaborative Study. *Journal of the American Medical Association, 283,* 756–762.

Wan, E. W., Davey, K., Page-Sharp, M., Hartmann, P. E., Simmer, K., & Ilett, K. F. (2008). Dose-effect study of domperidone as a galactagogue in preterm mothers with insufficient milk supply, and its transfer into milk. *British Journal of Clinical Pharmacology, 66,* 283–289.

Wardinsky, T. D., Montes, R. G., Friederich, R. L., Broadhurst, R. B., Sinnhuber, V., & Bartholomew, D. (1995). Vitamin B_{12} deficiency associated with low breast milk vitamin B_{12} concentration in an infant following maternal gastric bypass surgery. *Archives of Pediatrics and Adolescent Medicine, 149,* 1281–1284.

Watkins, S., Meltzer-Brody, S., Zolnoun, D., & Stuebe, A. (2011). Early breastfeeding experiences and postpartum depression. *Obstetrics and Gynecology, 118,* 214–221.

Webster, J., Moore, K., & McMullan, A. (1995). Breastfeeding outcomes for women with insulin dependent diabetes. *Journal of Human Lactation, 11,* 195–200.

Wei, L., Wang, H., Han, Y., & Li, C. (2008). Clinical observation on the effects of electroacupuncture at Shaoze (SI 1) in 46 cases of postpartum insufficient lactation. *Journal of Traditional Chinese Medicine, 28,* 168–172.

Weiss, R. F. (2001). *Weiss's herbal medicine* (Classic ed.). New York, NY: Thieme.

Whichelow, M. J., & Doddridge, M. C. (1983). Lactation in diabetic mothers. *British Medical Journal, 287,* 649–650.

Wiklund, P., Xu, L., Lvytikainen, A., Saltevo, J., Wang, Q., Volgyi, E., . . . Cheng, S. (2012). Prolonged breastfeeding protects mothers from later-life obesity and related cardio-metabolic disorders. *Public Health Nutrition, 15*(1), 67–74.

Williams, J., Auerbach, K., & Jacobi, A. (1989). Lateral epicondylitis (tennis elbow) in breastfeeding mothers. *Clinical Pediatrics, 28,* 42–43.

Willis, C., & Livingstone, V. (1995). Infant insufficient milk syndrome associated with maternal postpartum hemorrhage. *Journal of Human Lactation, 11,* 123–126.

Wittig, S. L., & Spatz, D. L. (2008). Induced lactation: Gaining a better understanding. *MCN: The American Journal of Maternal/Child Nursing, 33,* 76–81.

Wojcicki, J. M. (2011). Maternal prepregnancy body mass index and initiation and duration of breastfeeding: A review of the literature. *Journal of Women's Health, 20,* 341–347.

Woolridge, M. W., & Fischer, C. (1988). Overfeeding and symptoms of lactose malabsorption in the breastfed baby: A possible artifact of feeding management? *Lancet, 2,* 382–384.

World Health Organization. (1998). Relactation: Review of experience and recommendations for practice. Retrieved from http://whqlibdoc.who.int/hq/1998/WHO_CHS_CAH_98.14.pdf

Worthington, J., Jones, R., Crawford, M., & Forti, A. (1994). Pregnancy and multiple sclerosis: A three year prospective study. *Journal of Neurology, 241,* 228–233.

Yerby, M. S., Kaplan, P., & Tran, T. (2004). Risks and management of pregnancy in women with epilepsy. *Cleveland Clinic Journal of Medicine, 71*(suppl 2), S25–S37.

Yokoyama, Y., Ueda, T., Irahara, M., & Aono, T. (1994). Releases of oxytocin and prolactin during breast massage and suckling in puerperal women. *European Journal of Obstetrics and Gynecology and Reproductive Biology, 53,* 17.

Zanton, G. I., & Heinrichs, A. J. (2005). Meta-analysis to assess effect of prepubertal average daily gain of Holstein heifers on first-lactation production. *Journal of Dairy Science, 88,* 3860–3867.

Zapantis, A., Steinberg, J. G., & Schilit, L. (2012). Use of herbal galactagogues. *Journal of Pharmacy Practice, 25,* 222–231.

Zhao, Y., & Guo, H. (2006). The therapeutic effects of acupuncture in 30 cases of postpartum hypogalactia. *Journal of Traditional Chinese Medicine, 26,* 29–30.

Ziegler, A. G., Schmid, S., Huber, D., Hummel, M., & Bonifacio, E. (2003). Early infant feeding and risk of developing type 1 associated antibodies. *Journal of the American Medical Association, 290,* 1721–1728.

Zuppa, A. A., Sindico, P., Orchi, C., Carducci, C., Cardiello, V., Romagnoli, C., & Catenazzi, P. (2010). Safety and efficacy of galactogogues: Substances that induce, maintain, and increase breast milk production. *Journal of Pharmacy and Pharmaceutical Science, 13,* 162–174.

Zuppa, A. A., Tornesello, A., Papacci, P., Tortorolo, G., Segni, G., Lafuenti, G., . . . Carta, S. (1988). Relationship between maternal parity, basal prolactin levels and neonatal breast milk intake. *Biology of the Neonate, 53,* 144–147.

ADDITIONAL READING AND RESOURCES

Resource for Physically Challenged Mothers

Rogers, J. (2005). *Disabled woman's guide to pregnancy and birth.* New York, NY: Demos Medical Publishing.

Insufficient Milk

Mothers Overcoming Breastfeeding Issues (MOBI Motherhood International), http://www.mobimotherhood.org

Low Milk Supply

Low Milk Supply provides information and support for breastfeeding mothers concerned about low milk production: http://www.lowmilksupply.org

West, D., & Hirsch, E. M. (2008). *Breastfeeding after breast and nipple procedures: A guide for healthcare professionals.* Amarillo, TX: Hale Publishing.

West, D., & Marasco, L. (2008). *The breastfeeding mother's guide to making more milk.* New York, NY: McGraw-Hill.

Mood Disorders

Beck, C. T., & Driscoll, J. W. (2005). *Postpartum mood and anxiety disorders: A clinician's guide.* Sudbury, MA: Jones and Bartlett.

Kendall-Tackett, K. (2008). *Non-pharmacologic treatments for depression in new mothers.* Amarillo, TX: Hale Publishing.

Sichel, D., & Driscoll, J. W. (1999). *Women's moods: What every woman should know about hormones, the brain, and emotional health.* New York, NY: William Morrow.

Medications and Breastfeeding

Journals

Akus, M., & Bartick, M. (2007). Lactation safety recommendations and reliability compared in 10 medication resources. *Annals of Pharmacotherapy, 41,* 1352–1360.

American Academy of Pediatrics, Committee on Drugs. (2001). The transfer of drugs and other chemicals into human milk. *Pediatrics, 108,* 776–789.

Books

Briggs, G. R., Freeman, R. K., & Yaffe, S. J. (2014). *Drugs in pregnancy and lactation: A reference guide to fetal and neonatal risk* (10th ed.). Baltimore, MD: Lippincott, Williams & Wilkins.

Hale, T. W. (2014). *Medications and mothers' milk* (16th ed.). Amarillo, TX: Hale Publishing.

Hale, T. W., & Berens, P. (2010). *Clinical therapy in breastfeeding patients* (3rd ed.). Amarillo, TX: Hale Publishing

Hale, T. W., & Ilett, K. F. (2002). *Drug therapy and breastfeeding: From theory to clinical practice.* New York, NY: Parthenon.

Lawrence, R. A., & Lawrence, R. W. (2016). *Breastfeeding: A guide for the medical profession* (8th ed.). St. Louis, MO: Mosby.

Nice, F. (2011). *Nonprescription drugs for the breastfeeding mother.* Amarillo, TX: Hale Publishing.

Telephone Resources

Infant Risk Center at Texas Tech University, 806-352-2519

Breastfeeding and Human Lactation Study Center
University of Rochester School of Medicine and Dentistry
Box 777, Rochester, NY, 14642
For healthcare professionals: 585-275-0088, 8:00 am to 5:00 pm EST M-F
Breastfeeding warm line: 585-275-9575

Internet Resources

Dr. Hale's Breastfeeding Pharmacology Page, Infant Risk Center, Texas Tech University, http://www.infantrisk.com

LactMed, http://toxnet.nlm.nih.gov/cgi-bin/sis/htmlgen?LACT

Apps

Infant Risk Center for Health Care Providers app, http://www.infantrisk.com/apps

LactMed app, https://itunes.apple.com/us/app/lactmed/id441969514?mt=8

MommyMeds for Mothers app, http://mommymeds.com/mobile-apps

Maternal Employment

Berggren, K. (2006). *Working without weaning: A working mother's guide to breastfeeding.* Amarillo, TX: Hale Press. Available from http://www.ibreastfeeding.com

Department of Health, Oregon, http://public.health.oregon.gov/HealthyPeopleFamilies/Babies/Breastfeeding/Pages/workplace.aspx

Health Resources and Services Administration, The Business Case for Breastfeeding, http://mchb.hrsa.gov/pregnancyandbeyond/breastfeeding

Healthy Mothers, Healthy Babies, USA, http://www.hmhb.org

Massachusetts Breastfeeding Coalition, http://massbfc.org/workplace

Parenting in the Workplace Institute, http://www.parentingatwork.org

U.S. Breastfeeding Committee, http://www.usbreastfeeding.org

Vermont, http://healthvermont.gov/family/breastfeed/employer_project.aspx

Walker, M. (2011). *Breastfeeding and employment: Making it work.* Amarillo, TX: Hale Publishing.

Breastfeeding and working

Work and Pump, information about breastfeeding for working moms, http://www.workandpump.com

Child Care

"Breastfed Babies Welcome Here": This informational packet prepared by the U.S. Department of Agriculture promotes breastfeeding in childcare settings. It offers advice on feeding the breastfed infant; preparing for child care; and collecting, storing, and handling breastmilk. The packet is out of print at time of writing, but is available as a free ebook: https://play.google.com/store/books/details?id=eHgwAAAAYAAJ&rdid=book-eHgwAAAAYAAJ&rdot=1

Supplemental Food Programs
Food and Nutrition Service—USDA
3101 Park Center Drive
Alexandria, VA 22302
Telephone: 703-305-2680

California Department of Public Health, Women, Infants and Children Program, http://www.wicworks.ca.gov/breastfeeding/EmployeeResources/ReadyforChildcare.html

Massachusetts Department of Public Health, http://www.letsgo.org/wp-content/uploads/ECTAB03D05-How-To-Meet-the-Needs-Tab-5-DOUBLE-SIDED-COLOR.pdf

New York State Department of Health, http://www.health.state.ny.us/prevention/nutrition/cacfp/breastfeedingspon.htm

Vermont Department of Health, http://healthvermont.gov/family/breastfeed/childcare.aspx

Relactation/Induced Lactation/Adoptive Breastfeeding

The Protocols for Induced Lactation, Lenore Goldfarb and Jack Newman, http://www.asklenore.info/breastfeeding/induced_lactation/gn_protocols.shtml

Diabetes

Guidelines for managing diabetes with a section on breastfeeding, http://www.cdph.ca.gov/programs/cdapp/Pages/default.aspx

Slide presentation on diabetes and breastfeeding, http://lomalindahealth.org/medical-center/our-services/diabetes-treatment-center/resources/sweet-success/slides/growth-spurts/index.html

Epilepsy

Harden, C. L., Pennell, P. B., Koppel, B. S., Hovinga, C. A., Gidal, B., Meador, K. J., . . . Le Guen, C. (2009). Practice parameter update: Management issues for women with epilepsy: Focus on pregnancy (an evidence-based review): Vitamin K, folic acid, blood levels, and breastfeeding. *Neurology, 73,* 142–149.

Adoption

Schnell, A. (2013). *Breastfeeding without birthing: A breastfeeding guide for mothers through adoption, surrogacy, and other special circumstances.* Amarillo, TX, Praeclarus Press.

Index

Note: Page numbers followed by *f*, *t*, and *b* refer to figures, tables, and boxes respectively

B

C

I

M

O

P

T

U

V